Instructional Course Lectures

Volume 43 1994

American Academy
of Orthopaedic Surgeons

Instructional Course Lectures

Volume 43 1994

Edited by
Michael Schafer, MD
Ryerson Professor and Chairman
Department of Orthopaedic Surgery
Northwestern University Medical School
Chicago, Illinois

With 403 illustrations

American Academy
of Orthopaedic Surgeons

American Academy of Orthopaedic Surgeons

Instructional Course Lectures

Volume 43

Director, Division of Education: Mark W. Wieting
Director, Department of Publications: Marilyn L. Fox, PhD
Senior Editor: Bruce Davis
Associate Senior Editors: Joan Abern, Jane Baque
Production Manager: Loraine Edwalds
Assistant Production Manager: Kathy Brouillette
Editorial Assistants: Sharon Duffy, Sophie Tosta
Publications Secretaries: Geraldine Dubberke, Em Lee Lambos

Design: James Buddenbaum Design, Wilmette, Illinois
Typesetting: Media Graphics, Chicago, Illinois
Printing and binding: Rand McNally, Taunton, Massachusetts
Stock: Acid-free Resolve Gloss

The material presented in *Instructional Course Lectures Volume 43* has been made available by the American Academy of Orthopaedic Surgeons for educational purposes only. This material is not intended to present the only, or necessarily best, methods or procedures for the medical situations discussed, but rather is intended to represent an approach, view, statement, or opinion of the author(s) or producer(s), which may be helpful to others who face similar situations.

Some drugs and medical devices demonstrated in Academy courses or described in Academy print or electronic publications have Food and Drug Administration (FDA) clearance for use for specific purposes or for use only in restricted settings. The FDA has stated that it is the responsibility of the physician to determine the FDA status of each drug or device he or she wishes to use in clinical practice, and to use the products with appropriate patient consent and in compliance with applicable law.

Furthermore, any statements about commercial products are solely the opinion(s) of the author(s) and do not represent an Academy endorsement or evaluation of these products. These statements may not be used in advertising or for any commercial purpose.

Contributors

Roy K. Aaron, MD, Clinical Associate Professor, Department of Orthopaedics, Brown University, Providence, Rhode Island

A. Graham Apley, MB BS, FRCS, Consulting Surgeon, St. Thomas' Hospital, London, England

Steven P. Arnoczky, DVM, Wade O. Brinker Professor of Surgery, Director, Laboratory for Comparative Orthopaedic Research, College of Veterinary Medicine, Michigan State University, East Lansing, Michigan

Foster Betts, PhD, Associate Scientist, The Hospital for Special Surgery, New York, New York

J. Sybil Biermann, MD, Lecturer, Orthopaedic Surgery, The University of Michigan, Ann Arbor, Michigan

Jonathan Black, PhD, Principal, IMN Biomaterials, King of Prussia, Pennsylvania

J. Dennis Bobyn, PhD, Associate Professor, Department of Surgery, McGill University, Montreal General Hospital, Montreal, Quebec, Canada

Robert E. Booth, Jr., MD, Clinical Professor of Orthopaedic Surgery, Thomas Jefferson University, Philadelphia, Pennsylvania

Robert Barry Bourne, MD, FRCSC, Professor of Orthopaedic Surgery, University of Western Ontario, London, Ontario, Canada

Philip J. Branson, MD, Princeton Community Hospital, Princeton, West Virginia

C. Emerson Brooks, MD, Associate Professor, Department of Surgery, McGill University, Orthopaedic Surgeon-in-Chief, Montreal General Hospital, Montreal, Quebec, Canada

Bernard R. Cahill, MD, Clinical Professor, Orthopedic Surgery, University of Illinois College of Medicine, Peoria, Illinois

John J. Callaghan, MD, Professor, Department of Orthopaedics, University of Iowa College of Medicine, Iowa City, Iowa

W. Dilworth Cannon, Jr., MD, Professor of Clinical Orthopaedics, University of California, San Francisco, San Francisco, California

William N. Capello, MD, Professor, Department of Orthopaedic Surgery, Indiana University School of Medicine, Indianapolis, Indiana

James E. Carpenter, MD, Assistant Professor of Surgery, Section of Orthopaedic Surgery, University of Michigan Medical School, Ann Arbor, Michigan

T.J. Chandler, EdD, Director of Research and Education, Lexington Clinic Sports Medicine Center, Lexington, Kentucky

Mailine H. Chew, MD, Associate Clinical Professor of Medicine and Radiology, University of California at San Francisco, San Francisco, California

John P. Collier, DE, Professor of Engineering, Thayer School of Engineering, Dartmouth College, Hanover, New Hampshire

Henry R. Cowell, MD, PhD, Editor, *The Journal of Bone and Joint Surgery,* American Volume, Needham, Massachusetts

Walton W. Curl, MD, Director of Sports Medicine, Department of Orthopaedics, Bowman Gray School of Medicine, Winston-Salem, North Carolina

James A. D'Antonio, MD, Orthopaedic Surgeon, Sewickley Valley Hospital, Sewickley, Pennsylvania

Kenneth E. DeHaven, MD, Professor and Associate Chairman, Director of Athletic Medicine, Department of Orthopaedics, University of Rochester School of Medicine and Dentistry, Rochester, New York

Peter Devane, MB ChB, FRACS, MSc, Senior Lecturer, Department of Surgery, Wellington School of Medicine, Wellington South, New Zealand

David D. Dore, MD, Joint Reconstruction Fellow, Department of Orthopaedic Surgery, University of Pittsburgh Medical Center, Pittsburgh, Pennsylvania

Frederick Dorey, PhD, Associate Professor, Department of Orthopaedics, School of Medicine and Department of Biostatistics, School of Public Health, University of California, Los Angeles and Joint Replacement Institute, Los Angeles Orthopaedic Hospital, Los Angeles, California

Stephen B. Doty, PhD, Director, Analytical Microscopy Laboratory, The Hospital for Special Surgery, New York, New York

Clive P. Duncan, MD, FRCS(C), Professor (PT) of Orthopaedics, Department of Orthopaedics, Head, Division of Reconstructive Orthopaedics, University of British Columbia, Vancouver, British Columbia, Canada

Scott F. Dye, MD, Assistant Clinical Professor of Orthopaedic Surgery, University of California, San Francisco, California

Richard G. Eaton, MD, Professor, Clinical Orthopaedic Surgery, Columbia College of Physicians and Surgeons, Chief, Hand Surgery, Department of Orthopaedic Surgery, St. Luke's/Roosevelt Hospital Center, New York, New York

Edward Ebramzadeh, MS, Researcher, Biomaterials Group, Department of Handicap Research, University of Göteborg, Sweden, Instructor of Research Orthopaedics, J. Vernon Luck, Sr. Orthopaedic Research Center, Los Angeles Orthopaedic Hospital and the Department of Orthopaedics, University of Southern California, Los Angeles, California

Nas S. Eftekhar, MD, Professor of Orthopaedic Surgery, College of Physicians and Surgeons, Columbia University of New York, Attending Orthopaedic Surgeon and Chief of Hip and Implant Service at New York Orthopaedic Hospital Columbia-Presbyterian Medical Center, New York, New York

Brian G. Evans, MD, Attending Orthopaedic Surgeon, Department of Orthopaedic Surgery, Georgetown University Medical Center, Washington, DC

Henry A. Finn, MD, Associate Professor of Clinical Surgery, University of Chicago Medical Center, Department of Surgery, Section of Orthopaedic Surgery and Rehabilitation Medicine, Chicago, Illinois

Richard J. Friedman, MD, FRCS(C), Associate Professor of Orthopaedic Surgery, Medical University of South Carolina, Adjunct Associate Professor of Bioengineering, Clemson University, Charleston, South Carolina

Freddie H. Fu, MD, Professor of Orthopaedic Surgery, Vice Chairman/Clinical, Department of Orthopaedic Surgery, University of Pittsburgh, Pittsburgh, Pennsylvania

Jorge O. Galante, MD, Professor and Chairman, Department of Orthopedic Surgery, Rush-Presbyterian-St. Luke's Medical Center, Chicago, Illinois

Steven R. Garfin, MD, Professor, Department of Orthopedics and Rehabilitation, University of California-San Diego, San Diego, California

Richard H. Gelberman, MD, Professor of Orthopaedic Surgery, Harvard Medical School, Chief, Hand Surgery, Massachusetts General Hospital, Boston, Massachusetts

Harry K. Genant, MD, Chief, Musculoskeletal Radiology, Department of Radiology, University of California, San Francisco, California

Walter B. Greene, MD, Professor of Orthopaedic Surgery and Pediatrics, University of North Carolina Medical School, Chapel Hill, North Carolina

Edward N. Hanley, Jr., MD, Chairman, Department of Orthopaedic Surgery, Charlotte, North Carolina

Christopher D. Harner, MD, Assistant Professor, Department of Orthopaedic Surgery, University of Pittsburgh School of Medicine, Pittsburgh, Pennsylvania

William H. Harris, MD, Chief, Hip and Implant Unit, Massachusetts General Hospital, Boston, Massachusetts

Harry N. Herkowitz, MD, Chairman, Department of Orthopaedic Surgery, William Beaumont Hospital, Royal Oak, Michigan

Joseph H. Introcaso, MD, DMD, Assistant Professor, Department of Radiology, Northwestern University Medical School, Northwestern Memorial Hospital, Chicago, Illinois

Joshua J. Jacobs, MD, Assistant Professor, Department of Orthopaedic Surgery, Rush Medical College, Chicago, Illinois

Murali Jasty, MD, Surgeon, Massachusetts General Hospital, Clinical Assistant Professor in Orthopaedics, Harvard Medical School, Boston, Massachusetts

Darren L. Johnson, MD, Assistant Professor, Division of Orthopedics, Section of Sports Medicine, University of Kentucky, Lexington, Kentucky

John Paul Jones, Jr., MD, Medical Research Director, Diagnostic Osteonecrosis Center and Research Foundation, Kelseyville, California

Roberta Kasman, MD, Henry Ford Hospital, Detroit, Michigan

Robert B. Keller, MD, Executive Director, Maine Medical Assessment Foundation, Augusta, Maine

W. Ben Kibler, MD, Medical Director, Lexington Clinic Sports Medicine Center, Lexington, Kentucky

Patricia A. Kolowich, MD, Henry Ford Hospital, Center for Athletic Medicine, Detroit, Michigan

Matthew H. Liang, MD, MPH, Associate Professor of Medicine, Harvard Medical School, Boston, Massachusetts

James V. Luck, Jr., MD, President, Chief Executive Officer and Medical Director, Orthopaedic Hospital, Los Angeles, California

Theodore Malinin, MD, Department of Orthopaedics and Rehabilitation, University Miami - Jackson Memorial Medical Center, Miami, Florida

Larry S. Matthews, MD, Professor and Head, Section of Orthopaedic Surgery, Department of Surgery, University of Michigan Medical School, Ann Arbor, Michigan

Roy A. Maxion, PhD, Faculty, Department of Computer Science, Carnegie Mellon University, Pittsburgh, Pennsylvania

Michael B. Mayor, MD, Professor of Surgery in Orthopaedics, Dartmouth Hitchcock Medical Center, Dartmouth Medical School, Dartmouth Biomedical Engineering Center, Hanover, New Hampshire

Harry McKellop, PhD, Assistant Professor of Orthopaedics and Biomedical Engineering, University of Southern California, Director of Research, Los Angeles Orthopaedic Hospital, Los Angeles, California

Mark D. Miller, MD, Clinical Assistant Professor of Orthopaedic Surgery, Uniformed Services University of the Health Sciences, United States Air Force Academy Hospital/SGHST, US Air Force Academy, Colorado

Srdjan Mirkovic, MD, Assistant Professor of Orthopaedic Surgery, Reconstructive Spine Service, Northwestern University School of Medicine, Chicago, Illinois

Roby Mize, MD, Clinical Associate Professor, University of Texas, Southwestern Medical School, Dallas, Texas

Craig D. Morgan, MD, Associate Clinical Professor, Department of Orthopaedic Surgery, Thomas Jefferson University, Philadelphia, Pennsylvania

Philip C. Noble, MS, Director of Orthopaedic Research, Department of Orthopaedic Surgery, Baylor College of Medicine, Houston, Texas

James A. Nunley, II, MD, Professor of Orthopaedic Surgery, Duke University Medical School, Durham, North Carolina

Ronald E. Palmer, MD, Clinical Assistant Professor, University of Illinois College of Medicine at Peoria, Peoria, Illinois

Clayton R. Perry, MD, Associate Professor of Orthopaedic Surgery, Washington University School of Medicine, St. Louis, Missouri

Pasquale Petrera, MD, Joint Reconstruction Fellow, University of Pittsburgh Medical Center, Pittsburgh, Pennsylvania

Peter D. Pizzutillo, MD, Professor of Orthopaedic Surgery, Thomas Jefferson University, Philadelphia, Pennsylvania

Michael P. Recht, MD, Cleveland Clinic Foundation, Department of Radiology, Cleveland, Ohio

Donald Resnick, MD, Department of Radiology, Veterans Administration Medical Center, San Diego, California

Cecil H. Rorabeck, MD, FRCS(C), Professor and Chairman, Division of Orthopaedic Surgery, University Hospital, London, Ontario, Canada

Harry E. Rubash, MD, Associate Professor, Department of Orthopaedic Surgery, Chief, Division of Adult Reconstruction Surgery, University of Pittsburgh Medical Center, Pittsburgh, Pennsylvania

Sally A. Rudicel, MD, Assistant Professor of Orthopaedics, Tufts/New England Medical Center, Boston, Massachusetts

Jeffrey A. Russell, MS, Coordinator of Research and Education, Fondren Orthopedic Group L.L.P., Joe W. King Orthopedic Institute, Houston, Texas

Eduardo A. Salvati, MD, Clinical Professor, Orthopaedic Surgery, Cornell University Medical College, Chief of Hip and Knee Service, The Hospital for Special Surgery, New York, New York

Roy Sanders, MD, Director, Orthopaedic Trauma Services, Florida Orthopaedic Institute, Tampa, Florida

Augusto Sarmiento, MD, Professor, Department of Orthopaedics, University of Southern California, Vice President for Research, Los Angeles Orthopaedic Hospital, Los Angeles, California

Robert C. Schenck, Jr., MD, Assistant Professor, Department of Orthopaedics, The University of Texas Health Science Center at San Antonio, San Antonio, Texas

Michael A. Simon, MD, Professor of Surgery, Section of Orthopaedic Surgery and Rehabilitation Medicine, University of Chicago, Chicago, Illinois

Harry B. Skinner, MD, PhD, Professor, Orthopaedic Surgery and Mechanical Engineering, University of California, San Francisco, San Francisco, California

Daniel M. Spengler, MD, Professor and Chairman, Department of Orthopaedics and Rehabilitation, Vanderbilt University Medical Center, Nashville, Tennessee

Phillip G. Spiegel, MD, Attending Phusician, Spine Service, Orthopaedic Surgeon, Florida Orthopaedic Institute, Tampa, Florida

Jeffrey Spivak, MD, Hospital for Joint Diseases, Orthopaedic Institute, New York, New York

Dempsey S. Springfield, MD, Visiting Orthopaedic Surgeon, Department of Orthopaedics, Massachusetts General Hospital, Boston, Massachusetts

Lynn T. Staheli, MD, Professor, Orthopaedic Surgery, University of Washington School of Medicine, Seattle, Washington

Carl L. Stanitski, MD, Chief, Department of Orthopaedic Surgery, Children's Hospital of Michigan, Detroit, Michigan

Marvin E. Steinberg, MD, Professor and Vice Chairman, Department of Orthopaedic Surgery, University of Pennsylvania, School of Medicine, Philadelphia, Pennsylvania

Helene P. Surprenant, Laboratory Technician, Thayer School of Engineering, Dartmouth College, Hanover, New Hampshire

Victor A. Surprenant, Research Engineer, Thayer School of Engineering, Dartmouth College, Hanover, New Hampshire

Marc F. Swiontkowski, MD, Professor, Department of Orthopaedics, University of Washington, Chief of Orthopaedics, Harborview Medical Center, Seattle, Washington

Michael Tanzer, MD, Assistant Professor, Department of Surgery, McGill University, Montreal General Hospital, Montreal, Quebec, Canada

George H. Thompson, MD, Professor, Orthopaedic Surgery and Pediatrics, Director, Pediatric Orthopaedics, Case Western Reserve University, Cleveland, Ohio

James R. Urbaniak, MD, Virginia Flowers Baker Professor of Orthopaedic Surgery, Duke University Medical Center, Durham, North Carolina

Marnix van Holsbeeck, MD, Director, Section of Musculoskeletal Radiology and Section of Emergency Radiology, Department of Diagnostic Radiology, Henry Ford Hospital, Detroit, Michigan

Gordon A. Veale, MB ChB, FRACS, Orthopaedic Surgeon, Southland Base Hospital, Invercargill, New Zealand

James N. Weinstein, DO, Endowed Professor of Orthopaedic Surgery and Biomedical Engineering, University of Iowa, Iowa City, Iowa

Sam Wiesel, MD, Professor and Chairman, Department of Orthopaedic Surgery, Georgetown University Medical Center, Washington DC

Ian R. Williams, Research Assistant, Thayer School of Engineering, Dartmouth College, Hanover, New Hampshire

Savio L-Y. Woo, PhD, Ferguson Professor of Orthopaedic Surgery & Vice Chairman for Research, Department of Orthopaedic Surgery, University of Pittsburgh Medical Center, Pittsburgh, Pennsylvania

G. William Woods, MD, Medical Director, Fondren Orthopedic Group L.L.P., Joe W. King Orthopedic Institute, Houston, Texas

B. Mike Wroblewski, MB ChB, FRCS, Consultant Orthopaedic Surgeons, Wrightington Hospital, Professor of Orthopaedic Biomechanics, The University of Leeds, Centre for Hip Surgery, Wrightington Hospital, NR Wigan, United Kingdom

Marguerite Wrona, ME, Thayer School of Engineering, Dartmouth College, Hanover, New Hampshire

Preface

This 43rd volume of *Instructional Course Lectures* represents a collaborative accomplishment by individuals with varying expertise. We have attempted in this volume to capture an overview of the most pertinent topics in orthopaedics today and at the same time explore exciting new techniques and innovative methodologies. Each manuscript offers a unique approach or perspective that should prove to be a valuable resource for the specialist and generalist alike.

My experience as editor of this issue has been both rewarding and challenging. Interacting with all the participants offered an enjoyable learning opportunity. No doubt, the success of this publication is due to the combined efforts of the authors and the support of the American Academy of Orthopaedic Surgeons. We all applaud the Academy's continuing commitment to postgraduate medical education as well as the dedication exhibited by each of the contributors.

One-hundred and eighteen courses were presented at the Annual Meeting in San Francisco, February 1993. The resulting 63 chapters span a range of interests including sports, knees, pediatrics, implant fixation, total hip arthroplasty, spinal stenosis, diagnostic imaging, osteonecrosis, bone tumors, and methods of scientific publishing and presenting.

Selecting from so many excellent lectures proved to be a daunting, if not difficult, task. In keeping with the history of the *ICL*, we attempted to produce the most current and extensive information available. In so doing, we hope in some small way to have helped further the Academy's goal to educate and to promote orthopaedics, and to provide our readers with a national perspective on the topics selected.

I want to extend my gratitude to all members of the Committee on Instructional Courses and acknowledge the invaluable assistance of the staff of the Academy's Publications Department under the direction of Marilyn Fox, PhD. Copyediting was done by Bruce Davis, senior editor, and by Jane Baque and Joan Abern, associate senior editors. Production was overseen by Loraine Edwalds, production manager, with the able assistance of Kathy Brouillette, assistant production manager, and Sharon Duffy and Sophie Tosta, editorial assistants. Word processing was done by Geraldine Dubberke, Em Lee Lambos, and Sharon O'Brien. A special thanks is extended to Steven Stern, MD, Craig Torosian, MD, and June Wasser for their help in editing this volume and also to Caroline Fischer for her secretarial efforts.

Michael Schafer, MD
Chicago, Illinois
Chairman, Committee on Instructional Courses

James D. Heckman, MD
San Antonio, Texas

Richard H. Gelberman, MD
Boston, Massachusetts

Douglas W. Jackson, MD
Long Beach, California

Douglas J. Pritchard, MD
Rochester, Minnesota

Contents

SECTION X

Sports, Exercise, and Overuse Injuries

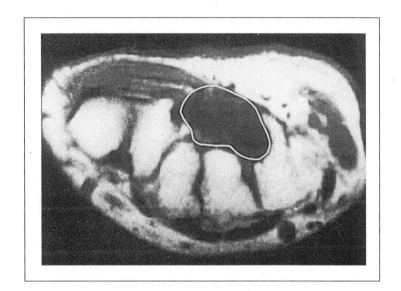

Physiology of Exercising Muscle

W. Ben Kibler, MD

Introduction

Information about the physiology of muscle during exercise is important for a variety of reasons in normal orthopaedic practice. The examples in Outline 1 present selected patient cases and suggest questions that relate to physiologic problems and their solutions. These case examples will provide an orientation to the first four chapters of this section, and will be discussed in a later chapter, on the clinical implications of exercise.

This section is oriented toward the physiology of muscle during more strenuous exercise, as in sports. However, many of the same concepts apply to the muscle in less strenuous situations, as in the workplace. Conditioning for those jobs and treatment of work-related injuries can proceed along the same lines.

Physiology of muscle during exercise should be considered in the context of both reaction to injury and enhancement of performance. Orthopaedic surgeons whose thinking about physiology is oriented only toward injury will not be able to provide the maximum benefit for their athletic patients. Most athletes are interested in performance and want to feel that their doctor is knowledgeable in this area. Also, because the muscle is a common denominator both in reaction to injury and in enhancement of performance, each of these aspects can be improved by proper rehabilitation and strength training of the muscle.

Performance

Optimum athletic performance is possible only when the athlete makes full use of the physiologic processes for motor recruitment, force production, flexibility, energy storage and release, and recovery. Similarly, any improvement in performance is based on improvement in these processes. No amount of skill can overcome a lack of training, because performance of such skills as running, throwing, and jumping is enhanced by proper conditioning (Fig. 1).[1] This conditioning has two components—general athletic fitness and sport-specific athletic fitness.

General athletic fitness reflects the body's baseline readiness for athletic activity. This level of fitness includes general body flexibility, large muscle strength for force production, and overall aerobic capacity for oxygen delivery and uptake into the cells as an aid in recovery following exercise.

Outline 1 Case examples

1. An athlete reports with recurrent ankle sprains and little residual ligamentous laxity. What physiologic variables may be contributing to recurrent sprains, how should they be evaluated, and how should they be rehabbed? When can the player return to play?

2. What weights should be lifted before the football season? Should weights be lifted during the football season? Should weights be lifted during the basketball season?

3. How many miles/day should be run as part of conditioning for soccer? For tennis?

4. A baseball pitcher with rotator cuff tendinitis symptoms is started on rotator cuff strengthening exercises, but the exercises make the symptoms worse. How should the rehab program be modified?

5. At what age can athletes start muscle strengthening? At what age should flexibility training be instituted for athletes?

6. A sprinter presents with a history of two hamstring muscle pulls in the last 6 months.

Sports-specific conditioning begins at this baseline level of fitness and orients the physiologic processes, the muscles, and the joints toward the athletic demands inherent in a particular sport. Flexibility, for example, is necessary in areas that are under maximum tensile stress, such as the hamstring and gastroc-

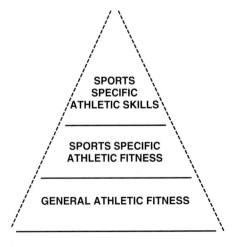

Fig. 1 Athletic skills, which result in performance, are based on general and sport specific athletic fitness. Optimum performance or improvement in performance will occur only if the athletic fitness base is intact.

nemius in runners or the wrist extensors in tennis players. Strength and power conditioning is focused on heavy weights and explosiveness in football players, and on lighter weights, more repetitions, and explosiveness in baseball players. Aerobic endurance is stressed in long distance runners or swimmers; anaerobic endurance is stressed in tennis players or soccer players.

The athlete and the doctor can maximize the athlete's performance by obtaining the best match between the demands required by the sport and the athlete's musculoskeletal ability to respond to those demands.[2] Similarly, evidence is accumulating that this musculoskeletal preparedness can also help decrease the risk of injury and modify the physiologic reaction to injury.[3,4] The relationship between these variables is shown in Figure 2. Performance and injury risk both come out of the same interaction between the sport's inherent demands and the response of the athlete's musculoskeletal base.

Reaction To Injury

Many types of physiologic alterations are observed when an athletic injury is evaluated. Some of these are caused by the injury, others—such as immobilization-induced muscle atrophy, capsular stiffness,[5] or decreased aerobic capacity—are the result of treatment. Some changes such as plantar flexor inflexibility in plantar fasciitis,[6] hamstring tightness in groin pulls,[7] or muscle weakness in lower extremity injuries,[8] accompany, or may even precede, the overt manifestations of the injury. Although it is not clear whether these are causes of the injuries or effects of the pathologic process, their recognition and treatment is mandatory for full functional recovery.

Some physiologic changes persist long after the cessation of symptoms, and these are often the limiting factor in functional return to competition[9,10] Some of these, such as ankle stiffness and peroneal muscle weakness after an ankle sprain, are relatively easy to recognize and treat. Others, such as posterior shoulder muscle weakness in lateral elbow epicondylitis, tight hip flexors and rotators,[11] weak abdominal muscles,[12] or scapular winging[13] in throwers with rotator cuff symptoms, may be more subtle and may occur in a location distant from the original injury. However, all must be recognized and treated.

In summary, an understanding of the physiology of exercising muscle will give the orthopaedic surgeon the knowledge needed to guide proper conditioning of muscle for performance and to evaluate correctly the athlete's reaction to injury. The following chapters in this section will detail anaerobic and aerobic capacity, the physiology of macrotrauma and microtrauma injury, and the physiology of conditioning. Review of the case histories will conclude the section and demonstrate clinical correlations.

References

1. Kibler WB, Chandler TJ: Sport specific conditioning. *Am J Sports Med*, in press.
2. Kibler WB: The sport preparticipation fitness examination. Champaign, IL, Human Kinetics Books, 1989.
3. Chandler TJ, Kibler WB: Strength training for prevention of injury, in Renstrom PA (ed): *IOC Encyclopedia of Sports Medicine*, vol 2, in press.
4. Kibler WB, Chandler TJ, Stracener ES: Musculoskeletal adaptations and injuries due to overtraining. *Exerc Sport Sci Rev* 1992;20:99-126.
5. Harrelson GL: Physiologic factors of rehabilitation, in Harrelson GL, Andrews JR (eds): *Rehabilitation of Sports Injuries*. Philadelphia, PA, WB Saunders, 1992, pp 13-36.
6. Kibler WB, Goldberg C, Chandler TJ: Functional biomechanical deficits in running athletes with plantar fasciitis. *Am J Sports Med* 1991;19:66-71.
7. Jackson DL, Nyland J: Club lacrosse: A physiological and injury profile. *Ann Sport Med* 1990;5:114-117.
8. Knapik JJ, Bauman CL, Jones BH, et al: Preseason strength and flexibility imbalances associated with athletic injuries in female collegiate athletes. *Am J Sport Med* 1991;19:76-81.
9. Herring SA: Rehabilitation of muscle injuries. *Med Sci Sports Exerc* 1990;22:453-456.
10. Herring SA, Nilson KL: Introduction to overuse injuries. *Clin Sports Med* 1987;6:225-239.
11. Kibler WB: Analysis of sport as a diagnostic aid in shoulder disorders, in Matsen F, Fu F, Hawkins R (eds): *The Shoulder: A Balance of Mobility and Stability*. Rosemont, IL, American Academy of Orthopaedic Surgeons, 1993.
12. Watkins RG, Dennis S, Dillin WH, et al: Dynamic EMG analysis of torque transfer in professional baseball pitchers. *Spine* 1989;14:404-408.
13. Kibler WB: The role of the scapula in the throwing motion. *Contemp Orthop* 1991;22:525-532.

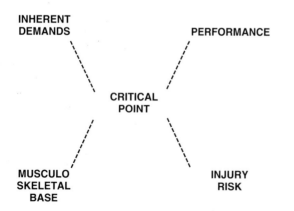

Fig. 2 The "critical point" framework. Every sport has inherent demands that must be met by the athlete's musculoskeletal base. This meeting place is the "critical point," out of which comes performance and injury risk.

The Anaerobic Energy System in Human Performance

B. R. Cahill, MD

Introduction

For the clinician interested in human performance enhancement, the results of a treatment program are more important than the exact details of the pathway necessary to reach these beneficial biologic adaptations. To the clinician, the ultimate measure of success is the patient's/athlete's response to the treatment. This channelized perspective is not unique. The medical profession has adopted established scientific information and has incorporated these advances into medical practice for years. Often, this was done without knowing in detail the exact biochemical/physiologic processes associated with these advances.

In the physical performance professions there has been a slow and reluctant adaptation of the scientific discoveries pertinent to human performance. Sports medicine clinicians, instead of being apologetic about a perceived gulf between them and exercise physiologists, should adopt the attitude of their medical colleagues by becoming more familiar with the physiologist's work, and, where appropriate, they should incorporate these practices into their profession. The purpose of this chapter is to present established anaerobic scientific principles as they should apply to the clinical practice of sports medicine.

The Clinical and Scientific Neglect of Anaerobics and the Emphasis on Aerobics

Early scientific interest in biologic energy systems focused on the aerobic with a relative disregard for the anaerobic process.[1-6] There were three principle reasons for this attention to the aerobic system.

That two distinct energy systems existed, that the aerobic was the work system and that the anaerobic was the power system had been recognized since the early 1900s. In 1923 Barr[7] established that there were two levels of exercise intensity provoking different acid-base balances, the more intense (anaerobic) causing an accumulation of lactate.[7,8] Hill[9] in 1924 discussed the oxygen debt and explained that this debt was due to lactate accumulation caused by exercise. In spite of this duality of biologic energy, the principle interest of early researchers was the human ability to perform work.

A method of measuring the aerobic system ($\dot{V}O_2$max) was reported by Robinson in 1938,[10] and was popularized by Åstrand.[11] The $\dot{V}O_2$max became the gold standard for measuring the aerobic system and fueled further interest in aerobic energy processes. No such anaerobic assessing test had yet reached this level of acceptance. In summary, the interest in aerobics and the lack of anaerobic incentive were due to the early researchers' interest in physiologic work, to an accepted method of assessing aerobic ability, and to the absence of an assessment test for the anaerobic system.

The Importance of the Anaerobic Energy System (AES) in Human Performance

At the most fundamental level, the primal importance of the AES is illustrated by the fact that all biologic activity is initiated with anaerobic energy. This means that the initiation of all movement is an anaerobic process.[12] In our evolution, the anaerobic capacity of all species has been an essential component of our survival.[13]

In 1986, de Vries stated, "Relatively few sports events in the United States require a sustained effort longer than 30 to 60 seconds. Consequently the vast majority of events depend upon anaerobic power, which has been given very little attention by researchers in physiology of exercise."[14]

In power sports, energy is derived almost exclusively from the AES.[1,13-16] While AES dependence is easily recognized in sports such as football and Olympic weight lifting, few clinicians realize that baseball is nearly entirely reliant on the AES. Because the AES is responsible for the initiation of all movement, the semi-sedentary sports of baseball, cricket, and dart throwing are anaerobic sports. The importance of the AES to military activities has been emphasized by Sharp[17] and Patton,[18] and the high degree of AES dependency of high-performance aircraft pilots by Tesch[16] and Bain.[19] Recent emphasis on the importance of enhancement of anaerobic ability in the geriatric population and the work of Bar-or[20,21] with children have emphasized the life-long importance of the AES.

Although the critical importance of anaerobic rehabilitation is obvious, little work has been done in this field. Few clinicians stress the anaerobic system in rehabilitation, and no reports indicate the degree of anaerobic rehabilitation attained, reporting instead isokinetic data.

The Physiologic Distinctions of the Two Biologic Energy Systems

From a practitioner's viewpoint the most important distinction between the two systems is the way they are used in human performance. The aerobic is the work system and the anaerobic is the power system. Table 1 outlines the salient features that distinguish the two energy systems.

The two energy systems are also distinguished by the anatomic extent of involvement of the body as a whole. The expression of anaerobic ability is a local phenomenon.[22] High anaerobic ability of the lower extremity does not imply similar ability in the arms or torso. Aerobic training provokes a more systemic than local adaptation of the organism as a whole. Because the cardiovascular and respiratory systems are intimately linked with aerobic processes, related changes occur that are both functional and dimensional.[12]

The aerobic system is configured for long-term, steady work, requiring from that system an efficient production of the energy source, adenosine triphosphate (ATP), by oxidative pathways. The anaerobic system is much less efficient but can provide short-term power for intense exercise by non-oxidative pathways. Histochemically and histologically, muscle fiber types reflect both the utilitarian and oxidative character of the two energy systems.[12,14]

Type I (slow twitch/aerobic) fibers have a higher percentage of oxidative enzymes and capillaries and a slower speed and strength of contraction than Type IIb (fast twitch/anaerobic). Conversely, the fatigability of Type IIb is higher than Type I. Fiber type IIa is an intermediate fiber type that exhibits characteristics of both Types I and IIb.

Motor units within a muscle are energy-system specific. Each motor unit is comprised of fibers of similar metabolic and contractile properties. Anaerobic motor units are innervated by large motor neurons with fast conduction times; aerobic units possess smaller and slower innervating neurons. As the intensity of exercise increases, Type I fibers are the first to be recruited, followed by IIa and finally IIb.[12]

The Assessment of the Anaerobic Energy System (AES)

The evaluation of physical fitness cannot be summarized by the measure of maximal oxygen uptake alone. Anaerobic metabolism, speed, strength, and maximal power are also determinant factors in many athletic activities.[23] Assessing anaerobic working capacity is of relevance to athletes and coaches, because anaerobic performances can be altered in response to anaerobic training.[24] Williams[25] has emphasized the importance of physiologic measurement in sport and points out the value of such data in physiologic profiling, assessment of training programs and evaluating the physiologic

Table 1
Distinguishing features of the two energy systems

	Aerobic	Anaerobic
Biologic utility	Work	Power
Biologic adaptation	Systemic	Local
Formula	F x D	F x D/T
Units	Joules	Watts
ATP production	Oxidative	High-energy phosphates, Anaerobic glycolysis
Fiber Types*	Type I (slow twitch)	Type IIb (fast twitch)

*Type IIa is intermediate.

demands of a sport. The physiologic rationale for using a short-term maximal exercise test in the evaluation of an athlete's anaerobic power and capacity is obvious.[16]

It is usual to divide anaerobic assessment into field and laboratory tests. For excellent reviews see Vandewalle[23] for laboratory tests and Bouchard and associates[1] for field tests. This article will consider only one of the laboratory tests, bicycle ergometry.

Of the laboratory tests, bicycle ergometry has emerged as the method of choice since its first report by Cumming[26] in 1973. Maud[3] states that, "the most popular test modality appears to be the cycle ergometer." Serresse,[24] Tesch,[16] and Vandewalle[23] also support the widespread use of bicycle ergometry to assess the AES.

Since Cumming's[26] report of the Wingate Anaerobic Test (WAT) in 1967, the WAT has grudgingly been accepted as the test methodology of choice.[1,3,16,18,21,23,24,27-29] The WAT is an "all out" bicycle ride of 30s duration against a fixed resistance calculated from body weight. The parameters reported by the WAT are: (1) peak power (PP), (2) mean power (MP), and (3) fatigue index (FI).

Bar-or,[21] himself a product of the Wingate Institute, while not the originator of the WAT, has researched, published, and nurtured the WAT to its present position of acceptance. His 1987 paper on WAT methodology, reliability, and validity is the best analysis of this anaerobic assessment test.[21]

Historically, there have been two principle dissensions related to the WAT—whether anaerobic capacity is measured by a 30s test,[1,13,30-35] and a corollary of this, ie, the appropriate length of the test. Depending on whether the alactic, lactacid, or anaerobic capacity is to be assessed, various authors have recommended test durations from 10s to 120s.[1,21,23,24,31,33,36-39] It is now generally agreed that the WAT does not fully assess anaerobic capacity, instead measuring another spectrum of the anaerobic energy system. According to Bar-or,[21] the WAT does assess peak power and local muscular endurance to supramaximal exercise, both valuable elements of the anaerobic athlete. While the WAT is considered a laboratory test, we have used it in the field, assessing over 1000 high school and college football players and over 400 female athletes.

In his paper, Williams[25] states "...physiological measurements of sportsmen during their participation in exercises which are part of their sport provides them, their coaches and sports medicine with a better understanding of the demands of their sport, a measure of their fitness and the basis for the biological adaptations to training. However, the link between the description of the physiological demands of a sport and the prescription of appropriate training loads is, as yet, not as strong as the layman would believe it to be."

Training the Anaerobic Energy System

Sports-specific training, which was introduced in the mid 1970s, proved to be more successful than generalized training in enhancing athletic performance. Over the past ten years there has been a growing trend toward energy system specific training. Energy system training recognizes the value of concentrating training on the predominant energy system used in an individual sport.

Aerobic researchers are confident with terming their "endurance" training programs aerobic, but anaerobic researchers and clinicians are less confident with designating their programs anaerobic. According to Knuttgen and Komi,[40] lack of preciseness has led to the misuse of terms and has resulted in confusion in reported anaerobic training results. This problem may be resolved with an accepted definition of anaerobic exercise.

Although no definition of anaerobic exercise has been elucidated, there are a number of criteria existing. The first is the acknowledgment that aerobic exercise is not anaerobic. The second is that anaerobic exercise is carried out at an intensity above the top limit of steady-state exercise (aerobic) of VO_2max. The third is that recovery between bouts of exercise in a training session must be incomplete. Fourth, the principle of progression must be followed or the program will stagnate.[41] Finally, combining aerobic and anaerobic training produces mixed results, with neither energy system significantly improving its efficiency.[42] Adhering to these principles and using existing training programs[41-45] will ensure that the anaerobic energy system is stressed to provide the desired biologic adaptations and performance improvement.

The practice of anaerobic training is illustrated in

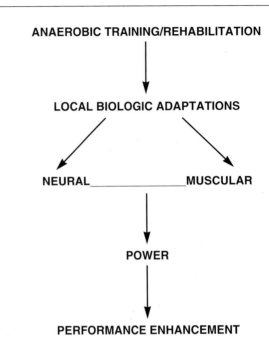

ANAEROBIC TRAINING/REHABILITATION

↓

LOCAL BIOLOGIC ADAPTATIONS

NEURAL_____MUSCULAR

↓

POWER

↓

PERFORMANCE ENHANCEMENT

Fig. 1 The practice of anaerobic training.

Figure 1. The local biologic adaptations that occur are either neural or muscular. It is well known that anaerobic training at intensities of 60% to 70% of maximal force-generating capacity (strength) results in adaptations that provoke an increase in total muscular size (cross-sectional area) and strength.[22,46] De Lorme,[14] over 40 years ago, recognized that the initial event in improvement in strength was a neural and not a muscular adaptation, and Moritani[15] and Sale[47] have confirmed this finding. The increased muscular cross-sectional area is accounted for by the increased myofibrillar protein, ie, fiber hypertrophy. The existence of fiber hyperplasia in humans is not generally accepted.[48]

Although morphologic adaptations are a consistent response to anaerobic training,[12,15,43,46,49] biochemical alterations are not. It is generally agreed that muscle glycogen storage is elevated by training.[12,42,43,49] Few authors report increased enzymatic activity of the anaerobic system.[12,42,50,51] According to Dudley,[50] "A large proportion of the power output spectrum (anaerobic) of humans has not been extensively studied...and this provides great opportunity in the bioenergetics of exercise." The physiology and energetics of the anaerobic energy system is less well known than the aerobic, but there is no doubt among researchers, clinicians, and coaches that the anaerobic system responds to appropriate training with biologic adaptations that result in increased performance.[52]

Anaerobic Rehabilitation After Injury

A literature search on the extent of anaerobic rehabilitation after injury produced no citations. Although the importance of the anaerobic energy system in human performance is recognized, this energy system may also play a more decisive role in returning the injured athlete to pre-injury participation form than is generally acknowledged.

Most traditional rehabilitation programs for lower extremity injuries include elements of anaerobic training, specifically heavy resistance training, plyometrics, and sprint training. However, these exercises may not reach supra-maximal intensities and may not adequately stress the AES.

There is no existing literature on anaerobic assessment after rehabilitation. Most traditional rehabilitation programs rely on isokinetic testing and functional progression performance to determine return to competition status. Since 1989 we have been assessing lower extremity injuries for their degree of anaerobic rehabilitation. We have used a traditional program, not the aggressive method that stresses rapid return to competition. In a study of 51 consecutive ACL reconstructions in young athletes, using the WAT to assess the extent of anaerobic rehabilitation, we were surprised to discover that 37% of the athletes were not anaerobically rehabilitated although they met all of our traditional criteria for return to competition.

Isokinetic testing is nearly a gold standard for return to playing status in traditional rehabilitation programs. Patton[18] and Smith[53] have stated that, in normal subjects, there is a high degree of correlation between high anaerobic and isokinetic abilities. In our ACL reconstructions study, no such correlation existed. We believe that normal isokinetic values do not reflect normal anaerobic ability, especially in subjects undergoing rehabilitation.

Since 1992 we have used principles of anaerobic training in our rehabilitation program. More importantly, we assess all lower extremity injuries monthly, beginning at month three. Assessment is by both the Wingate anaerobic test and isokinetic testing. Individuals with deficient anaerobic ability, demonstrated by the WAT, have their programs modified to include a higher proportion of anaerobic exercises. The preliminary results are encouraging.

References

1. Bouchard C, Taylor A, Simoneau J, et al: Testing anaerobic power and capacity, in MacDougall JD, Wenger HA, Green HJ (eds): *Physiological Testing of the High-Performance Athlete*, ed 2. Champaign, IL, Human Kinetics Books, 1991, pp 175-221.
2. Crielaard JM, Pirnay F: Anaerobic and aerobic power of top athletes. *Eur J Appl Physiol* 1981;47:295-300.
3. Maud PJ, Shultze BB: Norms for the Wingate anaerobic test with comparison to another similar test. *Res Q Exerc Sports* 1989;60:144-151.
4. Patton JF, Duggan A: Upper and lower body anaerobic power: Comparison between biathletes and control subjects. *Int J Sports Med* 1987;8:94-98.
5. Serresse O, Lortie G, Bouchard C, et al: Estimation of the contribution of the various energy systems during maximal work of short duration. *Int J Sports Med* 1988;9:456-460.
6. Watson RC, Sargeant TL: Laboratory and on-ice test comparisons of anaerobic power of ice hockey players. *Can J Appl Sport Sci* 1986;2:218-224.
7. Barr DP, Himwich HE: Studies in the physiology of muscular exercise: III. Development and duration of changes in acid-base equilibrium. *J Biol Chem* 1923;55:539-555.
8. Wasserman K, Koike A: Is the anaerobic threshold truly anaerobic? *Chest* 1992;101(suppl 5):211S-218S.
9. Hill AV, Long CNH, Lupton H: Muscular exercise, lactic acid, and the supply and utilisation of oxygen: VI. The oxygen debt at the end of exercise. *Proc R Soc Lond* 1924;97:127-138.
10. Robinson S: Experimental studies of physical fitness in relation to age. *Arbeitsphysiologie* 1938;10:251-323.
11. Åstrand PO: Human physical fitness with special references to sex and age. *Physiol Rev* 1956;36:307-335.
12. McArdle WD, Katch FI, Katch VL: *Exercise Physiology: Energy, Nutrition, and Human Performance*, ed 2. Philadelphia, PA, Lea & Febiger, 1986.
13. Saltin B: Anaerobic capacity: Past, present and prospective, in Taylor AW, Gollnick PD, Green HJ, et al (eds): *Biochemistry of Exercise VII*. Champaign, IL, Human Kinetics Books, 1990, pp 387-412.
14. de Lorme TL, Watkins AL: *Progressive Resistance Exercise: Technical and Medical Application*. New York, NY, Appleton Century-Crofts, Inc, New York, NY, 1951.
15. Moritani T: Time course of adaptations during strength and power training, in Komi PV (ed): *Strength and Power in Sport*. The Encyclopedia of Sports Medicine, IOC Medical Commission Publication. Oxford, Blackwell Scientific Publications, 1992, chap 9B, pp 266-278.
16. Tesch PA: Anaerobic testing: Research basis. *NSCA Journal* 1984;125-128.
17. Sharp O, Wright J, Vogel J, et al: Screening for physical capacity in U.S. Army: An analysis of measures predictive of strength and stamina. Natick, MA, U.S. Army Research Institute of Environmental Medicine, Tech. Rpt, T8/80, 1980.
18. Patton JF, Duggan A: An evaluation of tests of anaerobic power. *Aviat Space Environ Med* 1987;58:237-242.
19. Bain B, Jacobs I, Buick F: Effect of simulated air combat maneuvering on muscle glycogen and lactate. *Aviat Space Environ Med* 1992;63:505-509.
20. Bar-or O, Inbar O: Relationships among anaerobic capacity, sprint and middle distance running of school children, in Shepard RJ, Lavallee H (eds): *Physical Fitness Assessment: Principles, Practice and Application*. Springfield, IL, Charles C. Thomas, 1978, pp 142-147.
21. Bar-or O: The Wingate anaerobic test: An update on methodology, reliability and validity. *Sports Med* 1987;4:381-394.
22. Howald H: Malleability of the motor system: Training for maximizing power output. *J Exp Biol* 1985;115:365-373.
23. Vandewalle H, Peres G, Monod H: Standard anaerobic exercise tests. *Sports Med* 1987;4:268-289.
24. Serresse O, Simoneau JA, Bouchard C, et al: Aerobic and anaerobic energy contribution during maximal work output in 90-s determined with various ergocycle workloads. *Int J Sports Med* 1991;12:543-547.
25. Williams C: Value of physiological measurement in sport. *J R Coll Surg Edinb* 1990;35(suppl 6):S7-S13.

26. Cumming G: Correlation of athletic performance and aerobic power in 12 to 17-year-old children with bone age, calf muscle, total body potassium, heart volume and two indices of anaerobic power, in Bar-or O (ed): *Proceedings of the Fourth International Symposium on Pediatric Work Physiology*. Natanya, Wingate Institute, 1973, pp 109-134.

27. Nicklin R, O'Bryant H, Zenbauer T, et al: A computerized method for assessing anaerobic power and work capacity using maximal cycle ergometry. *J Appl Sport Sci Res* 1990;4:135-140.

28. Patton JF, Murphy MM, Frederick FA: Maximal power outputs during the Wingate anaerobic test. *Int J Sports Med* 1985;6:82-85.

29. Tharp GD, Newhouse RK, Uffelman L, et al: Comparison of sprint and run times with performance on the Wingate anaerobic test. *Res Q Exerc Sport* 1985;56:73-76.

30. Ayolon A, Inbar O, Bar-or O: Relationships among measurements of explosive strength and anaerobic power, in Nelson R, Morehouse C (eds): *International Series on Sport Sciences*. Baltimore, MD, University Press, 1974, vol 1, pp 572-577.

31. Boulay MR, Lortie G, Simoneau JA, et al: Specificity of aerobic and anaerobic work capacities and powers. *Int J Sports Med* 1985;6:325-328.

32. Jacobs I, Bar-or O, Karlsson J, et al: Changes in muscle metabolites in females with 30-s exhaustive exercise. *Med Sci Sports Exerc* 1982;14:457-460.

33. Medbo JI, Tabata I: Relative importance of aerobic and anaerobic energy release during short-lasting exhausting bicycle exercise. *J Appl Physiol* 1989;67:1881-1886.

34. Taunton JE, Maron H, Wilkinson JG: Anaerobic performance in middle and long distance runners. *Can J Appl Sport Sci* 1981;6:109-113.

35. Vandewalle H, Kapitaniak B, Grun S, et al: Comparison between a 30-S all-out test and a time-work test on a cycle ergometer. *Eur J Appl Physiol* 1989;58:375-381.

36. Gastin P, Lawson D, Hargreaves M, et al: Variable resistance loadings in anaerobic power testing. *Int J Sports Med* 1991;12:513-518.

37. Serresse O, Ama PF, Simoneau JA, et al: Anaerobic performances of sedentary and trained subjects. *Can J Sport Sci* 1989;14:46-52.

38. Simoneau JA, Lortie G, Boulay MR, et al: Tests of anaerobic alactacid and lactacid capacities: Description and reliability. *Can J Appl Sport Sci* 1983;8:266-270.

39. Vandewalle H, Peres G, Heller J, et al: All out anaerobic capacity tests on cycle ergometers: A comparative study on men and women. *Eur J Appl Physiol* 1985;54:222-229.

40. Knuttgen HG, Komi PV: Basic definitions for exercise, in Komi PV (ed): *Strength and Power in Sport*. The Encyclopedia of Sports Medicine, an IOC Medical Commission Publication. Oxford, Blackwell Scientific Publications, 1992, chap 1, pp 3-6.

41. Schmidtbleicher D: Training for power events, in Komi PV (ed): *Strength and Power in Sport*. The Encyclopedia of Sports Medicine, an IOC Medical Commission Publication. Oxford, Blackwell Scientific Publications, 1992, pp 381-395.

42. Stone M, Wilson D, Rozenek R, et al: Bridging the gap: Anaerobic: Physiologic. *NSCA Journal* 1984;40:63-65.

43. Cadefau J, Casademont J, Grau JM, et al: Biochemical and histochemical adaptation to sprint training in young athletes. *Acta Physiol Scand* 1990;140:341-351.

44. Fleck SJ, Kraemer WJ: *Designing Resistance Training Programs*. Champaign, IL, Human Kinetics Books, 1987.

45. Plisk S: Anaerobic metabolic conditioning: A brief review of theory, strategy and practical application. *J Appl Sports Sci Res* 1991;5:22-34.

46. MacDougall JD: Hypertrophy or hyperplasia, in Komi PV (ed): *Strength and Power in Sport*. The Encyclopedia of Sports Medicine, an IOC Medical Commission Publication. Oxford, Blackwell Scientific Publications, 1992, pp 230-238.

47. Sale DG: Neural adaptation to strength training, in Komi PV (ed): *Strength and Power in Sport*. The Encyclopedia of Sports Medicine, an IOC Medical Commission Publication. Oxford, Blackwell Scientific Publications, 1992, chap 9A, pp 249-265.

48. Matoba H, Gollnick PD: Response of skeletal muscle to training. *Sports Med* 1984;1:240-251.

49. Tesch PA: Skeletal muscle adaptations consequent to long-term heavy resistance exercise. *Med Sci Sports Exerc* 1988;20(suppl 5):S132-S134.

50. Dudley GA: Metabolic consequences of resistive-type exercise. *Med Sci Sports Exerc* 1988;20(suppl 5):S158-S161.

51. Roberts AD, Billeter R, Howald H: Anaerobic muscle enzyme changes after interval training. *Int J Sports Med* 1982;3:18-21.

52. Spriet L: Anaerobic metabolism in human skeletal muscle during short-term, intense activity. *Can J Physiol Pharmacol* 1992;70:157-165.

53. Smith DJ: The relationship between anaerobic power and isokinetic torque outputs. *Can J Sport Sci* 1987;12:3-5.

Physiology of Aerobic Fitness/Endurance

T. Jeff Chandler, EdD, CSCS, FACSM

Introduction

Aerobic exercise is one of the most widely researched, discussed, and used forms of exercise. Yet our knowledge in the area of aerobic metabolism is incomplete, particularly the role of the muscle in aerobic metabolism. Previous terminology and research in the area of aerobic metabolism may be inadequate in the face of new knowledge and concepts. Previous tests for aerobic efficiency, most notably the gold standard, $\dot{V}O_2$max, may provide only one part of the complex picture of true aerobic fitness. This being the case, a large volume of research that uses maximal oxygen uptake as a measure of fitness should be interpreted in light of this new line of thought.

A review of the terminology related to aerobic metabolism is necessary for a complete understanding of the concept. The typical bout of steady state aerobic exercise is depicted in Figure 1. When the supply of oxygen is sufficient to meet the demand, the predominant energy system is the aerobic system. In steady state exercise, lactate is removed at a rate equal to the rate of production. Two commonly used terms of aerobic fitness are aerobic power and aerobic capacity. Aerobic power is the oxygen uptake at maximal exercise intensity. This is often measured with a maximal treadmill or cycle ergometer test, resulting in a measure of $\dot{V}O_2$max expressed in terms of milliliters of oxygen per kilogram of body weight per minute (ml/kg/min). Aerobic power is limited by the ability of the heart and lungs to pump oxygenated blood to the working muscles. Aerobic capacity is the oxygen uptake at maximal effort expressed in liters of oxygen per minute (L/min).

Recently, measures of anaerobic threshold have been proposed as a way of measuring the body's ability to delay fatigue and perform endurance work (Fig. 2). Lactate threshold and ventilatory threshold have each been studied as performance indicators in terms of the body's ability to rid itself of lactic acid, an important metabolic intermediate linked to fatigue and decreased performance. With trained individuals, it appears that performance can improve without subsequent improvement in $\dot{V}O_2$max through positive changes in blood lactate response, ventilation, and the oxidative capacity of the muscle cells.

Sharkey[1] has proposed that aerobic metabolism should have two components, aerobic fitness and aerobic endurance. Aerobic fitness is defined as the ability of the athlete to take in, transport, and use oxygen. $\dot{V}O_2$max, the test upon which most of our decisions regarding exercise prescriptions for health and for performance are based, is a test for aerobic fitness.

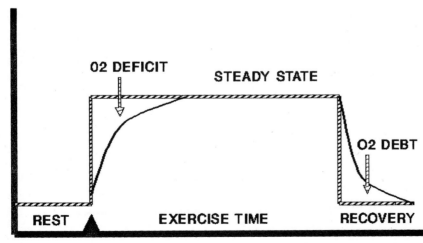

Fig. 1 A steady state of aerobic exercise where the oxygen supply is sufficient to meet the demand.

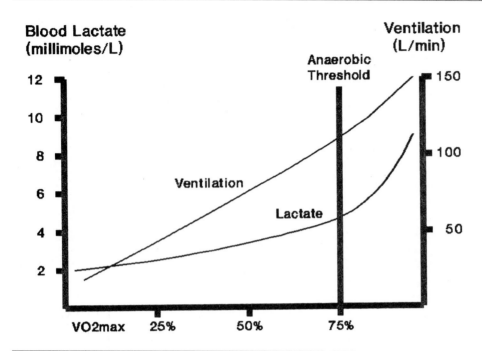

Fig. 2 Lactate threshold and ventilatory threshold as measures of anaerobic threshold. (Adapted from Sharkey B: *New Dimensions in Aerobic Fitness.* Champaign, IL, Human Kinetics Publishers, 1991, p 54.)

Aerobic endurance involves the ability of the muscle, using the aerobic enzymes, to perform prolonged work. Measures of aerobic endurance are not very prevalent, largely because of the importance previously placed on $\dot{V}O_2$max.

Energy Sources

The aerobic oxidative system can use proteins, fats, or carbohydrates as substrates. The substrate used to fuel the production of adenosine triphosphate depends on the availability of carbohydrates and fats. During the initial phases of aerobic exercise, and at exercise intensities of 95% of maximum and higher, carbohydrates are the preferred fuel. After 30 minutes of aerobic exercise of moderate intensity, the oxidation of fats increases in terms of contribution to energy production. Triglycerides stored in fat cells can be broken down, and free fatty acids released into the blood. Free fatty acids can be taken up by muscle and used for energy. Muscle tissue also contains small amounts of stored triglycerides as an intramuscular source of free fatty acids.

According to Sharkey,[1] health-related fitness may in the future be more closely related to aerobic endurance than to aerobic fitness as measured by $\dot{V}O_2$max, and it is possible that it may be related to the enhanced ability of the muscle to utilize fat.

Proteins, particularly skeletal muscle, can be broken down into amino acids, which can be converted into carbon skeletons, which can be converted to glucose by gluconeogenesis. Evidence suggests that protein may be used as a substrate to a greater extent than previously thought. Costill[2] reports that as much as 9% of the energy requirements for running a marathon may come from protein. This points to the need for endurance athletes to maintain an adequate protein intake, and may partially explain a comparative lack of muscle bulk in endurance athletes.

Conditioning

Conditioning the aerobic system for performance must be specific to the sport in which the athlete participates. Conditioning for predominately anaerobic sports, aerobic fitness will be the priority (Table 1). Conditioning for predominately aerobic sports, training for aerobic endurance will be the priority (Table 2). For the majority of sports that fall in between aerobic and anaerobic, specificity must be the key compo-

Table 1
General guidelines for a sample aerobic training program for primarily anaerobic sports

Time	Frequency	Intensity	Duration
Off-season	3-5 x week	Moderate-high	20 minutes
Preseason	2-3 x week	Moderate	20 minutes
In-season	1-2 x week	Moderate-low	20 minutes

Table 2
General guidelines for a sample aerobic training program for primarily aerobic sports

Time	Frequency	Intensity	Duration
Off-season	5-6 x week	Moderate	45-60+ minutes
Preseason	5-6 x week	Moderate-high	45-60+ minutes
In-season	3-5 x week	High	30-45 minutes

Table 3
General guidelines for a sample aerobic training program for mixed aerobic/anaerobic sports

Time	Frequency	Intensity	Duration
Off-season	3-5 x week	Moderate	30 minutes
Preseason	2-3 x week	Moderate-high	30 minutes
In-season	1-2 x week	Moderate	30 minutes

nent to guide the aerobic conditioning program. For sports that use both aerobic and anaerobic metabolism, work/rest intervals should be determined, along with the relative intensity of the work intervals. General guidelines for aerobic training of sports using mixed energy systems is presented in Table 3. For many mixed energy system sports, interval training in sport-specific work, rest, and intensity levels is the ideal form of aerobic training. Sports that are more aerobic in terms of work intervals can be of longer duration and lower intensity. Sports that are more anaerobic require work intervals of higher intensity and shorter duration.

A guiding principle for planning an aerobic conditioning program in seasonal sports is to progress from general aerobic fitness conditioning in the off-season to sport-specific aerobic fitness/endurance conditioning in the in-season. Typically, an "aerobic base" specific to a particular sport is built during the off-season. Preseason conditioning becomes more specific to the actual sporting activity, closely resembling the length and intensity of sport-specific work/rest intervals. Volume will decrease during the in-season phase to allow more time to be spent on sport-specific skills. Maintenance of the aerobic endurance gained during the off-season is the goal of most in-season programs.

Performance

The role of aerobic metabolism in performance of prolonged endurance activities is, without question, very important. The classic measurement of aerobic fitness is $\dot{V}O_2$max. When expressed in ml/kg/min, $\dot{V}O_2$max is a measure of aerobic power, and is generally thought to be highly related to performance in endurance running events. When expressed in liters per minute, $\dot{V}O_2$max is a measure of aerobic capacity, and is related to performance in such nonweightbearing activities as cycling and swimming. According to Noakes,[3] $\dot{V}O_2$max may predict performance in a heterogeneous group of athletes, but in a homogeneous group, this measurement does not predict performance among athletes of similar abilities. $\dot{V}O_2$max gen-

erally correlates at 0.7 to 0.8 with running performance, accounting for 50% to 64% of the variance in performance.[1] In one study, distance runs of 1, 2, and 6 miles correlated most strongly with $\dot{V}O_2$max, less strongly with percentage of slow twitch muscle fibers, and poorly with muscle enzyme patterns.[4]

Holloszy[5] demonstrated the importance of the role of aerobic enzymes on training. It seems that $\dot{V}O_2$max does not adequately explain the improvement in endurance relative to the peripheral factors, the oxidative enzyme changes in the muscle. In this study, $\dot{V}O_2$max improved only 14%, while endurance increased 500%, and cellular oxidative capacity increased 400%. It is clear that performance is related to other factors in addition to $\dot{V}O_2$max.

Of particular importance to athletes in a variety of sports is the level of aerobic fitness necessary for optimum performance in that particular sport. Traditional thought is that the higher the level of aerobic fitness in any sport, the better the performance. However, it is possible to improve performance without subsequent increases in $\dot{V}O_2$max.

The role of aerobic fitness in sports that are not primarily aerobic is a subject of some disagreement. Aerobic fitness likely has little predictive value in sports such as tennis, football, and soccer. The reasons for this are twofold. (1) In sports with a significant skill component, skill will be the best predictor of performance. (2) The aerobic system is used in these sports in recovery. The mechanisms of aerobic recovery from anaerobic events are not clear at the present time. It may be that other measures, in addition to $\dot{V}O_2$max, are necessary to predict the ability of the body to recover aerobically from short intense bouts of anaerobic exercise. Our knowledge in this area is incomplete. If an athlete recovers at an oxygen consumption of 40 ml/kg/min, is there an advantage to having a $\dot{V}O_2$max of 60 to 70 ml/kg/min? Are there any disadvantages of having a high $\dot{V}O_2$max?

Some evidence in the literature does suggest the possibility of a decrease in strength and power with extensive aerobic training.[6] This could occur because of an increase in the utilization of protein as a fuel for aerobic exercise. It has also been documented that dis-

Table 4
Strength and power deficits in prolonged endurance-trained athletes*

Athlete/Control	Measurement
	Grip Strength
Cross-country runners	106 kg
Average male student	117 kg
	Vertical Jump
Distance runners	13.5 in
Untrained controls	20.9 in

*Adapted with permission from Costill DL: *Inside Running: Basics of Sports Physiology*. Indianapolis, IN, Benchmark Press, 1986.

tance runners have lower levels of strength and power than other athletes (Table 4). This could be due to the percentage of slow twitch muscle fibers in the distance athlete, but is likely also a result of specificity of training.

Injury Risk

It has been hypothesized that by maintaining a high level of aerobic fitness, the athlete has a decreased risk of musculoskeletal injuries. Although this seems likely to be true, no studies have been found using only aerobic training that support this hypothesis. There is support for the possible mechanisms by which this could occur. By having a higher aerobic metabolic capacity, less energy may be spent on respiration and cardiac output, allowing more energy to be directed to performance in a particular sport. The ability to delay fatigue by having a high capacity for both aerobic fitness and aerobic endurance would seem to be very beneficial in this respect.

Muscular endurance is likely to play a large role in the decrease in injury risk with aerobic training. In terms of joint stability and injury prevention, strength of the muscles that cross the joint are important factors. Fatigue decreases the ability of a muscle to produce force and may have a factor in both traumatic and repetitive stress injuries. It should be noted that muscle endurance and aerobic endurance, although related, are two separate entities. One mechanism of improving local muscle endurance is to improve the strength of the involved musculature.

Aerobic training also has a positive effect on the strength of ligaments and tendons.[7,8] Both the size and strength of ligaments and tendons are improved with aerobic exercise. Increases in the size and strength of the muscle have not been reported with aerobic training. This may be related to protein utilization in the muscle for energy with long-term aerobic work.

Rehabilitation

Aerobic fitness/endurance can decrease very rapidly with bed rest. This decrease is likely caused by decreases in both central and peripheral factors of oxygen utilization. A summary of the effects of detraining are presented in Outline 1. Generally speaking, the athlete who remains relatively active, even when not training, will maintain aerobic fitness for about two weeks without a significant reduction of aerobic fitness. Tapering before a big event actually has positive benefits to performance.

The loss of aerobic fitness can be decreased by having the athlete perform some type of aerobic exercise during the rehabilitation process. With an upper body injury, this is not difficult, because the athlete can generally walk, jog, cycle, or perform stair-climbing exercises fairly early in the rehabilitation process. With a lower body injury, this is not as easy, because the athlete has to use a substitute or modified form of aerobic exercise. Swimming can be used in many cases and cycling may be appropriate with some stress fractures and ankle injuries. In some instances, an arm cycle ergometer may be used. The arm cycle, because it uses a smaller muscle mass, is not as demanding on the cardiorespiratory system, and is therefore generally not as effective in maintaining aerobic fitness.

The athlete who undergoes a forced layoff from training, such as surgery, will benefit from a high aerobic fitness/endurance level. After a layoff, the aerobically fit athlete will regain his aerobic fitness/endurance at a faster rate.[2]

Methods of Measurement

The most popular method of measuring of aerobic fitness is the $\dot{V}O_2$max test on a treadmill or cycle ergometer. As mentioned previously, this measurement is mistakenly seen by many as a measurement of complete aerobic fitness. The $\dot{V}O_2$max test measures primarily the ability of the body to take in, transport, and utilize oxygen. It does not adequately measure aerobic endurance, or the ability of the muscles to func-

Outline 1
The effect of inactivity on aerobic fitness/endurance parameters. Detraining of the aerobic system*

10% to 50% decline in muscles' aerobic capacity in 1 week
Mitochondrial enzymes may begin to decline within 48 hours
Muscle capillarization may decrease 10% to 20% within 5 to 12 days
Cardiac output begins to decline within 5 to 12 days
Lactate levels approach the untrained level after 4 weeks

*Reprinted with permission from Costill DL: *Inside Running: Basics of Sports Physiology*. Indianapolis, IN, Benchmark Press, 1986.

tion repeatedly for prolonged periods of time. It does provide important information in regards to aerobic fitness. Submaximal tests can also be performed on a cycle or treadmill, with the data being used to predict maximal performance. Step tests and 1.5-mile run tests are popular field tests of aerobic fitness.

Measurements of aerobic endurance should be an important part of testing the endurance athlete, and may prove in the future to have health-related benefits. Because aerobic endurance is, by definition, a result of a prolonged effort, tests of aerobic endurance will be of a prolonged nature. These tests will be used to devise shorter laboratory and field tests to predict aerobic endurance. Muscle biopsies to validate the oxidative capacity of muscle may be necessary to validate the predictive and field tests. Two concepts discussed earlier, blood lactate threshold measurements and ventilatory threshold measurements, are controversial predictors of endurance fitness and will require further validation.

Onset of blood lactate accumulation, the point where lactate reaches a specific range of from 2 to 4 millimoles, is one measure of blood lactate. Another measure of lactate is called maximal steady state and is defined by LaFontaine[9] as the treadmill velocity associated with a fixed blood lactate level of 2.2 millimoles. Long duration training may decrease postexercise lactate levels, making lactate measurement a possible measure of aerobic endurance.

Ventilatory threshold is a noninvasive measure that may prove to be helpful in the measurement of aerobic endurance. The respiratory system begins to increase in frequency to compensate for metabolic acidosis. Diet and protocol choices must be standardized if ventilatory threshold measures are to be of consistent value in measuring aerobic endurance.

Sharkey[1] proposes that tests of aerobic endurance should be of longer duration than the typical $\dot{V}O_2$max test, so that the aerobic enzyme system in the muscles is stressed. It may be necessary, according to Sharkey, to develop a 20-minute jog test or a 20-minute bike test for this purpose. Field tests to measure aerobic endurance should be based on longer duration tests, with shorter predictive tests being developed based on these tests. Weltman[10] who demonstrated that endurance capacity is closely related to blood lactate, has developed a 3,200-meter field test to predict lactate accumulation and $\dot{V}O_2$.

DeVries[11] proposed a test he terms Physical Work Capacity Fatigue Threshold. The equipment necessary for this test is a cycle ergometer and a stop watch, resulting in an estimate of both lactate threshold and $\dot{V}O_2$max from a single test of two or three short work bouts of one to four minutes in duration at heavy, moderate, and light workloads. The test correlates well with anaerobic threshold (r = .93) and with EMG measures of fatigue (r = .87).

Summary

Aerobic fitness and aerobic endurance are two separate components of aerobic metabolism. Aerobic fitness, best measured by $\dot{V}O_2$max, is a measure of oxygen transport and utilization. Aerobic endurance is not measured in a $\dot{V}O_2$max test because it does not measure the ability of the muscle to perform prolonged work. Endurance fitness may be a complementary measurement to $\dot{V}O_2$max, providing additional information regarding the capacity of the muscle for long-term work. The muscle is the primary site where increases in mitochondrial enzymes improve aerobic endurance capacity. Aerobic endurance may be more closely related to health-related fitness than aerobic fitness.

Conditioning must be specific to the sport or activity, progressing from general aerobic fitness in the off-season to sport-specific aerobic fitness/endurance during the playing season. Aerobic fitness/endurance decreases rapidly with detraining. Adequate aerobic fitness/endurance specific to a particular sport may help prevent injury in terms of delaying fatigue and improving the strength of the tendons and ligaments. A properly initiated sport-specific aerobic conditioning program is essential for maximal performance to be reached in most any sport.

References

1. Sharkey BJ: *New Dimensions in Aerobic Fitness.* Champaign, IL, Human Kinetics Publishers, 1991.
2. Costill DL: *Inside Running: Basics of Sports Physiology.* Indianapolis, IN, Benchmark Press, 1986.
3. Noakes T: *Lore of Running.* Cape Town, Oxford University Press, 1985.
4. Foster C, Costill DL, Daniels JT, et al: Skeletal muscle enzyme activity, fiber composition and VO_2 max in relation to distance running performance. *Eur J Appl Physiol* 1978;39:73-80.
5. Holloszy JO: Biochemical adaptations in muscle: Effects of exercise on mitochondrial oxygen uptake and respiratory enzyme activity in skeletal muscle. *J Biol Chem* 1967;242:2278-2282.
6. Hickson RC: Interference of strength development by simultaneously training for strength and endurance. *Eur J Appl Physiol* 1980;45:255-263.
7. Tipton CM, James SL, Mergner W, et al: The influence of exercise on strength of medial collateral knee ligaments of dogs. *Am J Physiol* 1970;218:894-902.
8. Tipton CM, Matthes RD, Maynard JA, et al: The influence of physical activity on ligaments and tendons. *Med Sci Sports Exerc* 1975;7:165-175.
9. LaFontaine TP, Londeree BR, Spath, WK: The maximal steady state versus selected running events. *Med Sci Sports Exerc* 1981;13:190-192.
10. Weltman A: The lactate threshold and endurance performance, in Granna W, Lombardo J, Sharkey B, et al (eds): Chicago, IL, Yearbook Medical Publishers, 1989, pp 91-116.
11. DeVries, HA: *Physiology of Exercise for Physical Education and Athletics.* Dubuque, IA, William C Brown, 1966, chap 16, pp 268-281.

Clinical Implications of Exercise: Injury and Performance

W. Ben Kibler, MD

Physiology of Muscle Response to Soft Tissue Injury

The physiologic responses of muscle to injury, and the physiologic alterations that are seen in muscle in injury evaluation and treatment, vary with the type of pathologic process that produces the injury. The two main types of pathologic processes in athletic injuries are macrotrauma and chronic microtrauma (Table 1).

Macrotrauma

Macrotrauma injuries are the result of an event—a one-time, high-force injury that produces overt clinical symptoms. Examples are acute lateral ankle sprain, fractures, or muscle contusions. In most cases, the muscles, tendons, bones, and ligaments are normal both at a cellular and tissue level before the event, and are abnormal after the event. The athlete can usually pinpoint the time of onset of the injury. The physiologic alterations in muscle are most frequently the result of immobilization or other treatment, or from disuse imposed because of the injury. A small proportion may occur as a result of the injury itself.

Immobilization can occur as a result of casting, splinting, or wrapping of the injury or as a consequence of protection after surgery.

Tissue stiffness, muscle weakness, and neurologic alterations are the most prominent alterations. Tissue stiffness following immobilization is largely caused by changes in the ground substance supporting tendons, muscles, ligaments and capsules.[1] There is reduction of glycosaminoglycan content and water which results in a reduction of collagen mass.[2] Random orientation of new collagen fibers and irregular cross-links between adjacent fibers occur due to lack of motion.[3] All connective tissues that are immobilized sustain these changes, not just the injured tissues. This results in generalized joint stiffness or arthrofibrosis, muscular inflexibility, and decreased range of motion.

Muscle weakness is an inevitable consequence of immobilization. Normal and injured muscle are immediately adversely affected by immobilization, leading to dramatic loss of fiber size[4] and strength[5] within three to seven days. Fiber size declines up to 15% after three days, and strength declines 15% after seven days. Muscle strength continues to decrease with longer immobilization, but muscle mass does not continue to decline as rapidly. Intracellular changes also reflect this process. Mitochondral size and number, and glyco-

Table 1
Difference in muscle physiologic response after macrotrauma or microtrauma injury

Macrotrauma	Microtrauma
Result from event	Result from process
Normal cellular and tissue structures before overt symptoms, abnormal after	Cellular and tissue structures show change before overt symptoms
Physiologic alterations due to immobilization, disuse, or direct injury	Physiologic alterations due to adaptations to process

Flexibility alterations
    Generalized stiffness
    Arthrofibrosis
	Flexibility alterations
	    Specific tensile based
	    No arthrofibrosis

Strength alterations
    Generalized deficit
    No imbalances
    Neural injury
    Decreased neural drive
    Muscle inhibition
	Strength alterations
	    Specific muscles
	    Tensile based
	    Force couple imbalance
	    Altered motor firing

Mechanics
    Kinetic chain involved
    Few adaptations
	Mechanics
	    Kinetic chain involved
	    Many adaptations

gen and ATP levels are all decreased.[6,7] These factors result in increase in muscle contraction time, decreased muscle tension, and decreased muscle endurance. These changes are seen in all muscles subjected to immobilization, leading to generalized muscle strength deficits around injured areas. Some muscles, such as the quadriceps and especially its vastus medialis component, seem to be more adversely affected, but because all muscles are affected, large force couple imbalances are rare.

The intramuscular contributions to muscular weakness are compounded by the neurologic alterations that result from injury or immobilization. Nerves may be injured in the macrotrauma injury, such as the peroneal nerve in ankle sprains, the ACL receptors in ACL injury, or the axillary nerve in shoulder dislocations. In these cases, altered sensory input or motor output will produce a change in lower motor neuron firing patterns, resulting in muscle weakness. Another common neurologic alteration is a loss of neural drive, probably produced by direct cortical activity, which can be estimated by the integrated EMG (Fig. 1). The exact mechanism of loss of neural drive is not known,

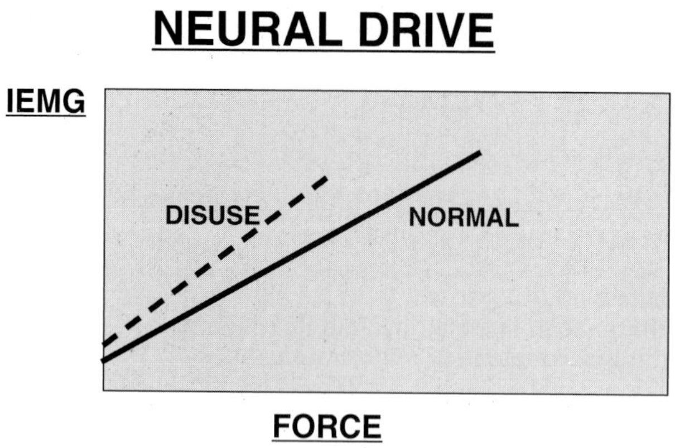

NEURAL DRIVE

IEMG

DISUSE   NORMAL

FORCE

Fig. 1 Loss of neural drive. Both force production and integrated EMG activity are decreased.

but probably reflects a series of central nervous system adjustments which include lack of motor unit recruitment, decreased motor unit firing rate, and asynchrony of firing patterns for specific movements. The net result is disordered motor firing which results in decreased force production.[8]

Muscle weakness also occurs as a result of disuse. The same type of cellular and intracellular alterations occur in disused as in immobilized muscle, but the magnitude and pace of changes is much less. The net result is generalized muscle strength and endurance weakness that involves all disused muscles, with asynchrony of motor firing patterns, but little force imbalance. Muscles subject to disuse may be relatively close to the injured area, such as the hamstrings and tensor fascia lata in quadriceps contusions, or they may be farther away, such as the deltoid in a severely sprained wrist or the gluteals in a severely sprained ankle. As a result of the distant muscle involvement in this latter category, these alterations enlarge the extent of the total injury to other areas of the kinetic chain.

Muscle inhibition is a potent cause of muscle weakness after macrotrauma. Traditionally, pain was thought to be the major cause of the inhibition, through a reflex modulated by small afferent pain fibers. However, many other factors have been shown to be involved. Capsular distension without a conscious level of pain, as in a chronic effusion or in a distended joint with applied anesthetic, can cause muscle inhibition.[9] A muscle displays higher levels of inhibition if it is immobilized in a shortened position.[9] Finally, other neurologic factors besides pain may cause inhibition. Proprioception is altered after immobilization,[10] and this is associated with alteration of muscle firing patterns. Also, the H reflex, which is concerned with maintenance of muscle tone and readiness to fire, is decreased by capsular distension. The loss of this prim-

ing mechanism for muscle contraction may cause inhibition of firing.[11]

Muscle inhibition appears to be more common after macrotrauma injury, probably because of the associated pain and acute tissue damage, with resulting swelling and immobilization. It should be recognized and treated at that time. However, if untreated or undertreated, it can appear as part of the spectrum of the chronic microtrauma injury. The quadriceps muscle that is inhibited secondary to thigh contusion or mild torn meniscus may allow enough force overload to bring about symptoms of patellar tendinitis.

Microtrauma

In contrast to macrotrauma, chronic microtrauma injuries are the result of a process, a gradual degeneration in the ability of the cells and tissues to maintain their integrity. This degeneration occurs before overt clinical symptoms appear. Examples of microtrauma injuries include plantar fasciitis, elbow epicondylitis, and patellar tendinitis. It is important to realize that acute exacerbations of chronic problems, such as a recurrent hamstring pull, or the acute symptomatic presentation of a chronic patellar tendinitis or rotator cuff tendinitis, should also be considered under the chronic microtrauma classification.[12] Degenerative changes in the cell include decrease in mitochondral enzyme levels,[13] change in RNA transcription,[14] and alterations in calcium release and uptake,[15] and result in decreased matrix production. This deficient matrix causes dysfunction of the tissue. The exact cause of this degenerative cycle is not known, but researchers have demonstrated that mechanical damage secondary to tensile loads can start this process.[14-16] These cellular alterations are not immediately manifest at a tissue or overt level because of the gradual nature of the process. However, by the time that overt clinical symptoms appear, the tissues around the area of injury already have associated physiologic alterations that are different in nature and location from those found in macrotrauma injuries.

The low-grade inflammatory process that has been demonstrated to occur in tensile strain muscle injuries[16] tends to heal with fibrotic tissue. This inflammatory-based fibrosis is particularly prone to scar contracture,[17] resulting in inflexibility of the specific muscles involved in the tensile process. Inflexibility of tensile muscles has been demonstrated in plantar fasciitis[18,19] and Achilles tendinitis (gastrocnemius/soleus),[19] lateral epicondylitis (wrist extensors),[20] and rotator cuff tendinitis (posterior deltoid and infraspinatus/teres minor).[21,22]

Muscle strength deficits are also seen in the specific muscles subjected to repetitive tensile loads. These deficits are probably caused by the tensile-based mechanical damage, some degree of selective inhibition of the particular muscle, failure of matrix and fibril production, and altered motor firing patterns.[23] The gastrocnemius/soleus complex in plantar fasciitis,[18] wrist extensors[20] and shoulder external rotators[24] in lateral epicondylitis, the subscapularis in chronic shoulder instability,[23] the scapular stabilizers in rotator cuff tendinitis[25,26] or instability,[26] and the quadriceps in leg injuries[27] have been shown to be abnormal.

Specific strength deficits in certain muscles also may set up force couple imbalances, since the paired muscle on the opposite side of the force couple is usually normal.[28] Imbalances are thought to be more important as predictors of further injury,[29] because properly balanced force couples are important in constraining the forces around the joint, maintaining anatomic integrity and mechanical efficiency. Force couple imbalances have been demonstrated in symptomatic baseball pitchers[30] and tennis players (shoulder internal/external rotators),[31] patellar tendinitis (knee flexors/extensors), and lacrosse players.[32]

Because of the process of microtrauma injury, the athlete often develops mechanical adaptations to compensate for the inflexibility, strength deficit, or force couple imbalance, in an attempt to maintain relatively normal force production or performance. These adaptations may be local, such as a racquet grip change and increased forearm supination in a tennis player with lateral epicondylitis or decreased stance phase on the affected foot in a runner with plantar fasciitis. The adaptations also may be distant, such as increased muscle firing patterns and muscle activation by arm muscles during throwing in a pitcher who has a pulled groin muscle and decreased leg strength or change in service motion in a tennis player with low back pain and trunk inflexibility. These adaptations, which are common in chronic microtrauma injury patterns,[22,33] must be identified in the evaluation and included in the rehabilitation process.

In summary, acute macrotrauma and chronic microtrauma injuries have different pathophysiologic mechanisms and different effects on the physiology of exercising muscle. These differences are listed in Table 1. Even though deficits in strength, flexibility, and mechanics exist in both instances, and often shade from one type to another, these deficits are sufficiently distinct to be evaluated and treated as separate entities. The orthopaedic surgeon should be aware of the different modes of injury presentation, so that proper evaluation can be carried out.

Physiology of Conditioning

Sport-Specific Conditioning

Maximum performance in athletic activities can be best obtained by conditioning the body by a sport-specific series of exercises designed to maximize the body's ability to withstand the demands inherent within a sport. This conditioning program, which will include an understanding of the inherent demands of the sport, an adequate preconditioning fitness examination, and conditioning for both performance enhancement and injury risk reduction, will be constructed and conducted under the framework of periodization.[34]

Different sports place different demands on the physiologic apparatus in the muscle. While all athletes in all sports need a general athletic base of adequate strength, flexibility, and endurance, certain key areas of muscle function are more heavily stressed for maximum performance with minimal injury risk. Football places more demands on muscles for absolute concentric strength, or maximal force production, than does basketball. Running has little demands for large force production, but does require eccentric strength, or force absorption. Force couple balance of concentric and eccentric strength around the shoulder is the key to maintenance of anatomic integrity and biomechanical efficiency in throwing athletes. Gymnastics and swimming have optimum demands for flexibility in key anatomic areas. Long distance runners have maximum need for aerobic endurance, while down linemen in football, track sprinters, or tennis players need mainly anaerobic endurance, and soccer players need a combination of both types of endurance. Knowledge of these and other differential demands[35] can guide the formulation of the sport-specific conditioning program.

The conditioning program needs to have a definite starting point and a firm goal. The goal is usually defined as optimum sport-specific fitness. The starting point, defined as the state of fitness before initiation of the conditioning process, should be measured by an adequate preconditioning examination. The examination may be as simple as some field tests, such as a timed mile run, push-ups, sit-ups, and a touch-your-toes flexibility exam, or as comprehensive as a complete preparticipation fitness examination.[35] However, because this examination will be the starting point for the conditioning process, it is suggested that as much data about sport-specific flexibility, strength, strength balance, and endurance should be obtained as possible.[34] The exercise prescription for the best pathway to sport-specific fitness can then be constructed (Fig. 2). A guide to constructing a battery of tests to check these sport-specific parameters has been published.[35]

The strength-conditioning process has traditionally been viewed as being devoted to building maximum strength for performance. Many studies have shown that the goals of improved force production, increased muscle bulk, and increased power can be achieved. These goals are accomplished by emphasis on large muscle training, concentric muscle work, maximum

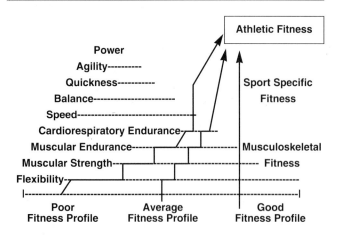

Fig. 2   The goal of a sport-specific conditioning program is optimum sport-specific fitness. The best pathway to that goal depends on the fitness level at the beginning of the process.

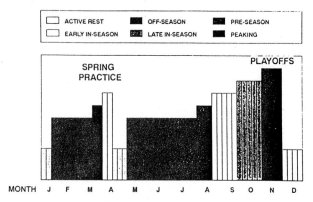

Fig. 3   Phases of a football periodization plan.

force production, and agonist muscle firing patterns. However, more work is now emerging that also views conditioning as a process for reduction in injury risk. In this situation, emphasis is placed on smaller muscle training, eccentric muscle work, force absorption, and antagonistic muscle firing patterns. Conditioning programs can be developed to incorporate both of these aspects of conditioning into the same program.[8,34,36] The framework for this development is the principle of periodization.

Similarly, the endurance-conditioning process has usually focused on aerobic endurance. However, many sports are more dependent on anaerobic activity for performance and on aerobic activity for recovery. Some studies have shown that uncoordinated conditioning of different endurance systems, or of endurance and strength, will not produce desired results, and that coordination of these activities under a periodization program will produce the best results.

Periodization

Periodization is a plan that matches the volume, intensity, and content of a conditioning program with the different phases of the training cycle so that optimal sport-specific preparedness is reached.[8,34,36] The training cycle is divided into separate phases related to an athletic season. The phases are the off-season, preseason, in-season, peaking, and recovery, or active rest, phases. For athletic activities with definable seasons, such as football, basketball, or baseball, the phases are easily defined and established (Fig. 3). For athletic activities with ill-defined seasons, such as tennis or long-distance running, the phases are more difficult to identify or establish. In these situations the phases of the training cycle should be based on important events

during the year (Fig. 4). Different aspects of muscle physiology and different aspects of general athletic fitness or sport-specific fitness are developed or stressed during each phase.

Active Rest

Active rest is the phase an athlete would go into immediately after the competitive season. In this stage the athlete has a brief period of total rest (1 or 2 days) followed by a period of remaining physically active by participating in a variety of activities unrelated to the primary sport. Cross-training, participation in enjoyable activities, and participation in activities that do not fit into the competitive year are key components of this phase. This phase is designed to give athletes a

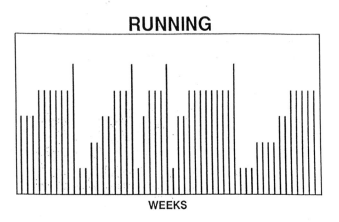

Fig. 4   Phases of a running periodization plan. The following phases are shown: active rest, off season, preseason, early season, and late season peaking.

mental and physical break from their sport for a period of up to several weeks.

Off-season Phase or General Preparation Phase

This phase, which marks the start of the conditioning process, prepares the body for more intense training. General athletic fitness is emphasized, with general flexibility exercises and heavy weight training, and running or other aerobic work appropriate to the sport. This is the best time to correct any musculoskeletal deficits, and the preconditioning evaluation should be done at this time. There may be some occasional sport-specific play, but ideally, no competition. Flexibility exercises would involve total body flexibility. Running, bicycling, stair climbing, or other aerobic work would emphasize improvement in $\dot{V}O_2$max and heart rate recovery from intense activity.

Weight training will focus more on performance and force generation, and will involve the large muscle groups, such as the quadriceps, gluteals, pectorals, and latissimus dorsi. The frequency should be two to five times per week. The duration varies, usually beginning with an endurance component (sets of 8 to 15 repetitions), progressing to a strength component (heavier weights at 4 to 6 repetitions), and ending with a power component (5 repetitions or less at high velocities). The intensity varies with the number of repetitions, but it is generally recommended that resistance be set to make the last 1 to 2 repetitions difficult but achievable.

This phase may need to be relatively long in young players who need to build their general fitness base. It may be shorter in athletes who are at the peak of their career, particularly in sports where participation takes up a large part of the calendar year. Recovery periods should be built into the schedule. Heavy weight training, plyometrics, intense running, and skill work should be arranged in the training schedule in a manner to allow recovery and repair.

Preseason or Specific Preparation Phase

The preseason phase is a period of high intensity and sport-specific work, in which total work volume remains high. There is a transition from general to sport-specific work in flexibility, strength, and endurance. General fitness drills, such as high-intensity weight training, are continued but are decreased in volume. Sport-specific skills are practiced and refined, and limited competitive play, such as exhibitions, is allowed. Flexibility emphasis is shifted to areas that are at maximal risk of maladaptation such as the gastrocnemius and hamstring in runners, or the back and posterior shoulder in throwing athletes. Endurance training becomes specific for sports demands. Tennis players run 5- to 20-yard dashes and practice hitting balls for 5 to 25 seconds at a time. Soccer players run 10- to

40-yard dashes, and do run intervals of 40 to 60 yards with 15 to 20 seconds of rest.

Weight training takes on an additional focus of injury reduction and force regulation involving the muscles used in a particular sport, for example, the back muscles, hamstrings, rotator cuff, and posterior shoulder and scapular stabilizing muscles in throwing or overhead athletes. The frequency of training these muscle groups in this manner is up to five times per week performed in sets of 8 to 15 repetitions. Because these muscles are generally smaller in cross-sectional area, the absolute amount of resistance may be smaller, but still should be set so that the last one to two repetitions are difficult. Plyometrics and rubber tubing are important means of exercise during this phase. Because of the high intensity of work, recovery periods should be emphasized and scheduled. Plyometrics should generally be done no more than two times per week to allow time for recovery.

Early In-season or Early Competitive Phase

This phase occurs in sports that have a long regular season, such as football or basketball. This is a holding phase, in which conditioning is high but not maximal, in preparation for the extra effort for peaking. Maintenance of conditioning level is the most important goal of this phase for most athletes, although young athletes may continue to experience some gains in strength and power. Competition is frequent in this phase. Sport-specific flexibility and endurance work is continued on a regular basis, but with less intensity as competition increases.

Weight training is maintained to counteract the tendency to lose strength during the season. The frequency of intense work should be one to two times a week, and the duration should continue to emphasize the endurance component of 8 to 15 repetitions. Adequate recovery periods must be planned after competitions. In sports that have weekly or biweekly competitions, hard practices and conditioning should come early in the week, with tapering one to two days before competition.

Late In-season or Peaking Phase

The goal of this phase is maximum efficiency of performance for intense competition. Conditioning work is usually at a minimum, emphasizing sport-specific flexibility and light weight training. Other conditioning work is usually tapered before competition if the volume of competition will be high. This high level of intensity and competition cannot be maintained indefinitely. Studies have shown that a high level of performance can be maintained for about 5 to 21 days. If total workload is maintained at a high level due to maintenance of training during intense competition, or is maintained over too long of a time, overload injuries and overtraining are distinct possibilities.

In summary, periodization is the best method of integrating the conditioning process with the demands of the sport to allow optimum readiness to play the sport. It is based on knowledge of the physiology of strength, flexibility, anaerobic endurance, and aerobic endurance. In addition to achieving maximal performance with minimal injury risk, it also helps to decrease the chances of overtraining. Overtraining is a continual risk in high performance conditioning or athletic activity, but periodized conditioning, by adjusting the volume, intensity, and content of the program or activity, minimizes the risk.

Overtraining

Overtraining is the down side of athletic activity, competition, and conditioning. It can be thought of as an imbalance between stress and recovery (Fig. 5), leading to a loss of homeostasis in the athlete's body. Overtraining is not one particular set of physical findings and one particular set of abnormal performance parameters. Rather, the athlete exhibits varying physical and psychological characteristics that will decrease performance and predispose to injury (Table 2). Overtraining usually presents as a series of nagging injuries, as decreased performance in the face of increased training, or as decreased motivation in the face of increased competition.

Musculoskeletal alterations include easy fatigability, muscle weakness, muscle imbalance, and repeated injuries, either to the same area, or areas distant in the kinetic chain.[37] Fatigability is probably related to alteration in sympathetic/parasympathetic tone,[38] and strength and strength balance are decreased when the muscles are overworked.[8] These two factors, in the face of continued athletic activity, create an overload situation on muscles, tendons, or bones that can lead to such injuries as shin splints, muscle strains, tendinitis, and stress fractures. If treatment is only directed towards the clinical symptoms, and the overtraining component is not addressed, these injuries can recur.

Any athlete who presents with a series of nagging, overload-related injuries that do not improve with normal therapy should be considered for the diagnosis of overtraining. Prompt recognition of the symptoms of overtraining can lead to proper diagnosis and institution of treatment programs that will decrease the chances of further overload. After the diagnosis is made, education about overtraining should be instituted. Treatment should be based on resolving the symptoms and correcting any strength or flexibility deficits that have occurred. As rehabilitation progresses towards return to play, periodization should be used to keep the volume of training below the overtraining threshold. More rest intervals should be employed, and the balance between conditioning and playing should be monitored. The athlete in peak training should be shown how to take a resting heart rate in the morning so that any abnormal elevation can be noticed as an early warning sign of overtraining. Many athletes, both at a professional and recreational level, are at risk of overtraining. A high index of suspicion, early institution of changes in training, and proper rehabilitation of musculoskeletal alterations are the most important factors in treating the frustrating performance loss and injuries associated with the overtraining syndrome.

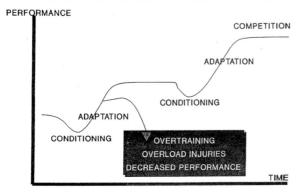

THE GENERAL ADAPTATION SYNDROME APPLIED TO ATHLETIC COMPETITION

Fig. 5 Overtraining is the result of inadequate adaptation to a conditioning response, an imbalance between stress and recovery.

Table 2
Physical and performance parameters associated with overtraining

Physical	Increased resting heart rate
	Easy fatigability
	Muscle weakness
	Recurrent injuries
	Alteration in hormone levels
	(plasma cortisol, thyroid, 24-hour epinephrine)
Psychological	Insomnia
	Irritability
	Lack of cooperation
	Decreased goals
	Lack of motivation
Performance	Increased times
	Increased perceived effort
	Alteration in mechanics

Discussion of Case Examples

Case 1

An athlete reports with recurrent ankle sprains and little residual ligamentous laxity. What physiologic variables may be contributing to recurrent sprains, how should they be evaluated, and how should they be rehabilitated? When can the player return to play?

This athlete represents an acute exacerbation of a chronic overload process, and has accompanying physiologic and mechanical alterations that predispose to further injury. A comprehensive examination of the surrounding supporting structures should be done to evaluate their competence. Physiologic alterations may include abnormalities of proprioception, peroneal and/or gastrocnemius muscle weakness, and decreased ankle dorsiflexion. Mechanical alterations may include decreased stance time, running and landing on the heels, and jumping and cutting off the opposite foot. Rehabilitation should include strengthening of all the supporting musculature, specific flexibility exercises for the gastrocnemius/soleus group, and proprioceptive exercises, such as agility work and the B.A.P.S. board. The athlete may return to play when adequate strength and flexibility are present, and the athlete can jump off the affected foot and complete a figure eight course with the obstacles two feet apart.

Case 2

What weights should be lifted before the football season? Should weights be lifted during the football season? Should weights be lifted during the basketball season?

A periodized conditioning program for football would include heavy weights for force generation in large muscle groups of the legs, trunk, and shoulders in the off-season phase. The preseason phase would continue weights for the same areas, but would work more on the power component by emphasizing lighter weights lifted rapidly. Plyometric activities would supplement weight lifting to help build power. The in-season phase should be a maintenance phase, with weight lifting for power once per week. Strength and power decline in the course of a football season, and this can be modified by weight lifting. Similarly, weight lifting can modify the strength and power decline that occurs during the basketball season. However, the emphasis on weight lifting for basketball should be strictly on power, because massive strength is less important in basketball.

Case 3

How many miles per day should be run as part of conditioning for soccer? For tennis?

Both soccer and tennis have been shown to demand mainly alactic anaerobic metabolism during sporting activities. Work/rest intervals in tennis show the average professional point to last 8 to 12 seconds, and the average recreational point to last 12 to 18 seconds. Most soccer runs are bursts of less than 10 seconds. Most (80% to 90%) of the activities of both sports are within these intervals. However, recovery from these activities takes place through aerobic mechanisms, so there is a role for training this component. Aerobic training, with running of 2 to 3 miles, should be emphasized during the off-season conditioning phase, but most endurance training in the preseason and in-season phases should consist of sprints, intervals, and agility drills, at an intensity, frequency, and duration that approximates those that occur during the matches.

Case 4

A baseball pitcher with rotator cuff tendinitis symptoms is started on rotator cuff strengthening exercises, but the exercises make the symptoms worse. How should the rehabilitation program be modified?

Rotator cuff tendinitis is classified as a chronic microtrauma process, so there usually will be some physiologic alterations accompanying the clinical symptoms. Weakness of the scapular stabilizing muscles is one of the most common alterations. If these muscles are weak, the scapula will not elevate properly, causing continued impingement. Also, weakness will allow abnormal scapular mobility, with consequent loss of a firm base for the origins of the rotator cuff musculature. These muscles cannot work properly to depress the humeral head off this base, leading to abnormal translation or impingement. In this situation, initial rehabilitation has to be focused on the scapular stabilizers before the rotator cuff rehabilitation will be completely successful.

Case 5

At what age can athletes start muscle strengthening? At what age should flexibility training be instituted for athletes?

A proper strength and flexibility program can be instituted at an early age, probably around 10 years old. Flexibility exercises should be emphasized to counteract the tendency to tightness that develops in growing athletes. Strength exercises are good as a general concept, but should be modified in several ways. First, most of the machines and other devices for strengthening are not built to the dimensions of young athletes. Second, significant strength gains cannot occur until after puberty. Third, muscular endurance is low until after puberty. Therefore, the major goals of a strength program for prepubertal athletes should be toning of the muscles and a proper introduction to the role of strengthening in the total athletic program. The available data shows that strength and flexibility programs organized along these guidelines do not pose a risk of injury or growth plate disturbance.

Case 6

A sprinter presents with a history of two hamstring muscle pulls in the last six months. What type of evaluation is appropriate? What type of rehabilitation should be instituted?

This case is one of an acute exacerbation of a chronic injury, and brings up the question of the completeness of the rehabilitation from the first injury. A complete evaluation of bilateral hamstring, quadriceps, iliotibial band, and gastrocnemius flexibility and strength should be done. In addition, there should be investigations of the athlete's running mechanics and the composition of the training program. Rehabilitation should be constructed around normalizing any musculoskeletal deficits that are present, and then creating normal force couples in the muscles and normal mechanics of the running activity. Imaging or other diagnostic evaluations should be used in recalcitrant cases that fail to respond to appropriate guided rehabilitation.

References

1. Harrelson GL: Physiologic factors of rehabilitation, in Harrelson GL, Andrews JR (eds): *Rehabilitation of Sports Injuries.* Philadelphia, PA, WB Saunders, 1992, pp 13-36.
2. Akeson WH, Amiel D, Abel MF, et al: Effects of immobilization on joints. *Clin Orthop* 1987;219:28-37.
3. Akeson WH, Amiel D, Woo SL: Immobility effects on synovial joints: The pathomechanics of joint contracture. *Biorheology* 1980;17:95-110.
4. Lindboe CF, Platou CS: Effect of immobilization of short duration on the muscle fibre size. *Clin Physiol* 1984;4:183-188.
5. Herring SA: Rehabilitation of muscle injuries. *Med Sci Sports Exerc* 1990;22:453-456.
6. Rifenberick DH, Max SR: Substrate utilization by disused rat skeletal muscles. *Am J Physiol* 1974;226:295-297.
7. Booth FW: Physiologic and biochemical effects of immobilization on muscle. *Clin Orthop* 1987;219:15-20.
8. Stone MH: *Weight Training: A Scientific Approach.* Minneapolis, MN, Bell Weather Press, 1987.
9. Tardieu C, Tabary JC, Tabary C, et al: Adaptation of connective tissue length to immobilization in the lengthened and shortened positions in cat soleus muscle. *J Physiol (Paris)* 1982;78:214-220.
10. Barrett DS: Proprioception and function after anterior cruciate reconstruction. *J Bone Joint Surg* 1991;73B:833-837.
11. Iles JF, Stokes M, Young A: Reflex actions of knee-joint receptors on quadriceps in man. *J Physiol* 1985;360:48P.
12. Kibler WB: Clinical aspects of muscle injury. *Med Sci Sports Exerc* 1990;22:450-452.
13. Physiology of tissue repair, in *Athletic Training and Sports Medicine,* ed 2. Park Ridge, IL, American Academy of Orthopaedic Surgeons, 1991, chap 8, pp 96-123.
14. Russell S: Biochemical alterations in muscle injury. ACSM Annual Meeting, Dallas, TX, May 1992.
15. Armstrong RB: Initial events in exercise-induced muscular injury. *Med Sci Sports Exerc* 1990;22:429-435.
16. Garrett WE Jr, Lohnes J: Cellular and matrix response to mechanical injury at the myotendinous junction, in Leadbetter WB, Buckwalter JA, Gordon SL (eds): *Sports-Induced Inflammation: Clinical and Basic Science Concepts.* Park Ridge, IL, American Academy of Orthopaedic Surgeons, 1990, chap 12, pp 215-224.
17. Steindler A: The theory of contractures, in *Kinesiology of the Human Body Under Normal and Pathological Conditions.* Springfield, IL, Charles C Thomas Pub, 1955, Lecture VI-II, pp 92-94.
18. Kibler WB, Goldberg C, Chandler TJ: Functional biomechanical deficits in running athletes with plantar fasciitis. *Am J Sports Med* 1991;19:66-71.
19. Clancy WG: Tendinitis and plantar fasciitis in runners, in D'Ambrosia R, Drez D Jr (eds): *Prevention and Treatment of Running Injuries.* Thorofare, NJ, CB Slack, 1982, pp 77-87.
20. Nirschl RP, Pettrone FA: Tennis elbow: The surgical treatment of lateral epicondylitis. *J Bone Joint Surg* 1979;61A:832-839.
21. Silliman JF, Hawkins RJ: Current concepts and recent advances in the athlete's shoulder. *Clin Sports Med* 1991;10:693-705.
22. Kibler WB: Concepts in exercise rehabilitation of athletic injury, in Leadbetter WB, Buckwalter JA, Gordon SL (eds): *Sports-Induced Inflammation: Clinical and Basic Science Concepts.* Park Ridge, IL, American Academy of Orthopaedic Surgeons, 1990, chap 52, pp 759-769.
23. Glousman R, Jobe FW, Tibone JE, et al: Dynamic electromyographic analysis of the throwing shoulder with glenohumeral instability. *J Bone Joint Surg* 1988;70A:220-226.
24. Kibler WB: Racquet sports, in Fu F, Stone DA (eds): *Sports Injuries—Mechanisms, Prevention and Treatment,* ed 2, in press.
25. Kibler WB: Physical examination of the shoulder, in Pettrone FA, Nirschl R (eds): *The Athlete's Shoulder,* in press.
26. Warner JJP, Micheli L: Scapulothoracic motion in normal shoulders and shoulders with glenohumeral instability and impingement syndrome: A study using moire topographic analysis. *Clin Orthop* 1992;285:191-199.
27. Knapik JJ, Bauman CL, Jones BH, et al: Preseason strength and flexibility imbalances associated with athletic injuries in female collegiate athletes. *Am J Sports Med* 1991;19:76-81.
28. Chandler TJ, Kibler WB, Stracener EC, et al: Shoulder strength, power, and endurance in college tennis players. *Am J Sport Med* 1992;20:455-458.
29. Knapik JJ, Jones BH, Bauman CL, et al: Strength, flexibility, and athletic injuries. *Sports Med* 1992;14:277-288.
30. Hinton RY: Isokinetic evaluation of shoulder rotational strength in high school baseball pitchers. *Am J Sports Med* 1988;16:274-279.
31. Winge S, Jorgensen U, Lassen Nielsen A: Epidemiology of injuries in Danish championship tennis players. *Int J Sport Med* 1989;10:368-371.
32. Jackson DL, Nyland J: Club lacrosse: A physiologic and injury profile. *Ann Sports Med* 1990;5:114-117.
33. Kibler WB, Chandler TJ, Pace BK: Principles of rehabilitation after chronic tendon injuries. *Clin Sport Med* 1992;11:661-671.
34. Kibler WB, Chandler TJ, Uhl T, et al: A musculoskeletal approach to the preparticipation physical examination: Preventing injury and improving performance. *Am J Sport Med* 1989;17:525-531.
35. Kibler WB: *The Sport Preparticipation Fitness Examination.* Champaign, IL, Human Kinetics Books, 1990.
36. Chandler TJ, Kibler WB: Strength training for injury prevention, in Renstrom PA (ed): *IOC Encyclopedia of Sports Medicine,* vol 2, in press.
37. Kibler WB, Chandler TJ, Stracener ES: Musculoskeletal adaptations and injuries due to overtraining. *Exerc Sport Sci Rev* 1992;20:99-126.
38. Kuipers H, Keizer HA: Overtraining in elite athletes: Review and directions for the future. *Sports Med* 1988;6:79-92.

Sports Injuries of the Hand

Ronald E. Palmer, MD

Introduction

Injuries to the hands of athletes are very common. Fortunately, most of them are relatively minor and rarely lead to permanent problems. However, certain injuries of the hand and wrist, when left untreated or inadequately treated, can lead to major disability and loss of function.

Athletes are active people, who are used to jamming and other minor hand injuries that cause swelling and stiffness. Many of these injuries are treated by themselves, their trainer, or their coach. Often, the individuals from whom they seek medical advice are not accustomed to taking care of significant hand injuries. What initially appears to be a relatively minor injury can turn out to have a significantly bad result.

To avoid later problems, one should always suspect that the injury may be worse than it seems. A careful evaluation and early treatment can avoid the risk of severe functional impairment.

Injuries to the digits of the hand occur most commonly in the ball-handling sports. These occur with a jamming or glancing blow to the digit or a forced injury against resistance. In this article, I will consider mallet fingers, avulsions of the flexor digitorum profundus, hyperextension injuries to the proximal interphalangeal (PIP) joint of the fingers, and dislocations. Injuries to the mid portion of the hand usually occur with a direct blow to the hand. These are not uncommonly seen in baseball players sliding into a bag with their hand extended, and they can result in fractures of the metacarpals.

Wrist injuries occur most commonly in contact sports and stick-handling sports. They usually involve hyperextension injuries of the wrist or injuries in the extremes of motion about the wrist. Scaphoid fractures and instability or dissociative problems of the wrist are the result.

General Evaluation

Clinical Examination

Perhaps the most important way to avoid missing a serious problem of the hand is to conduct a careful clinical evaluation. This can be done in a relatively short period of time. The history of the mechanism of the injury may be helpful, although many people are unable to relate the actual mechanism of injury. One should never forget to talk to the patient and particularly to ask them "exactly where does it hurt?" The most common complaints are of swelling, pain, limitation of motion, and local tenderness.

The evaluation begins with direct palpation to the local areas of tenderness. I believe any swelling and tenderness that continues more than a few days justifies a thorough evaluation. Any areas of swelling should be palpated for local tenderness to identify the specific area to be evaluated more closely. Range of motion should be evaluated at the outset, noting any loss of motion. If the hand or wrist is extremely tender or swollen, it may be best to consider radiographic evaluation before continuing with the clinical evaluation to rule out fracture or bony disruption. Stability of the bones and joints should also be evaluated and compared with the uninjured hand.

Palpation of the hand will identify precisely the local areas of tenderness. These tender spots usually identify the area of injury accurately. These may be in areas of the collateral ligaments, the supporting ligamentous structures, the volar plate, insertion of the tendons about the joints, or areas of bony architecture and disruption.

Radiographic Evaluation

It is important when obtaining a radiograph that the technician be advised of the specific area of tenderness and suspected area of pathology. When one is looking for a fracture or evaluating an injury about a PIP joint, a radiograph of the hand may miss a significant injury. Therefore, the evaluation should be ordered specifically for the area of clinical findings (ie, anteroposterior, lateral, and obliques of the PIP joint of the ring finger).

In most cases, I initially order anteroposterior and lateral evaluations only. If obliques are necessary, they can be added to the evaluation later, particularly if the original radiographs fail to show a suspected injury.

Radiologic evaluation of the wrist can be more difficult. I will usually begin with anteroposterior and lateral views of the wrist. If the problem seems to be on the radial side of the wrist, a navicular view is also included.

Mallet Fingers

The mechanism of injury of mallet fingers is usually a direct blow to the distal phalanx of the digit, which forcibly pushes the distal interphalangeal (DIP) joint into flexion as the extensor tendon is retracting. This causes either a disruption of the extensor tendon at its insertion or a small avulsion fracture. Injury can occur by either a direct or indirect method. Because the extensor tendon cannot act on its insertion, the DIP joint remains in a flexed position. The patient is unable to actively extend the DIP joint; however, passive extension is possible. The amount of clinical deformity or flexion at the DIP joint varies. It is usually associated with some local swelling and tenderness over the area. Most of the time the diagnosis is clear. The PIP joint should be observed for evidence of hyperextension (swan-necking). Radiographic evaluation, with anteroposterior and lateral views of the DIP joint, is important in evaluating dorsal avulsion fractures in order to determine the size of the fragment and the amount of displacement and to look for evidence of volar subluxation of the distal phalanx on the middle phalanx.

Treatment

For almost all mallet finger deformities, I recommend treating the injury with an extension or slight hyperextension splint of the DIP joint only. If treated correctly, the hyperextension of the PIP joint will resolve. There are a number of types of splints available for treatment of mallet finger deformities. However, none of these will work unless the patient has been properly advised of the treatment plan and objectives. It is imperative that the patient wear the splint, in order to keep the DIP joint in full extension or hyperextension. No flexion of the DIP joint can be allowed to occur during the entire treatment period. I advise the patient that any amount of flexion allowed to occur during the treatment period will result in a permanent flexion deformity after splinting has been discontinued. I recommend that the patients remove their splint daily for local skin care and, when they do, they must keep the DIP joint in hyperextension, usually with the PIP joint in flexion. The splint is then reapplied and kept in place until the next retaping and skin care procedure. If this treatment protocol fails, it is because the patient has not adhered to the instructions of never allowing flexion of the DIP joint. Loss of flexion following treatment in an extension splint for an appropriate amount of time is not a problem of the DIP joint.

I routinely treat mallet fingers with six weeks of immobilization of the DIP joint in extension or slight hyperextension. I generally keep a number of different types of splints in my office and give patients a choice of what they feel is most comfortable (Fig. 1). "Link" splints, which are commercially available, can be very effective. However, some people find these bulky. Small mallet finger splints are commercially available, or simple 1/2-inch aluminum splints can be cut to fit either dorsally or volarwards. I often advise patients that they may wish to change the splints from volar to dorsal to aid in skin care. The dorsal splints are cut somewhat larger. Both allow PIP motion. The dorsal splints are bent to keep the DIP joint in slight hyperextension with a piece of tape just distal to the PIP joint and another tape distal to the DIP joint. The volar splints can be worn with a single piece of tape over the DIP joint, bent to keep the finger in full extension.

After six weeks of splinting, I begin the patient on warm water soaks and gentle active range of motion. I recommend three weeks of continued night splinting

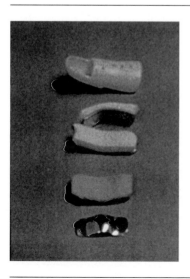
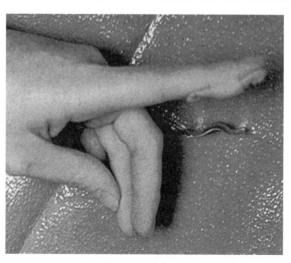

Fig. 1 Left, Depicts various types of splints available for the treatment of mallet finger. **Right,** The splint that I prefer for the treatment of mallet finger. Under the finger is the metal splint. Taped to the finger is the same splint with the concave portion of the splint facing towards the palmar aspect of the DIP joint and taped into place with one piece of tape about the DIP joint. There has also been mole skin applied to the splint.

of the DIP joint. Passive range of motion is discouraged until night splinting has been discontinued. Usually, passive range of motion is not necessary, but, if some stiffness persists, flexion taping for 20 minutes three times a day of the PIP and DIP joints in full flexion and passive stretching are begun.

I do not use Kirschner-wire fixation of the DIP joint in acute or chronic mallet fingers, although some sports medicine physicians do use K-wires, which they cut under the skin, to allow early return to sport. In my opinion, finger splints can be modified to accommodate most any sport. One must remember that even old mallet fingers, which occurred six to eight weeks prior to being evaluated, can be treated with the above described splinting protocol. Before surgical treatment of a chronic mallet finger deformity is begun, I would recommend a six-week trial of splinting in extension. In my experience, the exception to this is an old open mallet finger deformity, which may require excision of the scar and approximation of the edges of the tendons.

In the treatment of mallet finger deformity associated with dorsal chip fractures, I am accepting more and more volar subluxation (Fig. 2). Certainly, mild degrees of volar subluxation of the DIP joint can be accepted. I usually warn the patient that, although full function will return, there may be some enlargement dorsally about the joint. However, I also advise them that, if I surgically treat the finger, there will also be enlargement from the resultant scar. Consequently, surgical intervention is probably not justified.

Certainly, when there is a significant amount of volar subluxation, which will interfere with the mechanism of the joint and cause a decrease in flexion, one should consider surgical treatment. My preferred method of treatment is reapproximating the fragment with a Bunnell pull-out wire. Small fragments can be impossible to reinsert and the surgical treatment of trying to fix small fragments with pins or K-wire can cause more trauma and damage than accepting conservative treatment. With the larger fragments, one must take care to avoid nailbed injuries. The pull-out wire is put through the extensor tendon, brought through bone or about the bones on each side and tied to a felt pad and button on the volar aspect of the digit. I also routinely put a K-wire across the DIP joint, holding it in extension. Both of these are removed at five weeks and active and passive range of motion begun at that time.

Avulsions of the Flexor Digitorum Profundus Tendon

This is a commonly missed diagnosis, which is usually seen six to nine months after the injury because the finger is "getting in the way" or because of weakness. Although tendon surgery should never be taken lightly, the results of early treatment within two or three weeks

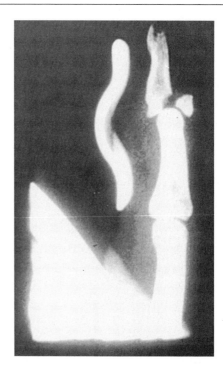

Fig. 2 Radiograph of a mallet finger with a dorsal avulsion fracture with volar subluxation. Small amounts of volar subluxation can be well treated with splinting only.

of injury gives the best prognosis. Results of late repair are less predictable. This is an injury that, if missed or is misdiagnosed, can cause substantial functional disability.

This injury is most common in football players. The injury occurs as one player lunges toward another and attempts to grasp the opponent's jersey or belt. As the athlete grasps at the nearly out-of-reach opponent, the distal phalanx is forcibly hyperextended as the player tries to flex the digit. This causes an avulsion of the flexor profundus tendon from its insertion, and may or may not involve a small avulsion fracture. Usually, the ring finger is involved and, rarely, the little finger. This injury can also occur in older people when trying to lift heavy weights.

Initially, the clinical findings in this injury are often somewhat subtle. There is local swelling, tenderness, and stiffness in the area, common complaints for football players and others who play contact sports. Unfortunately, they are often accepted and ignored. As mentioned earlier, I recommend that any swelling and stiffness that persists over a few days should be thoroughly evaluated. The findings are local tenderness over the area of the DIP joint and over the area of the distal end of the profundus tendon at the level to which it retracted. The flexor profundus tendon will either retract to the level of the PIP joint, where it is caught by the venculi at the chasm of Camper, or into the palm at about the level of the MCP joint. This area of tenderness is important to the treating physician, because it gives a preoperative determination of the level of the tendon retraction. Of course, the key to diagnosis of flexor profundus rupture is inability to flex the DIP joint. The patient should be asked to try to close all of the fingers of the hand into the palm in a closed fist fashion. With flexor profundus rupture, the DIP joint will not flex into the palm. The digits should also be examined with the PIP joint in extension and the patient asked to flex the DIP joint only.

A radiograph should be taken to evaluate for small avulsion fractures. When a small avulsion fracture is seen about the PIP joint, DIP joint function must be checked to make sure this is not a hyperextension injury or volar plate injury of the PIP joint, but a missed flexor profundus tendon rupture (the bone fragment is displaced more volarwards in flexor profundus ruptures).

Treatment

The treatment of ruptured flexor profundus tendons in athletes is surgical. In acute injuries, normal function of the finger is possible with surgical treatment. Flexor tendon surgery should be done only by a surgeon who is highly skilled in tendon surgery in the hand. Excessive injuries to the pulley system (the fibro-osseous system of the flexor tendons), or the flexor sublimis tendon can result in persistent limitation of motion and can even increase disability.

The surgical treatment is reattachment of the flexor profundus tendon into its avulsed area of attachment in the distal phalanx. I prefer a Bunnell pull-out wire for reattachment. Early motion should be started. I remove the Bunnell pull-out wire at five weeks postoperatively.

Missed flexor profundus ruptures are an extremely difficult surgical problem. Normally, the fibro-osseous sheath has not collapsed. Consequently, reconstruction of the pulley system and fibro-osseous sheath are generally not necessary. However, the flexor profundus can usually not be brought distally back into its bony insertion. Difficulty occurs because of contracture that develops in the flexor profundus muscle at five to six weeks following avulsion. However, I usually attempt to reattach the tendon, if possible, remembering that the flexor profundus does not insert into the proximal portion of the distal phalanx, but more toward its mid portion. If reinsertion is not possible, I generally treat this injury with a tendon graft. As this is usually an injury of a young athlete, in my opinion, the results are better with a tendon graft, which will restore some function to the DIP joint, than with a tenodesis of the DIP joint or creation of a sublimis finger by fusing the DIP joint. However, one must take care not to compromise the function which already exists.

Hyperextension Injuries of the PIP Joint

Acute dorsal PIP hyperextension injuries of the hand are extremely common injuries, which occur in sporting activities when a hyperextension force is applied to the digit. The finger is usually struck by a movable object or the finger strikes an immovable object and is hyperextended. These injuries are seen most frequently in the ball-handling sports.

The classification for acute dorsal PIP hyperextension injuries of the digits offers three types.[1] Type I (hyperextension) is an injury associated with volar plate avulsion from the base of the middle phalanx and a minor longitudinal split in the collateral ligaments. In this group, the articular surfaces remain intact. The middle phalanx articulates with the distal third of the condyle of the proximal phalanx. Type II (dorsal dislocation), an avulsion of the volar plate accompanied by a major split in the collateral ligament system, results in complete dorsal displacement of the middle phalanx. When reduced, type II dorsal dislocations are rarely unstable.

Type III (fracture dislocations) occurs when compressive forces are sufficient to shear away or impact the volar plate of the middle phalanx, producing a fracture dislocation. This is an injury that occurs in association with dislocations with a volar chip fracture of varying sizes. Fracture dislocations of the PIP joint are subdivided into stable and unstable. It is my experience that the size of the fragment, up to approximately 40% of the articular surface, has little relationship to whether the fracture dislocation is stable or unstable. Usually, very small chip fractures are stable. Certainly, the fractures that involve greater than 40% of the articular surface are more unstable fractures.

Treatment

Type I Type I injuries are best treated with buddy taping alone until swelling and symptoms have resolved, which ranges from a few days to three weeks. Even if symptoms resolve earlier, I usually recommend three weeks of buddy taping to protect the collateral ligaments.

Type II Type II injuries, which are dorsal dislocations, should be treated with closed reduction and buddy taping. Most dorsal dislocations of the PIP joint are reduced by the injured patient, a friend, or a coach. In acute dislocations, I rarely use a digital nerve block. It is my opinion that the nerve block hurts more than the gentle traction required to reduce the digit. If the digit does not easily reduce with gentle traction, I generally perform a nerve block. Attempted gentle reduction with distal traction and perhaps some increased hyperextension and distal traction usually reduces the digit. If it does not reduce easily after a complete nerve block, there is no reason to continue to attempt closed reduction. This is true for any dislocation, particularly irreducible dislocations around the MCP joint.

After the joint has been reduced, I recommend a radiograph, with a second radiograph approximately one week later to ensure that there is no instability or subluxation.

I recommend three weeks of buddy taping for all dislocated PIP joints. I encourage removing the buddy tapes early for warm water soaks and gentle active range of motion, but I recommend that the buddy tapes be worn day and night, except for periods of hand exercise. They should definitely be worn for all sporting activities during this three-week period and usually for another two to three weeks for contact sports afterwards.

Type III Type III fracture dislocations must be subdivided into the stable group and the unstable group. By far, the vast majority of these injuries are stable. In my opinion, stable fracture dislocations with avulsion fractures of the volar aspect are best treated with buddy taping alone. Extension block splints, casts, and, certainly, surgical procedures are not necessary. The important point in dealing with type III fracture dislocations is to check frequently for instability, not with manipulation or motion but with radiographs. Stability is determined by a lateral radiograph centered at the PIP joint. Any dorsal subluxation indicates instability (Fig. 3). Usually, after an acute fracture dislocation or type III injury of the PIP joint, I advise a protection splint in flexion for two to five days, until the local symptoms have subsided enough to allow buddy taping alone. At that time, radiographs are taken to check for any evidence of dorsal subluxation. As stated, by far the vast majority of these will be stable with no evidence of dorsal subluxation. Consequently, the patient is placed in buddy tapes and advised to avoid hyperextension. I usually allow return to any sporting activity with buddy tapes in place when symptoms allow. Radiographs are checked again one week following the application of buddy tapes and again two to three weeks later. In my experience, I have not had an acutely stable type III injury go on to dorsal subluxation with buddy taping alone.

Type III fracture dislocations with initial instability are a very difficult problem. They are much rarer and, although they normally involve more than 40% of the articular surface, they may involve only small chip fractures. In my opinion, dorsal subluxation is present initially and, too often, is not recognized. If the PIP joint is left subluxed, it will remain unstable and will become stiff and painful. Results of late treatment are not good. Therefore, this injury must be recognized early.

Type III unstable fracture dislocations of the PIP joint are treated with closed reduction and checked radiographically to make sure that the PIP joint is sta-

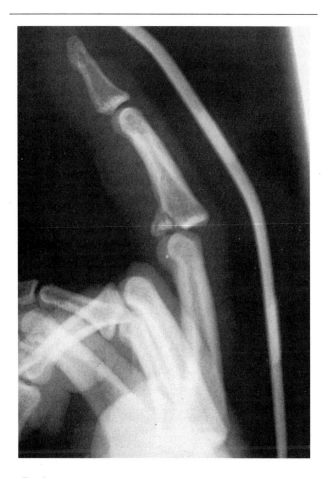

Fig. 3 Dorsal subluxation of the middle phalanx on the proximal phalanx. This subluxation denotes instability of this hyperextension injury. This is a type 3 unstable hyperextension injury of the PIP joint.

ble in flexion. If the PIP joint is stable in flexion, the injury is treated with an extension block splint, blocking extension greater than 40° or as needed to control stability (Fig. 4). Frequently radiographs are made of the PIP joint to ensure no evidence of dorsal subluxation. Active flexion is encouraged early.

If type III unstable fracture dislocations of the PIP joint are not stable in flexion and cannot be treated adequately in a hyperextension splint, surgical treatment is indicated. My choice for surgical treatment is reinsertion of the volar plate into the proximal portion of the middle phalanx with a Bunnell pull-out wire. If there is a fracture fragment, it is reduced and held with a Bunnell pull-out wire. I also place a pin across the PIP joint, to hold it in approximately 35° to 40° of flexion. Postoperatively, radiographs of the PIP joint must be taken to ensure reduction. The pins must be kept free of infection with prophylactic antibiotic treatment and local pin care. The pins and wires are removed at five weeks and a rehabilitative program begun.

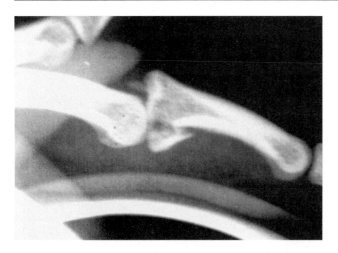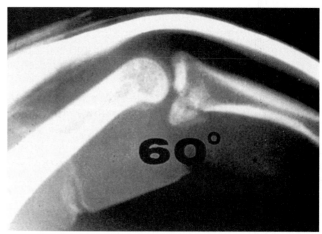

Fig. 4   **Left**, A type III unstable hyperextension injury of the PIP joint with subluxation. **Right**, A correction of the dorsal subluxation with flexion of the PIP joint at approximately 60°.

The key to a good result in type III unstable hyperextension injuries of the PIP joint is anatomic reduction of the dorsal subluxation and maintenance of that reduction until the joint is stable.

ment early, one can expect a good result. Over-treatment, with prolonged immobilization, can lead to as poor a result, with residual loss of function, as undertreatment or lack of treatment.

Conclusion

Athletic hand injuries are common. If problem cases are recognized and receive appropriate treat-

Reference

1. Green DP: *Operative Hand Surgery*, ed 2. New York, NY, Churchill Livingstone, 1988, vol 3, chap 18, p 779.

Peripheral Nerve Compression

Richard H. Gelberman, MD

Richard G. Eaton, MD

James R. Urbaniak, MD

The objective of this chapter is to provide the reader with a current, comprehensive review of fundamental clinical issues surrounding the most commonly encountered compressive neuropathies of the upper extremity. Relevant new data on the pathophysiology of neural compression introduce more specific discussions of the currently favored methods for the evaluation and treatment of carpal tunnel syndrome, cubital tunnel syndrome, and radial nerve entrapment in the proximal part of the forearm.

Pathophysiology of Nerve Compression

Recent experimental studies have demonstrated that a consistent sequence of events takes place when external compression forces are elevated around a peripheral nerve. Mechanical deformation has been found to be greatest in the superficial regions of the nerve and in the zones between compressed and uncompressed segments. External pressures of 20 to 30 mm of mercury (2.66 to 4.00 kPa) have been shown to impair venular flow in the epineurium and to retard intracellular axonal transport.[1-3] Pressures as low as 30 mm of mercury (4.00 kPa) cause changes in the permeability of intraneural blood vessels, further increasing intraneural interstitial fluid pressure. Patients with carpal tunnel syndrome have been shown to have intracarpal tunnel interstitial pressures at levels that are within this range (30 mm of mercury with the wrist in neutral position, increased to 90 mm of mercury [12 kPa] with the wrist in palmar flexion).[4] Experimentally induced higher pressures (130 to 150 mm of mercury [17.32 to 20.00 kPa]) cause an acute block of conduction,[5-7] and higher pressures cause marked changes in intraneural blood flow, vessel permeability, and fiber morphology (epineurial and perineurial thickening and eccentric positioning of nuclei and dispersion of Nissl substance within nerve cell bodies), leading to rapid deterioration of nerve function.[8-11]

Clinically, the presentation of acute and chronic nerve-compression lesions appears consistent with the sequence of events that has been identified experimentally. Low-level compression forces of relatively brief duration appear to cause changes in intraneural microcirculation that are intermittent and rapidly reversible on decompression. Higher levels of compression, maintained for longer periods of time, impair axonal transport and cause changes in the structure and function of peripheral nerves and nerve cell bodies, so that a longer period of time after decompression is required before recovery should be anticipated.

Carpal Tunnel Syndrome

The most commonly encountered peripheral neuropathy, carpal tunnel syndrome, occurs most frequently during middle or advanced age. (In a study performed at the Mayo Clinic,[12] the mean age of 1,215 patients was 54 years and 83% of the patients were more than 40 years old.) Occurring twice as frequently in women as in men, median nerve compression[12,13] causes symptoms of paresthesias and numbness in the median nerve distribution or in the entire hand, symptoms that frequently awaken patients from sleep. Motor abnormalities, including weakness and atrophy of the abductor pollicis brevis and opponens pollicis muscles, occur in advanced stages of compression.

While a precise cause for symptoms of median nerve compression may not be identifiable in many patients, a number of associated conditions should be considered during routine evaluation. In a useful classification of the causes of median nerve compression, Szabo and Madison[14] considered anatomic, physiologic, and patterns-of-use factors. Anatomic factors include conditions leading to a decrease in the size of the carpal tunnel (for example, acromegaly and osseous abnormalities of the wrist and distal radius) and those causing an increase in the contents of the carpal canal (for example, benign tumors, abnormal muscle bellies, non-specific synovitis, and hematomas). Physiologic factors include neuropathic conditions (for example, diabetes mellitus, alcoholism, amyloidosis, infection, gout, and tenosynovitis) and conditions altering fluid balance (for example, pregnancy, use of oral contraceptives, hypothyroidism, and long-term hemodialysis). Patterns-of-use factors range from repetitive flexion and extension of the wrist and digits to weightbearing on the carpal canal with the wrist extended (for example, while walking with a cane or crutch).

Insight into the relationship between mechanical factors and median nerve symptoms has been provided by recent findings in patients who used crutches and canes for walking. Gellman and associates[15] demonstrated that 38 (49%) of 77 paraplegics had signs and symptoms of carpal tunnel syndrome and that this prevalence increased with age. They found that, while baseline interstitial pressure was lower in paraplegic patients with carpal tunnel syndrome than in nonparaplegic patients with carpal tunnel syndrome, direct pressure on the hand combined with forced extension of the wrist caused very high elevations of interstitial pressure in the former group. Similarly, Waring and Werner[16] found a high prevalence of carpal tunnel syndrome in a group of patients who had had poliomyelitis and who used assistive devices.

The establishment of a diagnosis of carpal tunnel syndrome has two components: localization of nerve compression to the wrist level and elucidation of an underlying cause. Median nerve compression at the wrist is confirmed by the physician obtaining a history of characteristic symptoms and recording relevant sensory, motor, provocative, and electrophysiologic data. Although the wrist is the most frequent site of compression of the median nerve, proximal lesions should be considered, including nerve-root compression in the cervical spine as well as compressive neuropathies at the thoracic outlet, distal arm, and proximal forearm regions. Of the physical examination maneuvers and tests that can be used to rule out other sites of compression, the most frequently performed are physical and radiographic examinations of the cervical spine and the Roos overhead exercise test for thoracic outlet syndrome. (For the Roos test, the fingers are flexed and extended repeatedly with the arms held up. The response is considered positive when the patient experiences fatigue and paresthesias in the forearm and hand.) In addition, three provocative tests for median nerve compression in the proximal part of the forearm are performed (flexion of the flexor digitorum superficialis of the long finger and pronation and supination of the wrist against resistance).

Anteroposterior and lateral radiographs of the wrist are always made for patients who have suspected distal median nerve compression. While computed tomography and magnetic resonance imaging have provided useful information clinically and experimentally, these studies are not recommended for routine evaluation.

The most commonly encountered conditions associated with distal median nerve compression are peripheral neuropathy, diabetes mellitus, rheumatoid arthritis, hypothyroidism, and gout. The history and physical examination guide the selection of an appropriate laboratory evaluation, which can include tests for thyroid function, the level of antinuclear antibody, the level of rheumatoid factor, the erythrocyte sedimentation rate, and the level of fasting blood glucose in selected patients.

Physical Examination and Electrodiagnostic Studies

A sensory examination has a central role in the establishment of the diagnosis of carpal tunnel syn-drome. Although two-point discrimination (an innervation density test that measures the innervation of multiple overlapping peripheral receptor fields) is of little value for the diagnosis of early mild or moderate compression, it is useful for the confirmation of severe or chronic carpal tunnel syndrome. Recently, it has been shown that threshold tests (those evaluating single nerve fibers innervating a receptor or a group of receptor cells) are more effective in the detection of early compression effects on peripheral nerves. The specificity of the Semmes-Weinstein monofilament test, the most frequently used threshold test, is improved when values obtained in the gravity-assisted palmar-flexion position are compared with those obtained in the neutral position. Worsening of values obtained with 60 seconds of wrist flexion correlates well with increased nerve-conduction values and is indicative of median nerve compression at the wrist.[17]

Gellman and associates[18] evaluated the most commonly used provocative tests in patients with electrodiagnostically proved carpal tunnel syndrome and in normal subjects. The Phalen test, performed with the wrist in the gravity-assisted flexed position and the elbow extended, was found to be the most sensitive (71% sensitivity) and the Tinel sign, the most specific (94% specificity). Both tests are recommended for the routine assessment of patients with suspected carpal tunnel syndrome. Weakness of the abductor pollicis brevis and opponens pollicis brevis is indicative of an advanced stage of nerve compression.

Nerve-conduction studies are useful both for confirming the diagnosis and for determining the severity of the compression. Evidence of abnormal conduction values (decreased sensory amplitude being the initial finding) is considered the most specific single finding of median nerve compression at the wrist level. Signs of denervation are obtained by electromyographic studies in hands with the advanced stages of compression.

Nonsurgical Treatment

The most frequently used type of conservative treatment consists of a trial of splinting of the wrist in neutral position and injection of corticosteroids into the carpal canal (Fig. 1). While as many as 80% of patients have obtained temporary relief with this method,[19,20] a recent prospective clinical study demonstrated that less than one-fourth (11) of 50 patients were symptom-free 18 months after injection.[19] Green[21] performed carpal tunnel injections in 222 patients and noted that 180 (81%) obtained relief, which lasted one day to 40 months. Symptoms recurred frequently after two to four months and led to surgical treatment in 82 (46%) of the 180 patients. Green noted a correlation between the results of steroid injection and those of surgical

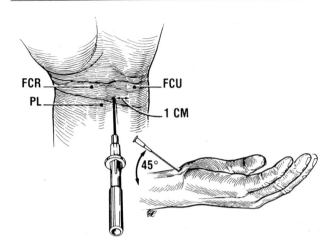

Fig. 1 Drawings showing the technique of carpal tunnel injection. **Left**, A 22-gauge needle, originally inserted 1 cm proximal to the distal wrist flexion crease through the flexor carpi radialis (FCR) tendon, is now inserted just lateral to the ulnar artery for a greater margin of safety. FCU = flexor carpi ulnaris and PL = palmaris longus. **Right**, The needle is angled 45° to 60° distally, advanced 2 cm through the flexor retinaculum, and the solution is injected.

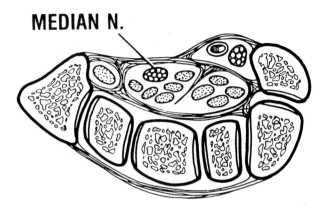

Fig. 2 Drawing showing the cross section of the carpal tunnel and the distal ulnar tunnel. The transverse carpal ligament forms the volar surface of the carpal tunnel and the dorsal boundary of the distal ulnar tunnel. The palmar carpal ligament forms the volar boundary of the proximal aspect of Guyon's canal. Nine flexor tendons and the median nerve extend through the carpal tunnel, with the nerve lying palmar-radially. The ulnar nerve lies dorso-ulnar to the ulnar artery within Guyon's canal.

treatment, with a good response to injection constituting an excellent prognostic sign with respect to operative treatment (77 [94%] of the 82 patients with a good response to the injection obtained relief from a subsequently performed carpal tunnel release). If an underlying disorder, such as rheumatoid arthritis, diabetes mellitus, or hypothyroidism, is noted, medical treatment should be initiated. For symptoms that are provoked by repetitive activities, ergonomic measures (for example, lowering of a computer keyboard, adjustment of the back and height of a seat, and alteration of the patient's work shift) may be helpful.

Carpal tunnel syndrome was noted in 56 (2%) of 2,358 pregnant women who were tested with sensory and motor examinations in one large series.[22] Of those patients, 46 (82%) had relief with nocturnal splinting, nine (16%) had no benefit from splinting, and one (2%) needed a carpal tunnel release. While most pregnant women recover from carpal tunnel symptoms within six weeks after delivery, release of the transverse carpal ligament is indicated for patients with persistent symptoms.

Carpal Tunnel Release

Anatomically, the narrowest segment of the carpal canal, a width of 10 mm, is located over the middle of the distal carpal row, an area that corresponds to the palmar-oriented prominence of the capitate (Fig. 2).[23] The number of fascicles in the median nerve in this region ranges from 13 proximally to 35 distally. The motor portion of the nerve, forming the thenar branch distally, is located in either the radial-palmar or the central portion of the nerve. Most frequently, it exits the radial-palmar aspect of the nerve in one of three branching patterns.

Schmidt and Lanz[23] noted that 46 of 100 thenar motor branches were extraligamentous, 31% were subligamentous, and 23% extended through the ligament (Fig. 3). To protect the lateral branches, they suggested that median nerve decompression be performed along a plane ulnar to the nerve, with division of the flexor retinaculum adjacent to the hook of the hamate.

In a study of 12 cadaveric hands, Taleisnik[24] described the course and variations of the palmar cutaneous branch of the median nerve as it relates to carpal tunnel release. He found that the palmar cutaneous nerve originates from the palmar-radial quadrant of the median nerve 5 cm proximal to the proximal wrist crease. The palmar cutaneous nerve remains bound to the main body of the median nerve for a distance of 16 to 25 mm; it then separates and courses to the wrist between the flexor carpi radialis and the palmaris longus tendons. The nerve enters a short tunnel, 9 to 16 mm long, within the transverse carpal ligament, immediately medial to the flexor carpi radialis tendon. Noting that accidental division of the palmar cutaneous branch of the median nerve is a frequent cause of postoperative dysesthesias, Taleisnik advised that avoidance of nerve injury is ensured only by specific isolation of the nerve or by transection of the transverse carpal ligament along its ulnar margin, at a point medial to the region where the final fibers of the cutaneous nerve exit the transverse carpal ligament.

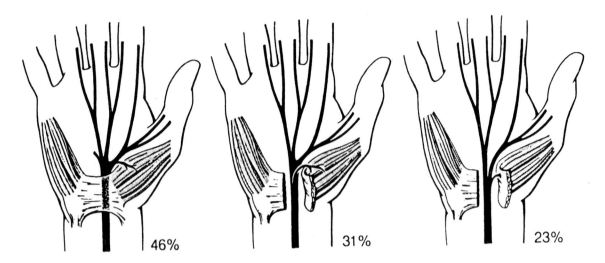

Fig. 3 Drawings showing the frequency of the extraligamentous, **left,** subligamentous, **center,** and transligamentous, **right,** course of the thenar branch. (Reproduced with permission from Schmidt H-M, Lanz U: Anatomy of the median nerve in the carpal tunnel, in Gelberman RH (ed): *Operative Nerve Repair and Reconstruction.* Philadelphia, PA, JB Lippincott, 1991, vol 2, pp 889-898.)

Surgical decompression of the carpal canal is performed under local or intravenous regional anesthesia. With the ring finger flexed to the palm, a mark is made on the distal wrist crease in line with the ulnar aspect of the ray of the ring finger. The skin incision and subsequent deeper dissection are carried lateral to the longitudinal plane created by this point and the ulnar aspect of the ring finger (Fig. 4). An incision is created from Kaplan's oblique line just ulnar to the thenar crease distally and extended to the wrist crease proximally, and the skin edges are retracted. (Kaplan's line, extending from the first web space, parallels the proximal transverse crease obliquely across the palm.) The transverse carpal ligament is identified and divided longitudinally, proximally to distally, in line with the ray of the ring finger. The antebrachial fascia is then divided proximally for 2 to 3 cm under direct vision. A bulky, below-the-elbow dressing is applied to the arm and hand, with the wrist in extension, and is worn for seven to nine days to prevent flexor tendon herniation. The sutures are removed, and active use is initiated at this point.

In 1985, Silver and associates[25] reported the effects of carpal tunnel release on numbness of the little finger. Of 16 patients with carpal tunnel syndrome and total hand numbness and paresthesias, 15 noted spontaneous improvement of symptoms related to the little finger after carpal tunnel release alone. As no patient had additional surgical treatment, and as the percentage of patients with mild residual symptoms was very small, the authors advised against the performance of routine decompression of Guyon's canal unless there is specific electrophysiologic evidence of ulnar nerve compression at the wrist.

A recent study involving volumetric measurements and magnetic resonance imaging showed the changes in the carpal tunnel and in Guyon's canal caused by

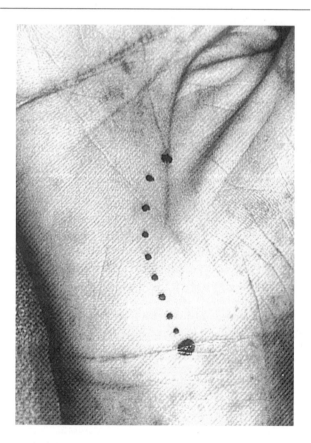

Fig. 4 Photograph showing that the incision for surgical decompression of the carpal canal parallels the thenar crease.

carpal tunnel release.[26] A 24% increase in the volume of the carpal canal following carpal tunnel release was observed, and a consistent change in shape (from oval to circular) took place because of an increase in the anteroposterior dimension (Fig. 5). A smaller increase in the mediolateral dimension was also seen. The median nerve displaced palmarly an average of 3.5 mm and Guyon's canal increased in size and changed from triangular to oval. As the importance of the 3.5 mm of anterior displacement of the median nerve and flexor tendons has not been determined, reconstruction of the transverse carpal ligament is not currently recommended.

Endoscopic Carpal Tunnel Release

In a recent prospective, blind-assessment, randomized study of 169 hands in 145 patients being managed with endoscopic or open carpal tunnel release, the functional outcomes (for example, a resumption of the activities of daily living and a return to work) were achieved more rapidly after the endoscopic method.[27] Overall satisfaction with the two procedures was not significantly different, and quantitative outcomes (for example, sensibility testing values, motor strength, carpal canal interstitial pressure, and electrophysiologic data) were nearly identical. More complications were noted with the endoscopic carpal-tunnel release. These included transection of digital nerves or of the superficial palmar arch, wound hematomas, and ulnar-nerve irritation at the wrist. The authors concluded that, until intraoperative safety is improved, they could not recommend widespread use of endoscopic carpal tunnel release.

Severe Compression of the Median Nerve at the Wrist

With severe or long-term compression of the median nerve at the wrist, progressive intraneural changes have included perineurial thickening, myelin thinning, and degeneration of small fibers. Intrafascicular neurolysis has been recommended for patients with constant sensory loss, thenar atrophy, and increased two-point discrimination in the median nerve distribution.[28] Neurolysis, performed under magnification, requires dissection of fascicular groups through regions of intrafascicular fibrosis. The posterior fascicles of the epineurium are not disturbed. In 1985, Rhoades and associates[29] reported on a series of patients with severe median nerve compression treated with the technique of neurolysis recommended by Curtis and Eversmann.[28] Rhoades and associates concluded that neurolysis was safe and effective in patients with severe carpal tunnel syndrome. In 1987, Gelberman and associates[30] reported on a similar group of patients with evidence of severe median nerve compression who had been managed with carpal tunnel release alone. With the numbers available, the authors found no significant difference ($p > 0.05$) between the results in the two groups and concluded that intrafascicular neurolysis was not beneficial for patients with severe median nerve compression. In 1988, Lowry and Follender[31] reported on two comparable groups of 25 patients each with severe carpal tunnel syndrome. One group was treated with transverse carpal-ligament release alone and the other, with ligament division and intrafascicular neurolysis. As the results indicated no difference between the two groups, the authors concluded that internal neurolysis

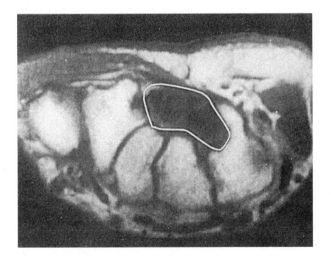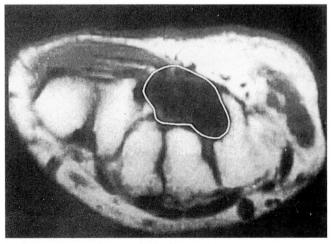

Fig. 5 **Left**, Preoperative magnetic resonance image of the carpal tunnel in a patient with carpal tunnel syndrome. Note the oval shape, with the greatest dimension in the mediolateral direction. **Right**, After a carpal tunnel release, the shape of the tunnel is circular, because of an increase in the anteroposterior dimension.

was not useful in patients with severe median nerve compression. At the present time, internal neurolysis is not considered an effective adjunct in the surgical treatment of hands with severe compression of the median nerve.

Acute Carpal Tunnel Syndrome

Acute compression of the median nerve at the wrist is being recognized with increasing frequency in patients with a fracture of the distal radius. Recently, specific criteria for the establishment of a diagnosis of acute carpal tunnel syndrome and for the determination of the need for surgical treatment have been provided.[32] The two factors most often associated with increased carpal canal pressure following trauma are use of a circular cast and immobilization of the wrist in a position of marked flexion. Interstitial pressure studies, showing that the critical pressure threshold for nerve fiber viability is 45 mm of mercury (6.00 kPa) (30 mm of mercury [4.00 kPa] below diastolic blood pressure) in normotensive patients, have helped physicians to distinguish nerve contusion at the wrist from acute carpal tunnel syndrome. When a patient has increased two-point discrimination in the median nerve distribution following fracture of the distal radius and application of a circular cast, the cast should be removed and the wrist should be extended to neutral. If symptoms do not improve within two to four hours, direct measurement of carpal canal interstitial pressure is recommended. If the interstitial pressure is elevated, open release of the carpal canal is carried out, with extension of the incision into the forearm, 4 cm proximal to the transverse wrist crease. The antebrachial fascia is divided proximally, and the median nerve is isolated as it emerges from the lateral border of the flexor digitorum superficialis muscle. The nerve is visualized throughout its course in the carpal canal. The motor branch of the median nerve is also visualized, and the floor of the carpal canal is inspected for osseous fragments.

Complications of Treatment

Complications of the treatment of carpal tunnel syndrome can usually be avoided if the surgeon is well trained and skillful; obtains a detailed, relevant history; and performs a thorough physical examination. Sound clinical judgment and knowledge of the appropriate anatomy, with appreciation of possible anomalous structures, influence the rate of success of treatment. Some hand surgeons have reported that 25% of the carpal tunnel procedures that they performed were done to correct complications of treatment of this syndrome. A rational treatment plan is available for each type of complication.

The major complications of treatment of carpal tunnel syndrome are: incorrect diagnosis, injection into

the median nerve, incomplete decompression, severance of the palmar cutaneous branch of the median nerve, a hypersensitive incision, reflex sympathetic dystrophy, severance of the recurrent motor branch of the median nerve, injury from neurolysis, a tender median nerve, adherence of nerves to the skin or to the flexor tendons, hematoma, and bow-stringing of the flexor tendons.[33,34]

Incorrect Diagnosis

Although carpal tunnel syndrome is the best understood and most frequently diagnosed compression neuropathy, it is also the most often overdiagnosed. The most prevalent management error related to this entity is an incorrect or incomplete diagnosis, which all too often leads to an inappropriate or unnecessary operation.

The important components of history recording, physical examination, diagnostic modalities, and differential diagnosis have already been described. However, some points deserve emphasis because the correct diagnosis of carpal tunnel syndrome must be established before surgical treatment is instituted.[35]

Once the diagnosis of carpal tunnel syndrome has been ascertained, an effort should be made to determine the exact cause of the condition. For example, is it tenosynovitis (the most common cause), and why? Is there a metabolic cause (for example, pregnancy, rheumatoid arthritis,[35] or hypothyroidism)?[36] Is a space-occupying lesion the culprit (for example, an osseous lesion, a ganglion, or an anomalous muscle)?[28,37-45]

Electrodiagnostic tests are not necessary in a patient with clearly defined symptoms and physical findings. However, when the presentation is equivocal, and in all compensation-related cases, these studies are strongly recommended. Although occasionally electrodiagnostic recordings are normal despite clinical compression of the median nerve in the carpal tunnel,[46] the surgeon should use restraint before operating on patients with normal electrodiagnostic findings, particularly if compensation or another source of secondary gain is involved. A useful diagnostic test in these situations is steroid and Xylocaine (lidocaine) injection into the carpal canal.[19]

An Allen test to determine the flow through the radial and ulnar arteries should be performed on the hand of every patient who is examined for suspected carpal tunnel syndrome because an occlusion of either of the major vessels can mimic symptoms of compression neuropathy.[12,19,47] To perform the Allen test, the examiner occludes the radial and ulnar arteries and then has the patient exsanguinate the hand actively by making three tight fists. The patient then opens the hand to a resting position, avoiding hyperextension of the wrist and finger joints. The radial and ulnar arteries are alternately released, and the completeness of a blush is noted in all digits of the hand.

Compression neuropathy of the lateral antebrachial cutaneous nerve[13,48] or of the superficial radial nerve[49] must be distinguished from carpal tunnel syndrome. In addition to seeking more proximal lesions, such as compression of the fifth and sixth cervical roots or compression by the pronator teres muscle, the diagnostician must appreciate that concomitant lesions (the so-called double-crush syndrome) can be the underlying cause of failure of carpal tunnel release.[50]

Injection into the Median Nerve

Prevention In appropriately selected patients (those without profound sensory loss, thenar atrophy, or severely prolonged nerve conduction latencies), injection of corticosteroids into the carpal canal is an effective method of treatment, but the efficacy of injection remains controversial.[19,21,23,40,51] If the steroid is injected directly into the median nerve, dysesthesias may occur and persist for several weeks. An effective way to avoid direct injection of the median nerve is to practice needle placement at the time of open operations for carpal tunnel release.[52] A 25-gauge needle should be inserted ulnarly to the palmaris longus tendon (or in line with the ring finger if the palmaris longus is absent), at an angle of 30° to the skin. If paresthesias are elicited, the needle should be withdrawn and repositioned.

Treatment If, when the median nerve is being surgically decompressed, the carrying agent from a previous cortisone injection is visible in the sheath of the median nerve, this material should be removed carefully with the use of microsurgical techniques.

Incomplete Decompression

One of the most common complications of carpal tunnel release is incomplete transection of the transverse carpal ligament.[19,53]

Prevention Adequate tourniquet ischemia for clear visualization of the border of the ligament is mandatory. Undoubtedly, the exposure is compromised if a short, longitudinal palmar incision or a transverse wrist incision is used. The transverse carpal ligament must be transected from the forearm fascia to the superficial palmar arch. If a short, longitudinal palmar incision in the thenar crease is used, adequate traction must be added to expose both the proximal and the distal border clearly. Endoscopic carpal tunnel release has added another dimension to incomplete decompression.

Treatment If the clinical and physical findings, especially abnormal electrodiagnostic studies, confirm the persistence of median nerve compression after a previous carpal tunnel release, the cause is usually incomplete transection of the ligament. An adequate incision

that extends across the wrist crease should be used to provide sufficient exposure for thorough re-exploration of the carpal tunnel canal, complete release of the ligament, and release of any fascial bands at the proximal wrist flexion crease.[54] Eversmann[54] emphasized that a remaining transverse band of forearm fascia at the proximal wrist flexion crease may perpetuate the compression of the median nerve.

Severance of the Palmar Cutaneous Branch of the Median Nerve

Prevention A common complication of surgical exposure of the carpal tunnel is severance of the palmar cutaneous branch of the median nerve.[39,55,56] Taleisnik documented the anatomy of this structure. To avoid the median nerve, the surgeon should make an incision in line with the ulnar aspect of the ring finger. The surgeon must decide whether or not he or she prefers to extend the incision proximally across the wrist flexion crease. A more radially placed incision or a transverse incision of the wrist flexion crease is more likely to injure the main branch of the palmar cutaneous nerve. In addition, the subcutaneous tissue over the transverse carpal ligament should be sectioned on the ulnar border to prevent injury to the terminal branches of the nerve.[24,57] The disturbance of these small terminal branches can result in a painful scar. The surgeon must also realize that an ulnarly placed incision can sever the cutaneous branch of the ulnar nerve or injure the ulnar nerve itself.[58] Therefore, an appropriately placed incision as well as an excellent exposure for visualization of the transverse carpal ligament are a must, and any blind cutting is to be condemned. If the palmar cutaneous nerve is severed, the patient will have dysesthesias and tenderness in the thenar area. The sensitivity usually prohibits normal use of the hand. Percussion of the operative scar in the thenar area will elicit pain and dysesthesias. The diagnosis can be confirmed by a local injection of Xylocaine (lidocaine) into the tender area; this should relieve the pain caused by an injured nerve.

Treatment It is difficult to treat a severed palmar cutaneous branch of the median nerve successfully. Usually, the distal portion of the severed nerve, or the terminal branch, is too small to locate, or it is too small for repair either with direct methods or with nerve-grafting. Occasionally, a large neuroma in continuity is located in the nerve proximal to the palm, and this may be repairable with direct means or with grafting techniques. The preferred method of management is isolation of the neuroma, mobilization of the proximal branch, and burial of the proximal branch more proximally and deeply beneath the soft and bulky forearm muscles. Resection of the nerve at its point of exit from the median nerve is not always effective, as this can result in another neuroma that is more painful than the first.

Hypersensitive Incision

A major source of complications in the release of the transverse carpal ligament is an inappropriate skin incision. A surgical incision that crosses the wrist flexion crease usually produces more inflammation and postoperative sensitivity than does one that does not cross the crease. However, there is no question that an incision that crosses the crease is the safest, because it allows the median nerve to be exposed proximally before the nerve begins to branch. Certainly, this curved longitudinal incision should be used in all re-explorations of the median nerve at the wrist. The incision must cross the wrist flexion crease obliquely, in line with the ulnar border of the ring finger.[24] Currently, the most popular approach is use of a short, curved incision adjacent to the ulnar aspect of the thenar crease, in line with the ulnar border of the ring finger and not crossing the wrist flexion crease. If careful retraction is used, this incision allows adequate exposure in patients who have not been operated on previously and results in a minimum of inflammation and scarring.

Prevention Undoubtedly, it is best to prevent a hypersensitive incision in the first place. Because the skin of the palmar side of the wrist is thin and immobile, revision of the scar is not easy. After excision of the scar, a well designed z-plasty is the least complicated approach, and it may be adequate. If the skin is not directly adherent to the median nerve, a split-thickness or, preferably, a full-thickness skin graft can be used for coverage. A local muscle-pedicle flap, such as the abductor digiti minimi, lumbrical muscle, or pronator quadratus, should be used if the scar is large. The management of involvement of the scar with the underlying median nerve will be discussed later.

Reflex Sympathetic Dystrophy

Prevention Reflex sympathetic dystrophy may follow decompression of the median nerve by any method. However, certain precautions can definitely diminish the chances of this complication occurring. A properly placed incision that allows good exposure minimizes trauma to the median nerve during the dissection. Internal neurolysis increases irritation of the nerve and should be avoided. Release of the tourniquet and thorough hemostasis before wound closure is strongly recommended. Perhaps the most important component of postoperative management is the application of a comfortable, bulky compressive dressing. Any type of constrictive elastic bandage should be avoided.

Treatment Early recognition and immediate treatment of this complication are essential to curtail symptoms. When swelling, redness, warm skin, hyperesthesias, and pain on motion occur within the first few weeks after surgery, corticosteroids (a Medrol Dosepak [methyl-prednisolone tablets]) should be administered orally.

Active range-of-motion exercises, closely supervised by a hand therapist, are beneficial, and a comfortable non-constricting supportive dressing should be used. Other medications such as Stelazine (trifluoperazine) or Elavil (amitriptyline) may be helpful in early management of this complication. Chronic and persistent symptoms of reflex sympathetic dystrophy should be treated with the use of stellate ganglion blocks.

Severance of the Recurrent Motor Branch of the Median Nerve

Prevention A knowledge of the anatomic variations of the recurrent motor branch of the median nerve is essential for a surgeon who performs carpal tunnel release. Although the recurrent motor branch usually exits from the radial side of the median nerve, in a small tunnel at the distal margin of the transverse carpal ligament, there are multiple variations of the branching.[59,60] The recurrent motor branch or even the median nerve proper can be injured unless the surgeon clearly exposes the transverse carpal ligament and visualizes it in a bloodless field. All neighboring structures must be observed carefully as the transverse carpal ligament is severed along its ulnar border.

Treatment If the recurrent motor branch is acutely transected (an event often signified by a twitch of the thenar muscles), it must be immediately repaired by microsurgical technique. Functional recovery usually can be expected if the distal branch can be located, which is not always easy, and a good repair is achieved. Excellent functional recovery has been reported even after repairs delayed as long as 14 months after the injury.[61]

Injury from Neurolysis

Prevention Since Curtis and Eversmann[28] popularized the technique of internal neurolysis combined with release of the transverse carpal ligament in the early 1970s, this procedure has been overused. The indications for neurolysis, even in conditions of severe scarring of the median nerve, remain controversial. With the numbers available, one of us (RHG) and coworkers demonstrated no significant difference ($p < 0.05$) between patients with severe carpal tunnel syndrome treated with ligament release alone and those treated with neurolysis combined with ligament release.[30] If internal neurolysis is chosen as an adjunct, it must be done with microinstruments and a microscope. This extensive dissection may cause direct mechanical injury and also may result in excessive postoperative intra-neural and perineural scarring. For these reasons, internal neurolysis of the median nerve at the wrist is rarely indicated.

Treatment Many patients complain of pain and dysesthesias for a few months after internal neurolysis. Persistent symptoms may be the result of transection of one or more nerve fascicles. This complication is difficult to treat successfully, because an additional operation may result in more scarring. If a fascicle has been severed, it should be repaired primarily, with 10-0 nylon and the use of a microscope. Despite repair, focal dysesthesias may persist as a result of individual fascicles being trapped in the scar tissue. If the dysesthesias are localized to one digit or to one area of a digit, microsurgical re- exploration is performed by location of the involved nerve or nerve branch distally, and its contributing fascicles are traced proximally through the median nerve in the carpal canal. The involved fascicles are isolated and freed from their surrounding intraneural tissue without disturbing the remainder of the nerve. If involvement of the main trunk of the median nerve by scarring produces symptoms of direct hypersensitivity or distal pain or dysesthesias, repeat neurolysis usually will not relieve the symptoms. In this situation, coverage of the involved area of the median nerve with a fat graft, as described in a subsequent section, is recommended.

Tenderness of the Median Nerve

Frequently, the median nerve is tender beneath the skin and subcutaneous tissue following carpal tunnel release. The causes of the tenderness include incomplete decompression, a neuroma in continuity (secondary to internal neurolysis or to fascicular severance from a dissection), scarring about the nerve, or a superficial position of the nerve (especially if the palmaris longus is absent).

Prevention The location of the skin incision influences the postoperative sensitivity of the median nerve. An incision that crosses the wrist flexion crease and extends proximally is more likely to cause scarring over the median nerve. An ulnarly placed skin incision allows the median nerve to be protected by undamaged subcutaneous tissue. In general, the less the nerve is disturbed, the better it responds to decompression. For this reason, the use of epineurotomy and, particularly, of internal neurolysis should generally be avoided. Attainment of hemostasis prior to wound closure and the inclusion of a small suction drain to diminish hematoma formation both decrease scar formation. To minimize scarring about the nerve, the only tissue that should be sutured is the skin. Finally, splinting of the wrist in slight dorsiflexion for five to seven days helps to maintain the median nerve in a deeper position.

Treatment There are several ways to manage a tender median nerve. A simple z-plasty of the skin, which may be combined with a silicone sheeting placed beneath the skin (and removed at three weeks), on occasion provides better superficial protection of the nerve. Various flaps from a distance, or even free tissue transfers, have been used successfully, but they usually create too much bulk. A small, local muscle-pedicle flap, such

as the pronator quadratus, abductor digiti minimi, or lumbrical muscle, provides good soft-tissue coverage for the median nerve, although mobilization of some of these flaps may be difficult. It is important not to injure the vascular pedicle of the muscle when it is transferred. These muscles usually must be covered with split-thickness skin graft to avoid tight skin. Subcutaneous fat, harvested from a separate incision in the proximal part of the forearm, provides excellent, immediate soft-tissue coverage with minimum additional dissection. However, the long-term survival of the transplanted adipose tissue has not been determined. A convenient, reliable, and uncomplicated procedure is coverage of the median nerve with a hypothenar fat flap.[34] With the use of subcutaneous dissection, the flap of hypothenar fat is mobilized, based on a radial vascular pedicle. The flap can then be folded over the critical portion of the median nerve (Fig. 6). If insufficient

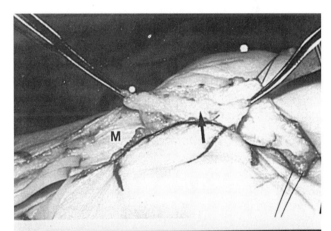

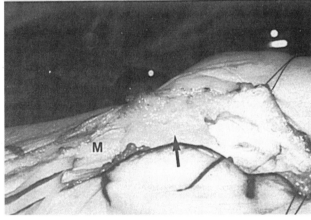

Fig. 6 Photographs demonstrating treatment of the complication of a tender median nerve (M) after a carpal tunnel procedure. **Top,** The hypothenar fat (arrow) is undermined by dissection of the ulnar border from the skin and maintenance of the radial-based pedicle. **Bottom,** The hypothenar fat flap (arrow) based on a radial pedicle is positioned over the sensitive median nerve. (Reprinted with permission from Urbaniak JR: Complications of treatment of carpal tunnel syndrome, in Gelberman RH (ed): *Operative Nerve Repair and Reconstruction.* Philadelphia, PA, JB Lippincott, 1991, vol. 2, p 976.)

fat is available, additional free fat from the proximal part of the forearm can be added. This technique does not sacrifice any vital tissue and generally provides reliable soft-tissue protection of the nerve.

Nerve Adherence to the Flexor Tendons

Prevention As tenosynovitis is the most common cause of carpal tunnel syndrome, hypertrophy of the tenosynovial sheath is a common finding at the time of carpal tunnel release. Excision of the synovial tissue is not recommended during most carpal tunnel releases because it promotes increased bleeding and scar formation, which may result in adherence of the nerve to the tendons as well as in restricted tendon excursion. Tenosynovectomy should be limited to patients in whom the abnormal synovial tissue is extremely bulky, inflamed, or invasive (such as in rheumatoid arthritis) or when a diagnostic biopsy is indicated. Thorough hemostasis diminishes peritendinous scar formation, and therefore the tourniquet should be released prior to wound closure to enable one to obtain more reliable hemostasis. The use of a small suction drain (which may be removed prior to discharge, as an outpatient procedure) is recommended. The most important step in the prevention or diminution of adherence of the flexor tendons to the median nerve is immediate, comfortable motion of the digits. This is accomplished by application of a short dorsal splint that extends from the mid-part of the forearm to the distal palmar crease. The wrist is held in slight dorsiflexion, but all digits have a free, full, active range of motion. An active range of motion is encouraged immediately after the operation, in order to keep the tendons and the median nerve mobile.

Treatment Hand therapy plays a major role in the management of nerve adherence to the flexor tendons. Active and passive assistive range-of-motion exercises and dynamic splinting are the most important ingredients of the therapy program to achieve painless, functional motion and to improve grip strength. Tenolysis is rarely indicated.

Hematoma

Prevention Hemorrhage can be a cause of acute carpal tunnel syndrome, but residual hematoma after carpal tunnel release is a more common problem. The steps that should be taken to avoid this complication have been discussed in the preceding sections. In addition to the attainment of good hemostasis, use of a suction drain, and application of a bulky compressive (but not constrictive) dressing, the surgeon must always be aware of the superficial palmar arch. The release of the transverse carpal ligament should be extended distally to the arch, which must be identified and protected during the decompression. Blind sectioning of the ligament has resulted in injury to the artery with secondary hematoma formation, skin slough, and circulatory deficiency of the hand.[56]

Treatment If a serious hematoma occurs, it should be evacuated promptly.

Flexor-Tendon Bow-Stringing

Prevention Although the transverse carpal ligament has been described as an important retinacular pulley for the digital flexors,[62] bow-stringing of the flexor tendons after complete release of this ligament is rare. While some have advocated methods of surgical treatment that include repair of the ligament by such means as z-lengthening,[63] the surgeon should be concerned about residual nerve constriction and additional scar formation, which can result from these procedures. An alternative, reliable method for the prevention of bow-stringing is sectioning of the ligament along its ulnar border to retain some of its pulley effect and immobilization of the wrist in slight dorsiflexion for a few days postoperatively.

Treatment In the rare situation when bow-stringing of the flexor tendons becomes symptomatic, the transverse carpal ligament can be reconstructed by use of a free tendon graft, such as the palmaris longus.[56] After ligament reconstruction, the surgeon's small finger must be able to pass beneath the ligament, to ensure that there is adequate space for the median nerve deep to the ligament.

Endoscopic Carpal Tunnel Release

This section would not be complete without a brief discussion of endoscopic carpal tunnel release. This technique has been gaining increasing popularity, but, unfortunately, the number of complications of carpal tunnel release has increased with its use. The stated advantages of this procedure are decreased discomfort in the palm of the hand and an earlier return to work and to the normal activities of daily living. However, direct injury to the median nerve, ulnar nerve, digital nerves, and superficial palmar arch have all been described.[27,64] In addition, visualization of mass lesions within the carpal tunnel may be difficult when the procedure is performed as recommended.

Cubital Tunnel Syndrome

The term cubital tunnel was proposed in 1958 by Feindel and Stratford.[65] They used it to identify a specific anatomic site for entrapment of the ulnar nerve and thus suggested a new idiopathic syndrome, distinct from tardy ulnar palsy, which had been associated with post-traumatic skeletal deformities such as cubitus valgus. The ulnar nerve, in its passage around the medial aspect of the elbow, is vulnerable to compromise from compression, scar fixation, or traction. The anatomic cubital tunnel through which it passes is a fibro-osseous ring formed by the medial epicondyle and the proximal part of the ulna and bridged by a specific fascial sheet (described by Osborne[66] in 1957). Because of the somewhat eccentric origin of this fascial roof, the cubital tunnel, unlike the carpal tunnel, changes contour and volume during elbow flexion and extension.[67] In flexion, the cross-sectional contour changes from slightly ovoid to elliptical.[68] Therefore, any swelling within the canal, or inflammation and thickening of this fascial sheet, may compress the ulnar nerve and its vasculature.[69]

The nerve is also vulnerable at several other sites, proximal and distal to the cubital tunnel. Most proximal is the most often mentioned, but rarely involved, arcade of Struthers, which lies 8 cm proximal to the epicondyle and through which the ulnar nerve passes from the anterior into the posterior brachial compartment.[53] Next is the thick medial intermuscular septum, which fans medially, bridging the concavity formed by the flare of the medial epicondyle. Because the nerve normally lies posterior and parallel to this septum, it is not a problem unless the nerve subluxates anteriorly across it or unless it is not excised adequately when the nerve is transposed anteriorly.

Distal to the cubital tunnel, the nerve enters the hiatus between the humeral and ulnar origins of the flexor-pronator muscles. With scarring or with congestion from vigorous wrist or finger flexor-muscle activity, the nerve may become compressed, particularly if the overlying fascia, a distal expansion of Osborne's fascia, becomes thickened or inelastic. As the nerve continues through the substance of the flexor-pronator mass, it may be compressed by fascial bands that represent the proximal origins of the epimysial envelopes of the individual muscles as they begin to separate into distinct bellies distal to the elbow.[70]

Pathomechanics

The ulnar nerve at the elbow is not only subcutaneous but is partially fixed within a narrow fibro-osseous tunnel. Prolonged elbow flexion, which stretches the nerve and narrows this tunnel, combined with resting on the elbow, such as when using a telephone, may produce paresthesias in the ring and little fingers of normal individuals. With swelling and minimum elbow inflammation or congestion of the flexor-pronator muscles, this stretch-compression compromises the vasculature of the ulnar nerve. Musicians who must maintain prolonged elbow flexion, particularly while vigorously exercising the wrist and finger flexors, are somewhat predisposed to ulnar nerve symptoms, ranging from tingling in the ring and little fingers to clumsiness and a lack of coordination. The throwing athlete places special stress on the ulnar nerve in the cubital tunnel at the peak of a wind-up, when the elbow is in flexion and slight varus angulation, at the same time that the shoulder is in abduction and maximum external rotation (Fig. 7).[71] With the

nerve under such stretch, a momentary lancinating pain from the elbow to the hand may occur, and when this motion is repeated regularly, it produces edema in the ulnar nerve at the medial aspect of the elbow. The same mechanism applies to the serving of a tennis ball. In these athletic patients, physical findings other than local tenderness may be minimum, and electrodiagnostic tests are rarely positive; however, complete relief may be obtained by anterior transposition of the nerve.[72,73]

Clinical Findings

The symptoms of cubital tunnel syndrome include medial elbow pain and a spectrum of complaints indicative of compromised ulnar nerve function. There may be sensory symptoms, progressing from tingling and burning in the fourth and fifth fingers to sensory loss and ultimately to anesthesia of these fingers. Motor problems may range from clumsiness to weakness of intrinsic muscle strength and pinch to middle phalanx claw deformity and gross intrinsic atrophy.

Specific physical findings include direct tenderness at, or posterior to, the medial epicondyle and a Tinel sign radiating to the fourth and fifth fingers on minimum manipulation of the nerve from 2 cm proximal to 2 cm distal to the cubital tunnel. Anterior subluxation of the nerve may occur with flexion; however, unless the nerve is specifically sensitive and symptoms are reproduced by light palpation while the nerve is subluxated, subluxation per se may not be a meaningful finding, as it occurs commonly in asymptomatic individuals. Sensory examination can be performed with two-point discrimination or the von Frey technique. Pinch and grip testing are excellent objective assessments of motor function. One of the earliest signs of muscular weakness is weakness of the third palmar interosseous muscle on comparative testing.

Electrodiagnostic examination is helpful in cases in which localization to the cubital tunnel is not well defined or the diagnosis is not clear-cut. False-negative electrodiagnostic examinations, however, are not uncommon, and it is not unusual for surgical intervention to provide complete relief of severe dysesthesias in patients with negative conduction studies.[72]

The differential diagnosis for cubital tunnel syndrome is extensive. Diagnoses range from systemic metabolic disorders such as diabetes and leprosy to the Guyon canal syndrome to the essentially epidemic malady, cervical radiculitis. The ability to elicit a Tinel sign radiating to the ulnar aspect of the wrist or to the fourth and fifth fingers by manipulation of the nerve over the mid-part of the brachium, proximal to the epicondyle, is strong evidence of radiculitis of the seventh or eighth cervical nerve root. Thoracic outlet syndrome also must be ruled out.

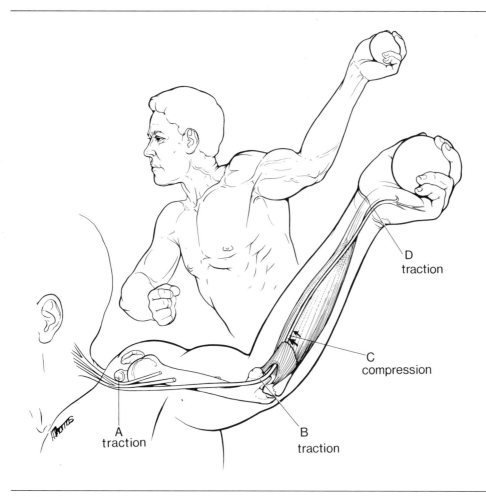

Fig. 7   The posture of a thrower's arm at the peak of wind-up creates traction or compresses the ulnar nerve in four places. A = axilla. There is traction on the medial cord of the plexus as the arm is abducted, extended, and externally rotated at the shoulder. B = elbow. The nerve is stretched as it passes behind the epicondyle with the elbow flexed in slight valgus. Adhesions secondary to previous elbow synovitis may increase this traction. C = flexor pronator insertion. Fixation and compression of the nerve occur due to flexor-pronator muscle engorgement after repetitive gripping of the ball and snapping of the wrist. D = wrist. Additional traction on the nerve occurs as the wrist is extended. (Reprinted with permission from Eaton RG: Anterior subcutaneous transposition, in Gelberman RH (ed): *Operative Nerve Repair and Reconstruction.* Philadelphia, PA, JB Lippincott, 1991, vol 2, p 1080.)

Conservative Treatment

Initial treatment involves rest of the elbow musculature and strict avoidance of external pressure when the elbow is flexed more than 90°. Adjustment of the arm posture that the patient assumes while holding a telephone and avoidance of resting on the flexed elbow during daytime activities or sleeping are helpful in early and mild cases. Cradling of the head on a flexed elbow in sleep is a frequent cause of finger paresthesias. Use of a flexible splint, such as a spandex-rubber basketball elbow-guard during sleep, both protects the medial aspect of the elbow and discourages excessive elbow flexion (Fig. 8). On occasion, use of a rigid splint at night may prove beneficial. Anti-inflammatory medications are occasionally helpful, but injections of steroid directly into the cubital tunnel are not advised.

Surgical Indications

Intractable symptoms after four to six weeks of conservative care or evidence of ulnar intrinsic motor loss are an indication for surgical decompression. It is essential to establish that the nerve compromise is clearly localized to the medial epicondyle area. In metabolic or granulomatous processes such as tubercu-

losis or leprosy, surgical decompression or relocation of the nerve to a less fixed or better vascularized area, or both, may improve nerve function even though it

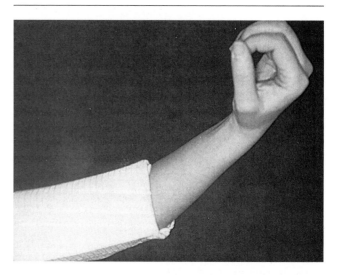

Fig. 8   The spandex-rubber elbow-guard used in conservative treatment of cubital tunnel syndrome. The guard restricts flexion and provides loose padding over the medial epicondyle.

does not completely reverse the intrinsic nerve damage. In diabetics, in addition to the metabolic peripheral neuropathy, a concomitant local compressive neuropathy may develop; thus, diabetics may be candidates for decompression and anterior transposition.[72]

Surgical Procedures

Surgical treatment involves either local decompression or anterior transposition. Local decompression procedures include posterior in situ release of Osborne's fascia or removal of the epicondyle, which acts as a capstan around which the nerve is stretched during flexion. In situ release, although simple, does not address fixation of the nerve to the periosteum or to the medial collateral ligament, and there is a risk of anterior subluxation of the nerve. The procedure is best reserved for patients with early, minimum nerve compression; normal elbow anatomy; and no subluxation.

Epicondylectomy takes local decompression one step further by removing one of the osseous walls of the cubital tunnel. It involves a great deal more tissue manipulation (a portion of the flexor-pronator origin) as well as periosteal stripping, and thus, theoretically, it may produce additional scarring and fixation of the nerve. Instability of the medial collateral ligament may occur when an excessive amount of the epicondyle is removed. Epicondylectomy is most commonly indicated for patients without post-traumatic scarring or known structural damage to the elbow joint. It is not advisable in high-performance athletes.

The most commonly performed cubital-tunnel procedure involves lysis with mobilization and anterior transposition of the nerve.[74] Anterior transposition allows the nerve to be positioned in a less scarred bed and to be functionally lengthened by the surgeon returning it to the anterior compartment, eliminating its short detour around the elbow in the posterior compartment. Three to 4 cm of length are gained by anterior rerouting, which also makes the procedure ideal for the elimination of tension during ulnar nerve repair in the elbow region.

Three methods of anterior transposition have been advocated, each with a different technique for stabilizing the nerve in an anterior position. The submuscular technique positions the nerve deep to the flexor-pronator muscle mass; the intramuscular technique reroutes the transposed nerve through a superficial channel in these muscles; and the subcutaneous technique stabilizes the nerve anteriorly by constructing a new short medial septum or sling posterior to the nerve, thus preventing its return to a retrocondylar position.

Submuscular Transposition

The submuscular method of anterior transposition was described by Learmonth[75] in 1942 and has had many advocates.[73,76,77] This technique includes detachment of the flexor-pronator origins from the humeral head, placement of the mobilized ulnar nerve beneath the flexor-pronator origins, and reattachment of these muscles to the epicondyle. In addition to maintaining the nerve anteriorly, this provides muscular padding over the nerve to protect it from trauma. Two to three weeks of immobilization are required for the muscles to heal sufficiently to withstand elbow motion, particularly extension. It cannot be disputed that this technique securely stabilizes the nerve anteriorly, and it has therefore been recommended for use even in high-performance athletes. Because of the need for muscle healing and restoration of elbow motion and power, the time for a return to full activity is longer than for the other two anterior transposition procedures. Due to the interdigitation of muscle fibers at the medial epicondyle, atraumatic separation of the common origins is not always possible, and a nerve may not always be in a well-defined intermuscular interval as described by Learmonth.[75] There is a potential for perineural scar formation, particularly when the elbow is immobilized in flexion to allow muscle reattachment.

Intramuscular Transposition

Maintenance of the transposed ulnar nerve anteriorly by intramuscular stabilization was proposed by Adson[78] in 1918. This technique has evolved into placement of the nerve in a 5-mm trough in the surface of the flexor-pronator muscle and closure of its superficial fascia over the nerve.[79] Great care must be exercised to avoid angulation of the nerve as it passes distal to this channel to enter the flexor-pronator hiatus and to continue its distal course deep to the flexor carpi ulnaris. There is a potential for persistent compression if the closure of the flexor-pronator fascia is tight or if muscle swelling develops, transfixing the nerve in this position while the elbow is flexed at 90° during the three weeks of postoperative immobilization.

Subcutaneous Transposition

In 1898, Curtis[80] described subcutaneous transposition but gave no technical details of his method for stabilization of the nerve in its new position. Over the years, subcutaneous transposition has been the most frequently performed procedure, although there have been no large studies analyzing the results of a specific technique. Complications are not uncommon; however, it is not clear whether untoward results are related to any single method of securing the nerve anteriorly. Suturing of a subcutaneous fat flap around the nerve,[81] suturing of the nerve deep to subcutaneous fascia, and fixing of epineurium to muscle fascia have all been described; however, such techniques each carry a potential for further compression and fixation of the nerve.

Stabilized Subcutaneous Transposition

In 1980, a technique was described that created a new medial septum posterior to the transposed nerve.[72] This technique does not secure the transposed nerve to any fixed structure, nor does it place any tissue other than normal cubital fat superficial to the nerve. Due to complete superficial dissection, immediate elbow motion is permitted and, indeed, is encouraged.[82,83] Thus, there is little potential for nerve fixation or entrapment. No muscles are disturbed or reattached. The results have been quite satisfactory,[83] although patients with chronic, intrinsic nerve-compression changes have not always had as complete a reversal of symptoms as have patients with neurapraxia or less axonal damage. It is axiomatic that transposition of the nerve eliminates extrinsic compression and improves the neurocirculation but does not specifically address advanced intraneural fibrosis.

Subcutaneous anterior transposition includes, as do all transposition procedures, complete release of the ulnar nerve from the distal 4 cm of the humerus to well into the flexor-pronator muscle mass. Preoperatively, with the elbow extended, the apex of the epicondyle is marked on the skin. A second mark is placed 1 cm anterior to this mark, and it represents the site for the subsequent dermal attachment of the new medial septum (Fig. 9, *top left*).[82] The incision is made midway between the olecranon and the medial epicondyle, extending 5 cm proximally and distally. Special care must be used to identify and preserve the posterior branches of the medial brachial and antebrachial cutaneous nerves, which cross the incisions almost perpendicularly from anterior to posterior. Injury to these nerves can create major postoperative dysesthesias.

The ulnar nerve is easily identified just proximal to the epicondyle, and the dissection is then extended proximally. When the nerve is mobilized, with use of extremely gentle dissection, the accompanying venous plexus, which usually runs in close proximity, must also be mobilized to ensure optimum postoperative microcirculation. Immediate postoperative dysesthesias appear to be greatly reduced when these vessels can be mobilized and transposed with the nerve. Feeder vessels into these longitudinal venous plexuses are ligated.

Proximal dissection is continued to 4 to 5 cm above the epicondyle. At this level, the nerve is relaxed and free to bow-string anteriorly, so that fixation by fibrous bands proximal to this level will not cause angulation or kinking. In the process of mobilization, the cord-like edge of the intermuscular septum is easily seen. This septum must be excised from the medial epicondyle flare to a point 3 to 4 cm proximally. Persistence of this ligament, over which the anteriorly transposed nerve must pass, may cause secondary compression of the nerve and is one of the most common causes of postoperative pain and paresthesias.

The nerve and accompanying venous plexus may be atraumatically retracted with a Penrose drain as dissection is continued distally. The fascia covering the cubital tunnel (Osborne's fascia) is sectioned, and the nerve is followed into the flexor-pronator hiatus by splitting the overlying muscle fascia and teasing the muscles apart. This dissection must continue for 2 to 3 cm into the muscle mass, preserving any motor branches along the way. Digital palpation identifies any additional fibrous cords deeper within the muscles. The transposed nerve should enter this hiatus somewhat more distally than normally, approaching from anterior to the epicondyle at a 40° to 45° angle with the elbow extended. With the nerve fully mobilized, it is possible to detect any area of local intrinsic compression by the presence of a persistent short segmental constriction. In such situations, a local epineurotomy may be performed to provide maximum decompression of the nerve. Extensive internal neurolysis is not justified.

The new medial septum or sling is created by using methylene blue to outline a 1.5-cm-wide square on the thickened anterior fascia of the flexor-pronator muscle mass (Fig. 9, *top right*). The medial margin lies at the medial limit of this fascia on the epicondyle. The fascia is incised with this single medial margin left intact and this flap is reflected medially, as in the opening of a book cover. The 1.5-cm-wide square flap is thus hinged medially, and the nerve is placed anterior to it. The free corners of this square are then sutured to the dermis, deep to the mark placed preoperatively on the skin 1 cm anterior to the epicondyle, using 3-0 nonabsorbable sutures. In its new anterior position, the nerve and its accompanying longitudinal venous plexus are bounded by muscle fascia posteriorly and by subcutaneous fat anteriorly (Fig. 9, *bottom*). It should not be compressed in its new routing, and it should be easily slid proximally and distally across the new medial septum. When the skin has been closed, the new septum lies slightly anterior to the horizontal plane of the epicondyle and maintains the nerve anteriorly, where it is protected medially by the flare of the epicondyle (Fig. 10).

A soft dressing is applied, and the patient is encouraged to flex and extend the elbow on the evening of the operation (Fig. 11). Rapid progression to full motion within three, four, or five days is the rule. Return to all but the most stressful activities is encouraged. The elbow should not be allowed to become stiff and, because the dissection is superficial, local pain with motion is brief and rarely severe.

Complications Stabilized subcutaneous transposition rarely leads to complications. Careful hemostasis should prevent hematoma formation, especially

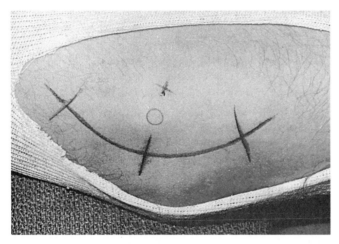

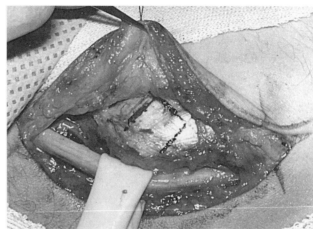

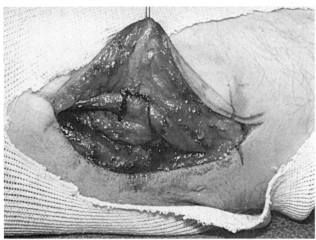

Fig. 9 Subcutaneous anterior transposition for the treatment of cubital tunnel syndrome. **Top left,** The skin incision is marked with the elbow in maximum extension. The markings include one (0) at the medial epicondyle and another (+) one centimeter anterior to this — the site for dermal attachment of the new medial septum. **Top right,** The 1.5-cm-wide flap is outlined on the flexor-pronator fascia. The medial edge is in the long axis of the humerus. **Bottom,** The reflected flap is sutured to the dermis at the premarked site (+, above) anterior to the epicondyle. Note that, with adequate proximal and distal mobilization, the nerve lies completely relaxed even with the elbow extended. It is covered only by subcutaneous fat. (Reprinted with permission from Eaton RG: Anterior subcutaneous transposition, in Gelberman RH (ed): *Operative Nerve Repair and Reconstruction.* Philadelphia, PA, JB Lippincott, 1991, vol 2, p 1082-1083.)

because only subcutaneous bleeding is produced. Injuries to the medial brachial and antebrachial cutaneous nerves may occur. Should these produce marked symptoms, they can be treated by an anterior transposition of the specific neuromata so that they are removed from areas of scar or traction with elbow motion. Direct sensitivity of the nerve to external trauma in its subcutaneous position is rarely seen. The anteromedial aspect of the elbow is protected by the projecting medial epicondyle, and direct trauma rarely reaches the nerve. Specific tenderness directly over the nerve is not common. Fixation of the nerve to the fascial flap or to its donor site has not been observed. Permanent restriction of elbow motion virtually never occurs when a motion program has been started immediately postoperatively. Assuming that the classic sites of compression described in the introduction to this paper have been released, persistent neural compromise is not a problem. Complete decompression and transposition to a noncompressible relaxed position may not always result in a complete return of motor and sensory function, due to intrinsic scarring within the nerve trunk. Internal microneuroanalysis of a limited, indented portion of the nerve may be considered at the time of the operation, but such dissection should be used only in patients with severe compromise and a well-localized narrowing of the nerve trunk.

Expanded applications The ulnar nerve in the cubital tunnel is inherently vulnerable to compression or fixation following external trauma or surgical dissection around the elbow. Because subcutaneous anterior transposition using a fascial sling is quite simple, it can be included in most juxtacubital reconstruction procedures, as well as in open reductions of fractures or dislocations. The length gained by anterior transposition facilitates nerve repair and positions the nerve in a favorable bed.

Radial Nerve Compression in the Forearm

The literature on entrapment of the radial nerve in the forearm is confusing to the clinician. Two separate syndromes have been defined for compression of the posterior interosseous nerve in the radial tunnel: (1)

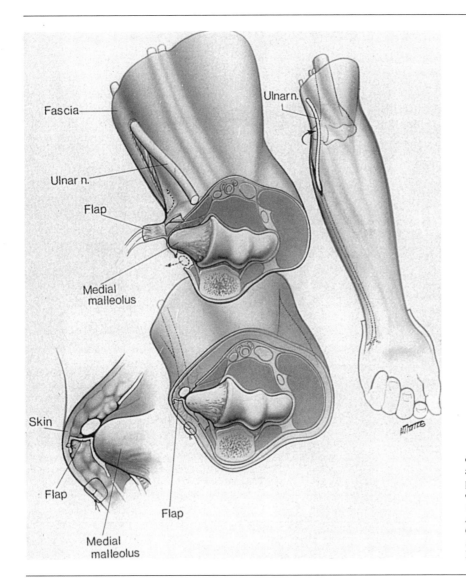

Fig. 10 The reflected fascial flap that connects the epicondyle to the dermis forms a stable medial septum or floor for the transposed nerve. The nerve is fully mobile, with only subcutaneous fat lying superficial to it. (Reprinted with permission from Eaton RG: Anterior subcutaneous transposition, in Gelberman RH (ed): *Operative Nerve Repair and Reconstruction*. Philadelphia, PA, JB Lippincott, 1991, vol 2, pp 1082-1083.)

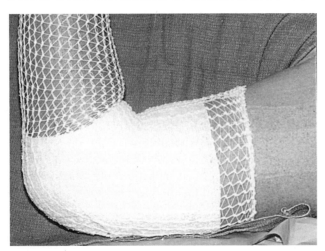

Fig. 11 The postoperative dressing is held in place with a loose mesh sleeve, which encourages the maintenance of normal elbow motion. (Reprinted with permission from Eaton RG: Anterior subcutaneous transposition, in Gelberman RH (ed): *Operative Nerve Repair and Reconstruction*. Philadelphia, PA, JB Lippincott, 1991, vol 2, pp 1082-1083.)

radial tunnel syndrome, which is compression of the posterior interosseous nerve in the radial tunnel that results in pain but no motor weakness, and (2) posterior interosseous nerve compression, which is compression of the posterior interosseous nerve in the radial tunnel that produces motor weakness but no pain. It is difficult for the conscientious diagnostician to accept the reality that the same nerve compressed in the same anatomic site can result in two entirely different symptom complexes. These compressive neuropathies are not common in comparison with those of the other major nerves in the upper extremity; therefore, caution must be exercised so as not to overdiagnose them. A clear understanding of the anatomy, the obtainment of an appropriate history, and the performance of a thorough physical examination enable the clinician to diagnose these uncommon syndromes accurately.

Radial Tunnel Syndrome

The condition that associates pain with compression of the posterior interosseous nerve was labeled radial tunnel syndrome, or resistant tennis elbow, in 1972 by Roles and Maudsley.[84] Since then, other authors have discussed this dubious syndrome with various degrees of enthusiasm.[85-90]

Anatomy In the distal third of the brachium, the radial nerve passes through the spiral groove of the humerus, from the posterior aspect to the anterior region of the arm. It pierces the intermuscular septum to enter the anterior compartment of the arm. The nerve divides into two terminal components, the motor posterior interosseous nerve and the sensory superficial radial nerve. In the anterior or ventral location, the nerve lies between the brachioradialis laterally and the brachialis medially. The extensor carpi radialis longus overlaps it anterolaterally, and the capitellum of the humerus is posterior. The radial tunnel begins at the level of the radiohumeral joint and extends through the arcade of Frohse.

The superficial radial nerve remains on the deep surface of the brachioradialis muscle to the mid-part of the forearm and is not subject to compression in the radial tunnel. The posterior interosseous nerve may be compressed by several structures as it enters the extensor aspect of the forearm.

Pathologic Findings The mnemonic FREAS can help one to remember the structures that have the potential to compress the posterior interosseous nerve in the radial tunnel: Fibrous bands, Recurrent radial vessels (the leash of Henry), Extensor carpi radialis brevis, Arcade of Frohse, and Supinator (the distal border). The potential sites of compression are described in the order of their location by dissection, from the superficial to the deep layers, during the surgical exposure of the posterior interosseous nerve. The fibrous bands are anterior to the radial head at the entrance of the radial tunnel (Fig. 12, *top left*). They are the least likely

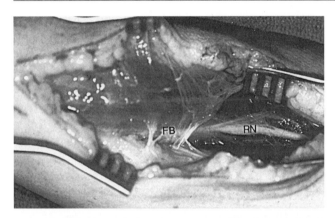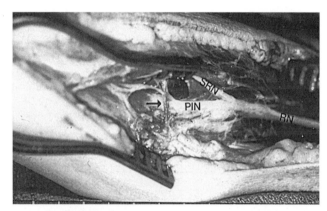

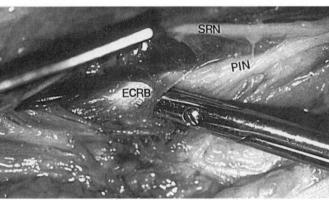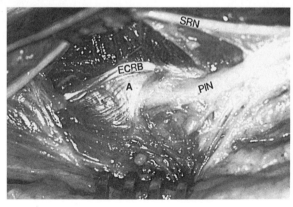

Fig. 12   These photographs show the structures that have the potential to compress the posterior interosseous nerve in the radial tunnel, causing radial tunnel syndrome. **Top left,** The superficial fibrous bands (FB) are anterior to the radial head, at the entrance of the radial tunnel. The radial nerve (RN) is seen before it enters the radial tunnel. **Top right,** The recurrent radial vessels (the leash of Henry) (arrow) cross the posterior interosseous nerve (PIN) to supply the brachioradialis and extensor carpi radialis muscles. Also seen are the radial nerve (RN) and the superficial radial nerve (SRN). **Bottom left,** The surgical scissors are interposed between the extensor carpi radialis brevis (ECRB) and the posterior interosseous nerve (PIN). The superficial radial nerve (SRN) does not enter the radial tunnel. **Bottom right,** The fibrous proximal border of the superficial belly of the supinator. The arcade of Frohse (A) is just deep to the reflected extensor carpi radialis brevis muscle (ECRB). The posterior interosseous nerve (PIN) may be compressed by the arcade of Frohse. The superficial radial nerve (SRN) is superficial to the radial tunnel.

cause of compression neuropathy. The second site of potential constriction is the fan-shaped recurrent radial vessels (the leash of Henry) (Fig. 12, *top right*). The recurrent radial artery has several branches with their venae comitantes, which cross the posterior interosseous nerve to supply the brachioradialis and extensor carpi radialis muscles. It has been postulated that they may become engorged with exercise and compress the nerve.

The tough, thin, tendinous margin of the extensor carpi radialis brevis muscle is the third structure encountered during the surgical exposure that may induce the neuropathy (Fig. 12, *bottom left*). The surgeon who is inexperienced in the exposure of the posterior interosseous nerve may mistakenly identify this structure as the arcade of Frohse, which lies directly deep to the proximal margin of the extensor carpi radialis brevis muscle.

The arcade of Frohse[91] is the free, strong, fibrous proximal border of the superficial belly of the supinator (Fig. 12, *bottom right*). It is the most common site of compression and should always be released in the exposure.

It is worthwhile to continue the exploration to the distal border of the superficial supinator muscle as, rarely, it may compress the nerve.[92] More frequently, a mass, such as a ganglion, may be found beneath the superficial belly of the supinator.[93]

Symptoms The pain in radial tunnel syndrome is similar to that of tennis elbow or lateral epicondylitis and therefore it is difficult to differentiate from those conditions. The pain occurs in the lateral elbow or extensor area and often radiates distally to the wrist. Because the pain is secondary to compression of a motor nerve, the character of the pain is a deep ache or similar to a muscle cramp. The pain is frequently nocturnal, occurs after exercise, and is relieved with rest. Specific activities, such as passive wrist flexion and pronation and active wrist dorsiflexion and supination, provoke the pain.

Physical Examination There are no sensory disturbances or loss of motor function in radial tunnel syndrome. Point tenderness is localized 5 cm distal to the lateral epicondyle over the extensor wad. Because this area is tender in the asymptomatic extremity, the tenderness must be compared with that of the uninvolved side. The so-called middle-finger test, which has been reported[88] to be pathognomonic of radial tunnel syndrome, is overrated. The test involves extension of the long finger with the elbow in extension and the wrist in neutral. This maneuver is positive if pain is provoked at the proximal area of the extensor carpi radialis brevis, which inserts distally on the third metacarpal. However, it may be positive in tennis elbow and is frequently absent in both syndromes.

To an extent, the physical examination may be correlated with the area of anatomic compression although, admittedly, the findings are not totally reliable. If the symptoms are reproduced with the elbow in full flexion, the forearm in supination, and the wrist in neutral, the fibrous bands are suspect. Reproduction of the symptoms by passive pronation of the forearm with the elbow in 45° to 90° of flexion and the wrist in full flexion indicates entrapment by the extensor carpi radialis brevis. This is further supported if the symptoms are relieved with passive wrist flexion. Compression by the arcade of Frohse is suspected if the symptoms are reproduced by isometric supination of the forearm in the fully pronated position.[85]

Diagnostic Tests Electrodiagnostic studies are generally not helpful in the diagnosis of radial tunnel syndrome. Electromyographic recordings are normal, because there are no motor palsies, and assessments of conduction velocities across the radial tunnel have not been a reliable aid in the diagnosis.

The most reliable test for diagnosis is a local anesthetic block. A local injection of 3 ml of 1% Xylocaine (lidocaine) into the radial tunnel, with relief of pain and creation of a posterior interosseous nerve palsy, confirms the diagnosis. A posterior interosseous nerve palsy must be produced for a reliable test. A prior injection into the lateral epicondylar region without relief of pain supports the diagnosis.

Conservative Treatment

Rest and avoidance of provocative activities or positions may relieve symptoms of radial tunnel syndrome. Non-steroidal anti-inflammatory agents are occasionally helpful. Splinting of the elbow in flexion, with the forearm in supination and the wrist in dorsiflexion, is a method of ensuring rest and providing relief of symptoms in some individuals.

Surgical Approaches

Three surgical approaches have been described for exposure of the posterior interosseous nerve in the radial tunnel. Henry's mobile wad (the brachioradialis, extensor carpi radialis longus, and extensor carpi radialis brevis)[94] serves as the focal area for orientation. One approach is anterior to it, the second is posterior, and the third is through the muscle mass. All approaches are performed under tourniquet ischemia.

Anterolateral Approach This is an excellent approach for exposure of all possible compressive structures. This generalized approach is especially recommended for the surgeon who is not thoroughly familiar with the regional anatomy or when the exact area of compression is unclear from the preoperative evaluation. The incision begins on the anterolateral aspect of the arm, 4 cm proximal to the elbow flexion crease, and extends to the flexion crease, where it is directed ulnarward for 2 to 3 cm. It then continues in a curved or z fashion, along the ulnar border of the mobile wad. The dissection proceeds between the brachialis and the brachioradialis to locate the radial nerve in the distal aspect of the arm, just proximal to the elbow flexion crease. Once located, the radial nerve is traced from proximal to distal to inspect the five potential sites of compression (FREAS). The fibrous bands are just anterior to the radial head. The fan-like radial recurrent vessels must be severed and ligated. Pronation of the forearm and flexion of the wrist may demonstrate compression of the posterior interosseous nerve by the fibrous margin of the extensor carpi radialis brevis muscle, and it should be released. The arcade of Frohse, which forms the tough, fibrous proximal border of the superficial belly of the supinator, must be transected. Complete division of the superficial belly of the supinator is recommended, because there can be a compressive fibrous band at its distal border. Full passive pronation of the forearm is helpful for visualization of the distal border of the supinator through this approach.

Posterolateral Approach This approach is best used to expose the distal portion of the supinator. It has the disadvantage of limited anatomic exposure proximally. If the lesion is not localized to the area of the arcade of Frohse, the posterolateral approach should not be used. The incision begins just distal to the lateral epicondyle and extends distally about 8 cm. The dissection is between the muscle bellies of the extensor carpi radialis brevis and the extensor digitorum communis. It is easier to begin the superficial dissection distally and expose the proximal border of the superficial belly of the supinator and decompress the nerve by division of the muscle to include the arcade of Frohse.

Transbrachioradialis Approach This is the most favored and direct approach to the radial tunnel (Fig. 13). A longitudinal 6-cm-long incision is made directly over the brachioradialis muscle in the region of the neck of the radius. (For cosmetic purposes, Lister suggested a transverse incision.[87]) The fascia of the brachioradialis is incised longitudinally, and the underlying muscle fibers are split along the same line with blunt dissection. The longitudinal, blunt muscle-splitting is carried deeper until fat is seen at the depth of the incision, identifying the location of the superficial radial nerve. Beneath this branch is the arcade of Frohse and the posterior interosseous nerve. The dissection is extended both proximally and distally to decompress the five areas of potential compression previously described. With experience, this approach becomes the most accessible, but, because proximal exposure is limited, the surgeon should be confident of the preoperative determination of the location of the lesion.

Postoperative Care

After all three approaches, the elbow is splinted in flexion and the wrist in dorsiflexion for a few days. An early range of motion is encouraged within the first week, although splinting of the wrist in dorsiflexion for 10 to 14 days may be necessary for comfort in some patients.

Results

This syndrome is frequently overdiagnosed, especially in patients with cumulative trauma or when there is the issue of secondary gain. The difficulty with diagnosis and outcome evaluation is that the clinical presentations are subjective and the surgical findings are often sparse. If the diagnosis is not confirmed by the local anesthetic block, as previously described, the surgeon and patient are often disappointed in the outcome of a surgical release. Because this entity is caused by dynamic compression, frequently the nerve does not show evidence of compression, such as narrowing, changes of color, or proximal swelling.

Pain relief has been reported in 67% to 95% of patients who have had surgical management of this syndrome (Table 1). Realistically, surgical treatment fails to relieve pain in close to 33% of patients.

Posterior Interosseous Nerve Syndrome

Agnew[96] described posterior interosseous nerve compression in 1863, when he found what he called a "bursal tumour" compressing the nerve with resulting motor weakness of the finger extensors. As stated, posterior interosseous nerve syndrome is the loss of motor function of all or some of the muscles innervated by this nerve.

Symptoms In this true motor palsy, the diagnosis is frequently delayed for many months, because the patient has no pain or paresthesias. The patient may complain of weakness of finger and thumb extension and of grip. The patient may have sustained trauma to the forearm in the past, but usually there is no associated injury.

Physical Examination With complete posterior interosseous nerve palsy, patients can actively extend the wrist in slight radial deviation, but they are unable to extend the wrist at neutral or in ulnar deviation. They can extend the digits at the interphalangeal joints, but not at the metacarpophalangeal joints. Perhaps more commonly, patients have an incomplete

Table 1
Results of Surgical Treatment of Radial Tunnel Syndrome

Series	Year	No. of Patients	Percentage of Patients Relieved of Pain
Roles and Maudsley[84]	1972	38	92
Lister et al[88]	1979	20	95
Ritts et al[89]	1987	42	74
Steichen et al[95]	1988	139	67

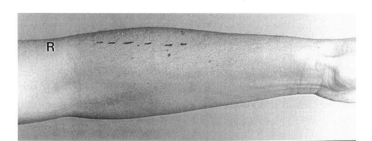

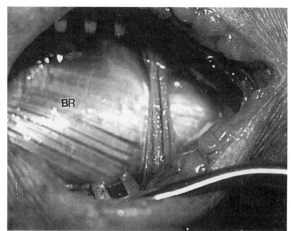

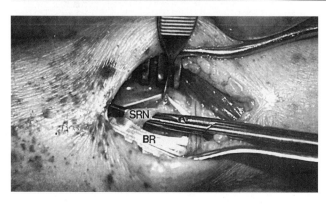

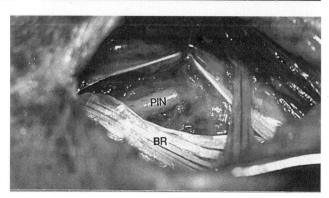

Fig. 13 These photographs show the transbrachioradialis surgical approach for treatment of radial tunnel syndrome. **Top left,** The skin incision is placed on the proximal part of the forearm, anterior to the brachioradialis. **Top right,** The fascia of the brachioradialis muscle (BR) beneath the subcutaneous layer. **Bottom left,** The superficial radial nerve (SRN) is initially located in the split brachioradialis muscle (BR). **Bottom right,** The superficial radial nerve is traced to the posterior interosseous nerve (PIN), which is deeper (BR = brachioradialis muscle).

motor palsy, with lack of extension of the long and ring fingers or other combinations, or even an isolated palsy of thumb extension.[96] Weakness of the supinator may be detected, and weakness of both power grip and wrist extension occurs.

Sensory function is intact. There may be tenderness in the radial tunnel or, occasionally, a mass may be palpable. Again, the tenderness should be compared with that of the contralateral forearm.

Diagnostic Tests Electromyography of the muscles innervated by the posterior interosseous nerve is helpful in establishing the diagnosis. Routine radiographs are nearly always normal, except when there is a history of osseous injury. A computed tomography scan or magnetic resonance image may show a mass in the radial tunnel.

Pathologic Findings The potential areas of compression are identical to those in radial tunnel syndrome. However, in addition to the compression by structures that are normally present, there are several other etiologies for motor neuropathy. These include trauma (for example, Monteggia fracture or dislocation of the radial head), inflammation (for example, a rheumatoid nodule or synovitis of the radiohumeral joint), masses (for example, a lipoma, ganglion, or fibroma), iatrogenic causes (for example, resection of the radial head or application or removal of a plate from the radius), and local injections.

Differential Diagnosis Rupture of the extensor tendons to the thumb or fingers, or both, may be confused with posterior interosseous nerve palsy. They may be differentiated by the tenodesis effect of passive flexion of the wrist: if the tendons are intact, the digits will extend. Another differentiation test is the succinylcholine test described by Doyle and associates.[97] Succinylcholine is a useful diagnostic aid for differentiation of loss of function due to nerve injury from muscle or tendon rupture. Succinylcholine, commonly used in anesthesia, paralyzes normal skeletal muscles by blocking transmission at the myoneural junction, but in denervated muscle, it produces sustained muscle contractions lasting several minutes (so-called denervation hypersensitivity). After the anesthesiologist has given succinylcholine, sustained contraction of the denervated muscle occurs and lasts for two to four minutes or longer. If the injury is caused by muscle or tendon disruption, fasciculations last only a few seconds.

Conservative Treatment The etiology of the posterior interosseous nerve palsy and the time of onset determine whether nonsurgical treatment is advisable. If the patient is seen soon after the onset of the weakness (which is unusual), then several weeks of rest with splinting may result in recovery.

Surgical Management If the weakness has been present for many months, if it follows acute trauma or a surgical procedure, or if it is progressive, then surgical exploration is indicated. The surgical approaches are the same as for radial tunnel syndrome except that the anterolateral approach is preferred, for more thorough exposure, when the site of the lesion cannot be pinpointed preoperatively. Naturally, in addition to relieving the compression by any of the five potentially compressive structures, the surgeon must remove any local masses. An osseous prominence that might cause impingement must also be corrected. If the nerve has been severed or has a neuroma in continuity, then interfascicular nerve grafting is usually indicated; direct repair is usually not feasible because of the multiple branching of the nerve at this level.

Results Decompression of the posterior interosseous nerve usually results in motor recovery if an anatomic lesion is found and the fascicles are intact. However, the surgeon and the patient must be patient, for it is not unusual for recovery of muscle function to be delayed for five to seven months. Tendon transfers are seldom indicated but are used if no recovery occurs after 12 to 18 months.

References

1. Dahlin LB, McLean WG: Effects of graded experimental compression on slow and fast axonal transport in rabbit vagus nerve. *J Neurol Sci* 1966;72:19-30.
2. Dahlin LB, Sjostrand J, McLean WG: Graded inhibition of retrograde axonal transport by compression of rabbit vagus nerve. *J Neurol Sci* 1986;76:221-230.
3. Dahlin LB, Rydevik B, McLean WG, et al: Changes in fast axonal transport during experimental nerve compresson at low pressures. *Exper Neurol* 1984;84:29-36.
4. Gelberman RH, Hergenroeder PT, Hargens AR, et al: The carpal tunnel syndrome: A study of carpal canal pressures. *J Bone Joint Surg* 1981;63A:380-383.
5. Dahlin LB, Shyu BC, Danielsen N, et al: Effect of nerve compression or ischaemia on conduction properties of myelinated and non-myelinated nerve fibres: An experimental study in the rabbit common peroneal nerve. *Acta Physiol Scand* 1989;136:97-105.
6. Fowler TJ, Ochoa J: Unmyelinated fibres in normal and compressed peripheral nerves of the baboon: A quantitative electron microscopic study. *Neuropathol Appl Neurobiol* 1975;1:247-265.
7. Gasser HS, Erlanger J: The role of fiber size in the establishment of a nerve block by pressure or cocaine. *Am J Physiol* 1929;88:581-591.
8. Berthold CH: Morphology of normal peripheral axons, in Waxman SG (ed): *Physiology and Pathobiology of Axons.* New York, NY, Raven Ress, 1978, pp 3-63.
9. Gilliatt RW: Acute compression block, in Sumner AJ (ed): *The Physiology of Peripheral Nerve Disease.* Philadelphia, PA, WB Saunders, 1980, pp 287-315.
10. Ochoa J, Fowler TJ, Gilliatt RW: Anatomical changes in peripheral nerves compressed by a pneumatic tourniquet. *J Anat* 1972;113:433-455.
11. Rydevik B, Nordberg C: Changes in nerve function and nerve fibre structure induced by acute, graded compression. *J Neurol Neurosurg Psychiatry* 1980;43:1070-1082.
12. Yamaguchi DM, Lipscomb PR, Soule EH: Carpal tunnel syndrome. *Minn Med* 1965;48:22-33.
13. Phalen GS: The carpal-tunnel syndrome: Seventeen years' experience in diagnosis and treatment of six hundred fifty-four hands. *J Bone Joint Surg* 1966;48A:211-228.
14. Szabo RM, Madison M: Carpal tunnel syndrome. *Orthop Clin North Am* 1992;23:103-109.
15. Gellman H, Chandler DR, Petrasek J, et al: Carpal tunnel syndrome in paraplegic patients. *J Bone Joint Surg* 1988;70A:517-519.
16. Waring WP III, Werner RA: Clinical management of carpal tunnel syndrome in patients with long-term sequelae of poliomyelitis. *J Hand Surg* 1989;14A:865-869.
17. Koris M, Gelberman RH, Duncan K, et al: Carpal tunnel syndrome: Evaluation of a quantitative provocational diagnostic test. *Clin Orthop* 1990;251:157-161.
18. Gellman H, Gelberman RH, Tan AM, et al: Carpal tunnel syndrome: An evaluation of the provocative diagnostic tests. *J Bone Joint Surg* 1986;68A:735-737.
19. Gelberman RH, Aronson D, Wesman MH: Carpal-tunnel syndrome: Results of a prospective trial of steroid injection and splinting. *J Bone Joint Surg* 1980;62A:1181-1184.
20. Goodman HV, Foster JB: Effect of local corticosteroid injection on median nerve conduction in carpal tunnel syndrome. *Ann Phys Med* 1962;6:287-294.
21. Green DP: Diagnostic and therapeutic value of carpal tunnel injection. *J Hand Surg* 1984;9A:850-854.
22. Ekman-Ordeberg G, Salgeback S, Ordeberg G: Carpal tunnel syndrome in pregnancy: A prospective study. *Acta Obstet Gynecol Scand* 1987;66:233-235.
23. Schmidt H-M, Lanz U: Anatomy of the median nerve in the carpal tunnel, in Gelberman RH (ed): *Operative Nerve Repair and Reconstruction.* Philadelphia, PA, JB Lippincott, 1991, vol 2, pp 889-898.
24. Taleisnik J: The palmar cutaneous branch of the median nerve and the approach to the carpal tunnel: An anatomical study. *J Bone Joint Surg* 1973;55A:1212-1217.
25. Silver MA, Gelberman RH, Gellman H, et al: Carpal tunnel syndrome: Associated abnormalities in ulnar nerve function and the effect of carpal tunnel release on these abnormalities. *J Hand Surg* 1985;10A:710-713
26. Richman JA, Gelberman RH, Rydevik BL, et al: Carpal tunnel volume determination by magnetic resonance imaging three-dimensional reconstruction. *J Hand Surg* 1987;12A:712-717.
27. Brown RA, Gelberman RH, Seiler JG III, et al: Carpal tunnel release: A prospective, randomized assessment of open and endoscopic methods. *J Bone Joint Surg* 1993;75A:1265-1275.
28. Curtis RM, Eversmann WW Jr: Internal neurolysis as an adjunct to the treatment of the carpal tunnel syndrome. *J Bone Joint Surg* 1973;55A:733-740.
29. Rhoades CE, Mowery CA, Gelberman RH: Results of internal neurolysis of the median nerve for severe carpal-tunnel syndrome. *J Bone Joint Surg* 1985;67A:253-256.
30. Gelberman RH, Pfeffer GB, Galbraith RT, et al: Results of treatment of severe carpal tunnel syndrome without internal

neurolysis of the median nerve. *J Bone Joint Surg* 1987;69A:896-903.

31. Lowry WE Jr, Follender AB: Interfascicular neurolysis in the several carpal tunnel syndrome: A prospective, randomizd, double-blind, controlled study. *Clin Orthop* 1988;227:251-254.

32. Gelberman RH: Acute carpal tunnel syndrome, in Gelberman RH (ed): *Operative Nerve Repair and Reconstruction.* Philadelphia, PA, JB Lippincott, 1991, vol 2, pp 939-948.

33. Kessler FB: Complications of the management of carpal tunnel syndrome. *Hand Clin* 1986;2:401-406.

34. Urbaniak JR: Complications of treatment of carpal tunnel syndrome, in Gelberman RH (ed): *Operative Nerve Repair and Reconstruction.* Philadelphia, PA, JB Lippincott, 1991, vol 2, pp 967-979.

35. Spinner M: Management of nerve compression lesions, in Murray JA (ed): *American Academy of Orthopaedic Surgeons Instructional Course Lectures XXXIII.* St. Louis, MO, CV Mosby, 1984, pp 498-512.

36. Purnell DC, Daly DD, Lipscomb PR: Carpal-tunnel syndrome associated with myxedema. *Arch Intern Med* 1961;108:751-756.

37. Aghasi MK, Rzetelny V, Axer A: The flexor digitorum superficialis as a cause of bilateral carpal-tunnel syndrome and trigger wrist: A case report. *J Bone Joint Surg* 1980;62A:134-135.

38. Butler B Jr, Bigley A, Bigley EC Sr: Aberrant index (first) lumbrical tendinous origin associated with carpal-tunnel syndrome: A case report. *J Bone Joint Surg* 1971;53A:160-162.

39. Das SK, Brown HG: In search of complications in carpal tunnel decompression. *Hand* 1976;8:243-249.

40. Duncan KH, Lewis RC Jr, Foreman KA, et al: Treatment of carpal tunnel syndrome by members of the American Society for Surgery of the Hand: Results of a questionnaire. *J Hand Surg* 1987;12A:384-391.

41. Harvey FJ, Bosanquet JS: Carpal tunnel syndrome caused by a simple ganglion. *Hand* 1981;13:164-166.

42. Lavey EB, Pearl RM: Patent median artery as a cause of carpal tunnel syndrome. *Ann Plast Surg* 1981;7:236-238.

43. Lourie GM, Levi LS, Toby B, et al: Distal rupture of the palmaris longus tendon and fascia as a cause of acute carpal tunnel syndrome. *J Hand Surg* 1990;15A:367-369.

44. Subin GD, Mallon WJ, Urbaniak JR: Diagnosis of ganglion in Guyon's canal by magnetic resonance imaging. *J Hand Surg* 1989;14A:640-643.

45. Touborg-Jensen A: Carpal tunnel syndrome caused by an abnormal distribution of the lumbrical muscles: Case report. *Scand J Reconstr Surg* 1970;4:72-74.

46. Grundberg AB: Carpal tunnel decompression in spite of normal electromyography. *J Hand Surg* 1983;8:348-349.

47. Richards RR, Urbaniak JR: Spontaneous retrocarpal radial artery thrombosis: A report of two cases. *J Hand Surg* 1984;9A:823-827.

48. Bassett FH III, Nunley JA: Compression of the musculocutaneous nerve at the elbow. *J Bone Joint Surg* 1982;64A:1050-1052.

49. Braidwood AS: Superficial radial neuropathy. *J Bone Joint Surg* 1975;57B:380-383.

50. Upton AR, McComas AJ: The double crush in nerve entrapment syndromes. *Lancet* 1973;2:359-362.

51. Kulick MI, Gordillo G, Javidi T, et al: Long-term analysis of patients having surgical treatment for carpal tunnel syndrome. *J Hand Surg* 1986;11A:59-66.

52. Wood MR: Hydrocortisone injections for carpal tunnel syndrome. *Hand* 1980;12:62-64.

53. Spinner M, Kaplan EB: The relationship of the ulnar nerve to the medial intermuscular septum in the arm and its clinical significance. *Hand* 1976;8:239-242.

54. Eversmann WW Jr: Complications of compression or entrapment neuropathies, in Boswick JA (ed): *Complications in Hand Surgery.* Philadelphia, PA, WB Saunders, 1986, pp 99-115.

55. Louis DS, Green TL, Noellert RC: Complications of carpal tunnel surgery. *J Neurosurg* 1985;62:352-356.

56. MacDonald RI, Lichtman DM, Hanlon JJ, et al: Complications of surgical release for carpal tunnel syndrome. *J Hand Surg* 1978;3:70-76.

57. Rietz K-A, Önne L: Analysis of sixty-five operated cases of carpal tunnel syndrome. *Acta Chir Scand* 1976;133:443-447.

58. Favero KJ, Gropper PT: Ulnar nerve laceration: A complication of carpal tunnel decompression: Case report and review of the literature. *J Hand Surg* 1987;12B:239-241.

59. Johnson RK, Shrewsbury MM: Anatomical course of the thenar branch of the median nerve: Usually in a separate tunnel through the transverse carpal ligament. *J Bone Joint Surg* 1970;52A:269-273.

60. Lanz U: Anatomical variations of the median nerve in the carpal tunnel. *J Hand Surg* 1977;2:44-53.

61. Lilly CJ, Magnell TD: Severance of the thenar branch of the median nerve as a complication of carpal tunnel release. *J Hand Surg* 1985;10A:399-402.

62. Kaplan EB: *Functional and Surgical Anatomy of the Hand,* ed 2. Philadelphia, PA, JB Lippincott, 1965.

63. Braun RM: The dynamic diagnosis of carpal tunnel syndrome and treatment by surgical release without complete transection of the transverse carpal ligament. Read at the Annual Meeting of the American Society for Surgery of the Hand, San Antonio, Texas, Sept. 10, 1987.

64. Feinstein PA: Endoscopic carpal tunnel release in a community-based series. *J Hand Surg* 1993;18A:451-454.

65. Feindel W, Stratford J: The role of the cubital tunnel in tardy ulnar palsy. *Can J Surg* 1958;1:287-300.

66. Osborne GV: The surgical treatment of tardy ulnar neuritis, in Proceedings of the British Orthopaedic Association. *J Bone Joint Surg* 1957;39B:782.

67. Apfelberg DB, Larson SJ: Dynamic anatomy of the ulnar nerve at the elbow. *Plast Reconstr Surg* 1973;51:79-81.

68. Adelaar RS, Foster WC, McDowell C: The treatment of the cubital tunnel syndrome. *J Hand Surg* 1984;9A:90-95.

69. Pechan J, Juli I: The pressure measurement in the ulnar nerve: A contribution to the pathophysiology of the cubital tunnel syndrome. *J Biomech* 1975;8:75-79.

70. Amadio PC, Beckenbaugh RD: Entrapment of the ulnar nerve by the deep flexor-pronator aponeurosis. *J Hand Surg* 1986;11A:83-87.

71. Jobe FW, Nuber G: Throwing injuries of the elbow. *Clin Sports Med* 1986;5:621-636.

72. Eaton RG, Crowe JF, Parkes JC III: Anterior transposition of the ulnar nerve using a non-compressing fasciodermal sling. *J Bone Joint Surg* 1980;62A:820-825.

73. Zemel NP, Jobe FW, Yocum LA: Submuscular transposition/ulnar nerve decompression in athletes, in Gelberman RH (ed): *Operative Nerve Repair and Reconstruction.* Philadelphia, PA, JB Lippincott, 1991, vol 2, pp 1097-1105.

74. Dellon AL: Review of treatment results for ulnar nerve entrapment at the elbow. *J Hand Surg* 1989;14A:688-700.

75. Learmonth JR: A technique for transplanting the ulnar nerve. *Surg Gynecol Obstet* 1942;75:792-793.

76. Janes PC, Mann RJ, Farnworth TK: Submuscular transposition of the ulnar nerve. *Clin Orthop* 1989;238:225-232.

77. Leffert RD: Anterior submuscular transposition of the ulnar nerves by the Learmonth technique. *J Hand Surg* 1982;7:147-155.

78. Adson AW: The surgical treatment of progressive ulnar paralysis. *Minn Med* 1918;1:455-460.

79. Kleinman WB, Bishop AT: Anterior intramuscular transposition of the ulnar nerve. *J Hand Surg* 1989;14A:972-979.

80. Curtis BF: Traumatic ulnar neuritis. Transplantation of the

nerve. *J Nerv Ment Dis* 1898;25:480-481.

81. Murphy JB: Cicatrical fixation of the ulnar nerve in its groove sequential to ancient fracture of olecranon process: Release and transference of nerve to new site: Resection of olecranon tip. *Clin JB Murphy* 1915;4:1095-1108.

82. Eaton RG: Anterior subcutaneous transposition, in Gelberman RH (ed): *Operative Nerve Repair and Reconstruction.* Philadelphia, PA, JB Lippincott, 1991, vol 2, pp 1077-1085.

83. Townsend PF, Eaton RG: Long-term follow-up of stabilized anterior subcutaneous transposition of the ulnar nerve. Read at the Annual Meeting of The American Academy of Orthopaedic Surgeons, Washington, DC, Feb 22, 1992.

84. Roles NC, Maudsley RH: Radial tunnel syndrome: Resistant tennis elbow as a nerve entrapment. *J Bone Joint Surg* 1972;54B:499-508.

85. Eversmann WW Jr: Entrapment and compression neuropathies, in Green DP (ed): *Operative Hand Surgery,* ed 3. New York, NY, Churchill Livingstone, 1993, vol 2, pp 1341-1385.

86. Hagert CG, Lundborg G, Hansen T: Entrapment of the posterior interosseous nerve. *Scand J Plast Reconstr Surg* 1977;11:205-212.

87. Lister GD: Radial tunnel syndrome, in Gelberman RH (ed): *Operative Nerve Repair and Reconstruction.* Philadelphia, PA, JB Lippincott, 1991.

88. Lister GD, Belsole RB, Kleinert HE: The radial tunnel syndrome. *J Hand Surg* 1979;4:52-59.

89. Ritts GD, Wood MB, Linscheid RL: Radial tunnel syndrome: A ten-year surgical experience. *Clin Orthop* 1987;219:201-205.

90. Spinner M: *Injuries to the Major Branches of Peripheral Nerves of the Forearm,* ed 2. Philadelphia, PA. WB Saunders, 1978, pp 147-154.

91. Frohse F, Frankel M: Die Muskeln des menschlichen Armes, in *Bardelben's Handbuch der Anatomie des Mensch.* Jena, Fisher, 1908.

92. Hirayama T, Takemitsu Y: Isolated paralysis of the descending branch of the posterior interosseous nerve: Report of a case. *J Bone Joint Surg* 1988;70A:1402-1403.

93. Spinner M: *Injuries to the Major Branches of Peripheral Nerves of the Forearm.* Philadelphia, PA, WB Saunders, 1972, p 55.

94. Henry AK: *Extensile Exposure,* ed 2. New York, NY, Churchill Livingstone, 1973, pp 100-107.

95. Steichen JB, Mulbry LW, Christensen AW: Radial tunnel syndrome: Clinical experience and results of treatment. *Orthop Trans* 1988;12:4.

96. Agnew DH: Bursal tumour producing loss of power of forearm [abstract]. *Am J Med Sci* 1863;46:404-405.

97. Doyle JR, Semenza J, Gilling B: The effect of succinylcholine on denervated skeletal muscle. *J Hand Surg* 1981;6:40-42.

Office Treatment of Elbow Injuries in the Athlete

Walton W. Curl, MD

Introduction

Athletes of all ages are prone to elbow injuries. These injuries can be as varied as the young Little League player with a medial epicondyle avulsion, the gymnast with osteochondritis dissecans of the elbow, or the pitcher with a chronic overload syndrome of the arm. Perhaps the most common elbow injury seen in athletes is lateral epicondylitis, or "tennis elbow."

Slocum[1] has classified elbow injuries in baseball players into three categories: (1) medial tension overload injuries, including medial epicondylitis and medial epicondyle fractures; (2) lateral compression injuries, such as osteochondritis dissecans of the capitellum; and (3) extensor overload injuries, primarily involving the posterior aspect of the elbow. These categories are useful in describing most of the other common injuries that occur in athletes.

Lateral Epicondylitis

Lateral epicondylitis is generally diagnosed by eliciting tenderness over the lateral epicondyle. The athlete often complains of pain on attempting to grip with the wrist and on pronating and supinating. Additionally, there is pain at the elbow with resisted extension. The neurologic examination should be normal. Magnetic resonance imaging (MRI) is helpful in identifying areas of inflammation in lateral epicondylitis (Fig. 1).

In the treatment of lateral epicondylitis, anti-inflammatory medications and counterforce bracing are the mainstays of treatment. Anti-inflammatories are generally given orally for approximately two to three weeks, depending on the type prescribed. Caution should be exercised in prescribing these medications because of the side effects—gastrointestinal upset or increased bleeding problems. Corticosteroid injections can be useful. Up to three injections are considered appropriate; after that one should be cautious in the amount of corticosteroid injections that are given. Counterforce bracing, or "tennis elbow bands," are quite effective in reducing symptoms and allowing individuals to continue normal activity (Fig. 2). These Velcro straps are placed approximately 2 to 3 cm distal to the epicondyle over the bulk of the extensor muscle group to act as a counterforce on the action of the extensor muscles as they pull on the lateral epicondyle.

Abnormal biomechanics can also play a role in the onset of lateral epicondylitis. In tennis, for example,

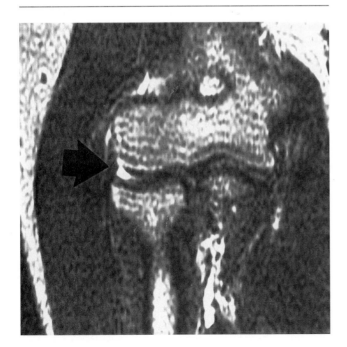

Fig. 1 MRI scan of the elbow, demonstrating increased signal intensity in the extensor communis tendon over the lateral epicondyle.

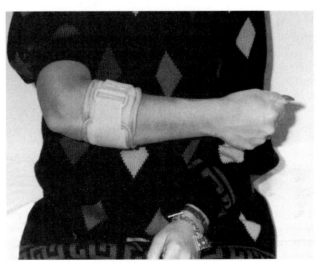

Fig. 2 Tennis elbow band placed firmly over the mid forearm to apply pressure or counterforce on the extensor tendon.

hitting off the back leg and hurrying a backhand, or hitting the ball with the wrist not locked can put an undue overload stress on the extensor mechanism and can lead to epicondylitis (Fig. 3). The tennis swing should be performed with the wrist locked, forming an "L" with the racquet and the forearm while hitting the ball (Fig. 4). The newer lighter graphite racquets with

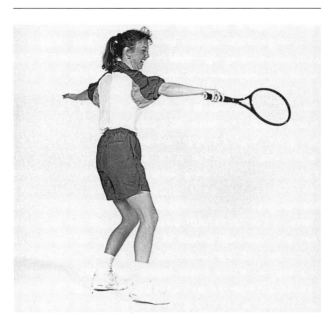

Fig. 3 Tennis player hitting off the back leg with the tennis racket dropped down and the wrist not locked.

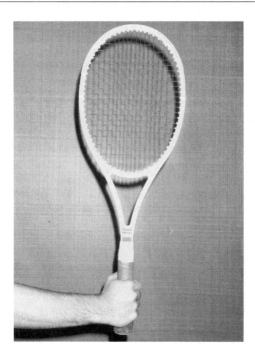

Fig. 4 When hitting the ball, the tennis racquet should form an "L" with the forearm.

a large "sweet" spot often can help unload the lateral epicondyle. Hitting with both hands, getting the weight to the front foot, and stroking the ball low instead of having to reach with the elbow more extended also are useful in decreasing the load on the elbow. The string tension also should be reduced to between 50 and 55 lb to help increase the amount of shock absorbed by the racquet. The size of the grip can be a contributing factor in lateral epicondylitis. The grip should be comfortable, but not too small. The distance from the proximal palmar crease to the end of the ring finger is generally considered the appropriate size for the racquet grip (Fig. 5).

Surgical intervention is a last resort. When lateral epicondylitis has not responded to conservative measures after six to eight months, or if it significantly alters a patient's lifestyle, surgery can be quite useful. Leach and Miller[2] point out that the primary problem in lateral epicondylitis is usually degeneration of the origin of the extensor carpi radialis brevis. Several procedures have been described in the literature. Perhaps one of the more successful of the procedures is to make an incision over the lateral epicondyle, identify the extensor mechanism at its origin on the lateral epicondyle, subperiosteally elevate it away from the bone, and then debride the extensor carpi radialis brevis tendon origin. Following this debridement, the extensor radialis brevis longus tendon is loosely reattached to its periosteal origin and the arm is splinted for ten days, increasing activities as tolerated and starting on an elbow rehabilitation program. Andrews and Wilk[3] have described an elbow rehabilitation program that has proven to be quite effective and can provide a therapist with a basic outline for designing a rehabilitation program for elbow injuries.

Medial Tension Overload

Medial tension overload syndromes generally occur during the acceleration phase of throwing. A valgus

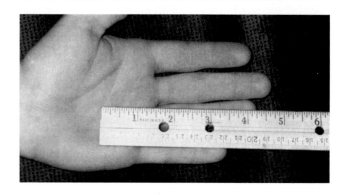

Fig. 5 Appropriate grip is measured as the distance from the proximal palmar crease to the tip of the ring finger.

load on the elbow is produced during throwing, causing increased tensile forces across the medial epicondyle. This becomes a problem when the elbow is subjected to prolonged valgus overload, particularly in repetitive sports such as tennis or baseball pitching. Medial tension overload can also occur in a sport such as golf when the club hits the ground before the ball and causes an undue valgus stress on the elbow (Fig. 6).

Medial Epicondylitis

Medial epicondylitis, inflammation of the origin of the wrist flexors at the elbow, is characterized by ten-

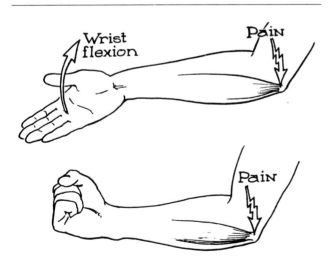

Fig. 6 Hitting the ground before the ball can place an undue stress on the medial aspect of the elbow.

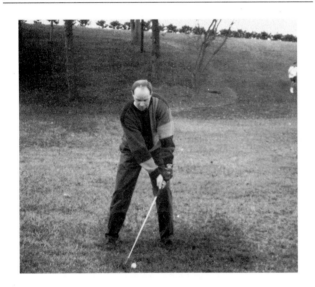

Fig. 7 Tenderness over the medial epicondyle and medial pain on forced flexion of the wrist are common clinical signs of medial epicondylitis.

derness over the medial epicondyle and medial pain on forced flexion of the wrist (Fig. 7). Radiographs are generally negative, but MRI may show an increased signal in the flexor tendon origin.

The treatment for medial epicondylitis is similar to that used for lateral epicondylitis. Anti-inflammatories and counterforce bracing are the mainstays of treatment. With this treatment, the symptoms of tendinitis generally can be relieved, allowing the individual to participate in sports. If the symptoms become chronic or recur, poor biomechanics may be contributing to the medial epicondylitis. The athlete's throwing mechanism, racquet swing, or golf swing may need to be analyzed. Corticosteroid injections into the origin of the flexor tendons on the medial epicondyle may be indicated. Because of the close proximity of the ulnar nerve, the local anesthetic that is used with the corticosteroid may cause a temporary paralysis of the ulnar nerve. Therefore, these injections should be performed judiciously. In chronic inflammatory conditions, multiple corticosteroid injections must be used with caution. Generally, up to three corticosteroid injections are considered therapeutic. If a good response is not obtained, further injections are usually counterproductive.

As a last resort, surgical intervention may be necessary. The surgery is accomplished through a medial incision and the flexor origin is identified and dissected free of the medial epicondyle. Occasionally, an area of inflammation may be seen; most of the time there are no obvious degenerative changes in the tendon. Releasing the tendon and scraping the tendon insertion on the epicondyle can be helpful in trying to induce a healing response. The flexor group is then loosely reattached to the periosteum of the bone. The arm is splinted in flexion with the wrist at neutral for approximately ten days, after which range of motion and strengthening exercises are started.

Medial Epicondyle Fractures

Medial epicondyle fractures are most common in children and adolescents and are generally considered epiphyseal avulsion injuries. The clinical signs generally involve pain, swelling, and, possibly, ecchymosis about the medial epicondyle. These fractures occur commonly in Little League pitchers, who, after throwing for a while, feel a sharp pain in the elbow. A valgus stress test performed with the elbow at 20° can sometimes elicit medial instability (Fig. 8). Radiographs can be helpful in distinguishing between a stable and an unstable elbow fracture. The gravity stress radiograph is perhaps the best test to determine elbow instability. This radiograph is taken with the patient supine, the elbow flexed 20°, and the thumb pointed down (Fig. 9). An anteroposterior radiograph of the elbow is

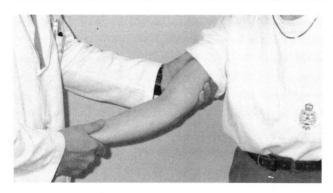

Fig. 8 The valgus stress test is performed with the elbow at 20° while stabilizing the upper arm. A valgus stress is placed across the medial aspect of the elbow to determine instability.

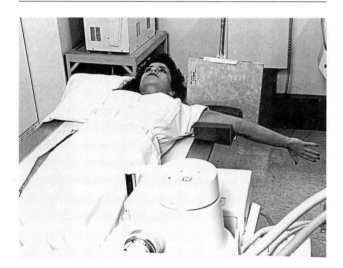

Fig. 9 Gravity stress radiographs of the elbow are taken with patient supine and the thumb pointed down, which allows gravity to open the medial side of the elbow.

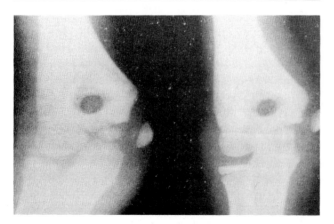

Fig. 10 Radiograph demonstrating a medial avulsion fracture, which is more displaced with the gravity stress radiograph.

taken to determine the amount of opening that occurs with gravity (Fig. 10). In larger athletes it may be necessary to add 1 to 2 lb of weight on the arm to increase the amount of stress and replicate the pathology.

In considering treatment of medial epicondyle fractures, it is generally agreed that a nondisplaced epicondyle fracture that does not open up on valgus stress testing or during a gravity stress radiograph can be splinted for three weeks and then started on range of motion and strengthening exercises, progressing through a strengthening program as the symptoms allow (Fig. 11). There is debate about how much displacement is acceptable before surgical intervention must be undertaken. Most authors agree that displacement between 0.5 and 1 cm is acceptable if the elbow is otherwise stable.[4] Generally, any displacement over 1 cm is significant and surgical intervention should be considered (Fig. 12). If surgery is indicated, a medial approach is used, the epicondyle is reduced under direct vision, and two Kirschner wires (K-wires) are placed across the fracture site (Fig. 13). The elbow is splinted in flexion for three to four weeks to allow healing. If, in addition to the avulsion fracture, there is ligamentous disruption, a ligamentous repair may be performed at the same time.

Lateral Compression Injuries

Lateral compression injuries of the elbow also occur during the acceleration phase. They occur primarily when compressive forces between the radial head and capitellum are increased during a valgus moment on the arm.

Osteochondritis Dissecans

Osteochondritis dissecans occurs in athletes who constantly overload and hyperextend the elbow. Gymnasts who are constantly loading their elbows on the balance beam and high bars are particularly susceptible.[5] Clinical symptoms of osteochondritis dissecans are locking, giving way, and crepitus on range of motion. Often radiographs will reveal a loose body (Fig. 14) within the joint and radiographic confirmation of osteochondritis dissecans also can be demonstrated (Fig. 15). MRI is often helpful in suspicious cases where the radiographs are negative. Treatment of osteochondritis dissecans is conservative unless there are indeed loose bodies within the joint or mechanical problems. Conservative treatment for acute exacerbations generally consists of splinting the elbow for three to four days, anti-inflammatory medications, and the application of heat. If mechanical symptoms occur and persist, then arthroscopic intervention can be useful in debriding loose bodies. If a nondisplaced fragment is present, the area may be drilled to encourage revascularization of the fragment.

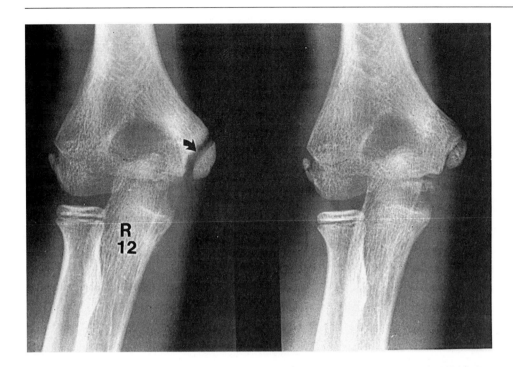

Fig. 11 Comparative radiographs demonstrating a minimally displaced medial epicondyle avulsion fracture.

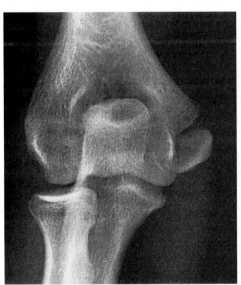 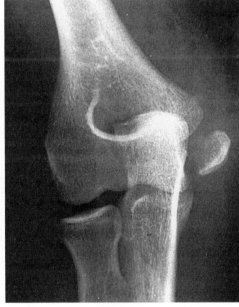

Fig. 12 **Left,** A normal medial epicondyle. **Right,** A medial epicondyle on the opposite elbow, which is displaced greater than 1 cm.

Extensor Overload

Extensor overload generally happens after the acceleration phase and occurs when compression and shear forces are applied to the posterior aspect of the elbow. These are frequently seen as chronic injuries in pitchers.[6] Clinical symptoms generally are pain on the posterior aspect of the elbow, especially with extension of the elbow, crepitus on range of motion, swelling, and occasional locking. Radiographs often show osteophyte formation (Fig. 16) in the olecranon fossa and on the proximal portion of the olecranon.[7]

Treatment is generally conservative, with heat and anti-inflammatories; however, if loss of motion or locking occurs, surgical intervention can be useful to debride the osteophytes on the tip of the olecranon and the olecranon fossa (Fig. 17).

Rehabilitation of Elbow Injuries

Rehabilitation of elbow injuries involves symptomatic treatment with anti-inflammatory medications, followed by gentle range of motion exercises and light

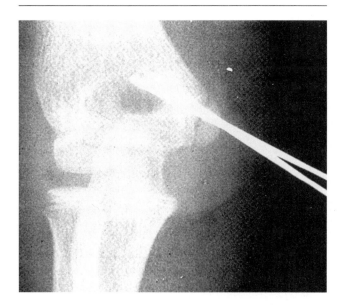

Fig. 13   Radiograph demonstrating fixation of medial epicondyle fracture with two K-wires.

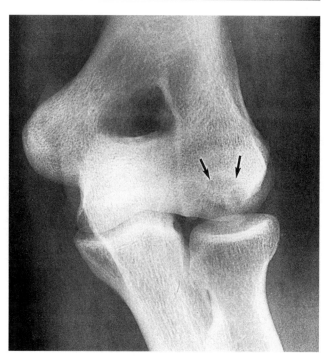

Fig. 15   Radiograph demonstrating osteochondritis dissecans of capitellum.

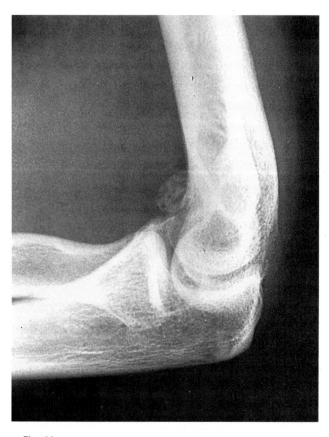

Fig. 14   Osteochondritis dissecans of the capitellum with loose body in anterior aspect of joint.

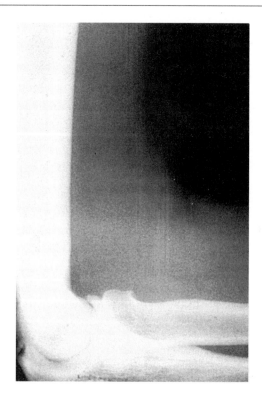

Fig. 16   Radiograph demonstrating osteophyte formation in olecranon fossa in the proximal portion of the olecranon.

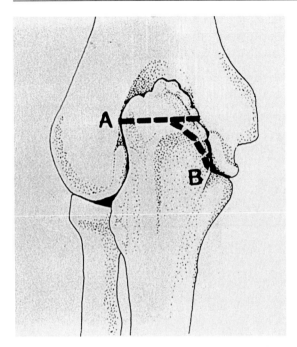

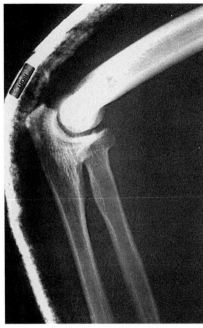

Fig. 17 **Left**, A drawing, showing posterior osteophytes to be surgically debrided. (A = line of resection of proximal ulnar osteophytes; B = line of resection of proximal medial osteophytes.) **Right**, A postoperative radiograph demonstrating excision of the posterior aspect of the olecranon process.

strengthening exercises. Deep friction massage can often be useful on medial or lateral epicondylitis. Often individuals with chronic elbow problems have a very subtle loss of grip strength, and grip strengthening exercises using putty or a rubber ball can be helpful. Additionally, stretching exercises are quite important to stretch out the extensor and flexor mechanisms and decrease overloading during exercise.

References

1. Slocum DB: Classification of elbow injuries from baseball pitching. *Tex Med* 1968;64:48-53.

2. Leach RE, Miller JK: Lateral and medial epicondylitis of the elbow. *Clin Sports Med* 1987;6:259-272.

3. Andrews JR, Wilk KE, Arrigo CA, et al: *Preventive and Rehabilitative Exercises for the Shoulder and Elbow.* Birmingham, AL, American Sports Medicine Institute, 1993.

4. Woods GW, Tullos HS: Elbow instability and medial epicondyle fractures. *Am J Sports Med* 1977;5:23-30.

5. Jackson DW, Silvino N, Reiman P: Osteochondritis in the female gymnast's elbow. *Arthroscopy* 1989;5:129-136.

6. Wilson FD, Andrews JR, Blackburn TA, et al: Valgus extension overload in the pitching elbow. *Am J Sports Med* 1983;11:83-88.

7. Andrews JR, Craven WM: Lesions of the posterior compartment of the elbow. *Clin Sports Med* 1991;10:637-652.

Knee

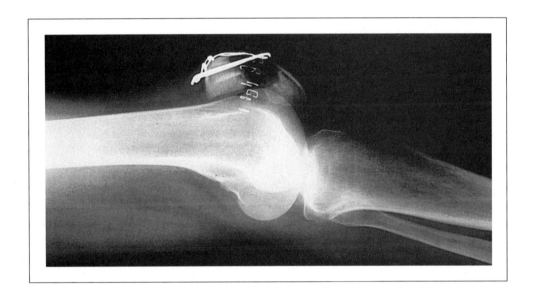

Meniscus Repair: Basic Science, Indications for Repair, and Open Repair

Kenneth E. DeHaven, MD

Steven Paul Arnoczky, DVM

Meniscal repair is not a new concept; the first known repair was performed more than a century ago by Annandale in Edinburgh, Scotland.[1] Despite this report, this procedure attracted little or no attention, and clinical management was directed toward excision, because the meniscus was believed to be of little importance to knee function and to be incapable of healing. Classic laboratory research by King[2] in the 1930s documented that meniscal lesions that communicate with the peripheral blood supply do indeed heal, but this report also went virtually unnoticed, possibly because of the general acceptance at that time of total meniscectomy for the treatment of meniscal tears. Despite Fairbank's[3] warning, in 1948, that degenerative changes can follow meniscectomy, it was not until several studies[4-8] in the 1960s and 1970s more completely documented the disappointing long-term results following meniscectomy that this approach began to be seriously questioned. During the same period, several laboratory studies helped to clarify the functional importance of the menisci in force transmission,[9-17] stability,[18-25] and shock absorption.[26-29] These factors have collectively led to the emergence of a more conservative clinical approach to the management of meniscal tears over the past two decades. Appropriate treatment now may include leaving certain tears alone; partial meniscectomy; and, in selected patients, meniscal repair. This chapter summarizes current basic-science information, the indications for repair, both open and arthroscopic repair techniques, and the results of meniscal repair.

Basic Science of the Meniscus

The menisci are C-shaped disks of fibrocartilage interposed between the condyles of the femur and tibia. Although they were once described as the functionless remains of leg muscle,[30] it has been realized that the menisci are integral components in the complex biomechanics of the knee joint.[31,32] This realization has resulted in a renewed interest in the basic science of the meniscus in terms of its structure, physiology, and function.

Gross Anatomy

The menisci of the knee joints serve as extensions of the tibia to deepen the articular surfaces in the region of the tibial plateau and, thus, to better accommodate the condyles of the femur. The peripheral border of each meniscus is thick and convex and is attached to the inside of the joint capsule; the opposite border tapers to a thin, free edge.[33] The proximal surfaces of the menisci are concave and are in contact with the condyles of the femur; the distal surfaces are flat and rest on the head of the tibia (Fig. 1).

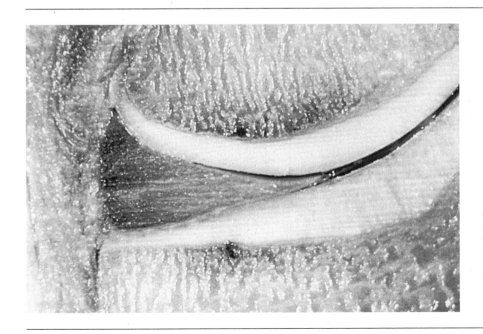

Fig. 1 Frontal section of the medial compartment of a knee, showing the articulation of the menisci with the condyles of the femur and tibia. (Reproduced with permission from Warren R, Arnoczky SP, Wickiewicz TL: Anatomy of the knee, in Nicholas JA, Hershman EB (eds): *The Lower Extremity and Spine in Sports Medicine*, St. Louis, MO, CV Mosby, 1986, p 686.)

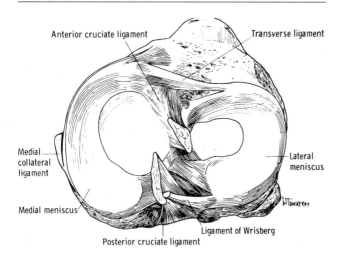

Fig. 2   Drawing of a tibial plateau, showing the shape and attachments of the medial and lateral menisci. (Reproduced with permission from Warren R, Arnoczky SP, Wickiewicz TL: Anatomy of the knee, in Nicholas JA, Hershman EB (eds): *The Lower Extremity and Spine in Sports Medicine*, St. Louis, MO, CV Mosby, 1986, p 687.)

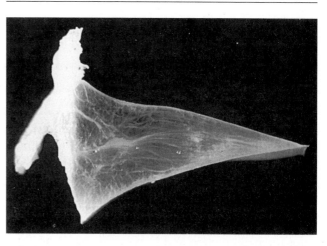

Fig. 3   Cross section of a lateral meniscus, showing the radial orientation of fibrous ties within the substance of the meniscus. (Reproduced with permission from Arnoczky SP, Torzilli PA: The biology of cartilage, in Hunter LY, Funk FJ Jr (eds): *Rehabilitation of the Injured Knee*. St. Louis, MO, CV Mosby, 1984, p 189.)

The medial meniscus is somewhat semicircular. It is approximately 3.5 cm long and is considerably wider posteriorly than it is anteriorly.[33] The anterior horn of the medial meniscus is attached to the tibial plateau in the area of the anterior intercondylar fossa, in front of the anterior cruciate ligament (Fig. 2). The posterior fibers of the anterior horn attachment merge with the transverse ligament, which connects the anterior horns of the medial and lateral menisci. The posterior horn of the medial meniscus is firmly attached to the posterior intercondylar fossa of the tibia between the attachments of the lateral meniscus and the posterior cruciate ligament. The periphery of the medial meniscus is attached to the joint capsule throughout its length. The tibial portion of the capsular attachment is often referred to as the coronary ligament. At its mid-point, the medial meniscus is more firmly attached to the femur and tibia through a thickening in the joint capsule known as the deep medial collateral ligament.

The lateral meniscus is almost circular, and it covers a larger portion of the articular surface of the tibia than does the medial meniscus; it is approximately the same width from front to back (Fig. 2). The anterior horn of the lateral meniscus is attached to the tibia, in front of the intercondylar eminence and behind the anterior extent of the attachment of the anterior cruciate ligament. The posterior horn of the lateral meniscus is attached behind the intercondylar eminence of the tibia, in front of the posterior end of the medial meniscus. While there is no attachment of the lateral meniscus to the fibular collateral ligament, there is a loose peripheral attachment to the joint capsule except in the region of the popliteus tendon.[33]

Several ligaments run from the posterior horn of the lateral meniscus to the medial femoral condyle, either just in front of or behind the origin of the posterior cruciate ligament. These are known as the anterior meniscofemoral ligament (the ligament of Humphry) and the posterior meniscofemoral ligament (the ligament of Wrisberg).[34]

Ultrastructure and Biochemistry

Histologically, the meniscus is fibrocartilaginous tissue composed, primarily, of an interlacing network of collagen fibers interposed with cells. The extracellular matrix consists of proteoglycan molecules as well as glycoproteins.

The extracellular matrix of the meniscus is composed primarily of collagen (60% to 70% of the dry weight).[35,36] It is mainly (90%) type-I collagen, although types II, III, V, and VI have been identified within the meniscus.[35,36] The circumferential orientation of these collagen fibers appears to be directly related to the function of the meniscus. In a classic study of the orientation of the collagen fibers within the menisci, it was noted that, although the principal orientation of the collagen fibers is circumferential, a few small, radially disposed fibers appear on both the femoral and the tibial surfaces of the menisci as well as within the substance of the tissue.[12] It has been theorized that these radial fibers provide structural rigidity and help to resist longitudinal splitting of the menisci, which could result from undue compression (Fig. 3).

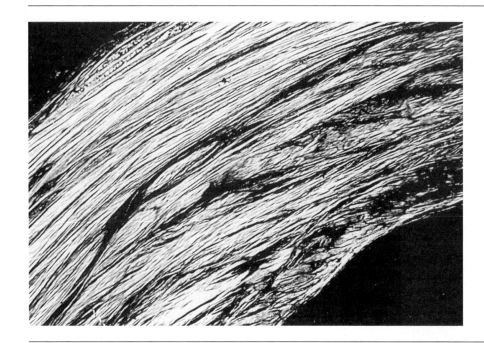

Fig. 4 Photomicrograph of a polarized longitudinal section of a medial meniscus, showing the circumferential orientation of the collagen fibers (hematoxylin and eosin, x 10).

Subsequent light and electron microscopic examinations of the menisci revealed three different collagen-framework layers: a superficial layer composed of a network of fine fibrils woven into a mesh-like matrix; a surface layer just beneath the superficial layer composed, in part, of irregularly aligned collagen bundles; and a middle layer in which the collagen fibers are larger and coarser and are oriented in a parallel, circumferential direction (Fig. 4).[37,38] It is this middle layer that allows the meniscus to resist tensile forces and to function as a transmitter of load across the knee joint.

Function

The function of the menisci has been inferred clinically from the degenerative changes that accompany their removal. Fairbank[3] described radiographic changes following meniscectomy that included narrowing of the joint space, flattening of the femoral condyle, and the formation of osteophytes (Fig. 5). These changes were attributed to the loss of the weight-bearing function of the meniscus. More sophisticated biomechanical studies have demonstrated that at least 50% of the compressive load of the knee joint is transmitted through the meniscus in extension and that approximately 85% of the load is transmitted in 90° of flexion.[9,39] In the meniscectomized knee, the contact area is reduced approximately 50%.[9,39] This greatly increases the load per unit area and results in damage and degeneration of the articular cartilage (Fig. 6). Partial meniscectomy has also been shown to increase contact pressures greatly.[40] In an experimental

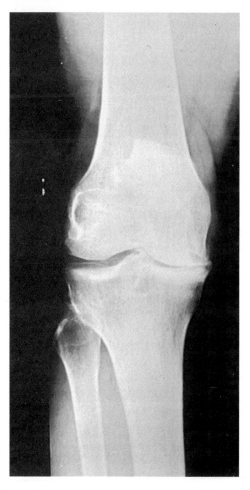

Fig. 5 Radiograph of a knee, showing the degenerative changes within the medial compartment of the joint secondary to meniscectomy. (Reproduced with permission from Arnoczky SP, Cooper DE: Meniscal repair, in Goldberg VM (ed): *Controversies of Total Knee Arthroplasty.* New York, NY, Raven Press, 1991, p 292.)

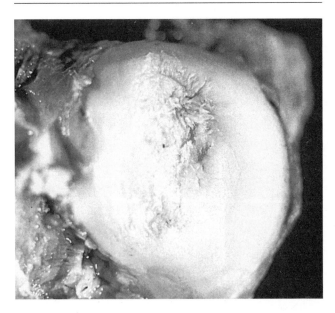

Fig. 6 Specimen of the lateral tibial plateau of a knee, showing the degeneration of the articular cartilage resulting from an absent lateral meniscus. (Reproduced with permission from Arnoczky SP, Cooper DE: Meniscal repair, in Goldberg VM (ed): *Controversies of Total Knee Arthroplasty.* New York, NY, Raven Press, 1991, p 292.)

study, resection of as little as 15% to 34% of the meniscus increased contact pressures by more than 350%.[41] Thus, even partial meniscectomy does not appear to be a benign procedure.[4,28,42]

Another proposed function of the meniscus is shock absorption. An examination of the compressive load-deformation response of normal and meniscectomized knees has suggested that the viscoelastic menisci may function to attenuate the intermittent shock waves generated by impulse-loading of the knee during gait.[29] Studies have shown that the shock-absorbing capacity of normal knees is about 20% higher than that of knees that have been treated with a meniscectomy.[29] Since the inability of a joint system to absorb shock has been implicated in the development of osteoarthrosis,[41] the meniscus appears to play an important role in the maintenance of the health of the knee joint.

In addition to their role in load transmission and shock absorption, the menisci are thought to contribute to knee-joint stability. While meniscectomy alone may not seriously decrease joint stability, studies have shown that performance of the procedure in association with insufficiency of the anterior cruciate ligament increases the anterior laxity of the knee.[20]

Because the menisci serve to increase the congruity between the condyles of the femur and the tibia, they contribute to overall joint conformity. It has been suggested that this function is also synergistic with the lubrication of the articular surfaces of the joint.[31]

Although this hypothesis has never been proved, it suggests another important function of the menisci.

Finally, it has been suggested that the menisci are proprioceptive structures providing a feedback mechanism for joint-position sense. This has been inferred from the observation of type-I and type-II nerve-endings in the anterior and posterior horns of the menisci.[43,44]

In summary, the proposed functions of the menisci include load-bearing, shock absorption, provision of joint stability, lubrication, and proprioception. Loss of the meniscus, in part or in total, greatly alters these functions and predisposes the knee joint to degenerative changes.

Vascular Anatomy

The menisci of the knee are relatively avascular structures; the limited peripheral blood supply originates predominantly from the lateral and medial geniculate arteries (both inferior and superior).[45] Branches from these vessels give rise to a perimeniscal capillary plexus within the synovial and capsular tissues of the knee joint. This plexus is an arborizing network of vessels that supplies the peripheral border of the meniscus throughout its attachment to the joint capsule (Fig. 7).[45] These perimeniscal vessels are oriented in a predominantly circumferential pattern, with radial branches directed toward the center of the joint. Anatomic studies have shown that the degree of vascular penetration is 10% to 30% of the width of the medial meniscus and 10% to 25% of the width of the lateral meniscus.[45]

The middle geniculate artery, along with a few terminal branches of the medial and lateral geniculate arteries, also supplies vessels to the meniscus through the vascular synovial covering of the anterior and posterior horn attachments. These synovial vessels penetrate the horn attachments and give rise to endoligamentous vessels that enter the meniscal horns for a short distance and end in terminal capillary loops. A small reflection of vascular synovial tissue is also present throughout the peripheral attachment of the medial and lateral menisci on both the femoral and the tibial articular surfaces. (An exception is the posterolateral portion of the lateral meniscus adjacent to the area of the popliteus tendon.) This synovial fringe extends for a short distance (1 to 3 mm) over the articular surfaces of the menisci and contains small, terminally looped vessels. While this vascular synovial tissue adheres intimately to the articular surfaces of the menisci, it does not contribute vessels into the meniscal tissue.[46]

Healing

Experimental studies of the vascular response of the meniscus to injury have demonstrated that the peripheral meniscal blood supply is capable of producing a

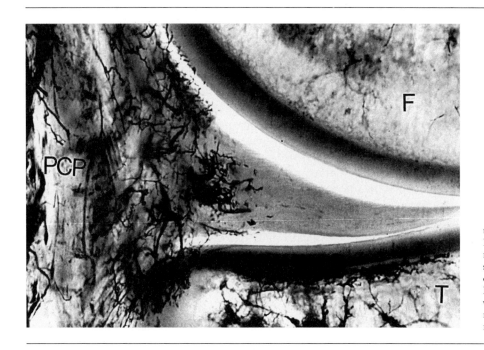

Fig. 7 Frontal section (5 mm thick) of the medial compartment of the knee. Branching radial vessels from the perimeniscal capillary plexus (PCP) can be seen penetrating the peripheral border of the medial meniscus (Spaltholz, x 3). F = femur and T = tibia. (Reproduced with permission from Arnoczky SP, Warren RF: Microvasculature of the human meniscus. *Am J Sports Med* 1982;10:91.)

reparative response (exudation, organization, vascularization, cellular proliferation, and remodeling) similar to that observed in other connective tissues.[2,46,47] Following injury within the peripheral vascular zone of the meniscus, there is formation of a fibrin clot that is rich in inflammatory cells. Vessels from the perimeniscal capillary plexus proliferate into this fibrin scaffold and are accompanied by the proliferation of undifferentiated mesenchymal cells. Eventually, the lesion is filled with a cellular, fibrovascular scar tissue that glues the wound edges together and appears continuous with normal adjacent meniscal fibrocartilage.[46] Vessels from the perimeniscal capillary plexus and a proliferative vascular pannus from the synovial fringe penetrate the fibrous scar to support this healing response. Experimental studies have shown that lesions within the vascular portion of the meniscus are completely healed by a fibrovascular scar by ten weeks (Fig. 8).[46,47]

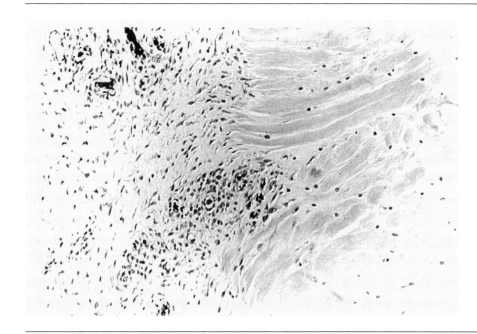

Fig. 8 Photomicrograph of a healing meniscus at the junction of the fibrovascular scar and the normal adjacent meniscal tissue (hematoxylin and eosin, x 100).

Modulation of this scar tissue into normal-appearing fibrocartilage, however, requires several months. The strength of this repair tissue as a function of time has not been delineated, and further study is needed to document its material properties.

The ability of meniscal lesions to heal has provided the rationale for the repair of peripheral meniscal injuries, and several reports[48-50] have demonstrated excellent results following primary repair of these injuries. Postoperative examination of these peripheral repairs has revealed a process of repair similar to that noted in experimental models.[51]

In the examination of injured menisci for potential repair, lesions are often classified by the location of the tear relative to the blood supply of the meniscus and by the vascular appearance of the peripheral and central surfaces of the tear. The so-called red-red tear (peripheral capsular detachment) has a functional blood supply on the capsular and meniscal sides of the lesion and obviously has the best prognosis for healing. The red-white tear (in the meniscal rim through the peripheral vascular zone) has an active peripheral blood supply, while the central (inner) surface of the lesion is devoid of functioning vessels. Theoretically, this lesion should have sufficient vascularity to heal by the aforementioned fibrovascular proliferation. The white-white tear (completely in the avascular zone) is without a blood supply and theoretically cannot heal.

While meniscal repair has generally been limited to the peripheral vascular area of the meniscus (red-red and red-white tears), many lesions occur in the central, avascular portion of the meniscus (white-white tears). Experimental and clinical observations have shown that these lesions are incapable of healing and have thereby provided the rationale for partial meniscectomy. In an effort to extend the level of the repair into these avascular areas, techniques that provide vascularity to white-white tears have been developed. These techniques include vascular access channels[46] and synovial abrasion.[51]

The concept of vascular access channels stems from the fact that lesions connected to the peripheral vascularity of the meniscus heal by the aforementioned process. Experimental studies have shown that connection of a lesion in the avascular portion of the meniscus to the peripheral blood supply via a vascular access channel can result in healing of the lesion. However, because the creation of a large enough access channel may disrupt the normal peripheral architecture of the meniscus, other methods for the stimulation of vascular ingrowth have been proposed.[51] The technique of synovial abrasion involves stimulation of the synovial fringe on both the femoral and the tibial surfaces of the meniscus. This stimulation is intended to produce a vascular pannus that will migrate into the lesion and, it is hoped, support a reparative response. An experimental study has demonstrated that, in addition to the described methods for provision of vascular access, an exogenous fibrin clot placed in a stable lesion in the avascular portion of the meniscus can support a reparative response similar to that seen in the vascular area.[52] The clot provides a potent chemotactic and mitogenic stimulus as well as a scaffold on which the cellular response is supported. This technique may allow the repair of avascular lesions anywhere in the meniscus or optimize the repair of lesions in areas of marginal vascularity. Clinical studies are currently under way to determine the applicability of this repair technique.

On the basis of these basic-science investigations, surgical repair has been widely accepted as the treatment of choice for certain meniscal lesions. This acceptance has led to the development of a number of surgical techniques with which to accomplish this goal.

Indications for Repair Versus Excision

The choice between repair and excision of a specific meniscal lesion is simplified by separation of the lesions that are definitely repairable from those that are questionably repairable. Tears known to be definitely repairable are traumatic, are within the vascular zone of the meniscus, and have caused minimum damage to the meniscal body fragment. These are most commonly vertical-longitudinal, peripheral, or nearly peripheral tears of 1 cm in length or longer.

Tears that should be considered questionably suitable for repair are those in the avascular zone or in an area where the vascularity is in doubt. When repair of such tears is attempted, it is important to add healing-enhancement techniques, such as rasping of the superior and inferior synovial fringes and the insertion of a fibrin clot. Tears that are not suitable for repair include those involving moderate or severe damage of the meniscus and complete radial tears. Even if successful repair and healing of those tears could be achieved, there is no evidence that the menisci would be capable of biomechanical function.

Preoperative information can alert both the surgeon and the patient that a meniscal tear is potentially repairable. Patients with a repairable meniscus are typically young (12 to 45 years old, with the average age being 21 years old)[49] and active (approximately 80% have an acute or chronic tear of the anterior cruciate ligament). Both medial and lateral menisci can be suitable for repair; over the years, the repair ratio of one of us (KD) has been three medial to two lateral. Preoperative diagnostic studies can also be helpful. Double-contrast arthrography is useful for the assessment of chronic lesions involving the medial meniscus. A vertical tear near the meniscosynovial junction with minimum staining of the meniscus indicates a high suitability for repair. However, extensive staining of the meniscus probably indicates that damage is severe and that the meniscus would most likely not be suitable for repair. More recently, the resolution and reliability of magnetic resonance imaging have improved, and, where available, this modality has largely supplanted arthrography for the evaluation of meniscal tears. When clearly positive, magnetic resonance imaging studies are almost always reliable, but many false-negative findings continue to be encountered, particularly regarding tears of the meniscosynovial junction.

Regardless of the amount of preoperative information that indicates that a meniscal tear is repairable, the final decision is made on the basis of arthroscopic assessment. This requires careful evaluation with use of a probe from anterior approaches to determine the exact type, location, and extent of the tear as well as the degree of damage to the meniscus. Even in tight knees, it is possible to visualize the inferior surfaces of both the medial and the lateral menisci out to the meniscosynovial junction. It is also usually (but not always) possible to see the superior surface of the lateral meniscus all of the way to the meniscosynovial junction from the front. However, it is usually not possible to evaluate the superior surface of the medial meniscus all of the way to the meniscosynovial junction, from an anterior approach, except in unusually lax knees. Therefore, it is recommended that posterior visualization be carried out when necessary for the lateral meniscus and routinely for the medial meniscus, either by placement of an arthroscope, angled 70°, through the intercondylar notch and into the posteromedial or posterolateral compartment, or by viewing through a posterior portal.

The other critical step in the arthroscopic determination of repairability is the assessment of vascularity at the site of the tear. The pneumatic tourniquet should not be inflated during the arthroscopic examination, because the presence of bleeding at the site of the tear is a crucial factor. In subacute and chronic lesions, the presence of vascular granulation tissue at the site of the tear is also indicative of vascularity. It is important to note, however, that the absence of observable bleeding at the site of the tear should not rule out the possibility of repair because the distention pressure of the arthroscopic irrigation-fluid system can be sufficient to close down the small capillary circulation. Under these circumstances, when bleeding or vascularity is not seen, a clinical judgment regarding whether or not to perform a repair must be based on the location of the tear relative to the meniscosynovial junction. Vascular injection studies[46] have indicated that a tear within 3 mm of the meniscosynovial junction is considered to be within the vascular zone of the meniscus, even when no bleeding is observed. If the tear is 5 mm or more from the meniscosynovial junction, it can be consid-

ered to be avascular unless there is direct evidence of vascularity (active bleeding or granulation tissue). The vascularity of tears 3 to 5 mm from the meniscosynovial junction is variable, and if repair is elected, enhancement of healing with insertion of a fibrin clot should be considered.

Open Meniscal Repair

Indications

The primary indication for open meniscal repair is a peripheral or nearly peripheral tear (within 1 to 2 mm of the meniscosynovial junction) of the posterior one-third of the medial or lateral meniscus. The length of the tear is also an important factor, because short tears (less than 7 mm) usually do not need to be repaired, as they frequently heal spontaneously or are asymptomatic even if they persist. Most tears that are repaired are considerably more than 1 cm long. Ideally, there should be little or no damage to the meniscal body. When there is considerable damage to the body fragment, effective function would be doubtful even if successful healing were to occur.

Open repair of a meniscosynovial tear that extends from the posterior third of the meniscus into the middle or even anterior third requires such extensive exposure that these tears are better handled by arthroscopic techniques. While unusual, peripheral tears confined to the anterior third of either meniscus are also suitable for open repair. It is important to recognize that it is difficult, if not impossible, to perform a satisfactory open repair of any tear that is not within 1 or 2 mm of the meniscosynovial junction, and that arthroscopic repair techniques are preferable for those lesions. It should also be noted that approximately 80% of repairable menisci are found in knees with an acute or chronic tear of the anterior cruciate ligament, and management decisions need to be linked to considerations of how this ligament is to be treated. If the anterior cruciate ligament is to be reconstructed, the sutures for the meniscal repair are not tied until the end of the reconstruction, so as to prevent damage to the meniscal repair from the motion and stability testing carried out during the ligament reconstruction.

Since all repairs of meniscal tears can be done with arthroscopy, one can question why any tears should be repaired with an open procedure if one is skilled in arthroscopic repair techniques. I (KD) continue to prefer the open technique whenever appropriate because of the ease of preparation of the meniscal rim and capsular bed, because of the ability to place vertically oriented sutures, and because the completed repair has been consistently more anatomic than the arthroscopic repair in my experience. Accordingly, there is at least the theoretical concern that arthroscopic repair of these tears might not be as reliable as the open technique has proved to be for me over the past 16 years. However, the all-inside technique described by Cannon and Morgan in their chapter may prove to allow the same type of repair, with comparable results, to be carried out with arthroscopic rather than open means.

Another factor to consider is that the morbidity associated with meniscal repair is primarily related to the protection needed for both initial healing and maturation, which is the same regardless of the type of technique used. This constraint tends to negate some of the usual advantages of arthroscopic procedures (decreased morbidity and an earlier return to function). In addition, I (KD) always use posterior skin incisions to retract and protect neurovascular structures while performing arthroscopic repair (essentially the same incisions as those used for open repair), which means that there is no substantial difference between the cosmetic results of open and arthroscopic repairs. However, there obviously is a difference between the cosmetic results of the all-inside approach and an open repair, and if the all-inside technique proves to be as reliable as an open repair, it may emerge as the preferred alternative.

Technique

The open technique of one of us (KD) has been previously reported.[49] Once it has been documented arthroscopically that open repair is suitable, one can proceed directly to the repair procedure. With current approaches to asepsis for arthroscopes and video equipment, reprepping and redraping are no longer recommended. Prophylactic antibiotics are used routinely. If there is no history of allergy, one gram of a cephalosporin is given intravenously before administration of anesthesia, and a second gram is administered intravenously after deflation of the tourniquet. When there is a history of allergy to penicillin or cephalosporins, clindamycin (600 mg) is administered intravenously before administration of anesthesia and after deflation of the tourniquet. Vancomycin (500 mg) is sometimes slowly administered intravenously before administration of anesthesia, when there is a history of allergy. The knee is flexed 90° and the pneumatic tourniquet is inflated.

Medial Meniscal Repair (Posterior) A 5- to 6-cm vertical posteromedial skin incision is centered at the level of the joint line and carried through the deep fascia to expose the posteromedial aspect of the capsule. An oblique capsular incision is made just posterior to the posterior border of the medial collateral ligament to expose the posterior meniscal tear. The peripheral rim of the meniscus is debrided of any unstable tags of meniscal tissue and freshened with a curet or a rasp. The capsular bed is also carefully prepared and fresh-

ened to ensure vascularity all along the capsular surface of the repair. It is not necessary or desirable to excise any intact and stable meniscal tissue that is still attached to the capsular bed.

Double-armed sutures (with a smaller needle on one end) are used to place vertical sutures that anatomically reapproximate the capsular bed back to the complete height of the meniscal rim. The smaller needle is passed from below upward through the meniscal rim, and the larger needle is passed from below upward through the corresponding portion of the capsular bed (Fig. 9, *top*). Sutures are placed 3 to 4 mm apart, and as many as necessary are used to complete the repair (Fig. 9, *bottom*). Absorbable or non-absorbable sutures may be used, and they can be tied inside or outside the capsule. I (KD) prefer to use small (4-0) absorbable suture and to tie the knots inside the capsule. Others[48,50] have preferred heavier, non-absorbable suture placed through the capsule and tied outside the capsule. Heavier (2-0) suture is used to repair the capsule securely back to the meniscal rim at the site of the capsular incision, and plicating sutures are used to complete the capsular repair proximal to the joint line. If a ligamentous procedure is being carried out simultaneously, the sutures for the meniscal repair are tagged to be tied later, after the ligamentous procedure has been completed.

Lateral Meniscal Repair (Posterior) The exposure and technique for the lateral meniscus (Fig. 10, *top*) are somewhat different and slightly more difficult than those for the medial meniscus because of the differences in anatomy and the necessity to work around the popliteus tendon. A 5- to 6-cm posterolateral vertical skin incision is made parallel to the posterior border of the fibular head. The iliotibial band is split in line with its fibers at the level of the joint line and retracted to expose the underlying capsule. An oblique posterolateral capsular incision is made parallel to the posterior border of the popliteus tendon to expose the lateral meniscal tear. The meniscal rim and capsular bed are prepared in a fashion similar to that described for the medial meniscus, and the same type of vertically oriented repair sutures are placed.

Because there is less space in which to work without damaging the popliteus tendon, the technique for placement of the sutures is different for the lateral meniscus. A small (4-0) absorbable suture with a small needle is used. First, the suture is passed from above downward through the meniscal rim and then it is passed from below upward through the capsular bed (two separate passes). It is helpful to use a nerve-hook or a comparable retractor to pull posteriorly on the capsular bed and popliteus tendon complex, in order to make sufficient room to pass the sutures. The first pass through the capsular side of the repair includes the deeper and strong (but relatively avascular) layer,

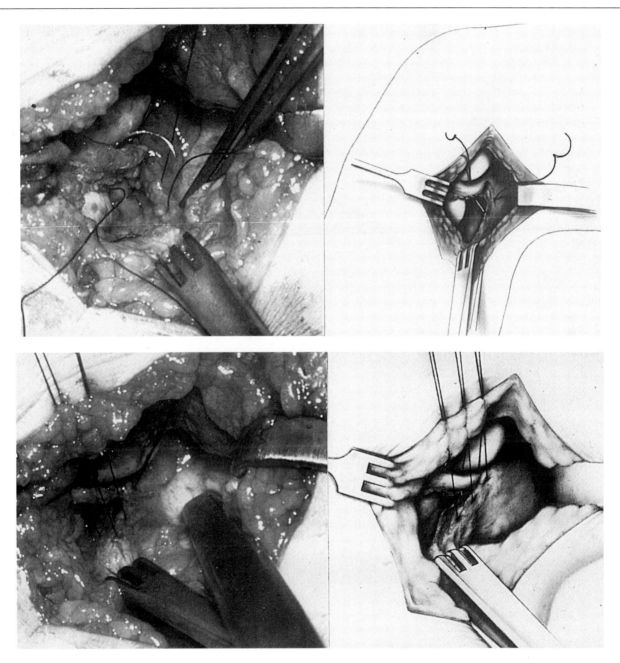

Fig. 9 The technique of medial meniscal repair. **Top,** After the vertical capsular incision has been made, the meniscal rim is sutured to its detached synovial bed with vertically placed absorbable 4-0 mattress sutures. A double-armed suture is used. First, the small needle is passed from the inferior to the superior surface of the meniscus, and then the larger needle is passed from below up through the capsular bed. **Bottom,** Individual sutures are placed 3 to 4 mm apart and tied intracapsularly. As many sutures are used as are necessary to achieve a strong repair. (Reproduced with permission from DeHaven KE, Black KP, Griffiths HJ: Open meniscus repair: Technique and two to nine year results. *Am J Sports Med* 1989;17:789.)

and the second pass is through the more superficial (but vascular) synovial membrane. Frequently, only two or three sutures are required to complete the repair around to the posterior border of the popliteus tendon, re-establishing the normal posterior border of the popliteus hiatus. The repair sutures are tied inside the capsule, and the capsular incision is closed careful-

ly with plicating sutures similar to the method described for the medial meniscus. Similarly, if the anterior cruciate ligament is being reconstructed during the same procedure, the sutures for the meniscal repair are tagged and tied later, after the ligamentous procedure has been completed. If the tear extends anterior to the popliteus tendon, the exposure

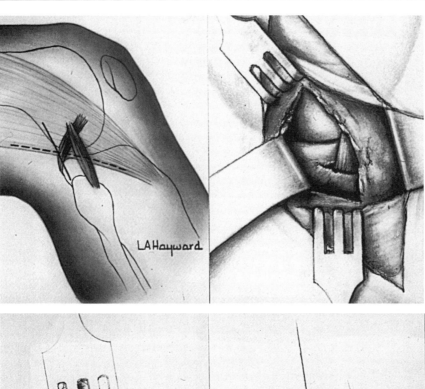

Fig. 10 The technique of lateral meniscal repair. **Top left,** The vertical skin incision is made just posterior to the fibular collateral ligament, and the iliotibial band is split in line with its fibers at the level of the joint line and retracted. **Top right,** The iliotibial band has been split in line with its fibers and retracted, and the capsule has been opened vertically just posterior to the popliteus tendon. This drawing demonstrates normal anatomy at the junction of the popliteus and meniscal rim with a normal popliteus hiatus. **Bottom left,** A peripheral tear of the posterior horn of the lateral meniscus, which extends to the popliteus hiatus. **Bottom center** and **right,** The suture is passed first from superior to inferior through the meniscus, then through the strong fibers that run from the medial belly of the popliteus to the lateral meniscus, and then through the synovial bed. (Reproduced with permission from DeHaven KE, Black KP, Griffiths HJ: Open meniscus repair: Technique and two to nine year results. *Am J Sports Med* 1989;17:790-791.)

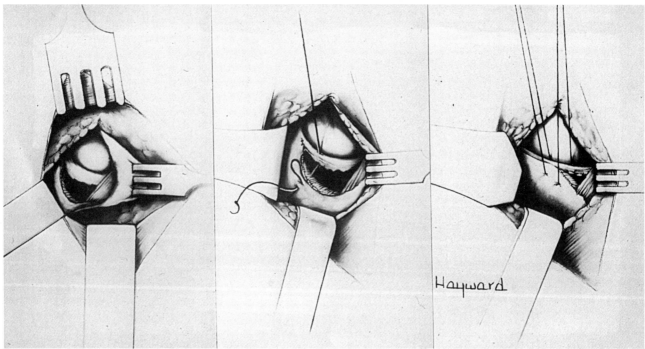

required for open repair, anterior as well as posterior to the popliteus tendon, is quite extensive, and in this case arthroscopic repair is preferable.

Aftercare

It is important to provide a six-week period of maximum protection, to allow initial healing, and a subsequent six-month interval of protection from vigorous stresses (which can cause early failure), to allow for maturation of the healing collagen tissue. Since 1976, my (KD) aftercare program has become more liberal in terms of motion, but it remains conservative with regard to early weightbearing. Minimum touch-down weightbearing with crutches is recommended for the first six weeks. Others[53] have employed early weightbearing with the knee held in extension in a splint, without any apparent deleterious effect on healing rates. It appears that it is possible to have either early motion or early weightbearing, but there is concern that the combination of the two could compromise the healing response.

For an isolated meniscal repair, a hinged knee splint is applied, with the hinges locked at 0° for the first two weeks, and it is worn until the wounds have healed and the sutures are removed. Isometric quadriceps and hamstrings-setting exercises, as well as straight-leg-raising exercises, are initiated immediately. Limited motion between 30° and 70° (with the hinges set for that range) is started after two weeks, and the splint is removed four weeks following surgery so that gentle stretching exercises can be added to increase the range of motion as tolerated. More vigorous stretching is initiated at six weeks, to regain any lost motion. At the same time, more strenuous strengthening exercises are begun. Weightbearing is progressively increased, as tolerated, after six weeks, and use of crutches is normally discontinued seven to eight weeks following surgery.

Low-impact and non-agility athletic activities are initiated three months following surgery if there is adequate motion and muscle strength and if there is no pain, tenderness, or effusion. These limited activities include bicycling, use of a Stair-Master, use of a rowing machine, swimming, and straight-line jogging. Full squats, hard running, and agility activities are not recommended until six months have passed, to allow maturation of the meniscal repair site. When meniscal repair is carried out in conjunction with reconstruction of a ligament (typically, the anterior cruciate ligament), the standard ligament-rehabilitation protocol is followed, except that weightbearing is limited until after six weeks. Doing so has provided adequate protection for the meniscal repair.

Results

The intermediate results (average, five years) and long-term results (minimum, ten years) of these open repair techniques have been assessed previously.[49] The survival rate for repaired menisci was 89% at five years and 79% at ten years or more. Both studies documented a higher failure rate in unstable knees (38% at five years and 54% at ten years). The long-term survival rate in stable knees and nearly stable knees (a difference of as much as 4.5 mm between the right and left knees under maximum manual stress) was 94%. This should be considered a best-case scenario for meniscal repair, because these tears were all very peripheral in location, the meniscal body had sustained minimum damage, and the knees were stable or only slightly unstable. Others have also reported favorable early and intermediate results of open repair techniques.[48,50,54-56]

While it is reassuring to know that these repaired menisci heal and remain healed, the most important issue is how well they function. The five-year study[49] revealed radiographic evidence of effective biomechanical function of knees that had had a successful meniscal repair, and the radiographic results of the long-term study are even more compelling. Radiographs were made, with the patient standing and

the knee in extension and in 45° of flexion, for the entire series. In 85% of the knees in which the repair had been clinically successful, the involved compartment was radiographically normal, compared with only 43% of the knees that had sustained a second tear and had been treated with a partial meniscectomy. This was a statistically significant difference (p = 0.04).

These results support the conclusion that not only are suitable meniscal tears repaired by these open techniques capable of healing, but also most remain healed over time (10 to 13 years) in stable or nearly stable knees that demonstrate biomechanical function.

References

1. Annandale T: The classic: An operation for displaced semilunar cartilage. *Clin Orthop* 1990;260:3-5.
2. King D: The healing of semilunar cartilages. *J Bone Joint Surg* 1936;18:333-342.
3. Fairbank TJ: Knee joint changes after meniscectomy. *J Bone Joint Surg* 1948;30B:664-670.
4. Cox JS, Nye CE, Schaefer WW, et al: The degenerative effects of partial and total resection of the medial meniscus in dogs' knees. *Clin Orthop* 1975;109:178-183.
5. Huckell JR: Is meniscectomy a benign procedure?: A long-term follow-up study. *Can J Surg* 1965;8:254-260.
6. Jones RE, Smith EC, Reisch JS: Effects of medial meniscectomy in patients older than forty years. *J Bone Joint Surg* 1978;60A:783-786.
7. Moskowitz RW, Davis W, Sammarco J, et al: Experimentally induced degenerative joint lesions following partial meniscectomy in the rabbit. *Arthritis Rheum* 1973;16:397-405.
8. Tapper EM, Hoover NW: Late results after meniscectomy. *J Bone Joint Surg* 1959;51A:517-526,600,603.
9. Ahmed AM, Burke DL: In-vitro measurement of static pressure distribution in synovial joints: Part I. Tibial surface of the knee. *J Biomech Eng* 1983;105:216-225.
10. Armstrong CG, Mow VC: Variations in the intrinsic mechanical properties of human articular cartilage with age, degeneration, and water content. *J Bone Joint Surg* 1982;64A:88-94.
11. Bourne RB, Finlay JB, Papadopoulos P, et al: The effect of medial meniscectomy on strain distribution in the proximal part of the tibia. *J Bone Joint Surg* 1984;66A:1431-1437.
12. Bullough PG, Munuera L, Murphy J, et al: The strength of the menisci of the knee as it relates to their fine structure. *J Bone Joint Surg* 1970;52B:564-567.
13. Fukubayashi T, Kurosawa H: The contact area and pressure distribution pattern of the knee: A study of normal and osteoarthrotic knee joints. *Acta Orthop Scand* 1980;51:871-879.
14. Kettelkamp DB, Jacobs AW: Tibiofemoral contact area: Determination and implications. *J Bone Joint Surg* 1972;54A:349-356.
15. Mathur PD; McDonald JR, Ghormley RK: A study of the tensile strength of the menisci of the knee. *J Bone Joint Surg* 1949;31A:650-654.
16. Shrive NG, O'Connor JJ, Goodfellow JW: Load-bearing in the knee joint. *Clin Orthop* 178;131:279-287.
17. Walker PS, Erkman MJ: The role of the menisci in force transmission across the knee. *Clin Orthop* 1975;109:184-192.
18. Fukubayashi T, Torzilli PA, Sherman MF, et al: An in vitro biomechanical evaluation of anterior-posterior motion of the knee: Tibial displacement, rotation, and torque. *J Bone Joint Surg* 1982;64A:258-264.
19. Hsieh HH, Walker PS: Stabilizing mechanisms of the

loaded and unloaded knee joint. *J Bone Joint Surg* 1976;58A:87-93.

20. Levy IM, Torzilli PA, Warren RF: The effect of medial meniscectomy on anterior-posterior motion of the knee. *J Bone Joint Surg* 1982;64A:883-888.

21. Markolf KL, Mensch JS, Amstutz HC: Stiffness and laxity of the knee: The contributions of the supporting structures: A quantitative in vitro study. *J Bone Joint Surg* 1976;58A:583-594.

22. Markolf KL, Bargar WL, Shoemaker SC, et al: The role of joint load in knee stability. *J Bone Joint Surg* 1981;63A:570-585.

23. Oretorp N, Gillquist J, Liljedahi SO: Long term results of surgery for non-acute anteromedial rotatory instability of the knee. *Acta Orthop Scand* 1979;50:329-336.

24. Shoemaker SC, Markolf KL: The role of the meniscus in the anterior-posterior stability of the loaded anterior cruciate-deficient knee: Effects of partial versus total excision. *J Bone Joint Surg* 1986;68A:71-79.

25. Wang CJ, Walker PS: Rotatory laxity of the human knee joint. *J Bone Joint Surg* 1974;56A:161-170.

26. Krause WR, Pope MH, Johnson RJ, et al: Mechanical changes in the knee after meniscectomy. *J Bone Joint Surg* 1976;58A:599-604.

27. Kurosawa H, Fukubayashi T, Nakajima H: Load-bearing mode of the knee joint: Physical behavior of the knee joint with or without menisci. *Clin Orthop* 1980;149:283-290.

28. Seedhom BB, Hargreaves DJ: Transmission of the load in the knee joint with special reference to the role of the menisci: Part II. Experimental results, discussion and conclusions. *Eng Med* 1979;8:220-228.

29. Voloshin AS, Wosk J: Shock absorption of meniscectomized and painful knees: A comparative in vivo study. *J Biomed Eng* 1983;5:157-161.

30. Sutton JB: *Ligaments: Their Nature and Morphology*. London, MK Lewis, 1897.

31. Arnoczky SP, Adams ME, DeHaven K, et al: Meniscus, in Woo SL-Y, Buckwalter J (eds): *Injury and Repair of the Musculoskeletal Soft Tissues*. Park Ridge, IL, American Academy of Orthopaedic Surgeons, 1988, pp 487-537.

32. Mow VC, Arnoczky SP, Jackson DW (eds): *Knee Meniscus: Basic and Clinical Foundations*, New York, NY, Raven Press, 1992, pp 37-89, 107-115.

33. Arnoczky SP: Gross and vascular anatomy of the meniscus and its role in meniscal healing, regeneration and remodeling, in Mow VC, Arnoczky SP, Jackson DW (eds): *Knee Meniscus: Basic and Clinical Foundations*. New York, NY, Raven Press, 1992, pp 1-14.

34. Warren R, Arnoczky SP, Wickiewicz TL: Anatomy of the knee, in Nicholas JA, Hershman EB (eds): *The Lower Extremity and Spine in Sports Medicine*. St. Louis, MO, CV Mosby, 1986, pp 657-694.

35. Adams ME, Hukins DWL: The extracellular matrix of the meniscus, in Mow VC, Arnoczky SP, Jackson DW (eds): *Knee Meniscus: Basic and Clinical Foundations*. New York, NY, Raven Press, 1992, pp 15-28.

36. Eyre DR, Koob TJ, Chun LE: Biochemistry of the meniscus: Unique profile of collagen types and site-dependent variations in composition. *Trans Orthop Res Soc* 1983;8:56.

37. Aspden RM, Yarker Y E, Hukins DW: Collagen orientations in the meniscus of the knee joint. *J Anat* 1985;140:371-380.

38. Yasui K: Three-dimensional architecture of human normal menisci. *J Japanese Orthop Assoc* 1978;52:391-399.

39. Ahmed AM: The load-bearing role of the knee menisci, in Mow VC, Arnoczky SP, Jackson DW (eds): *Knee Meniscus: Basic and Clinical Foundations*. New York, NY, Raven Press, 1992, pp 59-73.

40. Baratz ME, Fu FH, Mengato R: Meniscal tears: The effect of meniscectomy and of repair on intraarticular contact areas and stresses in the human knee: A preliminary report. *Am J Sports Med* 1986;14:270-275.

41. Radin EL, Rose RM: Role of subchondral bone in the initiation and progression of cartilage damage. *Clin Orthop* 1986;213:34-40.

42. Cox JS, Cordell LD: The degenerative effects of medial meniscus tears in dogs' knees. *Clin Orthop* 1977;125:236-242.

43. O'Connor BL, McConnaughey JS: The structure and innervation of cat knee menisci, and their relation to a "sensory hypothesis" of meniscal function. *Am J Anat* 1978;153:431-442.

44. Wilson AS, Legg PG, McNeur JC: Studies on the innervation of the medial meniscus in the human knee joint. *Anat Rec* 1969;165:485-491.

45. Arnoczky SP, Warren RF: Microvasculature of the human meniscus. *Am J Sports Med* 182;10:90-95.

46. Arnoczky SP, Warren RF: The microvasculature of the meniscus and its response to injury: An experimental study in the dog. *Am J Sports Med* 1983;11:131-141.

47. Cabaud HE, Rodkey WG, Fitzwater JE: Medical meniscus repairs: An experimental and morphologic study. *Am J Sports Med* 1981;9:129-134.

48. Cassidy RE, Shaffer AJ: Repair of peripheral meniscus tears: A preliminary report. *Am J Sports Med* 1981;9:209-214.

49. DeHaven KE, Black KP, Griffiths HJ: Open meniscus repair: Technique and two to nine year results. *Am J Sports Med* 1989;17:788-795.

50. Hamberg P, Gillquist J, Lysholm J: Suture of new and old peripheral meniscus tears. *J Bone Joint Surg* 1983;65A:193-197.

51. Henning CE, Lynch MA, Clark JR: Vascularity for healing of meniscus repairs. *Arthroscopy* 1987;3:13-18.

52. Arnoczky SP, Warren RF, Spivak JM: Meniscal repair using an exogenous fibrin clot: An experimental study in dogs. *J Bone Joint Surg* 1988;70A:1209-1217.

53. Morgan CD, Wojtys EM, Casscells CC, et al: Arthroscopic meniscal repair evaluated by second-look arthroscopy. *Am J Sports Med* 1991;19:632-637.

54. Dolan WA, Bhaskar G: Peripheral meniscus repair: A clinical pathological study of 75 cases. *Orthop Trans* 1983;7:503-504.

55. Hanks GA, Gause TM, Sebastianelli WJ, et al: Repair of peripheral meniscal tears: Open versus arthroscopic technique. *Arthroscopy* 1991;7:72-77.

56. Sommerlath K, Gillquist J: Knee function after meniscus repair and total meniscectomy: A 7-year follow-up study. *Arthroscopy* 1987;3:166-169.

Meniscal Repair: Arthroscopic Repair Techniques

W. Dilworth Cannon, Jr, MD

Craig D. Morgan, MD

Modified Henning Inside-to-Outside Technique Including Use of a Fibrin Clot

Over the past two decades, advances in arthroscopic techniques have contributed to technological advancements in meniscal repair. Ikeuchi[1] apparently performed the first arthroscopic meniscal repair in Tokyo in 1969 and reported on his first four patients in 1976. The first two repairs failed within four months after the operation. In 1978, Price and Allen[2] reported the results of 36 repairs of peripheral tears of the medial meniscus associated with disruption of the medial collateral ligament. To my (WDC) knowledge, Henning[3] performed the first arthroscopic repair in the United States in 1980. Other arthroscopic suturing techniques quickly followed. Three repair techniques have evolved: the inside-to-outside technique,[4-9] the outside-to-inside technique,[10,11] and the all-inside technique.[12] The limitation of the third technique is that, like open meniscal repair, it can be used only to repair tears that have a rim that is less than 2.5 mm wide. In the more popular, inside-to-outside technique, single and double-barreled instruments have been developed to enable the surgeon to pass either horizontal or vertical mattress sutures through the meniscus. Because vertically oriented sutures encompass more of the circumferentially oriented collagen bundles, those sutures have become more popular than the horizontal mattress sutures. Although it is easier to place a vertically oriented suture with use of a single-barreled meniscal-repair technique, a surgeon can achieve nearly the same result by turning and reorienting a double-barreled cannula after the first needle has been inserted but before the second needle is inserted at the other end of the suture. The surgeon should be proficient in more than one repair technique, because an occasion may arise when a specific meniscal tear can best be repaired with use of a technique other than that usually used by the surgeon.

In this paper, the Henning[3] technique will be described in detail. Its chief advantage over other techniques is that it enhances the surgeon's ability to place sutures precisely through complex meniscal tears, producing excellent coaptation of the meniscus. The most difficult aspect of the technique is retrieval of the 2.5-in (approximately 6-cm) needles through the posterior incisions. Other instrument sets that use longer needles have an advantage in this regard.

Preoperative Planning

While the final decision regarding the need to repair a meniscus is made at the time of the arthroscopy, I (WDC) prefer to obtain a preoperative magnetic resonance image (MRI) for young patients who may be candidates for repair. If the MRI suggests that a meniscal repair can be done, then enough time can be scheduled for surgical repair. The various surgical options, including meniscal repair, should be discussed thoroughly with the patient preoperatively. The surgeon should never be faced with the need to make a decision regarding meniscal repair in the middle of an arthroscopy without having discussed this procedure with the patient.

I (WDC) believe that the criteria for meniscal tears that are amenable to repair are broader than those outlined by DeHaven. Not only are vertical longitudinal tears in the peripheral 3 mm-wide vascularized zone of the meniscus repairable, but it is also possible to repair certain tears in the avascular zone, including some radial split and oblique flap tears, especially those close to the origins of the posterior horns of the medial and lateral menisci. In addition, surgeons should be more willing to repair tears that are noted during reconstruction of a torn anterior cruciate ligament (ACL), because these repairs have a greater likelihood of healing successfully than do repairs of isolated meniscal tears.

Medial Meniscal Repair

If a surgeon prefers to be seated during an operation, the involved leg of the patient can be flexed over the end of the table, with the involved hip abducted 20° to 30° to allow access to the posteromedial and posterolateral corners of the knee. When this technique is used, the uninvolved leg should be placed in a stirrup to prevent a nerve palsy. A second technique, which I (WDC) prefer, places the involved thigh in a thigh-holder distal to the tourniquet, with the hip flexed approximately 40°. A thick gel pad should be placed under the posterior aspect of the thigh to alleviate pressure on the sciatic nerve. The leg is abducted to allow the surgeon to stand between it and the table. There is ample access to the posteromedial and posterolateral corners of the knee for needle retrieval, and reconstruction of the ACL can be done without a change in limb position. The tourniquet should be placed around the proximal aspect of the thigh, but the use of the tourniquet should be saved for ligament reconstruction, if necessary.

Diagnostic arthroscopy indicates whether a meniscal repair is needed. If a repairable medial meniscal tear is found, a 6- to 7-cm long longitudinal incision is made at the posteromedial corner of the knee, centered at the joint line. To help determine the precise location of this incision, the arthroscope is passed through the intercondylar notch from the anterolateral portal. The light from the arthroscope illuminates the posteromedial corner of the knee. Deeper dissection should be done with the knee flexed 90°, in order to allow the saphenous nerve to fall posteriorly along with the pes anserinus. The direct head of the semimembranosus should be palpated, and dissection should be continued anterior to this tendon and halfway across the medial head of the gastrocnemius. A popliteal retractor from the Henning system (Stryker, San Jose, California) is placed in this location to deflect the meniscal repair needles. A small spoon or half of a pediatric vaginal speculum also can be used for this purpose. If the meniscal tear extends anterior to the site of the posteromedial incision, dissection should be done anteriorly, just superficial to the medial collateral ligament. If a long bucket-handle tear is to be repaired, it may be necessary to make a small secondary incision midway between the posteromedial incision and the anteromedial portal to retrieve anteriorly placed sutures.

The original Henning[3] system included a medial joint distractor, and its use is recommended if more than two or three sutures are to be employed in the repair. The distractor is attached to two 3/16-in (0.48-cm) Steinmann pins, one placed just proximal to the adductor tubercle on the femur and the other through the anteromedial flare of the tibia (Fig. 1). If visualization of the posterior horn of the medial meniscus remains unsatisfactory, additional joint distraction can be done by placing several transverse stab wounds through the superficial portion of the medial collateral ligament, to gain an additional 2 to 4 mm of joint-space opening. In Henning's experience, this release did not lead to chronic laxity, because the medial collateral ligament tightened as the meniscal repair healed.

A stab wound is made through the synovial membrane at the posteromedial corner, to allow introduction of a 2 to 3-mm rasp or burr. Introduction of a spinal needle through the posteromedial synovial membrane allows the surgeon to determine the best site for this incision. A burr, rasp, or small motorized shaver can be introduced through this small opening and used to abrade the meniscosynovial junction over the superior surface of the posterior horn of the medial meniscus. Abrasion should also be done on both

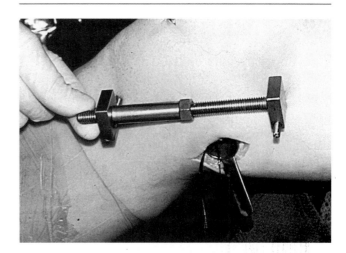

Fig. 1   A knee distractor is used for medial meniscal repairs to obtain better visualization of the posterior horn. The Henning popliteal retractor can be seen in the posteromedial incision. (Reproduced with permission from Cannon WD: Arthroscopic meniscal repair, in McGinty JB (ed): *Operative Arthroscopy*. New York, NY, Raven Press, 1991, p 239.)

sides of the tear site. The importance of abrasion of the handle side of the tear site was demonstrated by Henning. Histologic analysis of biopsy material showed that amorphous hypocellular material builds up on the surface of the handle after a tear. This material can impede the healing process and is best abraded away. The anterior surface of the posterior horn may be abraded either by introducing a burr or rasp through the anteromedial portal and directing it posteriorly, or by making a second posteromedial stab wound inferior to the first with direction of the burr or rasp under the meniscus to the inferior surface of the tear site.

In the Henning system, all suturing of the meniscus is done with non-absorbable 2-0 Ethibond (special order D-6702; Ethicon, Somerville, New Jersey), with double-armed taper-ended Keith needles. Approximately 4 mm from the tip of the needle, a 10° to 15° bend is made, and a second 10° to 15° bend is made in the same direction 10 mm from the first bend. These two bends in the needle not only enable the surgeon to perform ipsilateral placement of the suture near the origin of the posterior horn of the medial meniscus with posteromedial retrieval of the needle, they also allow better needle passes through the tear site.

The first needle to be passed is press-fitted into the special needle-holder that accompanies the Henning set of instruments (Stryker). Medial meniscal tears should be sutured with the knee flexed approximately 15° to 20°. A small cannula is placed through the anteromedial portal, as close to the medial edge of the patellar ligament as possible. If this portal is placed more medially, it is extremely difficult to suture from the ipsilateral approach because the needles pass into the middle of the popliteal fossa. The first suture should be placed through the inferior surface of the meniscus at the posterior horn origin of the tear (Fig. 2). After the needle has been inserted into the meniscal substance up to the second bend in the needle, a third bend is created by levering the cannula and needle-holder into the intercondylar notch (Fig. 3). This third bend allows the needle to be aimed toward the posteromedial incision. The popliteal retractor should be in position behind the posterior horn of the medial meniscus when this maneuver is done. When the needle is approximately halfway through the substance of the meniscus, the surgeon can palpate posteriorly with his or her index finger to locate the point of the needle. The needle should not be advanced when the surgeon's finger is in the posteromedial wound. Flexion of the knee to approximately 50° to 60° may facilitate location of the tip. Once the tip of the needle has been secured with a standard needle-holder (Fig. 4), the knee can be re-extended to approximately 15° to 20°, and the needle can be withdrawn through the posteromedial incision. The end of the suture is tagged. The second needle of the first suture should be passed through the cannula with the tip directed superiorly while the previously placed suture is pulled taut on the

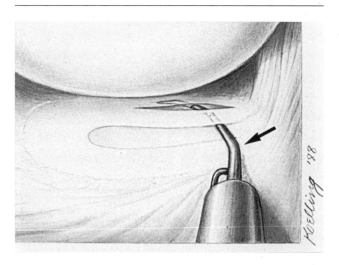

Fig. 3 The first suture, placed close to the posterior horn of either the medial or the lateral meniscus, can be difficult to retrieve posteriorly. A third bend in the needle (arrow) is made by levering the cannula and needle-holder into the intercondylar notch once the needle has engaged the meniscus. The additional bend allows the surgeon to guide the needle into the popliteal retractor with greater ease. (Reproduced with permission from Cannon WD: Arthroscopic meniscal repair, in McGinty JB (ed): *Operative Arthroscopy.* New York, NY, Raven Press, 1991, p 240.)

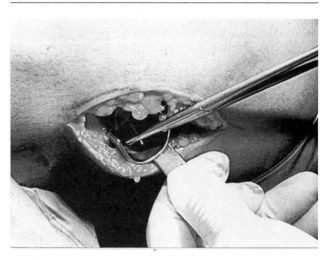

Fig. 4 Once the tip of the needle has penetrated the posterior horn and capsule, it is deflected off the popliteal retractor and is retrieved with a needle-holder. (Reproduced with permission from Cannon WD: Meniscal repair: The Henning technique. *Tech Orthop* 1993;8:95.)

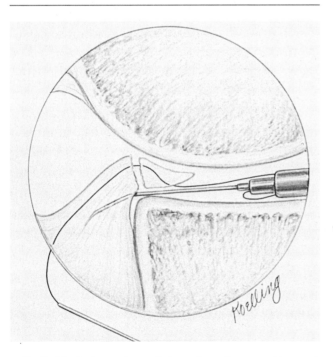

Fig. 2 The basic suturing technique, shown here, provides excellent meniscal tear coaptation. One pass of the suture is close to the superior surface of the meniscus, and the second pass is underneath the inferior rim and penetrates through the meniscosynovial junction. (Reproduced with permission from Cannon WD: Arthroscopic meniscal repair, in McGinty JB (ed): *Operative Arthroscopy.* New York, NY, Raven Press, 1991, p 240.)

inferior surface of the cannula. This prevents accidental skewering of the first suture. A vertical suture is made by passing the second needle under the meniscus, bypassing the tear site.

The second suture is placed through the superior surface of the meniscus, approximately 3 mm anterior to the first suture. This needle should go through as

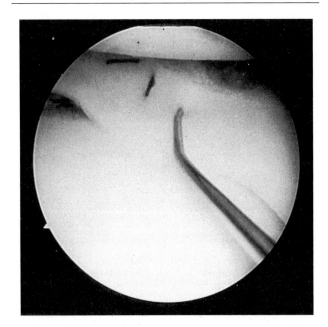

Fig. 5 This arthroscopic photograph shows the placement of a divergent vertically oriented mattress suture through the superior surface of the meniscus. (Reproduced with permission from Cannon WD: Arthroscopic meniscal repair, in McGinty JB (ed): *Operative Arthroscopy*. New York, NY, Raven Press, 1991, p 241.)

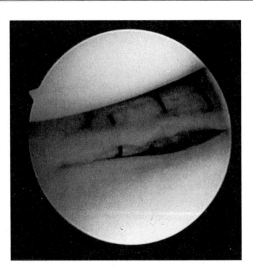

Fig. 6 Arthroscopic photograph showing the array of sutures alternating through the inferior and superior surfaces of the meniscus.

much of the meniscal substance as possible in an inferior direction (Fig. 5). The second needle of the second suture should pass over the top of the meniscus and exit at the meniscosynovial junction. Additional sutures are alternated between the superior and inferior surfaces every 3 to 4 mm (Fig. 6). Henning advocated the use of stacked sutures so that each inferior and superior suture lies in a vertical plane, with each suture securing approximately half of the substance of the

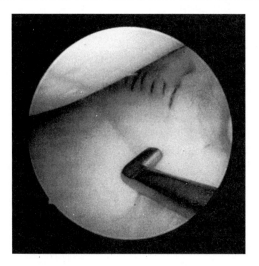

Fig. 7 The right medial meniscus of a patient 18 months after Henning had placed 42 sutures to repair a displaced bucket-handle tear.

meniscus. He believed that the use of stacked sutures in large numbers to coapt the meniscal fragment completely back to the segment of the rim produced a higher rate of success than did the use of staggered sutures. On one occasion, Henning used 42 sutures to repair a displaced bucket-handle tear of the medial meniscus (Fig. 7).

Sutures positioned anterior to the posteromedial corner of the meniscus are placed more easily by moving the cannula to the anterolateral portal and the arthroscope to the anteromedial portal. Needles that are passed through the most anterior extent of a bucket-handle tear are difficult to direct to the posteromedial incision, and a second short incision midway between the anteromedial portal and the posteromedial incision may help in needle retrieval.

If the anterior cruciate ligament is to be reconstructed, meniscal repair sutures are tied after the reconstruction to prevent displacement of the repair. Two-inch (5-cm) segments of sterile intravenous tubing are placed over each suture and snugged against the posterior part of the capsule. The tubing can be clamped, thus securing the meniscus in its orthotopic position during the reconstruction.

In a tight medial compartment, needles that are directed through the posterior horn of the meniscus have a tendency not to penetrate through much of the meniscal substance. This problem can be obviated by the surgeon placing a nerve-hook through an accessory anteromedial portal, approximately 1 to 2 cm from the anteromedial portal, and directing it to the posterior horn. The nerve-hook can be used to deflect the meniscus upward and downward, providing a more direct approach through its substance. Needles that are directed inferiorly through the posterior horn of the meniscus may exit through the direct head of the semimembranosus. If the needle cannot be easily redirected, it is acceptable to tie the suture over the direct head of the semimembranosus.

Arnoczky and associates[13] demonstrated that the use of a fibrin clot stimulates the repair process in the avascular zone of the canine meniscus. I (WDC) use a fibrin clot for all isolated meniscal repairs as well as for complex tears that are repaired in association with reconstruction of the ACL. I do not use a fibrin clot for simple tears that are repaired in conjunction with a reconstruction of the ACL. To prepare the clot, the anesthesiologist withdraws approximately 50 to 75 ml of venous blood, under sterile conditions, approximately 30 minutes before the clot is to be used. The blood is placed in a sterile plastic or glass container and stirred with a pair of sintered glass barrels from a pair of 20-ml syringes for approximately five to eight minutes (Fig. 8). After the fibrin clot adheres to the glass barrels, it is removed and washed in Ringer lactate. The clot is shaped into a tube-like structure, and meniscal repair sutures are passed through either end of the clot and tied. One suture with the attached needle should be at each end of the clot (Fig. 9). A 5 to 7-mm cannula is placed through the anteromedial portal, and the two needles that are attached to the clot are passed individually through the inferior surface of the meniscus at the most anterior and posterior poles of the tear (Fig. 10). Tension on the two sutures is adjusted evenly through the posteromedial incision,

and the clot is introduced into the cannula and is simultaneously pushed with a blunt obturator and pulled by the two posterior sutures. Once the clot is in the medial compartment, a nerve-hook and a Freer elevator can be used to tease the clot into its final resting position, under the inferior surface of the meniscus (Fig. 11). The meniscal repair sutures, which are loosened at the time of the insertion of the clot, are pulled tight, trapping the clot in the tear. The sutures are tied, starting at the origin of the posterior horn and working anteriorly. Before the sutures are cut, the single throws from the fibrin clot insertion are tied to one of the adjacent ends of the suture. It is good prac-

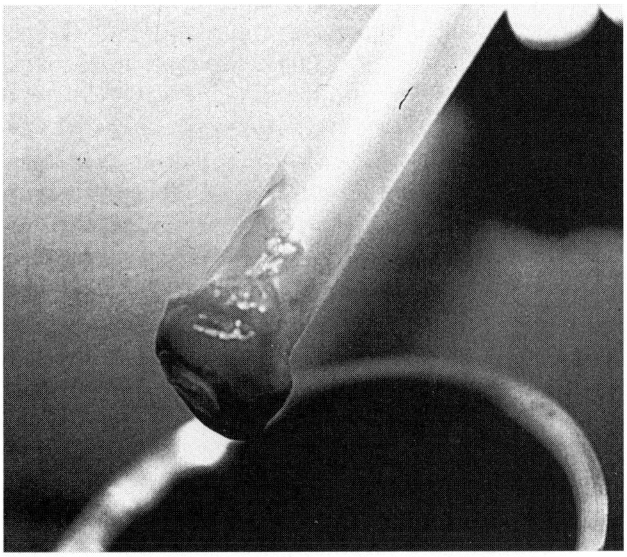

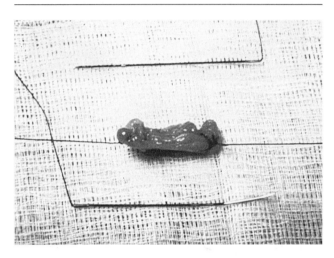

Fig. 9 A 2-0 Ethibond suture (Ethicon) has been placed through either end of the fibrin clot to facilitate its stable placement under the inferior surface of the meniscus at the tear site. (Reproduced with permission from Cannon WD, Vittori JM: Meniscal repair, in Aichroth PM, Cannon WD (eds): *Knee Surgery: Current Practice.* London, England, Martin Dunitz, 1992, p 80.)

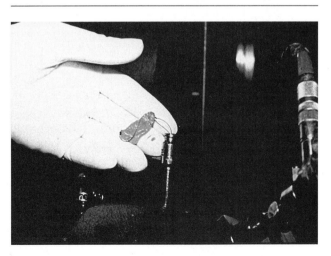

Fig. 10 The two sutures attached to either end of the clot have been placed under the meniscus at the anterior and posterior poles of the tear. The clot is about to be pulled into the joint through the cannula.

Fig. 8 A fibrin clot is collected on a sintered glass barrel after stirring venous blood for five to eight minutes. (Reproduced with permission from Cannon WD: Meniscal repair: The Henning technique. *Tech Orthop* 1993;8:96.)

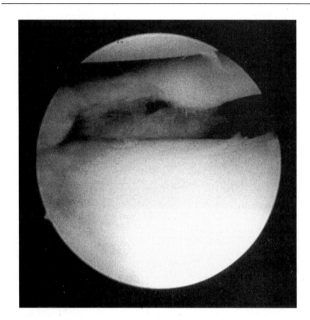

Fig. 11   The two sutures securing the fibrin clot have pulled the clot through the cannula into the joint space. This arthroscopic photograph shows the final appearance after the fibrin clot has been tucked under the meniscus and trapped as the meniscal repair sutures were pulled tight and tied. (Reproduced with permission from Cannon WD: Meniscal repair: The Henning technique. *Tech Orthop* 1993;8:97.)

tice to probe the meniscus before the suture is cut. If any of the sutures are loose, adjacent tied sutures can be tied together to tighten them.

Lateral Meniscal Repair

A 6- to 7-cm-long longitudinal incision is made at the posterolateral corner of the knee with its proximal pole at the posterior border of the iliotibial band. The biceps is split from the iliotibial band and retracted posteriorly, thus protecting the peroneal nerve, which lies behind it. This dissection should be done with the knee flexed 90°. The lateral head of the gastrocnemius is dissected free of the posterior aspect of the capsule; the dissection is started inferiorly and moved superiorly. A nerve-hook, passed through the anteromedial portal, through the intercondylar notch, and over the posterior horn of the lateral meniscus, can be palpated with a finger through the posterolateral incision. This ensures proper location of the incision. While the intercondylar notch is viewed through an anteromedial portal, the surgeon does a parameniscal abrasion and freshens the tear site in a fashion similar to that described for the medial site.

With the knee flexed approximately 60° to 90°, a cannula is placed through the anteromedial portal, and the first needle is placed through the inferior surface of the origin of the posterior horn. Again, it is very

helpful to make a third bend in the needle to direct it to the posterolateral incision. Because the popliteal artery lies just posterior to the origin of the posterior horn of the lateral meniscus, the surgeon should be certain that the needles are heading to the posterolateral corner of the knee and not straight posteriorly. The suturing technique is the same as that described for the medial side. The surgeon should try to avoid passing sutures directly through the popliteus tendon, because to do so may occasionally cause mild pain postoperatively. However, in my (WDC) experience, if suturing through the popliteus cannot be avoided, usually there will not be serious complications.

Postoperative Rehabilitation

If a meniscal repair and a reconstruction of the anterior cruciate ligament were done at the same time, an early return of a full range of motion of the knee should be emphasized. Because arthrofibrosis is extremely rare after an isolated meniscal repair, a more gradual return of range of motion may be recommended after this procedure. A brace may be worn at a fixed angle between 20° and 40° of flexion for the first three weeks postoperatively to lessen the possibility of fibrin clot disruption due to early motion. A full range of motion should be obtained by six weeks postoperatively. Weightbearing is not permitted for the first four weeks after an isolated meniscal repair or after a combined reconstruction of the ACL and meniscal repair. Progressive weightbearing to full weightbearing is encouraged by eight weeks for patients with a reconstruction of the ACL and by six weeks for patients with an isolated meniscal repair. Closed kinetic-chain quadriceps exercises, such as stationary bicycling, use of a stair-climbing exercise machine, and leg-presses, are begun at four weeks in both groups. An unrestricted program of progressive-resistance hamstring exercises may be begun after one week by patients who had a repair with a reconstruction and after three weeks by patients who had an isolated repair. Both groups of patients should be taught to avoid a fully squatted position and to be cautious about flexing the knee more than 135° to reduce stress on the repair site in the posterior horn.[14] Straight-ahead running can begin at five months and participation in non-contact sports at six months. Participation in contact sports is delayed until nine months postoperatively.

Results

The most common method used to assess the results of meniscal repair is clinical; it is based on pain, tenderness, clicking, and locking. An absence of these symptoms and signs suggests that the meniscus has healed. Scott and associates[9] developed a more precise technique based on anatomic assessment at least six months after the meniscal repair. They encouraged their patients to have an arthrogram performed after a medial meniscal repair and to have a second-look arthroscopy under local anesthesia if a lateral meniscal repair had been done. They considered the meniscus to be healed if the residual cleft at the site of the tear was less than 10% of the meniscal thickness (Fig. 12). A partially healed meniscus had less than a 50% residual cleft at the site of the tear. A residual cleft that was more than 50% of the thickness of the meniscus at any point along the tear indicated that the meniscus had failed to heal. Henning[3] noted that patients who had a partially healed meniscus had a satisfactory clinical outcome. Hence, he considered patients to have a satisfactory outcome if the anatomic assessment was in the healed or partially healed category. Interestingly, Henning found that two-thirds of the anatomic failures in his series were clinically asymptomatic. The clinical criteria for healing are less stringent than the anatomic criteria. This helps to explain the much higher prevalence of clinical healing in the literature compared with the results of the anatomic assessment of healing.

Of 160 arthroscopic meniscal repairs performed by one of us (WDC) between 1982 and 1992, 117 repairs were assessed with arthrography or second-look arthroscopy. Ninety-two (79%) of the meniscal repairs were done in conjunction with reconstruction of the ACL, and 25 (21%) of the isolated meniscal repairs were done in cruciate-stable knees. Sixty-six medial meniscal repairs (56%) and 51 lateral meniscal repairs (44%) were done. Forty-one repairs (35%) were of acute tears (the repair was done less than eight weeks after the injury) and 76 (65%) were of chronic lesions. To assess the status of healing, arthrography was done for 30 patients (26%) and arthroscopy for 87 patients (74%).

According to the anatomic assessment, the meniscal repair had a satisfactory outcome (the healed and incompletely healed categories) in 88 knees (75%), and 29 (25%) of the repairs had failed. There was a significant difference in the results (healing) between the knees that had had meniscal repair with synchronous reconstruction of the ACL compared with those who had meniscal repair in cruciate-stable knees. In the former group, there were 75 successful outcomes (82%), whereas in the isolated meniscal repair group, only 12 tears (48%) had a successful outcome anatomically (p<0.05) (Fig. 13).

There was a relationship between the width of the rim and healing in these two groups, with an increased rate of failure as rim widths increased to 4 to 5 mm, the avascular zone of the meniscus. Overall, the rate of failure increased from three (10%) of 29 repairs when the rims were less than 2 mm wide, to 19 (26%) of 74 for rims that were 2 to less than 4 mm wide, and to seven of 14 for rims that were 4 to 5 mm wide. There were no failures in the four patients in the isolated repair group with rims that were less than 2 mm wide (the upper limit of rim width that could be approached by open meniscal repair) (Fig. 14).

The rate of failure was directly related to the length

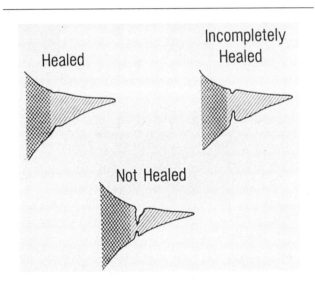

Fig. 12 Illustration demonstrating the various degrees of healing. Six months after the repair, the degree of healing is determined by arthrography for the medial side and by arthroscopy for the lateral side. A tear is classified as healed if it is healed over its full length and has a residual cleft of less than 10% of the meniscal thickness. A tear is classified as incompletely healed if it is healed over its full length with a residual cleft that is less than 50% of its vertical height. A tear is classified as not healed (failed) if there is a residual cleft of more than 50% of the thickness of the meniscus at any point over the length of the tear. (Reproduced with permission from Cannon WD: Arthroscopic meniscal repair, in McGinty JB (ed): *Operative Arthroscopy*. New York, NY, Raven Press, 1991, p 245.)

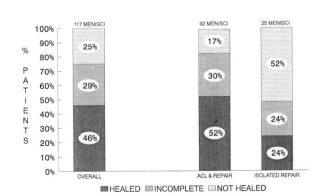

Fig. 13 Graph showing the overall results of meniscal repair. The results of the isolated meniscal repairs and those of the meniscal repairs with concurrent reconstruction of the anterior cruciate ligament are also compared. The sum of the healed and incompletely healed categories represents a satisfactory outcome.

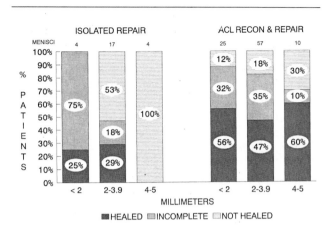

Fig. 14 Graph showing the relationship of rim width to healing of the meniscal repairs.

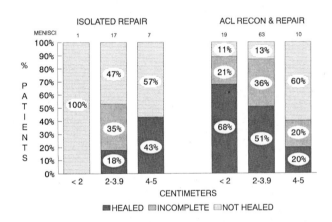

Fig. 15 Graph showing the relationship of meniscal tear length to healing of the meniscal repairs.

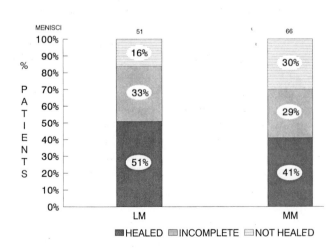

Fig. 16 Graph comparing the results of lateral and medial meniscal repairs. (LM = lateral meniscus and MM = medial meniscus).

of the meniscal tear. When both groups (isolated repair and repair with reconstruction) were combined, the rate of failure was three of 20 when the length of the tear was less than 2 cm. It increased to 16 (20%) of 80 for tear lengths of 2 to less than 4 cm and to 10 of 17 for tear lengths of 4 to 5 cm, the typical length of a bucket-handle tear (Fig. 15).

Overall, repairs of the lateral meniscus did better than repairs of the medial meniscus (Fig. 16). Acute meniscal repairs (done eight weeks or less after the injury) had a rate of satisfactory healing of 34 (83%) of 41, compared with 55 (72%) of 76 for the repairs that were done later than eight weeks after the injury (Fig. 17).

Surprisingly, patients who were older than 36 years of age did as well as younger patients (Fig. 18). There were few complications. One patient had a partial peroneal-nerve palsy, which resolved after six months.

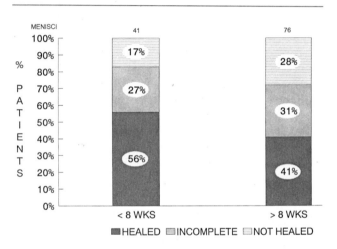

Fig. 17 Graph showing the effect of the time from the injury to the operation on the results of meniscal healing. Repairs of acute meniscal tears (eight weeks or less after the injury) did slightly better than repairs of chronic tears (more than eight weeks after the injury).

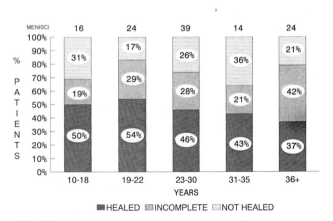

Fig. 18 Graph showing the relationship of age to meniscal healing.

Two patients had transient phlebitis. There were no infections, problems with wound healing, or vascular complications.

Discussion

Although arthroscopic meniscal repair is a difficult, technically demanding procedure, it does have advantages over open meniscal repair in that tears with a rim width of more than 2 mm and certain flap, radial split, and displaced bucket-handle tears can be repaired. As others have found,[9,15] most meniscal repairs are done in knees in which there is an associated disruption of the anterior cruciate ligament (92 tears [79%] in the present study). When in doubt, the surgeon should attempt to repair a meniscal tear in knees in which the ACL is being reconstructed. Even complex flap and radial split tears near the origin of the posterior horn of the lateral meniscus are amenable to successful repair. Some surgeons attempt to repair tears only in the outer 3-mm vascularized zone of the meniscus. However, in this study, seven of ten tears that were associated with ligament reconstruction and had a rim width of 4 to 5 mm had satisfactory healing.

A statistically significant increase in the rate of successful healing was noted in meniscal repairs done in conjunction with reconstruction of the ACL compared with isolated meniscal repairs ($P < 0.05$).[16] This difference may be explained by the following: (1) reconstruction of the ACL protects the repair site from the biomechanical forces accompanying the anterior tibial translation that originally caused the tear, and (2) surgical reconstruction leads to more intra-articular bleeding, resulting in fibrin-clot formation, which enhances meniscal healing. In one series of 28 patients in whom the site of a meniscal tear was biopsied within 12 days after the injury, with the sections stained with hematoxylin and eosin and examined under electron microscopy, it was found that all 16 of the isolated tears were associated with degenerative changes, whereas none of the 12 tears associated with reconstruction of the ACL had these changes (T. Tilling, personal communication, 1991). Previously, I (WDC) believed that meniscal tears that were associated with tears of the ACL were more peripheral than isolated tears, but a subsequent study found the rim widths of the two groups to be identical.[16]

At present, I use a fibrin clot in all isolated meniscal repairs and in repairs of complex tears associated with reconstruction of the ACL. As of 1992, I found a slightly higher rate of healing when a fibrin clot was used, although the numbers were too small to be statistically significant. Henning[15] found a statistically significant increase in the rate of healing with use of a fibrin clot in repairs of isolated meniscal tears. Before the use of fibrin clots, satisfactory healing occurred in only ten of 17 patients. After he began to use them, satisfactory healing occurred in 12 of 13 patients.

The Arthroscopic Outside-to-Inside Technique

The outside-to-inside suturing technique for arthroscopic meniscal repair was developed in the early 1980s in an attempt to avoid posterior neurovascular complications by use of a percutaneous approach. At that time, neurovascular complications were associated with arthroscopic inside-to-outside repairs of the posterior horns that were done without an open posterior exposure, in order to protect the posterior neurovascular structures (the saphenous nerve medially and the popliteal artery and peroneal nerve laterally). The concept of outside-to-inside suturing originated with Warren[11] and, as far as I (CDM) know, the clinical use of the procedure was first reported by Morgan and Casscells.[10]

In general, the outside-to-inside method delivers suture through the lumen of a standard 18-gauge spinal needle, directed percutaneously from a known safe-zone suturing portal outside the knee, through the capsule and the meniscal tear, and into an intra-articular location inside the knee under arthroscopic control; hence, the term outside-to-inside suturing.

In my (CDM) experience, the major advantage of this method over other arthroscopic or open techniques is that it is a rapid way of suturing a meniscal tear. Suturing of a 2-cm peripheral meniscal tear adds approximately ten minutes to routine diagnostic arthroscopy. In addition, the outside-to-inside technique is particularly suited for suture of the rather rare peripheral anterior-horn tears, which cannot be approached readily with the inside-to-outside method.

Indications

The type of tear for which the outside-to-inside meniscal repair is indicated is the same as that suitable for any type of meniscal repair: a mobile, single, vertical, longitudinal tear of the meniscus limited to the vascular outer one-third of the meniscal substance (Fig. 19). In my (CDM) experience, this type of tear has constituted between 10% and 20% of all meniscal lesions encountered in patients younger than 35 years of age and is rarely seen in patients older than 35. I do not repair flap tears, radial tears, cleavage tears, or vertical tears with secondary lesions that extend into the avascular inner two-thirds of the meniscus, because these tears have no vascular basis for healing. There is one exception to these contraindications: in the under-15 age-group, I repair mid-width single vertical tears in which bleeding is visualized arthroscopically.

In my (CDM) experience, two-thirds of all repairable meniscal tears (as just defined) are associated with instability of the ACL, with 90% of these tears

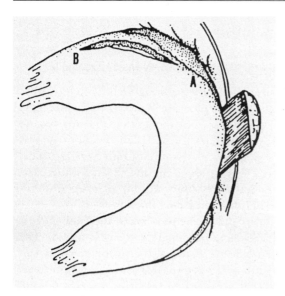

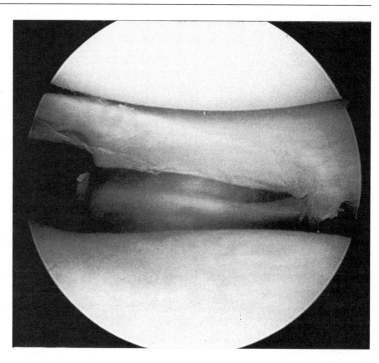

Fig. 19 **Left,** Drawing of a tear for which meniscal repair is indicated. The tear is a single, vertical, longitudinal rupture limited to the outer one-third of the meniscal substance. Ninety percent of such tears are limited to a location that involves the posterior horns. **Right,** An arthroscopic view of a displaced peripheral tear of the posterior horn of a left lateral meniscus.

limited to the posterior horns. If the figures are looked at another way, repairable meniscal tears occur in about 20% of all knees with an acute rupture of the ACL. This figure rises to approximately 30% in the under-20 age-group with an acute rupture. On the basis of these statistics, it is imperative that the surgeon who performs reconstructions of the ACL develop the skills and techniques necessary for the repair of indicated peripheral meniscal tears, rather than treating all meniscal lesions with excision.

Operative Technique

The patient is positioned supine on the operating table, with the end of the table flexed 120° at the mid-thigh level so that the uninvolved limb hangs over the padded break in the table with the knee flexed 90°. The involved limb is prepped and draped free from mid-thigh to mid-calf, allowing sterile circumferential access to the knee. A high thigh tourniquet is applied but is not inflated during the meniscal repair; use of an inflow pump obviates the need for a tourniquet during this procedure. The tourniquet is inflated after the meniscal repair, when the reconstruction of the anterior cruciate ligament is done. This approach avoids lengthy tourniquet times when a meniscal repair is performed with a reconstruction of the ligament under one period of anesthesia.

After arthroscopic confirmation of a peripheral tear

in the outer third of the meniscal substance, a local healing environment is created at the tear site with a meniscal repair rasp (Fig. 20). With the arthroscope placed from a contralateral anterior portal and the rasp placed from an ipsilateral anterior portal, the tear is debrided of any hypovascular, abortive repair tissue, and the local synovial tissue is excoriated to stimulate a vascular response.

Suturing Techniques

Suturing with the outside-to-inside method begins with direction of a standard 18-gauge spinal needle from a percutaneous suturing portal outside, through the capsule and both sides of the meniscal tear, while the inside is visualized with the arthroscope placed from a contralateral anterior viewing portal. Once the sharp tip of the needle is seen spanning the tear, monofilament absorbable suture (0-gauge PDS [polydioxanone]; Ethicon) is delivered across the tear through the lumen of the 18-gauge needle and is brought out through an ipsilateral anterior portal (Fig. 21). At this point, an interference knot (a knot thrown three times) is created on the end of the suture extending from the anterior portal. Next, the spinal needle is removed from the suturing portal, and the suture, with its interference knot at the end, is retrograded back into the knee by the surgeon pulling on the suture tail through the original suturing portal.

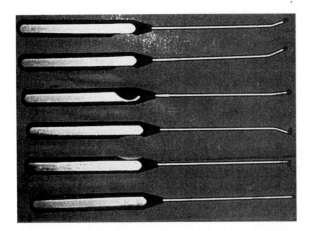

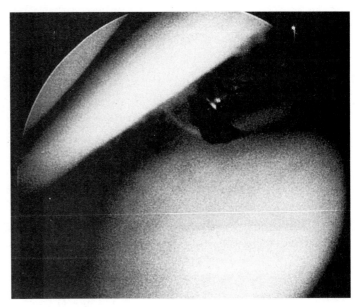

Fig. 20 **Left**, Meniscal repair rasps (Bowen, Rockville, Maryland). The rasps have a 2 mm diameter burr attached to a semimalleable shaft that facilitates the placement to the posterior horns from either anterior or posterior portals. **Right**, Intra-articular arthroscopic view of the terminal end of a meniscal repair rasp.

This results in apposition of the tear at the site of the interference knot. This process is repeated two or more times through the single suturing portal until the entire tear is stabilized (Fig. 22).

When this method of suturing is used, sutures may be placed on either the femoral or the tibial surface of the meniscus by directing the needle either proximally or distally. It is recommended that interference knots be placed on both the femoral and the tibial surfaces of the mobile meniscal fragment to create a vertically oriented suture pattern, which is important to balance the repair (Fig. 23).

The repair is completed by tying all suture tails together over the joint capsule through the single suturing portal. It has been my (CDM) experience, when viewing the more common posterior-horn tears with a 70° arthroscope through the intercondylar notch, that these tears separate with the knee in flexion and reduce with the knee in extension. Therefore, to avoid tension on the repair, I tie the repair sutures and immobilize the knee in full extension. This approach also minimizes the risk of entrapping the posterior part of the capsule in flexion at the repair site and of creating a flexion contracture.

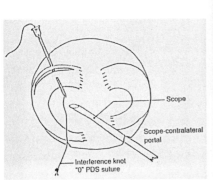

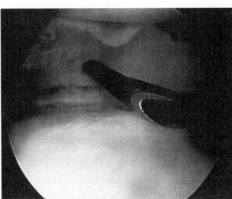

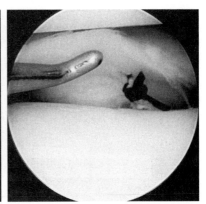

Fig. 21 Outside-to-inside suturing. **Left**, Placement of an 18-gauge spinal needle with suture delivered from outside to inside. The suture is brought out through an ipsilateral anterior portal for creation of an interference knot. PDS = polydioxanone. **Center**, Arthroscopic photograph of a spinal needle with suture in its lumen penetrating far posterior in the posterior horn of a medial meniscus. **Right**, Arthroscopic photograph of an interference knot, which was retrograded into the knee, apposing the tear at the suture site.

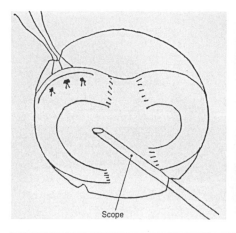 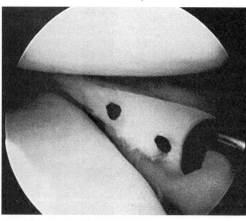

Fig. 22 A completed repair. **Left,** Completed repair of the posterior horn of the medial meniscus with three outside-to-inside sutures placed through a single posterior suturing portal. **Right,** Arthroscopic intra-articular photograph.

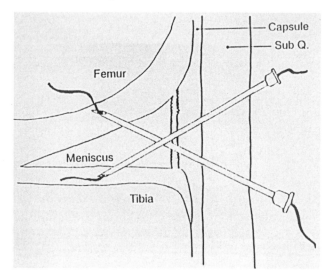

Fig. 23 Sutures can be placed on either the femoral or the tibial surface of the meniscus by angling the 18-gauge needle either distally or proximally. (Sub Q = subcutaneous tissue).

Creation of a Safe Suturing Portal

Knee position, and an understanding of topographic anatomy as it relates to knee position, are critical in the creation of safe suturing portals to repair tears of the posterior horns. Posterolaterally, as with any approach to suturing of the posterior horn of the lateral meniscus, the peroneal nerve must be avoided. With the knee in 90° of flexion or more, the peroneal nerve falls well below the level of the joint line and always lies posterior to the biceps femoris tendon, which is readily palpable. A safe window for the creation of the suture portal is located above the biceps tendon, at the level of the joint line, with the knee flexed 90° (Fig. 24). In contrast, with the knee in extension, the peroneal nerve crosses the lateral joint line just behind the posterolateral corner, directly in the path of approach for suturing with either the inside-to-outside or the outside-to-inside method. Therefore, extension of the

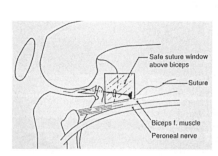 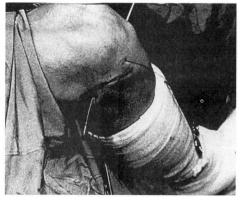 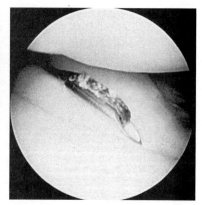

Fig. 24 Safe zone for creation of the suture portal. **Left,** Line drawing illustrating the safe zone for placement of the posterolateral suture portal above the biceps tendon with the knee flexed 90°. **Center,** Operative photograph showing proper placement of the posterolateral suture portal illustrated at left. **Right,** Arthroscopic photograph of needle placement far posterocentral in a lateral meniscus, outside the posterolateral portal seen in the center photograph.

knee should be avoided during suturing of the posterior horn of the lateral meniscus.

When suturing the posterior horn of the medial meniscus, the surgeon must take care to avoid the saphenous nerve. The main trunk, or sartorial branch, of the saphenous nerve is located along the posterior border of the sartorius, and the variably located infrapatellar branches come off anterior to the posterior border of the sartorius. The position of the saphenous nerve in relation to the posteromedial joint line changes greatly with knee motion. In extension, the saphenous nerve and all infrapatellar branches cross the medial joint line anterior to the posteromedial corner and are located 2 to 3 cm anterior to the semitendinosus tendon, which is palpable and may be used as a reference point. However, in the flexed knee, the main sartorial trunk and all infrapatellar branches of the saphenous nerve cross the medial joint line at, or slightly behind, the posteromedial corner and are in jeopardy of injury when an outside suturing portal is created. Thus, to avoid injury to the saphenous nerve, it is recommended that the outside suture portal to the posterior horn of the medial meniscus be made with the knee in full extension, at the level of the joint line, and at or behind the palpable semitendinosus tendon (Fig. 25). It is extremely important to note that the recommended position of extension for suturing on the medial side is exactly the opposite of the 90° flexed position recommended for suturing on the lateral side.

Postoperative Regimen

For isolated meniscal repairs in cruciate-stable knees, I (CDM) immobilize the knee in an inexpensive knee immobilizer in full extension for four weeks and allow immediate weightbearing as tolerated. Pivoting and collision athletics are to be avoided for four months postoperatively. When a meniscal repair is done in conjunction with a reconstruction of the anterior cruciate ligament, the knee is immobilized for two weeks in full extension and immediate weightbearing is permitted. However, during the first two weeks, the patient also does active range-of-motion exercises from 0° to 90° of flexion for 20 minutes twice a day with the immobilizer removed. Thus, after meniscal repair combined with reconstruction of the anterior cruciate ligament, weightbearing and a range of motion are allowed early, but not at the same time.

Results

Both clinical and second-look arthroscopic results of large series of outside-to-inside meniscal repairs have been reported with one to six years of follow-up.[10,17] The clinical rate of failure in a multicenter study of 353 outside-to-inside repairs was 3% (12 repairs). The low rate of failure in this study may in part be because of very conservative indications for repair.

In a separate study, 74 outside-to-inside repairs (all from the larger clinical series) were evaluated with second-look arthroscopy, and 12 failures (16%) were found. While 62 knees (84%) had stable healing at the repair site, only 48 (65%) had complete healing without a partial residual defect. On the basis of the data from this second-look study, it was concluded that (1) failure was always symptomatic, (2) incomplete healing (a partial defect) was asymptomatic if the repair was stable to probing, (3) failure was most commonly associated with an original tear located in the posterior horn of the medial meniscus in a knee with ACL deficiency that was not stabilized surgically, and (4) menis-

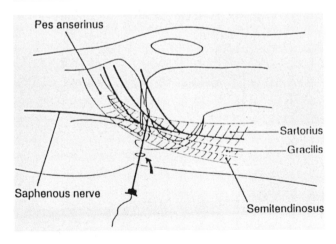
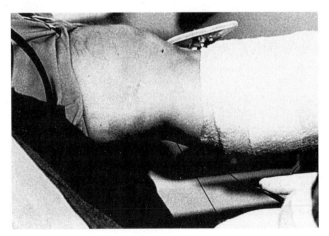

Fig. 25 Line drawing, **left**, and operative photograph, **right**, showing proper placement of the posteromedial suture portal behind the semitendinosus tendon in the fully extended knee.

cal repairs performed in conjunction with reconstruction of the ACL healed as well as, or better than, meniscal repairs done in cruciate-stable knees.

Complications

Ten complications (3%) occurred in the clinical series of 353 outside-to-inside repairs. The complications included three deep infections, which resolved with arthroscopic debridement; four symptomatic adhesion problems, which led to arthroscopic resection; one non-fatal pulmonary embolus; one saphenous neuroma, which occurred before we learned to go behind the pes-group tendons; and one semitendinosus ganglion.

All-Inside Arthroscopic Meniscal Repair

The all-inside meniscal repair recreates arthroscopically the open method of vertically oriented suture repair initially described and popularized by DeHaven.[18,19] As with the open method, this arthroscopic technique allows visualization and repair of the lesion where it appears — in the posterior compartment of the knee. Specifically, a posterior horn tear is viewed from the posterior compartment with a 70° arthroscope advanced from anterior through the intercondylar notch while operative instrumentation is introduced through a cannula placed into the posterior compartment from a posterior-corner approach. With both viewing and triangulating from a posterior approach into the posterior compartment, access is gained to all areas of the posterior aspect of the meniscus, particularly the far posterocentral area near the root attachment, which cannot be approached (technically or safely) with use of other (inside-to-outside or outside-to-inside) arthroscopic suturing methods.

The all-inside method introduces new arthroscopic instrumentation that places vertically oriented sutures across the meniscal tear and allows suture knots to be tied intra-articularly under arthroscopic control. This posterior approach results in a balanced anatomic posterior-horn repair that approximates both the meniscotibial and the meniscofemoral portions of the coronary ligament complex to the meniscus at the site of disruption, while excluding the posterior aspect of the capsule from the repair. The term all-inside is used to distinguish this entirely intracapsular arthroscopic suturing technique from arthroscopic methods that require extracapsular exposures or extracapsular knot-tying, or both.

Indications

The all-inside method is indicated for suturing of mobile, single, vertical longitudinal tears of the posterior horn of either meniscus located at or within 3 mm of the meniscocapsular junction (Fig. 26). In my (CDM) experience with more than 400 repairs, this type of tear, limited to the posterior horns, constitutes 90% of all outer-third, single, vertical longitudinal lesions. Only 10% present as isolated anterocentral tears or posterior horn tears that extend anterior to the posterior corner of the meniscus. The ratio of

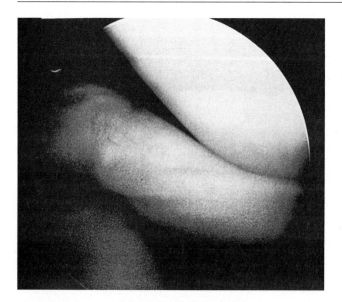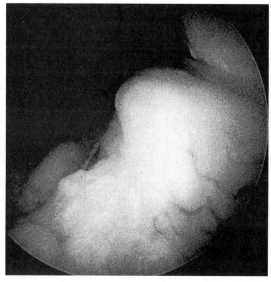

Fig. 26 **Left,** A displaced, peripheral tear of the posterior horn of the lateral meniscus, viewed with a 30° arthroscope from anterior. **Right,** A reduced peripheral tear of the posterior aspect of the medial meniscus, similar to the tear seen in Fig. 19, left, viewed from posterior with a 70° arthroscope advanced through the intercondylar notch.

medial-to-lateral repairable tears is approximately two to one. The repairable posterior-horn tears suitable for the all-inside repair constitute about 15% of all meniscal lesions encountered in my (CDM) practice in patients who are younger than 35 years old. This lesion is rarely seen in patients older than thirty-five years. Two-thirds of these repairable posterior-horn tears are associated with an ACL-deficient knee, and 20% of all patients with an acute rupture of the ACL who have an arthroscopy have a peripheral, repairable tear of the posterior horn. This figure increases to 35% in patients who are younger than 20 years old. For technical reasons, the all-inside method is indicated for posterior-horn tears only. Because of the lack of space for the instrumentation that is necessary for this technique, this method cannot be used readily to suture tears located anterior to the posterior corners of the meniscus. When posterior horn tears extend anterior to the posterior corners (peripheral bucket-handle tears), it is recommended that another suturing method be used to repair that portion of the meniscus.

Operative Technique

The set-up and patient-positioning for these procedures are similar to what I (CDM) use for arthroscopic reconstruction of the ACL, because most meniscal repairs are done concomitantly with a reconstruction of the ACL. When the two procedures are done together, the meniscal repair is done first without tourniquet control and is followed by the reconstruction of the ligament, which is done with the tourniquet inflated. This approach avoids a tourniquet time of longer than 90 minutes, as often occurs if both procedures are performed under tourniquet control. Use of an arthroscopic inflow pump obviates the need for a tourniquet during meniscal repair.

The patient is positioned supine on a standard operating table, with the table flexed at the mid-thigh level approximately 120°. The uninvolved knee is allowed to flex to 90° and to hang free over the padded end of the table. The involved limb is prepped and draped free from mid-thigh to mid-calf,

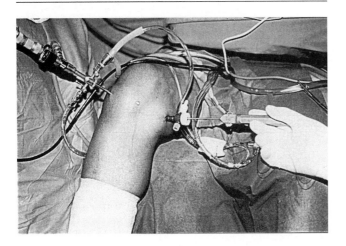

Fig. 27 Intraoperative photograph of a right knee during a posteromedial all-inside meniscal repair. Note the position of the patient and the draping, which allow circumferential access with the knee flexed 90°.

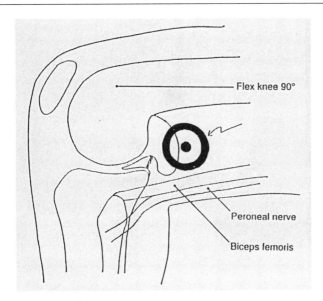
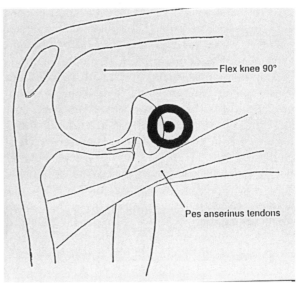

Fig. 28 **Left,** Proper placement of the posterolateral operative cannula, which begins outside, above the biceps tendon and above and behind the posterolateral joint line, and aims for the center of the joint with the knee flexed 90°. **Right,** Proper placement of the posteromedial operative cannula, which begins outside, above the medial hamstring tendons and above and behind the posteromedial joint line, and aims for the center of the joint with the knee flexed 90°.

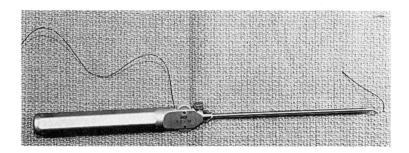

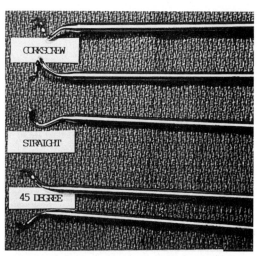

Fig. 29 Suture-hooks. **Left,** A suture-hook that includes a cannulated handle and shaft with a hooked terminal end for delivery of the suture down the lumen (Linvotech, Largo, Florida). **Right,** The various terminal angular designs of the suture-hooks: straight, 45° right and left, and corkscrew right and left.

and the knee is allowed to flex 90° over the break in the table to allow circumferential sterile access to the knee without the need for an assistant to hold the knee in position (Fig. 27). A leg-holder is not needed and is not used, because its presence on the thigh distal to the tourniquet compromises adequate exposure of the thigh.

After a standard, comprehensive, diagnostic arthroscopy is performed from both anteromedial and anterolateral portals, with a 30° arthroscope and a probe confirming the presence of a peripheral posterior-horn tear, the tear is viewed with a 70° arthroscope placed through the intercondylar notch from either the anteromedial or the anterolateral portal. Placement of the arthroscope through the notch is facilitated by creation of the anterolateral and anteromedial portals close to the anteromedial and anterolateral margins of the patellar ligament. To advance the arthroscope into the posteromedial compartment, the arthroscope is inserted into an anterolateral portal and passed under the posterior cruciate ligament. Advancement of the arthroscope into the posterolateral compartment begins from an anteromedial portal and continues under the ACL (if present). These maneuvers are best accomplished with the knee in 90° of flexion, using an arthroscope sheath loaded with a semiblunt obturator to feel the way under the respective cruciate ligaments. Only after the sheath has been positioned is the obturator exchanged for the 70° arthroscope. Once the arthroscope has been positioned in the desired posterior compartment, it is rotated 90° so that the posterior horn tear is in view (Figs. 26 and 27).

Placement of the Posterior Operative Cannula

After the tear has been well visualized, an 8-mm operative cannula is placed from posterior into the posterior compartment. The knee is flexed 90°, and the cannula is placed through a portal made in the soft spot above the palpable biceps femoris tendon, on the lateral side behind and above the joint line. It is advanced from this point toward the center of the joint, while its entrance through the posterior aspect of the capsule is visualized through the arthroscope (Fig. 28, *left*). By going above the biceps femoris tendon with the knee flexed 90°, injury to the peroneal nerve, which always lies below the biceps tendon in the flexed knee, can be avoided. With the knee in exten-

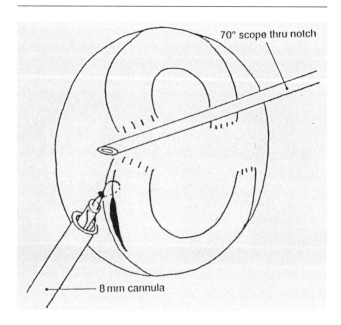

Fig. 30 Suture placement through a posterior operative cannula with a suture-hook; a 70° arthroscope was advanced through the intercondylar notch for viewing.

sion, however, the peroneal nerve crosses the postero-lateral joint line near the posterolateral corner and, in this position, is in jeopardy.

The cannula is placed into the posteromedial compartment in a similar fashion, beginning in the soft spot above the palpable medial hamstring tendons, behind and above the joint line, also with the knee in 90° of flexion (Figs. 27 and 28, *right*). On the medial side, the saphenous nerve is avoided by placing the operative portal above the medial hamstring tendons with the knee flexed 90°. The saphenous nerve is located at the posterior border of the sartorius, which falls well below the joint line in the flexed knee. In extension, however, the saphenous nerve and its infrapatellar branches all cross the medial joint line and are at risk of injury during placement of the operative cannula.

Creation of a Healing Environment Once the operative cannula is in place, both faces of the tear are debrided of any hypovascular, abortive repair tissue and the local synovial tissue is excoriated with a meniscal repair rasp to stimulate local bleeding (Fig. 20, *left*). The tear is usually prepared with a rasp placed through the posterior cannula while the meniscofemoral portion of the tear is viewed through the notch, and with

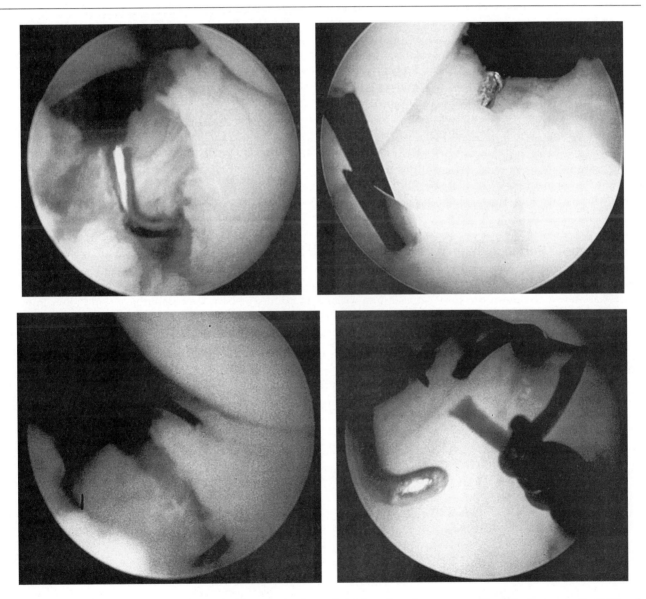

Fig. 31 A large meniscocapsular-junction tear of the posterior horn of a left lateral meniscus as seen with a 70° arthroscope placed through the intercondylar notch. The tear extends far posterocentral to the posterior root attachment of the meniscus. **Top left**, The tear, being probed through a posterolateral cannula. **Top right**, The tear, spanned by a straight suture-hook near the posterior root attachment, with the suture beginning to be introduced through the terminal end of the tool. **Bottom left**, A vertically oriented suture is left across the tear after removal of the suture-hook and bringing of the free end through the operative cannula. **Bottom right**, The completed repair with vertically oriented sutures after intra-articular knot-tying. Note the apposition of meniscus to meniscus at the tear site, with two suture knots evident.

the rasp placed from anterior while the meniscotibial portion of the tear is viewed from anterior (Fig. 20, *right*).

Suturing The sutures are placed with use of a meniscal repair suture-hook, delivered through the posterior operative cannula. The suture-hook is a cannulated 16-gauge needle with a hook-shaped terminal end interfaced to a shaft and handle with a roller device that feeds suture through it. Suture-hooks are available with three types of terminal angular designs to accommodate variable angles of approach and tear anatomy; these designs include a straight hook, 45° right and left hooks, and right and left corkscrews (Fig. 29). In general, when there is any degree of separation at the tear site, the tear is best spanned with the straight or 45° angled hooks, whereas anatomically reduced tears may be readily sutured with any of the hook designs.

Suturing is accomplished by manipulating the hook so that the sharp tip first penetrates the stable posterior-inferior rim and then advances across the tear into the mobile fragment from inferior to superior (Figs. 30 and 31 *top left*). After the hook has spanned both sides of the meniscal tear, approximately 31 to 36 cm (12 to 14 in) of monofilament suture (0- or 1-gauge PDS [polydioxanone]; Ethicon) are advanced into the posterior compartment (Fig. 31, *top right*). The tool is then withdrawn, leaving a vertical suture spanning the tear in a vertical orientation. The free end of the suture in the posterior compartment is then grasped and brought out through the posterior cannula, so that both ends of the suture are outside the cannula (Fig. 31, *bottom left*). Four sequential half-hitched throws are advanced down the posterior cannula with use of a double-holed knot-pusher, producing a double-stacked square knot that opposes the meniscal tear (Figs. 32 and 33). After the knot has been tied, the suture tails are cut intra-articularly, and the entire process is repeated as many times as necessary to stabilize the tear. Usually, three sutures are all that are

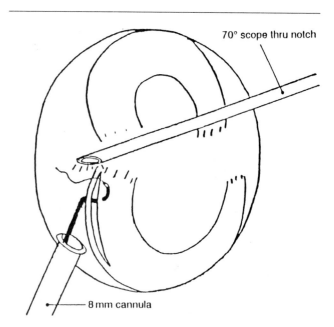

Fig. 32 Knot-tying done with an arthroscopic knot-pusher that advances sequential throws through the posterior cannula, with a 70° arthroscope advanced through the intercondylar notch for viewing.

needed to stabilize a large posterior-horn tear (Figs. 34 and 31, *bottom right*).

Postoperative Regimen

For isolated meniscal repairs in cruciate-stable knees, I (CDM) immobilize the knee in full extension in an inexpensive knee-immobilizer and allow immediate weightbearing. When a meniscal repair is done in combination with reconstruction of the ACL, the knee is immobilized for two weeks in full extension and immediate weightbearing is allowed. However, the patient is allowed an active range of motion, from 0° to 90° of flexion, twice a day for 20 minutes, beginning

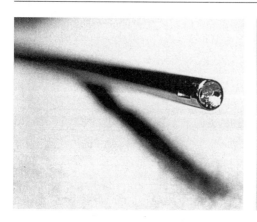
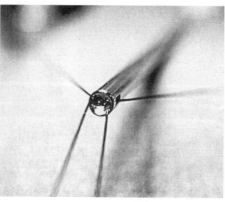

Fig. 33 Photographs of an arthroscopic knot-pusher (Arthrex, Naples, Florida). **Left,** Terminal end. **Right,** Terminal end advancing a surgeon's knot.

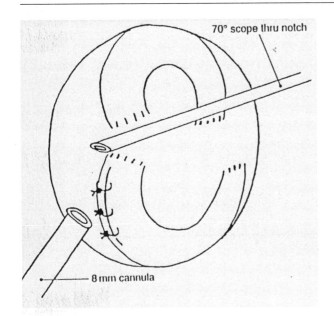
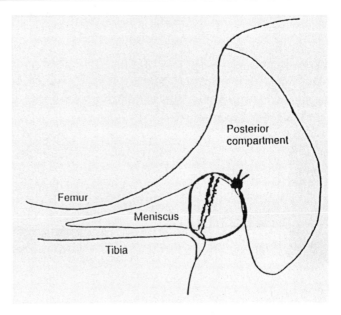

Fig. 34 Illustrations of a completed all-inside suture repair, which produces a vertically oriented, balanced repair that apposes meniscus to meniscus and excludes the posterior aspect of the capsule.

immediately postoperatively. After two weeks, progressive range-of-motion and strengthening exercises are instituted.

Advantages and Disadvantages

Some of the advantages of the all-inside arthroscopic meniscal-repair technique include safe placement of the suture far posterocentral in the posterior horn; a vertical orientation of the sutures that facilitates an anatomic, balanced repair; a meniscus-to-meniscus coaptation by sutures that avoids entrapment of the posterior part of the capsule; and avoidance of extracapsular posterior neurovascular injury by the sutures, because the sutures are placed and tied intra-articularly. The disadvantages of this technique are that it is technically demanding and requires the placement of a posterior operative cannula and visualization in the posterior compartment with a 70° arthroscope.

Clinical Experience

Between 1988 and 1991, I (CDM) performed and followed 47 all-inside meniscal repairs concurrently for one to four years. In this series, all associated instability of the ACL was stabilized as a concomitant procedure (30 knees). At the time of writing, no meniscal symptoms had recurred, and all patients were doing well clinically at their preinjury level of activity. No patient had had a second-look arthroscopy. With regard to perioperative complications, no neurovascular injury, infection, flexion contracture, or any other complication attributable to the all-inside meniscal repair procedure had developed in any patient.

References

1. Zkeuchi H: Surgery under arthroscopic control, in *Proceedings of the Socit International d'Arthroscopie.* Copenhagen, Denmark, 1975. *Rheumatologie* (special issue) 1976, pp 57-62.
2. Price CT, Allen WC: Ligament repair in the knee with preservation of the meniscus. *J Bone Joint Surg* 1978;60:61-65.
3. Henning CE: Arthroscopic repair of meniscus tears. *Orthopedics* 1983;6:1130-1132.
4. Barber FA, Stone RG: Meniscal repair: An arthroscopic technique. *J Bone Joint Surg* 1985;67B:39-41.
5. Cannon WD: Arthroscopic meniscal repair, in McGinty JB (ed): *Operative Arthroscopy.* New York, NY, Raven Press, 1991.
6. Cannon WD, Vittori JM: Meniscal repair, in Aichroth PM, Cannon WD (eds): *Knee Surgery: Current Practice.* London, Martin Dunitz, 1992, pp 71-84.
7. Clancy WG Jr, Graf BK: Arthroscopic meniscal repair. *Orthopedics* 1983;6:1125-1129.
8. Rosenberg T, Scott S, Paulos L: Arthroscopic surgery: Repair of peripheral detachment of the meniscus. *Contemp Orthop* 1985;10:43-50.
9. Scott GA, Jolly BL, Henning CE: Combined posterior incision and arthroscopic intra-articular repair of the meniscus: An examination of factors affecting healing. *J Bone Joint Surg* 1986;68A:847-861.
10. Morgan CD, Casscells SW: Arthroscopic meniscal repair: A safe approach to the posterior horns. *Arthroscopy* 1986;2:3-12.
11. Warren RF: Arthroscopic meniscus repair. *Arthroscopy* 1985;1:170-172.
12. Morgan CD: The "all-inside" meniscus repair. *Arthroscopy* 1991;7:120-125.
13. Arnoczky SP, Warren RF, Spivak JM: Meniscal repair using an exogenous fibrin clot: An experimental study in dogs. *J Bone Joint Surg* 1988;70A:1209-1217.
14. Dye SF, Cannon WD Jr: Anatomy and biomechanics of the anterior cruciate ligament. *Clin Sports Med* 1988;7:715-725.
15. Henning CE, Lynch MA, Yearout KM, et al: Arthroscopic meniscal repair using an exogenous fibrin clot. *Clin Orthop*

1990;252:64-72.

16. Cannon WD Jr, Vittori JM: The incidence of healing in arthroscopic meniscal repairs in anterior cruciate ligament-reconstructed knees versus stable knees. *Am J Sports Med* 1992;20:176-181.

17. Morgan CD, Wojtys EM, Casscells CD, et al: Arthroscopic meniscal repair evaluated by second-look arthroscopy. *Am J Sports Med* 1991;19:632-638.

18. DeHaven KE: Peripheral meniscus repair: An alternative to meniscectomy, in Proceedings of the Canadian Orthopaedic Association. *J Bone Joint Surg* 1981;63B:463.

19. DeHaven KE: Meniscus repair in the athlete. *Clin Orthop* 1985;198:31-35.

C H A P T E R   1 0

Fractures of the Patella

James E. Carpenter, MD

Roberta Kasman, MD

Larry S. Matthews, MD

Anatomy

The patella, the largest human sesamoid bone, lies within and is an important functional component of the knee extensor mechanism. Most of the quadriceps aponeurosis inserts directly into the superior pole of the patella, while the patellar ligament arises from its inferior pole. Some fibers, however, bypass the patella anteriorly and are confluent with the patellar ligament. Only the skin, a thin layer of subcutaneous tissue, and the prepatellar bursa overlie the patella. This subcutaneous location makes the patella prone to injuries from direct blows and falls. Posteriorly, the proximal three-quarters of the surface of the patella are covered with articular cartilage that is among the thickest found anywhere in the body. This surface only partially conforms to the anterior surface of the distal aspect of the femur and the trochlea. It has major medial and lateral facets.

Biomechanics

The patella is one link in the mechanism comprising the quadriceps muscle, the quadriceps tendon, the patella, and the patellar ligament. The mechanism serves two important biomechanical functions. First, as it is the principal site of insertion of the quadriceps muscle, it transmits the tensile forces generated by the quadriceps to the patellar ligament. Second, the patella effectively increases the lever arm of the knee extension mechanism from the axis of knee flexion-extension. This increases the knee extensor moment generated by contraction of the quadriceps. Kaufer[1] clearly documented this mechanical enhancing function of the patella. Using cadaveric knees, he balanced a simulated quadriceps force with a restraining force at the distal aspect of the tibia at 0° to 120° of knee flexion. By calculating the moment about the knee axis (the knee moment equals the tibial force multiplied by the tibial moment arm), he was able to determine the effective quadriceps moment arm (the quadriceps moment arm equals the knee moment divided by the quadriceps force). He found that the patella serves to increase the magnitude of the quadriceps moment arm and that the contribution made by the patella increases with progressive extension of the knee, being almost 30% at full extension. His findings have been confirmed by others[2] and they support the contention that total patellectomy should be avoided in the treatment of patellar disorders.

The patella is subjected to complex loading. With knee extension, it transmits almost all of the force of the quadriceps contraction and thus is loaded primarily in tension (Fig. 1). However, with knee flexion, its posterior surface contacts the distal aspect of the femur and is subjected to a compressive force, generally called the patellofemoral joint reactive force. Loading on this surface creates a three-point bending configuration in the patella (Fig. 2). This bending load results in tension at the anterior surface of the patella, which is additive to that naturally generated by distraction from contraction of the quadriceps. The relative contribution of these modes of loading of the patella depends primarily on the position of the knee joint. As the knee moves into greater flexion, the bending forces become increasingly important. The magnitude of tensile forces in the anterior surface of the patella reaches a maximum near 45° of knee flexion.[3]

Loads across the patella have not been precisely measured, but they probably are on the order of 3000

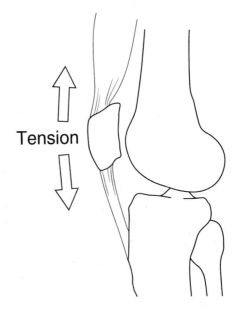

Fig. 1 The patella is loaded primarily in tension when the knee is in full extension. In this position, the patellofemoral contact force is minimum.

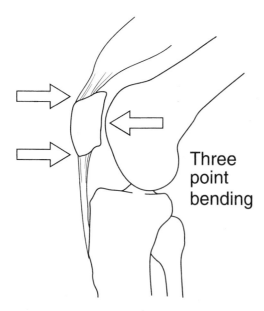

Fig. 2 With the knee in flexion, the patella is loaded in three-point bending as well as in tension. The bending moment increases with increasing knee flexion.

N of tensile load and may rise to 6000 N in young, trained men.[4] Considering the magnitude of tension, three-point bending stress, and compressive forces that occurs on the posterior surface of the patella in a loaded, flexed knee, the recognized prevalence of patellar fracture is not surprising. Studies in our laboratory of strain on the anterior patellar surface demonstrated that normal activities, such as stair-climbing, can generate magnitudes of surface strain that are dangerously close to values that result in a fracture (1000 to 2000 microstrain).[3] These large strains in the patella play a major role in the initiation of fractures and have an equally important effect on the efficacy of various methods of treatment of fractures.

The posterior articular surface of the patella is predominantly convex. The anterior articular surface of the femur is convex as well. Thus, the point of contact for the patellofemoral joint through much of the range of motion of the knee is a transversely linear band. We determined experimentally the contact area for the patellofemoral joint for a range of knee flexion angles and patellofemoral loads.[5] These studies showed small contact areas of approximately 2 to 4 cm² throughout most of the arc of flexion and extension (Fig. 3). The force with which the patella contacts the articular surface of the distal aspect of the femur can be estimated analytically with the use of the primary quadriceps force data reported by Smidt[6] and by Morrison[7] for a variety of activities and knee flexion angles. This provides the essential data for estimation

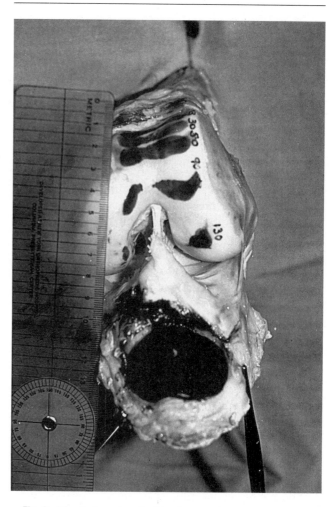

Fig. 3 The dark regions in this photograph of the knee indicate the contact area of the patella on the femur at different positions of knee flexion. These small areas in combination with high loads across the patellofemoral joint result in very high contact stresses (force divided by area).

of the patellofemoral contact stress. For virtually all activities and angles, the patellofemoral contact stresses (2 to 10 N per mm²) exceed those sustained by the tibiofemoral joint (2 to 5 N per mm²) and by other major weight-bearing joints. These high contact stresses magnify the importance of maintenance of articular congruity in the treatment of patellar fractures in order to facilitate and maximize stress distribution.

Classification of Patellar Fractures

Patellar fractures are classified according to both the mechanism of injury and morphology. There are two major mechanisms of injury: direct and indirect trauma. The patella may be fractured by a direct blow during a fall onto the knee or when it hits the dashboard in an automobile accident. Because of the small amount of prepatellar soft tissue and the direct contact with the distal aspect of the femur posteriorly, nearly all of the force of a direct blow is delivered to the patella. Such direct trauma frequently causes considerable comminution, but often there is little displacement of the fracture fragments. With certainty, the articular cartilage of the contact area is damaged by this mechanism of injury.

Indirect trauma that causes fractures can be caused by jumping or, more frequently, by unexpectedly rapid flexion of the knee against a fully contracted quadriceps. The natural anatomy and biomechanics of the knee, as previously described, create tension, three-point bending, and compressive strains in the patella that exceed values sufficient to cause a fracture. Fractures resulting from indirect injury tend to be less comminuted than those from direct trauma, but they are displaced and are often transverse. The articular cartilage is less damaged than with direct trauma.

Most patellar fractures occur as a result of a combination of direct and indirect trauma. Rarely does anyone hit a dashboard with a relaxed quadriceps. In addition, Thompson and associates[8,9] clearly demonstrated that direct blows to the patella of magnitudes less than those sufficient to cause patellar fractures predictably damage the contacting articular cartilage of the patella and femur and that early biochemical

and histologic changes after such blows are consistent with the initiation of post-traumatic osteoarthrosis.

In general, to facilitate treatment, patellar fractures are classified morphologically (Fig. 4). Fractures that occur in a medial-lateral direction are called transverse. These fractures are usually in the central or distal third of the patella. Vertical fractures are in the superior-inferior direction, and they are rare. Fractures of the edge of the patella that do not extend across the patella and that are not associated with disruption of the extensor mechanism are called marginal fractures. Displaced fractures are those with articular incongruity (step-off) of more than 2 mm or separation of the fragments of more than 3 mm.[10] Fractures with multiple fragments are called comminuted fractures. Some comminuted fractures can be characterized as stellate fractures. Some transverse fractures also demonstrate comminution of one or both poles.

Osteochondral fractures are primarily of two types. A direct blow, or more commonly a patellar dislocation, may cause an immediate fracture around the point of contact, separating a single fragment that includes articular cartilage, subchondral bone, and supporting trabecular bone. This piece may never displace, and in this case the fracture usually heals with time and causes little trouble. However, the fragment may displace and become a mechanically troublesome

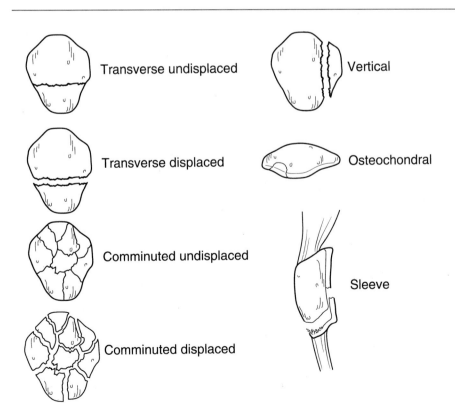

Transverse undisplaced

Transverse displaced

Comminuted undisplaced

Comminuted displaced

Vertical

Osteochondral

Sleeve

Fig. 4 Classification of patellar fractures on the basis of fracture morphology.

loose body. Excision has been recommended[11] in these situations but, for large fragments, stabilization by transosseous fixation with a Herbert screw has been described.[12] The other type of osteochondral fracture, a so-called sleeve fracture, occurs infrequently, when the inferior pole of the patella of a child or adolescent is pulled off together with a considerable amount of articular cartilage.[13] Such a fracture can be difficult to see on standard radiography. Clinical findings of local pain and tenderness, an extension lag (the inability to fully extend the knee actively), and radiographs showing a high-riding patella in comparison with the contralateral, uninjured side support this diagnosis. Houghton and Ackroyd[14] recommended surgical repair of these avulsion fractures. Other authors[13] have indicated that conservative or surgical treatment is appropriate, depending on the extent of the separation of the fragments and the functional capacity of the quadriceps mechanism. Heckman and Alkire[15] emphasized the importance of subluxation or dislocation of the patella in association with fractures and recommended treatment of patellar instability at the same time as the surgical repair of the extensor mechanism.

Evaluation of Patellar Fractures

A carefully recorded history, a thorough physical examination, and an accurate radiographic evaluation ensure diagnostic success. A history of a direct blow, an extraordinary muscle contraction, or unexpected, rapid knee flexion while the quadriceps was contracted, together with localized pain and the inability to strongly extend the knee, is nearly diagnostic. Weak voluntary extension, a palpable defect, and localized contusion, tenderness, and swelling help the examiner to make an accurate diagnosis. High-quality radiographs are necessary for classification of the fracture and facilitation of management decisions. The patella is difficult to see on some anteroposterior radiographs. More often than not, lateral radiographs reveal the comminution of the fracture or separation of the fragments, or both. Some vertical fractures are best seen on tangential or Merchant radiographs.[16] Rare marginal or peripheral fractures must be distinguished from secondary ossification centers that never fused with the body of the patella, creating a bipartite patella. Radiographs of the contralateral knee can help in this differentiation, because bipartite patella rarely occurs unilaterally. Computed tomography or other advanced imaging techniques are usually unnecessary. However, for occult and osteochondral fractures, computed tomography, with or without use of contrast medium, may be helpful. Bone scans have been used to help to identify stress fractures.

Treatment of Patellar Fractures

Conservative Treatment

For undisplaced vertical, peripheral, comminuted, or even transverse fractures associated with 2 mm or less of step-off incongruity in the articular surface, immobilization in a cylinder or an above-the-knee cast with the knee in extension has provided successful treatment.[10] Usually, the extensor mechanism is not totally disrupted at the time of such fractures. Four to six weeks of immobilization followed by gentle but progressive range-of-motion and, later, quadriceps-strengthening exercises produces good results. While a few degrees of extreme flexion are frequently lost, the overall result is a satisfied patient with little or no discomfort or disability. In a series of 212 fractures followed after non-surgical treatment, Boström[17] found slight or no pain in 89% of the patients and normal or slightly impaired function in 91%. The range of motion was 0° to 120° in more than 90%.

Surgical Treatment

Most patellar fractures should be treated surgically. Treatment should be aimed at the preservation of patellar function whenever possible, preferably through open reduction and internal fixation of the fragments. It is important to obtain secure fixation. If there is too much comminution for secure open reduction and internal fixation, but a major (usually superior) fragment with a substantial amount of normal articular cartilage is present, partial patellectomy is the appropriate approach. Occasionally, good distal and proximal pole fragments are present with comminution of the middle of the patella. In such situations, we have successfully removed the comminuted mid-portion, preserving both the proximal and distal poles, and created a smaller but functional patella.

General Surgical Principles

The soft tissue overlying the patella is often injured from direct compression or abrasion at the time of the fracture. In addition, a large fracture hematoma frequently develops, further compromising the soft tissues. Care should be taken to minimize additional injury to the soft tissues from compressive splints, excessive knee flexion, or direct contact with ice. If surgical treatment must be delayed, aspiration of a hematoma that is stretching the anterior skin should be considered. If there is severe compromise of the skin, so that postoperative wound-healing could be at risk, it may be necessary to postpone surgical repair; however, this is unusual. Open fractures of the patella are treated according to the same principles as open fractures of other parts of the skeleton are treated — with immediate irrigation and debridement followed by open reduction and internal fixation and delayed primary closure when the wound is clean.

The fracture can be approached via a midline longitudinal incision or a transverse incision. Although the cosmetic result is superior after a transverse incision, this incision can seldom be used for other procedures on the knee should these become necessary in the future; thus, we prefer a longitudinal incision. Once the fracture has been exposed, a defect in the extensor mechanism extending several centimeters medially or laterally, or both, is usually identified. The fracture site is then irrigated, and the integrity of the fragments is evaluated. Often there is comminution that was not recognized on the radiographs. The decision regarding whether to proceed with an open reduction and internal fixation, a partial patellectomy, or a total patellectomy is then re-evaluated.

Open Reduction and Internal Fixation

Transverse fractures with little or no comminution are the most amenable to treatment with open reduction and internal fixation. Fractures with a small amount of comminution can often be first converted to a simple transverse fracture by lag-screw fixation of the comminuted portion. The 3.5-mm cortical screws are best suited for this application. The most important aspect of surgical repair is assurance of a congruous reduction of the patellar articular surface. This goal should be achievable in the treatment of transverse fractures. However, once the fragments are reduced, there is no longer a large gap in the extensor mechanism and it is difficult to visualize or palpate the articular surface. Anatomic reduction of the anterior surface of the patella does not guarantee an anatomic reduction of the articular surface. It is not unusual for there to be some plastic deformation or comminution of the anterior aspect of the patella as a result of the injury, and this makes this surface unreliable for the judgment of the adequacy of the reduction of the articular surface. Therefore, we recommend extension of the exposure with a medial parapatellar capsular incision for a short distance proximally and medially. There must be enough release to allow adequate palpation and partial visualization of the fracture site to ensure anatomic reduction of the articular surface. It is not necessary to create a large medial arthrotomy, such as would be necessary for eversion and full visualization of the articular surface. The small arthrotomy can be closed after fixation.

Provisional stabilization of the fracture can usually be obtained with one or two bone-reduction forceps or with Kirschner wires. Definitive fixation can be achieved with wires and screws, either alone or in combination. Weber and associates,[18] in a biomechanical study, demonstrated that, of all of the wiring methods, the modified tension-band technique, as popularized

by the AO group, provided the best stability. Curtis[19] recommended use of the tension-band technique with additional circumferential wiring. The modified tension-band technique is currently the most widely accepted, and several studies have shown a high percentage of good results.[20-22] In a clinical series, Bostman and associates[23] found superior results with the modified tension-band technique compared with those obtained with screw fixation, circumferential wiring, and partial patellectomy. The contemporary orthopaedic literature supports the use of this technique whenever possible.[21-24]

The technique involves the use of two parallel 2.0-mm smooth Kirschner wires combined with an 18-gauge wire looped over the Kirschner wires and over the anterior aspect of the patella to act as a tension band (Fig. 5).[25] This anterior tension band neutralizes the large distraction force that occurs across the anterior surface with contraction of the quadriceps and also with flexion of the knee. As tension is resisted by this wire, compressive forces are generated at the posterior aspect of the fracture gap, improving stability at the articular surface. Failures are often directly attributable to errors in surgical technique.[21]

The parallel longitudinal Kirschner wires can be placed initially through the fracture site, brought flush with the fracture surface in a retrograde manner, and then placed across the fracture after reduction. This technique allows for more reliable placement of the longitudinal Kirschner wires in the mid-portion of the patella and is the method that we prefer. Alternatively, reduction may be obtained and secured with reduction forceps, after which the Kirschner wires can be placed

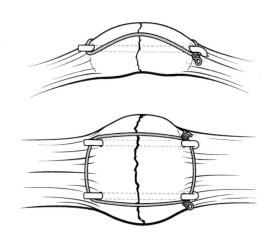

Fig. 5 The AO modified tension-band technique of fracture fixation. Two 2.0-mm Kirschner wires and an anterior tension band are used. As the knee is flexed, the fracture is compressed at the articular surface.

in an antegrade fashion through the patella and across the fracture. It is essential, when the tension band is being applied, that the anterior wire be placed directly adjacent to the patella as it courses posterior to the previously placed Kirschner wires. The most common error in this technique is the failure to bring the tension band directly into contact with the proximal and distal poles of the patella, leaving intervening soft tissue. When this happens and the fracture is then loaded, the fragments may slip apart on the Kirschner wires until the tension band becomes taut.

In an effort to overcome the problem of fragment separation, which can occur with use of the modified tension-band technique, interfragmentary screw fixation has been advocated (Fig. 6). Benjamin and associates,[26] in a biomechanical study, reported that screw fixation resulted in better stability than did the modified tension-band technique for simulated transverse fractures. However, it is not clear if this was a statistically significant difference. Screw fixation alone, however, may not be able to resist the large bending forces that occur with knee flexion, and the addition of a tension band has been advocated by some. Unfortunately, it is difficult to secure the tension band because the screws do not protrude sufficiently from the bone to allow interlocking with the wire. No clinical series of patients treated with the combination of screws and a tension band has been reported, to our knowledge.

At our institution, we evaluated a method in which interfragmentary screw fixation can be easily and securely combined with the use of an anterior tension band (Fig. 7). Theoretically, this construct should provide resistance to fracture displacement from anterior distraction when the knee is in extension as well as resistance to displacement as the knee moves into flexion. This technique was made possible by the development of appropriately sized (4.0 to 4.5-mm) cannulated screws. As with the modified tension-band technique, this method is most appropriate for simple, non-comminuted transverse fractures. As with other techniques of open reduction and internal fixation, reduction can be obtained and confirmed with the aid of a small extension of the arthrotomy on the medial side. Provisional fixation can be achieved with the cannulated-screw guide-wires or with reduction forceps. The screws are placed across the fracture in a lag fashion, with the threads engaging only the far side of the fracture. We found the 4.0 or 4.5-mm screws to be the most appropriate. Screws are best left 4 to 5 mm short of the measured length of the hole, to ensure that they will not protrude beyond the patella and cause stress concentration in the tension band. The 18-gauge tension-band wire is placed through one of the cannulated screws, then over the anterior surface of the patella, through the center of the other cannulated screw, and then back over the anterior surface of

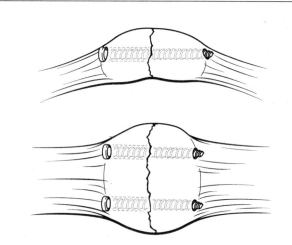

Fig. 6 Stabilization of a transverse patellar fracture with 4.5-mm lag screws alone.

the patella, where it is twisted to the other end of the wire. Two twists in the wire can be used to tighten each limb of the tension band symmetrically (Fig. 7, *bottom*).

Biomechanical analysis of cadaveric knees at our institution showed this construct to fail, on the average, with a quadriceps force of 732 N with the knee flexed 45°, while screws alone failed at 554 N ($p < 0.05$) and the modified tension-band technique alone failed at 395 N ($p < 0.05$). The sites of fractures that had been repaired with the modified tension-band technique and cannulated screws also demonstrated superior rigidity, displacing an average of 1.0 mm with simulated knee extension compared with 1.5 mm (p value not significant) when screws alone had been used and 4.4 mm ($p < 0.05$) when the modified tension-band technique alone had been used. Goings and Cole[27] reported 19 good or excellent results in a series of 21 patients who had been managed with a similar technique.

Partial Patellectomy

Unfortunately, not all patellar fractures are amenable to open reduction and internal fixation. We have found that, in most of the remaining cases, a large fragment of the patella can be preserved. This is most commonly the superior pole, but there are techniques to preserve the inferior pole as well. In a series of 40 patients with 78% good or excellent results reported by Saltzman and associates,[28] the size of the retained fragment was less than 4.1 cm^2 in only one patient. The minimum size of the patellar fragment below which partial patellectomy yielded poor results was not determined, and the minimum size of the patellar fragment needed to allow the performance of

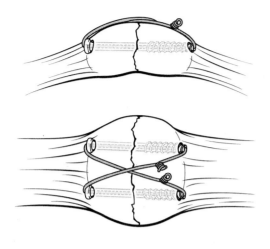

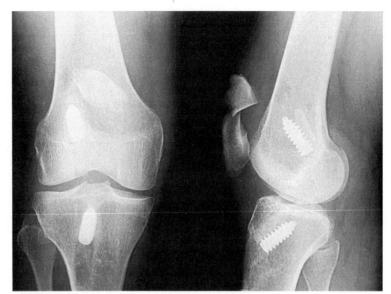

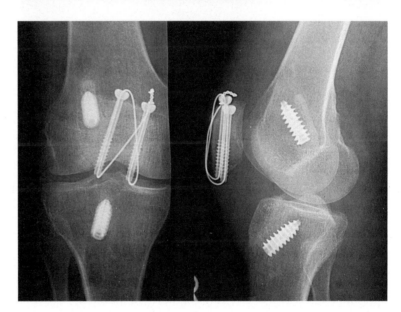

Fig. 7 A fixation technique in which cannulated screws as well as a tension band are used. This construct has proved to be stronger than that achieved with screws alone or with the modified tension-band technique alone in cadaveric knees. **Top left**, Drawing showing the technique. **Top right**, Radiograph showing a displaced, transverse patellar fracture after a reconstruction of the anterior cruciate ligament with a patellar-ligament autogenous graft. **Bottom**, Radiograph made after cannulated screws and tension-band wires were used to stabilize the fracture. The fracture subsequently united.

a partial patellectomy rather than a complete patellectomy has not been established, to our knowledge.

A standard partial patellectomy is performed by the surgeon removing all of the comminuted fragments. It is helpful to preserve as much of the length of the patellar ligament or the quadriceps tendon as possible. The ligament or tendon is then brought to the fractured surface of the patella through the use of multiple drill-holes and heavy non-absorbable sutures (for example, number-2 braided polyester) (Fig. 8). These holes through the fracture surface should enter near the articular surface so that there is a minimum step-off between the tendon and the remaining intact cartilage. The goal is to minimize any abrupt change in the articular surface that could lead to joint overload and

osteoarthrosis as well as to avoid rotation of the fragment anteriorly and posteriorly in the sagittal plane. It is important to try to maintain the length of the remaining ligament or tendon without excessive shortening. This is especially important with excision of the distal pole, which can shorten the patellar ligament markedly, lead to a low-riding patella, and create abnormal patellofemoral biomechanics.

Some surgeons have found it helpful to place a wire in parallel with the ligament repair to act as a check-rein. This wire or cable carries a portion of the load between the patella and the tibial tubercle, thus decreasing the load across the recently repaired patellar ligament-patella junction. Perry and associates[29] showed that this loadsharing cable improved the stabil-

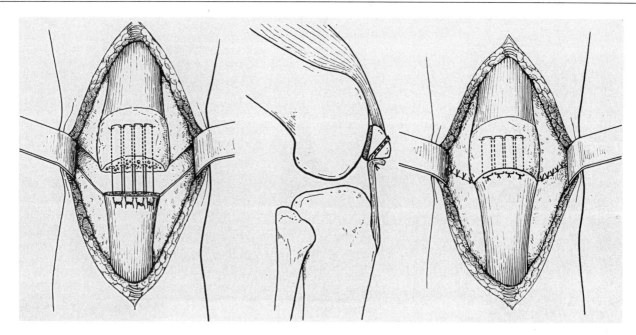

Fig. 8   The technique of partial patellectomy. This procedure is preferred to total patellectomy if open reduction and internal fixation is not possible.

ity of repairs in an experimental study. An 18-gauge wire is placed transversely through a drill-hole across the mid-portion of the remaining patella and through the tibial tubercle, and it is then secured as a loop. The tension on the wire should be adjusted so that the wire protects the ligament repair but is not so tight as to draw the patella distally. Use of this wire allows the patient to obtain a range of motion earlier postoperatively with less fear of disrupting the bone-to-ligament repair. The wire often undergoes fatigue failure, and it should be removed when the repair has healed, at approximately eight weeks. Although no comparable technique can be used when the inferior pole of the patella is repaired to the quadriceps tendon, a heavy suture (such as number-5 braided polyester) can be placed through a transverse patellar drill-hole and secured to the quadriceps tendon several centimeters proximal to the repair site to act as a checkrein and protect the repair. We do not find these techniques to be routinely necessary; however, they can help to protect a tenuous soft-tissue repair as well as to reassure one about the safety of beginning early motion.

In one long-term follow-up study of 40 patients who had been managed with partial patellectomy, the result was excellent in 20 patients (50%), good in 11 (28%), fair in 6 (15%), and poor in 3 (8%).[28] Quadriceps strength was, on the average, 85% of the strength on the uninjured side. Similar results were reported by Andrews and Hughston.[30] They recommended that total patellectomy be done only when the entire patel-

la is so severely comminuted that none of it can be used as part of the extensor mechanism of the knee.

Total Patellectomy

For patients with a severely comminuted fracture with separation of the fragments and no major articular fragment remaining intact, total patellectomy, despite its recognized limitations, may be the only reasonable treatment. The defect resulting from removal of the patella can be closed in a vertical, purse-string, or transverse fashion. There is no convincing evidence to recommend one method or another. After surgical repair, these patients should be managed with application of a cylinder or above-the-knee cast for six weeks, after which the cast is removed and range-of-motion and strengthening exercises are begun. Unfortunately, a loss of range of motion, a loss of knee extensor strength, an extension lag, and persistent discomfort are common after total patellectomy.

Einola and associates[31] found that, of 25 patients who had had a patellectomy, only seven had quadriceps power that was equal to or greater than 75% of the power of the intact knee. Jakobsen and associates[32] found quadriceps power to be, on the average, two-thirds that of the opposite limb. Three long-term studies[23,33,34] have evaluated the clinical results of patellectomy, and while this treatment was found to be better than no treatment at all, there were very few excellent results. When reported, the quadriceps strength was always markedly reduced.[31,32,35] Most authors concluded that an anatomic reduction and secure internal fixation, or partial patellectomy, were preferable to total patellectomy. Total patellectomy should be reserved for salvage treatment of fractures that cannot be fixed or treated with partial patellectomy.

Severe Comminution of the Mid-Part of the Patella with Adequate Poles

On rare occasions, adequate superior and inferior poles remain but the central portion of the patella is severely comminuted. A patella with this unusual frac-

ture pattern can sometimes be salvaged with an open reduction and internal fixation of the proximal pole to the distal pole (after removal of the intervening fragments) with use of either the modified tension-band or the screw technique already described (Fig. 9).

Postoperative Management

Because of the trauma that frequently is sustained by the thin overlying layer of soft tissue, as well as the swelling that occurs with these injuries, it is important

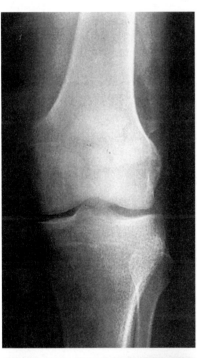
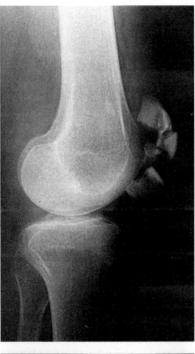

Fig. 9 A closed, comminuted patellar fracture with intact, large inferior and superior-pole fragments. **Top left and top right**, Preoperative radiographs. **Bottom left and bottom center**, Radiographs made after the smaller, comminuted fragments were removed from the mid-portion of the patella and the larger, pole fragments were secured to each other with screws and a tension band. This procedure was done as an alternative to partial patellectomy. **Bottom right**, Intraoperative photograph demonstrating the good alignment of the articular surfaces despite removal of the comminuted mid-portion of the patella.

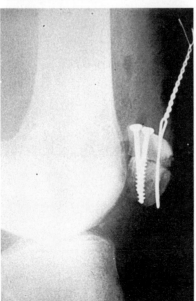
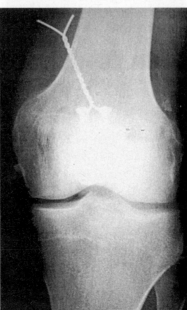
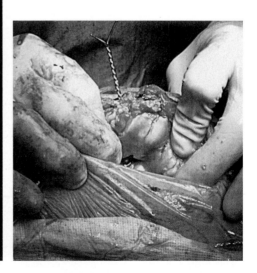

to monitor the wound closely after the operation. Placement of tight bandages or prolonged contact with ice may compromise wound-healing. Marked erythema and prolonged swelling commonly occur and are at times worrisome, as they may suggest infection; however, they usually resolve.

Postoperative continuous passive motion may reduce stiffness of the knee and improve healing of articular cartilage. This technique might be most effective when an osteochondral fracture has been treated with excision of fragments and there are remaining areas of exposed bone surface. However, the role of continuous passive motion after patellar fractures has not been determined.

It is generally impossible to maintain the patella in a mechanically unloaded state postoperatively. Even with the knee in full extension, the fracture is loaded with each contraction of the quadriceps. Weightbearing itself does not increase quadriceps force; it may actually reduce the force of the contraction of the quadriceps compared with the force that results from the limb being held up in a nonweightbearing state. Thus, weightbearing, with use of an external support for balance, should be permitted as tolerated.

Once wound healing is satisfactory, a range of motion can generally be permitted. The amount of motion that is allowed and the time that is needed before a range of motion is initiated depend on the stability of the surgical repair. With well-fixed, simple, transverse fractures, a range of motion can be initiated within the first several weeks. The ideal techniques for early range of motion have not been identified. Disruptive forces are minimized with active flexion followed by passive extension.

Patellar mobilization techniques can be safely performed early postoperatively. A removable splint may be used for protection between periods of rehabilitation. With rare exceptions, a range of motion should be initiated by six weeks to prevent prolonged stiffness of the knee. It is preferable for most patients who have had secure surgical repair to begin motion well before this time. Resistive exercises, however, should be delayed until there is evidence of fracture healing. Use of a protective splint and crutches can generally be discontinued when the range of motion has reached 90° and good quadriceps control has returned.

Complications

Infection

Fortunately, infection after a repair of a patellar fracture is uncommon; however, because the thin overlying skin is often damaged, wound healing can be delayed and infections may develop. Infection can be treated with local wound care and antibiotics or, occasionally, with open irrigation and debridement followed by delayed wound closure. Superficial infections can be managed initially with local wound care and antibiotics. However, if the infection extends below the subcutaneous tissue or if there is a question of septic osteoarthrosis, a formal incision and drainage should be performed, followed by delayed closure. Occasionally, joint aspiration through an uninfected area, with a cell count and culture of the fluid, helps to guide treatment.

Loss of Fixation

Loss of fracture fixation and reduction is a disheartening complication after open reduction and internal fixation of patellar fractures. This complication is most commonly due to unrecognized or underappreciated fragment comminution, usually involving the distal pole (Fig. 10). This condition allows the fixation

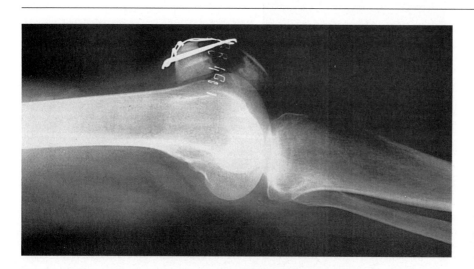

Fig. 10 Radiograph showing loss of fixation following modified tension-band repair because of comminution at the distal pole of the patella.

wires or screws to slide through the substance of the distal pole with contraction of the quadriceps. If it is recognized before there is marked displacement and the development of articular incongruity, immobilization with the knee in extension and suspension of motion may prevent further displacement while allowing for satisfactory healing. If, however, major displacement (more than 3 mm) occurs, further surgery may be necessary. Partial patellectomy is generally the most successful salvage procedure. This problem is best prevented by avoidance of open reduction and internal fixation when the quality of the bone is questionable.

Knee Stiffness

Some slight loss of knee motion after a patellar fracture is the rule rather than the exception. Generally, only a few degrees of flexion is lost while full extension is maintained. Early motion (within the first one or two weeks) may help to reduce the incidence of postoperative stiffness, so it is important to obtain secure fixation at the time of the repair. Prolonged immobilization of a knee that has been treated surgically can lead to postoperative contracture. If an extension contracture develops despite intensive physical therapy, secondary surgical treatment (removal of fracture fixation hardware and knee arthroscopy with lysis of adhesions) may be necessary. Depending on the severity of the patellar restriction, lateral or medial release, or both, may be necessary. Manipulation of the knee should be included as part of this procedure, but it should be done gently and with consideration for the compromised extensor mechanism. Quadricepsplasty is not indicated unless there has been an associated quadriceps or femoral injury.

Post-Traumatic Osteoarthrosis

Because of the magnitude of the loads across the patellofemoral joint, post-traumatic osteoarthrosis following patellar fracture is not uncommon.[10] Sørensen[36] evaluated patients 10 to 30 years after a patellar fracture and found that 45 (70%) of 64 knees demonstrated patellofemoral osteoarthrosis compared with 20 (31%) of the contralateral, uninjured knees. Osteoarthrosis may be caused by residual joint incongruity and the resulting increased contact stresses, which lead to overload and premature degeneration of the articular cartilage. Additionally, the articular surfaces are frequently injured at the time of the fracture, especially when the fracture resulted from a direct blow. This type of damage may lead to osteoarthrosis, even with good fracture reduction and repair.[37] Although there is no simple way to manage post-traumatic osteoarthrosis, symptoms may be reduced with partial patellectomy, elevation of the tibial tubercle, or even total patellectomy. Clearly, the goal in fracture management is avoidance of this complication by accurate fracture reduction and minimization of additional insults to the articular surface.

Nonunion

Presently, nonunion after a fracture of the patella is uncommon because of the frequent surgical management of displaced fractures. However, in the past, displaced patellar fractures were more often treated nonsurgically and nonunion was more common. In a long-term follow-up study of patients who had been managed from 1930 to 1951, Sørensen[36] found that 10% to 55% of the patellar fractures did not unite. Recently, the rate of nonunion was reported to be on the order of 1% or less.[20,23] If nonunion does occur, treatment should be based on the symptoms. A patient with a painless nonunion and a well functioning extensor mechanism does not need treatment. However, if the nonunion is painful or results in noticeable weakness of the extensor mechanism, the indicated treatment is open reduction and internal fixation with excision of intervening fibrous tissue and supplemental bone-grafting if it is needed to correct a large osseous defect. However, if adequate bone stock is not present, partial patellectomy is probably the procedure of choice.

Irritation From Hardware

Because the patella is a subcutaneous bone, hardware that has been used for fracture fixation is frequently palpable. Wires and wire knots seem to be particularly irritating to tissues; screws are less commonly bothersome. We do not think that routine removal is necessary, but we remove hardware readily after the fracture is solidly united if the patient has discomfort.

Summary

Patellar fractures usually occur from distraction and three-point bending of the patella as well as from direct blows. Surgical treatment is necessary for fractures that are displaced more than 2 mm and may include open reduction and internal fixation, partial patellectomy, or rarely, total patellectomy. We have presented a new technique for the stabilization of a simple transverse fracture that has provided superior results in laboratory tests. Postoperative complications can be minimized by good attention to wound care, accurate fracture reduction, secure fracture fixation, and an early range of motion. Despite the surgeon's best efforts, however, post-traumatic osteoarthrosis can develop and may require additional treatment.

References

1. Kaufer H: Mechanical function of the patella. *J Bone Joint Surg* 1971;53A:1551-1560.
2. Wendt PP, Johnson RP: A study of quadriceps excursion, torque, and the effect of patellectomy on cadaver knees. *J Bone Joint Surg* 1985;67A:726-732.

3. Goldstein SA, Coale E, Weiss A-P, et al: Patellar surface strain. *J Orthop Res* 1986;4:372-377.

4. Huberti HH, Hayes WC, Stone JL, et al: Force ratios in the quadriceps tendon and ligamentum patellae. *J Orthop Res* 1984;2:49-54.

5. Matthews LS, Sonstegard DA, Henke JA: Load bearing characteristics of the patello-femoral joint. *Acta Orthop Scand* 1977;48:511-516.

6. Smidt GL: Biomechanical analysis of knee flexion and extension. *J Biomech* 1973;6:79-92.

7. Morrison JB: The mechanics of muscle function in locomotion. *J Biomech* 1970;3:431-451.

8. Thompson RC Jr: An experimental study of surface injury to articular cartilage and enzyme responses within the joint. *Clin Orthop* 1975;107:239-248.

9. Thompson RC Jr, Oegema TR Jr, Lewis JL, et al: Osteoarthrotic changes after acute transarticular load: An animal model. *J Bone Joint Surg* 1991;73A:990-1001.

10. Edwards B, Johnell O, Redlund-Johnell I: Patellar fractures: A 30-year follow-up. *Acta Orthop Scand* 1989;60:712-714.

11. Rorabeck CH, Bobechko WP: Acute dislocation of the patella with osteochondral fracture: A review of eighteen cases. *J Bone Joint Surg* 1976;58B(2):237-240.

12. Rae PS, Khasawneh ZM: Herbert screw fixation of osteochondral fractures of the patella. *Injury* 1988;19:116-119.

13. Grogan, DP, Carey TP, Leffers D, et al: Avulsion fractures of the patella. *J Pediatr Orthop* 1990;10:721-730.

14. Houghton GR, Ackroyd CE: Sleeve fractures of the patella in children: A report of three cases. *J Bone Joint Surg* 1979;61-B:165-168.

15. Heckman JD, Alkire CC: Distal patellar pole fractures: A proposed common mechanism of injury. *Am J Sports Med* 1984;12:424-428.

16. Merchant AC, Mercer RL, Jacobsen RH, et al: Roentgenographic analysis of patellofemoral congruence. *J Bone Joint Surg* 1974;56A:1391-1396.

17. Boström A: Fracture of the patella: A study of 422 patellar fractures. *Acta Orthop Scand* 1972;143(suppl): S1–S80.

18. Weber MJ, Janecki CJ, McLeod P, et al: Efficacy of various forms of fixation of transverse fractures of the patella. *J Bone Joint Surg* 1980;62A:215-220.

19. Curtis MJ: Internal fixation for fractures of the patella: A comparison of two methods. *J Bone Joint Surg* 1990;72B:280-282.

20. Bostman O, Kiviluoto O, Nirhamo J: Comminuted displaced fractures of the patella. *Injury* 1981;13:196-202.

21. Hung LK, Chan KM, Chow YN, et al: Fractured patella: Operative treatment using the tension band principle. *Injury* 1985;16:343-347.

22. Levack B, Flannagan JP, Hobbs S: Results of surgical treatment of patellar fractures. *J Bone Joint Surg* 1985;67B:416-419.

23. Bostman O, Kiviluoto O, Santavirta S, et al: Fractures of the patella treated by operation. *Arch Orthop Trauma Surg* 1983;102:78-81.

24. Haajanen J, Karaharju E: Fractures of the patella: One hundred consecutive cases. *Ann Chir Gynaecol* 1981;70:32-35

25. Müller ME, Allgower M, Schneider R, et al: *Manual of Internal Fixation. Techniques Recommended by the AO Group*, translated by Schatzker J, ed. 2. New York, NY, Springer-Verlag, 1979, pp 248-252.

26. Benjamin J, Bried J, Dohm M, et al: Biomechanical evaluation of various forms of fixation of transverse patellar fractures. *J Orthop Trauma* 1987;1:219-222.

27. Goings GS, Cole JD: The use of cannulated screws and titanium cable for the fixation of patella fractures. Poster exhibit at the Annual Meeting of The American Academy of Orthopaedic Surgeons, San Francisco, CA, February 18, 1993.

28. Saltzman CL, Goulet JA, McClellan RT, et al: Results of treatment of displaced patellar fractures by partial patellectomy. *J Bone Joint Surg* 1990;72A:1279-1285.

29. Perry CR, McCarthy JA, Kain CC, et al: Patellar fixation protected with a load-sharing cable: A mechanical and clinical study. *J Orthop Trauma* 1988;2:234-240.

30. Andrews JR, Hughston JC: Treatment of patellar fractures by partial patellectomy. *South Med J* 1977;70:809-813,817.

31. Einola S, Aho AJ, Kallio P: Patellectomy after fracture: Long-term follow-up results with special reference to functional disability. *Acta Orthop Scand* 1976;47:441-447.

32. Jakobsen J, Christensen KS, Rasmussen OS: Patellectomy: A 20-year follow-up. *Acta Orthop Scand* 1985;56:430-432.

33. Sutton FS Jr, Thompson CH, Lipke J, et al: The effect of patellectomy on knee function. *J Bone Joint Surg* 1976;58A:537-540.

34. Wilkinson J: Fracture of the patella treated by total excision. A long-term follow-up. *J Bone Joint Surg* 1977;59B:352-354.

35. Peeples RE, Margo MK: Function after patellectomy. *Clin Orthop* 1978;132:180-186.

36. Sørensen KH: The late prognosis after fracture of the patella. *Acta Orthop Scand* 1964;34:198-212.

37. Donohue JM, Buss D, Oegema TR Jr, et al: The effects of indirect blunt trauma on adult canine articular cartilage. *J Bone Joint Surg* 1983;65A:948-957.

Treatment Options for Fractures of the Distal Femur

Roby Mize, MD

Introduction

Early attempts at internal fixation of distal femur fractures frequently gave unacceptably high rates of malunion, nonunion, and infection. Over the past 15 years, improved techniques of internal fixation have yielded results far superior to those achieved with traditional nonsurgical management. Meticulous internal fixation has been shown to yield good to excellent results in 60% to 80% of cases and allows immediate mobilization of the patient and the extremity, sparing the cardiopulmonary and other multisystem sequelae of long immobility.[1] A number of excellent devices are now available to provide the surgeon with improved techniques for fixation of these fractures. These include, but are not limited to: the 95° angled blade plate, the 95° condylar screw, the cloverleaf condylar plate, combined medial/lateral double plates, the locked intramedullary (IM) nail, and the Zickel supracondylar nail.

Mechanisms of Injury

Among young patients, fractures of the distal femur are usually a component of multiple trauma sustained in a high-velocity, high-impact injury, such as motor vehicle accidents or falls from a height. In particular, motorcycle accidents are a prime cause for these fractures in the patient aged 17 to 30 years. In the adult, fractures of the distal 15 cm of the femur account for only 7% of all femoral fractures, but as a result of our modern lifestyles and of high-velocity transportation, the incidence of these injuries is increasing.[2,3] The elderly patient may present with fractures due to trivial trauma, such as falling on the flexed knee.

Traditionally, skeletal traction followed by some type of external immobilization has been used to treat this injury.[4-6] Complications associated with closed management of this fracture led to the development of alternative methods of internal fixation.

Principles of Treatment

The objectives of surgical treatment of fractures of the distal femur are anatomic restoration and stable fixation. The Association for Study of Internal Fixation (AO/ASIF) developed the basic principles for successful surgical treatment of fractures. The distal femur fracture is difficult to treat. Regardless of which implant is used, in order to obtain the objectives the following basic principles must be upheld: (1) good preoperative planning; (2) careful atraumatic surgical technique; (3) accurate anatomic reduction; (4) stable internal fixation; (5) bone grafting of any defects; and (6) early, active rehabilitation of the injured limb and the patient.

Much of the credit for formulating and continuing to emphasize these basic principles should be given to the AO/ASIF Group from Switzerland. This unique group was organized in 1958 by Professor Martin Allgower of Basel and Maurice Müller of Bern.[7]

Classification

The classification of fractures traditionally serves to organize treatment approach and to provide a conceptual basis for comparing the results of various treatments. Charles Neer, MD was an early pioneer in the management of this injury. He developed a good classification, but one that did not address all the variables of a fracture of the distal femur.[8]

The AO/ASIF classification developed by Müller and associates[9] is an excellent anatomic classification system that differentiates between variations on three sets of circumstances. A_1, A_2, and A_3 are fractures proximal to the condyles with the condyles still basically intact. B_1, B_2, and B_3 are variations of a single condylar fracture. C_1, C_2, and C_3 are the more complex multicondylar fractures combined with associated supracondylar fractures (Fig. 1).

Although Müller presented an excellent classification, it, too, fails to describe all the complex and variable aspects of this injury. Other factors that may keep some fractures from falling comfortably into classification parameters play an important role in determining the approach to treatment and its outcome. These factors establish the "personality" of the fracture, and include: the presence of displaced fragments; the degree of comminution; the extent and degree of soft-tissue damage; associated neurovascular damage; the degree of articular involvement; bone quality; severity of multisystem injuries; and the presence of other fractures.

With the infinite variation in the type and degree of these contributing factors, many fractures are not easily comparable. Each case must be approached individ-

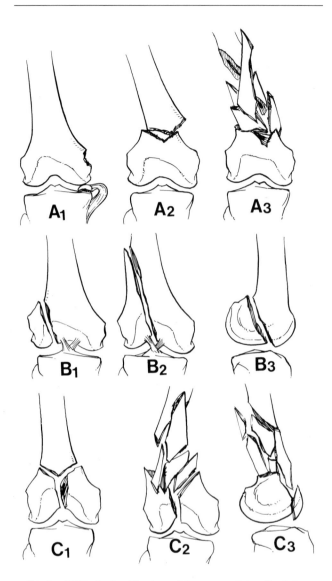

Fig. 1   Müller's classification of fractures of the distal femur. (Reproduced with permission from Müller ME: *Manual of Internal Fixation*, ed 2. New York, NY, Springer-Verlag, 1979.)

ually, and all factors must be considered when formulating a management plan.

As with most controversial fractures, there are basically two schools of thought concerning treatment: those who recommend closed, conservative treatment, and those who tend to operate.

Closed Treatment

Definite indications for the standard conservative closed treatment of this fracture include: the paraplegic or nonambulatory patient; the elderly patient with severe, massive comminution and/or osteopenia; and the rare, nondisplaced fracture.

In 1970, Mooney and associates[6] introduced the ambulatory cast/brace. This type of cast has contri-

buted significantly to overcoming many of the problems involved with closed methods. In 1974, Mays and Neufeld[10] introduced roller traction, which added another dimension to the closed method. It is similar to a cast/brace, but can be applied shortly after admission. The patient is allowed out of bed two to five days following injury. Cast/bracing and roller traction techniques are safe, but they are not free from major complications and the results are not always good. Associated problems with cast/bracing include shortening, angular and rotational deformities, restriction of joint motion, incongruity of the articular surfaces, residual traumatic arthritis, delayed unions and nonunions (infrequent), and the need for prolonged hospitalization. Meticulous attention to detail and high tolerance on the part of both the physician and patient are required with closed treatment of distal femur fractures.

Open Surgical Treatment

Choosing a Surgical Method

A prerequisite for the selection of the surgical method is adequate institutional support. Such support includes adequate instrumentation, skilled and experienced operating room personnel, and experienced physical medicine support.

Choosing a Fixation Device

The type of fixation device used depends on the type of fracture, available instrumentation, and the surgeon's experience and skill. Fractures of the distal femur may be repaired using cancellous screws, the condylar screw system, the angled blade plate, the cloverleaf condylar plate, combined medial/lateral double plates, the interlocking intramedullary nail, the supracondylar nail, or external fixation.[11,12]

Although the one-piece design and U-shaped blade of the angled blade plate provide the most stable fixation, the blade plate is technically much more difficult to use. Therefore, I recommend the AO/ASIF condylar screw system. This screw system is a refinement of the supracondylar plate and lag screw previously reported by numerous authors.[13-20] Simpler fixation devices have been reported, but most do not provide rigid fixation, thus negating the advantage of their simplicity. In dealing with the distal femur, the method of fixation and type of implant depends largely on the type of fracture.

The Angled Blade Plate   The condylar plate is a one-piece angled blade plate with a 95° fixed angle between the blade and the plate (Fig. 2, *top*). The blade is U-shaped, which contributes to the extreme strength of this device. Due to its one-piece construction and the broad flat blade, the blade plate provides stable fixa-

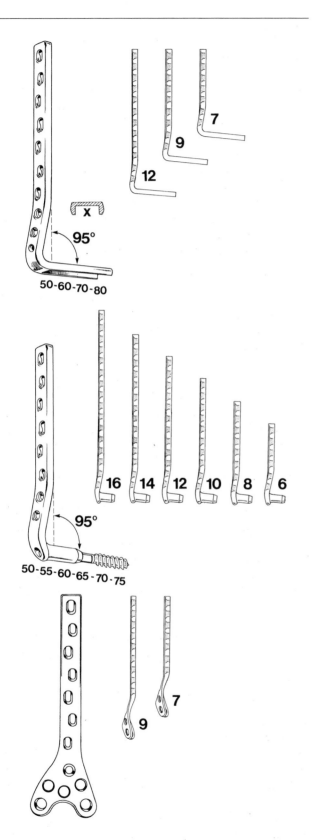

Fig. 2 Top, The angled blade plate. **Center,** The condylar screw system. **Bottom,** The cloverleaf condylar plate. (Reproduced with permission from Mize RD: Supracondylar and articular fractures of the distal femur, in Chapman MW (ed): *Operative Orthopaedics.* Philadelphia, PA, JB Lippincott, 1988, chap 45.)

tion for most fracture types. However, the one-piece characteristic of the plate also makes it difficult to use. Precision and correct alignment in all three planes is required for the insertion of this device.

The Condylar Screw System The condylar screw is basically a two-piece device connected with a small compressing screw (Fig. 2, *center*). It has a 95° angle between the screw and the side plate, and both the screw and side plate are available in a variety of lengths. Because it consists of two pieces, an advantage of the condylar screw is that, by rotating the screw, corrections may be made in the lateral or coronal plane after the lag screw has been inserted. Precise seating is also easier because the channel is precut directly over the guide wire. The cannulated triple reamer used for cutting the channel has less risk of disrupting split condyles than the seating chisel, especially in young, hard, cancellous bone. Another advantage of the condylar screw is its ability to compress condylar fragments.[21]

Both the condylar plate and screw must be inserted not only parallel to the knee joint, but also at a predetermined inclination and alignment to the femoral shaft. Proper alignment may prove difficult until the technique, which involves the use of K-wires and the available aiming devices, is mastered. With practice in the laboratory, experience with simple fractures, and good preoperative planning with close attention to detail, the technique can be mastered.

Cloverleaf Condylar Plate Regardless of the implant chosen, it is important to prepare a heavy cloverleaf condylar plate as a backup device (Fig. 2, *bottom*). For selected cases, this implant may be the only device that will succeed. For example, if the lateral condyle is comminuted or if there are multiple articular fracture lines in both the sagittal and coronal planes, both the condylar screw and the angled plate may be impossible to use. The cloverleaf condylar plate is an excellent device to salvage a failed condylar screw or a 95°-angled blade plate.

Although the cloverleaf condylar plate is technically easier to apply, it should not be used indiscriminately. A major problem with this device is its lack of a rigid interface between the heads of the screws and the plate; therefore, any deficiency of the medial cortex usually results in varus malalignment at four to six weeks postoperatively. If the fracture is not accurately reduced before this implant is introduced, distal fragment displacement into valgus alignment may result.

Because of its multipiece construction, when combined with the cancellous screws, the cloverleaf plate is not as strong as either the condylar screw system or the blade plate.

Medial/Lateral Double Plates A good solution for the fracture with severe deficiency on the medial side is the use of combined medial and lateral plates (Fig. 3). Both plates may be applied through separate incisions

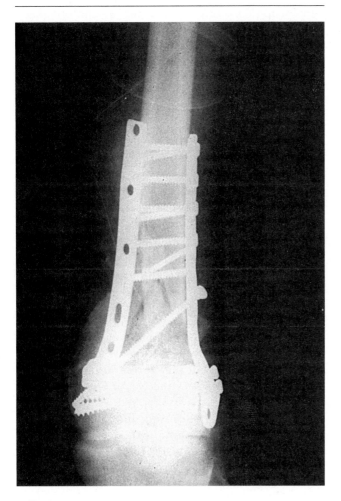

Fig. 3 The application of medial/lateral double plating.

during the primary procedure, or the additional plate may be applied secondarily. Any defects on the medial side should always be bone grafted. Sanders and associates[18] have discussed the use of double plating for unstable fractures of the distal femur.

The Interlocking Intramedullary Nail Some success has been reported with the interlocking intramedullary nail system.[22-26] Although the interlocking nail is a great improvement over traditional reamed intramedullary nailing and allows a greater number of comminuted and distal femoral fractures to be treated successfully, the risk of implant failure is great because of a high rate of nail breakage.[24,27] The nails are most likely to break when the screw holes are placed too close to the fracture site. Bucholz and associates[28] have stressed the importance of delayed weightbearing and suggest at least 5 cm of unobstructed bone around the nail hole to avoid breakage.

Although the interlocking nail allows early range of motion, once fracture union has occurred there is often unsatisfactory knee function.[29] Thus, a formal knee rehabilitation program is essential for good results. The interlocking screw system has an additional complication, in that effective screw placement is difficult. A freehand method of placement under fluoroscopic vision is generally employed, but it may require repeated drilling of the lateral cortex.[30] The drill tip can easily be directed toward a nail wall rather than through the interlocking holes and can contribute to nail breakage.[28,30] In osteopenic bone, screws may be completely misguided, resulting in thread damage and poor fixation.

Effective guiding systems have been explored, with some success being achieved using a laser-directed system. The intersection of perpendicular planes of a laser light can be aligned with the central X-ray beam. Once the correct line of entry is established, only the planes of light are needed to guide the drill, minimizing the surgeon's direct exposure to the X-ray. The image intensifier is then used to confirm the progression of the drill in anteroposterior and lateral views.[30]

The Supracondylar Nail Another interesting device that shows promise in selective cases is the supracondylar nail developed by Zickel and associates.[31] This device is particularly useful in the elderly patient with osteopenia. It is not suited for younger patients because of the frequent complication of shortening with any degree of comminution. Other technical problems surround the Zickel device.[32]

GSH Intramedullary Nail An internal fixation device that may become available for the treatment of distal femur fractures is the GSH intramedullary nail. This device, developed by Green, Seligson, and Henry, consists of a cannulated, single-piece, stainless steel implant that is produced in both 11 and 12 mm diameters. Henry believes that, when compared to traditional plate/screw devices, the intramedullary position of the GSH nail probably reduces operating time, decreases blood loss, and limits surgical dissection/exposure (Stephen Henry, personal communication, 1992).

External Fixation

Application of external fixation to the distal femur is quite limited. At least 10 cm of intact bone proximal to the articular joint line of the knee is a prerequisite for stable external fixation.

In my opinion, the only external fixation device that provides stable fixation for fractures of the femoral shaft is the Wagner apparatus.[33,34] Two Shantz screws placed proximally and two placed distally to the fracture site secure the device. This massive, telescopic, rectangular column maintains bone length without obstructing access to soft tissues.

The Wagner device allows immediate active mobilization with nonweightbearing crutch ambulation on the fourth postoperative day. Advantages include a unilateral configuration, a compact low profile, reduced surgical exposure, and the need for less metal than a large internal implant. Disadvantages of external fixation include a slow recovery of motion, pin-site infection, pin loosening or breakage, and the danger of nonunion.

Special Management Problems

The elderly patient with a fracture of the distal femur and the patient with an open fracture of the distal femur present special management problems in the treatment of this fracture.

The Elderly Patient Many orthopaedic surgeons consider advanced age and osteopenic bone contraindications for internal fixation. Usually, traction followed by cast/bracing is their treatment choice.[4-6] However, I believe that each case must be individualized. Advanced age alone should not be considered a contraindication to internal fixation. In certain cases, internal fixation for an osteopenic elderly patient may be the only solution. I have had good to excellent results in 20 of 25 elderly patients treated with internal fixation.[35] Surgical fixation is preferred in an attempt to avoid the complications of prolonged bed rest. However, with the presence of osteopenia, obtaining stable fixation is difficult, or perhaps impossible. Postoperative cast bracing or roller traction is frequently indicated.

Open fractures Patients with open fractures constitute another group that demands individual attention and considerable judgment. Critical factors include the condition of the soft tissues and any associated injuries. Soft tissues must be in sufficiently good condition to withstand major surgery. Surgical stabilization frequently eases the treatment of the soft tissues and mobilizes the patient earlier, and it facilitates the nursing care and decreases the hospital stay.[36] Regardless of the method of treatment chosen, wound debridement is mandatory and is the cornerstone of open fracture treatment.

Technique

The more technical aspects of management of this fracture include preoperative planning, surgical approach, bone grafting, and postoperative management.

Preoperative Planning

Once the decision for surgery has been made, preoperative planning is critical. For every periarticular fracture of the distal femur, a radiograph of the opposite normal femur is helpful. Accurate anteroposterior and lateral radiographs are centered on the joint. Also, a tunnel view of the intercondylar notch is helpful in judging the displacement of vertical fractures into the joint. Outlines of the normal femur, the fracture lines,

and the proposed position of the plate and screws are drawn on the radiograph with the aid of plastic templates. The chief surgeon must review and discuss the procedure step-by-step with the assistant surgeons. All necessary instruments, implants, and back-up devices should be obtained and prepared for use before surgery. This type of careful preoperative planning is instrumental in accomplishing an atraumatic surgical technique and a successful outcome.

The Surgical Approach

For the purposes of this explanation, I have chosen a Müller type C_1 injury, the so-called T or Y fracture with split condyles. The patient is positioned supine with a bolster under the knee to allow 90° of flexion. In the past, I recommended a lateral curvilinear incision to the level of the knee joint, extending distally and medially directly to the tibial tuberosity (Fig. 4, *top*). Several years ago, we modified this approach.[37] The basic incision is almost the same, but the distal portion ends *just lateral* to the tibial tuberosity (Fig. 4, bottom). If a more extensive exposure is required, the incision may be extended distally to the tibial tuberosity. The tuberosity may then be osteotomized with its attached patellar tendon and the entire quadriceps mechanism reflected. This exposure is easier for residents who have limited experience with this difficult fracture. With increased experience and expertise, it should rarely be necessary to osteotomize the tuberosity; however, this option should be retained when making the initial skin incision.

To accomplish this exposure (Fig. 4, *bottom*), the incision is extended to a point about 15 mm distal to the tibial tuberosity. The retinacular dissection is extended along the lateral margin of the patellar tendon. At this point, the tibial tuberosity should be fully exposed. A block of the tibial tuberosity is osteotomized. The block of tuberosity, with attached tendon and patella, is reflected medially to give complete exposure to the anterior and articular surfaces of the distal femur. Following the fixation of the fracture, the block of tuberosity is replaced in its bed and stabilized with a large 6.5-mm cancellous screw (Fig. 5). The screw should engage the posterior cortex.

Indications for the extensile surgical approach are quite limited. The most frequent indication for this approach is the inability to obtain an accurate reduction and stable fixation with the conventional lateral approach. Also, this approach is most useful for comminuted, displaced intra-articular fractures in multiple planes. Another definite indication for this approach is an intercondylar fracture of the femur associated with an ipsilateral displaced fracture of the tibial plateau.

With either surgical approach, care should be taken to remain anterior to the lateral collateral ligament. Lift the vastus lateralis upward and anteriorly, carefully

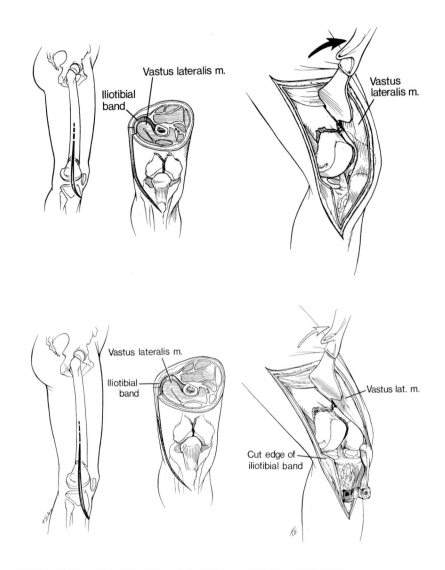

Fig. 4 **Top**, A lateral surgical approach to the distal femur. The incision is anterior to the lateral collateral ligament. The iliotibial band is opened in line with the skin incision. The distal femur is exposed by lifting the entire vastus lateralis muscle from the intermuscular septum by retracting anteriorly and medially. **Bottom**, A modified extensile surgical approach. The skin incision for the extensile approach extends to a point 15 mm distal to the tibial tuberosity. Proximally, the dissection is carried down to the femur, posterior to the vastus lateralis muscle, and anterior to the intermuscular septum. After the tibial tuberosity is elevated, a good exposure of all components of the fracture is achieved. (Reproduced with permission from Mize RD: Complex fractures of the distal end of the femur, in Meyers MH (ed): *The Multiply Injured Patient with Complex Fractures*. Malvern, PA, Lea & Febiger, 1984, chap 22, pp 275-290.)

ligate perforators to minimize blood loss, and avoid a transmuscular approach, because it leads to scarring and to binding down of the quadriceps.

Open the joint in front of the lateral ligament to gain a wide exposure of the joint so that the reduction of the articular surfaces is carried out under direct vision. Reduce the condyles with the knee flexed to 90°. Then, temporarily fix the condyles with a few crossed K-wires.

Bone Grafting

In 1989, we reported our first 68 cases, of which it was necessary to graft 59.[35] There is almost always medial instability with distal femur fractures because of compression forces on the medial aspect of the fracture site (Fig. 6). If a medial defect is present due to comminution, the femur will collapse under cyclic

axial loading from bending forces on the plate exactly opposite the defect (Fig. 7).

After the fracture is stabilized, the condition of the medial buttress can be assessed. If the medial buttress is found to be defective, autologous cancellous bone grafting is indicated. Failure to graft these defects can lead to possible implant failure, loss of reduction, and delayed union or nonunion. The graft may be taken from the anterior iliac crest or the ipsilateral trochanteric area. I prefer the anterior iliac crest as the donor site.

Closure and Postoperative Management

Suction drainage is recommended in all cases to prevent the formation of a hematoma. The synovial tissue, lateral retinaculum, and iliotibial band are closed in a routine fashion. The vastus lateralis muscle should

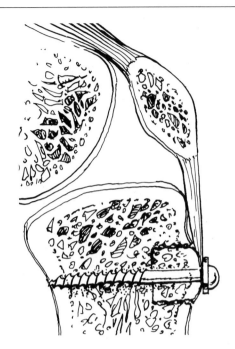

Fig. 5   Replacing the block of tuberosity. The stabilizing screw should engage the posterior cortex. (Reproduced with permission from Mize RD, Bucholz RW, Grogan DP: Surgical treatment of displaced, comminuted fractures of the distal end of the femur. *J Bone Joint Surg* 1982;64A:871-879.)

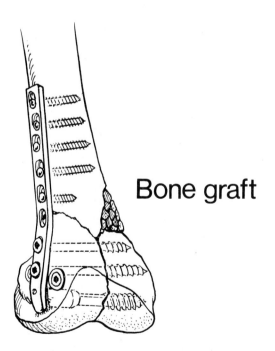

Fig. 6   Medial instability grafting. (Reproduced with permission from Mize RD: Complex fractures of the distal end of the femur, in Meyers MH (ed): *The Multiply Injured Patient with Complex Fractures.* Malvern, PA, Lea & Febiger, 1984, chap 22, pp 275-290.)

not be sutured to the intermuscular septum; doing so may retard recovery of knee motion. Meticulous closure of the skin is recommended.

Early active mobility of the patient and the limb with progressive, carefully staged weightbearing are the keys to successful postoperative management.

In the past, I recommended placing the limb in a Boehler frame with the hip and knee flexed to 90°. However, if available, I believe this type of injury is well suited for continuous passive motion (CPM), as popularized by Salter. The 90°/90° position, together with CPM, prevents quadriceps contracture, helps decrease swelling in the limb, and enhances postoperative range of motion. The CPM machine may be used with the suction drains in place. The drains usually are removed 24 to 48 hours postoperatively.

Without access to a CPM machine, the limb is maintained in the 90°/90° position for four to six days. While the limb is on the frame, the physical therapist may begin gentle, active, assisted range of motion. Early in the recovery period, the patient and the family should be educated on the danger of full weightbearing too soon, and reminded frequently thereafter. Early excessive weightbearing can lead to implant failure, resulting in deformity or delayed healing, and often resulting in the need for repeat surgery.

On about the fifth postoperative day, the patient is assisted in sitting on the side of the bed and dangling the legs. Gait training proceeds from parallel bars to the use of a walker or crutches. If fracture fixation is stable, the patient may begin partial weightbearing of about 10 kg. This can be practiced using ordinary bathroom scales. Complete nonweightbearing with the hip and knee flexed leads to circulatory stasis and rapid disuse osteoporosis.

The toe-touch gait using two crutches is maintained until there is clinical and radiographic evidence of

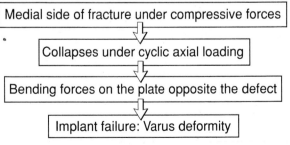

Fig. 7   The progression of a medial instability to varus deformity.

consolidation of the fracture. As a general rule, the patient should use two crutches for about two months, then may progress to one crutch for an additional one to two months. Full weightbearing is usually possible after about four months, when solid union is determined.

Complications

A wide range of complications has been reported with the surgical management of fractures of the distal femur. Associated neurovascular damage, delayed union, nonunion or malunion, joint contracture, knee instability, infection, posttraumatic arthritis, implant failure, thromboembolic disease, and refracture after removal of the implant have been cited as possible complications.

While some of these problems cannot be avoided, the incidence of most complications can be diminished by recognizing the potential pitfalls during various stages of treatment.

At the initial assessment, the physician must have a high index of suspicion for associated injuries of the head, chest, abdomen, and spine. The pelvis and all extremities should be evaluated carefully for possible occult injuries. Arteriography is indicated if vascular injury is suspected. Ligamentous instability of the knee can occur with fractures of the distal femur and often cannot be determined until after the fracture is stabilized.

The key to minimizing intraoperative and postoperative complications is good preoperative planning. During the planning phase, the surgeon can often determine the best surgical approach, type, position, and approximate size of the implants, and the need for bone grafting. Preparation of appropriate instrumentation will then result in a smoother surgical procedure with minimal exposure time.

During the surgical procedure, the basic principles of atraumatic technique, accurate reduction, stable fixation, and grafting of bony defects cannot be overemphasized. Strict adherence to these principles will decrease the incidence of implant failure, malunion or nonunion, infection, and delayed healing. Also, accurate reconstruction of the articular surfaces will help decrease posttraumatic arthritis, and suction drainage of the wound will decrease the incidence of hematoma and possible infection.

A common technical error while using the angled blade plate or the condylar screw system is incorrect placement of the blade or screw. Failure to insert the blade or condylar screw along the rhomboidal shape of the distal femur (Fig. 8), that is, the downward incline from the lateral to medial condyle, can cause the screw tip to break out the anterior surface of the medial femoral condyle.

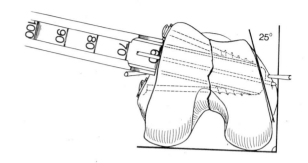

Fig. 8 The rhomboidal shape of the distal femur. (Reproduced with permission from Mize RD: Complex fractures of the distal end of the femur, in Meyers MH (ed): *The Multiply Injured Patient with Complex Fractures*. Malvern, PA, Lea & Febiger, 1984, chap 22, pp 275-290.)

Surgery may not be indicated for the fracture with severe osteopenia or comminution. Considerable judgment is required in these cases.

Patient education is stressed during the postoperative phase. Early excessive weightbearing may lead to implant failure, deformity, or delayed healing, and may necessitate additional surgery. Early active rehabilitation, however, helps to decrease swelling, enhance knee motion, avoid muscle contracture, and minimize the incidence of thromboembolic disease.

Prognosis

Good results can be expected in most cases if the basic principles are followed.[1,9,38] In 1979, Schatzker and Lambert[39] demonstrated the importance of strict adherence to these basic recommendations using instruments and implants developed by the AO/ASIF. Based on an evaluation of their results, two distinct groups emerged. The first group strictly adhered to the basic principles of accurate reduction and stable fixation and achieved good to excellent results in 71% of the cases. The second group did not follow the basic principles; and, despite using the same instruments and implants, only 21% of this group showed good to excellent results.[39] Merely using the AO/ASIF equipment does not guarantee good results. However, good results are achieved in most cases if the requirements of accurate reduction and stable fixation are met.

Summary

The correct use of the available implants is technically demanding, but the technique can be mastered if the surgeon follows a methodical approach to developing skills and confidence. If facilities are available, practice on artificial bones will improve your understanding of the instruments and your skills, as will assisting on as many cases as possible with experienced surgeons. Begin with relatively simple fractures and progress gradually to the more difficult ones.

In order to achieve a good result with surgical treatment of distal femur fractures, the basic principles developed by the AO/ASIF must be followed: good preoperative planning; careful surgical technique; accurate anatomic reduction; stable internal fixation; bone grafting of any defects; and early, active rehabilitation.

References

1. Radford PJ, Howell CJ: The AO dynamic condylar screw for fractures of the femur: Injury. *Br J Acc Surg* 1992;23:89-93.
2. Regazzoni P, Ruedi T, Allgower M: The dynamic condylar screw implant system for fractures of the distal femur. AO/ASIF Dialogue 1986; I:8.
3. Newman JH: Supracondylar fractures of the femur: Injury. *Br J Acc Surg* 1990;21:280-282.
4. Connolly JF, Dehne E, Lafollette B: Closed reduction and early cast-brace ambulation in the treatment of femoral fractures: II. Results in 143 fractures. *J Bone Joint Surg* 1973;55A:1581-1599.
5. Connolly JF, King P: Closed reduction and early cast-brace ambulation in the treatment of femoral fractures: I. An in-vivo quantitative analysis of immobilization in skeletal traction and a cast brace. *J Bone Joint Surg* 1973;55A:1559-1580.
6. Mooney V, Nickel VL, Harvey JP Jr, et al: Cast-brace treatment for fractures of the distal part of the femur: A prospective controlled study of one hundred and fifty patients. *J Bone Joint Surg* 1970;52A:1563-1578.
7. Allgower M: Cinderella of surgery: Fractures. *Surg Clin North Am* 1978;58:1071.
8. Neer CS II, Grantham SA, Shelton ML: Supracondylar fracture of the adult femur: A study of one hundred and ten cases. *J Bone Joint Surg* 1967;49A:591-613.
9. Müller ME, Allgower M, Schneider R, et al: *Manual of Internal Fixation Technique Recommended by the AO/ASIF Group*, ed 3. New York, NY, Springer-Verlag, 1992.
10. Mays J, Neufeld AJ: Skeletal traction methods. *Clin Orthop* 1974;102:144-151.
11. Mize RD: Treatment of fractures of the distal femur. *Ortho Surg Update Series* 1985;4:1.
12. Mize RD, Bucholz RW, Grogan DP: Surgical treatment of displaced, comminuted fractures of the distal end of the femur. *J Bone Joint Surg* 1982;64A:871-879.
13. Giles JB, DeLee JC, Heckman JD, et al: Supracondylar intercondylar fractures of the femur treated with a supracondylar plate and lag screw. *J Bone Joint Surg* 1982;64A:864-870.
14. Hall MF: Two-plane fixation of acute supracondylar and intracondylar fractures of the femur. *South Med J* 1978;71:1471-1479,1481.
15. Laskin R, Zimmerman J: The displaced intercondylar t-fracture of the distal femur: A simplified method of internal fixation. *Orthop Rev* 1975;4:49.
16. Pritchett JW: Supracondylar fractures of the femur. *Clin Orthop* 984;1984:173-177.
17. Sanders R, Regazzoni P, Ruedi TP: Treatment of supracondylar-intercondylar fractures of the femur using the dynamic condylar screw. *J Orthop Trauma* 1989;3:214-222.
18. Sanders R, Swiontkowski M, Rosen H, et al: Double-plating of comminuted, unstable fractures of the distal part of the femur. *J Bone Joint Surg* 1991;73A:341-346.
19. Shewring DJ, Meggitt BF: Fractures of the distal femur treated with the AO dynamic condylar screw. *J Bone Joint Surg* 1992;74B:122-125.
20. Zimmerman AJ: Intra-articular fractures of the distal femur. *Orthop Clin North Am* 1979;10:75-80.
21. Merchan EC, Maestu PR, Blanco RP: Blade-plating of closed displaced supracondylar fractures of the distal femur with the AO/ASIF system. *J Trauma* 1992;32:174-178.
22. Leung KS, Shen WY, So WS, et al: Interlocking intramedullary nailing for supracondylar and intercondylar fractures of the distal part of the femur. *J Bone Joint Surg* 1991;73A:332-340.
23. Winquist RA, Hansen ST Jr, Clawson DK: Closed intramedullary nailing of femoral fractures: A report of five hundred and twenty cases. *J Bone Joint Surg* 1984;66A:529-539.
24. Wu CC, Shih CH: Treatment of femoral supracondylar unstable comminuted fractures: Comparisons between plating and Grosse-Kempf interlocking nailing techniques. *Arch Orthop Trauma Surg* 1992;111:232-236.
25. Kyle RF, Schaffhausen JM, Bechtold JE: Biomechanical characteristics of interlocking femoral nails in the treatment of complex femoral fractures. *Clin Orthop* 1991;267:169-173.
26. Wu CC, Shih CH: Interlocking nailing of distal femoral fractures: 28 patients followed for 1-2 years. *Acta Orthop Scand* 1991;62:342-345.
27. Wu CC, Shih CH: Distal femoral nonunion treated with interlocking nailing. *J Trauma* 1991;31:1659-1662.
28. Bucholz RW, Ross SE, Lawrence KL: Fatigue fracture of the interlocking nail in the treatment of fractures of the distal part of the femoral shaft. *J Bone Joint Surg* 1987;69A:1391-1399.
29. Moore TJ, Campbell J, Wheeler K, et al: Knee function after complex femoral fractures treated with interlocking nails. *Clin Orthop* 1990;261:238-241.
30. Goulet JA, Londy F, Saltzman CL, et al: Interlocking intramedullary nails—an improved method of screw placement combining image intensification and laser light. *Clin Orthop* 1992;281:199-203.
31. Zickel RE, Hobeika P, Robbins DS: Zickel supracondylar nails of fractures of the distal end of the femur. *Clin Orthop* 1986;212:79-88.
32. Healey JH, Lane JM: Treatment of pathologic fractures of the distal femur with the Zickel supracondylar nail. *Clin Orthop* 1990;250:216-220.
33. Seligson D, Kristiansen TK: Use of the Wagner apparatus in complicated fractures of the distal femur. *J Trauma* 1978;18:795-799.
34. Stein H, Makin M: Use of the Wagner apparatus in fractures of the lower limb. *Orthop Rev* 1980;9:96-99.
35. Mize RD: Surgical management of complex fractures of the distal femur. *Clin Orthop* 1989;240:77.
36. Foster TE, Healy WL: Operative management of distal femoral fractures. *Orthop Rev* 1991;20:962-969.
37. Mize RD: Complex fractures of the distal end of the femur, in Meyers NH (ed): *The Multiply Injured Patient with Complex Fractures*. Philadelphia, PA, Lea & Febiger, 1984.
38. Yang RS, Liu HC, Liu TK: Supracondylar fractures of the femur. *J Trauma* 1990;30:315-319.
39. Schatzker J, Lambert DC: Supracondylar fractures of the femur. *Clin Orthop* 1979;138:77-83.

Fractures of the Tibial Plateau

Clayton R. Perry, MD

Fractures of the tibial plateau involve the proximal articular surface of the tibia. Plateau fractures are caused by the femoral condyle impacting into the articular surface as varus, valgus, or axial forces are applied across the knee.

Classification

There are several classifications of tibial plateau fractures (Fig. 1). These systems group different types of fractures along the same general lines, but they differ in minor details.[1-3] Tibial plateau fractures are classified into one of seven types: type 1, split fractures of the lateral plateau; type 2, depressed fractures of the lateral plateau; type 3, split depressed fractures of the lateral tibial plateau; type 4, low-energy fractures of the medial tibial plateau; type 5, high-energy fractures of the medial tibial plateau; type 6, bicondylar tibial plateau fractures; type 7, any of the above associated with a metaphyseal fracture.

Split Fractures

Split fractures of the lateral plateau (type 1) usually occur in young patients with relatively dense bone. The mechanism of injury is high energy (for example, a blow to the lateral side of the knee). The fracture, which is best seen on the anteroposterior projection, is vertical and seldom displaced more than 3 mm. We have seen several cases in which the lateral meniscus was torn peripherally and dislocated into the fracture site. Type 1 fractures are differentiated from type 3 fractures (split depressed fractures) in that there is no depression of the joint surface and the fracture line is more vertical.

Depressed Fractures

Depressed fractures (type 2) occur in elderly patients with osteopenic bone. The mechanism of injury is a low-energy valgus stress (for example, a minor fall). As the valgus stress is applied across the knee, the lateral

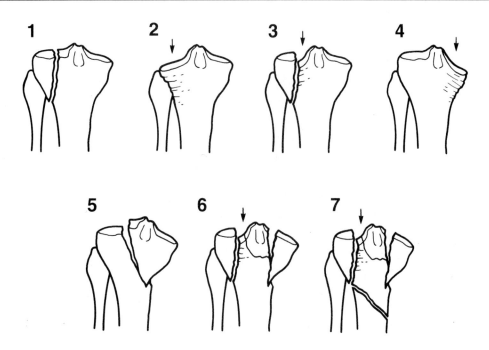

Fig. 1 Line drawings of the anteroposterior radiographs of the proximal tibia. (1) indicates a split fracture, (2) a depressed fracture of the lateral condyle, (3) a split depressed fracture of the lateral condyle, (4) a depressed, low-energy fracture of the medial condyle, (5) a high-energy fracture of the medial condyle, (6) a bicondylar fracture, and (7) a tibial plateau fracture associated with a fracture of the metaphysis.

femoral condyle sinks into and depresses the lateral plateau. Frequently no break in the cortex is seen radiographically; instead, the entire lateral plateau, including the metaphyseal cortex, is tilted laterally.

Split Depressed Fractures

Split depressed fractures (type 3) are the most common type of tibial plateau fracture. They occur in patients with normal or osteopenic bone. The mechanism of injury is a valgus stress, which impacts the lateral femoral condyle against the lateral tibial plateau. The lateral portion of the lateral plateau is fractured from the proximal tibia. As the femoral condyle continues to impact the remaining portion of the lateral plateau, it drives a segment of articular surface of the plateau into the metaphysis. The depressed segment is always on the medial side of the fracture, not on the split fragment. Whether the depressed segment is ante-

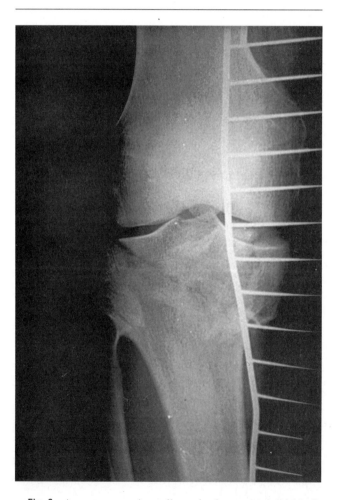

Fig. 2 An anteroposterior radiograph of a proximal tibia indicating a high-energy fracture of the medial tibial plateau. The lateral femoral condyle has been driven distally and medially into the tibial spines and the medial two thirds of the tibia has been sheered off.

rior or posterior depends on the degree of flexion at the time of injury (extension is associated with anterior depression, flexion with posterior depression).

Medial Tibial Plateau Fractures (Low Energy)

Fractures of the medial tibial plateau can be low energy (type 4) or high energy (type 5). Type 4 fractures are similar to depressed fractures of the lateral plateau (type 2 fractures) except that they are the result of a varus force across the knee. The varus force results in the medial femoral condyle being driven into the medial plateau. Like type 2 fractures, they occur in older osteopenic patients and are the result of low-energy trauma. Frequently a cortical break is not seen radiographically, and the entire medial plateau appears to be tilted medially.

Medial Tibial Plateau Fractures (High Energy)

Medial tibial plateau fractures caused by high energy (type 5 fractures) are distinct from type 4 fractures. These are fracture dislocations, and they are frequently associated with neurovascular injuries. Type 5 fractures are caused by an axial load and a valgus force across the knee. This results in the lateral femoral condyle impacting the tibial spines along a vector directed medially and distally (Fig. 2). The lateral collateral ligament is ruptured, the cruciates and medial collateral ligaments are intact.

Bicondylar Tibial Plateau Fractures

Bicondylar tibial plateau fractures (type 6) involve both medial and lateral condyles. These fractures are usually the result of complex high-energy trauma, although occasionally they are the result of simple axial loading in an osteopenic patient. Associated neurovascular injuries, ligamentous injuries, and compartment syndrome are common.

Tibial Plateau Fractures With Metaphyseal Dissociation

Tibial plateau fractures associated with a fracture of the proximal metaphysis (type 7) are rare injuries. They are similar to bicondylar fractures in that they are the result of high-energy trauma and frequently have associated neurovascular injuries. Because of the magnitude of the injury and the extensive surgical exposure necessary to reduce and stabilize them, these fractures have a high incidence of nonunion and postoperative infection.

Diagnosis and Initial Management

History and Physical Examination

There is a history of an injury to the knee. The patient complains of pain and swelling localized to the proximal tibia and knee. There is usually no discernible deformity, but there is a large knee effusion, which, when aspirated, consists of blood with fat in it. The presence of fat indicates an intra-articular fracture.

Radiographic Examination

Radiographs in the anteroposterior and lateral planes are of the most use, and should be carefully examined for fractures and evidence of joint depression. Tilting the x-ray beam 10° caudally, so that it profiles the articular surface, gives more accurate information regarding the amount of depression. Tomograms and CAT scans are also helpful in this regard.[4]

Initial Management

After the diagnosis of fracture of the tibial plateau has been made, the leg is placed in a toe to groin splint with the knee in 20° of flexion. Ice is applied to the anterior aspect of the knee.

Associated Injuries

Injuries frequently associated with fractures of the tibial plateaus are ruptures of the collateral ligaments, occlusion of the popliteal artery or its trifurcation, compartment syndrome, and stretching or laceration of the posterior tibial or common peroneal nerve. Any fracture of the lateral plateau may be associated with a rupture of the medial collateral ligament. Likewise, a fracture of the medial plateau may be associated with a rupture of the lateral collateral ligament. Tenderness over these ligaments indicates a possible injury. Apparent ligamentous laxity with varus and valgus stressing of the knee may be a misinterpretation of motion occurring through the fracture site. In questionable cases, the knee should be stressed under fluoroscopy.

Injuries of the popliteal artery or trifurcation are most likely to occur with high-energy medial tibial plateau and bicondylar fractures. Distal pulses should be carefully examined, and if they are absent an arteriogram must be obtained.

Compartment syndrome is indicated by the presence of the classic signs of increased intracompartmental pressure—swollen tense compartments, pain at rest, pain with passive stretch of muscles, and numbness in the first web space.

Injuries of the posterior tibial and peroneal nerves are identified by assessing sensation on the plantar aspect of the foot and in the first web space and active contraction of the flexor and extensor hallucis longus.

Definitive Management

The goals of management of tibial plateau fractures are to decrease the risk of post-traumatic osteoarthritis and to provide a stable knee with a normal axis of alignment. Management can be either surgical or nonsurgical. Relative indications for surgical management are reducible intra-articular incongruity (a step-off), intra-articular displacement (a gap without a step-off) of 3 mm or more, ligamentous instability, or a deviation in the alignment of the knee. Relative indications for nonsurgical management are a fracture which in the surgeon's judgment cannot be satisfactorily reduced and stabilized (usually because of extensive comminution), fracture blisters, and pre-existing osteoarthritis.

Nonsurgical Management

The nonsurgical management of tibial plateau fractures which are minimally displaced or in which there is pre-existing osteoarthritis consists of four to eight weeks of immobilization in a toe to groin cast, followed by four to eight weeks of nonweightbearing and protected mobilization in an ankle knee orthosis. Displaced fractures which are managed nonsurgically because of comminution or blisters are placed in balanced skeletal suspension with the knee at 45°. A sling supports the calf, and 10 to 20 pounds of traction is applied through a distal tibial pin. Alignment of the fracture is assessed radiographically every two to three days for the first two weeks, and the traction is adjusted accordingly. At two to three weeks, passive motion in the balanced suspension is initiated. At four to six weeks there is usually enough healing clinically and radiographically for balanced suspension to be discontinued and for a toe to groin cast brace to be applied. The cast is continued until eight to ten weeks from injury. Nonweightbearing is continued until twelve weeks from injury.[5]

Surgical Management

The goal of surgical management is anatomic alignment of the joint surface and sufficient stabilization to allow early motion. The surgical exposure and method of stabilization is based upon the type of fracture.

Split fractures (type 1) are managed operatively with attempted closed reduction under fluoroscopy and stabilization with percutaneous screws. The lateral plateau is displaced laterally and distally. To reduce the fracture the knee is flexed to 30° and a varus stress is applied. At the same time, the lateral plateau is pushed medially toward the proximal tibia. If this maneuver does not result in reduction, the fracture is exposed through a lateral parapatellar approach. The block to reduction (frequently the lateral meniscus) is identified and removed. Whether the fracture is reduced open or closed, it is stabilized with a minimum of two large cancellous screws (e.g., 6.5 mm

Synthes). The screws are inserted percutaneously using fluoroscopy to ensure accurate location. At least one screw should be within 5 mm of the joint surface. Postoperatively, the extremity is placed in a continuous passive motion machine and moved from 10° to 30°. When the patient can perform active range of motion, the continuous passive motion is discontinued. Nonweightbearing is maintained for six to eight weeks. If an open reduction was necessary because of a displaced lateral meniscus with a peripheral tear, the meniscus is repaired. Early postoperative motion is followed with a toe to groin cast for four weeks to allow healing of the meniscus.

Depressed fractures (type 2) are managed operatively through a straight anterior skin incision. This skin incision will facilitate total knee arthroplasty in the future, if it is necessary. The lateral plateau is either elevated with a bone tamp inserted through a window in the lateral metaphysis, or a vertical osteotomy of the lateral plateau is performed. This, in effect, converts the fracture to a split depressed fracture. If an osteotomy is performed, the anterior horn of the lateral meniscus is incised and the lateral plateau is "booked open" exposing the depressed condyle (Figs. 3, 4 and

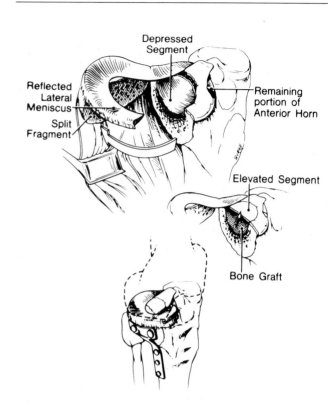

Fig. 4 After the anterior horn of the meniscus has been incised, the fracture is booked open. The depressed segment is elevated and the resulting cavity is packed with bone graft. A buttress plate is applied. (Reproduced with permission from Perry CR, Evans LG, Rice S, et al: A new surgical approach to fractures of the lateral tibial plateau. *J Bone Joint Surg* 1984;66A:1236-1240)

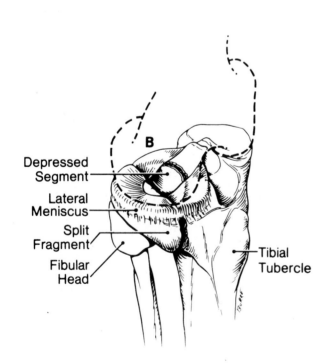

Fig. 3 Illustration of a split depressed fracture of the tibial plateau. (Reproduced with permission from Perry CR, Evans LG, Rice S, et al: A new surgical approach to fractures of the lateral tibial plateau. *J Bone Joint Surg* 1984;66A:1236-1240)

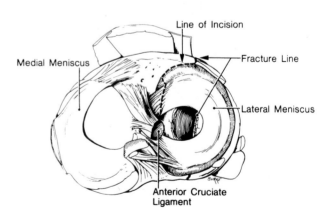

Fig. 5 The anterior horn of the lateral meniscus is incised as far medial as possible. (Reproduced with permission from Perry CR, Evans LG, Rice S, et al: A new surgical approach to fractures of the lateral tibial plateau. *J Bone Joint Surg* 1984;66A:1236-1240)

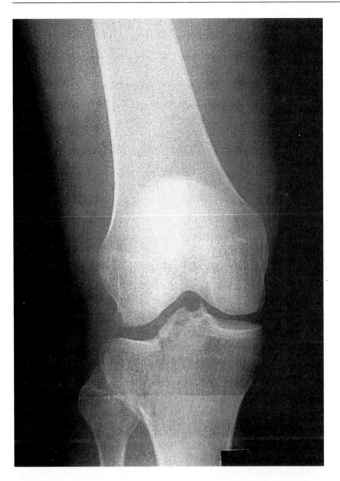 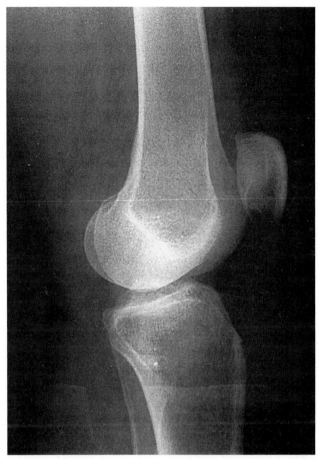

Fig. 6 **Left**, Anteroposterior and, **right**, lateral radiographs indicate a split depressed fracture of the medial plateau.

5). A group of patients in whom the anterior horn of the lateral meniscus was incised were arthroscoped six to 12 months following open reduction and fixation. In all cases the incised anterior horn of the lateral meniscus had healed.[6] If a metaphyseal window is used, the tibial attachment of the meniscus is incised and the meniscus is retracted superiorly to expose the plateau. Regardless of the surgical approach, the articular surface is elevated, and the resulting defect is packed with autogenous bone graft. A plate is applied laterally with two large cancellous screws within 5 mm of subchondral bone. These screws function to support the articular surface.

Split depressed fractures (type 3) are managed as described above. That is, the anterior horn of the lateral meniscus is incised and the fracture is "booked open" through the split component, exposing the depressed segment. The depressed segment is elevated, bone grafted, the split fragment is reduced and stabilized with a plate (Figs. 6 and 7).

Medial plateau fractures (type 4 and 5) are managed operatively through a straight anterior incision.

Depending on the location of the fracture, the anterior horn of the medial or lateral meniscus can be incised. There may be minimal compression with high-energy fractures, and in such cases bone grafting is not necessary. These fractures are always stabilized with a plate, because screws will not hold in the osteopenic bone of a patient with a low-energy fracture, and the high-energy fracture cannot be stabilized sufficiently with screws alone.

Bicondylar fractures (type 6) can be exposed by incising one or both anterior horns of the menisci. In addition the tibial tubercle can be osteotomized and the patellar tendon reflected.[7] Fragments are reduced, bone graft is used to fill defects, and medial and lateral plates are applied (Figs. 8 and 9).

Plateau fractures with an associated metaphyseal fracture (type 7) are managed by first addressing the intra-articular fracture and then the metaphyseal fracture. Either flexible intramedullary nails or a plate may be used to stabilize the metaphyseal fracture. Prolonged casting of the metaphyseal fracture is not an option, because a stiff knee will result.

Postoperative Management

The postoperative management of fracture types 2 through 7 is similar. Early postoperative motion is encouraged in all cases. Immobilization is not necessary unless a meniscus has been repaired. If a meniscus has been repaired, motion is encouraged postoperatively for one week. This is followed with four weeks of cast immobilization to allow the meniscus to heal. With the exception of split fractures (type 1), nonweightbearing is maintained for 12 weeks. Even with this extended period of nonweightbearing, late subsidence of the plateau is a frequent occurrence in osteopenic patients.

Complications

Complications of tibial plateau fractures include osteoarthritis, nonunion, infection, and late subsidence of a reduced plateau. Osteoarthritis is a result of articular incongruity, or injury to the articular cartilage that occurred at the time of fracture. Patients younger than 50 years of age who have osteoarthritis are managed conservatively with nonsteroidal anti-inflammatory medication and local steroid injections. If the symptoms warrant, an arthrodesis or a varus or valgus high tibial osteotomy designed to "unload" the involved condyle is performed. Patients older than 50 who have osteoarthritis are managed with an arthroplasty.

Nonunion of tibial plateau fractures is rare, and when it does occur it is often accompanied by infection. Nonunion more frequently follows a high-energy medial plateau fracture, a displaced bicondylar fracture, or a tibial plateau fracture associated with a metaphyseal fracture (types 5, 6, and 7). In evaluating the nonunion, it is important to determine if there is infection present, whether the knee joint is arthritic, and the amount of motion that is occurring through the joint as opposed to through the nonunion. If there is no evidence of infection and there is severe arthritis, the nonunion is managed with an arthroplasty in

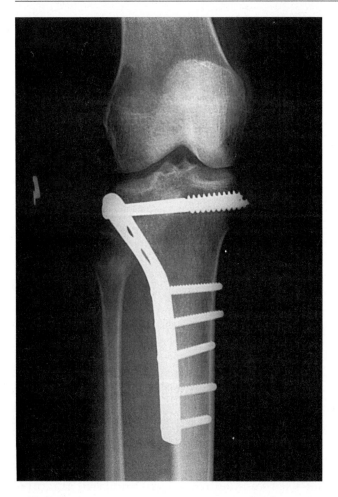 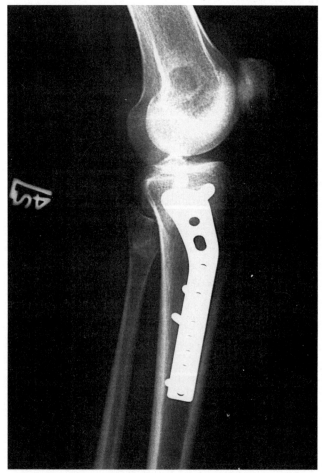

Fig. 7 **Left,** Anteroposterior and, **right,** lateral radiographs after reduction, bone grafting, and application of a buttress plate.

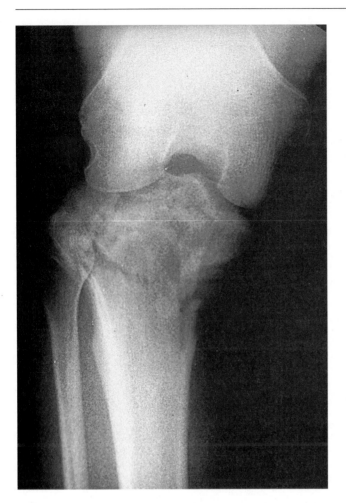 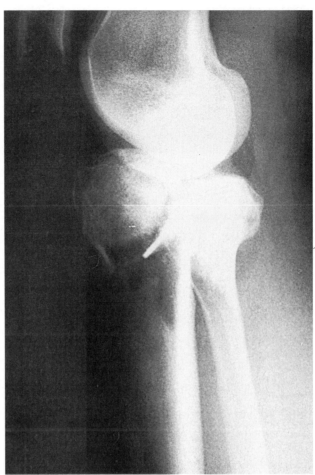

Fig. 8 **Left**, Anteroposterior and, **right**, lateral radiographs of the proximal tibia indicate a displaced and comminuted bicondylar tibial plateau fracture.

patients older than 50 years of age. A long stem tibial component is used. The unhealed bone fragments are reduced around the stem and held in place with wires, plates, and unicortical screws. The nonunion site is grafted with autogenous cancellous bone. In a patient under 50 years of age who has an aseptic arthritic nonunion, the nonunion is managed with an arthrodesis. We prefer to use an intramedullary nail, in conjunction with autogenous cancellous grafting. The nonunion is reduced around the nail and stabilized with screws and plates if necessary. Management of aseptic nonunions without arthritis consists of rigid stabilization in the form of plates and screws and autogenous cancellous bone grafting. In cases in which knee motion is restricted, there is a high incidence of failure of fixation. The principles of management of infected nonunions of tibial plateau fractures are debridement of necrotic tissue and foreign bodies, stabilization of the nonunion with screws and plates, management of dead space with antibiotic-impregnated beads or mus-

cle flaps, good soft tissue coverage with local or free tissue transfer, and antibiotic coverage based upon the sensitivities of the pathogenic organisms. Septic nonunions of the tibial plateau are frequently associated with destruction of the joint. In these cases knee arthrodesis is performed with an external fixator, not an intramedullary nail, to minimize the chance of converting localized osteomyelitis to intramedullary osteomyelitis of the tibia and femur.

Late subsidence of a reduced tibial plateau is seen most frequently in osteopenic patients who have sustained a depressed fracture of the lateral plateau or a low-energy fracture of the medial plateau (types 2 and 4). Late subsidence causes an alteration in the anatomic axis of the knee and results in arthritis and instability. Patients who are at risk must be followed closely after weightbearing has been initiated, because the most effective management starts with early recognition and prevention. The best way to recognize early subsidence is to examine serial radiographs in the

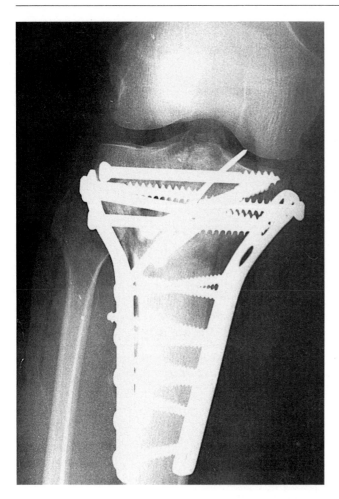 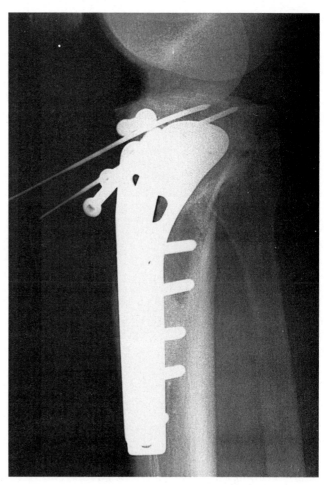

Fig. 9 **Left,** Anteroposterior and, **right,** lateral radiographs after reduction bone grafting and plating of the fracture. The primary risk of this procedure is skin necrosis and infection secondary to the high-energy injury and the extensive surgical exposure.

anteroposterior plane. To make the comparison between serial radiographs meaningful, the identical technique must be used. The beam must be centered over the knee and angled 10° distally to parallel the joint surface. Weightbearing is discontinued, and aggressive physical therapy, in particular strengthening and active range of motion, is instituted to increase bone mass. After two to four weeks partial weightbearing in a varus (lateral plateau) or valgus (medial plateau) knee brace is reinstituted. Weightbearing is increased gradually over the next two to four weeks. Radiographs are obtained weekly until after the patient is full weightbearing. If late subsidence has occurred and instability or the alteration in the axis of the knee is symptomatic, management consists of osteotomy or arthroplasty. Because this complication occurs primarily in osteopenic patients who are elderly, arthroplasty is frequently the best option.

References

1. Burri C, Bartzke G, Coldewey J, et al: Fractures of the tibial plateau. *Clin Orthop* 1979;138:84-93.

2. Hohl M: Tibial condylar fractures. *J Bone Joint Surg* 1967;49A:1455-1467.

3. Schatzker J, McBroom R, Bruce D: The tibial plateau fracture: The Toronto experience 1968-1975. *Clin Orthop* 1979;138:94-104.

4. Elstrom J, Pankovich AM, Sassoon H, et al: The use of tomography in the assessment of fractures of the tibial plateau. *J Bone Joint Surg* 1976;58A:551-555.

5. Scotland T, Wardlaw D: The use of cast-bracing as treatment for fractures of the tibial plateau. *J Bone Joint Surg* 1981;63B:575-578.

6. Perry CR, Evans LG, Rice S, et al: A new surgical approach to fractures of the lateral tibial plateau. *J Bone Joint Surg* 1984;66A:1236-1240.

7. Fernandez DL: Anterior approach to the knee with osteotomy of the tibial tubercle for bicondylar tibial fractures. *J Bone Joint Surg* 1988;70A:208-219.

The Dislocated Knee

Robert C. Schenck, Jr, MD

Introduction

Restoring ligament function of the dislocated knee remains a challenge for the orthopaedic surgeon. Unlike the clinician's frequent exposure to anterior cruciate ligament (ACL) injuries, the rarity of knee dislocations (less than 1.2% of orthopaedic trauma in one series) adds to the difficulty of treating an already devastating knee ligament injury.[1] Furthermore, many published series advocate surgical management of ligamentous injuries but give few details of the technique. Additionally, the risk of injury to the popliteal artery and the potential for postoperative complications underscore the difficulties encountered in the treatment of a knee dislocation.

Historical Review

Diagnosis

Several authors have questioned the long-standing opinion that both cruciate ligaments must be torn for a knee dislocation to occur. As early as 1975, Meyers and associates[2] referred to the knee dislocation with an intact posterior cruciate ligament (PCL). Shelbourne and associates[3] and Cooper and associates[4] have recently reported on patients with a radiographically defined knee dislocation, which, upon reduction or surgical exploration, demonstrated a functioning PCL. Some of these patients were noted to have had partial PCL tears.

In spite of joint position (that is, the dislocation), PCL integrity differentiates the injury from a classic knee dislocation. The presence of a functioning PCL directs surgical management to the treatment of the ACL. Immediate or delayed ACL reconstruction has been suggested by most authors as the treatment option for this type of knee dislocation.[3-5] Furthermore, a functioning PCL, in theory, would appear to protect the popliteal artery[4]; that is, the dislocated knee with a functioning PCL may have a decreased risk of arterial injury as compared to a classic knee dislocation. This final point has yet to be proved, as there are only limited reports of the PCL-intact knee dislocation. Nonetheless, the PCL-intact knee dislocation should be considered a distinct entity from that in which complete tears of both cruciate ligaments occurred. For the remainder of this discussion, the term "dislocated knee" refers to a complete bicruciate knee injury or a dislocation in which tears of both cruciate ligaments occurred.[5-8]

Vascular Injury

Numerous reports have documented the incidence of vascular injuries in association with knee dislocations, generally stated as 32%.[9-18] The incidence ranges from 16% as reported by Meyers and Harvey[15] to 64% as noted by Hoover.[10] The mechanism of arterial injury varies with the type of dislocation. When anterior dislocations injure the artery, it is usually by traction, resulting in an intimal tear. On the other hand, vascular injuries associated with posterior dislocations are frequently complete arterial tears.[9] Green and Allen[9] reported a higher incidence of vascular injury with posterior dislocations than with anterior dislocations (44% versus 39%, respectively). Others have noted a higher incidence of vascular injury with anterior dislocations.[12,19]

In general, regardless of the type of dislocation, the risk of arterial injury should be considered one in three. Furthermore, it is the orthopaedic surgeon, as the primary treating physician, who must initially evaluate the vascularity of the extremity. The difficulty in ensuring vascularity clinically has been well documented in many reports of knee dislocations.[2,9-12,15,20] Misdiagnosis of vascularity and delay in arterial repair based on adequate capillary refill and/or palpable peripheral pulses have been reported.[9] The presence of pedal pulses does not rule out an arterial injury. In a study by Jones and associates,[11] significant arterial injuries were discovered on arteriography in four (27%) of 15 limbs, despite the presence of postreduction pulses that were judged to be normal. These authors advocated the liberal use of arteriography in knee dislocations. Based on this and other reports, arteriography, even in the presence of palpable postreduction pulses, is justifiable in knee dislocations.[9,11,14] Obviously, during the clinical examination, the physician must look for any evidence of ischemia, diminished flow, or a compartment syndrome. Presence of ischemia requires immediate vascular reconstruction. However, the converse, a normal physical examination, does not completely rule out an injury to the vascular tree, and most authors recommend post-reduction arteriography.

The anatomy of the popliteal artery explains its susceptibility to injury. Because it is securely fixed proximally at the adductor hiatus and distally at the soleus arch, tibiofemoral displacement or hyperextension of the knee can result in injury to the artery. In Kennedy's[12] cadaveric study of complete knee dislocations, the anterior knee dislocation was produced by hyperextension: during hyperextension, the ACL was torn first, followed by rupture of the PCL at 30° hyperextension and by tearing of the popliteal artery at 50° hyperextension. With rupture of both cruciate ligaments, tibiofemoral displacement is unchecked and the popliteal artery is at risk for injury.

With respect to an established popliteal injury and resultant ischemia, blood flow must be reestablished within six to eight hours. Inadequacy of the collateral vessels in providing distal flow for limb survival was demonstrated clinically by experience in World War II. In the series by DeBakey and Simeone,[21] 80% of soldiers with a popliteal arterial injury without revascularization eventually required an amputation because of inadequate collateral circulation. Furthermore, the time to revascularization is critical, and the series by Green and Allen[9] in 1977 showed this critical period to be within six to eight hours after injury. These authors observed that patients with popliteal injuries whose limb was not revascularized in this time period required an amputation, nine out of ten times.[9]

Using the information reported by Green and Allen,[9] and Jones and associates,[11] a useful protocol for vascular management in knee dislocations can be derived:

1. The posterior tibialis and dorsalis pedis pulses should be evaluated in any patient with a knee dislocation.

2. Once the dislocation is reduced, the circulation should be reevaluated.

3. If the circulation is not normal after joint reduction, the popliteal artery should be explored immediately.

4. If arteriography is performed in the presence of abnormal circulation, surgical reanastomosis should not be delayed to obtain the study. Revascularization should be performed within six hours after injury or within an absolute maximum of eight hours. Vascular surgery consultation is needed for the appropriate management of such injuries. On-the-table arteriography in the operating room suite, followed by vascular exploration as indicated, is a safe and useful approach to such a clinical problem. Regardless, some authors recommend immediate exploration without arteriography. Thus the decision for arteriography in light of leg ischemia is controversial, as one does not want to delay arterial exploration and reconstruction. The decision for arteriography in leg ischemia should be made by the vascular surgeon, on the basis of his or her clinical experience.

5. Arteriography is justified after a knee dislocation when postreduction pedal pulses are normal.

6. It is unacceptable to suggest spasm as a cause for decreased or absent pedal pulses in an attempt to justify observation. If arterial insufficiency is present, there is a vascular injury.

7. Arterial injury is treated with excision of the damaged segment and reanastomosis with a reverse saphenous vein graft.

Neural Injury

The peroneal nerve is at greatest risk for injury in a knee dislocation. The incidence of injury to the peroneal nerve in knee dislocation has been reported to range from 14% to 35%.[20,22] Although frequently discussed as occurring with a posterolateral dislocation, peroneal nerve injury probably occurs most commonly in association with injury to the lateral ligamentous complex as would result with an adduction injury to the knee. The peroneal and tibial nerves are not as firmly fixed as the popliteal artery and are therefore less prone to injury. Nonetheless, nerve injury is usually a traction injury, with disruption precluding nerve repair.[19,20,23] Stocking paresthesia should alert the clinician to the possibility of a compartment syndrome in the differential diagnosis and not just simple neuropraxia of both tibial and common peroneal nerves. With respect to peroneal nerve palsy, Sisto and Warren[23] reported an improvement in nerve function in two of eight patients after late neurolysis. The authors recommended late peroneal nerve exploration and lysis if there was no evidence of neurotmesis or recovery.

Fractures and Avulsions

Fracture-dislocation of the knee as described by Moore[24] in 1981 involves a ligamentous injury to the knee in association with a fracture of the tibial or femoral condyles (Fig. 1). The fracture-dislocation is distinguished from the purely ligamentous definition of a knee dislocation, as discussed in this text. Avulsion injuries are frequently seen in knee dislocations (Segond's fractures, fibular head avulsion fractures, cruciate avulsions), but should be considered ligamentous injuries and not condylar injuries, unlike major fractures such as are seen in fracture-dislocations of the knee.

Two reports have documented a high incidence of cruciate ligament avulsions in knee dislocations. In separate series, Sisto and Warren[23] and Frassica and associates[25] noted similar percentages of PCL (88% and 77%, respectively) and ACL (63% and 46%, respectively) avulsions (Table 1). Combining both series, PCL avulsions were noted in approximately 80% of knee dislocations and ACL avulsions were noted in approximately 50% of dislocated knees. This is in con-

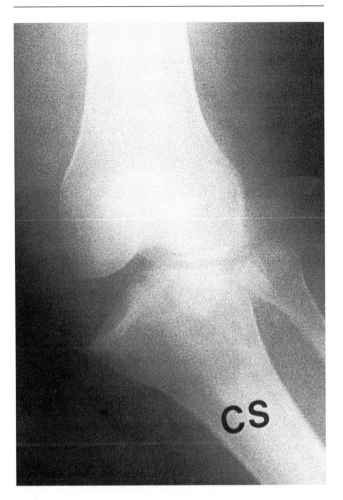

Fig. 1 Anteroposterior stress radiograph of a left knee fracture-dislocation showing fracture of the tibial plateau. (Reproduced with permission from Schenck RC Jr, Burke RL: The dislocated knee. *Perspect Orthop Surg* 1991;2:119-134.)

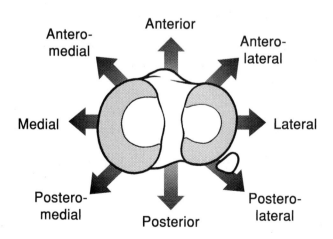

Fig. 2 Classification of knee dislocations based on displacement of the tibia on the femur.

trast to the high frequency of midsubstance tears that are seen in the isolated injuries to the ACL. As will be seen, the possibility of cruciate ligament avulsion directs and simplifies the treatment plan of the knee dislocation.

Classification

In 1963, Kennedy[12] classified knee dislocations in terms of tibial position with respect to the femur; that is, an anterior knee dislocation implies that the tibia is dislocated straight anterior to the femur. He noted five main types of dislocation: anterior, posterior, lateral, medial, and rotatory. Rotatory dislocations are classified into four groups: anteromedial, anterolateral, posteromedial, and posterolateral with posterolateral being the most frequently described type of rotatory knee dislocation.[9,20,22,26] This classification system has been utilized widely (Fig. 2).[2,9,11,15-19,22,23,25-28].

In one review of 245 knee dislocations, 61 (25%) were anterior, 45 (18%) were posterior, 31 (13%) were lateral, nine (4%) were rotatory, and eight (3%) were medial. In that series, 50 (20%) of the knee dislocations were unclassified as to the type.[9]

Although other series have documented varying incidences of the dislocation type, anterior displacement is considered the most common type of knee dislocation.[9,19] However, the least common type of knee dislocation, the posterolateral dislocation, is well described. The hallmark of this condition is that it cannot be reduced: the medial femoral condyle buttonholes through the medial capsule and the medial collateral ligament invaginates into the knee joint, preventing closed reduction.[20,22] A transverse furrow seen on the medial aspect of the knee is the sine qua non of this knee dislocation type and its irreducibility. The mechanism of injury as described by Quinlan and Sharrard[22] is that of an abduction force to the flexed knee coupled with internal rotation of the tibia. Peroneal nerve palsy frequently is associated with this type of dislocation, resulting from a traction injury to

Table 1
Presence of cruciate ligament avulsions in knee dislocations

Author	No. of Knees	Avulsed Ligament	
		Posterior	Anterior
Sisto and Warren[23]	16	14 (88%)	10 (63%)
Frassica and associates[25]	13	10 (77%)	6 (46%)
Total	29	24 (83%)	16 (55%)

(Reproduced with permission from Schenck RC Jr, Burke RL: The dislocated knee. *Perspect Orthop Surg* 1991;2:119-134.)

the nerve over the lateral femoral condyle. Skin necrosis secondary to pressure from the medially displaced femur has been reported.[20]

The position classification system of knee dislocations is well established and very useful in alerting the physician to the mechanism of injury, the reduction maneuver needed, and potential associated injuries (Outline 1). Nonetheless, the system has certain limitations. First, the direction of displacement occasionally is not known, because the knee may have spontaneously reduced at the time of injury or evaluation. Second, position classification only suggests possible ligamentous involvement. With the possibility of a PCL-intact knee dislocation, tearing of both cruciate ligaments is not guaranteed in a knee dislocation. Third, the exact status of the collateral ligaments also is not defined with an anterior or posterior knee dislocation. The ligamentous anatomy of the knee is complex, and many combinations of cruciate and collateral ligament disruptions are possible with a knee dislocation.

Thus, it is useful to further classify knee dislocations in terms of the ligaments involved. This is best performed at the time of injury (if tolerated) as well as during examination under anesthesia. One should be able to identify one of at least five possible injury patterns: (1) ACL/collateral ligament(s) torn, PCL intact (isolated case reports); (2) ACL/PCL torn, collateral ligaments intact (experimentally produced but clinically rare); (3) ACL/PCL/medial collateral ligament (MCL) torn, lateral collateral ligament (LCL), posterolateral corner (PLC) intact; (4) ACL/PCL/LCL-PLC torn, MCL intact; and (5) ACL/PCL/MCL/LCL-PLC torn. These subclassifications are based on ligament function and are very useful in deciding on treatment and surgical incision.

Knee dislocations have also been classified by the level of energy sustained, low or high. Although the term velocity has been most commonly used, most authors agree that energy most accurately describes an injury process. Nonetheless, the clinician should note that even with a low-velocity or low-energy knee dislocation, the possibility of a popliteal injury is present and arteriography is still recommended.[13,14]

Finally, the knee dislocation can be classified as open or closed, indicating the need for immediate attention to the soft tissues and joint. The degree of soft-tissue injury often determines the eventual ligamentous treatment.

Treatment

The literature is replete with clinical series of knee dislocations, and most authors advocate early operative repair of the damaged structures.[2,12,15,17,19,22,23,25,28-30] As Meyers and Harvey[15] noted in 1971, "It is . . . unlikely that any single physician personally cares for more than a few [knee dislocations] in a lifetime of practice." Therefore, it is useful to critically review the experience in the literature (Table 2).

In 1963, Kennedy[12] wrote the classic study on knee

Outline 1
Position classification of knee dislocations

Anterior
  Most common type
  Frequent arterial injury (traction)
  Hyperextension most common mechanism of injury
Posterior
  Frequent arterial injury (complete tears)
  High association with extensor mechanism disruption
Posterolateral
  Irreducible
  Medial femoral condyle buttonholed through medial capsule
  High incidence of peroneal nerve palsy
  Transverse skin furrow medially

Table 2
The dislocated knee: Literature review

Year	Author	No. of patients	Content
1955	O'Donoghue[26]	5	Advocated surgical ligament treatment
1958	Quinlan and Sharrard[22]	5	Mechanism of injury with posterolateral dislocation
1961	Hoover[10]	14	Eight of nine vascular injuries (89%) required an amputation
1963	Kennedy[12]	22	Classification system, cadaveric study, and advocated surgical treatment
1969	Shields and associates[17]	24	Advocated surgical ligament repair
1969	Reckling and Peltier[16]	15	Discussed associated injuries
1971	Meyers and Harvey[15]	18	Advocated surgical ligament repair
1975	Meyers and associates[2]	53	Reemphasized surgical ligament repair
1972	Taylor and associates[18]	41	Advocated nonsurgical ligament treatment for uncomplicated knee dislocations
1977	Green and Allen[9]	41	Defined an average incidence of popliteal arterial injury of 32% in knee dislocation
1979	Jones and associates[11]	22	Emphasized peripheral pulses as unreliable in verifying vascularity
1981	Hill and Rana[20]	1	Discussed posterolateral dislocations
1981	Moore[24]	132	Classified the fracture-dislocation of the knee
1985	Sisto and Warren[23]	19	Advocated surgical ligament repair; emphasized high incidence of ligament avulsions
1991	Frassica and associates[25]	17	Advocated surgical ligament repair

(Reproduced with permission from Schenck RC Jr, Burke RL: The dislocated knee. *Perspect Orthop Surg* 1991;2:119-134.)

dislocations, in which he followed 22 patients. He described a classification system, as noted previously, presented a cadaveric study attempting to reproduce dislocations, and advocated early ligament repair when severe damage is present. Kennedy also noted that nonsurgical treatment of uncomplicated cases may produce surprisingly good long-term results. He reported the high incidence of vascular injury with knee dislocations (27% in his series) and recommended immediate surgical treatment of such arterial injuries.

In 1969, two reports were published on knee dislocations and their sequelae.[16,17] Shields and associates[17] reported on 26 patients and concluded that closed reduction combined with open ligament repair was the method of choice for treatment. The incidence of vascular injury was 40% in this study with five (23%) of 22 patients who had arterial injury eventually undergoing an above-knee amputation.[17] Reckling and Peltier[16] analyzed 15 knee dislocations with five patients undergoing ligament repair. They noted good results with both surgical and closed treatment methods.

In 1971, Meyers and Harvey[15] noted difficulty in reconciling opinions on the need for surgical treatment for ligamentous injuries of knee dislocations based on the available literature. In their report, eight of nine knees (89%) treated nonsurgically were symptomatic at follow-up. In 1975, the same authors re-emphasized their initial impression that surgical treatment of all torn ligaments gives the best results. They again established the need for careful vascular observation and early arterial repair (before eight hours) to prevent gangrene of the leg.[15]

In 1972, Taylor and associates[18] reported on their experience with knee dislocations. They noted good results with nonsurgical treatment (26 knees) and recommended immobilization of the knee in slight flexion for a period of no greater than six weeks. These authors found that greater periods of immobilization produced a very stable, but unacceptably stiff knee; in contrast, shorter periods of immobilization (less than six weeks) produced a knee with full range of motion but with unacceptable laxity. In their series, 12 (75%) of 16 patients with surgical repair had fair or poor results. The authors acknowledged that a comparison between surgical and nonsurgical treatment was not possible in their study. Surgical repair was performed out of necessity (irreducibility, open joint, vascular injury) in ten patients. Their recommendation for closed treatment was for uncomplicated cases of knee dislocation only.[18]

In 1985, Sisto and Warren[23] reported on 19 patients, of whom 13 underwent acute complete ligamentous repair using the suture technique of Marshall and associates[31] (multiple looped ligament sutures of varying depths attached through bony tunnels). The authors recommended a surgical approach in young patients with knee dislocations but noted problems with continued pain and varying degrees of motion loss despite surgical intervention. They also reported the finding of frequent avulsions rather than midsubstance cruciate ligament tears in association with knee dislocations.[23]

In 1991 Frassica and associates[25] analyzed 17 patients treated for a dislocated knee. Of the 13 patients who underwent ligamentous repair, 12 had good or excellent results based on knee criteria developed by Meyers and Harvey.[15] In addition to recommending surgical treatment of the dislocated knee, the authors confirmed the high incidence of avulsed cruciate ligaments in knee dislocations.[25]

Also in 1991, Shelbourne and associates[28] report on their experience with 21 patients suffering low-velocity knee dislocations. These authors noted that one (4.8%) had a low incidence of arterial injury and four (19%) suffered a peroneal nerve palsy. Knee stiffness was noted in patients who underwent simultaneous ACL/PCL reconstructions. These authors advocated midthird patellar tendon reconstruction of the PCL as the initial ligamentous treatment in the knee dislocation.

Although most reports emphasize the importance of early surgical repair and the poor results obtained with closed treatment, no prospective trials to date have compared the two treatment options on similar types of knee dislocations. Yet with the recent advances in ligament reconstructions and repairs, it makes intuitive sense to perform acute ligamentous repairs. Shields and associates[17] noted in 1969 that multiple structures are found within the joint and "... it has been impossible... to always tell before surgery the exact magnitude of the internal derangement. Thus to predict satisfactory outcome with conservative treatment is difficult, if not altogether impossible." Despite this and numerous other arguments supporting acute ligamentous repair, a prospective study is needed to give further credence to the currently accepted surgical treatment rationale.[27] Unfortunately, the possibility of displaced intra-articular structures, such as collateral or cruciate ligaments or menisci, has influenced many authors to advocate early surgical treatment of the dislocated knee. Furthermore, rather than subjecting the patient to the documented adverse effects of immobilization on the knee, surgical repair allows early institution of range of motion exercises.

Surgery

With respect to specific surgical steps in treatment, Hughston and associates[32] emphasized the importance of PCL repair in the surgical management of ligamentous injuries when both cruciates were torn. Many authors agree with this approach (Jesse C. DeLee, personal communication, 1992; Frank R. Noyes, MD, personal communication, 1990).[23,26,28,31] In a report solely discussing knee dislocations, Shelbourne and associates[28] reinforced the need initially to reconstruct the PCL and advocated one delay ACL repair in the surgical approach to ligament repair of the dislocated knee.

Historically, many authors describe techniques to repair midsubstance tears or reattach avulsed cruciate and collateral ligaments. O'Donoghue[26] was the first to describe in a large series the use of suture reattachment or repair of knee ligament avulsions and midsubstance tears, respectively. Passing sutures through bony tunnels and then tying them over a "bony bridge" completed the reattachment or repair in his technique. As noted above, Marshall and associates[31] developed a looping suture technique for repair of midsubstance cruciate ligament tears. As well, Muller[30] discussed a suture reattachment technique using bony tunnels to reapproximate the ligament to its site of avulsion. He also described a technique of collateral ligament reattachment using a spiked washer and an AO screw.

With respect to the reattachment of an avulsed posterior cruciate ligament, Trickey[33,34] and Torisu[35,36] in separate reports showed good clinical results in reattaching an avulsed PCL (and bony fragment) with a screw. Krackow, in an attempt to restore PCL function in total knee arthroplasty, developed a locking whipstitch to reattach the posterior cruciate ligament to its bony site.[37,38] Reattachment of the cruciate or collateral avulsion is easily performed using screw or suture techniques. When a large bony fragment is present, screw techniques are useful, but when few or no fragments are present, sutures techniques are frequently needed.[39]

Preoperative Evaluation

Surgical decision making can be enhanced by use of magnetic resonance imaging (MRI). MRI is useful in identifying cruciate avulsions, as well as in predicting the finding of meniscal and chondral damage. The MRI can identify an avulsion or midsubstance injury of the PCL prior to arthrotomy, and will alert the clinician to a more likely need for reconstruction if a midsubstance tear is present (Figs. 3 and 4). Discussion with the radiologist before the study is useful to ensure an adequate MRI evaluation of the intercondylar notch and its contents. Lastly, stress radiographs with the patient under anesthesia in varus and valgus with the knee in extension can be important in the documentation of collateral integrity or disruption (Fig. 5).

Thus, with evaluation under anesthesia, stress radiographs, and preoperative MRI, an accurate preincision prediction of the damaged structures (both location and type) can be made. This assures the availability of a graft for a PCL reconstruction if a midsubstance tear is present and it clarifies the optimal placement of incisions of ligament surgery. As noted previously, initial evaluation of the neurovascularly intact knee dislo-

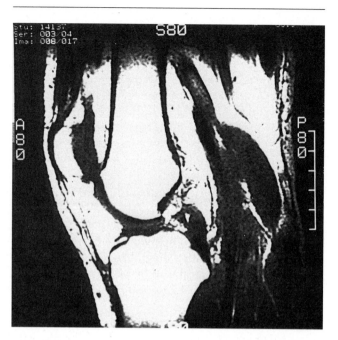

Fig. 3 Preoperative MRI showing the PCL avulsed from the femur. (Reproduced with permission from Schenck RC Jr, Robert C: Management of posterior cruciate ligament injuries in knee dislocations. *Oper Tech Sports Med* 1993;1:143-147.)

cation should always include arteriography to rule out a popliteal injury.

Surgical Decision Making

The term "repair" can be very confusing when discussing ligament surgery. For the purpose of clarity, the specific surgery and treatment techniques involved in knee dislocation will be discussed briefly. Thus, the terms "repair" of a midsubstance collateral tear, "reattachment" of a cruciate or collateral avulsion, and "reconstruction" of a midsubstance cruciate tear will be used. Although the selection of such terms appears to be elementary, any discussion of the wide spectrum of ligamentous injuries and appropriate treatments in knee dislocations requires such descriptions to provide clarity.

As stated earlier, the foundation of ligamentous management of the dislocated knee is the treatment of the torn PCL, whether it be PCL reattachment or reconstruction. The PCL is the primary concern for ligament surgery in the dislocated knee. Simultaneous PCL/ACL surgery is not recommended and ACL surgery is most commonly delayed. One exception is the presence of an ACL avulsion, where reattachment does not significantly increase surgical requirements. To avoid confusion of the term repair, the term reconstitute will be used generically to describe reattachment or reconstruction of the PCL. Repair of midsubstance cruciate tears is not advocated. In contrast to

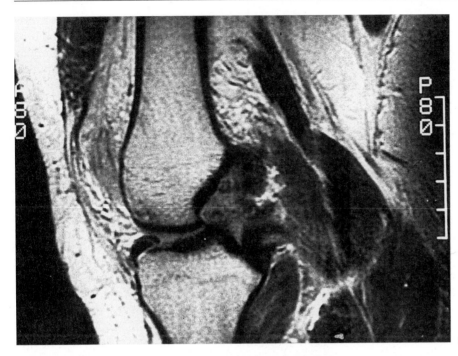

Fig. 4 Preoperative MRI showing a mid-substance tear of the PCL.

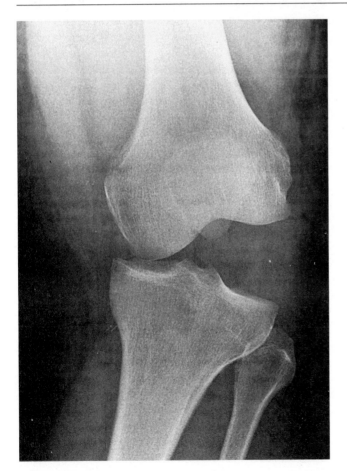

Fig. 5 Varus stress view of the knee in extension showing complete ACL/PCL/LCL-PLC disruption. (Reproduced with permission from Schenck RC Jr, Robert C: Management of posterior cruciate ligament injuries in knee dislocations. *Oper Tech Sports Med* 1993;1:143-147.)

Collateral Reattachment

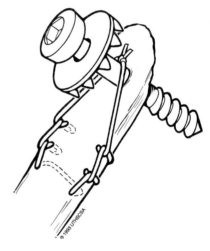

Fig. 6 The locking whipstitch suture is used in conjunction with an AO screw and spiked washer for ligament reattachment. (Reproduced with permission from Schenck RC Jr, Robert C: Management of posterior cruciate ligament injuries in knee dislocations. *Oper Tech Sports Med* 1993;1:143-147.)

the ACL/MCL injury pattern, repair or reattachment of collateral injuries is useful in the context of a knee dislocation (Fig. 6). The term reconstitute will be used in the context of collateral surgery as well. Lastly, midline incisions should be used if at all possible with respect to possible future procedures.

The following descriptions of surgical management of the dislocated knee are based on the ligaments involved.

ACL/Collateral Ligament(s) Torn, PCL Intact In this pattern, PCL integrity directs the treatment of this type of dislocation to the anterior cruciate ligament. One has two options in the treatment of the ACL tear. Either immediate surgery (reattachment or reconstruction) or a delayed reconstruction until range of motion is restored and collateral healing has occurred will lead to a successful result.

ACL/PCL Torn, Collateral Ligaments Intact Initial treatment requires reconstitution of the PCL and incisions are planned to approach the ligament injury. This injury pattern is rare, but treatment is simplified by collateral integrity.

ACL/PCL/MCL Torn, LCL-PLC Intact Again, the primary concern is reconstituting the PCL (Fig. 7). Using a straight midline or paramedian incision, the knee joint can be explored, meniscal cartilage inspected, and ligaments (PCL/MCL) treated. The PCL, if avulsed, can

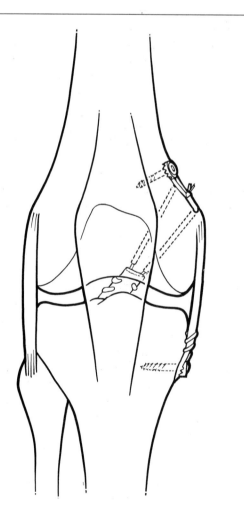

Fig. 7 Drawing depicting the initial surgical construct for tears of the ACL/PCL/MCL knee disorder. (Reproduced with permission from Schenck RC Jr, Robert C: Management of posterior cruciate ligament injuries in knee dislocations. *Oper Tech Sports Med* 1993;1:143-147.)

be reattached to the femur or tibia through this same incision. However, if a midsubstance PCL tear is present on MRI, preoperative selection of graft should be done; hence, the availability of allograft or of an intact extensor mechanism (based on physical examination and/or MRI) should be verified prior to surgery. With gentle dissection medially, the MCL can be easily identified and inspected, and repair or reattachment performed. Final tensioning and fixation of the PCL and MCL reconstitution should be performed in 20° flexion with the hip externally rotated, reducing the medial tibiofemoral compartment. The presence of a functioning posterolateral corner greatly simplifies the treatment of this type of knee dislocation.

ACL/PCL/LCL-PLC Torn; MCL Intact In this specific pattern, the finding of the torn LCL and posterolateral corner complicates treatment (Fig. 8). It is very important to reestablish the "corner" and associated tendinous injuries (biceps femoris and/or iliotibial band disruption) in addition to the PCL. The incision is placed posterolaterally. Once the peroneal nerve is isolated and gently retracted, the joint is inspected by subluxating the tibiofemoral joint (Fig. 9). The locking whipstitch described by Krackow[37,38] is used to reattach the lateral collateral ligament and associated posterolateral structures. Midsubstance tears of the posterolateral structures should be repaired as well. An additional small medial incision is used when the PCL is avulsed from the femur or if a femoral tunnel is required for reconstruction (Fig. 7). Tibial avulsions of the PCL can also be reattached through the posterolateral incision.

ACL/PCL/MCL/LCL-PLC Torn This pattern is most frequently associated with a high-energy injury. Reconstituting the posterior cruciate ligament and posterolateral corner is the early primary goal (Fig. 10). These two structures can be explored and treated using a primary posterolateral incision. As noted above, a small medial incision is frequently needed for PCL femoral reattachment or reconstruction.

Popliteal Artery Injury

Injury to the arterial tree requires immediate vascular reconstruction, with treatment of the ligaments being secondary. External fixation of the tibiofemoral joint is frequently required because of the degree of knee laxity and the potential risk of injury to the vascular repair. In such situations, external fixation and closed immobilization (if no ligamentous surgery is performed) for four to six weeks is frequently utilized. Olecranization of the patella as a stabilization technique is not recommended for knee dislocations. The ligamentous treatment of knee dislocations with vascular insufficiency continues to be debated because there are only isolated reports of such injuries. The primary goal of the surgeon in a vascular-insufficient knee dis-

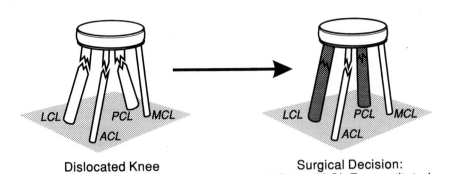

Dislocated Knee
ACL/PCL/LCL Torn

Surgical Decision:
PCL and LCL Reconstituted

Fig. 8 ACL/PCL/LCL-PCL torn. It is useful to reestablish the arcuate complex in conjunction with the approach to PCL reconstitution. (Reproduced with permission from Schenck RC Jr, Robert C: Management of posterior cruciate ligament injuries in knee dislocations. *Oper Tech Sports Med* 1993;1:143-147.)

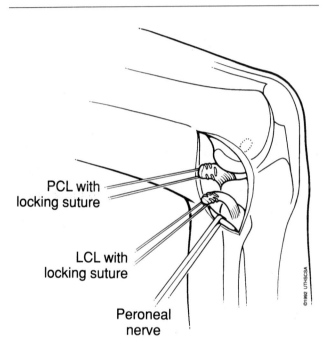

PCL with
locking suture

LCL with
locking suture

Peroneal
nerve

Fig. 9 Posterolateral exposure of the ACL/PCL/LCL-PLC injured knee dislocation, including initial exposure of the peroneal nerve.

location is to restore blood flow to the extremity, and to ensure that the repair is protected.

Rehabilitation

Despite the concern of stretching a PCL graft or reattachment, aggressive, early range of motion is required in any rehabilitation protocol for knee dislocation, because permanent flexion loss and fixed flexion contractures are significant risks with immobilization; more importantly, stiffness, once occurred, is a very difficult problem to correct in the knee dislocation that has been treated surgically. With reattachment or reconstruction of the PCL, early motion should be started, as should weightbearing and functional rehabilitation. If 90° of flexion has not been obtained by four weeks after surgery, manipulation under anesthesia and arthroscopic scar excision can be beneficial.

Summary and Future Directions

The management of the dislocated knee is complicated, because it involves both immediate identification of damaged neurovascular structures and a specif-

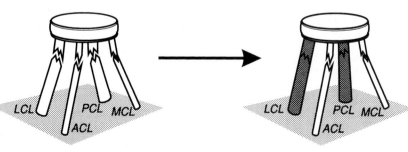

Dislocated Knee
ACL/PCL/LCL/MCL Torn

Surgical Decision:
PCL and LCL Reconstituted

Fig. 10 ACL/PCL/MCL/LCL-PLC. Significant knee injury requiring at least reestablishment of the PCL and LCL. Depending on stability obtained, repair of the MCL may be required. (Reproduced with permission from Schenck RC Jr, Robert C: Management of posterior cruciate ligament injuries in knee dislocations. *Oper Tech Sports Med* 1993;1:143-147.)

ic rationale for sequential ligamentous reconstruction, initially avoiding surgery on the ACL. Careful clinical vascular evaluation and arteriography are indicated in the dislocated knee. Evidence of ischemia requires immediate vascular exploration. Ligamentous management of the dislocated knee is, in effect, the management of the PCL; however, cruciate avulsions are frequently seen and can be reattached successfully. Preoperative MRI can identify avulsions and, equally important, indicate a possible need for a PCL reconstruction. Graft availability (extensor mechanism harvest or allograft) should be verified preoperatively and options (allograft, autograft) discussed with the patient. The collateral ligament injury should be treated surgically at the same time as the posterior cruciate ligament. Simultaneous cruciate reconstructions should be avoided, and treatment of the ACL should be delayed until full motion has been reestablished.

References

1. Bunt TJ, Malone JM, Moody M, et al: Frequency of vascular injury with blunt trauma-induced extremity injury. *Am J Surg* 1990;160:226-228.
2. Meyers MH, Moore TM, Harvey JP Jr: Follow-up notes on articles previously published in The Journal. Traumatic dislocation of the knee joint. *J Bone Joint Surg* 1975;57A:430-433.
3. Shelbourne KD, Pritchard J, Rettig AC, et al: Knee dislocations with intact PCL. *Orthop Rev* 1992;21:607-611.
4. Cooper DE, Speer KP, Wickiewicz TL, et al: Complete knee dislocation without posterior cruciate ligament disruption: A report of four cases and review of the literature. *Clin Orthop* 1992;284:228-233.
5. Schenck RC: *Management of PCL Injuries in Knee Dislocations. Techniques in Sportsmedicine.* Raven Press, 1993, vol 1, pp 143-147.
6. Schenck RC, Burke RL: The dislocated knee. *Perspect Orthop Surg* 1991;2:119-134.
7. Schenck RC, Burke R, Walker D: The dislocated knee: A new classification system. *South Med J* 1992;85:3S-61.
8. Schenck RC Jr, Nonweiler D, DeLee JC: The incomplete bicruciate ligament pattern: A report of two cases. *Orthop Rev* 1993;22:1249-1252.
9. Green NE, Allen BL: Vascular injuries associated with dislocation of the knee. *J Bone Joint Surg* 1977;59A:236-239.
10. Hoover NW: Injuries of the popliteal artery associated with fractures and dislocations. *Surg Clin North Am* 1961;41:1099-1112.
11. Jones RE, Smith EC, Bone GE: Vascular and orthopedic complications of knee dislocation. *Surg Gynecol Obstet* 1979;149:554-558.
12. Kennedy JC: Complete dislocation of the knee joint. *J Bone Joint Surg* 1963;45A:889-904.
13. McCoy GF, Hannon DG, Barr RJ, et al: Vascular injury associated with low-velocity dislocations of the knee. *J Bone Joint Surg* 1987;69B:285-287.
14. McCutchan JD, Gillham NR: Injury to the popliteal artery associated with dislocation of the knee: Palpable distal pulses do not negate the requirement for arteriography. *Injury* 1989;20:307-310.
15. Meyers MH, Harvey JP Jr: Traumatic dislocation of the knee joint: A study of eighteen cases. *J Bone Joint Surg* 1971;53A:16-29.
16. Reckling FW, Peltier LF: Acute knee dislocations and their complications. *J Trauma* 1969;9:181-191.
17. Shields L, Mital M, Cave EF: Complete dislocation of the knee: Experience at the Massachusetts General Hospital. *J Trauma* 1969;9:192-215.
18. Taylor AR, Arden GP, Rainey HA: Traumatic dislocation of the knee: A report of forty-three cases with special reference to conservative treatment. *J Bone Joint Surg* 1972;54B:96-102.
19. Rockwood CA Jr, Green DP: *Fractures in Adults*, ed 2. Philadelphia, PA, JB Lippincott, 1984, vol 2.
20. Hill JA, Rana NA: Complications of posterolateral dislocation of the knee: Case report and literature review. *Clin Orthop* 1981;154:212-215.
21. DeBakey ME, Simeone FA: Battle injuries of the arteries in world war II: An analysis of 2,471 cases. *Ann Surg* 1946;123:534-579.
22. Quinlan AG, Sharrard WJW: Posterolateral dislocation of the knee with capsular interposition. *J Bone Joint Surg* 1958;40B:660-663.
23. Sisto DJ, Warren RF: Complete knee dislocation: A follow-up study of operative treatment. *Clin Orthop* 1985;198:94-101.
24. Moore TM: Fracture-dislocation of the knee. *Clin Orthop* 1981;156:128-140.
25. Frassica FJ, Sim FH, Staeheli JW, et al: Dislocation of the knee. *Clin Orthop* 1992;263:200-205.
26. O'Donoghue DH: An analysis of end results of surgical treatment of major injuries to the ligaments of the knee. *J Bone Joint Surg* 1955;37A:1-13.
27. Montgomery TJ, White J, Roberts TS, et al: Orthopedic management of dislocations of the knee: A comparison of surgical reconstruction and immobilization. *Orthop Trans* 1992;16:225.
28. Shelbourne KD, Porter DA, Clingman JA, et al: Low-velocity knee dislocation. *Orthop Rev* 1991;20:995-1004.
29. Feagin JA Jr (ed): *The Crucial Ligaments: Diagnosis and Treatment of Ligamentous Injuries About the Knee.* New York, NY, Churchill Livingstone, 1988.
30. Muller W: *The Knee: Form, Function, and Ligament Reconstruction.* New York, NY, Springer-Verlag, 1983.
31. Marshall JL, Warren RF, Wickiewicz TL, et al: The anterior cruciate ligament: A technique of repair and reconstruction. *Clin Orthop* 1979;143:97-106.
32. Hughston JC, Bowden JA, Andrews JR, et al: Acute tears of the posterior cruciate ligament: Results of operative treatment. *J Bone Joint Surg* 1980;62A:438-450.
33. Trickey EL: Rupture of the posterior cruciate ligament of the knee. *J Bone Joint Surg* 1968;50B:334-341.
34. Trickey EL: Injuries to the posterior cruciate ligament: Diagnosis and treatment of early injuries and reconstruction of late instability. *Clin Orthop* 1980;147:76-81.
35. Torisu T: Isolated avulsion fracture of the tibial attachment of the posterior cruciate ligament. *J Bone Joint Surg* 1977;59A:68-72.
36. Torisu T: Avulsion fracture of the tibial attachment of the posterior cruciate ligament: Indications and results of delayed repair. *Clin Orthop* 1979;143:107-114.
37. Krackow KA, Thomas SC, Jones LC: A new stitch for ligament-tendon fixation: Brief note. *J Bone Joint Surg* 1986;68A:764-766.
38. Krackow KA, Thomas SC, Jones LC: Ligament-tendon fixation: Analysis of a new stitch and comparison with standard techniques. *Orthopaedics* 1988;11:909-917.
39. Schenck RC Jr, McGanity PLJ: Reattachment of avulsed cruciate ligaments: Report of a technique. *Orthop Trans* 1992;16:77.

Biomechanics of Knee Ligaments: Basic Concepts and Clinical Application

Freddie H. Fu, MD

Christopher D. Harner, MD

Darren L. Johnson, MD

Mark D. Miller, MD

Savio L-Y. Woo, PhD

The quest for improved techniques for the reconstruction of knee ligaments has led to a better understanding of the anatomy, biomechanics, and healing properties of these ligaments. The reconstructive surgeon of today must understand the key principles of normal ligament function in order to restore the injured knee to a satisfactory level of performance. In this chapter, we will review recent advances in knee ligament research, with an emphasis on pertinent clinical applications.

Functional Anatomy

The four important knee ligaments — the anterior cruciate, posterior cruciate, medial collateral, and lateral collateral ligaments — have been classified by a number of schemes. They can be defined, on the basis of their morphology, as flat (the medial collateral ligament) or cord-like (the anterior cruciate, posterior cruciate, and lateral collateral ligaments); they can be identified as intra-articular (the anterior and posterior cruciate ligaments) or extra-articular (the lateral collateral ligament and the superficial part of the medial collateral ligament); and they can be considered individually. Each of the ligaments, with the exception of the lateral collateral ligament, is divided into various bundles or components. The anterior cruciate ligament is composed of anteromedial and posterolateral bands[1] and possibly an intermediate band.[2] The posterior cruciate ligament is composed of anterolateral and posteromedial bands.[3] These divisions are important because each appears to have a separate function.[4] For both of the cruciate ligaments, the posterior portion is tight in extension and the anterior component is tight in flexion (Fig. 1).[5] The medial collateral ligament is composed of a superficial portion (also known as the superficial medial or tibial collateral ligament) and a deep portion (also known as the deep medial or middle capsular ligament).[6] The superficial portion of the medial collateral ligament can be divided into anterior and posterior portions; the anterior fibers of

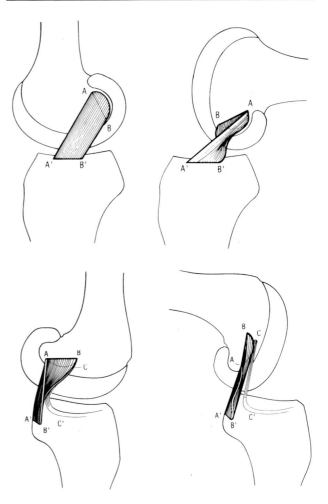

Fig. 1 Diagram illustrating tensioning of various bands of the anterior and posterior cruciate ligaments in extension and flexion. Note the tensioning of the posterior components of each ligament in extension and of the anterior components in flexion. For the anterior cruciate ligament (top), A-Á = the anteromedial band and B-Ḃ = the posterolateral band. For the posterior cruciate ligament (bottom), B-Ḃ = the anterolateral band and A-Á = the posteromedial band. C-C = the anterior meniscofemoral ligament (the ligament of Humphry). (Reproduced with permission from Girgis FG, Marshall JL, Monajem ARS: The cruciate ligaments of the knee joint: Anatomical, functional and experimental analysis. *Clin Orthop* 1975;106:229.)

the superficial portion of the ligament appear to tighten with knee flexion of 70° to 105°.[7] The deep portion of the medial collateral ligament can also be divided into two portions: the meniscofemoral and meniscotibial ligaments, which are defined by their respective insertions.[8]

The average length of the anterior cruciate ligament is 31 to 38 mm, and the average width is 11 mm; the average length of the posterior cruciate ligament is 38 mm and the average width is 13 mm.[5] The cross-sectional area of both of the cruciate ligaments varies along their lengths. The largest cross-sectional area of the anterior cruciate ligament is distal, and the largest cross-sectional area of the posterior cruciate ligament is proximal (Fig. 2).[9] The clinical importance of this finding is not yet understood. The anatomy of the insertion sites of the cruciate ligaments has been well described.[5,10] Particularly noteworthy is the fact that, although the posterior cruciate ligament is entirely intra-articular (as is the anterior cruciate ligament), the tibial attachment of the posterior cruciate ligament is 1 cm distal to the joint surface.[3,10,11]

Biochemically, the ligaments of the knee joint are composed primarily of type-I collagen, with variable amounts of elastin and reticulin. The collagen that makes up ligaments is grouped into bundles with a characteristic crimp — a sinusoidal, undulating waviness that allows the ligament to elongate or shorten slightly in an accordion-like fashion to adapt to external stresses. The crimp pattern of the cruciate ligaments has less amplitude (wave height and periodicity)

than the crimp pattern of the medial collateral ligament. Additionally, the width of the collagen bundles of the medial collateral ligament is about three times that of the anterior cruciate ligament.[12,13] Finally, recent electron-microscopy studies have confirmed that the medial collateral ligament has more collagen fibers per unit area than the anterior cruciate ligament has.[14] These findings may have important implications with regard to both the function and the healing of these ligaments.

Biomechanics

Biomechanics (the science of the action of forces on the living body[15]) can be somewhat intimidating to the uninitiated. Nevertheless, an understanding of a few key concepts can bring a new appreciation to the study of knee ligaments.

Although the function of the ligaments is somewhat complex, their primary role is to restrain abnormal motion. The anterior cruciate ligament is the primary restraint to anterior translation of the tibia relative to the femur; similarly, the posterior cruciate ligament serves as the primary restraint against posterior tibial displacement.[16] Both of the cruciate ligaments also regulate the screw-home mechanism of the knee.[17] The medial collateral ligament, particularly its superficial portion, acts as the primary restraint to valgus angulation, and the lateral collateral ligament serves as the primary restraint to varus angulation.[18] Both the medial and the lateral collateral ligament also serve in concert

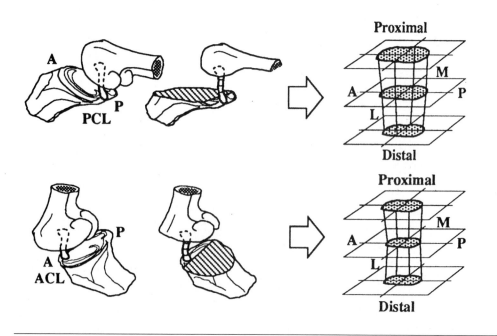

Fig. 2 Diagram illustrating the cross-sectional areas of the posterior cruciate ligament (PCL) and the anterior cruciate ligament (ACL). Note that the area does not remain constant for either ligament. A = anterior, P = posterior, M = medial, and L = lateral. (Reproduced with permission from Harner CD, Livesay GA, Choi NY, et al: Evaluation of the sizes and shapes of the human anterior and posterior cruciate ligaments: A comparative study. *Trans Orthop Res Soc* 1992;18:123.)

with their surrounding structures (the posteromedial corner and the posterolateral structures, respectively) to control axial rotation of the tibia on the femur.[19,20]

Strength of Materials

This branch of biomechanics deals with the relationships between externally applied loads and the resulting internal effects on a material.[15] Stress (forces per unit area) and strain (deformation of a body as a result of loading) can be represented on a stress-strain curve. The slope of this curve (Young modulus of elasticity or E) represents the stiffness of a material — that is, its ability to resist deformation. The tensile strength of a ligament is the maximum stress that the ligament can sustain before failure. A comparison of the mechanical properties of the anterior cruciate and medial collateral ligaments has revealed marked differences between the two ligaments (Fig. 3).[21] In the rabbit, the medial collateral ligament has approximately twice the stiffness and tensile strength of the anterior cruciate ligament. Unfortunately, similar data for the posterior cruciate and lateral collateral ligaments are not available, to our knowledge.

Ligament strain can be measured by a variety of methods, including a mercury gauge,[22,23] a Hall-effect strain transducer,[7] and a video dimension analyzer.[24] The advantages of this last method are that it avoids direct contact with the ligaments and it can measure strains independently of the insertion sites of the ligaments.

Tensile tests of ligaments have been done with use of the bone-ligament-bone complex because the ligaments are too short to be tested in an isolated fashion. The resulting load-elongation curve represents the structural properties of this complex. For the anterior cruciate ligament, the mean ultimate stiffness and ultimate failure load from testing of young human donors has been reported to be as high as 2,160 N/mm.[25] Because of anatomic complexity and variations with regard to the means of specimen preparation, the age of the donor, the orientation of the ligament during testing, and other factors, conflicting results have been previously reported.[26,27] The posterior cruciate ligament has been reported to be twice as strong as the anterior cruciate ligament on tensile testing in the laboratory,[28] but more recently its ultimate load was reported to be closer to that of the anterior cruciate ligament.[29] Nevertheless, it is widely accepted that the tensile strength of the posterior cruciate ligament is greater than that of the anterior cruciate ligament.

Viscoelasticity

Ligaments are viscoelastic — that is, their stress-strain behavior is time-rate dependent, with elongation of the ligament being more likely to occur with slower loading conditions. The rate of loading affects the ultimate load to failure. Ligaments also possess characteristic creep properties (progressive elongation with a constant load) and stress-relaxation properties (the amount of stress measured in a preloaded ligament decreases with time) (Fig. 4). For the anterior cruciate ligament, stress relaxation has been noted to stabilize at 80% of the initial stress over time.[30]

Kinematics

Kinematics (the study of body motion without regard to the cause of that motion[15]) is important to the understanding of the form and function of the knee. The main objective in knee ligament reconstruction is the restoration of joint stability with normal joint laxity and kinematics. Thus, we must gain an understanding of the role of the ligaments in the guiding of normal knee motion and the effects of ligament damage on this motion. The type of joint motion that results from reconstructive procedures about the knee must also be appreciated.

Motion of the knee can be described with the use of six degrees of freedom: three translations (anterior-posterior, medial-lateral, and cephalad-caudad) and three rotations (flexion-extension, internal-external rotation, and varus-valgus angulation). In knee motion, primary translation and rotation occur in the sagittal plane and are coupled with obligatory rotations about another axis: anterior-posterior rotation is coupled with internal rotation, and flexion-extension rotation is coupled with external rotation.

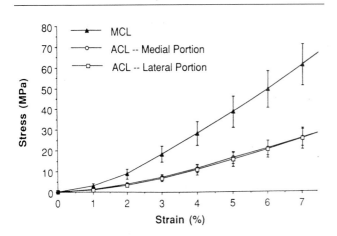

Fig. 3 A comparison of stress-strain curves for the medial collateral ligament (MCL) and the anterior cruciate ligament (ACL). Note the higher modulus of elasticity (E) and ultimate strength of the medial collateral ligament. (Reproduced with permission from Woo SL, Newton PO, MacKenna DA, et al: A comparative evaluation of the mechanical properties of the rabbit medial collateral and anterior cruciate ligaments. *J Biomech* 1992;25:377-386.)

The four major ligaments of the knee act in concert with the other static stabilizers (osseous geometry, capsular structures, and the menisci) and with the dynamic muscle stabilizers to define the limits of knee motion. The flexion-extension kinematic principles of the knee have been explained on the basis of a four-bar cruciate-linkage system (Fig. 5).[31] This model demonstrates the importance of the interaction between the cruciate ligaments and the osseous geometry and clarifies the central role of the anterior cruciate ligament in knee kinematics. The four bars represent the links formed between the tibial and femoral attachment sites of the anterior and posterior cruciate ligaments and the neutral fibers of the cruciate ligaments. During knee flexion, the instantaneous center of joint rotation (the

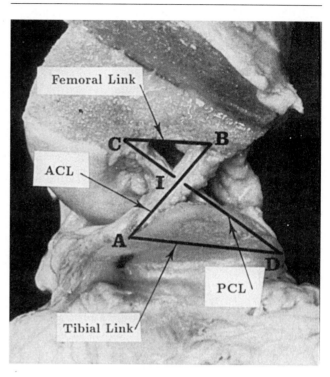

Fig. 5 Photograph showing four-bar linkage, which includes the anterior cruciate ligament (AB), the posterior cruciate ligament (CD), and the osseous links (CB = the femur and AD = the tibia). I = the instantaneous center of joint rotation. (Reproduced with permission from O'Connor J, Shercliff T, FitzPatrick D, et al: Geometry of the knee, in Daniel DM, Akeson WH, O'Connor JJ (eds): *Knee Ligaments: Structure, Function, Injury, and Repair.* New York, NY Raven Press, 1990, pp 163-199.)

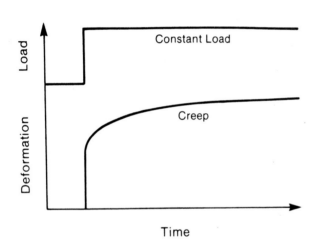

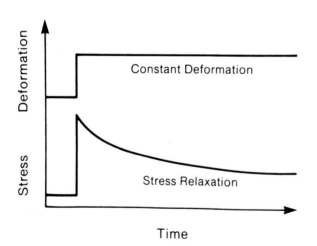

Fig. 4 Schematic representation of creep behavior (top) and stress relaxation (bottom). (Reproduced with permission from Woo SL-Y, Young EP: Structure and function of tendons and ligaments, in Mow VC, Hayes WC (eds): *Basic Orthopaedic Biomechanics.* New York, NY, Raven Press, 1991, p 203.)

point of intersection of the anterior and posterior cruciate ligaments) moves posteriorly, forcing a combination of rolling and sliding to occur between the articulating surfaces (Fig. 6). This unique mechanism prevents the femur from rolling off of the posterior aspect of the tibial plateau as the knee flexes.

The devices most frequently employed to quantify the amount of motion that occurs in a joint under external loading are linkage systems that include linear variable-differential transducers that measure translation and rotatory variable-differential transducers that measure rotation.[14,32,33] These two devices are attached to the two bones of a joint, and when the joint moves, the transducers translate or rotate and produce an output voltage proportional to the amount of translation or rotation. Hefzy and Grood[34] used a six-degrees-of-freedom electrogoniometer, known as an instrumented spatial linkage, which employs a kinematic chain of rotatory transducers and links connecting the two ends of the linkage to obtain much of the information that follows.

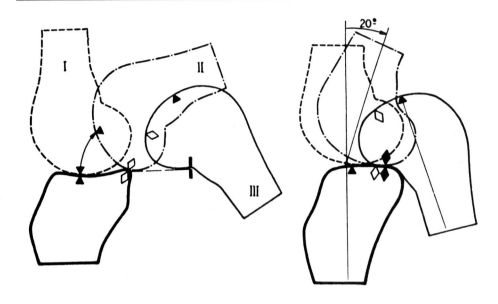

Fig. 6 Diagram illustrating the rolling and sliding in the normal knee. With pure rolling (**left**) the femur would roll off the posterior tibial plateau. The cruciates permit simultaneous rolling and sliding between the femur and the tibia (**right**). (Reproduced with permission from Kapandji IA: The knee, in *The Physiology of the Joints.* 1970, Paris, Editions Maloine, vol 2, p 72-135.)

Anterior Translation

The anterior cruciate ligament is the predominant restraint to anterior tibial displacement. The ligament accepts 75% of the anterior force at full extension and approximately 85% at 30° and 90° of flexion.[16,35] The observed loads within the anterior portion of the anterior cruciate ligament throughout knee flexion suggest that the posterior portion resists anterior tibial loading in only a limited range near full extension.[36] With the tibia in neutral rotation, the application of 100 N of anterior force produces anterior tibial translation of 2 to 5 mm at full extension and 5 to 8 mm at 30° of flexion.[17,19,20,37,38] As the flexion angle increases further, anterior translation decreases. Sectioning of the anterior cruciate ligament results in increased laxity at all flexion angles.[19,37,39] At 20° to 30° of flexion (where maximum anterior translation occurs) with a 100-N anterior force, 7 to 9 mm of increased translation is seen.[17,39] Large increases in anterior laxity are also seen after complete rupture of the deep and superficial fibers of the medial collateral ligament (a grade-III injury) in a knee with a torn anterior cruciate ligament[39,40]; however, isolated sectioning of the medial collateral ligament (in the presence of an intact anterior cruciate ligament) has little effect on anterior translation.[41] Isolated sectioning of the iliotibial band, the lateral collateral ligament, or the posterolateral and mid-lateral capsular structures in a knee with a torn anterior cruciate ligament also results in increased anterior translation, although to a lesser extent than in knees in which the medial collateral ligament has been sectioned.[16,39] Isolated sectioning of the posterior cruciate ligament results in no

change in anterior translation at any flexion angle.[42]

As noted, normal knee kinematics is a result of coupled motion, including internal rotation, valgus angulation, and anterior translation of the tibia.[17,19,37,39,41,43] Studies have demonstrated that prevention of rotation of the tibia decreases anterior and posterior displacement by as much as 30% and that, with loss of the cruciate ligaments, the normal coupled rotation decreases in magnitude.[17] This indicates the importance of the cruciate ligaments, not only in the restraint of anteroposterior translation but also in the initiation and control of internal and external tibial rotation during anteroposterior motion.

Loss of internal rotation and valgus angulation occurs with sectioning of the anterior cruciate ligament.[17,37] Combined sectioning of the anterior cruciate ligament, lateral collateral ligament, and posterolateral structures increases the coupled internal rotation associated with anterior displacement. Division of the posterior cruciate ligament, lateral collateral ligament, or posterolateral structures, individually or in combination, does not affect the coupling motion.[19] These observed coupled motions include true motion-coupling as well as the repositioning of the tibia that occurs following loss of the anterior cruciate ligament.[20,41]

Posterior Translation

The posterior cruciate ligament is the primary restraint to posterior tibial translation; it sustains 85% to 100% of the posterior force at both 30° and 90° of flexion.[16,35,44] The lateral collateral ligament and the posterolateral structures, including the popliteus tendon and arcuate ligament, are the secondary restraints, with the medial collateral ligament playing a lesser role.[19,20] The posterior aspect of the capsule makes an important contribution only near full extension.[19,20] Coupled external rotation and lateral translation accompanies posterior translation.[17,20]

Posterior translation of 4 to 5 mm is seen with the application of 100 N of posterior force.[17,19,38] Isolated loss of the posterior cruciate ligament results in an increase in posterior translation to a maximum of 15 to 20 mm at 90° of flexion[16,17,19] as well as a loss of coupled external rotation.[17,19,38] When the posterior aspect of the capsule, the posterolateral structures, and the lateral collateral ligament are sectioned, however, the coupled external rotation is increased.[19,20] This is maximum at 30° and diminishes with further flexion. Isolated loss of the anterior cruciate ligament results in no important change in posterior translation, coupled external rotation, or lateral translation at 90° of knee flexion.[17,20] Tibial rotation decreases anterior and posterior translation by tightening the secondary restraints. Internal tibial rotation reduces anterior and posterior laxity and increases the anterior and posterior stiffness of the joint by tightening the iliotibial band, the lateral aspect of the capsule, and the medial and lateral collateral ligaments, while external rotation tightens the medial and lateral collateral ligaments and the posterolateral structures. The strain in the fibers of the anterior and posterior cruciate ligaments increases during these rotations, with the amount being dependent on the flexion angle and the magnitude of the rotation.[23,45]

Varus Angulation

The lateral collateral ligament is the primary restraint to varus angulation; it resists approximately 55% of the applied load at full extension.[18-20] The lateral collateral ligament also acts to resist internal rotation forces. Its role increases with joint flexion, as the posterolateral structures become lax.[18] The cruciate ligaments (primarily the anterior cruciate ligament) resist approximately 25% of the moment at full extension. With joint flexion, resistance by the anterior cruciate ligament decreases, but large forces are found in the posterior cruciate ligament at 90° of flexion.[18] The capsular contribution to stability is three times greater in the posterior aspect than in the middle and anterior portions of the capsule. Coupled anteromedial translation and internal rotation occurs with a varus moment. Grood and associates[20] observed that coupled external rotation occurred during varus rotation when the posterolateral structures had been lost.

Isolated sectioning of the lateral collateral ligament results in an increase in varus opening, but this is a minimum increase unless the other lateral and posterolateral structures are also sectioned.[19,20] External rotation of the tibia also markedly increases after sec-

tioning of all of these structures. Subsequent cutting of the posterior cruciate ligament results in a further increase in varus angulation.[19] Isolated loss of the lateral and posterolateral structures or loss of the posterior cruciate ligament alone results in no increase in varus instability, but cutting of the lateral collateral ligament in combination with either the anterior or the posterior cruciate ligament results in a large increase in varus opening.[19,38] Coupled internal rotation is increased at full extension following sectioning of the anterior cruciate ligament, but the effect is minimum at 30° of flexion.

Valgus Angulation

The primary restraint to valgus rotation is the superficial portion of the medial collateral ligament.[41] At full extension, the medial collateral ligament resists about 50% of the applied valgus moment, whereas the anterior and posterior aspects of the capsule resist as much as 25%. The other 25% is shared between the anterior and posterior cruciate ligaments, with the posterior cruciate ligament resisting the most at full extension. The role of the medial collateral ligament increases with increasing flexion, as the posterior capsular structures become lax, but it decreases with increasing valgus moment and rotation, as the posteromedial aspect of the capsule becomes more involved.[18]

While isolated sectioning of the anterior cruciate ligament, posterior cruciate ligament, lateral collateral ligament, or posterolateral structures does not cause large increases in valgus angulation, sectioning of the medial collateral ligament increases valgus instability markedly.[18,38,41,46] Studies involving combined cutting have demonstrated that the largest increases in laxity follow combined sectioning of the medial collateral and posterior cruciate ligaments; this finding confirms that the primary restraint to valgus rotation is the medial collateral ligament, with the posterior cruciate ligament playing a secondary role.[38,46]

Normal coupled motions with an applied valgus load include lateral translation without noticeable internal-external rotation or anterior-posterior translation.[41] Isolated sectioning of the anterior cruciate ligament does not affect any of these coupled motions.[41]

Internal Rotation

Internal-rotation laxity increases with knee flexion, with the largest amount (25°) seen in the 20° to 40° range of knee flexion.[38,40,47] Of all of the structures around the knee, only the medial collateral and anterior cruciate ligaments play an important role in the restraint of internal rotation; isolated cutting of either of these ligaments results in a marked increase in internal-rotation laxity, with the medial collateral ligament playing a larger role.[20,38,40,47] Thus, the medial collateral ligament can be considered to be the major restraint to internal rotation.[19,48] Combined sectioning of the anterior cruciate and medial collateral ligaments results in much more laxity than does sectioning of either ligament alone. Loss of the anterior cruciate ligament in combination with loss of the lateral collateral ligament or the posterolateral structures, or both, also results in increased rotatory laxity of approximately 35°. Isolated cutting of the posterior cruciate ligament results in no increase in internal-rotation laxity.

Coupled anterior and medial translation occurs with internal rotation. Isolated loss of the anterior cruciate ligament results in an increase in the coupled anterior translation. Isolated loss of the posterior cruciate ligament, the lateral collateral ligament, or the posterolateral structures does not affect the coupled motion. Internal-rotation laxity is also increased following medial or lateral meniscectomy.

External Rotation

External-rotation laxity increases with knee flexion, with the largest amount (20°) being seen in the 30° to 40° range of flexion. External rotation is not directly limited by the cruciate ligaments. Only the posterior cruciate ligament, which becomes taut at 90° of flexion, would be expected to provide restraint should the posterolateral structures be injured.[19,45,49] External-rotation laxity is markedly increased only when the posterolateral structures or the lateral collateral ligament, or both, are cut.[20,47] Concomitant loss of the posterior cruciate ligament results in even greater increases in rotation laxity. The magnitude of this laxity varies directly with the flexion angle.

Coupled posterior and lateral translation occurs with external rotation. The only effect seen in studies involving cutting of the ligaments has been marked coupled posterior translations at all flexion angles following combined sectioning of the posterolateral structures and the posterior cruciate ligament.[19,20]

Effect of Joint-Loading on Muscle Action

The conditions of these in vitro tests are quite different from the functional conditions under which the joint performs in both normal and injured states. The knee and its ligaments are subjected to levels of force and displacement far beyond the envelope of passive motion commonly used in clinical testing. Several investigators have applied an axial load (either an externally applied static load or an internally applied load on the quadriceps or hamstring mechanism) to in vitro specimens during simulated laxity testing.[40,45,48-53] These studies have demonstrated that the stiffness of the knee is increased by loading of the joint and that the effect of sectioning of soft-tissue structures on joint motion is different from the effect seen in an unloaded joint. The quadriceps and hamstring mechanisms interact functionally with the knee ligaments as well. These are only two of the major muscle groups

around the knee, and they have just begun to be investigated.[48,54-56]

In general, in vivo clinical laxity tests demonstrate lower laxity levels than do in vitro simulations. These studies mark the beginning of our improved understanding of the complex kinematics of the knee during function and the synergistic role of the ligamentous and muscular structures.

Ligament Strain in Vivo

In order to determine the amount of strain on the anterior cruciate ligament in vivo, investigators at the University of Vermont measured strain in normal anterior cruciate ligaments using a sterile Hall-effect strain transducer placed arthroscopically after an operation for an unrelated condition.[57] They found that strain in the ligament was related to knee flexion, with the most strain occurring near full extension, especially with quadriceps contraction. Less strain occurred with co-contractions of both the quadriceps and the hamstring muscle groups and at greater degrees of flexion. Preliminary studies by the same investigators on reconstructions of the anterior cruciate ligament demonstrated similar strain patterns in anterior cruciate ligament grafts, with the levels of strain within the grafts one year postoperatively remaining higher than the levels in normal anterior cruciate ligaments.[57]

Healing of the Medial Collateral Ligament

An understanding of the physiology of healing of fibrous connective tissue is essential to the effective clinical management of ligament injuries. Ligaments are complex dynamic structures that exhibit biochemical heterogeneity along their length, and matrix composition changes with growth and maturation.[58] The healing response of intra-articular ligaments is very different from that of extra-articular ligaments. A torn anterior cruciate ligament often fails to show any healing response, while the medial collateral ligament seems to have a much better healing potential.[59-64] These differences have been attributed to local environment, sources of nutrition, the functions of the ligament, or intrinsic mechanical properties.[64,65]

The healing of extra-articular ligaments is analogous to other soft-tissue healing; there is evidence to suggest that periarticular ligaments heal through the production and remodeling of scar tissue.[59,66] Optimum healing of the medial collateral ligament occurs when the torn ends are in contact; the healing potential is directly related to the size of the gap between the torn ends.[67] Tension appears to have a positive effect on ligament healing.[68] Although it is still somewhat controversial, most authors have recommended nonsurgical management of isolated injuries of the medial collateral ligament.[69]

Extra-articular ligament repair occurs as a continuum, but it has been divided into three phases on the basis of morphologic and biochemical events.[70,71] While the timing and details of healing are probably ligament specific as well as model specific, these phases have been characterized for rabbit medial collateral ligaments, and the process is probably similar in human tissue.

Phase I (acute inflammation and reaction) occurs during the first 72 hours after an injury. Phase II (repair and regeneration) occupies the time period from 72 hours until approximately six weeks after the injury. Phase III (remodeling or maturation) occurs from six weeks to as long as 12 months or more after the injury. Even after 12 months, however, the ligament recovers only 50% to 70% of its original modulus and tensile strength,[64] although the stiffness and ultimate load of the entire bone-ligament complex may be totally recovered. This can occur because the healing tissue has a larger cross-sectional area.

Inflammatory Phase

Immediately after a mid-substance tear of the medial collateral ligament, the rupture gap fills in with erythrocytes and inflammatory cells. These inflammatory cells release potent vasodilators, such as histamine, serotonin, bradykinins, and prostaglandins.[66] These inflammatory mediators, the torn ligament ends, and the coagulum that fills the gap combine to initiate the healing process. Recent research has shown that the epiligament of the medial collateral ligament may be an important source of extracellular matrix, cells, and vasculature during this phase.[72] At the end of the inflammatory phase, fibroblasts originating from undifferentiated mesenchymal cells begin to produce an extracellular matrix of proteoglycan and collagen.[66] Most of the collagen that is synthesized at this stage is type III, which is thought to stabilize the extracellular collagen lattice. In contrast, type-I collagen, which predominates in healthy ligaments, is more important to long-term ligament function.[73] Biochemical studies have shown that the relative concentration of glycosaminoglycan, fibronectin, and DNA changes drastically during this first phase of repair.[60,66]

Repair and Regeneration Phase

This phase of the repair of the medial collateral ligament is heralded by organization of the original blood clot and is characterized by matrix and cellular proliferation.[58] Friable, highly vascular granulation tissue covers the ends of the torn ligament. Histologically, the tissue is highly cellular, and the fibroblast is the predominant cell type. Macrophages and mast cells are also abundant. Active synthesis of type-I collagen occurs in the proliferating scar and in adjacent normal-appearing tissue. Even though the ligament matrix contains more total collagen than it did preced-

ing the injury, the collagen concentration is lower because of the sparse, woven organization of the collagen framework. The biochemical changes (increased water, glycosaminoglycan, and DNA concentrations) that occur during this phase have been correlated with increasing modulus and tensile strength of the matrix.[58,63]

Remodeling and Maturation Phase

This phase of repair is characterized by decreased cellularity, vascularity, and synthetic activity. Collagen density increases and, histologically, collagen fibers appear to be aligned with the long axis of the ligament.[13,59,73] Transmission electron microscopy demonstrates that the collagen fibrils are slightly increased in diameter and are more densely packed than in the normal medial collateral ligament.[74] Biochemical changes include a decreased water content, slightly lower collagen concentration, and slightly increased total collagen content compared with the normal ligament. DNA content returns to a normal level, but proteoglycan content remains slightly increased. Throughout this phase, the ligament-scar matrix gradually matures into a tissue that is slightly more disorganized and hypercellular than normal tissue. This phase is variable in duration and is model and ligament specific.

Healing and Repair of Other Knee Ligaments

Lateral Collateral Ligament

Research on the healing of this ligament has not been as active as has investigation of healing of the medial collateral ligament. Early studies of canine models demonstrated that the lateral collateral ligament heals with less scar tissue when it has been repaired than when it has been treated nonsurgically.[75,76] A more recent, clinical study on the lateral ligament in humans demonstrated good success with nonsurgical treatment of grade-II sprains (5 to 10 mm of instability, an incomplete tear), but poor results with grade-III sprains (more than 10 mm of instability, a complete tear).[77] It should be noted, however, that the anterior cruciate ligament was also injured in association with many of the grade-III sprains in this study, and this may have affected the results. Clearly, healing of the lateral collateral ligament is an area in need of additional research.

Cruciate Ligaments

It has been well accepted that repair of an intrasubstance tear of the anterior cruciate ligament is clinically inferior to reconstructive options.[44] Like the anterior cruciate ligament, the posterior cruciate ligament heals poorly and suture alone is insufficient for restoration of the posterior cruciate ligament; it is not strong enough to withstand the applied forces on the knee.[78] Studies of animals have suggested that a limited intrinsic healing capacity may explain the poor healing of the anterior cruciate ligament, even when the torn ends of the injured ligament are held in close approximation by surgical repair.[79] This poor response may be related to the heterogeneity of the collagen fibrils of the cruciate ligaments (as opposed to those of the medial collateral ligament) or to a difference in fibroblast function within a synovial environment.[80] Fibroblasts from the anterior cruciate and medial collateral ligaments demonstrate different responses when evaluated in culture. Fibroblasts from the anterior cruciate ligament produce more type-I and less type-III collagen in repair than do fibroblasts from the medial collateral ligament.[71] This may help to explain, at least partially, the difference in the healing of these ligaments. The fact that the anterior cruciate ligament is intra-articular may not be enough, in and of itself, to explain the different healing responses, because, in one study, synovial fluid was actually found to stimulate cell proliferation.[81]

Autogenous and Allogeneic Grafts

Replacement of the medial collateral ligament with allograft has been studied in both rabbit[82] and dog models. In both studies, the tensile strengths of the allografts at one year were less than half of the values for the contralateral, control medial collateral ligaments.

Yasuda and associates[83] characterized the maturation of autogenous grafts composed of the anterior cruciate ligament in terms of four phases, on the basis of biopsies of specimens retrieved arthroscopically at specific periods of follow-up (Table 1). In animal models, patellar-ligament autogenous grafts have been shown to undergo a gradual change in cell morphology, collagen profile, cross-linking pattern, and glycosaminoglycan content. The process results in a graft with the morphology and biochemical profile approximating that of a normal anterior cruciate ligament.[84]

Unfortunately, the biomechanical properties of these grafts are less than ideal. Several studies of animal models have demonstrated structural properties of autogenous grafts composed of the anterior cruciate ligament to be approximately 30% to 40% of control values, with peak values attained between 30 weeks and two years.[85,86]

Structural properties of allografts may be affected by preservation processes. Freeze-drying and high-dose irradiation (three megarads) may adversely affect the strength and cause excessive crimping of the graft[87]; however, deep freezing, cold ethylene-gas sterilization, and low-dose irradiation (two megarads) do not markedly affect the mechanical properties of the graft.[88,89] Jackson and associates[90] evaluated the single effect of freezing by using an in situ freezing technique in an animal model. They found no difference between the frozen and the control tissues. Ethylene oxide sterilization of grafts, on the other hand, has been associated with complications and failure and is no longer recommended.[91,92] The adverse effects associated with ethylene oxide may be related to induced overproduction of interleukin-1 by synoviocytes.[93]

Fresh-frozen allografts from the anterior cruciate ligament have been shown to undergo a revascularization process similar to that of autogenous grafts.[94] Jackson and associates,[95] in a study of a goat model, demonstrated marked differences between allografts and autogenous grafts at six months. Unfortunately, the authors did not continue their study past the six-month point. Several investigators have recognized that the phases of healing of allografts lag behind those of autogenous grafts,[96] and the trends that Jackson and associates noted at six months might not have been present at the 12-month point. The same criticism is applicable to other animal studies that have demonstrated inferior strength of allograft tissues compared with that of autogenous graft tissues.[97]

In summary, an understanding of the biomechanics of the four pivotal knee ligaments — the anterior cruciate, posterior cruciate, medial collateral, and lateral collateral ligaments — provides the foundation for ligament reconstruction. The reconstructive surgeon must be as much a physician-scientist as a technician. The surgeon should strive to recreate the normal anatomy through accurate placement of grafts; use grafts with adequate material properties; eliminate abnormal translations, angulations, and rotations; understand the strains that affect ligaments; appreciate the capabilities of ligaments to heal; and have some fundamental knowledge about ligament grafts.

Table 1
Phases of maturation of autogenous grafts of the anterior cruciate ligament

Phase	Time Period (months)	Characteristics
1	<6	Synovial envelopment
2	6-12	Fibrous ingrowth
3	12-18	Transformation to ligament-like tissue
4	>18	Maturation

References

1. Furman W, Marshall JL, Girgis FG: The anterior cruciate ligament: A functional analysis based on postmortem studies. *J Bone Joint Surg* 1976;58A:179-185.

2. Norwood LA, Cross MJ: Anterior cruciate ligament: Functional anatomy of its bundles in rotary instabilities. *Am J Sports Med* 1979;7:23-26.

3. Hughston JC, Bowden JA, Andrews JR, et al: Acute tears of the posterior cruciate ligament: Results of operative treatment. *J Bone Joint Surg* 1980;62A:438-450.

4. Arnoczky SP: Anatomy of the anterior cruciate ligament. *Clin Orthop* 1983;172:19-25.

5. Girgis FG, Marshall JL, Al Monajem ARS: The cruciate ligaments of the knee joint: Anatomical, functional and experimental analysis. *Clin Orthop* 1975;106:216-231.

6. Warren LF, Marshall JL: The supporting structures and layers on the medial side of the knee: An anatomical analysis. *J Bone Joint Surg* 1979;61A:56-62.

7. Arms S, Boyle J, Johnson R, et al: Strain measurement in the medial collateral ligament of the human knee: An autopsy study. *J Biomech* 1983;16:491-496.

8. Warren LF, Marshall JL, Girgis F: The prime static stabilizer of the medial side of the knee. *J Bone Joint Surg* 1974;56A:665-674.

9. Harner CD, Livesay GA, Choi NY, et al: Evaluation of the sizes and shapes of the human anterior and posterior cruciate ligaments: A comparative study. *Trans Orthop Res Soc* 1992;17:123.

10. Harner CD, Kashiwaguchi S, Livesay GA, et al: Insertion site anatomy of the human anterior and posterior cruciate ligaments. *Trans Orthop Res Soc* 1993;18:341.

11. Cooper DE, Warren RF, Warner JJP: The posterior cruciate ligament and posterolateral structures of the knee: Anatomy, function, and patterns of injury, in Tullos HS (ed): *Instructional Course Lectures* XL, Park Ridge, IL, American Academy of Orthopaedic Surgeons. 1991, pp 249-270.

12. Amiel D, Billings E Jr, Akeson WH: Ligament structure, chemistry, and physiology, in Daniel DM, Akeson WH, O'Connor JJ (eds): *Knee Ligaments: Structure, Function, Injury, and Repair.* New York, NY, Raven Press, 1990, pp 77-91.

13. Amiel D, Frank CB, Harwood FL, et al: Collagen alteration in medial collateral ligament healing in a rabbit model. *Connect Tissue Res* 1987;16:357-366.

14. Hart RA, Woo SL-Y, Newton PO: Ultrastructural morphometry of anterior cruciate and medial collateral ligaments: An experimental study in rabbits. *J Orthop Res* 1992;10:96-103.

15. Miller MD: Biomechanics, in Miller MD (ed): *Review of Orthopaedics.* Philadelphia, PA, WB Saunders, 1992, pp 34-48.

16. Butler DL, Noyes FR, Grood ES: Ligamentous restraints to anterior-posterior drawer in the human knee: A biomechanical study. *J Bone Joint Surg* 1980;62A:259-270.

17. Fukubayashi T, Torzilli PA, Sherman MF, et al: An in vitro biomechanical evaluation of anterior-posterior motion of the knee: Tibial displacement, rotation, and torque. *J Bone Joint Surg* 1982;64A:258-264.

18. Grood ES, Noyes FR, Butler DL, et al: Ligamentous and capsular restraints preventing straight medial and lateral laxity in intact human cadaver knees. *J Bone Joint Surg* 1981;63A:1257-1269.

19. Gollehon DL, Torzilli PA, Warren RF: The role of the posterolateral and cruciate ligaments in the stability of the human knee: A biomechanical study. *J Bone Joint Surg* 1098;69A:233-242.

20. Grood ES, Stowers SF, Noyes FR: Limits of movement in the human knee: Effect of sectioning the posterior cruciate ligament and posterolateral structures. *J Bone Joint Surg* 1988;70A:88-97.

21. Woo SL, Newton PO, MacKenna DA, et al: A comparative evaluation of the mechanical properties of the rabbit medial collateral and anterior cruciate ligaments. *J Biomech* 1992;25:377-386.

22. Henning CE, Lynch MA, Glick KR Jr: An in vivo strain gage study of elongation of the anterior cruciate ligament. *Am J Sports Med* 1985;13:22-26.

23. Kennedy JC, Hawkins RJ, Willis RB: Strain gauge analysis of knee ligaments. *Clin Orthop* 1977;129:225-229.

24. Woo SL-Y, Gomez MA, Woo YK, et al: Mechanical properties of tendons and ligaments: II. The relationships of immobilization and exercise on tissue remodeling: Quasistatic and nonlinear viscoelastic properties. *Biorheology* 1982;19:397-408.

25. Woo SL-Y, Adams DJ: The tensile properties of human anterior cruciate ligament (ACL) and ACL graft tissues, in Danile DM, Akeson WH, O'Connor JJ (eds): *Knee Ligaments: Structure, Function, Injury, and Repair.* New York, NY, Raven Press, 1990, pp 279-289.

26. Noyes FR, Butler DL, Grood ES, et al: Biomechanical analysis of human ligament grafts used in knee-ligament repairs and reconstructions. *J Bone Joint Surg* 184;66A:344-352.

27. Woo SL-Y, Hollis JM, Adams DJ, et al: Tensile properties of the human femur-anterior cruciate ligament-tibia complex: The effects of specimen age and orientation. *Am J Sports Med* 1991;19:217-225.

28. Kennedy JC, Hawkins RJ, Willis RB, et al: Tension studies of human knee ligaments: Yield point, ultimate failure, and disruption of the cruciate and tibial collateral ligaments. *J Bone Joint Surg* 1976;58A:350-355.

29. Prietto MP, Bain JR, Stonebrook SN, et al: Tensile strength of the human posterior cruciate ligament (PCL). *Trans Orthop Res Soc* 1988;13:195.

30. Lyon RM, Lin HC, Kwan MK-W, et al: Stress relaxation of the anterior cruciate ligament (ACL) and the patellar tendon (PT). *Trans Orthop Res Soc* 1988;13:81.

31. Müller WW: Kinematics, in Müller WW (ed): *The Knee: Form, Function, and Ligament Reconstruction.* New York, NY, Springer, 1983, pp 8-28.

32. Hollis JM, Takai S, Adams DJ, et al: The effects of knee motion and external loading on the length of the anterior cruciate ligament (ACL): A kinematic study. *J Biomech Eng* 1991;113:208-214.

33. Takai S, Adams DJ, Livesay GA, et al: Determination of loads in the human anterior cruciate ligament. *Trans Orthop Res Soc* 1991;16:235.

34. Hefzy MS, Grood ES: Sensitivity of insertion locations on length patterns of anterior cruciate ligament fibers. *J Biomech Eng* 1986;108:73-82.

35. Piziali RL, Seering WP, Nagel DA, et al: The function of the primary ligaments of the knee in anterior-posterior and medial-lateral motions. *J Biomech* 1980;13:777-784.

36. Woo SL-Y, Livesay GA, Engle C: Biomechanics of the human anterior cruciate ligament: ACL structure and role in knee motion. *Orthop Rev* 192;21:835-842.

37. Levy IM, Torzilli PA, Warren RF: The effect of medial meniscectomy on anterior-posterior motion of the knee. *J Bone Joint Surg* 1982;64A:883-888.

38. Markolf KL, Mensch JS, Amstutz HC: Stiffness and laxity of the knee: The contributions of the supporting structures: A quantitative in vitro study. *J Bone Joint Surg* 1976;58A:583-594.

39. Sullivan D, Levy IM, Sheskier S, et al: Medial restraints to anterior-posterior motion of the knee. *J Bone Joint Surg* 1984;66A:930-936.

40. Shoemaker SC, Markhoff KL: Effects of joint load on the stiffness and laxity of ligament-deficient knees: An in vitro study of the anterior cruciate and medial collateral ligaments. *J Bone Joint Surg* 1985;67A:136-146.

41. Haimes JL, Grood ES, Blyski DI, et al: The effect of ACL and MCL sectioning on tibial displacement with applied valgus moment. *Trans Orthop Res Soc* 1988;13:196.

42. Stowers SF, Haimes JL, Suntay WJ, et al: The effect of tibial rotation on anterior-posterior laxity in the intact and injured knee. *Trans Orthop Res Soc* 187;12:242.

43. Torzilli PA, Greenberg RL, Insall J: An in vivo biomechanical evaluation of anterior-posterior motion of the knee: Roentgenographic measurement technique, stress machine, and stable population. *J Bone Joint Surg* 1981;63A:960-968.

44. Engebretsen L, Benum P, Sundalsvoll S: Primary suture of the anterior cruciate ligament: A 6-year follow-up of 74 cases. *Acta Orthop Scand* 1989;60:561-564.

45. Ahmed AM, Hyder A, Burke DL, et al: In-vitro ligament tension pattern in the flexed knee in passive loading. *J Orthop Res* 1987;5:217-230.

46. Mains DB, Andrews JG, Stonecipher T: Medial and anterior-posterior ligament stability of the human knee, measured with a stress apparatus. *Am J Sports Med* 1977;5:144-153.

47. Lipke JM, Janecki CJ, Nelson CL, et al: The role of incompetence of the anterior cruciate and lateral ligaments in antero-lateral and anteromedial instability: A biomechanical study of cadaver knees. *J Bone Joint Surg* 1981;63A:954-960.

48. More RC, Karras BT, Neiman R, et al: Hamstrings: An anterior cruciate ligament protagonist: An in vitro study. *Am J Sports Med* 1993;21:231-237.

49. Seering WP, Piziali RL, Nagel DA, et al: The function of the primary ligaments of the knee in varus-valgus and axial rotation. *J Biomech* 1980;13:785-794.

50. Biden E, O'Connor J: Experimental methods used to evaluate knee ligament function, in Daniel DM, Akeson WK, O'Connor JJ (eds): *Knee Ligaments: Structure, Function, Injury, and Repair*. New York, NY, Raven Press, 1990, pp 135-151.

51. Biden E, O'Connor J, Goodfellow J: Tibial rotation in the cadaver knee. *Trans Orthop Res Soc* 1984;9:30.

52. Blankevoort L, Huiskes R, DeLange A: The envelope of passive knee joint motion. *J Biomech* 1988;21:705-720.

53. O'Connor J, Biden E, Bradley J, et al: The muscle-stabilized knee, in Daniel DM, Akeson WH, O'Connor JJ (eds): *Knee Ligaments: Structure, Function, Injury, and Repair*. New York, NY, Raven Press, 1990, pp. 239-277.

54. Draganich LF, Vahey JW: An in vitro study of anterior cruciate ligament strain induced by quadriceps and hamstrings forces. *J Orthop Res* 1990;8:57-63.

55. Kalund S, Sinkjaer T, Arendt-Nielson L, et al: Altered timing of hamstring muscle action in anterior cruciate ligament deficient patients. *Am J Sports Med* 1990;18:245-248.

56. Renström P, Arms SW, Stanwyck TS, et al: Strain within the anterior cruciate ligament during hamstring and quadriceps activity. *Am J Sports Med* 1986;14:83-87.

57. Beynnon B, Howe JG, Pope MH, et al: The measurement of anterior cruciate ligament strain in vivo. *Int Orthop* 1992;16:1-12.

58. Frank C, McDonald D, Lieber R, et al: Biochemical heterogeneity within the maturing rabbit medial collateral ligament. *Clin Orthop* 1988;236:279-285.

59. Frank C, Amiel D, Akeson WH: Healing of the medial collateral ligament of the knee: A morphological and biomechanical assessment in rabbits. *Acta Orthop Scand* 1983;54:917-923.

60. Frank C, Woo SL-Y, Amiel D, et al: Medial collateral ligament healing: A multidisciplinary assessment in rabbits. *Am J Sports Med* 1983;11:379-389.

61. O'Donoghue DH, Rockwood CA Jr, Frank GR, et al: Repair of the anterior cruciate ligament in dogs. *J Bone Joint Surg* 1966;48A:503-519.

62. O'Donoghue DH, Frank GR, Jeter GL, et al: Repair and reconstruction of the anterior cruciate ligament in dogs: Factors influencing long-term results. *J Bone Joint Surg* 1971;53A:710-718.

63. Woo SL-Y, Gomez MA, Inoue M, et al: New experimental procedures to evaluate the biomechanical properties of healing canine medial collateral ligaments. *J Orthop Res* 1987;5:425-432.

64. Woo SL, Inoue M, McGurk-Burleson E, et al: Treatment of the medial collateral ligament injury: II. Structure and function of canine knees in response to differing treatment regimens. *Am J Sports Med* 1987;15:22-29.

65. Inoue M, McGurk-Burleson E, Hollis JM, et al: Treatment of the medial collateral ligament injury: I. The importance of anterior cruciate ligament on the varus-valgus knee laxity. *Am J Sports Med* 1987;15:15-21.

66. Frank C, Amiel D, Woo SL-Y, et al: Normal ligament properties and ligament healing. *Clin Orthop* 1985;196:15-25.

67. Frank C, Shrive N, Chimich D, et al: The effects of surface area and gap size on medial collateral ligament healing. *Trans Orthop Res Soc* 1991;16:138.

68. Gomez MA, Woo S L-Y: The advantages of applied tension on healing medial collateral ligament. *Trans Orthop Res Soc* 1989;14:184.

69. Hastings DE: The non-operative management of collateral ligament injuries of the knee joint. *Clin Orthop* 1980;147:22-28.

70. Ross R: The fibroblast and wound repair. *Biol Rev Camb Philos Soc* 1968;43:51-96.

71. Ross SM, Joshi R, Frank CB: Establishment and comparison of fibroblast cell lines from the medial collateral and anterior cruciate ligaments of the rabbit. *In Vitro Cell Devel Biol* 1990;26:579-584.

72. Chowdhury P, Matyas JR, Frank CB: The "epiligament" of the rabbit medial collateral ligament: a quantitative morphological study. *Connect Tissue Res* 1991;27:33-50.

73. Andriacchi T, Sabiston P, DeHaven K, et al: Ligament: Injury and repair, in Woo SL-Y, Buckwalter JA (eds): *Injury and Repair of the Musculoskeletal Soft Tissues*. Park Ridge, IL, American Academy of Orthopaedic Surgeons, 1988, pp 103-128.

74. Frank C, McDonald D, Bray D, et al: Collagen fibril diameters in the healing adult rabbit medial collateral ligament. *Connect Tissue Res* 1992;27:251-263.

75. O'Donoghue DH: An analysis of end results of surgical treatment of major injuries to the ligaments of the knee. *J Bone Joint Surg* 1955;37A:1-13.

76. O'Donoghue DH, Rockwood CA Jr, Zaricznyj B, et al: Repair of knee ligaments in dogs: I. The lateral collateral ligament. *J Bone Joint Surg* 1961;43A:1167-1178.

77. Kannus R: Nonoperative treatment of grade II and III sprains of the lateral ligament compartment of the knee. *Am J Sports Med* 1989;17:83-88.

78. Pournaras J, Symeonides PP: The results of surgical repair of acute tears of the posterior cruciate ligament. *Clin Orthop* 191;267:103-107.

79. Kleiner JB, Roux RD, Amiel D, et al: Primary healing of the anterior cruciate ligament (ACL). *Trans Orthop Res Soc* 1986;11:131.

80. Amiel D, Kuiper S, Akeson WH: Cruciate ligaments: Response to injury, in Daniel DM, Akeson WH, O'Connor JJ (eds): *Knee Ligaments: Structure, Function, Injury, and Repair*. New York, NY, Raven Press, 1990, pp 365-377.

81. Nickerson DA, Joshi R, Williams S, et al: Synovial fluid stimulates the proliferation of rabbit ligament: Fibroblasts in vitro. *Clin Orthop* 1992:274:294-299.

82. Sabiston P, Frank C, Lam T, et al: Transplantation of rabbit medial collateral ligament: II. Biomechanical evaluation of frozen/thawed allograft. *J Orthop Res* 1990;8:46-56.

83. Yasuda K, Tomiyama Y, Ohkoshi Y, et al: Arthroscopic observations of autogeneic quadriceps and patellar tendon grafts after anterior cruciate ligament reconstruction of the knee. *Clin Orthop* 1989;246:217-224.

84. Amiel D, Kleiner JB, Roux RD, et al: The phenomenon of "ligamentalization": Anterior cruciate ligament reconstruction with autogenous patellar tendon. *J Orthop Res* 1986;4:162-172.

85. Ballock RT, Woo SL-Y, Lyon RM, et al: Use of patellar tendon autograft for anterior cruciate ligament reconstruction in the rabbit: A long-term histologic and biomechanical study. *J Orthop Res* 1989;7:474-485.

86. Clancy WG Jr, Narechania RG, Rosenberg TD, et al: Anterior and posterior cruciate ligament reconstruction in rhesus monkeys: A histological, microangiographic, and biomechanical analysis. *J Bone Joint Surg* 1981;63A:1270-1284.

87. Paulos LE, France EP, Rosenberg TD, et al: Comparative material properties of allograft tissues for ligament replacement: Effects of type, age, sterilization and preservation. *Trans Orthop Res Soc* 1987;12:129.

88. Haut RC, Powlison AC: The effects of test environment and cyclic stretching on the failure properties of human patellar tendons. *J Orthop Res* 1990;8:532-540.

89. Woo SL-Y, Orlando CA, Camp JF, et al: Effects of postmortem storage by freezing on ligament tensile behavior. *J Biomech* 1986;19:399-404.

90. Jackson DW, Grood ES, Cohn BT, et al: The effects of in situ freezing on the anterior cruciate ligament: An experimental study in goats. *J Bone Joint Surg* 1991;73A:201-213.

91. Jackson DW, Windler GE, Simon TM: Intraarticular reaction associated with the use of freeze-dried, ethylene oxide-sterilized bone-patella tendon-bone allografts in the reconstruction of the anterior cruciate ligament. *Am J Sports Med* 1990;18:1-11.

92. Roberts TS, Drez D Jr, McCarthy W, et al: Anterior cruciate ligament reconstruction using freeze-dried, ethylene oxide-sterilized, bone-patellar tendon-bone allografts: Two year results in thirty-six patients. *Am J Sports Med* 1991;19:35-41.

93. Silvaggio VJ, Fu FH, Georgescu HI, et al: The induction of IL-1 by freeze dried ethylene oxide-treated bone-patellar tendon-bone allograft wear particles: An in vitro study. *Trans Orthop Res Soc* 1991;16:207.

94. Arnoczky SP, Warren RF, Ashlock MA: Replacement of the anterior cruciate ligament using a patellar tendon allograft: An experimental study. *J Bone Joint Surg* 1986;68A:376-385.

95. Jackson DW, Grood ES, Goldstein J, et al: Anterior cruciate ligament reconstruction using patella tendon autograft and allograft: An experimental study in goats. *Trans Orthop Res Soc* 1991;16:208.

96. Nikolaou PK, Seaber AV, Glisson RR, et al: Anterior cruciate ligament allograft transplantation: Long-term function, histology, revascularization, and operative technique. *Am J Sports Med* 1986;14:348-360.

97. Thorson E, Rodrigo JJ, Vasseur P, et al: Replacement of the anterior cruciate ligament: A comparison of autografts and allografts in dogs. *Acta Orthop Scand* 1989;60:555-560.

Office Pediatric Orthopaedics

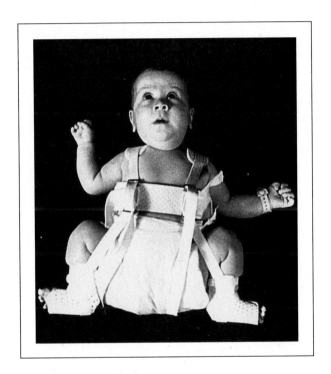

Genu Varum and Genu Valgum in Children

Walter B. Greene, MD

Introduction

For the orthopaedic surgeon, genu varum or genu valgum as a diagnostic question is most common in the 1- to 5-year-old child. Angular deformities that cause concern before that time occur in children who have either extremely short stature and an obvious skeletal dysplasia or some other systemic problem that has previously been evaluated and diagnosed. Likewise, angular deformities of the knee that occur after five years of age are usually related to trauma, infection, or some other systemic problem that has also been previously diagnosed.

Evaluation of the 1- to 5-year-old child with genu varum or genu valgum should start with measurement of the child's height. Plotting the height on standard growth charts identifies the child with short stature who needs further diagnostic evaluation. Certain skeletal dysplasias, such as pseudoachondroplasia and hypophosphatemic rickets, are not associated with short stature during infancy, but children with these conditions show decreasing height percentiles after they are 1 to 2 years old.[1,2] It is not enough to estimate a patient's height at this age, as it is the rare orthopaedic surgeon who can accurately categorize a young child's height by visual inspection (Fig. 1).

Motor development should also be assessed in these young children. Many elaborate developmental scales have been devised. They are useful for the developmental pediatrician but are too cumbersome for screening purposes. Development of motor milestones can be quickly assessed and effectively screened by checking the age-appropriate parameters listed in Tables 1 and 2. If developmental delay is suggested, a neurologic evaluation should be done and further consultation with a pediatrician or a pediatric neurologist should be considered.

Knee alignment changes as the child grows. It is necessary to understand these changes to distinguish normal from abnormal growth. Two studies have charted the normal development of the femoral-tibial angle. Salenius and Vankka[3] used radiographs to measure the femoral-tibial angle in a relatively homogeneous Finnish population. Engel and Staheli[4] derived measurements from clinical photographs of a more heterogeneous population of children in Seattle, Washington. Both studies demonstrated that normal knee alignment progresses from 10° to 15° of varus at birth to a maximum

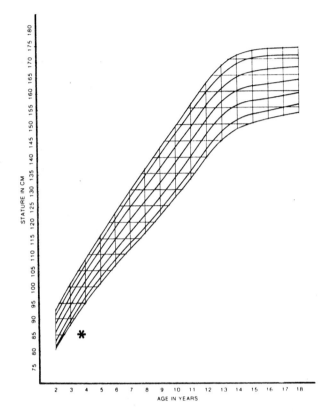

Fig. 1 Height of a 3-year, 8-month-old girl plotted on standard growth chart shows obvious short stature. Her mother was concerned about the child's "swaying gait pattern." Two previous evaluations had been done by orthopaedic surgeons who thought that the result of her examination were within normal limits. Physical examination showed only mild ligamentous laxity and slightly increased genu valgum, but the measurement of her height prompted radiographic studies that led to a diagnosis of pseudoachondroplasia.

Table 1
Gross motor developmental screen in infancy*

Age	Activity
4 months	Roll prone to supine
6 months	Sit alone
8 months	Get to sitting position, Crawl
12 months	Walk independently
15 months	Run

* Ages are rounded off and are the mean age at which the developmental milestone was achieved. Standard deviation was approximately 1.5 months in this study.
(Adapted with permission from Capute AJ, Shapiro BK, Palmer FB, et al: Normal gross motor development: The influences of race, sex, and socioeconomic status. *Dev Med Child Neurol* 1985;27:635-643.)

Table 2
Gross motor developmental screens during early childhood*

Age	Activity
2 years	Stairs, one step at a time
2.5 years	Jumps
3 years	Stairs, alternating feet
4 years	Hops on one foot
5 years	Skips

*Adapted with permission from Paine RS, Oppe TE: Neurological examination of children, Clinics in Developmental Medicine, Nos. 20/21. London, William Heinemann Medical Books.

or peak valgus angulation of 10° to 15° at the age of 3 to 3.5 years. The studies, however, differed in the time or age at which neutral femoral-tibial alignment was reached. Engel and Staheli[4] observed that neutral femoral-tibial alignment was reached at an average age of 12 to 14 months. Salenius and Vankka[3] recorded neutral alignment on their radiographic measurements when their patients were an average of 20 to 22 months old. My clinical observations, based on measuring knee alignment with a goniometer, indicate that neutral femoral-tibial alignment usually develops by the time the child is 14 months old.

Physical examination of a child with genu varum or genu valgum includes a survey of the entire lower extremity. The femoral-tibial angle, tibial torsion, and range of knee motion are specifically measured. Ligamentous laxity is assessed by observing the degree of knee and elbow hyperextension. Hip motion and stability also should be evaluated, because subtle abnormalities of gait associated with a dislocated hip may be incorrectly identified as a knee problem by concerned parents. Developmental dysplasia of the hip, however, is not associated with either excessive genu varum or genu valgum.

After completing the physical examination, the next decision in the evaluation process is whether radiographs of the knees are warranted. I obtain radiographs for the following reasons: (1) genu varum or genu valgum that is relatively severe for the child's age; (2) height less than the 25th percentile; (3) marked asymmetry of limb alignment; (4) excessive internal tibial torsion; (5) a positive family history for a bowleg deformity; and (6) genu varum that, according to the parents' history, has not improved or has worsened over the previous four months. These guidelines minimize acquisition of unnecessary radiographs, but are sensitive enough to include virtually all children who have a condition that requires ongoing evaluation and treatment.

Genu Varum

Genu varum as a diagnostic question for an orthopaedic surgeon is most common in the 14- to 36-month-old child. If there has been no history of previous trauma or infections, my differential diagnosis of genu varum in the 18- to 36-month-old child includes physiologic bowlegs, infantile tibia vara, hypophosphatemic rickets, metaphyseal chondrodysplasia, and focal fibrocartilaginous dysplasia. Physiologic bowlegs is the most common cause of genu varum in the 14- to 30-month-old child. These children have genu varum that persists after 18 months of age, but that will spontaneously resolve, usually before the age of three years. The primary consideration in these children is to rule out other disorders and to reassure the parents.

Typical radiographic characteristics of physiologic bowlegs include symmetrical involvement, a normal-appearing growth plate, and medial bowing of both the proximal part of the tibia and the distal part of the femur.[5] For a child who is younger than two years of age, the radiographic appearance and the femoral-tibial angle may be similar in physiologic bowlegs and infantile tibia vara. For a child of this age, the metaphyseal-diaphyseal angle can be helpful in the differentiation of these two conditions (Figs. 2 and 3). Levine and Drennan[6] noted that physiologic bowlegs was the ultimate diagnosis in 49 of 52 children who had a metaphyseal-diaphyseal angle of less than 11°; however, infantile tibia vara developed in all children with a metaphyseal-diaphyseal angle of 12° or more. Some orthopaedic surgeons now advocate that the metaphyseal-diaphyseal angle should be in the range of 14° to 16° before a diagnosis of infantile tibia vara is presumed and treatment prescribed.[7-9]

Infantile tibia vara is a developmental disorder of growth that affects the medial aspect of the proximal tibial physis. Children with infantile tibia vara have no apparent abnormality at birth, are generally healthy, and have early growth of the legs that is within normal limits. A typical history is that the genu varum has gotten worse since walking began. Infantile tibial vara is found more frequently in children who are black, female, and obese, and who started walking at an early age.[10-15]

The etiology of infantile tibia vara is best explained as abnormal compression on the medial aspect of the proximal tibial physis causing retardation of growth from that area and/or increased growth from the lateral aspect of the proximal tibial physis and proximal fibula.[16,17] If a child begins walking at an early age with the knees still aligned in marked varus, or if an obese child begins walking at the normal age with the knees in slight varus, the weightbearing compressive forces will be greater on the medial aspect of the physis. This initiates reduction in growth and progression of the genu varum. The persistent internal tibia torsion noted in

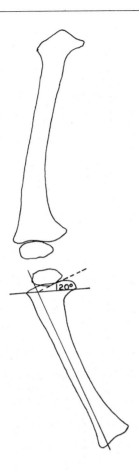

Fig. 2 Measurement of the metaphyseal-diaphyseal angle. The angle is made by a line drawn perpendicular to the axis of the tibia and a line drawn through the medial and lateral beak of the tibial metaphysis. (Adapted with permission from Levine AM, Drennan JC: Physiologic bowing and tibia vara: The metaphyseal-diaphyseal angle and the measurement of bow leg deformities. *J Bone Joint Surg* 1982;64A:1158-1163.)

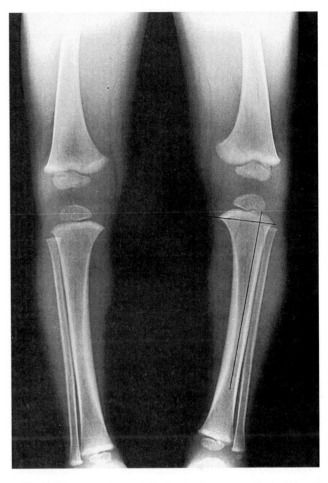

Fig. 3 A 2-year-old girl with persistent genu varum that measured 10° on clinical examination. On the radiograph, the metaphyseal-diaphyseal angle measures 3° on the right and 5° on the left. The growth plates have a normal appearance. The diagnosis was physiologic bowlegs, and no treatment was necessary. (Reproduced with permission from Greene WB: Infantile tibia vara, in Heckman JD (ed): *Instructional Course Lectures 42*. Rosemont, IL, American Academy of Orthopaedic Surgeons, 1993, pp 525-538.)

children with infantile tibia vara may be related to relative overgrowth of the fibula that blocks normal development of external tibial torsion.

Bracing is the treatment of choice for a 14- to 30-month-old child with infantile tibia vara (Fig. 4). When prescribing a brace for a 30- to 36-month-old child it is necessary to consider other factors, such as the medial physeal slope, the body weight, the gender, and the social situation. The medial physeal slope is the angle formed by the intersection of a line through the lateral aspect of the tibial physis and a line through the medial aspect of the physis (Fig. 5). In the study by Kling and associates,[18] a larger medial physeal slope correlated with a more advanced Langenskiold stage, but the medial physeal slope was a more objective measurement and easier to define. Experience with this mea-

surement is limited and has not been critically analyzed, but with a medial physeal slope of less than 50° in a 30- to 36-month-old child, I will prescribe a brace. With a medial physeal slope of 50° to 60°, orthotic treatment is selected only after consideration of other factors. Obesity, female gender, and a poor social situation are poor prognostic signs for successful brace treatment. For the 30- to 36-month-old child with a medial physeal slope of greater than 60°, a tibial osteotomy is the treatment of choice. With that degree of deformity, recurrent tibia vara is high even after osteotomy, and, therefore, it is presumed that brace therapy would be a failure even in a child younger than three years of age.

The orthosis that I prescribe for children with infantile tibia vara is a long leg brace with a free ankle, sin-

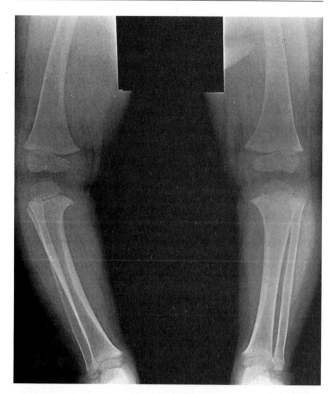

Fig. 4 1-year, 6-month-old girl with genu varum. The metaphyseal-diaphyseal angle was 20° on the right, and the medial aspect of the right proximal tibial physis has an inferior slope. The radiographic picture and abnormal metaphyseal-diaphyseal angle indicate that this patient has a high probability of having infantile tibia vara on the right side. A knee-ankle-foot orthosis was prescribed. (Reproduced with permission from Greene WB: Infantile tibia vara, in Heckman JD (ed): *Instructional Course Lectures 42.* Rosemont, IL, American Academy of Orthopaedic Surgeons, 1993, pp 525-538.)

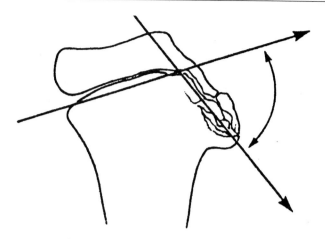

MEDIAL PHYSEAL SLOPE

Fig. 5 Measurement of the medial physeal slope. (Adapted with permission from Kling TF Jr, Volk AG, Dias L, et al: Infantile Blount's disease treated with osteotomy: Follow-up to maturity. *Orthop Trans* 1990;14:634.)

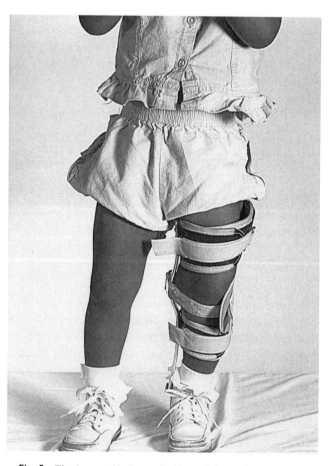

Fig. 6 The knee-ankle-foot orthosis used for patients with infantile tibia vara. The single medial upright has no knee joint. The lateral calf pulls the knee into valgus angulation. The brace can be easily adjusted as the genu varum corrects. (Reproduced with permission from Greene WB: Infantile tibia vara, in Heckman JD (ed): *Instructional Course Lectures 42.* Rosemont, IL, American Academy of Orthopaedic Surgeons, 1993, pp 525-538.)

gle medial upright and no hinge joint at the knee (Fig. 6). A cuff around the knee pulls the knee into valgus angulation. A hinge joint at the knee is not needed for sitting activities in these young children. Elimination of the knee joint makes it easier to align the cuff, allows easy adjustment of the medial upright as the deformity corrects, and makes the brace more adaptable for subsequent growth. Every six to 12 weeks, the medial upright can be bent to gain further valgus alignment at the knee.

Although some authors recommend only nighttime bracing in children with infantile tibia vara,[5,19] I believe that the brace should be worn 22 to 23 hours a day. This should maximize the potential for the brace to alter abnormal compressive forces so that normal growth will resume. In fact, if a child is not able to tolerate full-time brace wear, the time out of the brace should be while the child is sleeping, because standing and walking increase the compressive, growth-inhibiting forces, and the physis needs protection during these activities.

The radiographic parameters that permit early differentiation of physiologic bowlegs from infantile tibia vara are of relatively recent vintage. Therefore, the results of orthotic management in infantile tibia vara are still being defined. Early results have indicated that brace therapy for infantile tibia vara is successful in approximately 50% of the cases.[14] It is my impression that the results are even better if an above-the-knee brace is worn 23 hours a day. Most importantly, a trial with the brace before the child is 3 years old does not seem to compromise the results of subsequent tibial osteotomy.[5]

Osteotomy of the tibia is indicated for the child with infantile tibia vara who is first seen for treatment after age 3, for the child 30 to 36 months of age who is a poor candidate for brace therapy, and for the 3-year-old child who has persistent genu varum despite brace therapy.[20] Multiple techniques have been described for the performance of this procedure in children.[20-28] All involve placement of the osteotomy distal to the tibial tubercle to prevent damage to the tibial apophysis and subsequent genu recurvatum. Osteotomy of the fibula is also necessary to permit adequate correction of the genu varum and internal tibial torsion.

Hypophosphatemic rickets is probably the third most common cause of persistent genu varum in the 14- to 36-month-old child. Its unique sex-linked dominant inheritance pattern may lead to early recognition, but in many cases the diagnosis is delayed and is made after the child starts walking.[2] Parents initiate evaluation of these children because of short stature and/or genu varum. The height at diagnosis in a 1- to 5-year-old child with hypophosphatemic rickets is usually less than the 10th percentile, although occasionally it will be as much as the 25th percentile. Abnormal genu varum is observed in 95% of patients who have hypophosphatemic rickets.

Metaphyseal chondrodysplasia is an inherited disorder of bone growth that also causes bowing of the lower extremities. In the most common type of metaphyseal chondrodysplasia (Schmidt pattern), height and limb alignment are within normal limits at birth, but genu varum persists, and the retarded growth becomes obvious in the preschool years.[29]

Hypophosphatemic rickets and metaphyseal chondrodysplasia are often misdiagnosed. The key to identifying these disorders is the radiographic appearance of the physis. Both diseases show widening or rachitic-like changes at the physis (Fig. 7). The widening, however, is not as extreme as that seen in nutritional or vitamin D-deficient rickets. Hypophosphatemic rickets will be distinguished from metaphyseal chondrodysplasia by serum chemistry studies that show a low serum phosphorus.

Focal fibrocartilaginous dysplasia is a very uncommon disorder that causes a unilateral and progressive

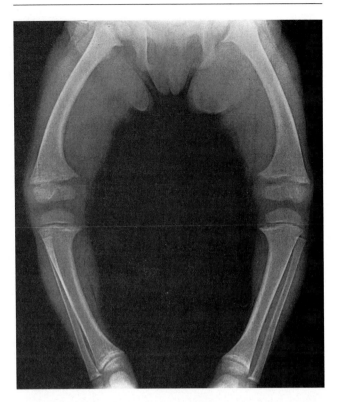

Fig. 7 Anteroposterior radiograph of the lower extremities of a 2-year, 8-month-old child with hypophosphatemic rickets. Note the widening of the physis, particularly at the "more active" distal femoral and proximal tibial growth plates. The child's height was less than the fifth percentile for age. (Reproduced with permission from Greene WB: Infantile tibia vara, in Heckman JD (ed): *Instructional Course Lectures 42.* Rosemont, IL, American Academy of Orthopaedic Surgeons, 1993, pp 525-538.)

tibia vara that is usually unilateral.[30] The radiographs are characterized by indentation of the medial aspect of the tibia at the junction of the metaphysis and the diaphysis (Fig. 8). Bone in this indented area shows dense fibrous tissue and a relatively greater amount of dense lamellar bone. Despite rather impressive radiographs, recurrent deformity is uncommon after a valgus, rotational osteotomy of the proximal tibia.

Genu Valgum

Genu valgum is a common concern of parents whose child has developed peak valgus knee alignment; that is, the 30- to 36-month-old child (Fig. 9). In the study by Salenius and Vankka,[3] the maximum or peak genu valgum averaged 12°±8°. When evaluating children with genu valgum, a hurried and brief inspection of the knees is neither adequate assessment nor adequate reassurance for the parents. On the other hand, measuring the height, asking questions concerning development of motor milestones, and examining

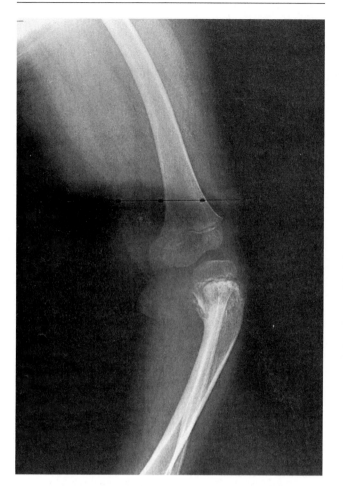

Fig. 8 Left lower extremity of a 3-year, 3-month-old white boy with progressive bowleg deformity. Abnormal genu varum was present bilaterally, although more severe on the left side. Height and serum phosphorus were within normal limits. Proximal tibial closing wedge osteotomy included a portion of the indented bone, which on gross and microscopic inspection, showed dense lamellar bone. Clinical and surgical findings were consistent with focal fibrocartilaginous dysplasia.

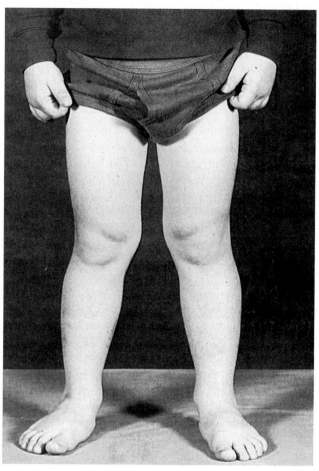

Fig. 9 A 3-year, 6-month-old boy referred for evaluation of "knock knees." Height was 70th percentile, and development was normal. Genu valgum measured 18° by clinical examination. The patient was considered to be within normal limits and an explanation was provided to the mother. No further follow-up was required.

the lower extremities as previously described can be done in a relatively short time. This degree of effort plus a brief explanation of normal knee development will reassure the parents, enhance the orthopaedic surgeon's reputation, and most importantly, largely eliminate the unnecessary second opinions that occur when a physician provides only cursory evaluation and explanation.

Radiographs are indicated for a child with genu valgum when short stature is present or when there is asymmetrical genu valgum. An anteroposterior (AP) standing radiograph on a 36×43 cm film is usually sufficient. The width of the physis and the height of the epiphysis are assessed, and the distal femoral-proximal tibial angle is measured to provide a baseline for a subsequent comparison. Children with normal height but asymmetric genu valgum often will have no obvious physeal or bony abnormalities (Fig. 10). With subsequent growth, spontaneous resolution of the asymmetrically increased valgus alignment typically occurs.

The differential diagnosis of genu valgum in a 2- to 5-year-old child includes hypophosphatemic rickets, previous proximal metaphyseal fracture of the tibia, multiple epiphyseal dysplasia, and pseudoachondroplasia. Although children with hypophosphatemic rickets typically develop genu varum, this disorder may be associated with increased genu valgum (Fig. 11). The short stature and widened growth plate will suggest the correct diagnosis, which can be confirmed by measuring serum phosphorus levels.

It is now well recognized that abnormal genu valgum may develop in children after fracture of the

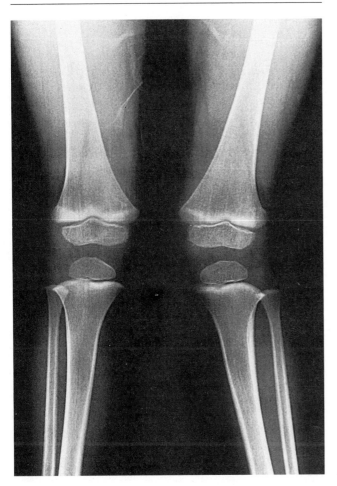

Fig. 10 Anteroposterior standing radiograph of a three-year, seven-month-old boy. Height and development were within normal limits. Radiographs showed asymmetric genu valgum with a femoral-tibial angle of 14° on the right and 24° on the left, but normal-appearing growth plates and bony structure. It is anticipated that this patient's genu valgum will spontaneously improve with growth, but observation was recommended.

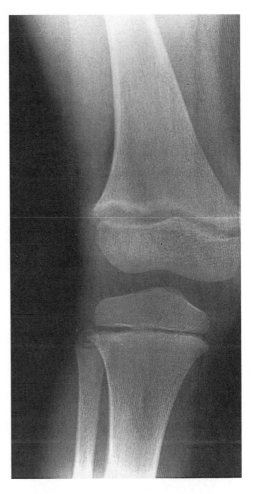

Fig. 11 A 6-year, 3-month-old boy with marked genu valgum of the right lower extremity associated with hypophosphatemic rickets. Note widening of the physis. Height was the 25th percentile for age, which is greater than most patients with hypophosphatemic rickets; however, compared to his unaffected parents, this child has relatively short stature.

proximal metaphysis of the tibia. This deformity typically occurs in a 2- to 8-year-old child with normal but pre-existent genu valgum.[31] In 40 consecutive fractures of the proximal tibial metaphysis in children, Skak and associates[32] found that valgus deformity developed in 15% of the greenstick and complete fractures but did not happen after buckle fractures. Observation of this deformity until early adolescence is recommended, as adequate correction occurred spontaneously in six of seven patients studied by Zionts and MacEwen.[33]

Multiple epiphyseal dysplasia is a disorder of ossification and growth of the epiphysis. Considerable clinical heterogeneity is seen in multiple epiphyseal dysplasia.[29] Some patients have extreme short stature and marked limitation of motion in multiple joints, whereas in other patients, the height is around the tenth percentile and the joint abnormalities are mild and not

disabling. Children with the milder form of the disease usually are evaluated between the ages of 2 and 8 years. The most common reason for referral in these patients is restricted hip motion and radiographs that simulate Legg-Perthes disease. Some children, however, are brought for evaluation of marked genu valgum. The relatively short stature in these patients should initiate radiographic evaluation. Radiographs of the knee in these children will demonstrate flattening of the distal femoral and proximal tibial epiphysis (Fig. 12). This finding should initiate further radiographic evaluation. An AP radiograph of the hand will show delayed skeletal maturation, and an AP radiograph of the pelvis will demonstrate fragmentation of the proximal femoral epiphysis.

Pseudoachondroplasia, another inherited skeletal dysplasia, is characterized by mild platyspondyly, rhi-

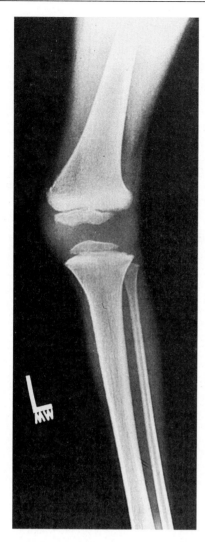

Fig. 12 Standing radiograph of a 4-year, 11-month-old boy referred for evaluation of increasing genu valgum. Height was just below the fifth percentile. Radiographs showed decreased vertical height of the epiphysis. Further evaluation confirmed a diagnosis of multiple epiphyseal dysplasia.

measurement of the child's height is critical in diagnosing these patients at an early age (Fig. 1).

Observation is the treatment of choice for the 30- to 36-month-old child with marked genu valgum who is otherwise normal. Unless the parents are overly concerned, I do not request follow-up evaluation of children who have genu valgum less than 20°. Admittedly, most children with genu valgum ≥ 20° will show spontaneous correction, but follow-up evaluation of these children not only reassures the parents, but also allows appropriately timed surgical intervention for the rare child who needs treatment. In addition, follow-up evaluation provides another opportunity to diagnose an unusual disease that has caused marked genu valgum.

Nonsurgical modalities such as medial heel wedges were at one time recommended for young children with genu valgum. It is now recognized that shoe modifications are ineffective in altering the biomechanics of growth at the knee. Long leg braces are totally impractical and unphysiologic for an otherwise normal child with a condition that will spontaneously correct more than 99% of the time.

If abnormal genu valgum persists into the second decade, correction by either hemiepiphysiodesis or stapling of the medial physis is an effective solution that has considerably less morbidity than a realignment osteotomy.[34,35] The distal femoral physis is usually the appropriate site for surgery in a patient with idiopathic genu valgum, but tracings and cutouts will demonstrate whether altering growth at the proximal tibial physis would provide more anatomic knee alignment. The advantage of stapling the physis is that the staples can be removed if excessive correction is occurring.[34] The advantage of a hemiepiphysiodesis is that this operation can be done percutaneously, and, therefore, the patient will have a smaller, more cosmetic scar. In addition, a hemiepiphysiodesis eliminates the necessity of a second operation to remove symptomatic metal. However, if the hemiepiphysiodesis causes overcorrection, a second operation will be required to arrest growth on the lateral aspect of the physis. Bowen and associates[35] have demonstrated that preoperative calculations usually can eliminate the problem of overcorrection after hemiepiphysiodesis. I perform a hemiepiphysiodesis when I am fairly certain that overcorrection will not occur, but I use staples in a child with atypical growth parameters.

Summary

Genu varum and genu valgum are often normal developmental changes in knee alignment that occur in a young child. Measuring the child's height and understanding normal development is the key to determining which children need further evaluation for a possible skeletal or metabolic bone dysplasia.

zomelic shortening of the extremities, flaring of the metaphysis, and delayed ossification of the epiphysis that progresses to articular surface deformities.[31] Although pseudoachondroplasia may cause severe short stature and early arthritic changes, this disorder usually is not diagnosed until the child is 2 or 3 years of age. During the first 1 or 2 years of life, the height of these children is relatively normal, and early motor milestones are attained at a normal age. Referral to an orthopaedic surgeon is typically initiated when the child is 2 or 3 years of age, with the parents expressing concern about any of the following: their child's short stature, genu valgum, genu varum, pes planus, or short digits. Because angular deformities and other musculoskeletal problems may not be extreme at this time,

References

1. Horton WA, Hall JG, Scott CI, et al: Growth curves for height for diastrophic dysplasia, spondyloepiphyseal dysplasia congenita, and pseudoachondroplasia. *Am J Dis Child* 1982;136:316-319.

2. Greene WB, Kahler SG: Hypophosphatemic rickets: Still misdiagnosed and inadequately treated. *South Med J* 1985;78:1179-1184.

3. Salenius P, Vankka E: The development of the tibiofemoral angle in children. *J Bone Joint Surg* 1975;57A:259-261.

4. Engel GM, Staheli LT: The natural history of torsion and other factors influencing gait in childhood: A study of the angle of gait, tibial torsion, knee angle, hip rotation, and development of the arch in normal children. *Clin Orthop* 1974;99:12-17.

5. Griffin PP: The lower limb, in Lovell WW, Winter RB (eds): *Pediatric Orthopaedics*, ed 1. Philadelphia, PA, JB Lippincott, 1978, vol 2, chap 20, pp 881-909.

6. Levine AM, Drennan JC: Physiological bowing and tibia vara: The metaphyseal-diaphyseal angle in the measurement of bowleg deformities. *J Bone Joint Surg* 1982;64A:1158-1163.

7. Drennan JC: Pediatric knee disorders. Presented at the 59th Annual Meeting of the American Academy of Orthopaedic Surgeons. Washington, DC, February 21, 1992.

8. Feldman MD, Schoenecke PL: Use of Drennan's metaphyseal-diaphyseal angle in evaluating bow legs. Presented at the 59th Annual Meeting of the American Academy of Orthopaedic Surgeons, Washington, DC, February 21, 1992.

9. Henderson RC, Lechner CT, DeMasi RA, et al: Variability in radiographic measurement of bowleg deformity in children. *J Pediatr Orthop* 1990;10:491-494.

10. Bathfield CA, Beighton PH: Blount disease: A review of etiological factors in 110 patients. *Clin Orthop* 1978;135:29-33.

11. Bateson EM: The relationship between Blount's disease and bowlegs. *Br J Radiol* 1968;41:107-114.

12. Ferriter P, Shapiro F: Infantile tibia vara: Factors affecting outcome following proximal tibial osteotomy. *J Pediatr Orthop* 1987;7:1-7.

13. Langenskiöld A, Riska EB: Tibia vara (osteochondrosis deformans tibiae): A survey of seventy-one cases. *J Bone Joint Surg* 1964;46A:1405-1420.

14. Loder RT, Johnson CE II: Infantile tibia vara. *J Pediatr Orthop* 1987;7:639-646.

15. Schoenecker PL, Meade WC, Pierron RL, et al: Blount's disease: A retrospective review and recommendations for treatment. *J Pediatr Orthop* 1985;5:181-186.

16. Cook SD, Lavernia CJ, Burke SW, et al: A biomechanical analysis of the etiology of tibia vara. *J Pediatr Orthop* 1983;3:449-454.

17. O'Neill DA, MacEwen GD: Early roentgenographic evaluation of bowlegged children. *J Pediatr Orthop* 1982;2:547-553.

18. Kling TF Jr, Volk AG, Dias L, et al: Infantile Blount's disease treated with osteotomy: Follow-up to maturity. *Orthop Trans* 1990;14:634-635.

19. Staheli LT: The lower limb, in Morrissy RT (ed): *Lovell and Winter's Pediatric Orthopaedics*, ed 3. Philadelphia, PA, JB Lippincott, 1990, vol 2, chap 20, pp 741-766.

20. Greene WB: Infantile tibia vara. *J Bone Joint Surg* 1993;75A:130-143, and in Heckman JD (ed): American Academy of Orthopaedic Surgeons Instructional Course Lectures 42. Rosemont, IL, 1993, pp 525-538.

21. Canale ST, Harper MC: Biotrigonometric analysis and practical applications of osteotomies of tibia in children, in Murray DG (ed): American Academy of Orthopaedic Surgeons Instructional Course Lectures XXX. St. Louis, MO, CV Mosby, 1981, chap 5, pp 85-101.

22. Dietz FR, Weinstein SL: Spike osteotomy for angular deformities of the long bones in children. *J Bone Joint Surg* 1988;70A:848-852.

23. Johnston CE II: Infantile tibia vara. *Clin Orthop* 1990;255:13-23.

24. Kruse RW, Bowen JR, Heithoff S: Oblique tibial osteotomy in the correction of tibial deformity in children. *J Pediatr Orthop* 1989;9:476-482.

25. Langenskiold A: Tibia vara: A critical review. *Clin Orthop* 1989;246:195-207.

26. Rab GT: Oblique tibial osteotomy for Blount's disease (tibia vara). *J Pediatr Orthop* 1988;8:715-720.

27. Richardson EG: Miscellaneous nontraumatic disorders, in Crenshaw AH (ed): *Campbell's Operative Orthopaedics*, ed 7. St. Louis, MO, CV Mosby, 1987, vol 2, chap 37, pp 1005-1088.

28. Smith CF: Tibia vara (Blount's disease). *J Bone Joint Surg* 1982;64A:630-632.

29. Bassett GS: Orthopaedic aspects of skeletal dysplasias, in Greene WB (ed): *Instructional Course Lectures XXXIX*. Park Ridge, IL, American Academy of Orthopaedic Surgeons, 1990, chap 48, 381-387.

30. Olney BW, Cole WG, Menelaus MB: Three additional cases of focal fibrocartilaginous dysplasia causing tibia vara. *J Pediatr Orthop* 1990;10:405-407.

31. Salter RB, Best TN: Pathogenesis of progressive valgus deformity following fractures of the proximal metaphyseal region of the tibia in young children, in Eilert RE (ed): *Instructional Course Lectures XLI*. Park Ridge, IL, American Academy of Orthopaedic Surgeons, 1992, pp 409-411.

32. Skak SV, Jensen TT, Poulsen TD: Fracture of the proximal metaphysis of the tibia in children. *Injury* 1987;18:149-156.

33. Zionts LE, MacEwen GD: Spontaneous improvement of post-traumatic tibia valga. *J Bone Joint Surg* 1986;68A:680-687.

34. Zuege RC, Kempken TG, Blount WP: Epiphyseal stapling for angular deformity at the knee. *J Bone Joint Surg* 1979;61A:320-329.

35. Bowen JR, Torres RR, Forlin E: Partial epiphysiodesis to address genu varum or genu valgum. *J Pediatr Orthop* 1992;12:359-364.

Metatarsus Adductus and Skewfoot

Walter B. Greene, MD

Introduction

Metatarsus adductus, a congenital deformity characterized by medial deviation of the forefoot, is the most common pediatric foot problem referred to an orthopaedic surgeon. In fact, at one large pediatric hospital, the number of children with metatarsus adductus exceeded the combined number of patients who were referred for clubfoot, flatfoot, calcaneovalgus, pes cavus, tarsal coalition, or vertical talus.[1] Despite its frequent occurrence, limited information is available concerning which children require treatment, the age at which treatment should be instituted, what constitutes effective nonsurgical therapy, and the role, if any, of surgical therapy. The management of metatarsus adductus, therefore, remains controversial. Indeed, I have often observed that when orthopaedic surgeons converse about metatarsus adductus, the number of different ways that are mentioned to manage this problem is usually equivalent to the number of orthopaedic surgeons in the group.

Skewfoot, on the other hand, is a very uncommon foot deformity that is characterized by forefoot adduction with marked heel valgus. Kite[2] observed only 12 cases of this "serpentine" foot deformity compared to 2,818 patients with metatarsus adductus, and, in 1986, Peterson[3] found only 50 cases of skewfoot previously reported in the literature. Despite the radical difference in frequency, it is appropriate to discuss these disorders in the same chapter, because skewfoot may actually represent one end of a spectrum of congenital forefoot disorders. Furthermore, many of the nonsurgical and surgical techniques of management used in metatarsus adductus can also be applied to a skewfoot.

Metatarsus Adductus

Nomenclature

The nomenclature for forefoot adduction disorders is confusing. Additional terminology includes metatarsus varus, metatarsus adductus et supinatus, complex metatarsus adductus, and metatarsus adductovarus. Some authors use the term "metatarsus adductus" and "metatarsus varus" interchangeably,[4-22] while others restrict the term "metatarsus varus" either to feet with a more severe form of metatarsus adductus[23,24] or to feet that also demonstrate supination of the forefoot.[1,25-28] During infancy, forefoot rotation may be more apparent than real, as many of these chubby infant feet that are apparently supinated will demonstrate a typical pes planus when standing and walking activities commence (Fig. 1).

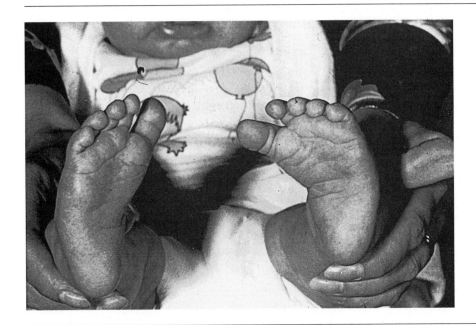

Fig. 1 Three-month-old infant with obvious metatarsus adductus. In this photograph, the foot appears to be supinated; however, when the foot was placed in weight-bearing position, the hindfoot alignment was normal.

I believe that metatarsus adductus most accurately describes the deformity and that subclassifications such as metatarsus varus should not be used until they are proven to be separate entities that can be objectively defined.

Incidence and Demographics

Inquiries to my colleagues who are pediatricians, concerning the incidence of metatarsus adductus at birth, bring statements such as "very common" or "frequently." Objective data, however, are very sparse. The oft-quoted figure found in the orthopaedic literature is one per thousand and comes from a report by Wynne-Davies.[22] This study was derived from children brought to a central hospital for treatment and, therefore, does not include children whose metatarsus adductus corrected spontaneously. Of note, a subsequent study by Wynne-Davies and associates[29] that examined the Edinburgh Register of the Newborn over a five-year period reported an even lower incidence of metatarsus adductus, the rate in this study being 0.2/1,000 live births.

In the only prospective analysis of metatarsus adductus, Hunziker and associates[30] evaluated 128 pre-term and 114 term children at birth, at age 1 year, and at 5 years of age. The pre-term children had a mean gestational age of 33.4 weeks (range, 27.1-36.8 weeks) and a mean birth-weight of 1,996 grams (range 1,030-2,450 grams). Therefore, the very low birth-weight infant is not included in this study. Twenty-five percent of the pre-term and 13% of the term infants had metatarsus adductus at birth. Twins accounted for the increased prevalence in the pre-term infants, as the percentage of children with metatarsus adductus was similar in single pre-term and term infants, but was significantly higher in twins compared to single infants (41% vs 16%). The higher prevalence of metatarsus adductus in twins has also been noted in another study.[29]

The number of children with metatarsus adductus that required treatment apparently increased after 1930, at least in North America. Kite[2,9] was the first to note this increase. Certainly, factors such as greater availability and knowledge of primary care physicians as well as the reputation of Dr. Kite, may have influenced his numbers; however, an increase in the number of children needing treatment for metatarsus adductus was also noted by other authors.[14,31] Placing infants in the prone position for sleeping became a common practice of North American mothers during that time. This sleeping posture usually positions the forefoot into adduction and may have contributed to the increased frequency of children requiring treatment for metatarsus adductus in the United States of America.[14,22,29] The recent recognition that the prone sleeping position is associated with Sudden Infant Death Syndrome[32] may change how newborn infants are positioned for sleeping and may decrease the number of children who have persistent metatarsus adductus.

Demographic data from three large series of patients referred for treatment of metatarsus adductus are summarized in Table 1. All three studies recorded a predominance of males, bilateral involvement, and affection of the left side in patients with unilateral involvement. The predominance of bilateral involvement has also been noted at birth, at least in term infants.[30] The preponderance of male and left-sided involvement may be secondary to other factors. Males attain motor skills and the ability to roll over at a later age.[33] A relative delay in being able to move from the prone position may explain the greater incidence of males needing treatment for metatarsus adductus. The greater number of patients with left side involvement may be related to asymmetrical tibial torsion. I have observed that internal tibia torsion usually persists longer on the left side than on the right. Persistent internal rotation of the left tibia may make it easier for a child sleeping in the prone position to position the forefoot into adduction. Therefore, metatarsus adductus would be less likely to resolve on the left side than on the right.

Etiology and Pathoanatomy

Intrauterine positioning is probably the most important factor in the etiology of metatarsus adductus. The high incidence in twin pregnancies,[29,30] the low inci-

Table 1
Metatarsus adductus: Demographic data

Reference	Number of Infants in Series	Bilateral Involvement	Side Involved in Unilateral Patients	Male Gender
Bleck[4]	152	60%	N.A.	60%
Kite[2]	2,818	56%	Left, 62%	53%
Kane[25]	720	57%	Left, 55%	34%

N.A. - not available

dence in very premature infants (gestational age < 30 weeks),[34] the greater incidence of bilateral involvement in term infants,[30] and, most importantly, the resolution of forefoot deformity with subsequent uninhibited growth in most children, support the role of intrauterine positioning.[14,16,17,30,35,36]

Some orthopaedic surgeons have indicated that metatarsus adductus may develop after birth. Ponseti and Becker[14] observed that metatarsus adductus was not recognized at birth in approximately one-third of their patients. Kite[9] noted that two thirds of his patients did not have metatarsus adductus at birth. The obvious deficiencies in these studies[9,14] is that the presence or absence of metatarsus adductus at birth was dependent on recall by the parents. Of note, the only prospective study of newborn infants did not record any children who subsequently developed metatarsus adductus.[30]

Anomalous muscle insertions as a cause of metatarsus adductus have been reported in two studies. In 14 of 15 feet undergoing surgery for metatarsus adductus, Browne and Paton[5] noted that the posterior tibialis tendon had only a small slip inserting into the navicular but a large slip inserting into the medial cuneiform and presumably into the second, third, and fourth metatarsals. These authors theorized that the anomalous posterior tibialis insertion pulled the foot into adduction and supination. Based on observation during surgery in 38 feet, Ghali and associates[37] thought that patients with metatarsus adductus had a preponderance of the anterior tibialis tendon inserting on the plantar aspect of the medial cuneiform. They theorized that this anomalous anterior tibialis insertion caused a greater supination force and, therefore, metatarsus varus. However, detailed dissection by Reimann and Werner[38] at autopsy of a newborn infant with pronounced unilateral metatarsus adductus and no other musculoskeletal deformities showed alterations in the shape of the medial cuneiform and subluxation of the metatarsals on the medial cuneiform, but did not demonstrate abnormal tendon insertions.

Kite[2] thought that metatarsus adductus was caused by muscle imbalance with initial overpull and then contracture of the tibialis anterior muscle. However, in anatomic dissections on stillborn fetuses, Reimann and Werner[15] could not achieve significant adduction of the forefoot by applying traction to the anterior tibialis, even after doing a capsulotomy of the first metatarsocuneiform joint. Metatarsus adductus occurred only after performing capsulotomies of the tarsometatarsal and midfoot intertarsal joints.

In my opinion, the evidence supporting anomalous tendon insertions or overactivity of the anterior tibialis muscle as a cause of metatarsus adductus is scant. The observations reported by Browne and Paton[5] and Ghali

and associates[37] were based on limited surgical dissection and have not been confirmed by other authors. The experimental studies by Reimann and Werner[15] do not support contracture of the anterior tibialis muscle as a cause of metatarsus adductus. In addition, hindfoot varus, rather than metatarsus adductus, is seen in children with cerebral palsy who demonstrate overactivity of either the anterior tibialis or posterior tibialis muscle during instrumented gait analysis.[39]

In summary, I believe that the etiology of metatarsus adductus is best explained by an intrauterine position that pushes the forefoot into adduction, causing deviant growth of the metatarsals and medial cuneiform. The deformity of the forefoot either resolves, persists, or worsens with subsequent growth. Contracture of the anterior tibialis muscle may develop, but this is a secondary phenomenon rather than a primary cause of metatarsus adductus. Forefoot adduction as a developmental problem probably occurs only in children with an underlying neuromuscular disorder or skeletal dysplasia.

Natural History and Timing of Treatment

The natural history of untreated metatarsus adductus has been analyzed in only one study. Rushforth[17] evaluated 179 untreated feet in 116 children before age 1 and then at ages ranging from 3 to 11 years. All feet at initial evaluation could be passively corrected to neutral. Therefore, this study included infants with typical metatarsus adductus, but excluded those with a relatively inflexible deformity. The feet were classified as mild, moderate, or severe using subjective clinical criteria. At final review, 58% had no deformity, 28% had mild and probably inconsequential metatarsus adductus, 11% had moderate residual deformity, and 4% had severe metatarsus adductus. Therefore, this study suggests that approximately 15% of children with metatarsus adductus need or would benefit from treatment.

The appropriate time to initiate treatment in metatarsus adductus is still debated. Kite[2] urged the obstetrician, pediatrician, or general practitioner to refer the child to an orthopaedic surgeon when he or she first suspected metatarsus adductus. Early referrals were thought to shorten the time required for correction and reduce the cost of treatment. Tachdjian[21] also advocated early treatment with serial casting. This author, however, believes that treating neonates and young infants with metatarsus adductus would result in unnecessary therapy for many children.

In a study of children prospectively evaluated at birth, Hunziker and associates[30] treated persistent metatarsus adductus starting at 3 months of age. Twenty-five percent of the affected feet in this study underwent cast correction. At age 5 years, none of the children born at term demonstrated residual deformity.

Nineteen percent of the preterm children had residual metatarsus adductus at age 5, but 75% of those with residual deformity had cerebral palsy.

By comparison, Ponseti and Becker[14] delayed initiation of cast therapy until an average age of 6 months and did not treat any child whose deformity remained passively correctable. By using these criteria, only 11.6% of this series required casting. The final result in the no treatment group was either a foot with normal alignment or a mild flat foot with a minimum degree of metatarsus adductus that was not handicapping.

On the other hand, two studies have demonstrated that the results of cast correction of metatarsus adductus are more difficult and less predictable when started after 8 to 9 months of age.[4,40] Bohne,[40] also noted a higher rate of recurrent deformities when cast correction was begun at 9 months of age or older, even when the feet had only moderate deformity.

In this author's opinion, corrective cast treatment of metatarsus adductus should be delayed for most children until approximately 6 months of age. In essence, the percentage of children requiring treatment at this age[14] is similar to the percentage of children who are left with residual deformity if untreated. In addition, starting treatment when a child is 6 months old does not seem to compromise the results of therapy and greatly minimizes unnecessary treatment. The exception to the 6-month guideline is the child that is born with a very rigid deformity, particularly one that has obvious increased heel valgus and a positive family history. These children are going to be more difficult to correct and, indeed, many of them do not obtain full correction by cast therapy.

Physical Examination and Differential Diagnosis

Most cases of metatarsus adductus are brought to an orthopaedic surgeon when the child is between the ages of 3 and 12 months. The parents express concern that "the feet or legs turn in." The physician should question the parents about the duration of pregnancy and whether any delivery or neonatal difficulties occurred. Motor development should also be assessed. The milestones that this author uses in screening motor development of children younger than 1 year of age are listed in Table 2. Premature delivery or a delay in development may indicate that the child has cerebral palsy. Treatment of the metatarsus adductus would, in that case, have a higher rate of recurrent or residual deformity.[30]

Obtaining a family history is important. It is the recalcitrant form of metatarsus adductus or a skewfoot deformity that typically has a positive history of an affected parent.[2] In addition, the usual sleeping posture of a younger child should also be ascertained, as the prone position with the feet turned in may be an important factor in metatarsus adductus that persists.

The most striking feature on physical examination of a foot with metatarsus adductus is the convex lateral border and the palpable prominence at the juncture of the fifth metatarsal and cuboid (Fig. 2). The higher arch described by Kite[10] is probably more apparent than real, but in severely affected feet a transverse crease is typically seen at the medial portion of the foot. Increased abduction of the great toe may be noted when the child is placed in the weight-bearing position.

In metatarsus adductus, the hindfoot is in neutral or increased valgus and never demonstrates a varus posture.[23] Normal ankle dorsiflexion is also present. These two findings are important, because some children with severe metatarsus adductus may, at first inspection, appear to have a clubfoot deformity.

The physical examination should also include a general survey of the spine and lower extremities. Earlier studies[8,12] indicated that metatarsus adductus was associated with developmental dysplasia of the hip, the incidence of hip dysplasia being approximately ten times higher in children with metatarsus adductus.[12] Subsequent studies[41,42] have demonstrated that there is no significant association of metatarsus adductus and development dysplasia of the hip. Therefore, the physical examination of children with metatarsus adductus should include tests that screen for hip pathology, just as an orthopaedic surgeon would do for any child at this age. Obtaining routine pelvic radiographs or ultrasound examinations, however, does not seem to be justified.

For the typical child with an adducted forefoot who is brought to an orthopaedic surgeon, the differential diagnosis would include metatarsus primus varus, hyperactive abductor hallucis, internal tibial torsion, mild clubfoot deformity, and skewfoot. Metatarsus adductus may also be found in generalized skeletal dysplasias. For example, metatarsus adductus by itself or

Table 2
Gross motor development screen - Infancy

Age	Activity
4 months	Roll prone to supine
6 months	Sit alone
8 months	Get to sitting position Crawl
12 months	Walk independently
15 months	Run

Ages are rounded off and are the mean age that developmental milestone was achieved. Standard deviation was approximately 1.5 months in this study.

and, in particular, the lateral part of the foot is straight. This problem resolves with subsequent growth and development.

In some infants with excessive internal tibial torsion, the foot on initial inspection will appear to have metatarsus adductus. Careful scrutiny of the different components of the foot and assessment of the tibial rotation, however, will demonstrate that this patient's intoeing is related to abnormal tibial torsion rather than metatarsus adductus.

A mild clubfoot deformity may be misdiagnosed as metatarsus adductus. The key to the correct diagnosis in these children is the position and movement of the hindfoot. Even a mild clubfoot will have limited dorsiflexion of the ankle. In a small child, this is most readily demonstrated by observing the heel as the foot is dorsiflexed. During this maneuver, the os calcis does not move inferiorly in a child with a clubfoot. In addition, the heel in these children cannot be placed in a valgus posture. In some clubfeet with mild equinus and relatively severe metatarsus adductus, a definitive diagnosis may not be possible by clinical examination. In this situation, a lateral radiograph with foot in maximum dorsiflexion will demonstrate the decreased talocalcaneal angle that is characteristic of a clubfoot deformity (Fig. 3).

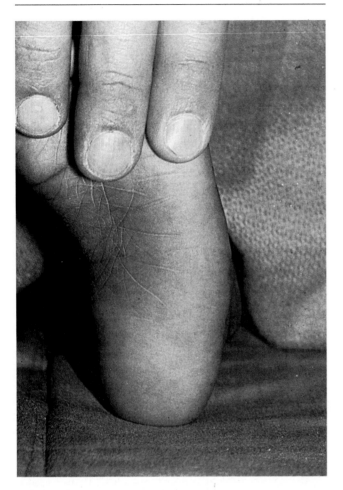

Fig. 2 Convexity along the lateral border of the foot is the most easily identified feature of metatarsus adductus on clinical examination.

metatarsus adductus with heel valgus is the most common foot deformity seen in diastrophic dwarfism.[43] These generalized skeletal dysplasias, however, are usually obvious at birth, and the diagnosis has usually been made before the child is 3 months old.

Metatarsus primus varus is rarely seen or diagnosed during early childhood, but in an older child, the key to differentiating this disorder from metatarsus adductus is the lateral border of the foot. Radiographs of a foot with metatarsus primus varus show medial deviation of the first metatarsal from the second metatarsal, but the lateral metatarsals are in normal alignment. By comparison, all metatarsals are adducted in metatarsus adductus.

The child with a hyperactive abductor hallucis or dynamic hallux varus typically presents to a physician after walking commences. These children are noted to have marked medial deviation of their great toe during ambulation. Their forefoot, however, is not deviated,

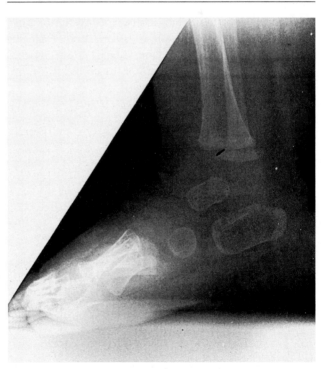

Fig. 3 Lateral radiograph of the foot in maximum dorsiflexion. This 8-month-old child was referred for evaluation of recurrent metatarsus adductus. The clinical examination was not definitive, but the decreased talocalcaneal angle seen on the radiograph indicates that this child has a clubfoot deformity.

Classification of Deformity by Clinical Criteria

All feet with metatarsus adductus are not the same and a reproducible classification scheme to guide treatment, to compare results of therapy, and to predict the possibility of recurrent deformity would be helpful. Limited progress has been made in devising such a grading system. The reasons for this include the difficulty in obtaining reproducible clinical measurements in a small child and the limited information that can be gleaned from radiographs of infant feet with their very limited ossification.

This author is aware of two systems that rate the severity of metatarsus adductus by clinical criteria. Neither has been correlated with radiographic measurements or observer reliability. The classification described by Bleck[4] seems to be the most widely used. Bleck noted that a line bisecting the weight-bearing ellipse of the heel normally crossed the forefoot between the second and third toes and rated metatarsus adductus as "mild" when the heel bisector crossed the third toe, as "moderate" when the heel bisector went between the third and fourth toe, and as "severe" when the heel bisector crossed between the fourth and fifth toe (Fig. 4). It is unclear whether the deformity should be rated as moderate or severe if the heel bisector crosses the fourth toe.

Bleck's[4] classification is useful and there may not be a better clinical rating system of metatarsus adductus. This author, however, has noted considerable intraobserver and interobserver variability in drawing or placing the heel bisector line and wonders whether Bleck's classification is anymore reliable than a "mild, moderate, or severe" visual assessment of the convexity on the lateral border of the foot.

Crawford and Gabriel's[44] classification of metatarsus adductus is based on flexibility and seems to extend Ponseti and Becker's[14] concept of which children do not require treatment. In their Type I metatarsus adductus, peroneal muscle stimulation actively pulls the forefoot past neutral. In Type II metatarsus adductus, the forefoot can be passively manipulated past neutral, but active correction is not observed, while Type III feet cannot be passively stretched to the neutral position. Type I feet are expected to resolve spontaneously, Type II are treated by stretching exercises, and Type III are casted. Crawford and Gabriel[44] did not describe the results of using their classification and I have no experience with this system.

Flexibility of the forefoot in determining outcome or treatment requirements needs further evaluation. Bleck[4] did not find that flexibility affected the result of therapy; however, virtually all of his patients were treated by serial casts, and in his study the flexibility index was not correlated with the duration of casting. Bohne[40] rated severity of the deformity by Bleck's heel bisector classification and only casted mild or moderate deformities if they were " rigid", which he defined as a foot where passive abduction failed to bring the second toe in line with the heel bisector. Thirty of the 165 feet in this study were classified as rigid, but the percentage of mild, moderate, or severe feet that had a rigid or inflexible metatarsus adductus was not delineated.

My classification of metatarsus adductus uses mild, moderate, or severe ratings that are based on correlating a visual gestalt of the convexity of the lateral border with Bleck's heel bisector system. Flexibility is rated by passive abduction of the forefoot, and a flexi-

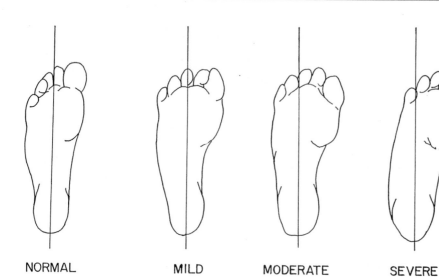

NORMAL   MILD   MODERATE   SEVERE

Fig. 4 Classification of metatarsus adductus as described by Bleck. (Reproduced with permission from Bleck, EE: Metatarsus adductus: Classification and relationship to all kinds of treatment. *J Pediatr Orthop* 1983;3:2-9.)

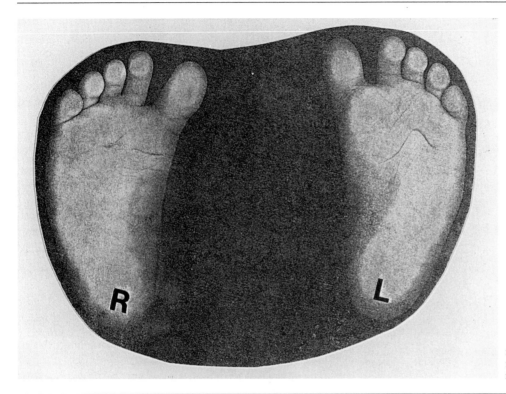

Fig. 5 Photocopy of feet in a 9-month-old child with bilateral metatarsus adductus. See Fig. 7 for comparison with radiographs.

ble foot is one in which the second toe can be brought in line with or past the heel bisector.[40]

Serial photocopies of the foot as a method of charting treatment of metatarsus adductus has recently been described (Fig 5).[45] This low cost, minimal risk idea is appealing, but Smith and associates[45] did not describe whether the photocopy could classify accurately the severity of the deformity. In limited experience with this technique, I have noted the following technical problems. The children may be scared by the bright light and noise of the photocopy machine. This apprehension can be minimized by having the child face the mother while she supports the child's trunk and a nurse positions the feet in a weightbearing posture. Because the photocopy is a reverse image, delineation of which image is the right or left foot can be confusing. This problem can be minimized by placing a marker on the photocopy machine.

Radiographs and Radiographic Classification

Radiographs demonstrate adductus of all metatarsals, but the medial deviation is most severe at the first metatarsal and progressively decreases from the second to the fifth metatarsal. In older children with severe deformity, the base of the metatarsal is medially angulated, the lateral cortex is thickened from being under tension, and the medial aspect of the first

cuneiform is irregular in shape.[46] The hindfoot shows normal or increased valgus.

The anteroposterior (AP) talo-first metatarsal angle is the radiographic measurement most often used to quantify the severity of metatarsus adductus. This angle is formed by a line drawn through the longitudinal axis of the talus and a line drawn through the longitudinal axis of the first metatarsal on an AP weightbearing radiograph (Fig. 6). The normal AP talo-first metatarsal angle in children younger than 4 years of age was initially reported to range from neutral to 20° valgus.[47] A subsequent larger study of children from infancy to 8 years of age found that the normal AP talo-first metatarsal angle progressively decreased as the child got older.[48] In this study,[48] the mean AP talo-first metatarsal angle for a 1-year-old child was 17° valgus ±12° (2 S.D.), for a 4-year-old was 10° valgus ±13° (2 S.D.), and for an 8-year-old child was 5° valgus ±13° (2 S.D.).

Radiographs are usually not necessary to make a diagnosis of metatarsus adductus. Furthermore, it is often difficult to position the feet of infants for reproducible AP and lateral radiographs. Therefore, many authors agree that routine radiographs are not required in children with metatarsus adductus.[4,21,24,44,49] Indeed, only two studies have examined the usefulness of radiographs in metatarsus adductus.[1,50]

In the primary study, Berg[1] described a radiographic classification of forefoot adduction in infants seen at

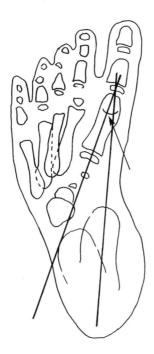

Fig. 6 Diagram of foot demonstrating AP talo-first metatarsal angle.

an average age of 5.5 months (range 2 to 17 months). Four patterns of deformity were described. A varus AP talo-first metatarsal angle was common to all groups, but they were differentiated by the midfoot and hindfoot alignment. Lateral translation of the midfoot was defined as the AP axis of the calcaneus crossing either the medial third of the cuboid or the base of the fourth metatarsal. Valgus alignment of the hindfoot, was defined as a lateral talocalcaneal angle of greater than 45°.

The four patterns of deformity in Berg's[1] study were simple metatarsus adductus, complex metatarsus adductus, simple skewfoot, and complex skewfoot. Simple metatarsus adductus had normal alignment of the mid and hindfoot. Complex metatarsus adductus had normal hindfoot alignment, but lateral translation of the midfoot. A simple skewfoot had increased valgus alignment of the hindfoot, but a normal relationship of the midpart of the foot. A complex skewfoot had abnormalities in all three components with forefoot adduction, lateral translation of the midfoot, and a valgus hindfoot.

Concerns have been raised about Berg's study. Mosca[51] had difficulty visualizing lateral shift of the midfoot without hindfoot valgus (complex metatarsus adductus) and hindfoot valgus without lateral shift of the midfoot (simple skewfoot). Another question is whether it is possible to determine heel valgus on a lat-

eral radiograph. If not, the parameters used to delineate simple and complex skewfoot deformity are unreliable. Furthermore, a subsequent study by Vanderwilde and associates[48] demonstrated that the lateral talocalcaneal angle in normal 1-year-old children was 40° ±15° (2 S.D.). Since Berg defined a valgus hindfoot as a lateral talocalcaneal angle > 45°, this may explain why his study had an unusually large number of children who were classified as having a simple or complex skewfoot deformity (25% in Berg's[1] study compared to 0.4% in Kite's[2] review).

A recent, well controlled study by Cook and associates[50] provides the most striking objection to Berg's radiographic classification. Their analysis demonstrated significant interobserver and intraobserver inconsistency when classifying metatarsus adductus by Berg's system. Furthermore, in contradistinction to the original study, Cook and associates[50] did not find that Berg's radiographic classification correlated with the length of time required for cast correction.

In summary, present evidence does not support the use of radiographs to subclassify different categories of metatarsus adductus. One, however, should use the concepts discussed by Berg[1] in analyzing radiographs of patients with metatarsus adductus (Fig. 7). These concepts include (1) measuring the severity of forefoot adduction by the AP talo-first metatarsal angle, (2) assessing the relationship of the midfoot on the hindfoot, and (3) determining whether there is excessive valgus of the hindfoot.

Treatment: Child Younger Than 1 Year of Age

For the typical 4- to 12-month-old child with metatarsus adductus, the treatment options are (1) continued observation, (2) stretching exercises, (3) splinting, and (4) serial casting. Surgical intervention is rarely, if ever, indicated for the child younger than 1 year of age.

I observe children younger than 6 months of age unless they meet the criteria that will be subsequently described for either stretching exercises or nighttime splinting. Even for the child 6 months or older, observation can be selected if the deformity has not gotten worse during the past 1 to 2 months and if the deformity is rated as either mild or moderate and is flexible.[40]

Stretching exercises are used by some[3,16,18,35,40,44] and railed against by others,[14,21,46] who think that the exercises, if done poorly, may cause harm. In his earlier publications, Kite[9,10] recommended selective use of stretching exercises for children who had milder deformities; however, in his last article on metatarsus adductus, it was emphasized that stretching exercises were ineffective.[2] Kite[2] noted that he would only let parents use a stretching program if the mother held the foot in the corrected position all day, and the father, taking over

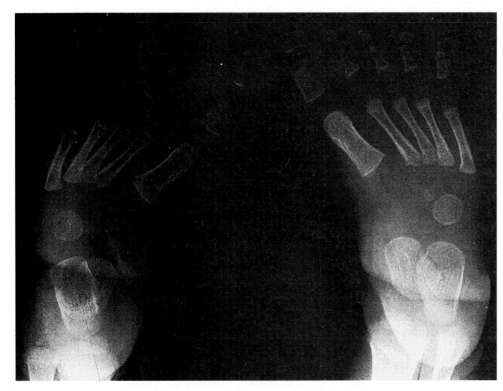

Fig. 7 AP radiograph of the feet taken of a 9-month-old male taken in a simulated weight-bearing posture. Compare with photocopy of same feet depicted in Fig. 5. AP talocalcaneal angle measures 22° varus on the right and 29° varus on the left. The cuboid and hindfoot alignment are within normal limits for the child's age.

immediately when he came home, held the foot all night. When given that choice, Kite[2] noted no difficulty in getting the parents to allow casting.

In my opinion, stretching exercises done by the parents are ineffective. The basis for this opinion is clinical observations and an experimental study that has evaluated the duration that a muscle must be stretched to prevent contracture in cerebral palsy.[52] In this study, no progression of the contracture occurred when the soleus muscle was stretched for at least six hours per day, but progressive contracture was noted when the stretching time was as short as two hours. This supports Kite's[2] observations that a typical program of stretching exercises will not influence the natural history of metatarsus adductus.

I use stretching exercises in children who would otherwise be treated by observation alone but whose parents or grandparents demand that something be done. It is doubtful that even poorly done exercises will cause excessive heel valgus, but I still instruct the parents to stabilize the heel with one hand while using the other hand to push the first metatarsal, but not the great toe, into abduction.

The use of night-time splints or shoes is controversial. Some authors think that a Dennis-Browne bar may increase heel valgus and may cause a severe flatfoot or a skewfoot deformity.[1,14,21,36,44] The contrary view is that night-time splints may be applied in a manner that will

not cause harm, but in a manner that will facilitate resolution of the metatarsus adductus.[16,23,24,35,49]

I advocate use of a Dennis-Browne splint at night-time and naptime for a flexible moderate or severe metatarsus adductus in the 4- to 7-month-old child who has a strong history of sleeping in the knee chest position. The splint is not used as a corrective device, but rather it is a means of preventing abnormal posture. Therefore, the feet are positioned in a physiologic position with open-toe, straight last shoes. To minimize the risk of applying abnormal torque at the ankle, the shoes are positioned on the bar in only 20° of external rotation. To prevent valgus thrust at the hindfoot, the bar is bent into an inverted V shape (Fig. 8). The effectiveness of a Dennis-Browne splint in altering the natural history of metatarsus adductus has not been proven; however, this author does think that selective use of this modality will obviate the need for serial casting in some children.

For a child younger than 3 months of age, Huurman[23] advocates positioning the feet in an externally rotated position. Two holes are punched through the medial side of the heel of a soft infant's shoe. A shoe lace is woven through the holes and tied so that a child will keep the legs externally rotated and the forefoot abducted while sleeping in the prone position. This author has not used this technique; however, it seems simple and might be a useful method of initiating

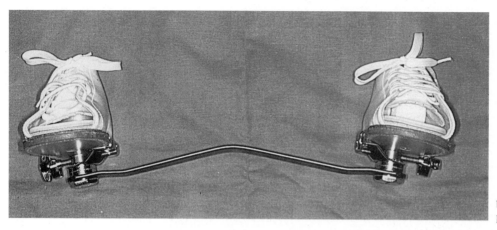

Fig. 8 Dennis-Browne splint bent in the inverted V position to prevent excessive heel valgus.

treatment for severe metatarsus adductus in the very young infant.

Of note, an orthotic bootee has been developed as an alternative to cast therapy in metatarsus adductus. The Bebax orthosis provides multi-directional hinge adjustments between the forefoot and hindfoot. Two studies on this brace have been presented, but at the time of this writing neither has been published. Allen and Weiner[53] reviewed 52 cases treated between 1 and 9 months of age and noted good parental acceptance of the brace. Only two patients required additional treatment beyond their protocol of three months in the Bebax bootee followed by two months in reverse last shoes. In a prospective, randomized study of 27 infants (age 3 to 9 months), Herzenberg and Greenfield[54] found that both casting and the Bebax orthosis were effective but that the orthosis was less costly and better tolerated by the parents. This author has no experience with this orthosis but questions whether this device would be equivalent to casting if its use was restricted to children who were 6 months of age or older.

Serial cast correction is the "gold standard" of nonsurgical therapy for metatarsus adductus. I reserve cast therapy, with the exceptions previously noted, for children who are at least 6 months or older. When casting a child with metatarsus adductus, the principals outlined by Kite[2] and Ponseti and Becker[14] should be followed. The key is to maximize the corrective force at the deformity but avoid accentuation of heel valgus and subsequent flat foot deformity. The position of the heel must be controlled while the forefoot is molded into abduction.

Some authors advocate a below knee cast for metatarsus adductus,[6,16,18,21,23] while other authors favor an above knee cast.[2,14,19,21,36,46,55] Certainly, a short leg cast is easier to apply and facilitates handling and mobility of the child. The rational of a long leg cast has various

explanations. Kite[2] extended the cast to the midthigh with the knee flexed in order to minimize problems with cast slippage. Ponseti and Becker[14] thought that a long leg cast maintained hindfoot position and allowed correction of internal tibial torsion. Recent experiments, however, indicate that correction of internal tibial torsion is not possible by splinting the foot in external rotation.[56] Turco[55] noted that an above-knee cast with the knee flexed would allow the foot to be immobilized in slight equinus, thereby inverting the calcaneus in relationship to the talus and allowing the heel to be maintained in a neutral position. This author has switched from using a short leg to applying a long leg cast for metatarsus adductus. My impression is that a long leg cast is more effective and shortens the duration of treatment. I also agree that keeping the ankle in slight equinus is helpful in avoding exacerbation of heel valgus.

The technique of casting a left-sided metatarsus adductus will be described. To prevent chafing of the skin, a strip of stockinette bandage is placed at the midthigh. A thin layer of cotton padding is wrapped around the leg with extra strips placed over the Achilles tendon and malleoli. Keeping the padding thin maximizes the corrective force, minimizes problems of cast slippage, and is feasible when the cast is removed by soaking rather than sawing. The wet plaster of Paris bandage is then applied to the foot and distal calf. After a quick smoothing of the layers, the hands are positioned to mold the forefoot into abduction while holding the heel in a neutral position. The left index and long finger apply pressure to the medial side of the first metatarsal. In these small feet, one should be careful to place the fingers so that they do not push the great toe into valgus. The right hand positions the ankle in slight equinus and cups the heel in a neutral position. The thenar eminence of the right hand must be positioned only over the calcaneus and cuboid. Otherwise, abduction of the metatarsals is impeded. After this portion has hardened, the cast is extended to the midthigh region with the knee flexed.

The cast should be applied with the idea that it will be soaked off by the parents on the evening prior to the next cast application. This allows the parents to bath the child and eliminates lingering infant distress from a noisy cast saw. To facilitate removal of the cast by the parents, the orthopaedic surgeon should "bunch up" a small amount of the plaster bandage at the end of each roll. This nodule of plaster will help the parent identify the starting point for unwrapping the cast.

Various guidelines have been proposed concerning the duration of casting. Kite[2] continued casting until (1) the convexity along the lateral border of the foot was replaced by a slight concavity, (2) the prominence at the base of the fifth metatarsal was barely palpable, and (3) muscle balance had been achieved, with active abduction clearly evident. Kite[2] advised erring on the side of under correction to minimize the risk of causing a flatfoot deformity. Approximately one-fifth of his patients required a few additional casts at a later date. Bleck[4] advocated that casting be continued until the heel bisector line was between the second and third toe or until no further progress was observed. The median duration of casting in his study was two months, with one patient necessitating 6.5 months of cast therapy. At completion of cast therapy, about half of his patients were placed in a night splint for a median of four months. Recurrent deformity was noted in approximately 12% of his patients. McCauley[13] observed that using a holding cast after correction of the metatarsus adductus reduced the recurrence rate from 37% to 8%.

The duration of casting that I use is six to twelve weeks. To correct a metatarsus adductus, the typical child will require three long-leg casts applied every two weeks. The metatarsus adductus is judged to be corrected when the lateral border of the foot is straight. An additional "holding" cast is used for two to three weeks. Less than nine weeks is required for some children, while others require a longer duration of casting; however, prolonged treatment, i.e., more than twelve weeks, is not well tolerated and, in my opinion, adds little to subsequent results. Therefore, if the metatarsus adductus is not completely corrected after twelve weeks, I will discontinue therapy. Some of these children develop recurrent deformity and require other therapy, but most show continued improvement with subsequent growth.

Cast therapy usually breaks the habit of the child sleeping in the knee-chest position. Therefore, subsequent night splinting is rarely indicated. I do, however, prescribe straight-last shoes at completion of cast therapy. These slightly modified shoes are actually "physio-logic" for an infant's foot and may minimize the risk of recurrent forefoot adduction.

Treatment: Child 1 to 3 Years of Age

For the 1- to 3-year-old child with resistant metatarsus adductus, the treatment options are (1) observation, (2) serial casting, (3) limited medial release followed by serial casting, or (4) a complete tarsometatarsal capsulotomy, better known as a Heyman-Herndon procedure. Observation is indicated for a child with a mild deformity. This degree of metatarsus adductus should not cause cosmetic or shoe wear problems.

In the 1- to 3-year-old child, serial casting may correct a moderate metatarsus adductus; however, at this age, casting is certainly more difficult and has a higher rate of recurrent deformity.[13] Long-leg casts are impractical in this age group. Fortunately, the leg is long enough at this age for heel alignment to be controlled in a short leg cast.

In 1975, Lichtblau[57] described sectioning of the abductor hallucis tendon in 20 patient with metatarsus varus; however, 19 of these patients had forefoot adduction associated with other disorders such as clubfoot or myelomeningocele. Bleck,[4] in 1983, recorded the results of tenotomy of the abductor hallucis at the head of the first metatarsal in ten patients (17 feet) with metatarsus adductus. The average age at operation was 20.9 months. The procedure was limited to feet that demonstrated flexibility of the forefoot on an AP radiograph. Postoperative examination demonstrated correction of all feet but no further details were provided.[4] Other authors have subsequently recommended a similar procedure for the child younger than 3 years of age but have not reported results of this treatment.[23,24]

In my opinion, a limited medial release followed by serial casting is a good option for the 1- to 3-year-old child with residual metatarsal adductus (Fig. 9). The limited medial release I perform is more extensive than that described by Lichtblau[57] and includes lengthening of the abductor hallucis tendon, releasing the portion of the anterior tibialis tendon that inserts on the first metatarsal, and a medial capsulotomy of the first metatarsal-cuneiform joint. The principle of this operation is that after release of the most contracted soft tissues, the subsequent duration of casting can be shortened and the results of therapy enhanced. The limited medial release should not cause the long-term problems associated with a Heyman-Herndon procedure.[58] The inability to passively abduct the forefoot to the midline is not a contraindication to this procedure; however, very rigid forefoot deformities should not be treated by this technique.

My technique of performing a limited medial release for metatarsus adductus is as follows. Beginning 1 cm proximal to the first metatarsocuneiform joint, a

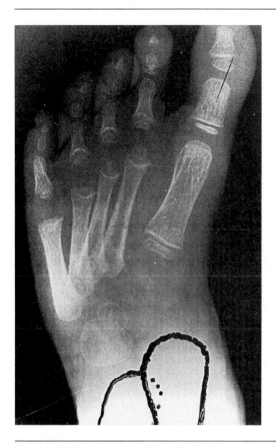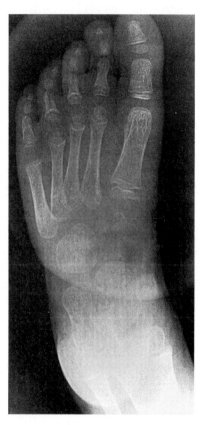

Fig. 9 **Left**, AP standing radiograph of the left foot of a 2-year, 10-month-old female with persistent metatarsus adductus following two previous trials of cast therapy, one initiated at 6 months of age and one when patient was 18 months old. AP talocalcaneal angle measures 20° varus. Patient underwent limited medal release followed by 3 months of serial casting. **Right**, AP standing radiograph at the age of 3 years, 9 months demonstrates normal forefoot alignment.

3-cm incision is made on the dorsomedial border of the foot. At the distal portion of the incision, the tendon of the abductor hallucis is identified and fractionally lengthened, that is, it is tenotomized in an area that has sufficient underlying muscle to prevent disruption of the muscle-tendon unit. This allows the tendon to heal in a lengthened position but prevents hallux valgus deformity. The sheath of the anterior tibialis tendon is opened, and the portion of the anterior tibialis tendon that inserts on the first metatarsal is released, but the attachment of the tendon on the medial cuneiform is left intact. Releasing this portion of the anterior tibialis tendon enhances correction of metatarsus adductus, provides clear access to the first metatarsocuneiform joint, and has not caused any apparent bony deformity or limitation of dorsiflexion. Capsulotomy of the first metatarsocuneiform joint is limited to the medial side and the medial one-half of the plantar and dorsal surface. The limited capsulotomy minimizes the risk of injuring the articular surface and subsequent dorsal bossing. At completion of the operation, the skin is closed by a subcuticular technique and a short-leg cast is applied with molding of the forefoot into abduction. The plantar surface of the cast is contoured to provide a good weight-bearing surface, as it is impossible to keep children of this age from

walking after the second or third post-operative day.

Serial felt wedges and serial cast changes are used to correct residual forefoot adduction that remains after the limited medial release. Inserting a wedge can be done without changing the cast and, therefore, is easier on the child and also eliminates the risk of losing good hindfoot position. The first felt wedge is inserted approximately one week after the operation. A rectangle of plaster is removed from the dorsum of the forefoot. The medial border of the cast is retained, but the "cast window" rectangle of plaster should include enough of the lateral wall to allow abduction of the forefoot. A wedge of felt is inserted between the medial border of the cast and the first metatarsal. The plaster rectangle is then replaced and secured with a roll of plaster. Either cast wedges or cast changes are continued on a weekly basis until the forefoot adduction is corrected. A holding cast is then used for an additional three to four weeks to allow further modeling of the tarsometatarsal joints and resumption of normal growth.

The limited medial release is a simple procedure that has not caused any apparent problems. In my experience the metatarsus adductus has corrected in a satisfactory fashion; however, there are a limited number of cases that satisfy the indications for this procedure. Further follow-up and critical review is certainly warranted.

Other procedures have been described for resistant metatarsus adductus in the younger child. Thompson[59] resected the entire abductor hallucis muscle and tendon. In 29 of his 82 cases, the procedure was performed before 1 year of age. Hallux valgus complicated the resection in 23%. Mitchell[27] released the origin of the abductor hallucis and noted good results in eight patients, but he also observed that the procedure was difficult. The extensive dissection and greater possibility of nerve injury would prevent this author from doing this operation for metatarsus adductus. Ghali and associates[37] released the portion of the anterior tibialis tendon that inserted into the medial cuneiform and did a capsulotomy of the medial, dorsal, and plantar aspects of the first metatarsocuneiform and naviculocuneiform joint. The median age at surgery was 1.7 years, and the authors reported uniformly excellent results. I, however, question the need and advisability of releasing the naviculocuneiform joint.

Treatment: Child 3 Years and Older

For the child who has residual moderate or severe metatarsus adductus and is 3 years of age or older, the treatment options are (1) complete tarsometatarsal capsulotomy (Heyman-Herndon procedure), (2) metatarsal osteotomies with or without open wedge osteotomy of the medial cuneiform, or (3) accept the deformity.

Heyman and associates,[7] in 1958, reported results of a tarsometatarsal capsulotomy for residual forefoot abduction. A subsequent follow-up series[60] from the same institution analyzed this procedure in 80 feet with metatarsus adductus and noted excellent results in 56 feet, good in 18, fair in two, and poor in four. At that time the authors[60] concluded that the Heyman-Herndon procedure was primarily indicated for a child 3 to 8 years of age with resistant metatarsus adductus and neutral hindfoot alignment, but they also used this procedure for selected children younger than 3 years of age. The following technical aspects were emphasized: (1) avoiding damage to the articular surface, (2) division of only the intermetatarsal and tarsometatarsal ligament, (3) retention of the lateral capsule at the fifth metatarsocuboid joint, (4) resecting only the medial two-thirds of the plantar aspect of the first metatarsal capsule, and (5) plaster cast immobilization for a minimum of four months.

For many years the Heyman-Herndon procedure was the treatment of choice for a "middle age" child with residual metatarsus adductus.[21] A recent long-term follow-up study, however, has raised concerns about this procedure. Stark and associates[58] noted a high incidence of failures that were characterized by dorsal bony prominences, difficulty with proper shoe fitting,

and degenerative changes at the tarsometatarsal joints. Results were worse in patients who also had clubfoot, but even in the group with uncomplicated metatarsus adductus, 40% of the feet were placed in the poor category. The findings of this study and the long duration of post-operative cast immobilization have caused many current authors to narrow their indications for the Heyman-Herndon procedure to the 3- and 4-year-old child and to proceed with metatarsal osteotomies at 5 years of age.[23,44,49] One author even implied that the best treatment for a 4-year-old child was to wait a year and perform metatarsal osteotomies.[49]

Osteotomy of the metatarsals for residual forefoot adduction in children was originally described by Steytler and Vanderwalt,[20] but the landmark series was the 1971 report by Berman and Gartland[61] on 119 feet, 18 of which had congenital metatarsus adductus. These authors performed a dome-shaped osteotomy at the base of each metatarsal and, for later patients in their series, internally fixed the forefoot with two smooth pins, one inserted across the first and one inserted across the fifth metatarsal osteotomy. Only six weeks of short-leg cast immobilization was typically required. In the group with congenital metatarsus adductus there were ten excellent, seven good, and one fair result. Compared to the Heyman-Herndon procedure, Berman and Gartland[61] thought that metatarsal osteotomies provided more satisfactory results in children 6 years of age or older.

Shortening of the first metatarsal is the unique complication of correcting metatarsus adductus by metatarsal osteotomies.[61-63] This complication is related to the proximal position of the first metatarsal physis and occurred in 5% of the patients in one series,[61] but was found in 30% of the cases reviewed by Holden.[63] In their series, the development of a short first metatarsal correlated with surgical technique. The osteotomy crossed the physis in two affected feet, and in the other six cases, the procedure was characterized either by extensive periosteal dissection and/or placement of the osteotomy close to the physis. The incidence of this complication was not increased in younger children; however, as expected, the amount of shortening was directly related to the age of the child at the operation. Holden and associates[63] recommended roentgenographic localization of the first metatarsal physis prior to any subperiosteal dissection and placement of the first metatarsal osteotomy at least 6 mm distal to the physis.

Present evidence supports metatarsal osteotomies as the preferred procedure for children 6 years of age or older (Fig. 10), but should we abandon the Heyman-Herndon procedure in the 3- to 5-year-old child? The theoretical advantage of tarsal-metatarsal capsulotomies in these younger children is that by repositioning the joints, subsequent growth will allow remodel-

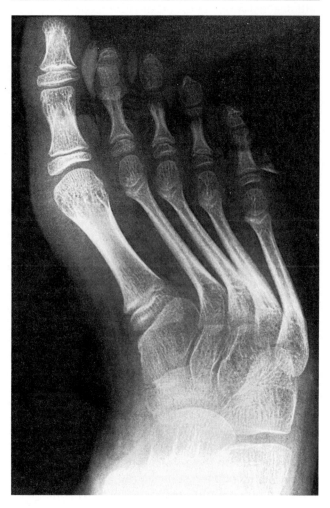

Fig. 10 AP nonweightbearing radiograph of the foot in an 8-year-old girl with mild mental retardation, tracheal stenosis, and residual metatarsus adductus compromising shoe wear. Longstanding forefoot deformity and bony changes require multiple metatarsal osteotomies as opposed to soft tissue releases. Note trapezoid shape of medial cuneiform. Open wedge osteotomy of the medial cuneiform and osteotomy of second, third, and fourth metatarsals as described by Kling and associates[11] could also be considered.

metatarsal osteotomies in the 3- to 5-year-old child, this author will continue to use the Heyman-Herndon procedure for moderate or severe metatarsus adductus in this age group.

My modifications to the Heyman-Herndon procedure[60] are relatively minor. I routinely lengthen the abductor hallucis tendon and release the anterior tibialis tendon as described for a limited medial release. I prefer three vertical incisions to improve cosmesis and to permit adequate exposure of the abductor hallucis tendon. The first incision is placed on the dorsomedial border of the foot as described for the limited medial release. The second incision is centered over the second metatarsal, and the third incision is centered over the fourth metatarsal. To avoid damaging the articular surfaces, careful technique and a blunt-ended blade should be utilized when making the capsulotomies.

In doing multiple metatarsal osteotomies, I also prefer three vertical incisions rather than a single transverse dorsal incision and routinely lengthen the abductor hallucis tendon. Accurate localization of the first metatarsal physis must be accomplished before subperiosteal exposure of that bone. Smooth pins through the first and fifth metatarsal, as described by Berman and Gartland,[61] are used to fix the forefoot in the abducted position. A smaller threaded pin, however, is first drilled retrograde through the osteotomy site and the diaphyseal cortex. The smaller threaded pin is easier to drill through diaphyseal bone. It can then be exchanged for a larger, smooth pin that is driven across the osteotomy site into metaphyseal bone at the base of the first and fifth metatarsal and into the cuneiform and cuboid bones if necessary.

Open wedge osteotomy of the medial cuneiform, combined with soft tissue releases or metatarsal osteotomies, have been described for metatarsus adductus in the older child with severe deformity.[11,26,51,64] These procedures will be discussed in the section on skewfoot deformity.

Skewfoot

Some authors think that a skewfoot deformity (forefoot adduction with heel valgus) is a complication of treating metatarsus adductus.[34] Cases without prior treatment, however, have been well-documented.[3] It would seem that a skewfoot should be classified as a congenital rather than a developmental disorder, but this has not been proven.

The clinical examination of an older child with skewfoot deformity is characteristic. The foot has an "S" or a "Z" shape with the heel in marked valgus, and the forefoot fixed in a rigid adduction. Medial deviation of the talus causes a fullness on the medial side of the foot that progresses to a concavity at the site of the

ing of the articular surfaces so that more normal joint alignment and weight-bearing forces are achieved. The theoretical disadvantages of multiple osteotomies in the 3- to 5-year-old child is that a second deformity is being created to compensate for abnormal joint alignment. It is possible, although not proven, that patients who underwent multiple osteotomies at this age would have a higher rate of recurrent deformity and a subsequent greater degree of tarsometatarsal degenerative arthritis in their adult years. Furthermore, the consequences of injuring the first metatarsal physis is certainly greater in a 3- to 5-year-old child than it is in one who is 6 years of age or older. Therefore, until subsequent studies demonstrate the superiority of laterally subluxated navicular.

By comparison, defining excessive hindfoot valgus and diagnosing skewfoot is very difficult in an infant. Their feet are small and chubby, which limits the clinical examination. Even radiographs do not permit differentiation of metatarsus adductus from a skewfoot in the child. Obtaining reproducible radiographs of the foot is a challenge at this age. Furthermore, measurement of heel valgus is inconsistent because only a small, relatively round portion of the talus and the calcaneus has ossified. Finally, lateral translation of the navicular, a cardinal sign of skewfoot, cannot be documented until that bone begins to ossify at around 2 to 4 years of age (Fig. 11).

I believe that the diagnosis of skewfoot deformity should be restricted to children whose foot deformity meets the criteria described by Kite,[2] that is, a fixed heel valgus and forefoot adduction that cannot be completely corrected by casting. Therefore, the 6-month-old boy with increased heel valgus and severe forefoot adduction described by Peterson[3] would not be classified by this author as having skewfoot, because this patient's foot deformity was successfully treated with four weeks of serial casting. I would have classified this patient's foot deformity as metatarsus adductus with increased heel valgus.

Even though a definitive diagnosis may not be possible during infancy, cast therapy is certainly warranted for the young child who presents with a possible skewfoot deformity. These children have an unusual degree of forefoot adduction and are the children that I start casting before 6 months of age. By my definition, cast treatment of a skewfoot deformity will not be curative; however, like the child with a clubfoot deformity, casting will help obtain partial correction of the foot adduction. Obviously, it is essential to keep the heel in neutral or varus while applying the cast. In my opinion, a long-leg cast, which permits enough ankle equinus to lock the heel into inversion while the forefoot is molded into abduction, is mandatory for these patients.

As described by Peterson,[3] a variety of operations have been recommended for skewfoot deformity. These include metatarsal osteotomy, excision of the base of the first metatarsal, excision of the bases of all the metatarsals, reduction of the subluxed first metatarsal-cuneiform joint, arthrodesis of the first metatarsal-cuneiform joint, tarsometatarsal capsulotomies, spread and strut bone graft of the first metatarsal-navicular joint, correction of the abnormal insertion of the anterior tibial tendon, excision of the adductor hallucis muscle and tendon, soft tissue release, incision through Chopart's joint, wedge tarsectomy, wedge resection of the cuboid, excision of the cuboid, calcaneocuboid arthrodesis, subtalar arthrodesis (Grice), calcaneal osteotomy (Dwyer), triple arthro-

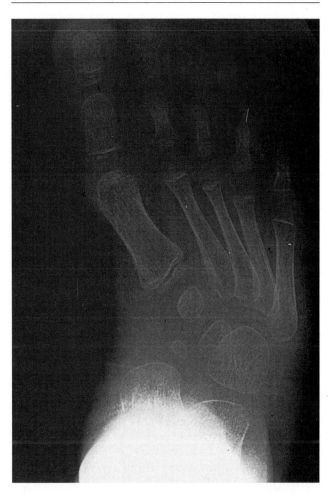

Fig. 11 AP standing radiograph of the foot in a 3-year, 3-month-old male with striking metatarsus adductus. No previous therapy had been performed. In addition to the severe forefoot adduction, early ossification of the navicular demonstrates lateral translation of the midfoot on the hindfoot. Radiographs are consistent with skewfoot deformity. A Heyman-Herndon procedure was performed. Significant subluxation of the first metatarsal on the medial cuneiform was noted at surgery. In addition, the medial cuneiform had a trapezoidal shape. The forefoot deformity recurred. At this age, observation of a skewfoot deformity is probably the best option with anticipation that more definitive bony procedures can be performed at a later age.

desis, and combinations of these procedures.

Kendrick and associates[60] confirmed the earlier observations of Heyman and associates,[7] who noted that tarsometatarsal capsulotomies were unsuccessful in patients with skewfoot deformity unless the forefoot release was combined with a Grice procedure (Fig. 11). Peterson[3] also noted recurrent deformity in two patients treated by a posterior medial release and temporary pin fixation of the realigned tarsals, but observed normal alignment of the foot, no pain, and normal activity levels when a subtalar extra-articular arthrodesis (Grice procedure) was combined with soft-tissue realignment of the tarsals.

In the older child, it is obvious that the medial cuneiform in a skewfoot has a trapezoidal shape, with the proximal and distal articular surfaces converging medially. Fowler,[65] in 1959, described an open-wedge osteotomy of the first cuneiform and plantar fascia release in selected patients with resistant metatarsus adductus. Lincoln and associates[26] described results of this procedure in a series of 19 feet that included patients with clubfeet and arthrogryposis, as well as primary metatarsus adductus. Lincoln and associates[26] made a vertical osteotomy through the first cuneiform with a sharp thin osteotome, opened the osteotomy medially, and inserted a wedge of bank bone or autogenous iliac bone graft. Kling and associates[11] combined an open wedge osteotomy of the first cuneiform with osteotomy of the second, third, and fourth metatarsal for patients with "resistant metatarsus adductus" secondary to treated clubfoot or untreated metatarsus adductus. In this series, the obliquity of the first metatarsal-cuneiform joint was reduced by a mean of 10° or 71%. Reducing the obliquity of the first metatarsal-cuneiform joint was thought to minimize the risk of recurrent forefoot adduction. The results in 32 feet were rated as good or excellent.[11]

Based on the premise that soft-tissue correction of forefoot adduction is ineffective and hindfoot arthrodesis is unnecessary, Mosca[51] advocated a new approach for skewfoot deformity. For the valgus heel deformity, Mosca performs an open wedge osteotomy of the calcaneus as described by Evans.[66] The calcaneal osteotomy corrects the malalignment at the talocalcaneal as well as the talonavicular joint. During the same procedure, the metatarsus adductus is corrected by performing a opening wedge osteotomy of the medial cuneiform. Tricortical iliac crest allograft bone is used at both sites. If increased midtarsal cavus was present, a dorso-lateral closing wedge osteotomy of the cuboid is also performed.

Although the best treatment for a child with a skewfoot deformity can still be debated, it is obvious that any operation that corrects only the metatarsus adductus or the hindfoot deformity will not succeed in realigning the foot. At the present time, this author thinks that surgical therapy for a skewfoot deformity should be delayed until the child is at least 6 years old and has either become symptomatic or demonstrates progressive deformity. The procedure advocated by Mosca[51] would then be recommended unless degenerative changes had already occurred at the talocalcaneal joint.

References

1. Berg EE: A reappraisal of metatarsus adductus and skewfoot. *J Bone Joint Surg* 1986;68A:1185-1196.
2. Kite JH: Congenital metatarsus varus. *J Bone Joint Surg* 1967;49A:388-397.
3. Peterson HA: Skewfoot (forefoot adduction with heel valgus). *J Pediatr Orthop* 1986;6:24-30.
4. Bleck EE: Metatarsus adductus: Classification and relationship to outcomes of treatment. *J Pediatr Orthop* 1983;3:2-9.
5. Browne RS, Paton DF: Anomalous insertion of the tibialis posterior tendon in congenital metatarsus varus. *J Bone Joint Surg* 1979;61B:74-76.
6. Gruber MA, Dee R: Congenital metatarsus varus, in Dee R, Mango E, Hurst LC (eds): *Principles of Orthopaedic Practice.* New York, NY, McGraw-Hill, 1989, pp 1148-1150.
7. Heyman CH, Herndon CH, Strong JM: Mobilization of the tarsometatarsal and intermetatarsal joints for the correction of resistant adduction of the fore part of the foot in congenital club-foot or congenital metatarsus varus. *J Bone Joint Surg* 1958;40A:299-310.
8. Jacobs JE: Metatarsus varus and hip dysplasia. *Clin Orthop* 1960;16:203-213.
9. Kite JH: Congenital metatarsus varus: Report of 300 cases. *J Bone Joint Surg* 1950;32A:500-506.
10. Kite JH: Congenital metatarsus varus: Report of 400 cases, in *American Academy of Orthopaedic Surgeons Instructional Course Lectures Volume VII,* Pease CN, Banks SW (eds). Ann Arbor, MI, JW Edwards, 1950, pp 126-129.
11. Kling TF Jr, Schmidt TL, Conklin MJ: Open wedge osteotomy of the first cuneiform for metatarsus adductus. *Orthop Trans* 11991;15:106.
12. Kumar SJ, MacEwen GD: The incidence of hip dysplasia with metatarsus adductus. *Clin Orthop* 1982;164:234-235.
13. McCauley J Jr, Lusskin R, Bromley J: Recurrence in congenital metatarsus varus. *J Bone Joint Surg* 1964;46A:525-532.
14. Ponseti IV, Becker JR: Congenital metatarsus adductus: The results of treatment. *J Bone Joint Surg* 1966;48A:702-711.
15. Reimann I, Werner HH: Congenital metatarsus varus: A suggestion for a possible mechanism and relation to other foot deformities. *Clin Orthop* 1975;110:223-226.
16. Renshaw TS (ed): The Foot, in *Pediatric Orthopedics.* Philadelphia, PA, WB Saunders, 1986, pp 123-139.
17. Rushforth GF: The natural history of hooked forefoot. *J Bone Joint Surg* 1978;60B:530-532.
18. Salter RB: Congenital Abnormalities, in *Textbook of Disorders and Injuries of the Musculoskeletal System,* ed 2. Baltimore, MD, Williams & Wilkins, 1983, pp 113-144.
19. Sharrard WJW: Congenital metatarsus varus and adductus, in *Pediatric Orthopaedics and Fractures.* Oxford, Blackwell Scientific Publications, 1971, pp 281-283.
20. Steytler JCS, Van der Walt ID: Correction of resistant adduction of the forefoot in congenital club-foot and congenital metatarsus varus by metatarsal osteotomy. *Br J Surg* 1966;53:558-560.
21. Tachdjian MO: The foot and leg, in *Pediatric Orthopedics,* ed 2. Philadelphia, PA, WB Saunders, 1990, pp 2405-3012.
22. Wynne-Davies R: Family studies and the cause of congenital club foot: talipes equinovarus, talipes calcaneo-valgus and metatarsus varus. *J Bone Joint Surg* 1964;46B:445-463.
23. Huurman WW: Congenital foot deformities, in Mann RA (ed): *Surgery of the Foot,* ed 5. St. Louis, MO, CV Mosby, 1986, pp 519-567.
24. Thompson GH, Simons GW III: Congenital talipes equinovarus (clubfeet) and metatarsus adductus, in Drennan JC (ed): *The Child's Foot and Ankle.* New York, NY, Raven Press, 1992, pp 97-133.
25. Kane R: Metatarsus varus. *Bull N Y Acad Med* 1987;63:828-834.
26. Lincoln CR, Wood KE, Bugg EI Jr: Metatarsus varus corrected by open wedge osteotomy of the first cuneiform bone. *Orthop Clin North Am* 1976;7:795-798.
27. Mitchell GP: Abductor hallucis release in congenital metatarsus varus. *Int Orthop* 1980;3:299-304.

28. Peabody CW, Muro F: Congenital metatarsus varus. *J Bone Joint Surg* 1933;15:171-189.

29. Wynne-Davies R, Littlejohn A, Gormley J: Aetiology and interrelationship of some common skeletal deformities: Talipes equinovarus and calcaneovalgus, metatarsus varus, congenital dislocation of the hip, and infantile idiopathic scoliosis. *J Med Genet* 1982;19:321-328.

30. Hunziker UA, Largo RH, Duc G: Neonatal metatarsus adductus, joint mobility, axis and rotation of the lower extremity in preterm and term children 0-5 years of age. *Eur J Pediatr* 1988;148:19-23.

31. McCormick DW, Blount WP: Metatarsus adductovarus: "Skewfoot." *JAMA* 194;141:449-453.

32. Hunt CE, Shannon DC: Sudden infant death syndrome and sleeping position. *Pediatrics* 1992;90:115-118.

33. Capute AJ, Shapiro BK, Palmer FB, et al: Normal gross motor development: The influences of race, sex and socio-economic status. *Dev Med Child Neurol* 1985;27:635-643.

34. Katz K, Naor N, Merlob P, et al: Rotational deformities of the tibia and foot in preterm infants. *J Pediatr Orthop* 1990;10:483-485.

35. Hensinger RN, Jones ET: Deformities of the foot and toes, in *Neonatal Orthopaedics*. New York, Grune & Stratton, 1981, pp 279-301.

36. Staheli LT: Rotational problems of the lower extremities. *Orthop Clin North Am* 1987;18:503-512.

37. Ghali NN, Abberton MJ, Silk FF: The management of metatarsus adductus et supinatus. *J Bone Joint Surg* 1984;66B:376-380.

38. Reimann I, Werner HH: The pathology of congenital metatarsus varus. A post-mortem study of a newborn infant. *Acta Orthop Scand* 1983;54:847-849.

39. Wills CA, Hoffer MM, Perry J: A comparison of foot-switch and EMG analysis of varus deformities of the feet of children with cerebral palsy. *Dev Med Child Neurol* 988;30:227-231.

40. Bohne W: Metatarsus adductus. *Bull N Y Acad Med* 1987;63:835-838.

41. Gruber MA, Lozano JA: Metatarsus varus and developmental dysplasia of the hip: Is there a relationship? *Orthop Trans* 1991;15:336.

42. Kollme, CE, Betz RR, Clancy M, et al: Relationship of congenital hip and foot deformities: A National Shriners Hospital survey. *Orthop Trans* 1991;15:96.

43. Ryoppy S, Poussa M, Merikanto J, et al: Foot deformities in diastrophic dysplasia: An analysis of 102 patients. *J Bone Joint Surg* 1992;74B:441-444.

44. Crawford AH, Gabriel KR: Foot and ankle problems. *Orthop Clin North Am* 1987;18:649-666.

45. Smith JT, Bleck EE, Gamble JG, et al: Simple method of documenting metatarsus adductus. *J Pediatr Orthop* 1991;11:679-680.

46. Turek SL: Congenital deformities, in *Orthopaedics: Principles and Their Application*, ed 4. Philadelphia, PA, JB Lippincott, 1984, pp 283-361.

47. Simons GW: Analytical radiography of club feet. *J Bone Joint Surg* 1977;59B:485-489.

48. Vanderwilde R, Staheli LT, Chew DE, et al: Measurements on radiographs of the foot in normal infants and children. *J Bone Joint Surg* 1988;70A:407-415.

49. Meehan P: Other conditions of the foot, in Morrissy RT (ed): *Lovell and Winter's Pediatric Orthopaedics*, ed 3. Philadelphia, PA, JB Lippincott, 1990, pp 991-1021.

50. Cook DA, Breed AL, Cook T, et al: Observer variability in the radiographic measurement and classification of metatarsus adductus. *J Pediatr Orthop* 1992;12:86-89.

51. Mosca VS: Flexible flatfoot and skewfoot, in Drennan JC (ed): *The Child's Foot and Ankle*. New York, NY, Raven Press, 1992, pp 355-376.

52. Tardieu C, Lespargot A, Tabary C, et al: For how long must the soleus muscle be stretched each day to prevent contracture? *Dev Med Child Neurol* 1988;30:3-10.

53. Allen W, Weiner DS: The treatment of metatarsus adductovarus with a hinged adjustable shoe orthosis. *Orthop Trans* 1989;13:245-246.

54. Herzenberg JE, Greenfield ML: Prospective randomized treatment trial for resistant metatarsus adductus. *Orthop Trans* 1993;17:79.

55. Turco VJ: Comments on metatarsus adductus. *Bull N Y Acad Med* 1987;63:837-838.

56. Barlow DW, Staheli LT: Effects of lateral rotation splinting on lower extremity bone growth: An in vivo study in rabbits. *J Pediatr Orthop* 1991;11:583-587.

57. Lichtblau S: Section of the abductor hallucis tendon for correction of metatarsus varus deformity. *Clin Orthop* 1975;110:227-232.

58. Stark JG, Johanson JE, Winter RB: The Heyman-Herndon tarsometatarsal capsulotomy for metatarsus adductus: Results in 48 feet. *J Pediatr Orthop* 1987;7:305-310.

59. Thomson SA: Hallux varus and metatarsus varus: A five-year study (1954-1958). *Clin Orthop* 1960;16:109-118.

60. Kendrick RE, Sharma NK, Hassler WL, et al: Tarsometatarsal mobilization for resistant adduction of the fore part of the foot: A follow-up study. *J Bone Joint Surg* 1970;52A:61-70.

61. Berman A, Gartland JJ: Metatarsal osteotomy for the correction of adduction of the fore part of the foot in children. *J Bone Joint Surg* 1971;53A:498-506.

62. Gamble JG, Decker S, Abrams RC: Short first ray as a complication of multiple metatarsal osteotomies. *Clin Orthop* 1982;164:241-244.

63. Holden D, Siff S, Butler J, et al: Shortening of the first metatarsal as a complication of metatarsal osteotomies. *J Bone Joint Surg* 1984;66A:582-587.

64. Anderson DJ, Schoenecker PL, Blair VP, et al: Combined lateral column shortening and medial column lengthening in the treatment of severe forefoot adductus. *Orthop Trans* 1991;15:768.

65. Fowler SB, Brooks AL, Parrish TF: The cavo-varus foot. *J Bone Joint Surg* 1959;41A:757.

66. Evans D: Calcaneo-valgus deformity. *J Bone Joint Surg* 1975;57B:270-278.

Developmental Dysplasia of the Hip

Peter D. Pizzutillo, MD

Introduction

The early detection of developmental dysplasia of the hip (DDH) has significantly improved since the inception of screening programs in the newborn nursery. Despite persistent efforts to improve screening techniques and protocols that allow for a large proportion of newborn infants to be examined by pediatric and orthopaedic physicians, the ideal goal of early detection of all hip pathology has yet to be attained.[1] While critics of the screening process may suggest lack of expertise on the part of the examiners as the primary cause for this problem, students of DDH recognize that this problem is multifaceted and not merely a unidimensional mechanical problem.[2-4] The degree of instability, the time of onset of instability, the association with extrinsic environmental factors, and the association with underlying systemic pathology of connective tissue, muscle, and neural tissue combine to form a complex of clinical findings that is not easily described by a single term.

Although office evaluation and management of children with this problem are frequently uncomplicated, a small percentage of infants with DDH will not respond to standard treatment protocols in the expected manner. These patients will require complex treatment programs and will have less favorable results.

The most problematic issue is the infant with a missed diagnosis of hip pathology. It is well known that delay of treatment is associated with complex treatments, more complications, and poorer long-term results.

Evaluation of the Newborn

Perinatal History

The initial evaluation of the child suspected of DDH includes a detailed review of the pregnancy and delivery.[5] Factors to be considered include maternal age, maternal health during the pregnancy, the occurrence of vaginal bleeding or leakage of amniotic fluid, maternal infection, and the use of drugs or alcohol during the pregnancy. Although many of these factors have no direct association with the idiopathic form of DDH, their importance lies in the exclusion of other etiologies of hip instability. Maternal exposure to infection as well as the use of drugs or alcohol may suggest the child's central nervous system as the cause of hip instability. Maternal diabetes is associated with sacral agenesis, and poor prenatal care with insufficient intake of folic acid is associated with the development of myelomeningocele. Myopathies such as central core disease and nemaline rod myopathy, in addition to nonspecific mitochondrial myopathies, are associated with hip dysplasia. A history of decreased frequency or vigor of intrauterine fetal motion may suggest an underlying myopathy as the primary process in creating an unstable hip. The history of weak sucking ability or of frequent choking while being nursed suggests myopathy.

Whether delivery is vaginal or by cesarean section, it is well recognized that the fetus in breech position is at considerably higher risk for hip pathology when compared to infants delivered with vertex presentation. A diligent review of family history is conducted to determine the presence of DDH, as well as neuromuscular diseases and connective tissue disorders, such as Ehlers-Danlos syndrome.

Clinical Examination

The physical examination requires that the child be completely undressed, including diaper, and be relaxed. If the diaper is left in place in order to speed the examination, mild degrees of asymmetry of hip abduction as well as midline defects of the lower spine may not be detected. A warm examining room with no outside stimulation and the use of a soft, warm blanket facilitate relaxation of the child. A crying child may be fully relaxed and merely protesting. Examining the crying, tight baby, however, is a pitfall that must be avoided, because even advanced degrees of hip displacement may be missed by the experienced examiner under these circumstances.

The formal orthopaedic examination is preceded by an estimation of development as well as a neurologic evaluation. It is important to make the diagnosis of significant motor delay or of central nervous system disorder, because either of these removes the existing hip problem from the idiopathic realm. Development is measured by the quality of head and trunk control and, later, by the ability to crawl, pull to stand, and walk. The presence of handedness in the infant or toddler, the detection of asymmetrical tone when limbs are compared to each other, or the persistence of primitive reflexes may indicate significant central nervous system problems.

A complete orthopaedic examination is necessary for comprehensive evaluation of the child. Examination of the head and neck may reveal congenital muscular torticollis which has an associated incidence of DDH of 20%. The remainder of the spine may exhibit midline defects, such as a hairy patch, hemangioma, or sinus, that may indicate the existence of congenital spinal anomalies such as diastematomyelia. The upper extremities may exhibit ligamentous laxity, as occurs in Ehlers-Danlos syndrome or dislocation of the radial head, as in Larsen's syndrome. Both of these conditions have a high incidence of DDH. A correlation has been noted between the existence of foot deformities, such as metatarsus adductus or clubfoot, and DDH; however, this association has not been confirmed by other investigators.

The formal evaluation of the hip is preceded by an overall impression of both lower extremities. The thigh and lower leg are examined for congenital limb deformities that may cause asymmetry in girth and length. The newborn infant with congenital short femur and coxa vara will typically present with shortening of the thigh, limited abduction of the involved hip, and a radiographic appearance suggestive of hip instability (Fig. 1).

The soft tissue components of the thigh and leg are examined for asymmetry, especially asymmetry of the thigh folds. The presence of asymmetrical thigh folds (Fig.2) should be a warning to further examine the hip with great diligence but is not pathognomonic of hip dislocation, because 10% of normal infants will display similar findings.

Hip Examination

With the child in a relaxed state, the hips may be reliably examined. Both hips should be widely abducted in a gentle manner with concomitant upward pressure on the greater trochanters to attempt a reductive maneuver of the hip. In the young infant under the age of 3 months, instability frequently persists, and the

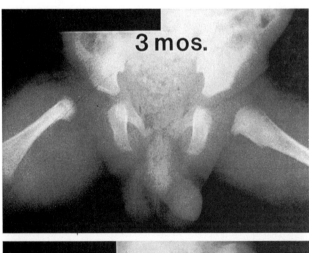

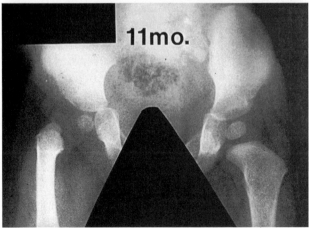

Fig. 1 Early radiograph of congenital coxa vara may suggest dislocation of the hip, however, continued ossification clarifies the diagnosis.

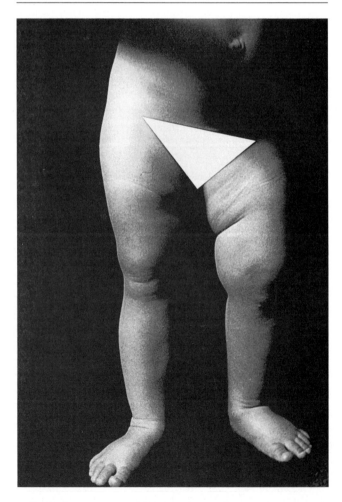

Fig. 2 Frontal view of child's lower extremities reveals asymmetric thigh folds.

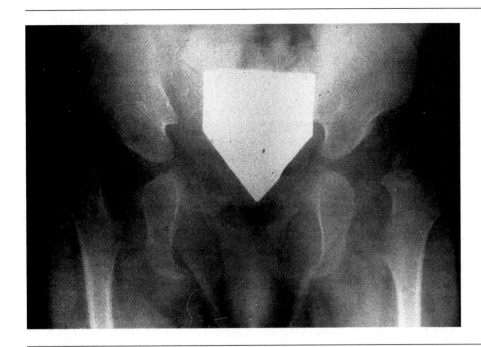

Fig. 3 Radiograph reveals bilateral dislocation of hips in child with Ehlers-Danlos syndrome.

described Ortolani maneuver will result in the palpable "thud" of reduction of the femoral head into the acetabulum. As the infant ages, instability becomes progressively less prominent, and the Ortolani maneuver will become negative. In this group of children, contracture will reveal marked asymmetry of hip abduction when the hips are examined at 90° of flexion. Even minor degrees of asymmetry need to be evaluated either by radiography or by realtime ultrasonography. In addition, if abduction of the hips is symmetrical but is less than 45°, imaging studies are strongly recommended to rule out the existence of bilateral hip dislocation. This is a difficult condition to diagnose by physical examination alone and, if suspected, requires diligent investigation. Unfortunately, bilateral hip dislocation is not uncommon in association with Ehlers-Danlos syndrome (Fig. 3). The difficulty of early diagnosis by physical examination alone is made more difficult in this group by their joint laxity, which may result in hip abduction far in excess of the 45° limit that has been stated. Ehlers-Danlos syndrome is more commonly detected after children begin to walk, when it is observed that they walk with a widened perineum and tend to have hyperlordosis of the lumbar spine.

The Ortolani maneuver is complemented by the provocative test of Barlow. As with the performance of the Ortolani maneuver, each hip should be examined in isolation, with the other hip being held in wide, fixed abduction to lock the pelvis. A much more critical evaluation of each hip can thus be accomplished. Once the hips have been flexed to 90° and one hip has been abducted to lock the pelvis, the hip to be examined is gently brought into adduction by grasping the distal thigh between the thumb and index finger while the fourth or fifth digit rests on the greater trochanter as a sensing finger. In the adducted position, a gentle pistoning motion is begun with slow but gentle regularity in an attempt to determine whether the femoral head is gliding within the acetabulum or can actually be displaced posteriorly out of the acetabulum. The pistoning motion should be done in varying degrees of flexion and extension for a complete examination of stability. If the Barlow test is only performed with the hip in flexion, instability may not be detected.

Hip Clicks

The performance of these tests may result in the production of "hip clicks." There are many soft tissue structures that may create a palpable and occasionally audible clicking sound. These may emanate from the child's knee joint or patella and be transmitted to the hip area or may occur about the hip region, for example, in the iliotibial band. It is of the utmost importance that these children have a definitive diagnosis made in order to avoid over-treatment. Although ultrasonographic studies may suggest the existence of mild, subclinical instability in the hips of these children, the clinical importance of this observation has yet to be established.[6]

It is strongly recommended that the term "hip click" as a diagnosis be eliminated from common usage by orthopaedic surgeons and pediatricians alike. As the result of a child's physical examination and imaging studies, there are only four terms that are helpful as diagnoses. If the examination and all studies are within normal limits, the hip is normal. If the infant's hip is reducible by the Ortolani maneuver, the hip is dislocated. In the older infant, if the Ortolani and Barlow tests are negative but there is marked limitation of hip abduction of one or both hips and imaging studies confirm displacement of the femoral head from the acetabulum, the hip is dislocated. If the Barlow test results in displacement of the femoral head out of the acetabulum, the hip is dislocatable. If the Barlow test results in pistoning or gliding of the femoral head within the confines of the acetabulum, the hip is subluxatable.

Radiography and Ultrasonography

The infant with a dislocatable or dislocated hip requires immediate treatment. Imaging studies are not helpful in the very young infant with these findings but are indicated in the young infant with teratologic hip dislocation in order to evaluate the secondary changes about the acetabulum. In the older infant with fixed dislocation of the hip, radiography will document acetabular changes and give a baseline study for future comparison. The infant with a subluxatable hip can be objectively evaluated by real-time, stress ultrasonography of the hips both at the initial evaluation and later, if treatment is required.[5,7]

Treatment

Hip Adduction Contractures

Occasionally, infants with normal imaging studies will be noted to have a mild (5° to 10°) asymmetry of hip abduction. These children, who essentially have normal hips, can be treated with gentle stretching of the adductors of the hip at diaper changes with expected good resolution of the asymmetry.

Subluxatable Hips

The newborn infant with a subluxatable hip may be observed for three weeks without any treatment. In the vast majority of these infants, the hips stabilize spontaneously with no expected sequelae. If the hip remains subluxatable at three weeks of age, treatment is indicated. The simplest and safest method of treatment at this stage is use of the Pavlik harness for up to six weeks. In this condition there is no contraindication to removal of the harness for bathing, but effective use requires continued use of the harness for the remainder of the day. The Pavlik harness treatment must be monitored by a knowledgeable physician, because a high incidence of complications results from faulty application of the harness.[8] Parents need to be instructed in the application, purpose, and pitfalls of use of the Pavlik harness. They should be informed of the fact that the harness can be applied incorrectly and cause damage to the hip joint, the blood supply of the

hip, or the femoral nerve. The parents must be actively involved in the management of this problem and be invited to call you or your office with any concerns. The infant in the harness will require weekly checks for harness fit and for correctness of application. By missing appointments, the parents risk hyperflexion of the hip in the rapidly growing infant, with the potential complications of fixed inferior dislocation of the hip and of femoral neuropathy (Fig. 4). Mothers especially are concerned about the appearance and cleanliness of their babies. With frequent diaper changes and placement of diapers under the harness straps, no skin problems should occur.

When you diagnose a child older than 4 weeks of age with a subluxatable hip, it is important to consider other disorders, such as myopathy or connective tissue disorders, as the cause. These infants can also be treated with a Pavlik harness. While their clinical instability may resolve with only three weeks of treatment, it is important to continue treatment until the residuals of acetabular dysplasia are resolved by imaging studies.

Dislocatable and Dislocated Hips

The infant with a dislocatable or dislocated hip requires immediate treatment. If the Ortolani maneuver results in easy relocation of the dislocated hip, the infant may be treated in a Pavlik harness.[9] Under these circumstances of greater instability, the harness should be considered as a cast substitute and be left in place at all times until your evaluation determines that it is safe to begin weaning from the harness. Children under the age of 6 months can usually be treated by the Pavlik harness. A flexion-abduction anteroposterior radiograph of the hips and pelvis is useful in determining whether the child can be treated by the harness. If this radiograph reveals that the dislocated hip reduces into the acetabulum or that the femoral head and metaphyseal axis are directed toward the triradiate cartilage but are not deeply seated in the acetabulum (the intermediate hip), the Pavlik harness may be used. In the latter case the femoral head will "dock" into the acetabulum by two weeks of harness wear. If the head does not reduce concentrically by that time, the harness treatment should be abandoned and traction initiated in preparation for either a closed or open reduction of the hip joint. Open reduction of the hip joint in the neurologically normal child under the age of 1 year is not frequently required.

If the flexion-abduction radiograph reveals that the femoral head and neck continue to point above the acetabulum (Fig. 5), the Pavlik harness will be of no help and the patient should be initiated into a traction program prior to closed versus open reduction. It is not within the scope of this discussion to determine the appropriateness or efficacy of traction techniques for reduction versus the use of immediate open reduction.[2,5]

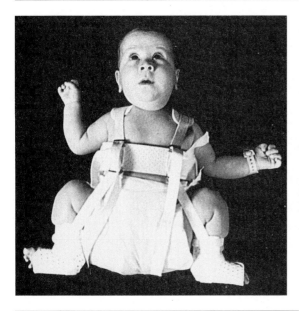

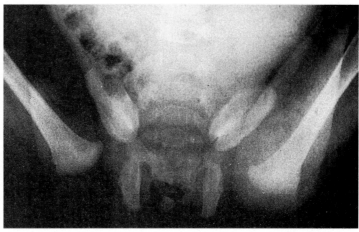

Fig. 4 Hyperflexion of anterior straps of Pavlik harness has resulted in secondary obturator dislocation of left hip.

If traction is elected for your patient, then a home traction program has proved to be economically sound, psychologically appealing to the families, and effective.[10] Inpatient traction can be accomplished but is limited by insurance coverage for nonacute problems and creates psychologic strains for the family and for the treating physician who is daily entreated by the family to hasten treatment. The home traction program can be directed by your office with commercially available Bradford frames, aluminum tubing, water weights, and pulleys that make for a lightweight and portable system for continuous traction through the day.

It should be emphasized that ongoing follow-up of these patients will be required throughout their growth, because recent studies have revealed a failure of normal development of the hip even in those patients previously thought to have concentric reductions of the hip. Quantification of development of the acetabulum by the acetabular index or by a variety of other radiographic or ultrasonographic measurements is part of this long-term evaluation.

Fig. 5 Attempted abduction of hips reveals persistent point of right femoral head and neck above the true acetabulum.

References

1. Bialik V, Fishman J, Katzir J, et al: Clinical assessment of hip instability in the newborn by an orthopedic surgeon and a pediatrician. *J Pediatr Orthop* 1986;6:703-705.
2. Bennett JT, MacEwen GD: Congenital dislocation of the hip: Recent advances and current problems. *Clin Orthop* 1989;247:15-21.
3. Hadlow V: Neonatal screening for congenital dislocation of the hip: A prospective 21-year survey. *J Bone Joint Surg* 1988;70B:740-743.
4. Ilfeld FW, Westin GW, Makin M: Missed or developmental dislocation of the hip. *Clin Orthop* 1986;203:276-281.
5. Coleman SS: *Congenital Dysplasia and Dislocation of the Hip*. St. Louis, MO, CV Mosby, 1978.
6. Clark NM, Clegg J, Al-Chalabi AN: Ultrasound screening of hips at risk for CDH: Failure to reduce the incidence of late cases. *J Bone Joint Surg* 1989;71B:9-12.
7. Graf R: Fundamentals of sonographic diagnosis of infant hip dysplasia. *J Pediatr Orthop* 1984;4:735-740.
8. Mubarak S, Garfin S, Vance R, et al: Pitfalls in the use of the Pavlik harness for treatment of congenital dysplasia, subluxation, and dislocation of the hip. *J Bone Joint Surg* 1981;63A:1239-1248.
9. Ramsey PL, Lasser S, MacEwen GD: Congenital dislocation of the hip: Use of the Pavlik harness in the child during the first six months of life. *J Bone Joint Surg* 1976;58A:1000-1004.
10. Mubarak SJ, Beck LR, Sutherland D: Home traction in the management of congenital dislocation of the hips. *J Pediatr Orthop* 1986;6:721-723.

Idiopathic Scoliosis and Kyphosis

Peter D. Pizzutillo, MD

Introduction

Abnormalities of spinal alignment are among the most common non-traumatic musculoskeletal problems of childhood and adolescence. These problems are typically encountered in the orthopaedist's office. Alterations in alignment in the anteroposterior or frontal plane are termed scoliosis and the majority are idiopathic (of unknown causation) in origin. Round back or kyphotic deformities are second only to idiopathic scoliosis as a cause of spinal deformity. The most common kyphotic disorder is Scheuermann's disease.

Idiopathic Scoliosis

In the past three decades, the level of awareness of the existence and incidence of scoliosis in the general population has been raised in the orthopaedic and pediatric communities as well as in the physical therapy and nursing disciplines. School screening has been primarily responsible for the dissemination of information.[1,2] Instead of being confronted with a young adolescent who has a spinal curvature in excess of 60° at the first medical evaluation, clinicians now are evaluating children and adolescents with spinal curvatures less than 20°. While the vast majority of these children may only require observation, difficulties exist in some communities regarding the availability of medical follow-up and care. With early detection, the patient with scoliosis now has more treatment options, such as bracing. In addition, affected families are alerted to the increased risk of scoliosis in other young family members.

Clinical Evaluation

The evaluation of the new patient with scoliosis should be comprehensive in order to eliminate less common forms of scoliosis and to formulate appropriate treatment programs. A detailed review of birth and developmental history provides information to rule out neurologic and myopathic causes of scoliosis.

History

It is important to know the circumstances that led to the initial clinical examination. Was back deformity detected in the asymptomatic individual during a routine physical examination, school screening, or by a parent? Was pain a factor that led to the evaluation by a physician? If so, what is the nature of the pain? Is it activity related? Does pain occur more frequently at night or does it wake the individual from a sound sleep? Is there a history of recent trauma to the back? Does pain radiate to other parts of the body? Is pain related to menses in the young female? Have there been any episodes of sphincter dysfunction? Is the scoliotic deformity a documented recent development in an individual who has been well cared for by a physician? A detailed history can help to eliminate traumatic, gynecologic, and neoplastic etiologies that require additional evaluation and consultation with nonorthopaedic colleagues.[3]

It is necessary to document the female patient's date of menarche to assist in the determination of skeletal maturity of the spine. The patient's past medical history may reveal information about recent trauma, repeated thoracotomy, congenital heart disease, neurologic conditions, such as hydrocephalus, neoplasms, such as Wilms' tumor, and adjunctive radiation therapy. All of these conditions are associated with considerable risk for the development of variants of scoliosis that differ from idiopathic scoliosis.[3]

While the precise onset of scoliosis is frequently difficult to determine, the existence of school screening and the annual screening of children by a pediatrician or family practitioner have established that a small group of children appear to have had an acute onset of rapidly progressive scoliosis. This scenario strongly suggests a neurologic cause for the developing scoliosis. Magnetic resonance imaging (MRI) is effective in evaluating the neuraxis and may reveal syringomyelia or intraspinal neoplasm, such as astrocytoma of the cord, in this group of patients. A rare problem that is being recognized more readily today is scoliosis secondary to axial dystonia. Early recognition of scoliosis due to dystonia is important, because the spinal deformity, which is refractory to brace treatment, may be treated successfully with pharmacologic agents before secondary structural changes develop in the spine.

A review of the family history is helpful. It is important to ask parents specific questions about any family history of myopathy or of neurologic disorders such as neurofibromatosis. In the past, family members of affected children with idiopathic scoliosis were not aware of the existence of scoliosis in the family. Public education has begun to reverse this problem and more families today have learned about scoliosis. With a posi-

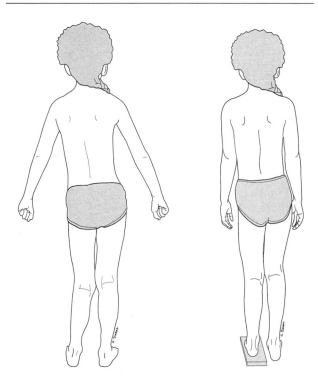

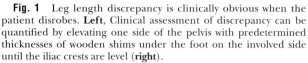

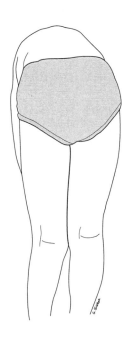

Fig. 1 Leg length discrepancy is clinically obvious when the patient disrobes. **Left,** Clinical assessment of discrepancy can be quantified by elevating one side of the pelvis with predetermined thicknesses of wooden shims under the foot on the involved side until the iliac crests are level (**right**).

Fig. 2 When the back is examined in forward flexion in the presence of uncorrected leg length discrepancy, the trunk on the side of the longer leg is higher at all vertebral levels than the trunk on the short limb side.

tive family history of idiopathic scoliosis, the diagnosis of idiopathic scoliosis in a new patient can be made with a greater degree of confidence.

Physical Examination

Physical examination is accomplished after the patient disrobes. Shorts are appropriate for boys, and a two-piece bathing suit or a back-opening gown is used for girls. A detailed evaluation of the skin is done to determine the existence of café au lait spots or midline defects of the spine, such as a hairy patch, hemangioma, or sinus. An appreciation of leg length discrepancy, hemihypertrophy, or hemiatrophy can only be reliably obtained with the patient disrobed. The presence of a member of your office staff as well as the patient's parent during the entire examination is prudent.

In addition to the orthopaedic examination, a neurologic assessment of motor and sensory function as well as cerebellar function should be accomplished. The orthopaedic assessment should be comprehensive and include the neck and both upper and lower extremities with the back examination performed last.

The examination of the back includes assessment of rib cage deformity and thus requires that the child be viewed from both sides and from the back. The presence of pectus carinatum or of pectus excavatum may be incidental but may also be a clue to the existence of Marfan's syndrome. When the patient is examined in the erect position in bare feet, the symmetry of the shoulders and of the scapulae, the truncopelvic alignment, the height of the iliac crests for determination of leg length discrepancy, and foot morphology can be determined. If leg length discrepancy is detected, wooden shims of various thicknesses can be placed under the foot of the short leg to clinically quantify the leg length difference and to level the pelvis for a more critical evaluation of the spine (Fig. 1). When leg length discrepancy results in apparent scoliosis (Fig. 2), the curvature can be fully corrected by leveling the pelvis. Scoliosis and leg length discrepancy may coexist as independent entities. Under this circumstance, it is necessary to level the pelvis at each examination to isolate the spine for scoliosis evaluation and to eliminate the effects of leg length discrepancy that may either mollify or accentuate the clinical appearance of the scoliosis.

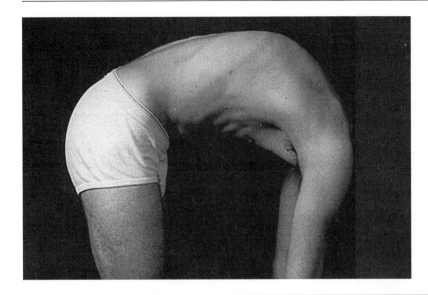

Fig. 3 The back is viewed from the side to assess the presence of kyphosis.

The patient is asked to stand erect with feet together and with knees in extension, and then is instructed to bend forward with both hands and arms hanging freely in a relaxed position. Frequently young patients will grasp one leg or the other or bend one knee during the examination. This invariably creates the spurious impression of scoliosis and can be avoided by having the office staff person who is present alert you if the patient does this. The back should first be viewed from the side to determine the existence of significant kyphosis (Fig. 3). The patient should be observed carefully during forward flexion to document fluidity of

motion and reversal of curve patterns. Back pain will prohibit a precise examination of the spine for determination of true scoliosis because secondary guarding or list may suggest scoliosis that will resolve as the pain subsides. If the trunk deviates to one side during repeated attempts at forward flexion and the patient is not able to forward flex in the midline, intraspinal lesion versus axial dystonia must be considered.

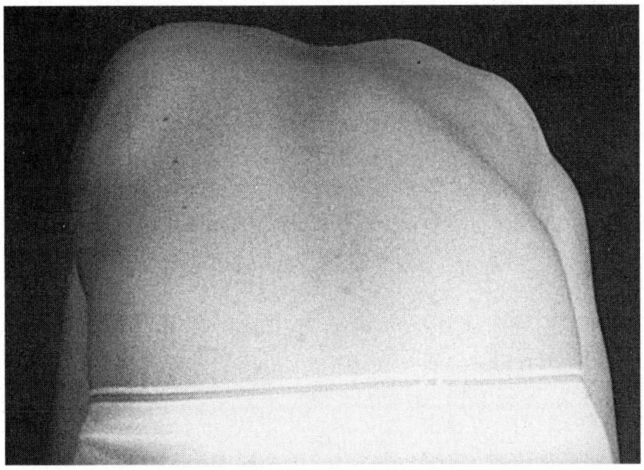

If the patient is able to forward flex in the midline, each region of the spine can be viewed with that segment parallel to the floor. The high thoracic, middle thoracic, thoracolumbar, and lumbar segments are viewed separately when parallel to the floor. Asymmetry at each region (Fig. 4) can be quantified using the scoliometer to determine the angle of trunk rotation. This instrument is a reliable guide and an objective means of documenting clinical observations. It has significantly reduced radiographic exposure in the follow-up of young patients with scoliosis.

Radiographic Assessment

The clinical examination of the child or adolescent with scoliosis will require radiographic analysis of the spine to document the curve pattern and magnitude, to determine skeletal maturity of the spine, and to rule out congenital anomalies or other lesions of the spine (Fig. 5). If congenital anomalies are discovered, the patient will require radiographs of the cervical spine to rule out concomitant congenital anomalies and renal ultrasonography to establish the anatomy and function of the kidneys. The initial radiographic studies include standing lateral and posteroanterior (PA) views of the thoracic and lumbar spine, including the top of the

Fig. 4 In forward flexion, asymmetry can be determined for each spinal segment.

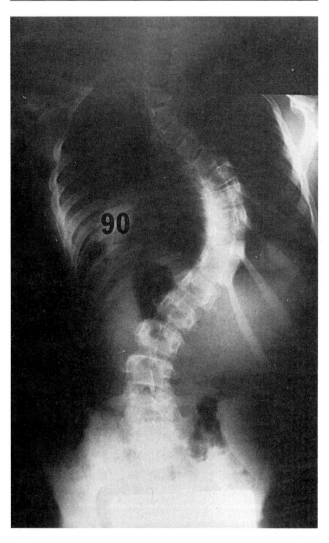

Fig. 5 Standing PA radiograph reveals a 90° right thoracic curve.

with a progressive spinal curve greater than 50° or with a cosmetically unacceptable curvature less than 50° should be evaluated for surgical correction and stabilization.[4,5]

The skeletally immature child or adolescent with a curve less than 30° and with good cosmesis can be observed at frequent intervals by physical examination and by serial radiographs until maturity and spine stability have been achieved.[6] When the patient exhibits acceptable cosmesis but has curve magnitude between 30° and 45°, bracing has been effective in improving the natural history of the untreated scoliotic spine.[7] The braced patient is followed every four months with physical examination and with radiographic evaluation on a less frequent schedule.

Follow-up radiographs should be done in the erect position after removal of the brace. If the scoliotic curve is maintained, the patient is allowed to complete the bracing program. If the patient displays progressive worsening of the scoliotic curve despite proper brace treatment, surgical correction and stabilization are indicated. The immature adolescent with a spinal curvature greater than 45° does not have a good likelihood of success by brace treatment and thus surgical correction and stabilization are indicated.[6,7]

Kyphosis

The examination of the young back may yield important information when viewed in the forward flexed position from behind or from the head of the patient but is not complete until it is also viewed from the side. Severe limitations of motion of the spine in flexion and extension suggest spinal pathology, such as symptomatic spondylolisthesis, intraspinal lesions (such as a large extruded fragment of disk material), congenital anomalies, and kyphosis. Rare clinical findings, such as full extension of the spine with no forward flexion, may be indicative of more generalized pathology, such as the rigid spine syndrome or myopathy.

Clinical Evaluation

Increased dorsal kyphosis is associated with increased lumbar lordosis. In the first decade of life, these clinical findings are usually asymptomatic and come to the clinician's attention because of parental concern with the child's posture. Radiographic evaluation includes erect PA and lateral views of the entire thoracic and lumbar spine. In those children with postural kyphosis, radiographic examination may reveal increased dorsal kyphosis and lumbar lordosis but no intrinsic bony pathology is noted in the vertebral body, the vertebral end-plates, or in the intervertebral disk. By voluntarily bringing the spine to a more erect position, these children are readily able to assume normal posture. When the child wishes to maintain a more

pelvis to determine Risser level. There is no indication for routine supine radiographs, and the use of bending radiographs is limited to preoperative evaluation. If the lateral view of the spine is normal, then a PA view of the spine is usually the only view required during follow-up evaluations. The PA view requires 25% of the radiation used to obtain a lateral view. If the lateral view reveals hypokyphosis of the thoracic spine, spondylolysis, or spondylolisthesis, then repeat lateral views of the spine will be needed in follow-up evaluations, but with less frequency than the PA view.

Treatment

The treatment of the skeletally mature adolescent with a curve of less than 50° and cosmetic acceptability involves repeated clinical and radiographic examinations two years later. The skeletally mature adolescent

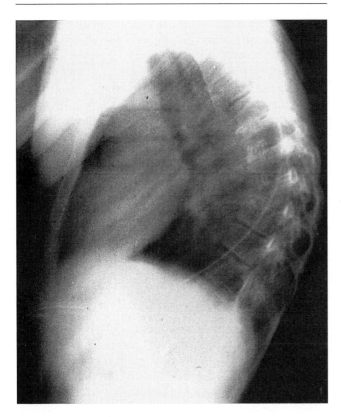

Fig. 6 Lateral radiograph of thoracic spine reveals increased dorsal kyphosis with wedging of vertebral bodies and end-plate irregularities.

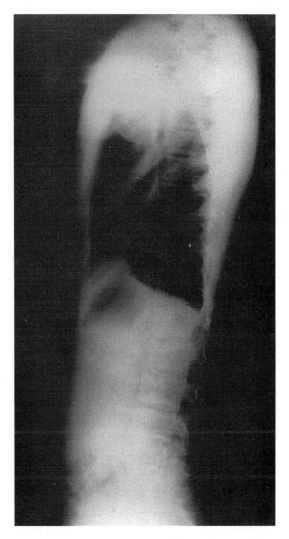

Fig. 7 Lateral radiographs of the spine reveal marked flattening of the lumbar spine.

normal posture, a physical therapy program involving strengthening the abdominal and paraspinal musculature with continued attention to the practice of good posture is successful. As these children enter the second decade of life, they tend to develop contracture of the pectoralis muscles as well as of the hamstrings. Stretching of these muscle-tendon groups becomes an integral component of the therapy program.

Early in the second decade of life, interscapular pain or increased spinal deformity may develop. Clinical examination of these individuals will frequently reveal weakness of the extensor muscles of the spine and of the abdomen. Hamstring and pectoral muscle tightness are more frequent than in younger populations. The neurologic examination is normal.

Radiographic Assessment

Erect PA views of the spine will reveal a mild thoracic scoliosis (usually less than 20°) and lateral views will reveal increased magnitude of dorsal kyphosis as well as relatively increased lumbar lordosis.[8] Close inspection of the lateral radiograph will reveal anterior wedging of vertebral bodies, disk space narrowing, end-plate irregularities, and Schmorl's nodes consistent with a diagno-

sis of Scheuermann's disease (Fig. 6). Although the natural history of this problem is generally benign, a small percentage of patients do suffer from increasing kyphotic deformity, and an even smaller percentage of patients have intractable pain. While the incidence of spondylolysis and spondylolisthesis is higher in this population, it is not common for the latter conditions to be significant contributing factors in pain production. The etiology of Scheuermann's disease remains elusive.

Treatment

In the skeletally immature individual, radiographic changes noted in the vertebral bodies, and the increased kyphosis and lordosis, have been treated successfully by a combined program using orthotics and exercise. As opposed to the orthotic treatment of scoliosis, the expected outcome of orthotic treatment of Scheuermann's disease is one of relief of pain and structural improvement in the alignment and development of the spine. The use of orthotics in this condition does not need to be as lengthy as that required for scoliosis. The beneficial effects of bracing are noted after 12 to 18 months of use, following which the brace can be safely weaned over a short period of time.[9]

The orthotic requirements demand the ability to flatten the lumbar lordosis. This is needed for reversal of the increased thoracic kyphosis. While this objective may be satisfactorily achieved by use of an underarm TLSO in the slim to average sized patient, heavier patients will require use of a modified Milwaukee brace with an anterior pusher pad. Concomitant exercises out of the brace are an integral part of the pro-

gram. The goals of the exercise program are the relief of hamstring contracture, stretching of the spine in extension, and strengthening of the paraspinal and abdominal musculature.

Follow-up evaluation involves checking the brace for good fit and examination of the patient without the brace. Hamstring tightness and abdominal strength are easily checked in the office. Erect lateral radiographs of the spine out of brace are repeated every six months to document curve magnitude and reversal of wedging. Radiographs should be obtained without the brace for a realistic evaluation of curve management. Surgical treatment of Scheuermann's kyphosis is infrequent and is indicated for the rarely occurring progressive kyphosis and for intractable back pain. Repeated PA radiographs of the spine are not indicated unless clinical examination indicates significant changes of the spine in the coronal plane.

Lumbar Scheuermann's Disease

Lumbar Scheuermann's disease differs significantly from Scheuermann's kyphosis. Adolescent patients will present more frequently with low-grade levels of low back pain with marked flattening of the lumbar lordosis (Fig. 7). Clinical examination usually will not reveal muscle spasm or localized tenderness; however, the flattening of the lumbar lordosis is quite rigid and is not clinically reversible by hyperextension maneuvers. Hamstring tightness is a frequent finding with a normal neurologic evaluation.

Lateral radiography of the lumbar spine reveals large defects of the lower thoracic and lumbar vertebral bodies at their anterosuperior borders. Focal enlargement of vertebral bodies also is noted occasionally (Fig. 8).

Back pain is quickly relieved by application of a TLSO with molded lumbar lordosis. Radiographic defects of the vertebral bodies resolve, but complete restitution of normal lumbar lordosis is rarely achieved. Brace use averages 12 to 18 months and should be complemented with hamstring stretching exercises.[10]

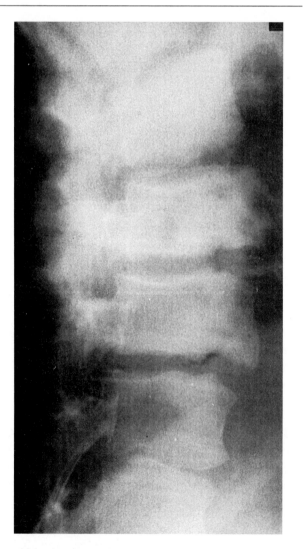

Fig. 8   Lateral radiograph of the lumbar spine reveals focal enlargement of vertebral bodies with anterior defects at the corners of the vertebral bodies.

References

1. Ashworth MA (ed): Symposium on school screening for scoliosis: Scoliosis Research Society and British Scoliosis Society. *Spine* 1988;13:1177-1200.
2. Lonstein JE, Bjorklund S, Wanninger MH, et al: Voluntary school screening for scoliosis in Minnesota. *J Bone Joint Surg* 1982;64A:481-488.
3. Bradford DS, Lonstein JE, Moe JH, et al (eds): *Moe's Textbook of Scoliosis and Other Spinal Deformities*, ed 2. Philadelphia, PA, WB Saunders, 1987.
4. Lonstein JE, Carlson JM: The prediction of curve progression in untreated idiopathic scoliosis during growth. *J Bone Joint Surg* 1984;66A:1061-1071.
5. Weinstein SL: Idiopathic scoliosis: Natural history. *Spine* 1986;11:780-783.

6. Bunnell WP: The natural history of idiopathic scoliosis before skeletal maturity. *Spine* 1986;11:773-776.

7. Winter RB, Lonstein JE, Drogt J, et al: The effectiveness of bracing in the nonoperative treatment of idiopathic scoliosis. *Spine* 1986;11:790-791.

8. Blumenthal SL, Roach J, Herring JA: Lumbar Scheuermann's: A clinical series and classification. *Spine* 1987;12:929-932.

9. Sachs B, Bradford D, Winter R, et al: Scheuermann's kyphosis: Follow-up of Milwaukee-brace treatment. *J Bone Joint Surg* 1987;69A:50-57.

10. Stagnara P, De Mauroy JC, Dran G, et al: Reciprocal angulation of vertebral bodies in a sagittal plane: Approach to references for the evaluation of kyphosis and lordosis. *Spine* 1982;7:335-342.

Footwear for Children

Lynn T. Staheli, MD

Introduction

The traditional approach to shoewear for children is being reevaluated.[1-5] Historically, supportive shoes were considered necessary for normal foot development.[6,7] Shoe modifications, or corrective shoes, were thought to correct flatfoot, and rotational and angulatory problems in infants and children.[8-10] Millions of children wore modified shoes that were functionally limiting, uncomfortable, and potentially embarrassing to the child.

With time, data have been compiled that challenge these traditional views. Studies have provided normative data, addressing the effects of shoewear and the effectiveness of shoe modifications and inserts. This accumulated information is now sufficient to allow an appraisal of footwear for children and judge the efficacy of shoe modifications.

The Bare Foot

The natural unshod state of the foot, studied by investigators[11-13] in Africa and the Solomon Islands, is characterized by (1) excellent mobility, especially of the forefoot; (2) thickening of the plantar skin by as much as 1 cm; (3) creases on the plantar and dorsal aspects of the foot, allowing considerable mobility of the forefoot; (4) alignment of the phalanges with the metatarsals, spreading the toes; and (5) no static foot deformities. Most foot problems were secondary to injury or infection. The unshod foot appears to function well with few deformities.

Normal Longitudinal Arch Development

Development of the longitudinal arch of the normal foot in children has been the subject of several studies.[8,14-17] Each study has shown that the longitudinal arch develops spontaneously with growth, and that the range of normal arches is very broad (Fig. 1). The development of the longitudinal arch is thought to be due to a reduction of subcutaneous fat and of ligamentous laxity with advancing age. The reduced incidence of flatfoot in barefoot populations[17] would suggest that muscle strength and mobility may be additional factors in arch development.

Radiographs of normal feet in children show that talar inclination as measured by the talar metatarsal angles decreases with increasing age and that the range of normal angles is very broad (Fig. 2).[18] The normal range includes values previously considered diagnostic of pes planus.

Both clinical and radiographic findings suggest that the longitudinal arch develops spontaneously during childhood. Just as in other human characteristics, the range of normal is very broad. In previous studies, feet that fell within the normal range by these newly elucidated definitions of normal often were treated.[19-21]

The Effect of Children's Shoewear on Normal Feet

The effects of shoewear have been described by many authors.[22-29] The harmful effects of shoewear have included deformity of the lesser toes[30] and hallux valgus.[31,32] Sim-Fook and Hodgson[32] compared 118 Chinese who wore shoes and 107 who did not. The feet of the unshod group showed greater mobility and fewer deformities than did those of the shoe wearers.

More recently, Rao and Joseph[17] studied the effects of wearing shoes on longitudinal arch development in 2,300 Indian children, of whom 1,555 wore shoes and 745 had never worn shoes. The authors found that the

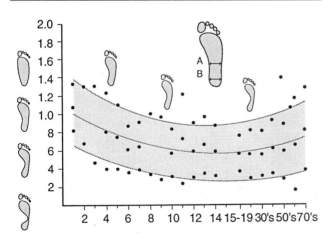

Fig. 1 Development of the longitudinal arch. Based on a study of 882 normal feet of children, the shaded area represents the + or -2 SD above and below the mean for arch development. Arch development is defined as a ratio of A/B. (Reproduced with permission from Staheli LT, Chew DE, Corbett M: The longitudinal arch: A survey of eight hundred and eighty-two feet in normal children and adults. *J Bone Joint Surg* 1987;69A:426-428.)

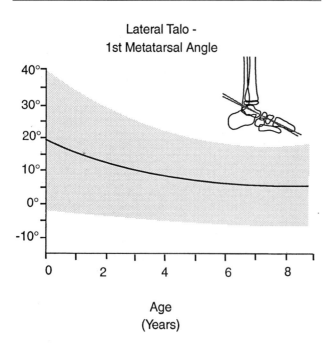

Fig. 2 Normal talo-1st metatarsal angles. These values are based on measurements from standing radiographs in normal feet in children. Note the wide range of normal as shown in the shaded areas. (Reproduced with permission from Vanderwilde R, Staheli LT, Chew DE, et al: Measurements on radiographs of the foot in normal infants and children. *J Bone Joint Surg* 1988;70A:407-415.)

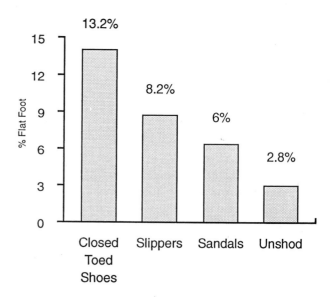

Fig. 3 Percentage of children with flatfeet related to shoeing practices, based on a study of 2,300 children from India. (Reproduced with permission from Rao UB, Joseph B: The influence of footwear on the prevalence of flat foot: A survey of 2,300 children. *J Bone Joint Surg* 1992;74B:525-527.)

Outline 1
Features of a good shoe for children

Flexible, to allow free mobility
Quadrangular, to conform to the normal shape of the foot
Flat, to avoid forcing the toes into the end of the shoe
Porous, to allow evaporation of moisture
Moderate sole friction, to avoid slippery or adhesive sole materials
Lightweight, to reduce energy expenditure
Acceptable appearance for the child
Reasonable price for the parents

---

prevalence of flatfoot declined with age, was increased in children who exhibited increased joint laxity, and was significantly greater in children who wore shoes (Fig. 3).

These studies suggest that the traditional view that the foot needs support is unfounded. The child's foot appears to fare best in an unrestricted environment with free mobility and with the toes uncompressed. The findings suggest that shoe construction should be based on the barefoot model, emphasizing flexibility and allowing normal positioning of the toes while protecting the foot.[5]

Shoes for Infants and Children With Normal Feet

The major purpose of the shoe is to protect the foot from injury or cold, while still allowing the foot the freedom and mobility provided in the barefoot state. Shoe design can be based on the barefoot model,[5] and healthy shoes are currently available. Parents often request guidelines in making the selection (Outline 1). Some shoes meet the criteria for healthy shoes better than others.[1,33-35]

The major problem parents face is selecting good shoes for girls. The conflict between fashion and function remains. Shoe designers often promote shoes for girls that repeat the problems in shoes for women. Poor design includes elevated heels, pointed toes, and small size. Such shoewear renders the foot mechanically unstable; compresses the toes, increasing the incidence of bunions[31,32]; and is often uncomfortable.

Shoewear and the Flexible Flatfoot

Modified shoes have been most commonly used to treat the flexible flatfoot.[36-40] For such treatment to be appropriate, two basic assumptions must be met. First, treatment should be necessary; that is, the flexible flatfoot causes disability. Second, treatment should be effective in developing an arch.[41]

The necessity of treating the flexible flatfoot can be traced to an era in which all flatfeet were lumped together. Flatfeet were simply considered abnormal and were thought to cause disability. The importance of separating the pathologic and physiologic forms was addressed in the classic foot study by the Canadian Army during World War II.[42] This study was undertaken to determine the appropriateness of disqualifying men from military service based on flatfeet. Harris and Beath[42] found that the flexible flatfoot was not a source of disability, in contrast with flatfeet associated with a heel cord contracture or tarsal coalitions. More recently, a foot study by the Israeli Army[43] showed that the low arch provided a protective effect in preventing stress injuries. The simple flexible flatfoot appears to be a variation of normal and not a source of any demonstrated disability. The data suggest that treatment of the flexible flatfoot is unnecessary.

The effectiveness of shoes for correcting the flexible flatfoot has an interesting history. In 1933, Mattison[44] estimated that 100 different arch supports and 50 "doctor's" shoes were being marketed. Unaware that the longitudinal arch develops spontaneously in the child, and noting that the arch appeared in the child after a shoe modification or insert such as the Thomas heel, Whitman plate, Helfet heelcup, University of Califor-nia Biomechanics Laboratory (UCBL) inserts, or various sole wedges, was prescribed, physicians concluded that the shoe modification was responsible for the change. These shoe modifications became known as corrective shoes. Despite some occasional objections,[45-47] the use of modified shoes became a major part of orthopaedic management of developmental variations in infants and children.

A number of studies have addressed the effectiveness of shoe modifications in correcting the flexible flatfoot. The immediate effect of shoe modifications on pes planus was studied by Penneau and associates,[48] who found no significant difference between radiographs taken with children standing in shoes or standing barefoot. In contrast, Bordelon[20] showed a reduction in the talometatarsal angle in children wearing custom-molded inserts.

Several longitudinal studies of children wearing a variety of shoe modifications have been reported. Mereday and associates[49] applied the UCBL inserts in ten children with flexible flatfoot over a period of two years. All showed an improvement in gait, comfort, and arch configuration that was maintained throughout a six-month follow-up period. Bleck and Berzins[19] also treated 71 children for pes planus with UCBL inserts or Helfet heelcups for more than a year and found that 79% showed clinical and radiographic improvement. Bordelon[20] reported a follow-up of six of 50 children treated for pes planus with inserts. In these six patients, he reported improvement in the talometatarsal angles following the use of customized orthotic inserts. The correction had been maintained in five of the six children seen at follow-up.

These three studies were performed without controls and with radiographic measures that often fell within the range of normal. The normal range of the tarsal metatarsal angle is very wide and changes with age, as shown by Vanderwilde and associates[18] (Fig. 2). Bordelon[20] had considered some values falling within this range to be abnormal. Furthermore, the wide range of normal makes the 3° of improvement cited as a threshold of significance[19] questionable.

In 1989, two prospective controlled studies evaluated the effectiveness of shoe modifications in correcting the flexible flatfoot. In a three-year prospective controlled study of 129 children, Wenger and associates[21] found that arch development was not altered by corrective shoes or inserts when compared with normal shoewear (Fig. 4). This finding was confirmed by Gould and associates.[8] These prospective studies showed no significant difference between modified and regular shoes in arch development. These findings suggest that shoe modifications make little or no change in the flexible flatfoot and that such treatment should be considered to be ineffective. These studies are consistent with the conclusion that treatment of the flexible flatfoot in the infant or child is both unnecessary and ineffective.

Corrective Shoes and Inserts on Lower Limb on Intoeing

Shoe modifications have also been prescribed for correcting rotational and angulatory problems in the infant and child. Various shoe wedges have been

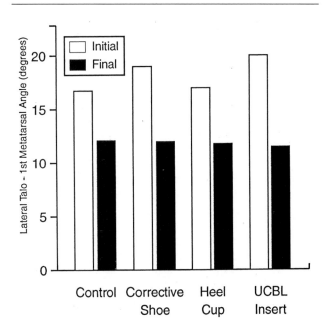

Fig. 4 Longitudinal arch development related to shoe corrections, based on controlled, prospective study. (Reproduced with permission from Wenger DR, Mauldin D, Speck G, et al: Corrective shoes as treatment for flexible flatfoot in infants and children. *J Bone Joint Surg* 1989;71A:800-810.)

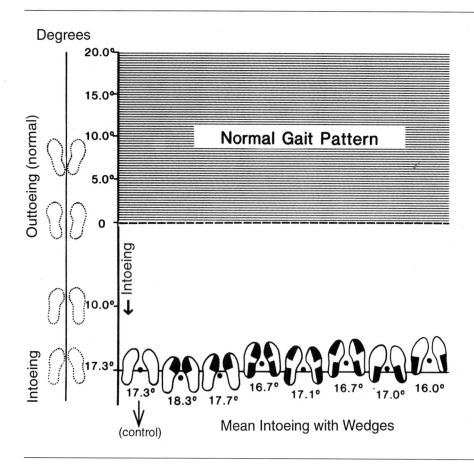

Fig. 5 Effects of shoe wedges. This study demonstrates the ineffectiveness of shoe wedges in changing the foot progression angle. Various wedges were placed (shown in black). Mean values for each wedge are shown compared with the unwedged controls. (Reproduced with permission from Knittel G, Staheli LT: The effectiveness of shoe modifications for intoeing. *Orthop Clin North Am* 1976;7:1019-1025.)

shown to have no effect on the foot progression angle of the child with intoeing (Fig. 5).[50]

Noncontroversial Shoe Modification for Current Use

Some shoe modifications may be of value. These modifications are not corrective but simply provide an immediate mechanical effect, which may be beneficial. Cushioned footwear may help reduce the incidence of overuse syndrome in the older child or adolescent. Shoe inserts, which redistribute loading on the sole of the foot, are useful in managing rigid foot deformities. Shoe lifts may improve gait in children with moderate or severe limb length discrepancies.

Conclusions

Shoewear for children should be considered as clothing, protecting the foot from exposure and injury. The supportive shoe is unnecessary and may be harmful to the growing foot. Shoe modification or inserts are not corrective; the term "corrective shoe" is a misnomer. Shoe design should be based on the barefoot model and should promote normal development of the foot by allowing freedom of movement and adequate space for normal toe position. Unfortunately,

the design of girls' shoes is often based on fashion at the expense of the health of the foot.

References

1. Bleck EE: The shoeing of children: Sham or science? *Dev Med Child Neurol* 1971;13:188-195.
2. Staheli LT, Griffin L: Corrective shoes for children: A survey of current practice. *Pediatrics* 1980;65:13-17.
3. Staheli LT: Corrective shoes for children. *J Cont Educ Pediatr* 1978;20:22-25.
4. Staheli LT: Lower positional deformity in infants and children: A review. *J Pediatr Orthop* 1990;10:559-563.
5. Staheli LT: Shoes for children: A review. *Pediatrics* 1991;88:371-375.
6. Andry N: *Orthopaedia: Or the Art of Correcting and Preventing Deformities in Children*. London, England, A Millar, 1961. Translated from the French.
7. Griffith JPC: *The Diseases of Infants and Children*. Philadelphia, PA, WB Saunders, 1919, pp 423-424.
8. Gould N, Moreland M, Alvarez, R, et al: Development of the child's arch. *Foot Ankle* 1989;9:241-245.
9. Polokoff MM: An approach to children's foot orthopedics. *J Am Podiatr Assoc* 1976;66:419-422.
10. Tax HR: Enough is enough: Tax answers Staheli. *J Curr Podiatr Med* 1987;36:6-12.
11. Engle ET, Morton DJ: Notes on foot disorders among natives of the Belgian Congo. *J Bone Joint Surg* 1931;13:311-318.
12. Hoffman P: Conclusions drawn from a comparative study of

the feet of barefooted and shoe-wearing peoples. *Am J Orthop Surg* 1905;3:105-136.

13. James CS: Footprints and feet of natives of the Solomon Islands. *Lancet* 1939;2:1390-1393.

14. Morley AJM: Knock-knee in children. *Br Med J* 1957;2:976-979.

15. Engel GM, Staheli LT: The natural history of torsion and other factors influencing gait in childhood: A study of the angle of gait, tibial torsion knee angle, hip rotation, and development of the arch in normal children. *Clin Orthop* 1974;99:12-17.

16. Staheli LT, Chew DE, Corbett M: The longitudinal arch: A survey of eight hundred and eighty-two feet in normal children and adults. *J Bone Joint Surg* 1987;69A:426-428.

17. Rao UB, Joseph B: The influence of footwear on the prevalence of flat foot: A survey of 2,300 children. *J Bone Joint Surg* 1992;74B:525-527.

18. Vanderwilde R, Staheli LT, Chew DE, et al: Measurements on radiographs of the foot in normal infants and children. *J Bone Joint Surg* 1988;70A:407-415.

19. Bleck EE, Berzins UJ: Conservative management of pes valgus with plantar flexed talus, flexible. *Clin Orthop* 1977;122:85-94.

20. Bordelon RL: Hypermobile flatfoot in children: Comprehension, evaluation, and treatment. *Clin Orthop* 1983;181:7-14.

21. Wenger DR, Mauldin D, Speck G, et al: Corrective shoes and inserts as treatment for flexible flatfoot in infants and children. *J Bone Joint Surg* 1989;71A:800-810.

22. Adams TD: Proper shoeing of the child. *JAMA* 1929;92:1753-1755.

23. Brooke COSB: *Foot Health Med Officer* 1948;80:146-147.

24. Camper P: The classic: Dissertation on the best form of shoe. *Clin Orthop* 1975;110:2-5.

25. Crandon LRG: Flexible balancing shoes. *Boston Med Surg J* 1906;155:505-507.

26. Didia BC, Omu ET, Obuoforibo AA: The use of footprint contact index II for classification of flat feet in a Nigerian population. *Foot Ankle* 1987;7:285-289.

27. McKee JJ: Baby needs new shoes! *Hygeia* 1942;20:142-143.

28. Souttier R: Shoes and feet. *Boston Med Surg J* 1906;154:40-42.

29. Wilkins EH: Feet: With particular reference to school children. *Med Officer* 1941;66:5-30.

30. Emslie M: Prevention of foot deformities in children. *Lancet* 1939;2:1260-1263.

31. Shine IB: Incidence of hallux valgus in a partially shoe-wearing community. *Br Med J* 1965;5451:1648-1650.

32. Sim-Fook L, Hodgson AR: A comparison of foot forms among the non-shoe and shoe-wearing Chinese population. *J Bone Joint Surg* 1958;40A:1058-1062.

33. Barnett CH: Footwear for healthy and disordered feet. *Physiotherapy* 1967;53:137-140.

34. Coughlin MF: Fitting children's shoes: What to tell the parents. *J Musculoskeletal Med* 1985;2:39-46.

35. Gould N: Shoes versus sneakers in toddler ambulation. *Foot Ankle* 1985;6:105-107.

36. Cote HP: Shoes for cure of flat foot. *Med World* 1908;26:207-209.

37. Helfet AJ: New way of treating flat feet in children. *Lancet* 1956;1:262-264.

38. Roehm HR: Weak, pronated and flat feet in childhood. *Arch Pediatr* 1933;50:380-394.

39. Whitman R: Importance of positive support in the curative treatment of weak feet and a comparison of the means employed to ensure it. *Am J Orthop Surg* 1913;11:215-230.

40. Wickstrom J, Williams RA: Shoe corrections and orthopaedic foot supports. *Clin Orthop* 1970;70:30-42.

41. Staheli LT: Philosophy of care. *Pediatr Clin North Am* 1986;33:1269-1275.

42. Harris RI, Beath T: Army foot survey: An investigation of foot ailments in Canadian soldiers. Ottawa, Canada: Ottawa National Research Council of Canada, 1947.

43. Giladi M, Milgrom C, Stein M, et al: The low arch: A protective factor in stress fractures: A prospective study of 295 military recruits. *Orthop Rev* 1985;14:709-712.

44. Mattison ND: What are "arch support" shoes anyway? *Am Med* 1933;39:582-585.

45. Dyment PG, Bogan PM: Pediatricians attitudes concerning infants' shoes. *Pediatrics* 1972;50:655-657.

46. Sofield HA: Care of the feet of normal children. *Illinois Med J* 1941;79:253-256.

47. Stewart SF: Footgear: Its history, uses, and abuses. *Clin Orthop* 1972;88:119-130.

48. Penneau K, Lutter LD, Winter RD: Pes planus: Radiographic changes with foot orthoses and shoes. *Foot Ankle* 1982;2:299-303.

49. Mereday C, Dolan CM, Lusskin R: Evaluation of the University of California Biomechanics Laboratory shoe insert in "flexible" pes planus. *Clin Orthop* 1972;82:45-58.

50. Knittel G, Staheli LT: The effectiveness of shoe modifications for intoeing. *Orthop Clin North Am* 1976;7:1019-1025.

Rotational Problems in Children

Lynn T. Staheli, MD

Rotational problems of the lower extremity affect a vast number of infants and children. Like flexible flat feet, bowed legs, and genu valgum, rotational problems fall into the category of physiological or postural problems that occur in normal infants and children.[1] Some deformities, such as metatarsus adductus, are secondary to intrauterine position. Most problems, such as medial tibial torsion, represent a variability during a stage of normal development, whereas problems such as medial femoral torsion are often inherited. Rarely, these problems persist into adolescence and, if they are severe, they can result in disability.

Rotational problems of the lower extremity in infants and children often concern parents enough to prompt them to seek a consultation with an orthopaedic surgeon. Optimum management is based on an understanding of the cause and natural history of the condition and of the effectiveness of various treatment options. Management ranges from simple observation to shoe modifications, bracing, physical therapy, and operative treatment. In this chapter, I will make suggestions concerning management on the basis of objective data rather than on the basis of tradition or speculation.

The normal range of rotation of the foot, leg, and hip was defined to include measurements that fall within two standard deviations of the mean. Rotation within the normal range is described as version; that outside the range of normal is described as torsion. For example, children normally have femoral anteversion. Those with hip rotation values that are outside the normal range are said to have medial or lateral femoral torsion.

Natural History

The lower limb bud develops during the fourth week in utero, with the great toe growing in a preaxial position. During the seventh week of gestation, the entire lower limb rotates medially, bringing the great toe to the midline. During the remainder of intrauterine life, the lower limb rotates laterally. In the newborn infant, the hips are flexed and the lower limbs are positioned in lateral rotation, since medial hip rotation is limited. The fact that the hips are in the most laterally rotated position at the same time as there is femoral anteversion creates a paradox. This is most likely explained by the presence of a lateral rota-

tion contracture of the hip, secondary to intrauterine position, that masks the effect of the anteversion.[2] With time, the contracture resolves, and the underlying anteversion becomes the major determinant of hip rotation (Fig. 1).

During infancy and childhood, the lower extremities continue to rotate laterally. The lateral rotation is due to a decrease of about 25° in femoral anteversion and about 15° of lateral rotation of the tibia. This range of normal is broad and includes both mild in-toeing and severe out-toeing during infancy and early childhood. Lateral rotation of the lower limb normally occurs during growth, and this explains why the in-toeing that is so common in toddlers is rarely seen in adults.[3]

Evaluation

The first step in the evaluation of a rotational problem is to understand the reason for the consultation. After this, the physician must make an accurate diagnosis, assess the severity of the rotational problem, and provide appropriate management.

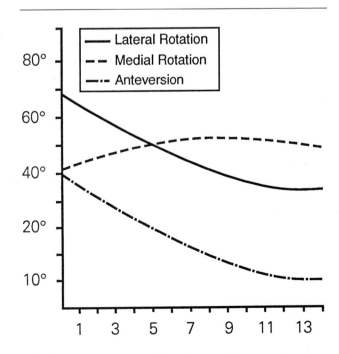

Fig. 1 Values for hip rotation and anteversion, according to age (horizontal axis).

Family Concerns

Identify the reason for the consultation. Who is most concerned? Is it the parents, the grandparents, or the referring physician? What is the primary cause of concern? Is it the child's present problem or the fear that the current problem will persist and cause some long-term disability, such as arthritis? Some families have been told that the rotational problem will cause secondary problems with regard to the feet, hip, or spine. Others imagine that the in-toeing will make it difficult for the child to participate in sports during adolescence or to function normally as an adult. Determine whether the family is concerned about the way that the child sits, stands, walks, or runs. Take their concerns seriously. Families are often deeply worried about their child and, by the time that they are seen in consultation, their fears for the child's future may be considerable. Finally, make certain that you understand what the parents mean when they describe a foot that is turned in or out. They may be describing a varus or valgus foot deformity rather than a rotational problem.

Family History

Inquire about any family history of rotational problems. Sometimes rotational problems, such as femoral torsion, are inherited. The mother of a girl with medial femoral torsion may recall that, as a child, she sat in the same manner as her daughter, with the lower limbs in the W position. Document the mother's rotational profile. The mother, who often has a similar but less pronounced pattern than that seen in the child, may not even notice that she has the same problem. Likewise, although the father of a boy with medial tibial torsion may have some reduction of the thigh-foot angle on the same side as his son has the rotational deformity, the father is seldom aware of any problem. Measurement of the parents' rotational profiles can aid in the assessment of how the child is likely to be affected as an adult. It also provides the physician with information with which to reassure the family that the child is likely to do well, with few functional problems.

Screening Examination

Sometimes a rotational problem is a manifestation of an underlying disorder. Mild in-toeing may be the presenting complaint in mild spastic hemiparesis secondary to cerebral palsy. Limb asymmetry is often seen in infants who have hip dysplasia. Medial tibial torsion is usually found to be associated with tibia vara. Out-toeing is a classic feature of slipped capital femoral epiphysis. Before you focus on the rotational problem, make certain that the rest of the musculoskeletal system is normal. Perform a careful examination to rule out more serious problems. Any suspicious clinical finding should prompt a more intensive evaluation.

Observe the child while he or she is walking and running.

The child who has hemiparesis elevates the affected arm and walks with a mild equinus gait in addition to mild in-toeing. An equinus gait requires a careful neurologic examination to rule out cerebral palsy, and it may be necessary to determine the creatinine phosphokinase level to rule out muscular dystrophy. Mild hemiparesis secondary to cerebral palsy is the most common serious problem seen in children in our torsion clinic.

The hips must be carefully evaluated to rule out hip dysplasia. Hip rotation and abduction should be symmetrical. Finally, note the alignment of the femur and tibia, and distinguish between frontal plane deformity from bowed legs or genu valgum and transverse plane deformity from rotational problems.

Rotational Profile

The rotational profile provides the information necessary to establish a diagnosis and to quantitate the severity of rotational problems. Compare measurements with the normal standards to determine the relevance of the findings. Several measurements must be made.

Estimate the foot-progression angle as the child walks toward the examiner (Fig. 2). This is the average amount of in-toeing or out-toeing and is expressed in degrees; the in-toeing values are preceded by a minus sign. Observe the child while he or she is running, as running often accentuates the problem. Be certain to observe any particular features of the way that the child walks or runs that concern the family.

Next, examine the child while he or she is prone with the knees flexed 90°. Avoid pushing down on the pelvis or applying force during the examination. Allow both hips to fall into maximum medial and lateral rotation as a result of gravity alone. The degree of medial and lateral rotation of the hip is determined by the vertical tibial angle. Hip rotation should be symmetrical. Asymmetrical rotation is often indicative of a disorder of the hip and, if it is present, a roentgenogram of the pelvis should be made. Medial rotation is normally less than 70° for girls and about 60° for boys. Higher values suggest a diagnosis of medial femoral torsion, which may be considered to be mild if the range is between 70° and 80°, moderate if it is between 80° and 90°, and severe if it is 90° or more.

Determine the degree of tibial rotation by measuring the thigh-foot angle or the transmalleolar angle. The thigh-foot angle is the angular difference between the axis of the foot and the axis of the thigh, and it provides a rapid and convenient means of assessing rotation of the tibia and hindfoot. This angle is assessed with the foot in the resting position that allows the subtalar and mid-tarsal joints to fall into a neutral position.

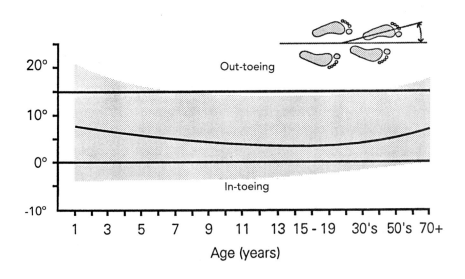

Fig. 2 The foot-progression angle changes with age (horizontal axis). The normal range is very broad (shaded area). Mild in-toeing is normal in childhood and out-toeing is more often seen in infants. (Reproduced with permission from Staheli LT, Corbett M, Wyss C, et al: Lower-extremity rotational problems in children: Normal values to guide management. *J Bone Joint Surg* 1985;67A:41-43.)

If the infant does not remain still but continues to move the feet, watch the foot for 15 to 30 seconds and average the readings for the different positions observed. With practice, the assessment will become reasonably reproducible and sufficiently accurate for clinical use. There are numerous methods for measurement of the transmalleolar axis. The easiest method for the assessment of rotation of the tibia and hindfoot is to draw a line across the sole of the foot, connecting dots placed over the center of the medial and lateral malleoli. A right angle to this line is compared with the axis of the thigh to provide the transmalleolar axis. This axis is important in the assessment of complex foot deformities, such as club feet, in which the axis is usually normal or laterally rotated while the thigh-foot angle is medially rotated. These measurements and findings demonstrate whether the rotational deformity involves the foot rather than the tibia.

Evaluate the shape and direction of the sole of the foot. The deformity may be assessed by projection of the midline axis of the hindfoot forward, through the forefoot, to quantitate forefoot adduction. In the normal foot, this line projects between the second and third toes. If the deformity is mild, the line falls along the longitudinal axis of the third toe; if it is moderate, it falls between the third and fourth toes; and if it is severe, the line falls between the fourth and fifth toes.[4] The shape of the foot can be recorded by imaging of the sole of the foot with a photocopy machine[5] or with photography. We use a Polaroid camera for this purpose.

Classification

The rotational profile provides the information necessary to establish a diagnosis. Torsional problems may be classified according to the direction of the deformity and the age of the child when the deformity is first seen.

In-toeing

During the first year of life, inward rotation of the foot is usually due to metatarsus adductus alone or combined with medial tibial torsion. Unilateral deformity is most common on the left side, for no known reason. In-toeing by a toddler is usually due to medial tibial torsion alone or combined with metatarsus adductus, and it may involve one or both sides. When in-toeing is first seen during early childhood, it is usually due to medial femoral torsion and it is nearly always bilateral and symmetrical, unlike medial tibial torsion. Some children have combinations of these deformities, which may result in severe in-toeing. Metatarsus adductus and medial tibial torsion are often combined, and medial tibial torsion and medial femoral torsion may exist together. Sometimes a child is seen, as a toddler, with medial tibial torsion, which persists as in-toeing into early childhood due to the development of medial femoral torsion. In-toeing that persists into late childhood may be due to medial tibial torsion or to medial femoral torsion.

Out-toeing

In early infancy, out-toeing is normal and is due to external rotation contractures. Out-toeing by the older child or adolescent is usually due to lateral tibial torsion and occasionally due to lateral femoral torsion. Lateral femoral torsion occurs more commonly in obese children and in association with slipped capital femoral epiphysis and, when it is unilateral, it is more common on the right side.

Management Principles

The challenges that the physician faces when managing rotational problems are the establishment of the correct diagnosis and the effective reassurance of the parents. A flowchart to determine the best management can be helpful (Fig. 3). There are several principles underlying the management of rotational problems that apply to all of the different entities.

First, treatment of tibial and femoral torsion is both unnecessary and ineffective, since the vast majority of medial tibial and medial femoral torsional problems resolve spontaneously. The major challenge is family management. Effective reassurance requires that the physician take the concerns of the family seriously. Some orthopaedists object to the management of rotational problems, which they consider problems of the "worried well." The parents' concerns are real and, when they are deprecated, the parents often feel humiliated. Reassurance of a worried family is an important part of treatment.

Perform a careful and thorough evaluation. This provides correct diagnosis and enhances the family's confidence in the plan of management.

Provide the parents with information about the natural history of rotational problems. Emphasize that these problems tend to resolve spontaneously, that disability-producing deformities persist in only about one child in a thousand, and that such deformities can be corrected effectively in late childhood if necessary. Discuss the concerns of the grandparents with the individuals who have brought the child for the evaluation. This is important whether or not the grandparents are present at the time of the examination. The grandparents' child-raising experience occurred during an era when developmental variations were often considered to be serious problems that could produce a disability. Rotational problems were usually treated with shoe modifications and braces. Update the education of the grandparents, verbally through the parents and, when possible, with written material. Reassure the parents that you will follow the child along with them to make sure that the problem resolves.

Resist the temptation to do something to the child to satisfy the family. Such intervention harms the child by interfering with sleep or play, by causing embarrassment, or by leading to a loss of self-esteem. Any adult who has worn braces or shoe modifications as a child recalls the experience as unpleasant. Why jeopardize the happiness of the child when the problem is parental anxiety and concern? Furthermore, we have a responsi-

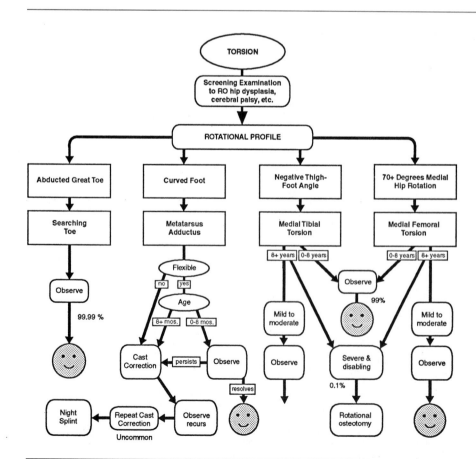

Fig. 3 Suggested management of torsional problems. RO = rule out.

bility to reduce the cost of medical care by avoiding unnecessary and ineffective interventions. Finally, such intervention sets a low standard for orthopaedic care.

Rotational osteotomy is effective, but it is very rarely indicated. Operative correction should be delayed until late childhood and it should be performed only for a severe deformity that is producing substantial disability. The parents should be aware that an osteotomy is not prophylactic and is performed only to correct a tangible functional problem.

Forefoot Adductus

Metatarsus Adductus and Varus

The most common congenital foot deformity is metatarsus adductus.[6] The deformity, which is caused by intrauterine position, is flexible and resolves spontaneously in more than 90% of children.[6-9] In contrast, metatarsus varus is rigid, causes a plantar crease, deforms the medial cuneiform,[10] and often persists so that it requires treatment. Persistent or rigid forefoot adductus can be readily corrected with a cast. Unlike the treatment of club foot, cast correction of the adducted forefoot can be delayed until it is clear that the deformity is not resolving. I prefer to wait until the child is 3 months old before I treat metatarsus varus and until the age of 6 to 9 months before I treat the unusual case of metatarsus adductus that has not resolved on its own. When treatment is necessary, a cast that extends above the knee corrects an adducted foot much more efficiently than does a below-the-knee cast or brace, since the above-the-knee cast can control tibial rotation. The cast is applied with the knee flexed 20° to 25°, as this allows the toddler to walk. Casts are changed biweekly, and correction is usually achieved after two to three changes. Correction with an above-the-knee cast is effective until the age of 4 or 5 years. Recurrence following correction is uncommon. If the deformity recurs or if it is first seen after the age of 2 years, night-splinting may reduce the risk of additional recurrences. The night splint is made by modification of the final corrective cast. The cast is split in half and lined with padding, and Velcro closures are applied. The splint is worn at night for three additional months. Operative correction of residual deformity is controversial. Release of the abductor hallucis,[11] capsulotomy,[12] and metatarsal osteotomy have been recommended. I believe that operative correction is not appropriate because complications are frequent.[13] Residual adductus is not a cause of bunion formation,[14] and no long-term disability has been reported.

Skew Foot

This condition, which has also been described as a z foot or serpentine foot,[15] is another manifestation of an adductus deformity. The skew foot is a rare disorder characterized by a valgus position of the heel, plantar flexion of the talus, and abduction of the midfoot. The foot is flexible. The diagnosis is confirmed by anteroposterior and lateral standing roentgenograms of the foot. In skew foot, a combination of abduction at the mid-tarsal joints and adduction of the metatarsals gives the foot a z configuration on the anteroposterior roentgenogram. The lateral projection shows a reduction in the calcaneal pitch and plantar flexion of the talus. Non-operative treatment of skew foot is ineffective, and operative correction is best delayed until after the age of 6 years. An opening wedge osteotomy of the calcaneus[16] is done to correct the mid-tarsal abduction deformity and to position the sustentaculum to elevate the neck of the talus. This is combined with an opening wedge osteotomy of the first cuneiform to correct the forefoot adductus.

Dynamic Hallux Abductus

This condition is seen during the stance phase of walking and is sometimes referred to as a spastic abductor hallucis syndrome or a searching toe. The deformity is due to a dynamic imbalance of the abductor and adductor muscles of the great toe. The deformity occurs in toddlers and resolves as fine motor coordination develops during early childhood. No treatment is necessary.

Tibial Torsion

Tibial torsion, which is common during infancy and early childhood, is defined by the angular difference between the transmalleolar axis and the bicondylar axis of the knee. Medial tibial torsion is the most common cause of in-toeing.

Clinical Features

Medial tibial torsion is most apparent when infants first begin to walk. It affects both sexes equally, and it is often asymmetrical. The condition is bilateral in about two-thirds of affected infants, and it is associated with metatarsus adductus in about one-third. Unilateral medial tibial torsion is seen twice as often on the left side as on the right side.[17] The feet are medially rotated, while the patella remains in a neutral position. The infant exhibits in-toeing and may trip and appear clumsy. Lateral tibial torsion is usually initially seen during late childhood or adolescence; sometimes it is first detected when an adolescent is evaluated for patellofemoral pain. It is often unilateral, and it is more common on the right side.

Cause

Prenatal factors may contribute to tibial torsion.[18] Medial tibial torsion does not occur in preterm infants,[19] suggesting that it is an intrauterine positional deformity. Preterm infants tend to exhibit out-toeing until late childhood.[20] Postnatal factors such as prone sleeping and sitting posture[21] have been suggested as causes of tibial torsion, but such relationships have not been documented. Tibial torsion is often found in children with tibia vara, myelodysplasia, or residual weakness following poliomyelitis. Less commonly, tibial torsion can be familial,[22] and it has also been seen in association with malunion of tibial fractures. I believe that most cases of tibial torsion, especially when associated with metatarsus adductus, are due to intrauterine position. Other cases simply represent an extreme of normal variability, and some persistent cases may have a genetic basis.

Measurement

The accuracy of all measurements of tibial torsion is affected by the changes that occur in the axis of rotation at the ankle and knee with varying degrees of flexion. Fortunately, this effect is minimum. For clinical purposes, a physical examination is adequate to evaluate and manage tibial version.[23] More complex and expensive methods of measurement involving the use of computerized tomographic scans,[24] ultrasound,[25,26] fluoroscope,[27-29] and clinical measuring aids[30] have been described, but their advantage over simpler clinical measurements remains to be demonstrated. At present, these special imaging techniques are appropriate only for the purposes of research.

Normal Values

Studies of cadavers[31,32] and those of live subjects[30,33-36] have demonstrated that the transmalleolar axis consistently rotates laterally during growth (Fig. 4). On the average, tibial version has been shown to range from 2° to 4° at birth and from 10° to 20° in adults. A wide range of normal (0 to 40°) has been recorded in adults. Recognition of the spontaneous lateral rotation of the tibia with growth and the wide range of normal are important considerations in the planning of appropriate management of tibial torsion.

Natural History

The natural history of medial tibial torsion is spontaneous resolution. This resolution is most rapid in infancy, but it appears to continue throughout growth.[36] Lateral tibial torsion appears to increase with growth, but it is seldom a problem until late childhood or adolescence.

Disability

Disability from medial tibial torsion in the older child or adolescent is rare. Because runners often demonstrate in-toeing, some claim that a mild degree of in-toeing may actually be beneficial. In an unpublished study that we performed on members of our university track team, the values for thigh-foot angles were usually in the lower-normal range as compared with our published control values. It is possible that mild in-toeing facilitates running by placing the toes in an optimum position to assist in ankle push-off. In contrast, disability from lateral tibial torsion has been documented: difficulty in parallel skiing,[37] an increased prevalence of patellofemoral instability,[38] and patellofemoral pain[39] have been reported.

Nonoperative Management

The management of tibial torsion is controversial. On the basis of clinical impressions, tibial torsion has been treated with night splints,[31] shoe wedges and orthotics, exercises, and attempts to control the sleep-

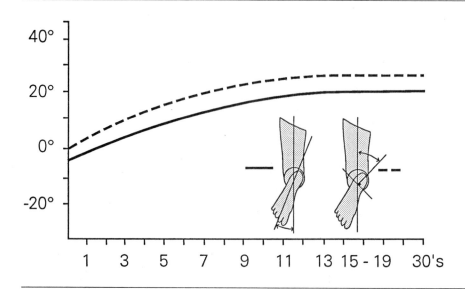

Fig. 4 Both the thigh-foot angle (solid line) and the transmalleolar angle (interrupted line) increase with age (horizontal axis). (Reproduced with permission from Staheli LT, Corbett M, Wyss C, et al: Lower-extremity rotational problems in children: Normal values to guide management. *J Bone Joint Surg* 1985;67A:41-43.)

ing, sitting, and walking patterns of infants and children. Others have believed that medial tibial torsion resolves with time and treatment is unnecessary.[40] Clinical studies suggest that non-operative treatment of tibial torsion is ineffective. In a controlled, prospective study of infants with medial tibial torsion, the outcome for the untreated control group was comparable with that for the infants treated with night splints.[41] In a rabbit model that included use of skeletal markers, simulated night-splinting produced no rotational change of the tibia or femur.[42] Likewise, the application of shoe wedges failed to reduce the in-toeing of children.[43] On the basis of these studies, it would appear that the improvement that has been observed in infants and children who were treated with various techniques was due to the normal, spontaneous lateral rotation of the tibia that occurs with growth and not to the treatment itself. I believe that any treatment of tibial torsion in the infant or child is both unnecessary and ineffective.

Tibial Osteotomy

Tibial rotational osteotomy is very rarely necessary for correction of tibial torsion. It should not be done until after the age of 10 years, as medial tibial torsion tends to improve with time and lateral tibial torsion is seldom a problem during the first decade of life. Proximal tibial rotational osteotomy has been associated with frequent complications, ranging from peroneal nerve injury to compartment syndromes.[44] In our experience, and those of others,[45-47] distal supramalleolar rotational osteotomy is equally effective and much safer when used to correct persistent lateral tibial torsion. To justify operative correction, the deformity should be severe, with a thigh-foot angle of less than −10° or more than +40°. The coexistence of femoral torsion will affect the indications for tibial osteotomy. For example, if the child has femoral retrotorsion, severe out-toeing, and a thigh-foot angle of +30°, the tibia may need to be derotated. In some cases, the rotational deformity of the tibia and femur may be roughly equal. In such cases, correction of one level is appropriate to bring the foot-progression angle to an acceptable level. A supramalleolar tibial osteotomy is the procedure of choice, since the morbidity of the procedure is less than that associated with a femoral osteotomy. The tibial osteotomy requires immobilization of the lower limb in a cast extending above the knee, and the fixation pins can be removed, without anesthesia, in the office or clinic. The technique for distal tibial rotational osteotomy has been described elsewhere.[46,48]

Femoral Torsion

Femoral version is defined as the angular difference between the axis of the femoral neck and the trans-

condylar axis of the knee. Medial femoral torsion is a common clinical problem during early childhood.

Clinical Features

Medial femoral torsion is the most common cause of in-toeing that first presents in early childhood. It is twice as common in girls as in boys, it is nearly always symmetrical, and it is often familial. The child sits with the limbs in the W position, walks with an in-toeing gait with the patella medially rotated, and runs in an awkward pattern. The appearance while running is characterized by medial rotation of the thighs during swing phase, producing an outward rotation of the legs and feet. This has been described as an egg-beater pattern. The gait appears clumsy and inefficient, and the in-toeing becomes more pronounced when the child is tired. Tripping as a result of crossing the feet may occur, and the child may be teased by other children because of the pigeon-toed gait and the peculiar running pattern.

Cause

Increased anteversion has been created in cats by application of casts with their limbs in maximum medial rotation.[49] Reduced anteversion is seen in obese adolescents. It has been suggested that the increased load causes remodeling of the femoral neck, which results in retroversion.[50] Increased anteversion has been found as a recessive trait in some rabbits.[51] Most cases of femoral torsion are probably inherited[40,52] or simply represent the extremes of normal variability.[36]

Measurement

There are several methods for the measurement of femoral anteversion. Roentgenographic techniques include fluoroscopy,[53] biplane imaging,[54-57] axial roentgenography,[58] axial tomography,[59] and computed tomographic scanning.[60] Most recently, ultrasound methods have also been used.[61] In addition to the inherent problems of imaging with ultrasound[62] and computed tomographic scanning,[63] such methods are not more accurate than the clinical methods.[64] Furthermore, these imaging techniques are expensive and may involve radiation exposure. The clinical means for the measurement of femoral anteversion include the assessment of hip rotation[65] and the prone rotation test for femoral anteversion.[64] With the child lying prone, the examiner medially rotates the thigh while palpating the greater trochanter. The degree of anteversion is determined by the degree of medial rotation that is necessary to bring the trochanter into greatest prominence. In this position, the femoral neck is horizontal. For these reasons, I believe that, for routine management of children with rotational problems, physical examination alone is sufficient and appropriate. Imaging is indicated only if hip rotation is asymmetrical, operative correction is planned, or anteversion must be measured for clinical studies.

Normal Values

On the average, femoral anteversion ranges from 30° to 40° at birth[66] and decreases progressively throughout growth. In adults, anteversion averages between 8° and 14°,[67] with an average of 8° in men and 14° in women.[68] The range of normal is broad, with specimens having shown as much as 36° of anteversion.

Natural History

Medial femoral torsion is usually first diagnosed after the age of 3 years. In-toeing secondary to medial femoral torsion becomes most pronounced between the ages of 4 and 6 years and then improves during late childhood.[67] This course parallels the pattern of hip rotation seen in normal children, in whom medial hip rotation is greatest during early childhood and then declines with increasing age.[69] In children with medial femoral torsion, femoral anteversion decreases about 1.5° per year and medial hip rotation decreases about 2° or 3° per year. This decrease results in spontaneous resolution of medial femoral torsion in more than 80% of affected children.[70]

Disability

Medial femoral torsion was once speculated to cause a variety of problems during adult life, including osteoarthrosis of the hip[71-73] and impaired running ability. However, clinical studies showed that adults with osteoarthrosis had values for femoral anteversion that were equivalent to control values.[74,75] The physical performance of women with medial femoral torsion was also found to be equivalent to that of control subjects.[76] The relationship between medial femoral torsion and knee pain is less clear. Adults who had medial femoral torsion as children were found to have a greater prevalence of knee pain than did control subjects.[77] In another study, knee pain was not significantly more common in subjects with medial femoral torsion.[78] In still another study of adults with medial femoral torsion, the patellofemoral characteristics (as determined with roentgenography) were found to be comparable with those of control subjects.[79] These conflicting reports suggest that the problem is complex. Possibly, knee pain is most likely to occur with medial femoral torsion if secondary or associated lateral tibial torsion is also present. Overall, however, these findings suggest that medial femoral torsion is a relatively benign condition.

In contrast, lateral femoral torsion may not be as benign, since it has been found to be associated with osteoarthrosis,[80] an increased risk of stress fracture of the lower limb,[81] and slipped capital femoral epiph-

ysis.[82] In fact, the disability from lateral femoral torsion may be considerably greater than has been generally appreciated.

Nonoperative Treatment

Several methods have been tried for the treatment of medial femoral torsion, but none have been demonstrated to be effective. Shoe wedges do not improve in-toeing,[43] and twister cables and night splints do not reduce measured femoral anteversion in children.[67] Although children are often harassed for sitting with the lower limbs in the W posture or for in-toeing, and orthotics are commonly prescribed for their shoes, it seems unlikely that these measures will change the course of the deformity. I believe that non-operative treatment of femoral torsion is ineffective.

Operative Treatment

In the past, some orthopaedists performed operative correction of medial femoral torsion in young children, as they believed that this would not only correct the child's in-toeing but also prevent osteoarthrosis and functional disability during adult life.[83] Rotational osteotomies effectively corrected the child's in-toeing, but complications were frequent. In two large series, complications such as nonunion, delayed union, malunion, and infection occurred in about 15% of the children.[52,84] In another study, valgus deformity requiring a second osteotomy developed in two of 14 patients who had had a distal femoral osteotomy. These deformities were thought to be due to unilateral overgrowth of the distal part of the femur.[85] I believe that the indications for rotational osteotomy for medial femoral torsion should be well defined.[52] The procedure should be performed only after the age of 8 to 10 years, for persistent, severe deformity. The child should have more than 50° of measured anteversion and more than 80° of medial hip rotation. The family should be aware that the procedure is not prophylactic and that it is not done to prevent osteoarthrosis. Considerable care should be taken with the technique as complications have been frequent. I prefer the intertrochanteric level because the bone surfaces are broad, which increases the stability of fixation and ensures better bone contact, and healing is rapid. Rotation of 45° is usually appropriate. The rotation should be monitored with guide pins to ensure accuracy. The procedure has been described in detail elsewhere.[48]

Acetabular Version

Histomorphometric study has shown that acetabular anteversion remains constant throughout the first half of intrauterine life.[86] As demonstrated by computerized tomographic imaging, acetabular version remains relatively constant throughout childhood, with a mean value of 13°.[87] These findings suggest that acetabular version is not a common factor in rotational problems.

Torsional Malalignment Syndrome

Torsional malalignment syndrome is a combination of medial femoral and lateral tibial torsion.[88] The axis of the knee is rotated medial to the line of progression. It is commonly believed that, in some children with medial femoral torsion, the reduction of in-toeing that occurs in late childhood is due, in part, to the development of lateral tibial torsion. In patients who had patellofemoral symptoms, medial hip rotation was increased.[89] In another study, of patients who had patellar instability, the combination of medial femoral torsion and lateral tibial torsion was more commonly observed.[90] In contrast, others[39] found that patients with chronic knee pain had lateral tibial torsion but no increase in femoral anteversion. In a study of women with medial femoral torsion, measured tibial version was not increased compared with a control group with normal anteversion.[91] These divergent findings suggest that the development of lateral tibial torsion in compensation for medial femoral torsion is inconsistent and that operative correction of medial femoral torsion to correct torsional malalignment is not justified. Despite the uncertainty of its pathogenesis, this malalignment can complicate the management of knee pain or patellar instability. Considering that correction of this torsional malalignment requires a four-level osteotomy, conservative management is appealing. When a conservative approach fails, operative correction may be considered. I have performed such a correction only twice—by a two-team approach, with the medial femoral torsion corrected by intertrochanteric osteotomy and the lateral tibial torsion corrected by supramalleolar osteotomy during the same operative session. Fixation was provided by a combination of cross-pin fixation and a spica cast. Fortunately, the deformities were corrected successfully, pain was eliminated, and no complications occurred.

Conclusions

Rotational problems are common in infants and children and rare in adolescents. They cause concern in parents and sometimes produce minor functional problems in children. The parents' concerns must be taken seriously. The child must be evaluated carefully, and an accurate diagnosis must be established. The most important part of care is reassurance of the parents. Persistent or rigid metatarsus adductus or varus can be treated with a cast, even late in the first year of life. Observational management is best for medial tibial or femoral torsion in toddlers and children. Perhaps, overall, only 0.1% of torsional deformities

persist and may necessitate osteotomy. Osteotomy should be delayed until late childhood and is only indicated if the deformity is very severe and produces functional disability.

References

1. Staheli LT: Lower positional deformity in infants and children: A review. *J Pediatr Orthop* 1990;10:559-563.
2. Pitkow RB: External rotation contracture of the extended hip: A common phenomenon of infancy obscuring femoral neck anteversion and the most frequent cause of out-toeing gait in children. *Clin Orthop* 1975;110:139-145.
3. Svenningsen S, Terjesen T, Auflem M, et al: Hip rotation and in-toeing gait: A study of normal subjects from four years until adult age. *Clin Orthop* 1990;251:177-182.
4. Bleck EE: Metatarsus adductus: classification and relationship to outcomes of treatment. *J Pediatr Orthop* 1983;3:2-9.
5. Smith JT, Bleck EE, Gamble JG, et al: Simple method of documenting metatarsus adductus. *J Pediatr Orthop* 1991;11:679-680.
6. Hunziker UA, Largo RH, Duc G, et al: Neonatal metatarsus adductus, joint mobility, axis and rotation of the lower extremity in preterm and term children 0-5 years of age. *Eur J Pediatr* 1988;148:19-23.
7. Ponseti IV, Becker JR: Congenital metatarsus adductus: The results of treatment. *J Bone Joint Surg* 1966;48A:702-711.
8. Rushforth GF: The natural history of hooked forefoot. *J Bone Joint Surg* 1978;60B:530-532.
9. Taussig G, Pilliard D: Congenital metatarsus varus: Value of orthopedic treatment and role of surgery: Apropos of 290 cases. *Rev Chir Orthop* 1983;69:29-46.
10. Reimann I, Werner HH: The pathology of congenital metatarsus varus: A post-mortem study of a newborn infant. *Acta Orthop Scand* 1983;54:847-849.
11. Mitchell GP: Abductor hallucis release in congenital metatarsus varus. *Int Orthop* 1980;3:299-304.
12. Heyman CH, Herndon CH, Strong JM: Mobilization of the tarsometatarsal and intermetatarsal joints for the correction of resistent adduction of the fore part of the foot in congenital club-foot or congenital metatarsus varus. *J Bone Joint Surg* 1958;40A:299-310.
13. Stark JG, Johanson JE, Winter RB: The Heyman-Herndon tarsometatarsal capsulotomy for metatarsus adductus: Results in 48 feet. *J Pediatr Orthop* 1987;7:305-310.
14. Kilmartin TE, Barrington RL, Wallace WA: Metatarsus primus varus: A statistical study. *J Bone Joint Surg* 1991;73B:937-940.
15. Jawish R, Rigault P, Padovani JP, et al: The z-shaped or serpentine foot in children and adolescents. *Chir Pediatr* 1990;31:314-321.
16. Mosca VS: Calcaneal neck lengthening for severe abducto-valgus (flat) hindfoot deformity in children. *Orthop Trans* 1992;16:653.
17. Katz JF: Behavior of internal tibia torsion in infancy. *Mt Sinai J Med* 1982;49:7-12.
18. Thelander HE, Fitzhugh ML: Posture habits in infancy affecting foot and leg alignments. *J Pediatr* 1942;21:306-314.
19. Katz K, Naor N, Merlob P, et al: Rotational deformities of the tibia and foot in preterm infants. *J Pediatr Orthop* 1990;10:483-485.
20. Katz K, Krikler R, Wielunsky, E, et al: Effect of neonatal posture on later lower limb rotation and gait in premature infants. *J Pediatr Orthop* 1991;11:520-522.
21. Knight RA: Developmental deformities of the lower extremities. *J Bone Joint Surg* 1954;36A:521-527.

22. Blumel J, Eggers GWN, Evans EB: Eight cases of hereditary bilateral medial tibial torsion in four generations. *J Bone Joint Surg* 1957;39A:1198-1202.

23. Stuberg W, Temme J, Kaplan P, et al: Measurement of tibial torsion and thigh-foot angle using goniometry and computed tomography. *Clin Orthop* 1991;272:208-212.

24. Reikeras O, Hoiseth A: Torsion of the leg determined by computed tomography. *Acta Orthop Scand* 1989;60:330-333.

25. Butler-Manuel PA, Guy RL, Heatley FW: Measurement of tibial torsion—a new technique applicable to ultrasound and computed tomography. *Br J Radiol* 1992;65:119-126.

26. Joseph B, Carver RA, Bell MJ, et al: Measurement of tibial torsion by ultrasound. *J Pediatr Orthop* 1987;7:317-323.

27. Clementz BG: Assessment of tibial torsion and rotational deformity with a new fluoroscopic technique. *Clin Orthop* 1989;245:199-209.

28. Clementz BG, Magnusson A: Assessment of tibial torsion employing fluoroscopy, computed tomography and the cryosectioning technique. *Acta Radiol* 1989;30:75-80.

29. Clementz BG, Magnusson A: Fluoroscopic measurement of tibial torsion in adults: A comparison of three methods. *Arch Orthop Traumat Surg* 1989;108:150-153.

30. Staheli LT, Engel GM: Tibial torsion: A method of assessment and a survey of normal children. *Clin Orthop* 1972;86:183-186.

31. Hutter CG Jr, Scott W: Tibial torsion. *J Bone Joint Surg* 1949;31A:511-518.

32. Le Damany P: La torsion du tibia: Normale, pathologique, expérimentale. *J de l'anat et physiol (Paris)* 1909;45:598-615.

33. Clementz BG: Tibial torsion measured in normal adults. *Acta Orthop Scand* 1988;59:441-442.

34. Khermosh O, Lior G, Weissman SL: Tibial torsion in children. *Clin Orthop* 1971;79:25-31.

35. Malekafzali S, Wood MB: Tibial torsion—a simple clinical apparatus for its measurement and its application to a normal adult population. *Clin Orthop* 1979;145:154-157.

36. Staheli LT, Corbett M, Wyss C, et al: Lower-extremity rotational problems in children: Normal values to guide management. *J Bone Joint Surg* 1985;67A:39-47.

37. Winter WG Jr, Lafferty JF: The skiing sequelae of tibial torsion. *Orthop Clin North Am* 1976;7:231-240.

38. Turner MS, Smillie IS: The effect of tibial torsion on the pathology of the knee. *J Bone Joint Surg* 1981;63B:396-398.

39. Cooke TDV, Price N, Fisher B, et al: The inwardly pointing knee: An unrecognized problem of external rotational malalignment. *Clin Orthop* 1990;260:56-60.

40. Weseley MS, Barenfeld PA, Eisenstein AL: Thoughts on in-toeing and out-toeing: Twenty years' experience with over 5000 cases and a review of the literature. *Foot Ankle* 1981;2:49-57.

41. Heinrich SD, Sharps C: Lower extremity torsional deformities in children: A prospective comparison of two treatment modalities. *Orthop Trans* 1989;13:554-555, 1989.

42. Barlow DW, Staheli LT: Effects of lateral rotation splinting on lower extremity bone growth: An in-vivo study in rabbits. *J Pediatr Orthop* 1991;11:583-587.

43. Knittel G, Staheli LT: The effectiveness of shoe modifications for intoeing. *Orthop Clin North Am* 1976;7:1019-1025.

44. Schrock RD Jr: Peroneal nerve palsy following derotation osteotomies for tibial torsion. *Clin Orthop* 1969;62:172-177.

45. Bennett JT, Bunnell WP, MacEwen GD: Rotational osteotomy of the distal tibia and fibula. *J Pediatr Orthop* 1985;5:294-298.

46. Krengel WF III, Staheli LT: Tibial rotational osteotomy for idiopathic torsion: A comparison of the proximal and distal osteotomy levels. *Clin Orthop* 1992;283:285-289.

47. McNicol D, Leong JCY, Hsu LCS: Supramalleolar derotation osteotomy for lateral tibial torsion and associated equinovarus deformity of the foot. *J Bone Joint Surg* 1983;65B:166-170.

48. Mosca VS, Staheli LT: Surgical management of torsional and angular deformities of the lower extremities, in Chapman MW, Madison M (eds): *Operative Orthopedics.* Philadelphia, PA, JB Lippincott, 1988, vol 3, pp 2227-2235.

49. Glauber A, Vizkelety T: The influence of the iliopsoas muscle on femoral antetorsion. *Arch Orthop* Unfall-Chir 1966;60:71-79.

50. Galbraith RT, Gelberman RH, Hajek PC, et al: Obesity and decreased femoral anteversion in adolescence. *J Orthop Res* 1987;5:523-528.

51. Arendar GM, Milch RA: Splay-leg—a recessively inherited form of femoral neck anteversion, femoral shaft torsion and subluxation of the hip in the laboratory lop rabbit: Its possible relationship to factors involved in so-called "congenital dislocation" of the hip. *Clin Orthop* 1966;44:221-229.

52. Staheli LT, Clawson DK, Hubbard DD: Medial femoral torsion: experience with operative treatment. *Clin Orthop* 1980;146:222-225.

53. Rogers SP: A method for determining the angle of torsion of the neck of the femur. *J Bone Joint Surg* 1931;13:821-824.

54. Dunlap K, Shands AR Jr, Hollister LC Jr, et al: A new method for determination of torsion of the femur. *J Bone Joint Surg* 1953;35A:289-311.

55. Lee DY, Lee CK, Cho TJ: A new method for measurement of femoral anteversion: A comparative study with other radiographic methods. *Int Orthop* 1992;16:277-281.

56. Magilligan DJ: Calculation of the angle of anteversion by means of horizontal lateral roentgenography. *J Bone Joint Surg* 1956;38A:1231-1246.

57. Ogata K, Goldsand EM: A simple biplanar method of measuring femoral anteversion and neck-shaft angle. *J Bone Joint Surg* 1979;61A:846-851.

58. Dunn DM: Anteversion of the neck of the femur: A method of measurement. *J Bone Joint Surg* 1952;34B:181-186.

59. Hubbard DD, Staheli LT: The direct radiographic measurement of femoral torsion using axial tomography: Technic and comparison with an indirect radiographic method. *Clin Orthop* 1972;86:16-20.

60. Weiner DS, Cook AJ, Hoyt WA Jr, et al: Computed tomography in the measurement of femoral anteversion. *Orthopedics* 1978;1:299-306.

61. Moulton A, Upadhyay SS: A direct method of measuring femoral anteversion using ultrasound. *J Bone Joint Surg* 1982;64B:469-472.

62. Terjesen T, Anda S, Ronningen H: Ultrasound examination for measurement of femoral anteversion in children. *Skeletal Radiol* 1993;22:33-36.

63. Murphy SB, Simon SR, Kijewski PK, et al: Femoral anteversion. *J Bone Joint Surg* 1987;69A:1169-1176.

64. Ruwe PA, Gage JR, Ozonoff MB, et al: Clinical determination of femoral anteversion: A comparison with established techniques. *J Bone Joint Surg* 1992;74A:820-830.

65. Crane L: Femoral torsion and its relation to toeing-in and toeing-out. *J Bone Joint Surg* 1959;41A:421-428.

66. Shands AR Jr, Steele MK: Torsion of the femur: A follow-up report on the use of the Dunlap method for its determination. *J Bone Joint Surg* 1958;40A:803-816.

67. Fabry G, MacEwen GD, Shands AR Jr: Torsion of the femur: A follow-up study in normal and abnormal conditions. *J Bone Joint Surg* 1973;55A:1726-1738.

68. Kate BR: Anteversion versus torsion of the femoral neck. *Acta Anat* 1976;94:457-463.

69. Engel GM, Staheli LT: The natural history of torsion and other factors influencing gait in childhood: A study of the

angle of gait, tibial torsion, knee angle, hip rotation, and development of the arch in normal children. *Clin Orthop* 1974;99:12-17.

70. Svenningsen S, Apalset K, Terjesen T, et al: Regression of femoral anteversion: A prospective study of intoeing children. *Acta Orthop Scand* 1989;60:170-173.

71. Alvik I: Increased anteversion of the femoral neck as sole sign of dysplasia coxae. *Acta Orthop Scand* 1960;29:301-306.

72. McSweeny A: A study of femoral torsion in children. *J Bone Joint Surg* 1971;53B:90-95.

73. Somerville EW: Persistent foetal alignment of the hip. *J Bone Joint Surg* 1957;39B:106-113.

74. Hubbard DD, Staheli LT, Chew DE, et al: Medial femoral torsion and osteoarthritis. *J Pediatr Orthop* 1988;8:540-542.

75. Wedge JH, Munkacsi I, Loback D: Anteversion of the femur and idiopathic osteoarthrosis of the hip. *J Bone Joint Surg* 1989;71A:1040-1043.

76. Staheli LT, Lippert F, Denotter P: Femoral anteversion and physical performance in adolescent and adult life. *Clin Orthop* 1977;129:213-216.

77. Stroud KL, Smith AD, Kruse RW: The relationship between increased femoral anteversion in childhood and patellofemoral pain in adulthood. *Orthop Trans* 1989;13:555.

78. Pizzutillo PD, Eidelson SG: Persistent femoral anteversion and knee pain in the second decade of life. *Orthop Trans* 1989;13:555.

79. Reikeras O: Patellofemoral characteristics in patients with increased femoral anteversion. *Skeletal Radiol* 1992;21:311-313.

80. Tonnis D, Heinecke A: Diminished femoral antetorsion syndrome: A cause of pain and osteoarthritis. *J Pediatr Orthop* 1991;11:419-431.

81. Giladi M, Milgrom C, Stein M, et al: External rotation of the hip: A predictor of risk for stress fractures. *Clin Orthop* 1987;216:131-134.

82. Pritchett JW, Perdue KD: Mechanical factors in slipped capital femoral epiphysis. *J Pediatr Orthop* 1988;8:385-388.

83. Somerville EW: Persistent foetal alignment of the hip: Treatment. *Acta Orthop Belg* 1977;43:552-556.

84. Svenningsen S, Apalset K, Terjesen T, et al: Osteotomy for femoral anteversion: Complications in 95 children. *Acta Orthop Scand* 1989;60:401-405.

85. Fonseca AS, Bassett GS: Valgus deformity following derotation osteotomy to correct medial femoral torsion. *J Pediatr Orthop* 1988;8:295-299.

86. Lee J, Jarvis J, Uhthoff HK, et al: The fetal acetabulum: A histomorphometric study of acetabular anteversion and femoral head coverage. *Clin Orthop* 1992;281:48-55.

87. Jacquemier M, Jouve JL, Bollini G, et al: Acetabular anteversion in children. *J Pediatr Orthop* 1992;12:373-375.

88. Staheli LT: Rotational problems of the lower extremities. *Orthop Clin North Am* 1987;18:503-512.

89. Hvid I, Andersen LI: The quadriceps angle and its relation to femoral torsion. *Acta Orthop Scand* 1982;53:577-579.

90. Airanow S, Zippel H: Femoro-tibial torsion in patellar instability. A contribution to the pathogenesis of recurrent and habitual patellar dislocations. *Beitr Orthop Traumat* 1990;37:311-316.

91. Reikeras O: Is there a relationship between femoral anteversion and leg torsion? *Skeletal Radiol* 1991;20:409-411.

Anterior Knee Pain Syndromes in the Adolescent

Carl L. Stanitski, MD

Adolescent patients with symptoms of pain about the anterior aspect of the knee are regular visitors to orthopaedists' offices. A variety of commonly occurring conditions that cause anterior knee discomfort will be discussed in this chapter, which emphasizes diagnosis and nonsurgical treatment modalities.

The parts of the patellofemoral mechanism develop in concert embryologically,[1,2] and the function of the mechanism must be considered in terms of the relationships between the patella, the femur, and the quadriceps. This unique articulation must also be considered as only one element of the elegant, integrated, articulated linkage system that makes up the lower extremity.

Overuse Problems

In addition to the common acute injuries that occur about the knee, such as patellar dislocation and ligamentous and meniscal damage, sports-related musculoskeletal injuries caused by overuse are seen frequently. Overuse injury results from unresolved, submaximal stress in previously normal tissues.[3-6] Normal physiologic adaptation occurs in response to use, and reasonable amounts of stress are essential for normal connective-tissue function. However, when this system is overwhelmed and an adequate time frame for stress resolution is not provided, overuse injuries occur. Stress injuries, at the extreme of the adaptation spectrum, are particularly common when the musculoskeletal system of an adolescent is not ready for the demands placed on it by parents, coaches, or peers.[7,8]

A common approach to the diagnosis and treatment of childhood and adolescent overuse injury is an interdependent, five-phase program that includes (1) factor identification, (2) factor modification, (3) pain control, (4) progressive rehabilitation, and (5) maintenance.[6]

In the diagnosis of overuse injury, a major effort should be made to identify the factor or factors that led to the condition. In broad terms, these often include environmental, anatomic, and training factors, with training abuses being the most common source of overuse. Once the proper diagnosis has been made, modification of the appropriate causative factors is undertaken. Pain control after a correct diagnosis allows a variety of rehabilitative techniques to be used, with progressive, functional, active rehabilitation leading to a return to full levels of activity. A maintenance program is then necessary to sustain rehabilitative gain and to prevent recurrent or new injury.

Osgood-Schlatter Disease

A presenting problem that is extremely common is Osgood-Schlatter disease. The patient, who is usually in the preteen or early teenage years, presents with activity-related discomfort around the tibial tubercle. Swelling and tenderness readily suggest the diagnosis of Osgood-Schlatter disease, although use of the term disease for this condition may impart an excessively ominous tone and perhaps should be avoided.

Boys are more commonly affected than girls, but the prevalence in girls is increasing because of their increased participation in sports activity. In girls, the condition tends to appear at an earlier age — that is, 11 to 13 years — as compared with boys, who commonly present one to two years later.[9] Kujala and associates[9] found a 21% prevalence of Osgood-Schlatter disease in a group of athletic adolescents, but only a 4.5% prevalence in a group of similar age who were non-athletic. The tibial tubercle may be prominent bilaterally, but usually one side is more symptomatic. Both sides are symptomatic in 20% to 30% of patients.

Osgood-Schlatter disease is thought to result from submaximal, repetitive, tensile stresses acting on the immature junction of the patellar ligament, tibial tubercle, and tibia, causing mild avulsion injuries followed by attempts at osseous repair.[10-12] The onset of symptoms usually occurs during a rapid growth phase, with pain being intermittent and aggravated by activities, especially ones that require kneeling, squatting, or repeated jumping.

Physical examination demonstrates swelling and prominence of the tibial tubercle, accompanied by exquisite local tenderness. Patellar ligament and peripatellar tenderness may also be found. The remainder of the examination is usually normal.

Radiographs are an essential part of the evaluation, particularly to show that a bone tumor or another rare disorder is not the cause of the pain. Varying patterns of tibial tubercle morphology are seen on radiographs. Progressive physiologic epiphysiodesis at the tibial tubercle occurs through centrifugal ossification from proximal to distal. In as many as 50% of reported cases, a discrete, separate ossicle is noted at the tibial tubercle (Fig. 1).[13]

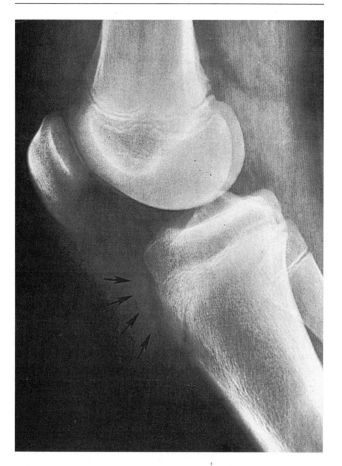

Fig. 1 Separate intratendinous ossification areas in a skeletally immature boy.

that 12 to 24 months are required for spontaneous resolution of symptoms by progressive physiologic epiphysiodesis. In the interim, treatment with ice, anti-inflammatory medication, and an appropriately contoured knee-pad usually controls symptoms. Hamstring and quadriceps flexibility should be maintained, and sports activity should be balanced according to the severity of the symptoms. Physical education instructors, coaches, and parents must understand and appreciate the variety of symptom intensity. If symptoms progress or are disabling during routine daily activities, a course of immobilization for seven to ten days will usually relieve the acute discomfort. Radiation treatment and steroid injections into the tibial tubercle should not be used.

When symptoms persist and are unrelieved by conservative measures, excision of a symptomatic ossicle or ossicles (Fig. 2) and the adjacent bursa will often fully relieve symptoms.[16,17] It is not necessary to await skeletal maturity to enucleate such an ossicle. In a skeletally mature patient, debulking of a prominent tubercle may also improve the appearance of the knee when it is done at the time of ossicle excision. The patient must be made aware, however, of the possibility of some residual tubercle prominence due to scar formation postoperatively.

Despite the common and benign clinical presentation of the condition, one should not be lulled into complacency, especially with regard to a patient who has unilateral involvement. Lewis and Reilly[14] cautioned against the misdiagnosis of so-called sports tumors. D'Ambrosia and MacDonald[15] reported two cases of so-called clinically obvious Osgood-Schlatter disease that, on further analysis, turned out to be osteomyelitis of the tibial tubercle in one patient and an arteriovenous malformation in the other. Osgood-Schlatter disease and slipped capital femoral epiphysis may present concurrently. It must be remembered that knee pain in a child may be caused by hip disease and, therefore, an examination of the hip must always be part of the evaluation of any child with symptoms of knee pain.

Few studies have analyzed the natural history of Osgood-Schlatter disease. Krause and associates[13] retrospectively reviewed the findings in patients with a history of Osgood-Schlatter disease. Most patients were found to be asymptomatic in adulthood.

Treatment of Osgood-Schlatter disease is usually nonoperative. The patient and family must understand

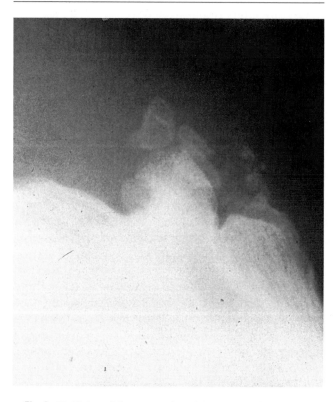

Fig. 2 Multiple ossicles as sequelae of Osgood-Schlatter disease in a symptomatic 23-year-old carpet installer.

Sinding-Larsen-Johansson Disease

Sinding-Larsen-Johansson disease is another cause of discomfort in the anterior aspect of the knee. This condition is believed to be caused by persistent traction at the cartilaginous junction of the patella and the patellar ligament, usually at the inferior patellar pole.[18-20] Occasionally, similar symptoms can occur proximally, at the junction of the quadriceps tendon and the patella.[21] Sinding-Larsen-Johansson disease is usually seen in an active preteen boy who complains of activity-related pain. Tenderness is found at the involved site, and the remainder of the knee examination is usually normal. Radiographs may show varying amounts and shapes of calcification or ossification at the junction of the patella and the ligament (Fig. 3). The differential diagnosis includes patellar stress fracture, sleeve fracture (an avulsion fracture through the region where the non-ossified cartilaginous portion of the patella meets the bone),[21] and a type-I bipartite patella. In the older adolescent, an adult-type of jumper's knee (proximal patellar-ligament tendinitis) must be considered.[22] The treatment program outlined for Osgood-Schlatter disease is also successful in the management of the Sinding-Larsen-Johansson condition. The symptoms usually resolve with progressive skeletal maturation over 12 to 18 months. In rare instances, surgical debridement of the necrotic intratendinous tissue causing a jumper's knee may be needed in patients who do not respond to non-operative management.[23]

Multipartite Patella

A multipartite patella may present a diagnostic dilemma in a child with anterior knee symptoms. These often incidental radiographic findings have been classified into three types by Saupe[24] (Fig. 4): type I — at the inferior pole (5% of all lesions) (Fig. 5), type II — at the lateral patellar margin (20%), and type III — at the superolateral pole (75%) (Fig. 6).

The exact prevalence of bipartite or multipartite patella is unknown. Bilaterality is uncommon. A strong nine-to-one male dominance has been a consistent finding in all series.[24,25] The junction sites of such varia-

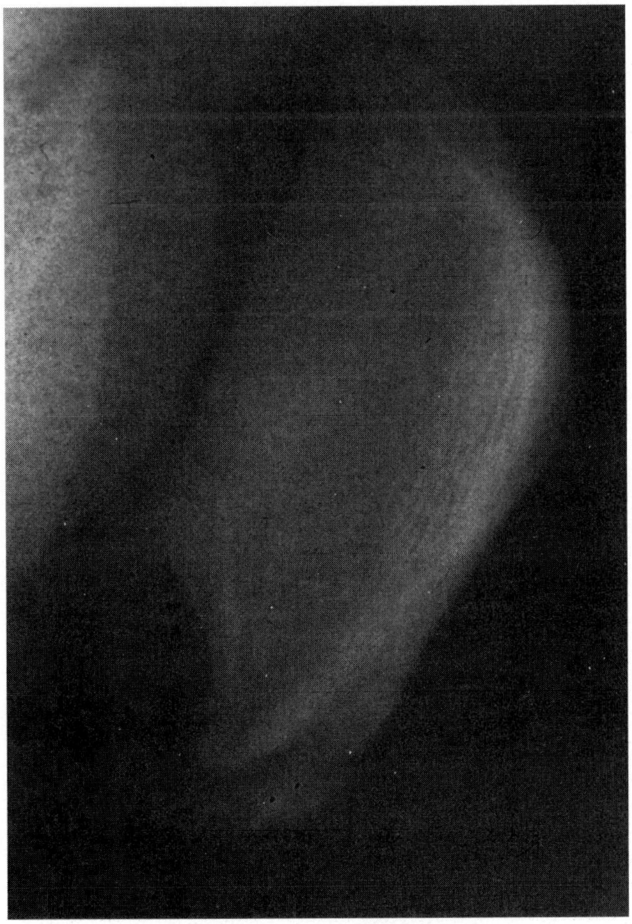

Fig. 3   Distal patellar-pole ossification in a symptomatic 10-year-old boy.

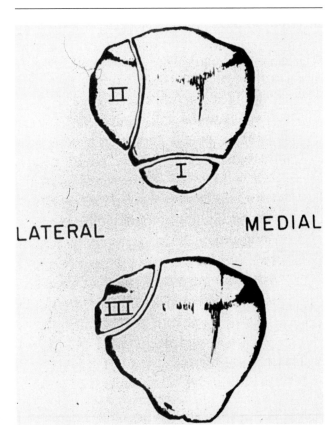

Fig. 4   Saupe's classification of bipartite patellae. (Reprinted with permission from Green WT, Jr: Painful bipartite patellae: A report of three cases. *Clin Orthop* 1975;110:199.)

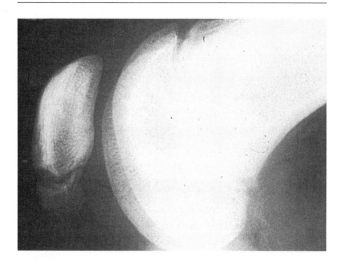

Fig. 5   Type I bipartite patellae in an asymptomatic 13-year-old gymnast.

tions in patellar formation may become symptomatic after acute or chronic stress.[26] The differential diagnosis of altered patellar configuration in a symptomatic child should include acute fracture, stress fracture, and a dorsal patellar defect (Fig. 7).

Examination of the symptomatic knee shows a slightly enlarged patella with tenderness at the junction of the main body of the patella and the fragment. Tomograms (Fig. 8), computed tomography scans, or magnetic resonance imaging may be needed to evaluate incongruity of the articular surface relationships of the fragment and the patellar body if the patient does not respond to initial treatment.

Treatment depends on the acuity and severity of the symptoms. In the acute situation, pain is usually due to a separation between the fragment and the main body of the patella, and knee immobilization for three weeks usually solves the problem.[26] In chronic cases, modification of activity over three to four weeks may be all that is required for resolution.[25] If symptoms persist, the entire fragment, through the region where the fragment meets the body of the patella, may be excised to eliminate the painful pseudarticulation.[25,27,28]

Pathological Plica

The plicae are normal synovial folds that, because they can be seen arthroscopically, have recently become the focus of attention during arthroscopy.[29,30] Patients with a symptomatic plica in the knee complain of pseudolocking and a pop or a snap of the knee at particular degrees of flexion. The patient often presents, particularly when the medial plica is involved, with symptoms similar to the anterior knee diseases already described. Physical findings are limited to localized tenderness at the involved site and snapping of the knee at the medial aspect of the patella as the knee passes actively from 30° to 60° of flexion. With a pathological medial plica, lateral patellar translation by the examiner increases tension on this medial band and increases the symptoms.[29,31] Care should be taken not to attribute such symptoms to an unstable patellofemoral mechanism. Similarly, the fact that the

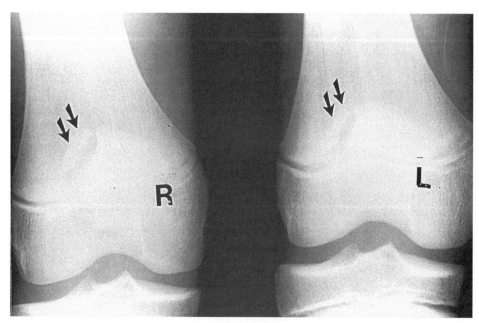

Fig. 6   Bilateral type III bipartite patellae (arrows) noted as an incidental radiographic finding.

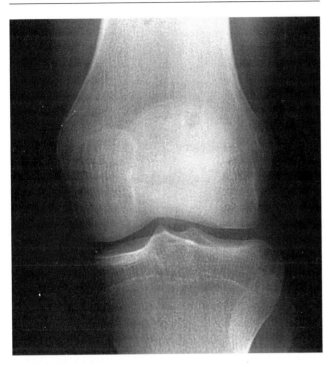

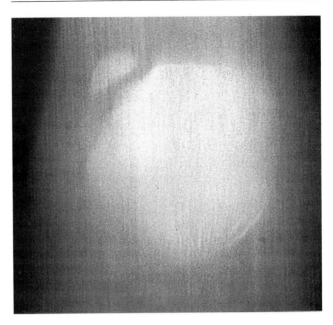

Fig. 8   Tomogram showing type III bipartite patella; there is chronic separation.

Fig. 7   A dorsal patellar defect in superolateral pole is a radiographic curiosity of unknown etiology. It most likely represents an abnormality of patellar ossification.

medial plica has an anterior extension to the fat pad or to the medial meniscus may result in the symptoms being referred to the anterior joint line; this condition should not be confused with meniscal pathology. Because of the dynamic nature of plica symptoms, static-imaging studies have not been particularly helpful. While a plica may be seen on magnetic resonance imaging, no criteria have been developed for the diagnosis of a pathological plica.

Two mechanisms may produce plica pathology.[32,33] The first involves a direct blow with resultant hemorrhage, edema, and progressive fibrosis of this synovial structure. The second mechanism involves overuse when task-specific demands, often associated with minor irregularities of knee mechanics, cause progressive inflammation with recurrent synovitis, edema, and fibrosis with thickening of the plica, which progressively irritates the surrounding tissue.

The diagnosis of symptomatic plica is made by exclusion. The presence of a plica, by itself, does not connote pathology. Other causes of anterior knee pathology must be sought and ruled out, and such pain should not be blithely ascribed to this often gossamer structure. When no other specific cause can be identified, most patients respond to a nonsurgical program that includes contrast therapy (alteration of heat and cold), quadriceps flexibility exercises, and anti-inflammatory medication.[32,33]

Arthroscopy has led to a markedly increased frequency of diagnosis and surgical excision of so-called pathological plicae. One must ask whether this is an arthroscopic wastebasket diagnosis that is made when no other obvious pathology is seen in the knee. This is not to say that a condition of pathological plica may not exist and may not be cured by arthroscopic resection. However, the frequency with which this diagnosis is presently made has increased disproportionately. As Patel noted, "the relationship between plica and disease and the relationship of plica and symptoms remain inconclusive and unclear."[30]

Reflex Sympathetic Dystrophy

Anterior knee pain in children and adolescents may be caused by reflex sympathetic dystrophy, a condition manifested by pain and autonomic dysfunction. In national surveys of complications of arthroscopy, procedures on the patellofemoral joint were reported to be associated with a high prevalence of reflex sympathetic dystrophy.[34-36] Despite recent increased emphasis on the recognition of reflex sympathetic dystrophy in the lower extremity,[34,37-43] it is commonly not considered in the differential diagnosis of knee pain (either preoperatively or postoperatively), especially in children and adolescents. In a series of children with reflex sympathetic dystrophy, reported by Wilder and associates,[43] the average delay from the injury to the correct diagnosis was one year.

The three classic stages — acute, dystrophic, and

atrophic — are temporally related.[41] The acute stage begins within three months after presentation; the dystrophic stage, more than three to six months after presentation; and the atrophic stage, more than six months after presentation.

The onset of reflex sympathetic dystrophy is commonly attributed to an antecedent injury or to activity that is often trivial or ill defined. The primary relevant finding in reflex sympathetic dystrophy is pain out of proportion with the magnitude of the initiating injury. Other symptoms may be swelling, stiffness, and cutaneous manifestations such as sweating and trophic changes.

Sensitivity to the slightest touch (allodynia) is the most common physical finding and is seen in almost 90% of the patients.[41,43] Trophic changes in the skin, mottling, cyanosis, and swelling may not be seen as commonly in children as in adults with reflex sympathetic dystrophy. Limitation of joint motion and diminished muscle strength are often present. Depending on the stage of the disease, focal patchy demineralization and osteoporosis may be seen on radiography, but, again, not with the frequency found in adults with reflex sympathetic dystrophy. Bone scan changes are also uncommon, but bone scans may help to rule out associated conditions such as a stress fracture.[44]

The response of reflex sympathetic dystrophy to treatment is variable, and a multidisciplinary approach is helpful. Treatment of children tends to involve the use of fewer invasive procedures than that of adults, with sympathetic blocks being used less frequently. In contrast to the result in adults, the outcome in children tends to be more favorable but resolution may take as long as three months.[39,41,42]

Wilder and associates[43] proposed a management algorithm specifically for the management of children and adolescents. It includes initial treatment with cognitive behavioral pain-management techniques, physical therapy, and use of transcutaneous electrical nerve stimulation. If the clinical outcome is not satisfactory, tricyclic antidepressant medication is added to the protocol. If improvement is not seen, sympathetic blocks are then included. If the symptoms still do not resolve, these treatments are continued with the addition of steroids, calcitonin, beta blockers, vasodilators, and other specifically indicated medications.

Idiopathic Anterior Knee Pain

The meaning of the term chondromalacia patellae has been changed from connoting a gross pathological observation made during an operation or at an autopsy to a clinical condition of ill-defined anterior knee pain. The cause of the anterior knee pain has been mistakenly ascribed to a deranged patellar articular surface. There is abundant evidence of the almost universal presence of asymptomatic articular cartilage changes in the medial facet of the patella, occurring from young adulthood onward.[39,45] Most preadolescents and early adolescents with anterior knee symptoms have pristine articular surfaces and normal synovial tissue. The cause of such peripatellar symptoms is unknown. Fulkerson and associates[46,47] suggested changes in the retinacular nerves as a cause of such pain, on the basis of histologic changes in the nerve similar to those seen in a Morton interdigital neuroma. Ficat and Hungerford[38] ascribed this pain to abnormal patellofemoral mechanics created by an abnormal insertion of the vastus lateralis causing lateral tightness, pressure along the lateral patellar border, and the excessive lateral pressure syndrome (tightness of the lateral extensor retinaculum with resulting impingement of the patella laterally).

The diagnosis of so-called chondromalacia patellae is nonspecific, and the term should be abandoned. If a child or adolescent has anterior knee pain, it should be called idiopathic anterior knee pain until a satisfactory etiology has been established. The use of the term chondromalacia is as nonspecific for such symptoms as internal derangement is for intra-articular disorders. Not all unexplained anterior knee pain should be simply written off as so-called chondromalacia patellae. Diagnostic efforts must be made to rule out specific causes of the pain, such as intra-articular disorders, patellar instability, overuse, malalignment, referred pain, tumor,[14,48] and infection.[49] A detailed history and a careful physical examination that includes the hip often lead to the correct diagnosis. When used prudently, various imaging studies help to complete the diagnostic picture.

When patients with poorly localized anterior knee pain are asked to indicate the location of the discomfort, they encompass the entire front of the knee with the hand; this is a sign that I refer to as the grab sign (Fig. 9). They may also complain of discomfort following prolonged sitting (the theater sign). Pseudolocking, as opposed to true mechanical locking, is a common symptom as well. Any sports-training program should be assessed to ensure that overuse factors (stair-running, full squats with weights, or the use of stair-climbing exercise equipment) are not contributing abnormal stress to the patellofemoral joint. A cautionary situation associated with adolescent knee pain is a parent who expresses more concern as evidenced by the parent talking more than the patient. Such a combination should make the orthopaedist extremely wary of the true source and nature of such complaints.

On physical examination, the following should be evaluated: gait, the range of motion and alignment of the lower extremity, knee joint stability, patellar tracking, focal tenderness, and the presence or absence of effusion. With patellofemoral problems, knee joint-line

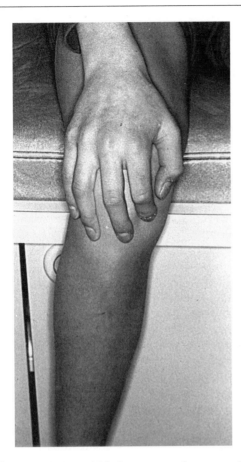

Fig. 9   The grab sign, which demonstrates the non-specific location of anterior knee pain.

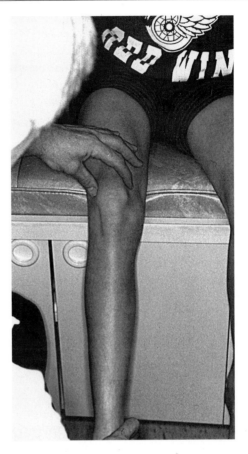

Fig. 10   Evaluation of active and passive patellar tracking by direct, *en face* observation.

tenderness is usually located anteriorly and not at the middle or posterior aspects, as is commonly seen with meniscal injuries. Quadriceps, hamstring, and hip muscle strength should be assessed. Patellar tracking is best seen when the examiner is seated in front of the patient and takes the knee through a full passive and active range of motion (Fig. 10). Much has been made recently of the concept of passive patellar tilt and glide. Because the patella follows an active toroidal path, and not simply one of flexion and extension, such motions are important, but normative values for each of these patellar motions have not been established.[50] Because anterior knee symptoms are usually bilateral, with the intensity varying from side to side, the contralateral knee should always be assessed as well.

Patellofemoral crepitus does not indicate knee pathology, especially in young people. In reviewing the findings in 123 young adult medical students, Abernethy and associates[51] found asymptomatic patellofemoral crepitus in more than 60%, with only four (3%) having true chronic anterior knee discomfort. Factors remote from the knee that can affect the

patellofemoral articulation include excessive tibial rotation and abnormal foot and ankle mechanics, particularly excessive foot pronation.[52]

Fairbank and associates[53] studied mechanical factors that affect the prevalence of knee pain in school children. Joint mobility, Q angle, genu varum, and femoral neck anteversion were not found to be different in patients with anterior knee pain when compared with age-matched control subjects. The single differentiating point between the patients and their symptom-free contemporaries was the increased vigor of participation in sports activities by the patients. In contrast to the patients in that series, many patients with anterior knee symptoms are overweight, unathletic teenagers with little interest in physical activity.

Standard radiographs are usually not helpful in the evaluation of the etiology of anterior knee pain but they do demonstrate patellar size and position. Determination of the patellar ligament-patella ratio to identify patella alta or patella infera may be difficult in skeletally immature patients.[54-56] It has been suggested that a variety of tangential patellar radiographs be used to ascertain the relationship between the patella and its femoral trochlea. Such radiographs are made with the knee in a static position, whereas most tracking abnormalities occur during dynamic use.[57,58]

Once other sources of anterior knee pain have been ruled out, the spectrum of therapy that has been suggested has ranged from nihilism to surgical intervention. Few studies have assessed the natural history of this condition. Goodfellow[59] called chondromalacia a "mythical disease" and equated anterior knee pain in adolescents with the pain of a headache. He believed that surgical intervention for this condition was no more rational than the drilling of burr holes in the skull for a headache. In his series, 94% of the patients without treatment complained of occasional mild knee discomfort but had no actual limitation at a two- to eight-year follow-up, and 45% had had spontaneous improvement of pain. He recommended reassurance of the patient and parents that the disorder is benign.

In most reported, controlled studies, nonsurgical treatment has been extremely successful in 75% to 90% of the patients.[39,45,60-66] Nonsurgical treatment does not mean no treatment. Possible treatment modalities include exercises, contrast therapies, orthoses, and anti-inflammatory medications (Outline 1). The general principles of the treatment of overuse, as already outlined, are used as initial management. The prescription for rehabilitation must be individually tailored, and a single approach for all patients should be avoided. Participation in sports activity is encouraged, and a carte blanche excuse for avoidance of physical education is not appropriate. Restoration of quadriceps and hamstring strength and flexibility with exercises specific for these muscles is an essential part of management. Use of orthotic devices to control abnormal foot and ankle mechanics can also play a role. Contrast therapy may be helpful, as are a variety of anti-inflammatory medications. A number of knee braces have been proposed for the management of anterior knee pain.[67,68] The exact mechanism of such bracing action is unknown, and a marked placebo effect must be considered. Lysholm and associates,[69] in an attempt to study the effect of patellar braces on quadriceps function (as measured by isokinetic testing), found that quadriceps power increased with brace use. However, the authors used extremely low test speeds that were not in the range of routine activity and certainly not as high as those demanded during sports activity. If a patient is unresponsive to a well-monitored program of treatment, one must begin to question the accuracy of the diagnosis and begin to search for other causes, including psychiatric as well as non-orthopaedic origins.[70,71]

So-called chondromalacia patellae appears to have been a disorder awaiting the invention of the arthroscope. Although the role of arthroscopy in the diagnosis and treatment of patellofemoral disorders is commonly discussed among arthroscopic and sports surgery specialty orthopaedists, few objective data are available. Lateral retinacular release, performed in an attempt to improve minor tracking abnormalities, has not been shown radiographically to change the patellar location, tilt, or translation.[51,62,72-74] Arthroscopic procedures about the patellofemoral joint should be done only for documented, objective, preoperative findings and not for pain alone.[75] Of all arthroscopic procedures of the knee, those involving the patella have the highest complication rate.[35,36,76,77] These complications include infection, persistent hemarthrosis, bleeding problems secondary to laceration of the geniculate artery, reflex sympathetic dystrophy, and neural injury.

A major factor in the management of idiopathic anterior knee pain is the reassurance of the patient and family that the nature of these symptoms is benign. For athletes who participate in high-demand sports activity, modification of the training schedule, development of a consistent therapy program, and understanding of the nature of the condition allow continued participation. Again, because of its lack of specificity, the term chondromalacia should not be used for the diagnosis of anterior knee pain. Such pain must be considered idiopathic until the true etiology is known. There is little evidence to suggest that anterior patellofemoral pain in the preteen or adolescent leads to progressive articular cartilage changes or early joint senescence.

In summary, adolescents with symptoms about the anterior aspect of the knee are common visitors to orthopaedic offices. Efforts must be made to diagnose

---

Outline 1
Conservative Treatment Modalities for Anterior Knee Pain

Flexibility Exercises
Quadriceps
Hamstrings
Tensor fascia femoris
Triceps surae

Strengthening Exercises
Quadriceps (short arc)*

Contrast Therapies
Ice massage
Heat

Orthoses
Knee sleeve
Shoe inserts

Medications
Aspirin
Non-steroidal anti-inflammatory drugs

---
* Eccentric quadriceps exercises should be avoided initially because they may cause pain.

the source of such pain; the pain should not be blithely dismissed as being the result of so-called chondromalacia. Such pain must be considered idiopathic until a more specific and accurate diagnosis can be made. The diagnosis of idiopathic chondromalacia patellae should be uncommon when accurate diagnostic methods are employed. The term chondromalacia is nonspecific and should be eliminated as a diagnosis except in circumstances where true gross changes of the patellar articular surface are seen and documented as the source of pain. The anterior knee pain of preadolescence should not be equated with the patellofemoral degenerative joint disease seen in middle-aged and older adults.

Sources of pain about the knee may include overuse, tendinitis, patellar instability and maltracking, pathological plica, abnormal (multipartite) patellar formation, and benign and malignant tumors about the knee. It must be remembered that knee pain in skeletally immature patients should be considered to have been caused by hip disease until proved otherwise. With the use of this approach, the diagnosis of slipped capital femoral epiphysis will not be missed. Reflex sympathetic dystrophy should also be considered in any child with knee pain, particularly when the severity of the pain is out of proportion with the injury. Most patients with anterior knee pain respond to diagnosis-specific nonsurgical treatment protocols that eliminate overuse.

References

1. Doskocil M: Formation of the femoropatellar part of the human knee joint. *Folia Morphol (Praha)* 1985;33:38-47.
2. Gardner E, O'Rahilly R: The early development of the knee joint in staged human embryos. *J Anat* 1968;102:289-299.
3. Herring SA, Nilson KL: Introduction to overuse injuries. *Clin Sports Med* 19876:225-239.
4. Leadbetter WB, Buckwalter JA, Gordon SL (eds): *Sports-Induced Inflammation. Clinical and Basic Science Concepts.* Park Ridge, IL, American Academy of Orthopaedic Surgeons, 1990.
5. Micheli LJ: Overuse injuries in children's sports: The growth factor. *Orthop Clin North Am* 1983;14:337-360.
6. Stanitski CL: Common injuries in preadolescent and adolescent athletes: Recommendations for prevention. *Sportsmed* 1989;7:32-41.
7. Stanitski CL: Repetitive stress and connective tissue, in Sullivan JA, Grana WA (eds): *The Pediatric Athlete.* Park Ridge, IL, American Academy of Orthopaedic Surgeons,1988, pp 203-209.
8. Woo SL, Buckwalter JA (eds): *Injury and Repair of the Musculoskeletal Soft Tissues,* ed 2. Park Ridge, IL, American Academy of Orthopaedic Surgeons, 1988, pp 3-13.
9. Kujala UM, Kvist M, Heinonen O: Osgood-Schlatter's disease in adolescent athletes: Retrospective study of incidence and duration. *Am J Sports Med* 1985;13:236-241,1985.
10. Ogden JA, Southwick WO: Osgood-Schlatter's disease and tibial tuberosity development. *Clin Orthop* 1976;116:180-189.
11. Osgood RB: Lesions of the tibial tubercle occurring during adolescence. *Boston Med Surg J* 1903;148:114-117.
12. Schlatter C: Verletzungen des schnabelförmigen Fortsatzes der oberen Tibiaepiphyse. *Beitr Klin Chir* 1903;38:874-887.
13. Krause BL, Williams JP, Catterall A: Natural history of Osgood-Schlatter disease. *J Pediatr Orthop* 1990;10:65-68.
14. Lewis MM, Reilly JF: Sports tumors. *Am J Sports Med* 1987;15:362-365.
15. D'Ambrosia RD, MacDonald GL: Pitfalls in the diagnosis of Osgood-Schlatter disease. *Clin Orthop* 1975;110:206-209.
16. Glynn MK, Regan BF: Surgical treatment of Osgood-Schlatter's disease. *J Pediatr Orthop* 1983;3:216-219.
17. Mital MA, Matza RA, et al: The so-called unresolved Osgood-Schlatter lesion: A concept based on fifteen surgically treated lesions. *J Bone Joint Surg* 1980;62A:732-739.
18. Johansson S: En förut icke beskriven sjukdom i patella. *Hydiea* 1922;84:161-166.
19. Medlar RC, Lyne ED: Sinding-Larsen-Johansson disease: Its etiology and natural history. *J Bone Joint Surg* 1978;60A:1113-1116.
20. Sinding-Larsen MF: A hitherto unknown affection of the patella in children. *Acta Radiol* 1921;1:171-173.
21. Batten J, Menelaus, MB: Fragmentation of the proximal pole of the patella: Another manifestation of juvenile traction osteochondritis? *J Bone Joint Surg* 1985;67B:249-251.
22. Blazina ME, Kerlan RK, Jobe FW, et al: Jumper's knee. *Orthop Clin North Am* 1973;4:665-678.
23. Roels J, Martens, Mulier JC, et al: Patellar tendinitis (jumper's knee). *Am J Sports Med* 1978;6:362-368.
24. Green WT Jr: Painful bipartite patellae: A report of three cases. *Clin Orthop* 1975;110:197-200.
25. Weaver JK: Bipartite patella as a cause of disability in the athlete. *Am J Sports Med* 1977;5:137-143.
26. Echeverria TS, Bersani FA: Acute fracture simulating a symptomatic bipartite patella: Report of a case. *Am J Sports Med* 1980;8:48-50.
27. Bourne MH, Bianco AJ Jr: Bipartite patella in the adolescent: Results of surgical excision. *J Pediatr* 1990;10:69-73.
28. Ogden JA, McCarthy SM, Jokl P: The painful bipartite patella. *J Pediatr Orthop* 1982;2:263-269.
29. Hardaker WT, Whipple TL, Bassett FH III: Diagnosis and treatment of the plica syndrome of the knee. *J Bone Joint Surg* 1980;62A:221-225.
30. Patel D: Arthroscopy of the plicae-synovial folds and their significance. *Am J Sports Med* 1978;6:217-225.
31. Patel D: Plica as a cause of anterior knee pain. *Orthop Clin North Am* 1986;17:273-277.
32. Broom MJ, Fulkerson JP: The plica syndrome: A new perspective. *Orthop Clin North Am* 1986;17:279-281.
33. Pipkin G: Lesions of the suprapatellar plica. *J Bone Joint Surg* 1950;32A:363-369.
34. DeLee J.: RSD following arthroscopic surgery. *Arthroscopy* 1985;1:214-218.
35. Small, NC: An analysis of complications in lateral retinacular release procedures. *J Arthroscopy* 189;5:282-286.
36. Youmans WT: Surgical complications of the patellofemoral articulation. *Clin Sports Med* 1989;8:331-342
37. Bernstein BH, Singsen BH, Kent JT, et al: Reflex neurovascular dystrophy in childhood. *J Pediatr* 1978;93:211-215.
38. Ficat RP, Hungerford DS: *Disorders of the Patellofemoral Joint.* Baltimore, MD, Williams & Wilkins, 1977.
39. Fulkerson J, Hungerford D: *Disorders of the Patellofemoral Joint.* Baltimore, MD, Williams & Wilkins, 1990.
40. Olsson GL, Arnér S, Hirsch G: Reflex sympathetic dystrophy in children, in Tyler DC, Krane EJ (eds): *Advances in Pain Research and Therapy.* New York, NY, Raven Press, 1990, vol 15, pp 323-331.
41. Ruggeri SB, Athreya BH, Doughty R; et al: Reflex sympathetic dystrophy in children. *Clin Orthop* 1982;163:225-230.

42. Schutzer SF, Gossling HR: The treatment of reflex sympathetic dystrophy syndrome. *J Bone Joint Surg* 1984;66A:625-629.

43. Wilder RT, Berde CB, Wolohan M, et al: Reflex sympathetic dystrophy in children: Clinical characteristics and follow-up of seventy patients. *J Bone Joint Surg* 1992;74A:910-919.

44. Goldsmith DP, Vivino FB, Eichenfield AH, et al: Nuclear imaging and clinical features of childhood reflex neurovascular dystrophy: Comparison with adults. *Arthritis Rheum* 1989;32:480-485.

45. Radin EL: A rational approach to the treatment of patellofemoral pain. *Clin Orthop* 1979;144:107-109.

46. Fulkerson JP: Evaluation of the peripatellar soft tissues and retinaculum in patients with patellofemoral pain. *Clin Sports Med* 1989;8:197-202.

47. Fulkerson JP, Tennant R, Jaivin JS, et al: Histologic evidence of retinacular nerve injury associated with patellofemoral malalignment. *Clin Orthop* 1985;197:196-205.

48. Kransdorf MJ, Moser RP Jr, Vinh TN, et al: Primary tumors of the patella: A review of 42 cases. *Skeletal Radiol* 1989;18:365-371.

49. Roy DR, Greene WB, Gamble JG: Osteomyelitis of the patella in children. *J Pediatr Orthop* 1991;11:364-366.

50. Kolowich PA, Paulos LE, Rosenberg TD, et al: Lateral release of the patella: Indications and contraindications. *Am J Sports Med* 1990;18:359-365.

51. Abernethy PJ, Townsend PR, Rose RM, et al: Is chondromalacia patellae a separate clinical entity? *J Bone Joint Surg* 1978;60B:205-210.

52. Fulkerson JP, Shea KP: Disorders of patellofemoral alignment. *J Bone Joint Surg* 1990;72A:1424-1429.

53. Fairbank JC, Pynsent PB, van Poortvliet JA, et al: Mechanical factors in the incidence of knee pain in adolescents and young adults. *J Bone Joint Surg* 1984;66B:685-693.

54. Grelsamer RP, Meadows S: The modified Insall-Salvati ratio for assessment of patellar height. *Clin Orthop* 1992;282:170-176.

55. Insall J, Salvati E: Patella position in the normal knee joint. *Radiology* 1971;101:101-104.

56. Koshino T, Sugimoto K: New measurement of patellar height in the knees of children. *J Pediatr Orthop* 1989;9:216-218.

57. Laurin CA, Dussault R, Levesque HP: The tangential x-ray investigation of the patellofemoral joint: x-ray technique, diagnostic criteria and their interpretation. *Clin Orthop* 1979;144:16-26.

58. Merchant AC, Mercer RL, Jacobsen RH, et al: Roentgenographic analysis of patellofemoral congruence. *J Bone Joint Surg* 1974;56A:1391-1396.

59. Goodfellow JW: Chondromalacia patella: A mythical disease?, in Proceedings of the South African Orthopaedic Association. *J Bone Joint Surg* 1984;66B:455-456.

60. Busch MT, DeHaven KE: Pitfalls of the lateral retinacular release. *Clin Sports Med* 1989;8:279-290.

61. Dehaven KE, Dolan WA, Mayer PJ: Chondromalacia patellae in athletes: Clinical presentation and conservative management. *Am J Sports Med* 1979;7:5-11.

62. Insall J: Current concepts review: Patellar pain. *J Bone Joint Surg* 1982;64A:147-152.

63. Micheli LJ, Stanitski CL: Lateral patellar retinacular release. *Am J Sports Med* 1981;9:330-336.

64. Sandow MJ, Goodfellow JW: The natural history of anterior knee pain in adolescents. *J Bone Joint Surg* 1985;67B:36-38.

65. Stougard J: Chondromalacia of the patella: Physical signs in relation to operative findings. *Acta Orthop Scand* 1975;46:685-694.

66. Yates C, Grana WA: Patellofemoral pain: A prospective study. *Orthopedics* 1986;9:663-667.

67. Bennett JG, Stauber WT: Evaluation and treatment of anterior knee pain using eccentric exercise. *Med Sci Sports Exerc* 1986;18:526-530.

68. Levine J, Splain S: Use of the infrapatella strap in the treatment of patellofemoral pain. *Clin Orthop* 1979;139:179-181.

69. Lysholm J, Nordin M, Ekstrand J, et al: The effect of a patella brace on performance in a knee extension strength test in patients with patellar pain. *Am J Sports Med* 1984;12:110-112.

70. Ehrlich MG, Zaleske DJ: Pediatric orthopedic pain of unknown origin. *J Pediatr* 1986;6:460-468.

71. Palumbo PM Jr: Dynamic patellar brace: A new orthosis in the management of patellofemoral disorders: A preliminary report. *Am J Sports Med* 1981;9:45-49.

72. Merchant AC, Mercer RL: Lateral release of the patella: A preliminary report. *Clin Orthop* 1974;103:40-45.

73. O'Neill DB, Micheli LJ, Warner JP: Patellofemoral stress: A prospective analysis of exercise treatment in adolescents and adults. *Am J Sports Med* 1992;20:151-156.

74. Pillemer FG, Micheli LJ: Psychological considerations in youth sports. *Clin Sports Med* 1988;7:679-689.

75. Joyce MJ, Mankin HJ: Caveat arthroscopos: Extra-articular lesions of bone stimulating intra-articular pathology of the knee. *J Bone Joint Surg* 1983;65A:289-292.

76. Ceder LC, Larson RL: Z-plasty lateral retinacular release for the treatment of patellar compression syndrome. *Clin Orthop* 1979;144:110-113.

77. Dugdale TW, Barnett PR: Historical background: Patellofemoral pain in young people. *Orthop Clin North Am* 1986;17:211-219.

Back Pain in Children

George H. Thompson, MD

Back pain in children (especially pre-adolescents) that persists for more than one to two weeks is often due to organic causes[1-6]; this is in contrast to back pain in adults, which is frequently mechanical or psychological in origin. Hensinger,[2] in a study of 100 skeletally immature patients who had back pain of at least two months' duration, found that 84 patients had evidence of underlying pathology: 33 had an occult fracture, spondylolysis, or spondylolisthesis; 33 had kyphosis or scoliosis; and 18 had an infection or a tumor. In the remaining 16 patients, there was no definitive diagnosis. In many of these children, the etiology of the back pain was not apparent on the first visit, and additional evaluations and studies were necessary to establish the diagnosis. A careful history should be elicited and a thorough physical examination should be performed on every child who presents with back pain.[1-4]

Initial Examination

History

When the history is elicited, many variables must be recorded: the nature of the onset of the pain; the location, character, and radiation of the pain; the duration of the symptoms; the normal level of activity; the antecedent factors, such as injuries; the general health and developmental history; the scholastic progress; the family history; and whether there are systemic symptoms, such as fever or weight loss, or neurologic symptoms, such as muscle weakness, sensory changes, or bowel or bladder dysfunction.

Physical Examination

Physical examination includes a complete musculoskeletal and neurologic evaluation. Spinal alignment, mobility, muscle spasm, and areas of tenderness are evaluated and recorded. The neurologic examination involves assessment of gait, balance, coordination, and muscle strength. It also includes sensory evaluation, such as reactions to pain and light touch, deep-tendon reflexes, and pathological reflexes such as the Babinski sign. It is important to record the presence of even the most subtle differences from normal. Physicians must thoroughly evaluate a child who presents with: (1) persistent or increasing pain; (2) systemic symptoms such as fever, malaise, or weight loss; (3) neurologic symptoms or findings; (4) bowel or bladder dysfunction; (5)

a young age, especially one of less than 4 years (a tumor should be suspected); or (6) a painful, left thoracic curvature of the spine.[2] Gynecologic consultation may be indicated in premenarchal adolescent girls with persistent low back pain, in order to rule out a diagnosis of hematocolpos due to an imperforate hymen, which has been reported as a rare cause of low back pain.[7]

Radiographic Assessment

Posteroanterior and lateral standing radiographs of the entire length of the spine should be made. In addition, right and left oblique views of the involved area are obtained. Additional views may be necessary, depending on the history, location of the pain, findings on physical examination, and differential diagnoses being considered. Flexion and extension views, especially when the pain is located in the cervical or lumbar spine, may be useful in the evaluation of mobility and instability. Other imaging procedures that can be used in the evaluation of back pain include: technetium bone scans, computed tomography scans, laminagrams, metrizamide myelograms, and magnetic resonance imaging scans. Magnetic resonance imaging is indicated when intraspinal pathology is suspected. Each of these five types of scans should be used only for very specific reasons—either to substantiate a particular diagnosis or in the face of persistent symptoms.

Laboratory Evaluation

Laboratory tests must include a complete blood-cell count and measurement of the erythrocyte sedimentation rate. Tests for rheumatoid factor, antinuclear antibodies, and human leukocyte antigen B27 are indicated only when an infection or an inflammatory disorder is suspected. Extensive initial laboratory testing as a routine procedure is unnecessary and not very useful. However, if a myelogram is obtained, the cerebrospinal fluid must be analyzed.[8]

Differential Diagnosis

The differential diagnosis of pediatric back pain includes congenital, developmental, traumatic, infectious, systemic, arthritic, neoplastic (benign and malignant), and psychogenic causes (Outline 1). Winter[6] stated that Scheuermann's disease is the most common cause of pain in the thoracic and thoracolumbar

Outline 1
Differential Diagnoses of Back Pain in Children

Congenital
    Diastematomyelia
    Cervical spine anomalies

Developmental
    Painful scoliosis
    Kyphosis (Scheuermann's disease)

Traumatic
    Occult fractures
    Muscle strain
    Spondylolysis and spondylolisthesis
    Herniated disk
    Slipped vertebral apophysis
    Upper cervical spine instability

Infectious
    Diskitis
    Vertebral osteomyelitis
    Tuberculosis

Systemic diseases
    Chronic infection
    Storage diseases
    Juvenile osteoporosis

Juvenile arthritis
    Rheumatoid arthritis
    Ankylosing spondylitis

Neoplastic (benign and malignant)
    Benign
        Osteoid-osteoma
        Osteoblastoma
        Aneurysmal bone cyst
        Eosinophilic granuloma
    Malignant
        Osteogenic sarcoma
        Spinal cord tumor
        Metastatic
    Psychogenic

regions of the back, while spondylolysis or spondylolisthesis is the most common cause in the lumbar and lumbosacral regions. However, all of the diagnostic categories must be considered in children and adolescents who have back pain.

Congenital

Back pain due to congenital abnormalities of the spine is uncommon. Occasionally, congenital defects in the cervical spine in association with Klippel-Feil syndrome,[9] diastematomyelia in the thoracic spine, and defects in the lumbar spine such as congenital absence of a pedicle[10] may be associated with pain. Pain associated with Klippel-Feil syndrome is usually due to hypermobility or instability of the adjacent vertebral segment or to degenerative osteoarthrosis.[11] Diastematomyelia, which is frequently associated with a cutaneous malformation overlying the defect, is more likely to present with neurologic abnormalities involving the lower extremities, such as a unilateral cavus foot or calf atrophy, rather than with back pain.[12] Plain

roentgenograms are only occasionally diagnostic, although widening of the interpedicular distance may be indicative of an associated diastematomyelia. Magnetic resonance imaging studies provide the most definitive evidence of the pathology.[13,14] Computed tomography combined with myelography can also be informative. Malformations of the sacrum or a lack of integrity of the posterior structures may also predispose to spondylolysis and pain.[15]

Developmental

Idiopathic Scoliosis Idiopathic scoliosis in children should be considered a painless disorder. Scoliosis associated with back pain should arouse suspicion of an underlying problem, such as infection, diskitis, or a tumor. The majority of idiopathic curvatures are right thoracic curves. Left thoracic curvatures are uncommon and are often associated with an underlying abnormality[16] (Fig. 1). Coonrad and associates[16] found only 27 left thoracic curve patterns in 1,662 consecutive patients with apparent idiopathic scoliosis; however, nine (33%) of the 27 patients were found to have a definite neurogenic etiology, including an occult syrinx, a spinal cord tumor, a neuromuscular disorder, or another condition. A patient who has a painful left thoracic curvature should have an extensive musculoskeletal and neurologic evaluation. Depending on the child's symptoms, a technetium bone scan or magnetic resonance imaging may be necessary. The former is indicated when an osseous abnormality is suspected. If a spinal cord tumor or an intraspinal abnormality is suspected, magnetic resonance imaging is the procedure of choice. An asymptomatic left thoracic curve in a patient who had normal findings on neurologic examination can be managed according to the magnitude of the curve.

Scheuermann's Disease Children who have Scheuermann's disease often present with pain, which is usually located over the apex of the kyphosis but which also can be in the lower lumbar spine, especially if marked lumbar lordosis is present. Scheuermann's disease is the most common cause of structural kyphosis of the thoracic or thoracolumbar spine in skeletally immature adolescents.[17-19] There is usually a strong hereditary tendency. The etiology is not known; it is possible that the kyphosis develops first and the vertebral changes, as seen on plain radiographs, are a secondary change.[17] Pain may be aggravated by standing, sitting, and physical activity, and it usually subsides with cessation of growth unless there is a severe residual deformity. The diagnosis of Scheuermann's disease is based on the physical findings of kyphosis, poor posture, and 5° of wedging or more of at least three vertebrae at the apex of the kyphosis, as seen on the lateral standing roentgenogram.[19] The apex of the deformity is usually located at the level of the disk space between

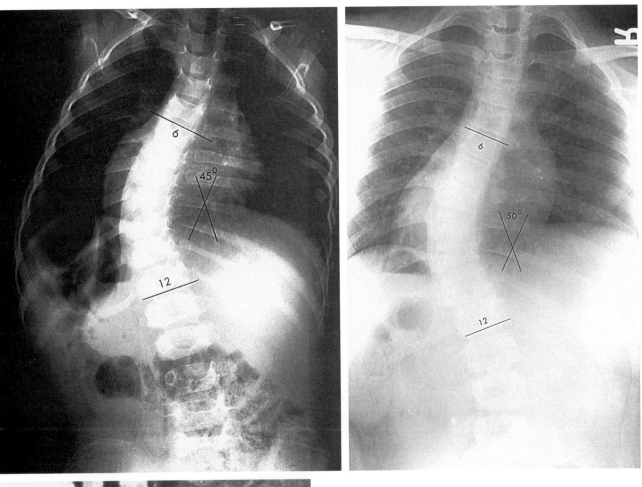

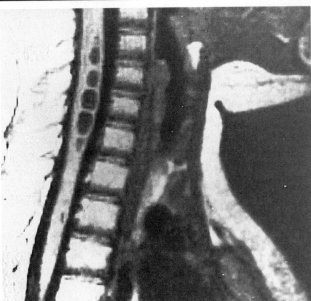

Fig. 1 A 15-month-old boy who had idiopathic infantile scoliosis and no pain. **Top left**, Standing posteroanterior radiograph of the spine, showing a 45° left thoracic scoliosis from T6 to T12. **Top right**, Ten years later and after prolonged orthotic management, the curve measures 50°. The patient remained asymptomatic and was neurologically normal. **Bottom**, A magnetic resonance imaging scan, made at the same time as the radiograph at top right, revealed a syrinx involving his cervical spinal cord. The syrinx did not expand, but the curve continued to progress slowly. The patient later underwent a successful posterior spinal fusion and Cotrel-Dubousset instrumentation.

the seventh and eighth thoracic vertebrae.[18] A kyphotic angle of greater than 45° is considered to be abnormal. Schmorl nodes are often present, along with irregularity and flattening of the vertebral end-plates and narrowing of the vertebral disk spaces. There is a varying degree of scoliosis in approximately one-third of patients.[18] A lateral roentgenogram, made with the patient lying supine over a bolster in order to hyperextend the spine, often reveals the deformity to be structural. Associated neurologic deficits are uncommon. The increased lumbar lordosis results in abnormal shear stress in the lower lumbar pars interarticularis, especially at the fifth lumbar level, causing an increased prevalence of spondylolysis in patients who have Scheuermann's disease.[15,20]

The treatment of Scheuermann's disease is based on the severity of the deformity, the presence of pain, and the age of the patient. Usually, skeletally immature adolescents with a kyphotic deformity of less than 50° and no evidence of progression need only observation.[17] Exercises to decrease lumbar lordosis, to correct hamstring-muscle contractures, and to correct the kyphosis by hyperextension of the thoracic spine may be effective in adolescents who are being treated with bracing and in those who have back pain.[18] Adolescents with a progressive deformity (usually greater than 60° or 65°) or persistent pain, or both[17] can usually be managed successfully with a Milwaukee brace, especially if the treatment is initiated before skeletal maturity. Partial reversal of the vertebral wedging may be noted on radiographs following 12 to 18 months of full-time bracing (22 hours per day). Sachs and associates[18] reported that 76 (69%) of 110 adolescents with Scheuermann's kyphosis who wore a Milwaukee brace consistently, who participated in an exercise program, and who were followed for at least five years had a permanent decrease of the deformity. There was no change in ten patients and, in 24 patients (22%), the deformity became worse. Patients who had an initial kyphosis of greater than 74° were most likely to have progression of the deformity.[18] Operative treatment is rarely necessary for patients who have Scheuermann's disease. Occasionally, patients with a severe deformity (75° or more), as well as those who have a deformity associated with persistent back pain that is unresponsive to conservative treatment, may be considered for operative intervention.[18]

Traumatic

Occult Fractures Occult fractures typically occur after minor injuries, such as falls during sports-related activities. They can also occur after more severe trauma, although they may not be readily apparent. The injuries usually involve the pars interarticularis or the transverse or spinous processes, and they are often not visible on plain radiographs. If the patient has persistent pain, additional studies, such as a technetium bone scan, may be useful for localization of an occult fracture. Additional information can be obtained with tomography or computed tomographic scanning. Treatment is usually conservative, with restriction of activities until the acute symptoms have resolved, followed by institution of a rehabilitation program. Occasionally, immobilization with an orthosis is neces-

sary to relieve pain. Although most occult fractures heal spontaneously, fractures of the facets may be potentially unstable. Therefore, it is important to make an accurate diagnosis. A word of caution: every injury does not have to be evaluated with use of all available studies. Care and discretion should be exercised when back pain in children is being evaluated.

Muscle Strain Muscle strain is easily diagnosed on the basis of the history, the physical examination, and a normal radiograph. The condition is usually the result of a direct contusion or of an overuse syndrome in sports-related activities. Improper conditioning and too-rapid advances in terms of the level of play are common causes of muscle strain. Recurrence is prevented by restriction of activities until the symptoms have resolved, followed by the use of proper training techniques.

Spondylolysis and Spondylolisthesis These are common causes of low back pain in adolescents.[6,15,21-27] The most widely accepted classification of the defect, which occurs in approximately 6% of the general population,[28] was proposed by Wiltse and associates,[27] in 1976. The dysplastic (type-I) and isthmic (type-II) forms occur most commonly in children and adolescents. The origin of spondylolysis is currently believed to be a stress or fatigue fracture of the pars interarticularis, which can occur at physiologic loads during cyclic flexion and extension movements of the lumbar spine. This may account for the increased prevalence of spondylolysis in female gymnasts or other athletes involved in repetitive hyperextension maneuvers. Female gender is associated with an increased risk of severe displacement, an earlier increase in the deformity, and more clinical symptoms. It is not known why gender is a risk factor.[15]

Back pain due to spondylolysis or spondylolisthesis commonly develops in late childhood or adolescence and is usually mild. When present, the pain is localized in the low back and, to a lesser extent, in the posterior aspect of the buttocks and thighs. Symptoms are usually initiated or aggravated by strenuous activities, particularly those that require repetitive flexion and extension of the lumbar spine, such as rowing, gymnastics, diving, playing hockey, and pitching a baseball. Symptoms are usually decreased by rest and by restriction of activities. Neurologic symptoms or deficits are uncommon except in severe spondylolisthesis.[22,23,25] Symptomatic adolescents often have tight hamstrings, which result in a gait that is peculiar to children who have spondylolisthesis.[15,21,25,29] Tight hamstring muscles tilt the pelvis backward and limit hip flexion, resulting in a stiff-legged gait with a short stride length. Physical examination may also demonstrate increased lumbar lordosis and tenderness to palpation over the lumbar spinous processes and paraspinous muscles.[25] Distortion of the pelvis and trunk becomes clinically apparent only when the degree of slippage is moderate or severe. Of adolescents who have symptomatic spondylolisthesis, 25% to 50% have an associated scoliosis.[21,23]

The diagnosis of spondylolysis or spondylolisthesis can usually be made on routine posteroanterior and lateral standing radiographs of the lumbar spine, with the lateral view being especially useful. The most common site of involvement is the area between the fifth lumbar and the first sacral segment. An associated spina bifida occulta is a common finding.[21,24,28] In spondylolysis, oblique radiographs of the lumbar spine are frequently necessary to allow visualization of the pars interarticularis. If there is a history of a previous injury, an acute fracture may be present (Fig. 2) and the defect in the pars interarticularis is narrow with irregular edges. In contrast, the edges of long-standing defects are smooth and rounded, and a pseudarthrosis is usually present. When a spondylolysis is suspected clinically but cannot be confirmed on radiographs, a technetium bone scan can be helpful for the determination of whether there is a lesion and, if there is, whether the lesion is acute or chronic.[30] Bodner and associates[31] found single photon emission computed tomography (SPECT) to be more sensitive than technetium bone scans in the diagnosis of stress fractures or stress reactions in the spine, such as spondylolysis. Computed tomography, magnetic resonance imaging, and myelography are rarely indicated except in severe spondylolisthesis or when the diagnosis is not known.[15,22]

Vertebral displacement in spondylolisthesis is usually measured according to the technique of Meyerding.[32] Grade I is displacement between 0 and 25%; grade II, between 26% and 50%; grade III, between 51% and 75%; and grade IV, between 76% and 100%. Other measurements, such as sacral inclination and slip angle, have been used in the assessment of spondylolisthesis.[33]

Symptomatic spondylolysis is treated on an outpatient basis. An acute fracture may heal after a period of immobilization in a Risser cast or a spinal orthosis. A unilateral pars interarticularis fracture is more likely to heal than a bilateral fracture. Restriction of activities, rest, and strengthening exercises for the muscles of the back and abdomen are relatively successful in controlling symptoms in adolescents who have long-standing spondylolisthesis associated with mild backache and tight hamstrings.[34] It is important that all children with spondylolysis be followed clinically and radiographically, usually at four- to six-month intervals, for possible progression to spondylolisthesis. The majority of children who have spondylolysis are asymptomatic, and the presence of back pain requires consideration of other causes of back pain. Development and progression of spondylolisthesis is more commonly seen in female patients, especially those with a dysplastic (type-I) spondylolisthesis; in adolescents with early onset of spondylolisthesis; in the presence of a severe degree of slippage (grade III or IV) at the time of the initial diagnosis; and in association with an increased sacral inclination.[15,22,26,28,35-37]

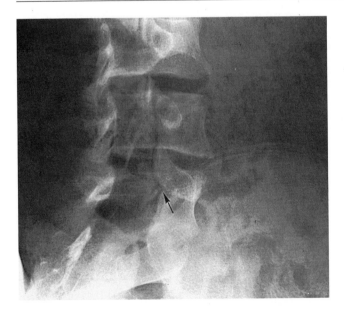 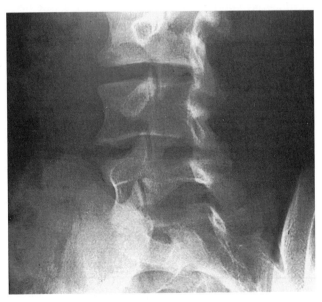

Fig. 2 Left, Left oblique radiograph of the lumbosacral spine in a 15-year-old boy with a one-week history of left-sided low back pain following an injury sustained during football practice. There is a fracture of the pars interarticularis at L5 (arrow) and a fracture of the inferior articular facet of L4. **Right,** A right oblique lumbosacral radiograph does not demonstrate a pars interarticularis fracture on this side.

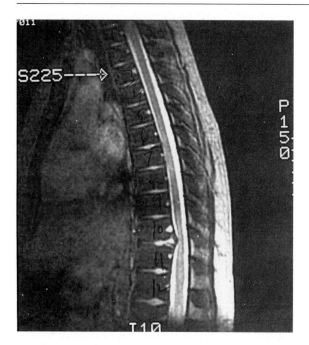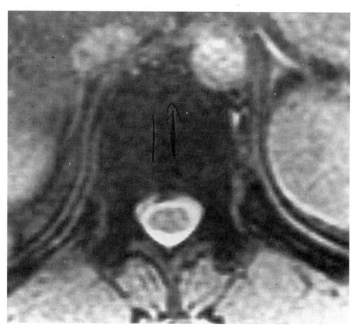

Fig. 3 **Left**, Magnetic resonance imaging of the thoracic spine in a 12-year-old boy who engaged in wrestling as a sports activity and who had a six-month history of lower thoracic back pain. The plain radiographs and neurologic examination were normal. There is slippage of the inferior ring apophysis of T10. **Right**, Axial view shows only slight narrowing of the spinal canal. The patient was treated with restriction of activities for two months followed by a conditioning program in physical therapy. One year later, he had no back pain.

Symptomatic treatment may be considered for grade-I and II spondylolisthesis.[21,24,34,36,37] Bell and associates[21] reported relief of pain and no evidence of progression in 28 patients who had grade-I or II spondylolisthesis and had been treated with an antilordotic total-contact orthosis and exercises for a mean of 25 months. They attributed the success of the treatment to a decrease in lumbar lordosis and sacral inclination when the patients were wearing the brace. However, with persistent symptoms or evidence of radiographic progression, operative intervention may be necessary.[22,23,25,34,38] Pizzutillo and Hummer[34] reported that adolescents who had painful grade-III or IV spondylolisthesis responded poorly to conservative management and often required operative intervention.

Herniated Disk A herniated disk can occur in children, although it is relatively uncommon. Back pain is the major symptom and a positive straight-leg-raising test (the Lasègue sign) is the most common physical finding.[38-42] The back pain is typically increased by activity and relieved by rest. Neurologic symptoms or findings are uncommon.[41] Herniations are most common at the disk spaces between the fourth and fifth lumbar vertebrae and between the fifth lumbar and first sacral vertebrae. Disk-space narrowing is uncommon, and plain radiographs are usually normal. There can be associat-ed congenital anomalies in the lumbosacral area in children with a herniated disk.[39-42] These include transitional vertebrae, spinal stenosis, lateral recess stenosis, and spina bifida. A herniated disk can be diagnosed with magnetic resonance imaging studies, computed tomographic scans, or myelography. Conservative management, including restriction of activities, bed rest, and administration of analgesic medication, should be tried initially. If there is no relief of the pain, or if there are persistent neurologic symptoms, then operative intervention may be necessary.[39-42] This is especially true when there are associated congenital anomalies.

Slipped Vertebral Apophysis This typically occurs in adolescents, especially boys, and is associated with heavy lifting and vigorous physical activities (Fig. 3). Typically, the ring apophysis with the adjacent disk is displaced into the vertebral canal. The patient typically has signs and symptoms of an acute herniated disk, and the radiograph may show a small bone fragment (which represents the edge of the ring apophysis) within the spinal canal. The diagnosis is best made with imaging studies or with myelography. The most common location of a slipped vertebral apophysis is in the lower lumbar spine. Conservative treatment is usually unsuccessful, and most patients require operative excision of the disk and ring apophysis.

Diskitis

Diskitis is a benign, self-limiting inflammation or infection of an intervertebral disk space or a vertebral end-plate.[43] Most authors have considered diskitis to be an osteomyelitis of the vertebral end-plate that invades the disk secondarily, without producing acute osteomyelitis of the vertebral body.[44-48] Other authors, however, have suggested that it is an inflammatory response secondary to trauma.[49,50] It occurs primarily in younger children, and the lumbar spine is the most common location. The child typically complains of back pain and refuses to flex the spine. Young children may also complain of hip or abdominal pain and may refuse to stand or walk.[43,48] They may be able to flex the trunk at the hips, but they will not flex the spine. Localized tenderness in the lumbar region is a common finding.

Diskitis differs from other types of osteomyelitis, as there are usually no systemic symptoms. Affected children are typically afebrile and have a normal white blood cell count.[43,45,48] The erythrocyte sedimentation rate is usually elevated, although not dramatically. Plain radiographs of the spine may not be diagnostic early in the disease process, as there may have been inadequate time for the development of the characteristic changes of disk-space narrowing or of irregularity involving the adjacent vertebral end-plates.[43,45] A technetium bone scan, which demonstrates increased uptake of the isotope in the infected disk space, may be useful in the early diagnosis of diskitis.[43,48,51] Computed tomography and magnetic resonance imaging scans may also be helpful.[43,52] Szalay and associates,[52] in 1987, reported that magnetic resonance imaging studies were more sensitive than technetium bone scans with respect to the demonstration of diskitis prior to the development of radiographic changes. Green and Edwards[45] recommended that, when abnormalities are visible on plain radiographs, lateral tomograms of the spine should be done, as they eliminate overlying bowel gas and other soft-tissue shadows that may obscure the lumbar spine.

When a causative organism can be identified, it is most commonly *Staphylococcus aureus*. Unfortunately, blood cultures to identify the infecting organism are infrequently done because of the morbidity associated with a needle biopsy of the spine. A biopsy is indicated only for children who fail to respond to nonoperative management, and for older children and adolescents in whom a different organism may be suspected.[43,45,48] Most children are treated empirically with systemic administration of antibiotics and with rest.[45,47,48] Use of spinal immobilization with a cast or orthosis depends on the severity of the symptoms. Crawford and associates[43] recommended that antibiotics be used only when symptomatic treatment, such as immobilization, has failed. They found that, in 36 consecutive children with diskitis, the infection healed satisfactorily, regardless of the treatment.

Juvenile Arthritis

Pain in the cervical spine may occasionally be the presenting symptom for juvenile rheumatoid arthritis, and pain in the thoracic spine, for juvenile ankylosing spondylitis.[51,53] However, the spine is rarely the only site of involvement, and careful evaluation frequently shows that other joints have been affected. Limitation of neck motion in juvenile rheumatoid arthritis and decreased chest expansion in ankylosing spondylitis are the common findings on physical examination and they may precede radiographic changes. Hensinger[51] reported that back pain was uncommon in children who had juvenile rheumatoid arthritis and that, when it was present, there were relatively few radiographic changes. They suggested that, if a child has severe pain, other causes of back pain must also be considered. Laboratory studies often help in the establishment of the diagnosis. A child who has juvenile arthritis should be treated by a pediatric rheumatologist. However, an increased prevalence of scoliosis has been reported in these children, and periodic orthopaedic evaluation is also indicated.[54]

Tumors

Back pain may be the presenting complaint in children who have a tumor involving the vertebral column or the spinal cord. However, other common presenting symptoms include weakness of the lower extremities, a limp, scoliosis, and loss of sphincter control. Benign and malignant tumors can be a cause of back pain, and the thoracic and lumbar regions are the most common sites of involvement in the spine. Fraser and associates[8] found changes on the radiographs of 22 of 40 children who had a spinal tumor. Common radiographic findings included erosion of the neural arch, erosion of the vertebral body, tumor shadow, paraspinal calcifications, and widening of the spinal canal.[8]

Benign Tumors The majority of tumors of the spine in children are benign, in contrast with spinal tumors in adults, which are most often malignant. Children who have a spinal tumor can present with back pain, with a painful non-structural scoliosis, and with or without neurologic deficits. In 1990, Delamarter and associates[55] reported that only 41 (2%) of 1,917 musculoskeletal lesions were primary osseous lesions of the spine (cervical, thoracic, and lumbar) and had been noted on plain radiographs. In this series, eight patients who had a thoracic or lumbar spinal lesion had open epiphyses, and seven of them had a benign lesion. The most common benign osseous tumors of the spine are osteoblastoma, osteoid-osteoma, solitary bone cyst, and eosinophilic granuloma.[29,56-60]

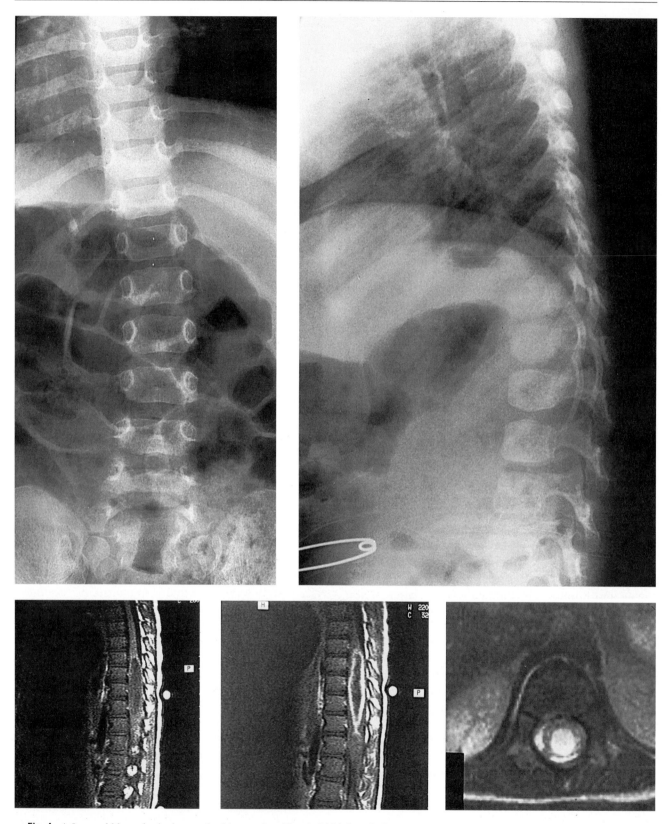

Fig. 4   A 2-year-old boy who had a two-day history of a stiff, painful back and who refused to stand or walk. He was afebrile and the neurologic examination was normal. **Top left**, Sitting anteroposterior radiograph showing mild thoracolumbar scoliosis without any signs of rotation. **Top right**, Lateral sitting radiograph showing mild straightening of the spine, especially in the lumbar region. **Bottom left**, Sagittal magnetic resonance imaging shows a large intramedullary tumor of the thoracic spinal cord. **Bottom center**, Enhanced magnetic resonance imaging following injection of gadolinium allows improved visualization of the tumor. **Bottom right**, Axial computed tomographic scan demonstrating diffuse expansion of the spinal cord. At surgery, the tumor was found to be a grade II astrocytoma.

Osteoid-osteomas, which can occur in the spine, are small and usually sclerotic and they involve the posterior elements. Osteoblastomas, which commonly occur in the spine, are larger and more destructive and they typically involve the pedicles of the thoracic and lumbar vertebrae.[29,31,56] Vertebral body involvement is uncommon. Osteoblastomas that occur in the cervical or thoracic spine can produce spinal cord compression, resulting in neurologic changes.[29] Eosinophilic granuloma typically produces vertebral collapse, resulting in vertebral plana.[58]

When a tumor is suspected but the plain radiographs are normal, a technetium bone scan may be helpful for localization of the lesion. Additional studies, such as laminagrams and imaging studies, may be necessary to further assess the precise location and size of the tumor as well as to determine whether the spinal canal has been compromised. Most benign spinal tumors require excision; however, the symptoms of an osteoid-osteoma are relieved by long-term use of salicylates, and the lesion may spontaneously resolve over time.[56]

Malignant Tumors Malignant tumors involving the spine of a child are uncommon. They can present as a primary osseous lesion, a neurogenic lesion arising from the spinal cord, or a metastatic lesion. Conrad and associates[61] suggested that neuroblastoma, sarcoma, and astrocytoma were the major primary malignant spinal tumors. Between 1970 and 1985, 29 children presented with symptoms suggestive of spinal cord compression that included back pain and neurologic defects.[61] Conrad and associates found that pain was the most consistent finding in children who had a sarcoma, whereas astrocytomas were more likely to be associated with motor weakness (Fig. 4). Gait disturbances and spinal deformity, such as scoliosis, were also commonly observed in children who had astrocytoma. The younger the child at the time of presentation, the higher the prevalence of neuroblastoma.

Most primary malignant tumors of bone can be detected on plain radiographs as areas of osseous destruction and possibly of vertebral collapse. However, Conrad and associates[61] found that soft-tissue tumors were best diagnosed with magnetic resonance imaging studies or computed tomographic studies with myelography. Technetium bone scans were not always helpful.

Acute leukemia can also present as back pain.[62] The most common radiographic abnormalities are osteopenia and compression fractures in the lumbar spine. Hematologic evaluation is usually diagnostic for acute leukemia.[62]

Conclusions

The diagnosis of back pain in children is based on a high index of suspicion of the various possible causes and on a careful evaluation. The question always arises as to how extensive an evaluation should be performed initially, particularly when the symptoms are mild and of short duration. There is no standardized sequence for evaluation, and each child must be assessed individually. The decision regarding testing is based on the history, physical examination, and plain radiographs. If there are no neurologic symptoms or findings and the range of motion and the radiographs of the spine are normal, Turner and associates[5] recommended conservative management with use of medication for relief of pain and a course of physical therapy. More extensive studies are indicated if the back pain persists for one or two months.

References

1. Bunnel WP: Back pain in children. *Orthop Clin North Am* 1982;13:587-604.
2. Hensinger RN: Back pain in children, in Brandord DS, Hensinger RN (eds): *The Pediatric Spine.* New York, NY, Theime Inc, 1985, pp 41-60.
3. King HA: Back pain in children. *Pediatr Clin North Am* 1984;31:1083-1095.
4. King HA: Evaluating the child with back pain. *Pediatr Clin North Am* 196;33:1489-1493.
5. Turner PG, Green JH, Galasko CSB: Back pain in childhood. *Spine* 1989;14:812-814.
6. Winter RB: Spinal problems in pediatric orthopaedics, in Morrissy RT (ed): *Lovell and Winter's Pediatric Orthopaedics,* ed 3. Philadelphia, PA, JB Lippincott, 1990, pp 625-702.
7. Letts M, Haasbeck I: Hematocolpos as a cause of back pain in premenarchal adolescents. *J Pediatr Orthop* 1990;10:731-732.
8. Fraser RD, Peterson DC, Simpson DA: Orthopaedic aspects of spinal tumors in children. *J Bone Joint Surg* 1977;59B:143-151.
9. Kalamchi A, Thompson GH: Congenital anomalies of the spine, in Dee R, Mango E, Hurst LC (eds): *Principles of Orthopaedic Practice.* New York, NY, McGraw-Hill, 1989, pp 838-860.
10. Polly DW Jr, Mason DE: Congenital absence of a lumbar pedicle presenting as back pain in children. *J Pediatr Orthop* 1991;11:214-219.
11. Hensinger RN: Congenital anomalies of the cervical spine. *Clin Orthop* 1991;264:16-38.
12. Rasool MN, Govender S, Naidoo KS, et al: Foot deformities in occult spinal abnormalities in children: A review of 16 cases. *J Pediatr Orthop* 1992;12:94-99.
13. Packer RJ, Zimmerman RA, Sutton LN, et al: Magnetic resonance imaging of spinal cord disease of childhood. *Pediatrics* 1986;78:251-256.
14. Szalay EA, Roach JW, Smith H, et al: Magnetic resonance imaging of the spinal cord in spinal dysraphisms. *J Pediatr Orthop* 1987;7:541-545.
15. Hensinger RN: Current concepts review: Spondylolysis and spondylolisthesis in children and adolescents. *J Bone Joint Surg* 1989;71A:1098-1107.
16. Coonrad RW, Richardson WJ, Oakes WJ: Left thoracic curves can be different. *Orthop Trans* 1985;9:126-127.
17. Lowe TG: Current concepts review: Scheuermann disease. *J Bone Joint Surg* 1990;72A:940-945.
18. Sachs B, Bradford D, Winter R, et al: Scheuermann kyphosis: Follow-up of Milwaukee brace treatment. *J Bone Joint Surg* 1987;69A:50-57.
19. Sorensen KH: *Scheuermann's Juvenile Kyphosis: Clinical*

Appearances, Radiography, Aetiology, and Prognosis. Copenhagen, Munsksgaard, 1964.

20. Ogilvie JW, Sherman J: Spondylysis in Scheuermann's disease. *Spine* 1987;12:251-253.

21. Bell DF, Ehrlich MG, Zalenske DJ: Brace treatment for symptomatic spondylolisthesis. *Clin Orthop* 1988;236:192-198.

22. Boxall D, Bradford DS, Winter RB, et al: Management of severe spondylolisthesis in children and adolescents. *J Bone Joint Surg* 1979;61A:479-495.

23. Burkus JK, Lonstein JE, Winter RB, et al: Long-term evaluation of adolescents treated operatively for spondylolisthesis: A comparison of in-situ arthrodesis only with in-situ arthrodesis and reduction followed by immobilization in a cast. *J Bone Joint Surg* 1992;74A:693-704.

24. Frennered AK, Danielson BI, Nachemson AL: Natural history of symptomatic isthmic low-grade spondylolisthesis in children and adolescents: A seven-year follow-up study. *J Pediatr Orthop* 1991;11:209-213.

25. Landholm TS, Ragni P, Ylikoski M, et al: Lumbar isthemic spondylolisthesis in children and adolescents: Radiographic evaluation and results of operative treatment. *Spine* 1990;15:1350-1355.

26. Seitsalo S: Operative and conservative treatment of moderate spondylolisthesis in young patients. *J Bone Joint Surg* 1990;72B:908-913.

27. Wiltse LL, Newman PH, Macnab I: Classification of spondylolysis and spondylolisthesis. *Clin Orthop* 1976;117:23-29.

28. Fredrickson BE, Baker D, McHolick WJ, et al: The natural history of spondylolysis and spondylolisthesis. *J Bone Joint Surg* 1984;66A:699-707.

29. Boriani S, Capanna R, Donati D, et al: Osteoblastoma of the spine. *Clin Orthop* 1992;278:37-45.

30. VanDenOever M, Merrick MV, Scott JHS: Bone scintigraphy in symptomatic spondylolysis. *J Bone Joint Surg* 1987;69B:453-456.

31. Bodner RJ, Heyman S, Drummond DS, et al: The use of single photon emission computed tomography (SPECT) in the diagnosis of low-back pain in young patients. *Spine* 1988;13:115-1160.

32. Meyerding HW: Spondylolisthesis. *Surg Gynecol Obstet* 1932;54:371-377.

33. Wiltse LL, Winter RB: Terminology and measurement of spondylolisthesis. *J Bone Joint Surg* 1983;65A:768-772.

34. Pizzutillo PD, Hummer CD III: Nonoperative treatment for painful adolescent spondylolysis or spondylolisthesis. *J Pediatr Orthop* 1989;9:538-540.

35. Danielson BI, Frennered AK, Irstram LKH: Radiographic progression of isthmic lumbar spondylolisthesis in young patients. *Spine* 1991;16:422-425.

36. Seitsalo S, Osterman K, Poussa M, et al: Spondylolisthesis in children under 12 years of age: Long-term results of 56 patients treated conservatively or operatively. *J Pediatr Orthop* 1988;8:516-521.

37. Seitsalo S, Osterman K, Hyvarinen H, et al: Progression of spondylolisthesis in children and adolescents: A long-term follow-up of 272 patients. *Spine* 1991,16:417-421.

38. Giroux JC, Leclercq TA: Lumbar disc excision in the second decade. *Spine* 1982;7:168-170.

39. Bradford DS, Garcia A: Herniation of the lumbar intervertebral disk in children and adolescents. *JAMA* 1969;210:2045-2051.

40. DeOrio JK, Bianco AJ Jr: Lumbar disc excision in children and adolescents. *J Bone Joint Surg* 1982;64A:991-996.

41. Epstein JA, Epstein NE, Marc J, et al: Lumbar intervertebral disk herniation in teenage children: Recognition and management of associated anomalies. *Spine* 1984;9:427-432.

42. Kurihara A, Kataoka O: Lumbar disc herniation in children and adolescents: A review of 70 operated cases and their minimum 5 year follow-up studies. *Spine* 1980;5:443-451.

43. Crawford AH, Kucharzyk DW, Ruda R, et al: Diskitis in children. *Clin Orthop* 1991;226:70-79.

44. Boston HC Jr, Bianc, AJ Jr, Rhodes KH: Disk space infection in children. *Orthop Clin North Am* 1975;6:953-964.

45. Green NE, Edwards K: Bone and joint infections in children. *Orthop Clin North Am* 1987;18:155-576.

46. McNeil TW: Spinal infections, in Green WB (ed): *Instructional Course Lectures XXXIX.* Park Ridge, IL, American Academy of Orthopaedic Surgeons, 1990, pp 515-524.

47. Scoles PV, Quinn TP: Intervertebral discitis in children and adolescents. *Clin Orthop* 1982;162:31-36.

48. Wenger DR, Bobechko WP, Gilday DL: The spectrum of intervertebral disc-space infection in children. *J Bone Joint Surg* 1978;60A:100-108.

49. Peterson HA: Disc-space infection in children, in Evarts CMcC (ed): American Academy of Orthopaedic Surgeons *Instructional Course Lectures XXXII.* St. Louis, MO, CV Mosby, 1983, pp 50-60.

50. Spiegel PG, Kengla KW, Isaacson AS, et al: Intervertebral disc-space inflammation in children. *J Bone Joint Surg* 1972;54A:284-296.

51. Hensinger RN, DeVito PD, Ragsdale CG: Changes in the cervical spine in juvenile rheumatoid arthritis. *J Bone Joint Surg* 1986;68A:189-198.

52. Szalay E, Green H, Heller R: Magnetic resonance imaging in the diagnosis of childhood discitis. *J Pediatr Orthop* 1987;7:164-167.

53. Kredich D, Patrone HA: Pediatric spondyloarthropathies. *Clin Orthop* 1990;259:18-22.

54. Ross AC, Edgar MA, Swann M, et al: Scoliosis in juvenile chronic arthritis. *J Bone Joint Surg* 1987;69B:175-178.

55. Delamarter RB, Sachs BL, Thompson GH, et al: Primary neoplasms of the thoracic and lumbar spine: An analysis of 29 conservative cases. *Clin Orthop* 1990;256:87-100.

56. Gitelis S, Schajowicz F: Osteoid osteoma and ostoblastoma. *Orthop Clin North Am* 1989;20:313-325.

57. Healey JH, Ghelman B: Osteoid osteoma and osteoblasoma: Current concepts and recent advances. *Clin Orthop* 196;204:76-85.

58. Makley JT, Carter JR: Eosinophilic granuloma of bone. *Clin Orthop* 1986;204:37-44.

59. Nemoto O, Moser RP, VanDam BE, et al: Osteoblastoma of the spine: A review of 75 cases. *Spine* 1990;15:1272-1280.

60. Tachdjian MD, Matsen DD: Orthopaedic aspects of intraspinal tumors in infants and children. *J Bone Joint Surg* 1965;47A:223-231.

61. Conrad EU III, Olszewski AD, Berger M, et al: Pediatric spine tumors with spinal cord compromise. *J Pediatr Orthop* 1992;12:454-460.

62. Rogalsky RJ, Black GB, Reed MH: Orthopaedic manifestations of leukemia in children. *J Bone Joint Surg* 1986;68A:494-501.

Implant Fixation

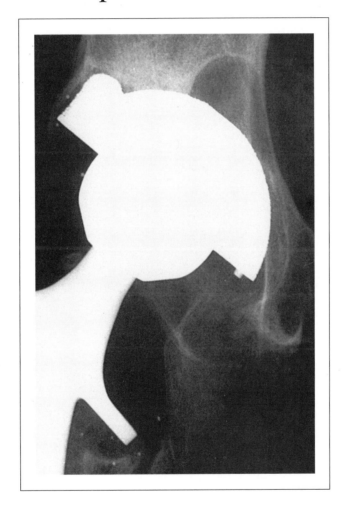

Current Concepts in Orthopaedic Biomaterials and Implant Fixation

Richard J. Friedman, MD, FRCS

Jonathan Black, PhD

Jorge O. Galante, MD, DMSc

Joshua J. Jacobs, MD

Harry B. Skinner, MD, PhD

The technological advances in orthopaedic surgery continue at an unprecedented rate. Many new designs and biomaterials represent not only practical improvements but also possible new problems. Current issues with regard to total joint arthroplasty relate to such topics as which biomaterial should be used in a particular situation, the systemic and remote-site effects of the various biomaterials that are used, and the local response (such as osteolysis) to orthopaedic biomaterials. Despite considerable success in the clinical application of biomaterials, many problems remain unsolved. Clinical and basic research continues in an effort to explore new methods for the enhancement of the bone-prosthesis interface and of long-term implant fixation.

Current Issues in the Design and Use of Biomaterials in Orthopaedic Surgery

Bearing Surfaces

The two early concerns regarding bearing surfaces in joint arthroplasty were the limited life expectancy of the prosthesis as a result of wear necessitating replacement and the loosening torque that results from friction. It is now apparent that the principal problem is the quantity of wear debris that is produced from the bearing surfaces. It has been well documented that this wear debris can be voluminous and that it stimulates cellular osteolysis in the vicinity of the joint, resulting in loosening of the prosthesis.[1-5] Wear debris is produced primarily through three mechanisms: abrasion, adhesion, and fatigue. Wear debris can also act as a stress concentrator, producing secondary three-body wear.

Adhesive wear results when interatomic forces between the mating wear surfaces become greater than the intrinsic forces between the molecules of the bulk material. By this means, material adheres to the opposite surface of the wear couple. This problem primarily affects ultra-high molecular weight polyethylene (UHMWPE), which is transferred to the harder surface with subsequent shedding into the joint space. The major attempt to solve this problem has been to alter the surface that bears on the polyethylene. Very little has been accomplished toward reducing the variability in mechanical or wear properties of medical-grade UHMWPE.[6]

Another aspect of adhesive wear is the adhesion of the passivated layer of oxide on the opposing implant surface to the UHMWPE, resulting in transfer of the passivated layer to the polymer. This material is then essentially a free oxide polishing powder that can accentuate the roughening process of the hard bearing surface. Thus, three-body wear develops, with titanium oxide or cobalt-chromium oxide—instead of cement—as the third body.

Abrasive wear is dependent on contact stress, surface hardness, and surface finish (roughness). Abrasive wear is analogous to the production of sawdust on the surface of wood by sandpaper. A soft surface is abraded by a rougher, harder surface, resulting in debris. Surface roughness is measured in terms of the asperities and depressions of a surface with a profilometer or with a laser technique. The roughness (R) is usually expressed in terms of the average roughness (Ra) or mean distance between peaks and valleys; the peak roughness (Rmax), which is the maximum distance between peaks and valleys; or the root mean square roughness (Rrms), which is the square root of the average of the squares of the peaks and valleys on a surface.[7] Obviously, different values of surface roughness can be obtained with the use of the different methods of calculation and measurement. The measurement of roughness that best predicts minimum wear is a matter of controversy. The surface hardness plays a role because the harder a material is, the longer a smooth surface finish will be maintained.[8] Surface hardness can be increased by various treatments, such as nitriding (the formation of a nitrogen compound on the surface) or ion implantation. For example, the hardness of Ti-6Al-4V (Table 1) can be increased more than twofold by this method. The acceleration of nitrogen ions into the surface to a depth of about 0.1 mm alters the structure, creating a local strain on an atomic level that hardens the surface.

Conformation of the bearing surfaces is important because it is a factor in the determination of contact stress. Higher contact stresses between UHMWPE and other biomaterials are thought to result in greater polymeric wear.[9] Therefore, an increase in the modulus of the polymer increases the contact stress and may result in increased wear. A recently released type of UHMWPE with higher strength also has a higher modulus, but its wear performance is unclear.[10]

The contact angle of the bearing surfaces can be important for the reduction of adhesive wear as well as for lubrication of the surfaces to prevent abrasive wear. A high contact angle of a fluid on a hard surface results in that liquid beading up on the surface, while a low contact angle results in the formation of a liquid film on the surface of the material. The contact angles for distilled water on polished implant surfaces range from 20° for titanium alloy to 100° for UHMWPE (Table 2).

Fatigue of the articulating surface can be a mechanism for the production of wear debris. High contact stress in UHMWPE, resulting from low conformation of the articulating surfaces, high loads, or both, can cause subsurface stress that exceeds the fatigue strength of the polyethylene. Multiple stress cycles can progress to crack formation and production of wear debris.

One can conclude, from an analysis of the cited factors, that a hard surface that is wet by physiologic fluids is probably the best surface to articulate against UHMWPE. At present, the most likely candidates for this surface seem to be ceramic materials, either aluminum oxide or zirconium oxide, while a cobalt-chromium alloy seems to be a close second. Ceramic materials may be optimum for bearing surfaces, as they are very hard, can be polished to smooth surfaces, and are wet by physiologic fluids.[11] However, at the present time in the United States, only cobalt-chromium alloy has an adequate history of use, and it is currently the preferred material for bearing surfaces.

Morse Tapers

Morse tapers are one of a number of machine tool tapers that have been used for more than 100 years to provide frictional rotatory coupling in drill presses, milling machines, and lathes.[12] These tapers vary in dimension, with different diameters and angles that range from 2° to 8°. The dimensions vary according to the company that initially introduced the specific taper. The orthopaedic industry has adapted these tapers, under the generic name of Morse tapers, as a means of reliably joining modular components at the operating table. They are now available in femoral and acetabular component designs, in humeral head component designs, and even as intramedullary rods.

Morse tapers are not standardized in the orthopaedic industry; they vary from company to company. Thus, the trunion (male portion) and the bore (female portion) may appear to be compatible but might be totally incompatible. Extreme care must be taken in the use of these tapers at the time of revision procedures to be sure that products from different manufacturers are not mixed, because to do so can lead to dissociation.

The surface finish, composition, and design tolerances may affect the fit of the trunion and bore and, therefore, the longevity of the connection. As in other materials applications in orthopaedic surgery, fretting and fretting corrosion can be a problem with Morse tapers. Such problems may be exacerbated by the presence of blood degradation products, by the chemical activity of oxygen at the interface, or by both, as compared with the general environment of the hip.

There is concern regarding the use of a cobalt-chromium alloy for the female portion of the Morse taper in contact with a titanium-alloy or a cobalt-chromium alloy male mating surface. It is currently unknown whether the use of zirconia or alumina, the two ceramic materials that are now available for use as Morse taper femoral heads, would eliminate this problem. Although the ceramic heads are not susceptible to electrochemical corrosion, the metal male portion may still undergo corrosion caused by differential oxygen concentrations at the trunion-bore interface, as compared with the outside of the prosthesis. Continuous and repeated removal of the passivating layer from the metallic material through fretting increases the tendency of the metal to corrode.

Zirconia is much stronger than alumina, and thus the risk of catastrophic failure from hoop stresses is

---

Table 1
Hardness of materials used to articulate against UHMWPE in joint replacement

Material	Surface Hardness
Ti-6Al-4V	330
Cobalt-chromium alloy	400
Nitrogen ion-implanted Ti-6Al-4V	770
Zirconia	1,430

Table 2
Contact angle of distilled water on polished surfaces of arthroplasty implant materials

Material	Contact Angle (°)
UHMWPE	100
Cobalt-chromium alloy	60
Zirconia	30
Alumina	30
Titanium alloy	20

This table reflects the results of a single study and may not be reproducible. Alteration of any of a number of variables could have a marked effect on the figures. (Reproduced with permission from Smith and Nephew Richards, Inc, Memphis, TN.)

lower with zirconia. However, the Food and Drug Administration has suggested standard dimensions for bores and trunions made of these materials to prevent excessive hoop stresses. Thus, when ceramic materials are used, it is particularly important that the bores be matched to the trunions. The load to failure of ceramic femoral heads can be reduced markedly with inappropriate selection of the trunion and bore or when particulate debris has been inadvertently left in the interface at the operation, especially when the weaker (alumina) ceramic has been employed.[13]

Choice of Biomaterials in Total Joint Arthroplasty

Advances in the design of total joint replacements have suggested that certain biomaterials are more appropriate for particular applications. Generally, these applications can be grouped according to anatomic location. Thus, we will describe the selection of biomaterials for particular applications according to the anatomic location and the type of application. The overriding variables are strength, modulus, hardness, biologic response, and use with or without cement. It should also be noted that choices of biomaterials are design-specific, and replacement of one material with another may require a compensatory change in design.

For a femoral component that will be cemented in place during a total hip or knee arthroplasty, only two materials—cobalt-chromium alloys and titanium alloys—are available commercially at the present time. In the near future, ceramic materials may be alternatives in total knee arthroplasty, as a result of the properties of their bearing surfaces. The variables that should be considered during the selection of a material for the femoral component of a total hip or knee arthroplasty are flexibility, fatigue strength, and surface hardness. Cobalt-chromium alloys are preferred at present because they have stood the test of time as bearing surfaces in the knee and hip. Titanium alloys have been found to generate large amounts of particulate metallic debris.[14-16] The potential for production of wear debris from contact between titanium alloy and cement, bone, or soft tissue may be diminished in the future with the application of coatings, such as titanium nitride, that materially increase the surface hardness. The stability of these coatings must be guaranteed to prevent three-body wear.

The flexibility of a prosthesis that has been cemented into the proximal part of the femur is a concern because of the poor mechanical properties of cement. Under the best conditions, bone cement has a fatigue endurance limit on the order of four to five megapascals in tension.[17] Previous studies have suggested that a more rigid prosthesis reduces stress in the cement and thus would prolong the service life of the cemented prosthesis.[18]

It must be remembered that the flexibility of a prosthesis depends on both material and geometric properties, as pointed out by Sarmiento and Gruen.[19] As the elastic modulus of titanium alloy is one-half that of cobalt-chromium alloy, a titanium prosthesis with the same geometry as a cobalt-chromium prosthesis is half as stiff. Axial, bending, and torsional stiffness must also be considered because the hip is subjected to all of these loads. Because the geometric stiffness in torsion and bending is proportional to the diameter to the fourth power, small changes in dimensions can have large effects on the geometric contribution to stiffness. Therefore, the stem of a 15-mm-diameter prosthesis made of titanium alloy is just as stiff as the stem of a 13.5-mm-diameter prosthesis made of cobalt-chromium alloy.[20] If one assumes that a uniform 2- to 3-mm-thick cement mantle is optimum, the upper limit on the size of a prosthesis that allows for this cement mantle can be determined. Construction of a prosthesis of that size with cobalt-chromium results in a stiffer implant, with the lowest stresses in the cement for that construct, but it might lead to increased stress-shielding.

On the basis of the premise that the lowest stress in the cement prolongs the life of the prosthesis, the material most suited for a femoral total hip component that is to be inserted with cement is cobalt-chromium alloy. To lessen the remote chance of fatigue failure, a forged cobalt-chromium alloy is optimum. Furthermore, because titanium alloy is associated with substantial production of wear debris, cobalt-chromium alloy is the preferred material for the femoral component in a total knee arthroplasty as well.

Different variables are important in the selection of biomaterials for a femoral component that is designed to be inserted without cement in a total hip or knee arthroplasty. While stress-shielding has been shown to be an important consideration in total hip arthroplasty, it has not been an issue with respect to total knee femoral components to date. No differences in terms of bone ingrowth in commercially available prostheses have been attributed to different metal materials or porous-surface morphology, suggesting that the selection of a femoral component designed to be inserted without cement in a total knee arthroplasty should be based on the properties of the bearing surface.[21] Thus, cobalt-chromium appears to be the metal of choice for this component.

The flexibility of the prosthesis and the selection of the material for a total hip arthroplasty performed without cement are important for different reasons. Flexibility has been inversely related to pain in the thigh[22,23] and stress-shielding.[24] Thus, material properties relating to these variables may be important factors in the success of a total hip arthroplasty done without cement. This phenomenon is less important in patients with thicker cortices and smaller medullary canals because of the relationship between the size of the prosthesis and the size of the bone. It must be remembered that the absolute flexibility of the prosthesis is not important; its flexibility in relation to the flexibility of the bone is the primary concern. The amounts of flexibility in axial, torsional, and flexural loading each depend on the intrinsic material property that relates to stiffness (the elastic modulus for axial and flexural loading and the shear modulus for torsional loading). These material properties for titanium alloy are approximately half those for cobalt-chromium alloy. Thus, to minimize stress-shielding and pain after a total hip arthroplasty done without cement, a titanium-alloy femoral component should be used.

There are similar limitations with regard to the materials that can be selected for an acetabular component in a total hip arthroplasty and for a tibial component in a total knee arthroplasty when the prostheses are to be cemented into place. Use of a metal-backed acetabular or tibial component introduces the possibility of the materials fracturing, and it creates two wear surfaces (the inner surface that articulates with the joint and the opposite surface between the UHMWPE and the metal shell or tray). Cost is also a factor: the use of a metal shell or tray may more than double the cost for the component.

The clinical superiority of metal-backed components has not been demonstrated, despite early theoretical arguments suggesting that there might be a benefit. The use of a metal shell or tray for arthroplasty components may compromise the thickness of the UHMWPE, resulting in increased contact stress and therefore decreased longevity. Potential advantages of the metal-backed tibial tray include the opportunity for the surgeon to fine-tune the ligamentous tension and to distribute load more evenly in a total knee arthroplasty by varying the UHMWPE insert after insertion.[25] The metal-backed acetabular component improves the stability of the arthroplasty because extended liners, offsets, and constrained inserts can be used.

Thus, for both tibial and acetabular components that are to be inserted with cement, the all-UHMWPE prosthesis has to be considered an adequate alternative because it is cost-effective and as effective as the metal-backed component. If, for some reason, a metal-backed component is selected, it can be made of either cobalt-chromium alloy or titanium alloy because the strengths of these two materials are similar.

Acetabular and tibial components that are to be inserted without cement should be constructed of cobalt-chromium alloy or titanium alloy to provide an ingrowth surface, with UHMWPE to provide a bearing surface. Because of the compressive loading on these prostheses, the material properties should have little

bearing on the selection. A prosthesis of either type of alloy can be made to be sufficiently strong, and other design considerations become more important than the choice of materials.

The selection of the material for a patellar component is relatively unambiguous at the present time.[26-29] An all-UHMWPE component is generally preferred.

Design Factors

The important parameters involved in the design of a femoral component that is to be cemented into place have evolved somewhat empirically over the years. The prosthesis should have relatively smooth surfaces, with no sharp edges, so that sites of stress concentration are eliminated from both the prosthesis and the cement. The prosthesis should also be somewhat broader laterally than medially to help to diffuse the compressive stress medially. This design may also increase the torsional and bending rigidity of the prosthesis. Generally, the surface should have a matte finish, which allows some mechanical interlock with the cement. Some surgeons are proponents of a smooth surface, which presumably allows subsidence and thereby keeps the cement in compressive loading. Other surgeons prefer a means for attachment of the cement to the prosthesis, such as precoating of the prosthesis with polymethylmethacrylate. In order to provide a uniform cement mantle, some method for centering of the prosthetic stem in the distal part of the canal is necessary, and this is usually a design consideration for the femoral stem.

The design of the femoral stem of a prosthesis that is to be used without cement raises other important considerations. The prosthesis should be minimally stiff and maximally stable, and it should prevent migration of particles from the articular surface to the stem of the prosthesis. It should include a means of attachment to the musculoskeletal system. In an attempt to minimize stiffness in the stem portion of the prosthesis, slots (clothespin design) as well as grooves have been utilized. These strategies are intended to reduce stress-shielding over the life of the prosthesis. Similarly, minimization of the stiffness of the prosthesis may result in less pain in the thigh.[20,22,23]

Strategies to maximize the stability of the prosthesis are controversial. Some clinicians prefer extensive porous coating, others prefer proximal fill of the canal, while others choose designs with distal flutes to provide rotational stability. Maximum initial stability is generally accepted as important for the achievement of a pain-free result. However, filling of the medullary canal, extensive porous coating, and proximal filling all tend to accentuate the stiffness of the prosthesis in relation to the bone and to transmit the load distally. Optimization of these two competing factors in order to achieve long-term stability with minimum stress-shielding is an unresolved issue in the design of femoral components that are to be inserted without cement. While the extent of the porous coating that is necessary for optimum results has not been determined, circumferential proximal porous coating appears to be necessary to prevent or minimize particle migration toward the stem of the prosthesis.

While the size of the pores necessary to permit ingrowth of bone has been determined, the necessity of ingrowth into a porous structure for a good long-term result is still controversial. Plasma-spraying of rough surfaces, use of smooth surfaces, and coating of smooth and porous surfaces with calcium hydroxyapatite are all techniques that potentially allow ingrowth. Presently available evidence suggests that porous ingrowth surfaces with beads or wires that create pore-interconnection sizes in the range of 100 to 500 μm are optimum. Improvements in initial bone ingrowth may be achieved through the application of calcium hydroxyapatite coatings. Some of these coatings have been approved by the Food and Drug Administration on the basis of promising results in both animal and clinical studies.

The choice of femoral head size seems to have settled on 26 or 28 mm. The 32-mm head produces too large a volume of wear debris, and the 22-mm head produces too much linear wear or creep.[30] Less acetabular strain and lower revision rates are associated with use of a 26 or 28-mm head.[31,32] Evidence for a lower prevalence of dislocation of the 32-mm head compared with that of the 26- or 28-mm head is lacking, except perhaps when a long neck is needed. In this situation, an extended neck sleeve may cause impingement on the cup, loosening of the acetabular component, or dissociation of the plastic component.

Design considerations for the femoral component of a total knee arthroplasty include the depth of the patellofemoral groove, the proximal extent of the anterior flange, left and right versus universal designs, and the contact area with the patellar and the tibial components. An adequate depth of the patellofemoral groove to provide patellar stability without compromise of the integrity of the prosthesis or removal of excessive bone stock is important. Left and right designs provide some degree of patellofemoral stability that is not possible with a design intended for either the left or the right limb. Adequate proximal extension of the anterior flange minimizes the chance that the patella will ride off the flange proximally in full extension. Perhaps the most important factor, however, is the contact area of the femoral condyles with the patella and the tibial plateaus. Point and line contact suggest excessive contact stress, which may lead to excessive wear of the tibial and patellar components.[9,33] The design of the patellar component has to be such that the contact area with the femoral component is maximized (thereby minimizing contact stress) when the prosthesis has been implanted correctly and aligned adequately. This contact area is maximized with a patellar design that conforms to the femoral surface,[34] especially during flexion (when higher stresses are encountered).

Acetabular components that are to be cemented in place should be designed so that there is enough mechanical interdigitation of the cement to provide fixation but not so much that areas of stress concentration are produced. Metal-backed components have theoretical advantages[18,35,36] and were shown early on to have clinical advantages.[37,38] However, later clinical studies appeared to refute these early reports.[39-41] As long as adequate polymer thickness (more than 6 to 8 mm) is maintained, use of all-UHMWPE acetabular components is probably justified on the basis of cost because the superiority of cemented metal-backed components has not been demonstrated.[42-44]

Acetabular components that are to be inserted without cement should be designed to be portions of spheres so that spherical reaming will optimize contact. These components should be thick enough so that adequate strength is obtained despite holes for fixation. Revisions in which hemispherical contact is not obtainable could lead to fatigue failure through the holes.[45] Fixation can be accomplished with press-fitting alone or with press-fitting and adjunctive use of screws or spikes. While undersized reaming and press-fitting by an experienced surgeon can generally result in consistent fixation, occasionally loosening that may have been prevented by a screw does occur, even when the operation was done with skill. Although screws may provide excellent initial fixation, later they may be sources of fretting, which could produce wear debris. Unfilled screw-holes provide access for wear debris from the UHMWPE liner to the area behind the ingrowth cup. Furthermore, UHMWPE may cold-flow (creep) into these holes, resulting in early failure of the polyethylene liner. Fixation of spikes to the outer surface of the cup may lead to difficulties with implantation, such as an inability to obtain proper alignment. The spikes may also make adequate seating of the cup difficult.

Another important design consideration is the congruence of the inner surface of the metal shell to the outer surface of the UHMWPE liner. Inadequate congruence of these surfaces can lead to excessive stress and fracture of the UHMWPE or, alternatively, to motion and wear between the components. Adequate provision for attachment of the plastic insert to the metal shell should be intrinsic to the design of the cup. Furthermore, an antirotation design is crucial for components with extended walls or offsets.

The design of the tibial component of a total knee arthroplasty is dependent on the biomaterial to some extent. An all-polymer tibial component should be a minimum of 8 to 9 mm thick, and it should have a surface that permits attachment of the cement to the plateau and to the stem surface.[46,47] A tibial prosthesis made of UHMWPE should have a stem to help reduce lift-off, and the stem should be designed to prevent flexion, extension, varus and valgus angulation, and rotation. Due to the mechanical properties of UHMW-PE, a stem length of more than 5 cm is probably minimally beneficial in terms of stability. A metal tibial tray should be at least 3 mm thick for strength.

The metal-backed tibial plateau initially was thought to be an advance, on the basis of theoretical and laboratory studies and of some clinical corroboration.[48-51] The metal-backed tibial plateau probably provides a greater margin of safety in that it distributes stresses to the two condyles of the tibia if the surgeon is unable to obtain perfect alignment.[25] The tibial plateau may lose its support due to the development of a fibrous membrane, osteolysis from wear debris, or resorption of bone graft. (Lack of support can also be caused by errors on the part of the surgeon.) In these cases, stem support of the tibial plateau is crucial to prevent fatigue failure of the cantilever plateau.[52-55] The UHMWPE insert should be at least 5 to 6 mm thick,[35] the component should lock in positively to minimize motion between the plateau and the plastic, and the bearing surface of the plastic should conform to the femoral component as much as possible. Conformation to the femoral component is an important aspect of the design, but it is controversial in that increased conformation constrains motion. Femoral roll-back, the posterior displacement of the femoral component on the tibial component during flexion, can be problematic with a conforming tibial component. Loosening is also a concern in constrained designs. The differences between the clinical results from designs that necessitate removal of the posterior cruciate ligament and those with which the ligament is retained are not definitive.[34]

Systemic and Remote-Site Effects of Biomaterials

Materials Systems

Although consensus is slowly emerging, there is no acknowledged best material for the fabrication of orthopaedic implants.[56-58] Each material has a particular combination of properties, determined by its composition and processing, and each set of properties produces both benefits and limitations within the bounds of any device design. Thus, some materials are better suited for load-bearing applications in bending while others are more suitable for articulating surfaces.

In general, at least in the short and middle range of service (up to ten years postoperatively), it has proved easier to meet the mechanical requirements than the biological requirements imposed by local, systemic, and remote-site responses to the material, its constituents, and their degradation products. Initial clinical applications and later laboratory experiments have tended to focus primarily on the device and its immediate surroundings. More recently, as partial and total joint replacements have routinely begun to exceed a decade in vivo, attention has turned to more subtle aspects of host responses: responses producing symptoms either systemically or at sites remote from the implant. These responses must be understood in terms of a coupling between the material in a prosthetic device and the human body. This coupling, in turn, depends on the fundamental chemical nature of the material, as reflected by its chemical constituents and their interatomic bonds (Table 3).

Interest in systemic and remote-site effects has tended to focus on metals, which possess the desirable properties of high strength, toughness, and ductility, but are all subject to chemical attack, principally by corrosion.[59] It must be emphasized that, as is the case for other prosthetic materials, modern metals, when properly manufactured, processed, and handled both before implantation and in the operating room, are stable and do not generally present biologic response problems in the short term. However, this success with metals has been obtained by severe limitation of the choices of materials from among all available engineering options (Table 4).[60]

Systemic and Remote-Site versus Implant-Site Host Responses

Two general observations apply to the issue of remote and systemic responses to biomaterials.[61] First, it is difficult to observe these responses; most symptoms attributable to systemic (and also to remote-site) effects can be expected to occur normally in any population of orthopaedic patients[62] or, for that matter, in populations being seen for other problems. Thus, the identification of implant-referable symptoms at a site other than that of the implant depends to a great degree on either the availability of comparative epidemiologic data or the ability to perform tests on the patient before and after removal of the device.[63] Second, there is a widespread lack of epidemiologic follow-up studies of any but selected aspects of orthopaedic procedures, such as pain and joint mobility, that are directly related to the implant procedure.

Nevertheless, on the basis of studies with animal models and limited clinical observations, we recognize the possibility of systemic or remote-site effects and can group them into four general classifications:[62] metabolic, bacteriologic, immunologic, and neoplastic.

In the discussion of either systemic or remote-site effects, it is necessary to adopt a standard of proof so as not to repeat hearsay or to draw incorrect conclusions. Black[56] proposed four criteria necessary and sufficient

Table 3
Coupling modalities of biomaterials

Material Class	Primary Chemical Bonds	Coupling Modality
Metal	Metallic	Corrosion and dissolution products; wear debris release (secondary)
Polymer	Covalent; van der Waals	Elution and dissolution; wear-debris release (in load-bearing situations)
Ceramic (nonabsorbable)	Ionic	Little or none; primarily wear-debris release
Ceramic (absorbable)	Ionic	Dissolution; particulate release
Polymer-matrix composites	Materials: as above; structure: van der Waals	Materials: as above; structure: particulate release

Table 4
Current biomaterials in clinical use*

Metals	Stainless steels (F 138, F 621, F 745, F 1314), cobalt-based alloys (F 75, F 90, F 562, F 563), titanium (F 67) and titanium-based alloys (F 136, F 620)
Polymers	UHMWPE (F 648), polymethylmethacrylate (F451)
Ceramics	Alumina (F 603), β-tricalcium phosphate (F 1088), calcium hydroxyapatite (F 1185)
Composite components	Polysulfone (F 702), polyetheretherketone, carbon fiber

* Standard designations of the American Society for Testing Materials[60] are given in parentheses.

to establish the clinical reality of such effects: (1) The basic mechanism of the biologic response must be demonstrated in at least one biologic model, either in vitro or in an animal model. (2) After the causative implant-related species (the particular element, molecule, or ion) has been identified, its release by a functional implant and its systemic distribution either in an animal model or in patients (preferably both) must be shown. (3) The putative biologic response must be identified either in an animal model or in patients (preferably both) with functional implants. (4) If demonstrated in patients, the biologic response must be recognized on the basis of a statistically sound epidemiologic study with suitable non-exposed controls

and, unless the response is of a threshold type, a dose-response or exposure-incidence relationship must be demonstrated.

For the effects discussed in the rest of this section, conditions 1 and 2 have been met in all cases and condition 3, in some cases. Evidence to satisfy condition 4 is mostly lacking. Thus, research continues on the reality and clinical importance of systemic and remote-site effects of implants. However, the release of degradation products from implants and the transport of these products, in soluble and particulate forms, to remote sites is now incontrovertible.[64-66]

Metabolic Effects The important roles played by the nonphysiologic metals—that is, those other than sodium, potassium, calcium, and iron—are now well recognized. Current dietary recommendations include a daily minimum intake of magnesium and zinc, and daily intakes of copper, manganese, molybdenum, and chromium are recognized as safe; at least one of the latter three metals is found in all stainless steels and cobalt-based super alloys.[67] All metallic elements in materials that are used in implant applications, with the possible exception of titanium, are recognized as playing either an essential or a toxic role in mammalian metabolism.[68] However, even in the case of essential elements, elevated doses can produce toxic effects,[69,70] which may be seen locally, systemically, or in remote organ systems.

Bacteriologic Effects Deep infections, whether immediate or delayed, remain a small but serious problem in patients with orthopaedic implants.[71] Foreign materials contribute to the cause and complicate the treatment of infections of the musculoskeletal system. They provide a protected surface that seems to favor colonization and growth,[72] as has been shown in animal models, by a reduction of the minimum titer of infectious organisms needed to propagate an infection and in clinical situations by the difficulty encountered in the treatment of an established infection in the presence of an implant. While initial infections may be ascribed to contamination during the procedure, infections that occur later are most likely caused by disturbance of a previously existing infectious nidus or to hematogenous seeding from an infected remote site.[73] With the exception of polymethylmethacrylate cement cured in situ, which has a particular propensity for supporting infection, no material for fixation of implants seems to present a better or worse risk of infection at the site of the prosthesis.[74] However, in the presence of such infection, it has been shown that increased corrosion of multipart metallic fracture fixation devices may occur.[75] Additionally, the observation of corrosion associated with modular joint-replacement devices, especially at the head-neck junction, suggests that other processes, in addition to infection, may render this design feature especially prone to the release of metallic material.[76,77] Such release may predispose to local infection, through ionic suppression of leukocyte chemotactic ability and particulate suppression of the respiratory burst ability of the leukocytes.[78-80] Concerns with regard to systemic infection have focused on the possibility of suppression of leukocyte activity at remote sites, as suggested by the dose-response promotion of lung infections in rats with large-area cobalt-alloy implants in remote soft-tissue locations.[81]

Immunologic Effects It has now been well established that many metallic ions, such as cobalt, chromium, and nickel, when released from implants, can serve as haptens and elicit type-IV delayed hypersensitivity reactions in previously sensitized individuals.[82] In addition, there is concern that a chronically loose implant, with its higher release rate of metallic material, may sensitize previously unsensitized individuals.[83] More recent evidence of previously unrecognized immune responses to titanium-alloy devices,[84] polymethylmethacrylate bone cement,[85] and silicone elastomers[86] has raised concern about a possible generality of response. However, as of now, despite growing case-report literature relating dermatitis, urticaria, eczematous reactions, and other, more subtle immunologic phenomena to implants and their degradation products, no clear picture has emerged of either the magnitude of the problem or its causal clinical development in the general case.[55]

Neoplastic Effects There can be little question of the carcinogenic potential of metallic species, particularly chromium, cobalt, and nickel, released from implants.[87] Increasing numbers of tumors are being reported in association with joint replacements, although the total incidence remains low.[88] Epidemiologic investigation of the incidence of remote-site and systemic tumors suggests an elevated risk of lymphoma and leukemia in patients after total hip arthroplasty.[89,90] Of perhaps greater concern is the emerging evidence that organometallic ions, produced in association with implants, constitute a chronic stress on the immune system.[79,89] While this may prove beneficial in the short term, there is the possibility of immune system depletion in the longer term (more than ten years postoperatively) and a resultant increasing incidence of tumors, caused by the innate carcinogenicity of the released materials, as well as increased progression of tumors arising from other sources. A preliminary survey of musculoskeletal tumors in American patients with joint replacement devices failed to show any elevation in incidence (leukemia and lymphoma incidences were not investigated in this study), but it was reported that tumors occurring in the same limb as the implant progressed quite rapidly.[91] As the life spans of patients continue to increase and the age at the time of joint replacement declines,

these concerns may well become more important. It is particularly in consideration of neoplasia that a close focus on the local implant site and on the short term may result in other sources of risk (both systemic and remote) being overlooked.

Research Issues

The mechanisms, including release and distribution, of the possible effects of implant degradation products on systemic and remote-site physiology have been reasonably well established. Current research is focusing on two unresolved aspects of the problem. Most of our knowledge about the function of biomaterials in humans has been gained by observation of clinical symptoms, primarily those associated with failed implants, and through retrieval and analysis of failed implants. This has given us a somewhat one-sided and incomplete view of a biomaterial's in vivo performance.[92] There is a developing interest in the definition and measurement of in vivo performance—that is, an attempt is being made to develop a true physiology of biomaterials. Related to this and in response to the previously noted gap, there is a renewed interest in postoperative follow-up, not simply for the determination of device performance but for the examination of overall patient outcome. Results of outcome studies can, and it is hoped will, cast further light on the reality and gravity of systemic and remote-site effects. Such studies are of great importance in view of the rapidly increasing patient populations with permanent implants and a perceived trend toward lower ages at the time of implantation.

Current Practice

It is difficult to make firm recommendations concerning systemic and remote-site effects in clinical practice. The following points are suggestions for the clinician to consider, both when evaluating patients for permanent implant procedures and when evaluating untoward responses that may be implant-related:

Metabolic Effects There is no reason for current concern.

Bacteriologic Effects It is important to recognize the role of infection in the acceleration of corrosion through promotion of local acidosis. This effect should be taken into account when removal of temporary implants or revision of permanent implants is being considered clinically, especially if the prostheses contain components known to be fabricated from stainless steel or cobalt-based alloys. Titanium-based alloys are somewhat more stable under acidic conditions and thus pose a lower relative risk in the presence of implant site infection.

Immunologic Effects There does not yet appear to be sound justification for routine preoperative testing for metal sensitivity of patients who are scheduled to receive implants. However, the medical history should include appropriate questions to determine if the patient has a history of suspicious allergy to metal or if he or she works in a setting that increases the risk of sensitization. Unexplained rashes (unassociated with food or medication); inflammation associated with jewelry; or industrial employment in printing, dye manufacture, leather-tanning, or mining, smelting, and fabrication or finishing of metals, especially electroplating, should arouse some suspicion of an established immune response to one or more metals. In such cases, selective use of dermal or intradermal allergen testing may be indicated. Documented allergy to either nickel or chromium, which are the most common metallic allergens, is a probable contraindication to the use of stainless steel or cobalt-based alloys. Although there are now a few reports of allergy to titanium-based alloy systems or their components, the picture is less clear.[84] Similarly, the results of tests for metal allergy may help to explain symptoms associated with loose, painful permanent implants that need to be revised without evidence of implant-site infection. Here again, positive test results are a probable contraindication to the use of stainless steel or cobalt-based-alloy components.

Neoplastic Effects The clinical consequences of neoplastic transformation are sufficiently severe to require caution. Clinical evidence of neoplastic transformation associated with stainless steel or cobalt-based alloys is extremely scant. However, it has been suggested that care be exercised in the use of large-surface-area cobalt-based-alloy components, particularly in younger patients.[61] Tissues recovered from the implant site during revision procedures should be studied with great care, especially in the case of rapidly changing clinical or radiographic appearance, to rule out the possibility of neoplastic transformation.

The era of recognition and study of systemic and remote-site effects of implants is just beginning. The practicing orthopaedic surgeon is advised to continue to follow the scientific and clinical literature and to carefully scrutinize his or her own patients with the possibility of systemic and remote-site effects of biomaterials well in mind.

Local Response to Biomaterials: Bone Lysis in Total Hip Arthroplasty

Bone loss has been recognized as a potential serious complication of the use of femoral stems without cement. Bone loss can become a clinical problem for several reasons, including failure of fixation of the implant, periprosthetic fracture of the host bone, pain, and disability. In addition, changes in the structure of the femur can present very serious problems if further reconstruction is needed.

In the absence of infection, bone loss can usually be ascribed to one of two major causes: bone remodeling and the phenomenon of osteolysis. While the process of stress-induced bone remodeling and the occurrence of stress-shielding have not, so far, produced widespread serious complications, focal osteolysis is currently a major clinical problem. Therefore, the following discussion will deal only with our current understanding of osteolysis.

Clinical Features

Osteolysis, or periprosthetic bone loss, is usually recognized radiographically either as diffuse femoral cortical thinning or as a focal cystic lesion. The focal lesion may involve the periacetabular or proximal femoral metaphyseal trabecular bone, the femoral diaphyseal cortical bone, or both. The focal cystic lesion is more problematic and more likely to result in clinical complications.

Osteolysis is frequently associated with loose cemented femoral components. In 1968, Charnley and associates[93] were probably the first to recognize the phenomenon of endosteal osteolysis, which they described at that time as an "alteration of texture of cortex." They found this in four of 190 hips with a cemented total prosthesis, at 3 to 8 years after the operation. Although Charnley and associates attributed these changes to chronic infection, most of the patients were asymptomatic and the radiographic appearance of the bone was quite similar to what later would be described as osteolysis. Several authors have since described the phenomenon of osteolysis in patients with loose femoral components.[1,94-96]

Focal osteolysis has also been described in conjunction with stable cemented femoral components. Jasty and associates[97] described four cases in a series of more than 3,000 total hip replacements. However, the prevalence was found to be higher in a subsequent review at the same center: of 106 cemented total hip prostheses with a minimum ten-year follow-up, seven were associated with an osteolytic lesion.[98] Maloney and associates[99] described 25 cases of focal femoral osteolysis in association with radiographically stable, cemented femoral implants. Three of these components were retrieved at autopsy, allowing a complete biomechanical analysis. The time interval between the arthroplasty and the radiographic appearance of the localized osteolysis ranged from 40 to 168 months. The rate of progression of these lesions was variable, and in one case, progression to gross loosening of the femoral implant was observed. In 15 (60%) of the patients, the area of osteolysis corresponded to either a defect in the cement mantle or an area of very thin cement. In addition to a deficiency in the cement mantle, direct communication between the joint and the focal lesion has been postulated as an important element in the pathogenesis of these lesions.[100]

The occurrence of osteolysis in association with both well-fixed and loose cemented total hip prostheses has given rise to the term cement disease.[101] Histologically, cement disease is characterized by the presence of variable amounts of cement, UHMWPE, and metal debris in tissue infiltrated with macrophages, giant cells, and vascular granulation tissue. Although initially it was thought that a reaction to particulate polymethylmethacrylate played a central role in the pathogenesis of these lesions, it has been accepted more recently that UHMWPE is a major contributor to the phenomenon of bone resorption. In addition, mechanical factors, hypersensitivity, and metal particles may be important in the etiology of these lesions. In the case of loose implants, the additional feature of cement-bone and cement-implant relative motion also may play an exacerbating role.

Focal femoral osteolysis has now also been recognized in association with loose implants that were inserted without cement. In a review of the results of 121 total hip arthroplasties in which a titanium fiber-metal prosthesis had been inserted without cement, at a minimum five-year follow-up the prevalence of femoral component loosening was 9%, with a total of 12 loose implants.[102] The prevalence of focal osteolysis in association with these 12 implants was 40%. Osteolysis has also been observed adjacent to loose cobalt-based-alloy porous-coated femoral stems that had been fixed without cement. Osteolysis in this setting is thought to be related to implant motion and tissue reaction to abraded particulate wear debris. The important observation is that the absence of acrylic cement does not preclude the occurrence of osteolysis in association with a loose implant. Furthermore, a loose implant that was inserted without cement can be as damaging to the surrounding tissues as a loose cemented implant.

Osteolysis has also been recognized as a complication in association with stable femoral components fixed without cement. Maloney and associates[103] reported a study of the results of 474 consecutive total hip arthroplasties that they had performed. Three series of patients were included: two separate groups with titanium-alloy implants and one group with cobalt-chromium-alloy implants. The overall prevalence of osteolysis, approximately 3%, was the same for femoral stems made of cobalt-chromium alloy and those made of titanium alloy. Of the 16 cases, 14 occurred in male patients.

In a recent review of the results after implantation of titanium-alloy implants, nine of 110 hips with a radiographically stable prosthesis showed focal femoral osteolysis, an overall prevalence of 8%.[102] The interval from implantation to the radiographic appearance of the lesion in the nine hips averaged 50 months (range, 36 to 63 months). Most of these patients were asymptomatic, with a Harris hip score of 94 points (range, 77 to 100 points). Only one patient had pain in the thigh. There was no difference in age, weight, gender, Harris score, canal fill, or any radiographic parameter between the patients with and those without femoral osteolysis. However, the diagnosis of osteonecrosis was more frequent among the patients with osteolysis (55%) than among those without osteolysis (29%). Most likely, a number of factors contributed to this relationship between osteolysis and osteonecrosis. The patients with osteonecrosis may have had a subtle underlying abnormality in bone metabolism because of steroid use or other intraosseous pathology. In addition, these patients tended to be younger and probably were more active than the total hip arthroplasty population at large. Radiographically, these lesions were most common in the vicinity of the distal aspect of the stem, in Gruen zones 3, 4, and 5. Typically, these patients also demonstrated endosteal scalloping of the proximal medial femoral cortex (Gruen zone 7), and these lesions were generally progressive.[104]

It appears that endosteal erosions in patients with stable femoral components that were fixed without cement are observed earlier than those in patients with cemented components. In addition, the prevalence appears to be higher, at least for this type of design without cement. In our experience, the prevalence of femoral osteolysis after a total of 484 arthroplasties with titanium-alloy hip prostheses was 9% at two years. However, at a minimum eight-year follow-up of 47 hips, the prevalence was 15%. This illustrates that the prevalence of femoral osteolysis in this patient population is increasing with time. Because osteolysis is usually asymptomatic, long-term radiographic follow-up of all patients with a total hip arthroplasty, and particularly those in whom the implant was inserted without cement, is necessary to identify osteolysis before the occurrence of major complications secondary to progressive bone loss. A 10% to 20% prevalence of focal femoral osteolysis at two to nine years has been described with other implant systems fabricated from both cobalt-chromium and titanium-based alloys.[104-107]

Acetabular osteolysis has received less attention in the literature, but it does occur in association with loose cemented acetabular components,[96,108] and recently it has emerged as a distinct clinical problem associated with both loose and well-fixed implants that had been inserted without cement. Although only limited reports have been presented thus far, the prevalence appears to differ depending on the type of acetabular component and the duration of follow-up. Stulberg and associates[109] reported a prevalence of 46% at the time of a five- to seven-year follow-up of cobalt-chromium-alloy implants. Beauchesne and associates[110] reported a 28% prevalence of acetabular osteolysis at a six-year follow-up of cobalt-chromium-alloy acetabular components. In a recent review of 83 titanium-alloy acetabular components by Schmalzried and Harris,[111] only one case of osteolysis was recognized with a minimum of five years of follow-up. In another experience with titanium-alloy acetabular components, osteolysis was suspected in association with two of 140 components at five to seven years.

Radiographically, it is possible to distinguish between two types of acetabular lesions. Periacetabular lesions are seen primarily in the periphery of the acetabulum, and retroacetabular lesions tend to be central and to infiltrate the body of the ilium, occasionally the body of the ischium, or both.

The severity of acetabular osteolysis in association with acetabular implants inserted without cement is not yet clear. The time following implantation is a critical variable, and because most current acetabular systems that do not include the use of cement were introduced less than ten years ago, not enough time has passed for the magnitude or importance of the problem to be ascertained.

Histologic Features

Tissue from ten patients with femoral osteolysis associated with implants that had been fixed with cement and later revised was examined by two of us (JOG and JJJ). The tissues were prepared with standard histologic techniques for examination under plain and polarized light microscopy. Five of these patients had a loose prosthesis at the time of the revision procedure, and the joint pseudocapsule revealed a hypertrophic synovitis with areas of necrosis. Areas of intense histiocytic infiltration were present, with occasional foreign-body giant cells and lymphocytes. Plasma cells were scarce, and there was no evidence of acute inflammation. Many of the histiocytes contained fine, opaque black granules; these granules were also present in extracellular locations. Under polarized light, strongly birefringent particles, which ranged in size from less than 1 µm to approximately 50 µm, were seen. The larger particles tended to be polygonal. Occasionally, the birefringent particles were associated with foreign-body giant cells, but more commonly they were associated with sheets of histiocytes.

Specimens obtained from the femoral membrane in the vicinity of the osteolytic lesions in the patients with loose implants demonstrated dense fibrous tissue with foci of intense histiocytic infiltration and foreign-body giant cells. Intermingled with the histiocytes were a small number of lymphocytes. Occasional areas of necrosis were observed, but there was no evidence of an acute inflammatory process. Isolated areas demonstrated fine, opaque black granules within the histiocytes, similar to but less numerous than those seen in the capsule. Under polarized light, minute, strongly birefringent particles characteristic of UHMWPE were observed within the cytoplasm of the histiocytes.

In spite of the fact that these implants were loose, back-scattered electron microscopy demonstrated bone ingrowth in four of the five components. In one case, a histiocytic infiltrate was present within the porous coating, associated with resorption lacunae in the ingrown bone. This suggests trabecular bone failure either as a result of, or aided by, the resorption process.

In the five patients in whom the components were well fixed at the time of the revision procedure, the histologic appearance of the joint pseudocapsule and interfacial membrane was qualitatively similar to that described for the patients with the loose prostheses. Quantitatively, there appeared to be more particulate debris in the patients with loose components. In one case, a fragment of cortical bone was obtained from an anterolateral window adjacent to an osteolytic lesion. Close to the endosteal surface of this cortical window were widened haversian spaces, occasionally filled by histiocytes. The endosteal surface was irregular with a serrated appearance, showed typical Howship lacunae and osteoclasts, and was covered by a fibrous membrane that, in many fields, had been completely replaced by sheets of histiocytes containing foreign materials of the same appearance as those in the capsule and femoral membrane, as seen under both plain and polarized light. On the membrane surface facing the endosteum, several mononucleated and multinucleated osteoclasts were found. All of these components demonstrated areas of extensive bone ingrowth on back-scattered electron microscopy, although the ingrowth was difficult to quantify due to the destruction of the pads during extraction of the component.

Particle Analysis

The joint pseudocapsule and interfacial membranes were evaluated with electron microprobe analysis, analytic electron microscopy, and Fourier transform infrared (FTIR) spectroscopy to determine the identity and amount of particulate wear debris. The joint pseudocapsule contained particles of titanium alloy ranging from less than 1 µm to 20 µm in size. In many fields, single particles were not discernible, although elemental maps demonstrated the presence of titanium, aluminum, and vanadium diffusely throughout the section, suggesting the presence of particles in the size range of less than 1 µm. The number of metallic particles was, in general, much smaller in the pseudocapsule around the components that were well fixed at the time of the revision procedure.

Electron microprobe analysis of the interfacial membrane revealed titanium-alloy particles up to 20 μm in size. Certain sections from around the loose implants had a heavy metallic load with non-discernible submicrometer-size particles. However, metal particles were scant around the well-fixed implants. Fourier transform infrared spectroscopy was employed to identify any polymeric particles, and while several particles with UHMWPE-like spectra were observed, this technique is only applicable to particles no smaller than 5 to 10 μm in size. The analytic electron microscope affords better resolution than the electron microprobe. This modality identified silicate particles and stainless-steel particles in addition to titanium-alloy particles.

Although these studies provided some important insight into the particulate milieu, the identity of the very fine intracellular particles that appeared birefringent under polarized light was not definitively ascertained. While the larger particles possessed the characteristic morphology of UHMWPE wear debris and were positively identified as that material by the Fourier transform infrared spectroscopy, the finer particles are beyond the sensitivity of that technique. Furthermore, although metal particles are not birefringent, very fine particles may reflect polarized light in such a way as to give the appearance of birefringence. Broad surveys of the literature failed to provide any definite guidance in the identification of these particles.

Recently, Shanbhag and associates[112] conducted a study to characterize the composition and morphology of debris extracted from interfacial membranes recovered at revision of titanium-alloy total hip prostheses that had been inserted without cement. Interfacial membranous tissue was obtained from 11 patients undergoing revision procedures a mean of 62 months (range, eight to 114 months) after implantation. The composition of the particulate debris was characterized with the use of scanning electron microscopy, quantitative energy dispersive x-ray analysis, and Fourier transform infrared spectroscopy. Particle-size analysis was accomplished with manual measurement of scanning electron microscope micrographs. The examination of these tissues revealed that most of the particles seen were submicrometer UHMWPE. In addition, a smaller number of titanium-alloy and unalloyed-titanium particles were identified, as were bone particles and occasional stainless-steel and silicate particles.

Pathogenesis

The pathogenesis of focal osteolysis has not been fully elucidated. In 1977, Willert and Semlitsch[4] were among the first to suggest that a macrophage response to particulate debris was an important factor leading to periprosthetic bone resorption and aseptic loosening. The findings of Goldring and associates,[113] in 1983, have proved to be a hallmark in our understanding of the nature of the interface between the implant and the host. They described a synovial-like membrane at the bone-cement interface in patients with loose total hip prostheses. This membrane had the capacity to produce large amounts of prostaglandin E_2 and collagenase and to lead to bone resorption. Since that time, many investigators have been studying the relationship of intercellular mediators to periprosthetic bone loss and aseptic loosening.[114-132]

In general terms, it has been hypothesized that the generation of particles and their migration into the synovial cavity and the periprosthetic space stimulates macrophage recruitment and proliferation, phagocytosis, and, subsequently, secretion of various cytokines and intercellular mediators such as interleukin-1 and prostaglandin E_2. These substances, in turn, stimulate osteoclastic bone resorption.

A study was undertaken to measure the secretion of five intracellular mediators (interleukin-1, interleukin-6, interleukin-8, tumor necrosis factor, and prostaglandin E_2) in explants of interfacial membranes of prostheses, inserted without cement, associated with femoral osteolysis. Only the concentration of interleukin-1 was significantly elevated ($p < 0.01$) in the culture media, compared with controls and explants from around failed cemented implants.[133] This suggests that, of the various cytokines that can cause bone resorption, interleukin-1 may play a central role in the process. Other investigators have also alluded to this.[134] Cell and organ culture models have been used to study particle-induced bone resorption and have demonstrated that phagocytosable particles of unalloyed titanium and polymethylmethacrylate (less than 10 μm) could stimulate the secretion of interleukin-1 and prostaglandin E_2 from peritoneal macrophages in a dose and time-dependent manner.[135] Furthermore, 1- to 3-μm particles of unalloyed titanium markedly enhanced the bone-resorbing activity of these macrophages. Prostaglandin-E_2 and interleukin-1 inhibition only partially blocked this effect, suggesting that a complex cascade of cytokine-mediator interactions governs this pathologic bone-resorptive process.

Two critical concerns regarding the pathogenesis of osteolysis need to be addressed: (1) the origin of the particles and (2) the relative contribution of the various particulates in inciting tissue reaction and secondary osteolysis of bone. The particles may originate at a number of different sites. At the level of the acetabular component, particles can originate on the articular surface of the UHMWPE, on the non-articular surface of the UHMWPE, at the metal shell, or at the fixation screws. In the femoral component, the stem, the porous coating, the articular surface, and the modular connections can produce particles. Surgical tools, bone, remnants from the surface-processing of the prosthetic device, and the catalyst used in processing the UHMWPE can all be sources of particulate debris.

The predominant particle appears to be UHMWPE. Most likely, the bulk of this debris originates from the articular surface. The debris has ready access to the proximal-medial femoral cortex and the trochanteric region, and localized osteolytic lesions in these areas are not uncommon. For the most part, their clinical importance is limited unless large granulomatous lesions develop.

In contrast, distal femoral osteolysis presents a more complex problem with regard to the determination of the pathway of particle migration. Two pathways to the femoral canal can be identified. In the case of a noncircumferential coating or a press-fit stem without a coating, a space can often be recognized between the neocortical shell that forms around the implant and the metallic surface of the implant. The space can be a real cavity or it can be occupied by loose connective tissue. In both instances, direct access of particulate material to the distal femoral canal is feasible. Autopsy retrievals in cases without demonstrable osteolysis have shown the presence of histiocytes in cavities surrounding the implant; the histiocytes have been associated with particulate birefringent intracellular material with the same characteristics as those identified in tissues from the joint capsule.[136] Another possible pathway to the distal aspect of the femoral canal is through the perivascular lymphatic system, as described by Willert and Semlitsch.[4] In the case of circumferential coatings, access to the distal aspect of the stem-bone interface is restricted. While the overall prevalence of femoral osteolysis may not be lower with circumferentially coated implants, the lesions that do develop tend to be proximal to the porous coating.

With regard to the two types of acetabular lesions, the peripheral lesion is probably related to wear debris originating from the joint cavity and is similar to the lesions seen in the area of the proximal-medial femoral cortex or the greater trochanter. On the other hand, the debris responsible for the retroacetabular lesions probably originates on the convex side of the acetabular insert. The debris migrates behind the metallic component, through holes in the shell created during the manufacturing process (Fig. 1). The volume of the debris is probably related to a number of variables, including the smoothness of the concave metallic surface of the acetabular component, the degree of tolerance between the polymer and the metal shell, and the relative stability of the insert.

Metallic debris may originate from the femoral stem as a result of stem-bone fretting. This is certainly true in the case of loose implants when gross motion is present between the prosthesis and the surrounding bone. This may also be the case for stable implants, as motion can nevertheless occur between the distal portion of a proximally coated porous stem and the surrounding bone.[137] Other sources of metal debris include the articular surface, the porous coating (often unalloyed titanium), the metal backing of the acetabular component, and acetabular fixation screws.

Fretting and corrosion at the Morse taper junction have recently been recognized as important sources of particulate debris. The phenomenon has been described in tapers and heads made from similar metals (cobalt-based alloy) as well as in tapers and heads made from the mixed metal combination of a cobalt-based-alloy head on a titanium-based-alloy neck.[138] The phenomenon is complex, and a number of variables related to the metallurgy and the dimensions of the Morse taper are involved. Tolerance, size, and shape have all been found to be meaningful variables in the production of fretting initially and of corrosion of the involved metallic elements secondarily.[138,139] Furthermore, the corrosion products formed at the junction of the head and neck have been identified in the joint pseudocapsule, in the articular surface of the UHMWPE insert, in the femoral membrane, and in osteolytic lesions within the femoral canal.[140]

In other investigations, a number of other anomalous particulate species were recovered, including silicate particles, which were probably remnants from the surface-processing that was used to finish the metallic stems. However, a subset of these silicates was observed in close association with the UHMWPE debris, and these were most likely remnants of the Ziegler-Nata catalyst used in the manufacture of the UHMWPE.[112] These particles have been recognized as inclusions within the UHMWPE and can occasionally be observed at the surface of the polymeric component. Their presence has been linked to excessive wear at the metallic counterface.[15] The stainless-steel particles observed are assumed to be contaminants introduced from the surgical instruments.[112] In some cases, these particles may represent debris from cerclage wires that were used to stabilize an intraoperative femoral fracture or a trochanteric osteotomy.

While the clinical relevance of the corrosion products and other anomalous particles is not fully understood, the particles are potentially biologically active, leading to macrophage stimulation. In addition, the particles can lead to three-body wear and thus can potentially be the source of increased UHMWPE wear.

The second major question regarding pathogenesis concerns the relative contribution of each of the particulate species to the overall process. In vitro cell-culture studies have demonstrated that the macrophage and fibroblast response to particulate debris was dependent on particle size, composition, and dose.[141] Several centers have been investigating these issues with the use of fabricated or retrieved particulate materials in cell cultures. While these studies are promising, a major limitation has been the unavailability of large amounts of particulate debris in the 0.1 to 2 μm size range. To draw

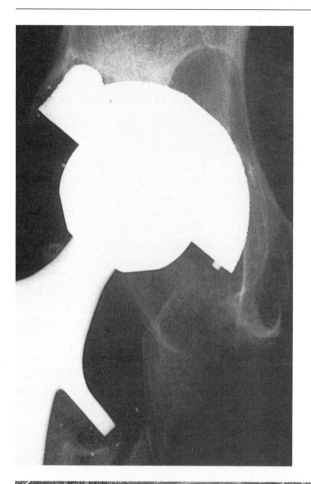

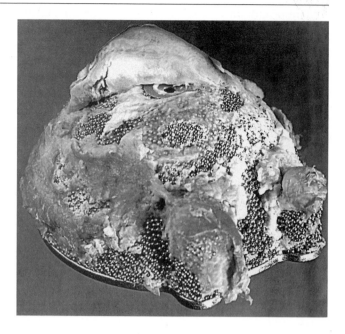

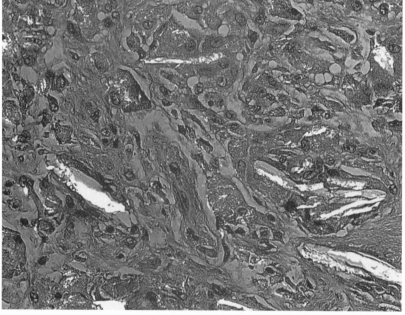

Fig. 1   Top left, Anteroposterior radiograph of the right hip made three years postoperatively, showing osteolysis adjacent to an acetabular cup fixed without cement. Note the large cyst-like defect in the ilium superior to the acetabular dome. The femoral head is eccentrically located, suggesting considerable wear of the UHMWPE. Note also the loose beads and bone loss subjacent to the collar of the femoral component. **Top right,** This photograph, made following component removal, shows a large granuloma adherent to the dome of the acetabular component, corresponding to the osteolytic lesion seen on the roentgenogram. The granuloma was sectioned to reveal its association with the hole in the metallic portion of the acetabular cup. **Bottom,** Polarized light microscopy of this section from the granuloma demonstrated a histiocytic infiltrate with prominent foreign-body giant cells, which are associated with large shards of UHMWPE up to several hundred μm in length. The more numerous submicron UHMWPE particles are noted within histiocytes (hematoxylin and eosin, original magnification, 500 X).

meaningful conclusions from in vitro cell-culture models, one needs to make sure that factors such as composition, particle size, size distribution, number, and shape are well characterized and controlled.

Another confounding factor is that certain particulates, such as cobalt-based alloy, may be cytotoxic when introduced in a bolus but may not be cytotoxic when introduced in smaller doses over a longer time-interval, which more closely simulates the clinical situation.[142] This precludes a direct comparison between the biologic effects of cobalt-based-alloy and titanium-based-alloy wear particles in short-term cell-culture experiments, for example. In addition, freshly generated in vivo wear particles are likely to be more chemically active than their fabricated or retrieved counterparts. These freshly generated particles would be expected to interact rapidly with the periprosthetic fluids and to be coated with organic molecules such as proteins. This situation is difficult to model with the use of fabricated or retrieved wear debris, because the latter has been extracted with enzymatic digestion, which destroys any organic coating. In spite of these limitations, there is a growing consensus that UHMW-PE particles are the most biologically active, if for no other reason than that their sheer number creates an enormous surface area for interaction with the surrounding tissues.

Solutions

The basic strategy designed to address the problem of osteolysis should incorporate methods to decrease the periprosthetic particulate burden. Polymeric wear remains the most serious and elusive problem. A number of factors govern the rate of the UHMWPE wear, including femoral head diameter and polymer thickness. Femoral heads with a diameter of 32 mm have been associated with increased volumetric UHMWPE wear, so it is common practice to use 28-mm heads.[30] With smaller metal-backed acetabular components (less than 51 mm), the use of a 22-mm head becomes advisable to maintain an adequate thickness of polymer.

Ceramic heads have been introduced as another means of decreasing UHMWPE wear. While their performance in laboratory environments has indicated that UHMWPE wear can be decreased, ceramics may create different problems, particularly fracture of the ceramic component.[143] Furthermore, the utility of ceramic heads in the clinical setting has not been demonstrated conclusively.

A modified UHMWPE, fabricated with a proprietary process including treatment with heat and pressure, has recently been introduced in the hope that the performance of the polymer would be improved. While the mechanical properties of this modified polyethylene appear to be better in many respects, initial reports have suggested that the wear performance does not appear to be improved.[10,144]

The elimination of UHMWPE is another approach being investigated clinically in various centers. There has been a renewed interest in the application of metal-metal bearings, with initial reports indicating some potential advantages to this approach.[145] Ceramic-ceramic bearings are being used clinically in

some centers, but their extensive clinical application is still several years away.

Metallic wear is also being addressed. Nitriding and nitrogen-ion implantation have been introduced to decrease the potential for abrasive wear and fretting in titanium-alloy stems. This approach may also be of value for cobalt-alloy stems. Polishing of the stem removes surface asperities and decreases particle generation from stem-bone fretting. In addition, polishing minimizes silicate contamination. Forthcoming are improvements in the design of modular connections that will address manufacturing tolerances, taper geometry, and metallurgic processing in order to minimize the prevalence and severity of the mechanically assisted crevice-corrosion process that has been demonstrated.[138] In order for surgeons and manufacturers to continue to benefit from the advantages of modular designs, a great deal of attention needs to be directed toward the optimization of these designs. In general terms, the number of modular designs should be increased only with caution.

Improvements in the design of acetabular prostheses should include improved tolerances between the UHMWPE insert and the metal backing, improved finish on the metallic concave surfaces, secure locking mechanisms, and the avoidance of holes on the convex portion of the acetabular prosthesis.

Implant fixation is also an important variable. It is believed that circumferential, more extensive porous coatings will improve fixation as well as reduce the likelihood of transport of UHMWPE particles to the distal portion of the femoral canal. Surgical technique has an important role in the development of osteolysis, in that initial rigid fixation facilitates bone ingrowth and thereby minimizes relative motion between the bone and the implant. Furthermore, the surgeon needs to pay careful attention to the intraoperative assembly of modular connections.

Osteolysis associated with total hip arthroplasty performed without cement generally is an adverse local response to foreign particulate material. It has serious clinical consequences, including prosthetic loosening, periprosthetic fracture, and severe bone-stock deficiency. All of these factors pose serious problems if further reconstruction must be done. In the next several years, considerable effort should be directed toward increasing our understanding of this phenomenon and ultimately preventing it.

Advances in Biomaterials to Enhance Implant Fixation

A prerequisite for the success of any orthopaedic arthroplasty is permanent fixation of the components to the surrounding osseous environment with no intervening soft tissue. This process, known as osseointegration, occurs at the interface between the bone and the implant surface. It is affected by both biomechanical forces and biomaterial properties. The forces transmitted between the prosthesis and the bone depend on the design and geometry of the implant, the materials used, and the mechanical characteristics of the surrounding bone. The biomaterial properties of the surface determine the relative biocompatibility of the material, the surface biochemistry, and therefore the degree of fixation. Of the materials that are currently in use for implant fixation, commercially pure titanium and calcium hydroxyapatite are associated with the best result in terms of osseointegration.

Bioactive Ceramic Coatings

The fixation of metal prostheses to bone can occur in a number of ways, including the formation of a microinterlock or osseointegration. In the former situation, the metal substrate is covered with pores of an optimum size for mineralized bone to grow into the porous surface, thus achieving a microinterlock.[146,147] However, there is no chemical bonding of the metal to the bone, and histologic studies of retrieved porous hip and knee prostheses have shown variable ingrowth.[148,149] A considerable number of pores are filled with fibrous tissue, and the pores that are filled with bone have a fibrous membrane separating bone from metal.

Bioactive calcium-phosphate ceramics such as calcium hydroxyapatite have been studied for more than 15 years. They have been shown to be biocompatible, non-toxic, and capable of bonding directly to bone, thus allowing for true osseointegration.[150-152] This is because the synthetic form of calcium hydroxyapatite resembles the apatitic mineral component of human bone and can be made essentially non-resorbable for long-term application.

Basic Science Research

Numerous animal studies have shown that a calcium hydroxyapatite coating increases the amount of bone-implant contact through the preferential deposition of new bone both on the surface of the implant and on the host bed, with no intervening fibrous tissue.[153] The maximum fixation strength is increased, and the time required to achieve adequate fixation strength is decreased. Plasma-sprayed calcium-hydroxyapatite coatings applied to roughened or porous titanium or cobalt-chromium surfaces enhance bone apposition to the implant and interface attachment strengths.[154,155]

The bond between the metal substrate and the calcium hydroxyapatite is critical to the success of a coated prosthesis, and the developmental process is complex.[156] Not all calcium hydroxyapatite coatings are the same, nor are they applied to the metallic components in the same way. The coatings can fail if they are improperly applied, controlled, used, or formulated.

Calcium hydroxyapatite can be characterized by its calcium-phosphate ratio, crystallinity, grain size, density, dissolution properties, and strength. Techniques such as x-ray diffraction provide much more comprehensive information than does infrared spectroscopy in the characterization (identification of the biochemical properties) of calcium hydroxyapatite.[157]

Although there are many techniques for the application of a calcium hydroxyapatite coating to a metal surface, the most extensively used has been plasma spraying. The ceramic powder is introduced into a flame that directs the particles for deposition onto the metal surface. Newer techniques such as low-pressure plasma spraying are being developed to provide a coating that is both stronger and more resistant to dissolution or degradation of bond strength between the metal and the coating.[158] Thinner coatings have been recommended because they do not affect the mechanical properties of the substrate metal.[159] A 50-μm-thick calcium-hydroxyapatite coating remains highly adherent to the substrate metal without affecting its fatigue properties. Thicker coatings (120 and 240 μm) are more susceptible to delamination and fatigue, because of the mechanical mismatch between the ceramic coating and the metal substrate.

Other studies have examined even thinner coatings over porous cobalt-chromium-alloy implants in dogs.[160] A 25-μm-thick coating increased both the interface attachment strength and the percentage of bone ingrowth, as demonstrated with the use of paired comparisons, which minimize biologic variability. While push-out tests such as those used in this study are commonly used to determine interface shear strengths, a number of confounding variables can make their interpretation difficult. Tensile testing of the interface may provide a more direct measure of bone-implant attachment. Interface testing performed in this manner has suggested that the strength is determined not only by the bond between the calcium hydroxyapatite and the substrate metal, but also by the intrinsic tensile strength of the calcium hydroxyapatite coating itself.[161]

In a canine titanium-alloy femoral component model, a 50-μm-thick calcium-hydroxyapatite coating demonstrated significantly ($p < 0.05$) increased fixation strength as early as three weeks. The fixation strength was increased at six weeks and then remained stable.[162] At 12 weeks, the coated prostheses had three times greater pull-out strength than the uncoated controls. Histologic examination showed nearly circumferential osseointegration. Another study demonstrated similarly encouraging results in a canine model.[163]

Regardless of the technique used to achieve it, initial stable fixation is required for a successful outcome. Excessive motion inhibits bone ingrowth by producing a reactive fibrous membrane.[153] The quality of the initial press-fit in an arthroplasty done without cement is an important factor for initial stability and subsequent long-term fixation.[164] Micromotion of as little as 100 to 500 μm between the bone and the implant is sufficient to inhibit bone ingrowth and to result in the formation of a fibrous membrane between the bone and the mechanically unstable implant.[165] In one study, a membrane formed around both titanium and calcium hydroxyapatite-coated implants, but the fibrous tissue that formed around the coated implants consisted mainly of fibrocartilage, with a higher concentration of collagen fibers arranged in a radial pattern.[166] This resulted in stronger fibrous anchorage of the unstable coated implants compared with the stable uncoated implants. Mechanically stable coated implants had the best fixation with the greatest amount of bone apposition, and this occurred relatively early.

Recent studies examining the fibrous membrane have suggested that a calcium hydroxyapatite coating has the capability to replace a motion-induced fibrous membrane with bone when subjected to a continuous load.[167] Thus, calcium hydroxyapatite may be able to stabilize the interface through a number of different mechanisms.

An increased amount of bone apposition means a larger interface between the prosthesis and the bone, producing a stronger and more stable bond that may last for a longer period of time. However, even in a stable environment, there is a limit to the amount of contact that can be achieved with a press-fit. When a femoral stem is press-fit into the femoral canal, only 10% to 20% of the prosthesis comes into direct contact with bone, thus limiting the size of the interface.[168] Recent studies have shown that mineralized bone can span gaps as large as 2 mm adjacent to a stable implant with a calcium hydroxyapatite coating.[169-171] This occurs in both normal and osteopenic bone.[172] Initial stability is a necessary but not a sufficient factor in the prediction of long-term fixation. Calcium hydroxyapatite appears to enhance the interface between the prosthesis and the bone by compensating for an imprecise press-fit caused by surgical inaccuracies and physical limitations.[173] The coating acts as a substrate for new-bone formation and can compensate for a lack of direct osseous contact with the metal surface. However, for an arthroplasty to be successful, precise, meticulous techniques by the surgeon are still required; calcium hydroxyapatite will not compensate for poor surgical technique. Hydroxyapatite may be able to make a well-done arthroplasty a little better by providing a larger interface that is stronger and more stable, and therefore may last for a longer period of time, but a weak bond between the metal prosthesis and the hydroxyapatite coating may lead to loosening and failure of the implant.

Clinical Results

Clinical trials of calcium hydroxyapatite-coated total hip prostheses began in 1986; present ongoing investigations are involving a variety of implant substrates and designs, not only for total hip arthroplasty but also for total knee and total shoulder arthroplasty.

Two large multicenter trials of total hip prostheses coated with calcium hydroxyapatite, with follow-up of two years or more, have recently been reported, both with encouraging early results; these have led to Food and Drug Administration approval of a calcium hydroxyapatite coating for certain indications.[174,175] Numerous other clinical trials with early follow-up[176-179] support the basic science data indicating that calcium hydroxyapatite appears to enhance and accelerate the formation of a bond between the bone and the prosthesis, as judged by encouraging early clinical and radiographic findings. In the short-term, the pain ratings and mean Harris hip scores have been comparable with, or superior to, those that have been reported for cemented or porous-coated press-fit prostheses.

Retrieval Studies

Recently, investigators have reported retrieval data from well-functioning calcium hydroxyapatite-coated femoral stems obtained at autopsy.[180-185] Components that had been in situ for three weeks to 25 months showed no evidence of an inflammatory reaction or fibrous tissue formation between the bone and the calcium hydroxyapatite. In most cases, no clear boundary between the newly formed bone and the coating was visible by scanning electron microscopy. Biologic osseointegration appeared to have taken place, and the coating enhanced early skeletal fixation secondary to its osteoconductive properties. The implants were mechanically stable, with bone-remodeling seen at the bone-implant interface according to Wolff's law. However, all results are not uniform and some interfaces show regional loss of the calcium hydroxyapatite coating because of osteoclastic resorption. Concerns exist regarding possible delamination and the formation of particulate debris with longer follow-up.

The long-term clinical durability of the interface between the calcium hydroxyapatite and the prosthesis remains unknown. The potential for degradation of the coating raises concern regarding the subsequent release of calcium hydroxyapatite particles into the joint space, which could damage the implant surfaces through third-body wear or stimulate an inflammatory reaction with possible osteolysis and loosening. Two recent retrieval studies have demonstrated calcium hydroxyapatite particulate debris and wear of the UHMWPE in total hip prostheses with titanium femoral heads.[186,187] Although the evidence is indirect, these studies suggest that separation and migration of calcium hydroxyapatite particles may be a cause of component wear, osteolysis from the generation of additional particulate debris, and subsequent implant loosening. While the short-term results are encouraging and justify continued study of calcium hydroxyapatite-coated hip implants, caution should be exercised. Longer follow-up is necessary to determine the long-term status of the coating, because failure may occur at the hydroxyapatite-prosthesis interface.

Future Applications

As previously mentioned, clinical trials of calcium hydroxyapatite-coated total knee and shoulder prostheses are currently ongoing, but the results have yet to be published. Early follow-up data for calcium hydroxyapatite-coated proximal humeral implants have shown encouraging results, with good radiographic evidence of osseointegration and excellent clinical outcomes at one to two years.[188] Calcium hydroxyapatite can also be used to coat other types of implants to improve their fixation strength. Coating of either titanium or stainless-steel screws with calcium hydroxyapatite has been shown to substantially improve the interface shear strength in dogs at six weeks.[189] With a stronger bond between the screw and bone, micromotion of a component fixed with screws may be minimized early on when the patient is undergoing rehabilitation, thus allowing for osseointegration and a stable implant.

Another use for bioactive ceramics is as a biodegradable cement or component of cement that can bond with bone. Calcium phosphate cements have been developed that set up rapidly in situ, are not exothermic or damaging to the surrounding tissues, attain high compressive strengths, and are highly biocompatible compared with polymethylmethacrylate.[190-193] To provide initial stabilization, the prosthesis is embedded in a biodegradable calcium-phosphate cement that can bond directly with the host bone to provide improved fixation. Over time, there is slow resorption of the cement as new bone is laid down, with subsequent remodeling. In addition, these active cements can be used to fill gaps between a prosthesis fixed without cement and bone, thereby increasing the size and stability of the interface.

Conclusions

The use of orthopaedic implants is growing rapidly in terms of both number and sophistication. As new designs move through development and into clinical use, problems arise with the use of traditional biomaterials in new roles, and new biomaterials are required to achieve the desired therapeutic goals. The use of modular components, while affording potential technical and cost advantages, has produced concerns about fretting and corrosion. Because wear produces biologically active debris, which has been implicated as the major cause of osteolysis, wear is emerging as the principal limit on successful long-term fixation of total joint components, implanted either with or without cement. Longer durations of the prostheses in situ, due both to greater clinical success of devices and to younger patient age at implantation, increase concerns about the biologic consequences of long-term local exposure to biomaterials and about systemic exposure to their degradation products. A wide range of new materials and processes, including bioactive coatings, wear-resistant surface modifications, modified bone cements, and composite and resorbable materials, are the subjects of laboratory and early clinical evaluation.

Orthopaedic surgery has been, and should always be, a conservative discipline, because it deals more with enhancement of patient life experience than with life preservation or extension. Therefore, however exciting and promising new technological developments may seem, their general adoption should proceed through the traditional practices of continuing clinical observation and the review and selection of devices and therapeutic approaches best suited to each individual patient. Only in this way can progress in biomaterials contribute to progress in orthopaedic surgery without sacrifice of the enormous gains already made.

References

1. Harris WH, Schiller AL, Scholler J-M, et al: Extensive localized bone resorption in the femur following total hip replacement. *J Bone Joint Surg* 1976;58A:612-618.
2. Howie DW, Vernon-Roberts B, Oakeshott R, et al: A rat model of resorption of bone at the cement-bone interface in the presence of polyethylene wear particles. *J Bone Joint Surg* 1988;70A:257-263.
3. Skinner HB, Mabey MF: Soft-tissue response to total hip surface replacement. *J Biomed Mater Res* 1987;21:569-584.
4. Willert H-G, Semlitsch M: Reactions of the articular capsule to wear products of artificial joint prostheses. *J Biomed Mater Res* 1977;11:157-164.
5. Willert H-G, Ludwig J, Semlitsch M: Reaction of bone to methacrylate after hip arthroplasty: A long-term gross, light microscopic, and scanning electron microscopic study. *J Bone Joint Surg* 1974;56A:1368-1382.
6. Collier JP, Mayor MB, Surprenant VA, et al: The biomechanical problems of polyethylene as a bearing surface. *Clin Orthop* 1990;261:107-113.
7. Davidson JA: Characteristics of metal and ceramic total hip bearing surfaces and the effect on long-term UHMWPE wear. Read at the *20th Open Scientific Meeting of The Hip Society*, Washington, DC, Feb. 23, 1992.
8. McKellop HA, Rostlund TV: The wear behavior of ion-implanted Ti-6Al-4V against UHMW polyethylene. *J Biomed Mater Res* 1990;24:1413-1425.
9. Rostoker W, Galante JO: Some new studies of the wear behavior of ultrahigh molecular weight polyethylene. *J Biomed Mater Res* 1976;10:303-310.
10. McKellop H, Lu B, Li S: Wear of acetabular cups of conventional and modified UHMW polyethylenes compared on a hip joint simulator. *Trans Orthop Res Soc* 1992;17:356.

11. Weightman B, Light D: The effect of the surface finish of alumina and stainless steel on the wear rate of UHMW polyethylene. *Biomaterials* 1986;7:20-24.

12. Carmichael C (ed): *Kent's Mechanical Engineers' Handbook Design and Production Volume,* ed 12. New York, NY, Wiley & Sons, 1950, pp 8-18.

13. Skinner HB: Current biomaterial problems in implants, in Eilert RE (ed): *Instructional Course Lectures XLI.* Park Ridge, IL, American Academy of Orthopaedic Surgeons, 1992, pp 137-144.

14. Agins HJ, Alcock NW, Bansal M, et al: Metallic wear in failed titanium-alloy total hip replacements: A histological and quantitative analysis. *J Bone Joint Surg* 1988;70A:347-356.

15. Black J, Sherk H, Bonini J, et al: Metallosis associated with a stable titanium-alloy femoral component in total hip replacement: A case report. *J Bone Joint Surg* 1990;72A:126-130.

16. McKellop HA, Sarmiento A, Schwinn CP, et al: In vivo wear of titanium-alloy hip prostheses. *J Bone Joint Surg* 1990;72A:512-517.

17. Davies JP, Burke DW, O'Connor DO, et al: Comparison of the fatigue characteristics of centrifuged and uncentrifuged Simplex P bone cement. *J Orthop Res* 1989;5:366-371.

18. Crowninshield RD, Pedersen DR, Brand RA, et al: Analytical support for acetabular component metal backing, in *The Hip: Proceedings of the 11th Open Scientific Meeting of The Hip Society.* St. Louis, MO, CV Mosby, 1983, pp 207-215.

19. Sarmiento A, Gruen TA: Radiographic analysis of a low-modulus titanium-alloy femoral total hip component: Two-to six-year follow-up. *J Bone Joint Surg* 1985;67A:48-56.

20. Skinner HB: Isoelasticity and total hip arthroplasty. *Orthopedics* 1991;14:323-328.

21. Hulbert SF, Cooke FW, Klawitter JJ, et al: Attachment of prostheses to the musculoskeletal system by tissue ingrowth and mechanical interlocking. *J Biomed Mater Res* 1973;7:1-23.

22. Franks E, Mont MA, Maar DC, et al: Thigh pain as related to bending rigidity of the femoral prosthesis and bone. *Trans Orthop Res Soc* 1992;17:296.

23. Skinner HB, Curlin FJ: Decreased pain with lower flexural rigidity of uncemented femoral prostheses. *Orthopedics* 1990;13:1223-1228.

24. Bobyn JD, Glassman AH, Goto H, et al: The effect of stem stiffness on femoral bone resorption after canine porous-coated total hip arthroplasty. *Clin Orthop* 1990;261:196-213.

25. Hsu HP, Garg A, Walker PS, et al: Effect of knee component alignment on tibial load distribution with clinical correlation. *Clin Orthop* 1989;248:135-144.

26. Bayley JC, Scott RD, Ewald FC, et al: Failure of the metal-backed patellar component after total hip replacement. *J Bone Joint Surg* 1988;70A:668-674.

27. Lombardi AV Jr, Engh GA, Volz RG, et al: Fracture/dissociation of the polyethylene in metal-backed patellar components in total knee arthroplasty. *J Bone Joint Surg* 1988;70A:675-679.

28. Stulberg BN, de Swart RJ, Reger S, et al: Factors influencing wear of all-polyethylene patellar components: A retrieval study. Read at the American Society for the Testing of Materials Symposium on Biocompatibility of Particulate Implant Materials, San Antonio, Texas, Oct. 31, 1990.

29. Sutherland CJ: Patellar component dissociation in total knee arthroplasty: A report of two cases. *Clin Orthop* 1988;228:178-181.

30. Livermore J, Ilstrup D, Morrey BF: Effect of femoral head size on wear of the polyethylene acetabular component. *J Bone Joint Surg* 1990;72A:518-528.

31. Hoeltzel DA, Walt MJ, Kyle RF, et al: The effects of femoral head size on the deformation of ultrahigh molecular weight polyethylene acetabular cups. *J Biomech* 1989;22:1163-1173.

32. Morrey BF, Ilstrup D: Size of the femoral head and acetabular revision in total hip-replacement arthroplasty. *J Bone Joint Surg* 1989;71A:50-55.

33. Wright TM, Bartel DL: The problem of surface damage in polyethylene total knee components. *Clin Orthop* 1986;205:67-74.

34. Bindelglass DF, Cohen JL, Dorr LD: Current principles of design for cemented and cementless knees. *Tech Orthop* 1991;6:80-85.

35. Carter DR: Finite-element analysis of a metal-backed acetabular component, in *The Hip: Proceedings of the 11th Open Scientific Meeting of The Hip Society.* St. Louis, MO, CV Mosby, 1983, pp 216-228.

36. Carter DR, Vasu R, Harris WH: Stress distributions in the acetabular region: II. Effects of cement thickness and metal backing of the total hip acetabular component. *J Biomech* 1982;15:165-170.

37. Harris WH: Advances in total hip arthroplasty: The metal-backed acetabular component. *Clin Orthop* 1984;183:4-11.

38. Harris WH, White RE Jr: Socket fixation using a metal-backed acetabular component for total hip replacement: A minimum five-year follow-up. *J Bone Joint Surg* 1982;64A:745-748.

39. Cohen MG, Hays MB, Garcia JJ, et al: Fracture of a metal-backed acetabular cup: A case report. *J Arthroplasty* 1988;3:263-265.

40. Dorr LD, Takei GK, Conaty JP: Total hip arthroplasties in patients less than 45 years old. *J Bone Joint Surg* 1983;65A:474-479.

41. Ritter MA, Keating EM, Faris PM, et al: Metal-backed acetabular cups in total hip arthroplasty. *J Bone Joint Surg* 1990;72A:672-677.

42. Collins DN, Chetta SG, Nelson CL: Fracture of the acetabular cup: A case report. *J Bone Joint Surg* 1982;64A:939-940.

43. Harley JM, Boston DA: Acetabular cup failure after total hip replacement. *J Bone Joint Surg* 1985;67B:222-224.

44. Salvati EA, Wright TM, Burstein AH, et al: Fracture of polyethylene acetabular cups: Report of two cases. *J Bone Joint Surg* 1979;61A:1239-1242

45. Burton DT, Skinner HB: Stress analysis of a total hip acetabular component: An FEM study. *Biomater Artif Cells Artif Organs* 1989;17:371-383.

46. Dorr LD: Polyethylene versus metal-backed tibial components. Read at State-of-the-Art in Total Joint Replacement. Scottsdale, AZ, Nov. 21, 1988.

47. Ranawat CS, Boachie-Adjei O: Survivorship analysis and results of total condylar knee arthroplasty: Eight- to 11-year follow-up period. *Clin Orthop* 1988;226:6-13.

48. Bartel DL, Burstein AH, Santavicca EA, et al: Performance of the tibial component in total knee replacement: Conventional and revision designs. *J Bone Joint Surg* 1982;64A:1026-1033.

49. Ewald FC, Jacobs MA, Miegel RE, et al: Kinematic total knee replacement. *J Bone Joint Surg* 1984;66A:1032-1040.

50. Reilly D, Walker PS, Ben-Dov M, et al: Effects of tibial components on load transfer in the upper tibia. *Clin Orthop* 1992;165:273-282.

51. Walker PS, Greene D, Reilly D, et al: Fixation of tibial components of knee prostheses. *J Bone Joint Surg* 1981;63A:258-267.

52. Mendes DG, Brandon D, Galor L, et al: Breakage of the metal tray in total knee replacement. *Orthopedics* 1984;7:860-862.

53. Paganelli JV, Skinner HB, Mote CD Jr: Prediction of fatigue failure of a total knee replacement tibial plateau using finite element analysis. *Orthopedics* 1988;11:1161-1168.

54. Scott RD, Ewald FC, Walker PS: Fracture of the metallic tibial tray following total knee replacement: Report of two cases. *J Bone Joint Surg* 1984;66A:780-782.

55. Skinner HB, Mabey MF, Paganelli JV, et al: Failure analysis of PCA revision total knee replacement tibial component: A preliminary study using the finite element method. *Orthopedics* 1987;10:581-584.

56. Black J: *Biological Performance of Materials: Fundamentals of Biocompatibility*, ed 2. New York, NY, Dekker, 1992, pp 110, 184, 275.

57. Ducheyne P, Cohn CS: Biomaterial: Structure processing and mechanical properties, in Steinberg ME (ed): *The Hip and Its Disorders*. Philadelphia, PA, WB Saunders, 1991, pp 905-928.

58. Galante JO, Lemons J, Spector M, et al: The biologic effects of implant materials. *J Orthop Res* 1991;9:760-775.

59. Black J: Does corrosion matter? *J Bone Joint Surg* 1988;70B: 517-520.

60. American Society for Testing Materials: 1992 Annual Book of ASTM Standards. Section 13: Medical Devices and Services. Philadelphia, PA, American Society for Testing Materials, 1992.

61. Black J: Biomaterials: Biocompatibility, in Steinberg ME (ed): *The Hip and Its Disorders*. Philadelphia PA, 1991, pp 929-944.

62. Black J: Systemic effects of biomaterials. *Biomaterials* 1984;5:11-18.

63. Fraker AC, Griffin CD: *Corrosion and Degradation of Implant Materials: Second Symposium*. Philadelphia, PA, American Society for Testing Materials STP 859 1985, p 195.

64. Jacobs JJ, Skipor AK, Black J, et al: Release and excretion of metal in patients who have a total hip-replacement component made of titanium-base alloy. *J Bone Joint Surg* 1991;73A:1475-1486.

65. Langkamer VG, Case CP, Heap P, et al: Systemic distribution of wear debris after hip replacement. *J Bone Joint Surg* 1992;74B:831-839.

66. Michel R: Trace metal analysis in biocompatibility testing. *CRC Crit Rev Biocompat* 1987;3:236-317.

67. National Research Council Subcommittee: *Tenth Edition of the RDAs Food and Nutrition Board Commission on Life Sciences: Recommended Dietary Allowances*, ed 10. Washington, DC, National Academy Press, 1989.

68. Mertz W (ed): *Trace Elements in Human and Animal Nutrition*, ed 5. Orlando, FL, Academic Press, 1986.

69. Friberg L, Nordberg GF, Vouk VB (eds): *Handbook on the Toxicology of Metals*. Amsterdam, Elsevier, 1986.

70. Luckey TD, Venugopal B: *Metal Toxicity in Mammals. Physiologic and Chemical Basis for Metal Toxicity*. New York, NY, Plenum Press, 1977, vol 1.

71. Esterhai JL Jr, Gristina AG, Poss R (eds): *Musculoskeletal Infection*. Park Ridge, IL, American Academy of Orthopaedic Surgeons, 1992.

72. Gristina AG, Naylor PT, Myrvik QN: Biomaterial-centered infections: Microbial adhesion versus tissue integration, in Wadström T, Eliasson I, Holder I, et al (eds): *Pathogenesis of Wound and Biomaterial-Associated Infections*. New York, NY, Springer, 1990, pp 193-216.

73. Schmalzried TP, Amstutz HC, Au MK, et al: Etiology of deep sepsis in total hip arthroplasty: The significance of hematogenous and recurrent infections. *Clin Orthop* 1992;280:200-207.

74. Petty W, Spanier S, Shuster JJ, et al: The influence of skeletal implants on the incidence of infection: Experiments in a canine model. *J Bone Joint Surg* 1985;67A:1236-1244.

75. Hierholzer S, Hierholzer G, Sauer KH, et al: Increased corrosion of stainless steel implants in infected plated fractures. *Arch Orthop Trauma Surg* 1984;102:198-206.

76. Collier JP, Surprenant VA, Jensen RE, et al: Corrosion at the interface of cobalt-alloy heads on titanium-alloy stems. *Clin Orthop* 1991;271:305-312.

77. Mathiesen EB, Lindgren JU, Blomgren GG, et al: Corrosion of modular hip prostheses. *J Bone Joint Surg* 1991;73B:569-575.

78. Pascual A, Tsukayama D, Wicklund BH, et al: The effect of stainless steel, cobalt-chromium titanium alloy and titanium on respiratory burst activity of human polymorphonuclear leukocytes. *Clin Orthop* 1992;280:281-288.

79. Rae T: Cell biochemistry in relation to the inflammatory response to foreign materials, in Williams DF (ed): *Fundamental Aspects of Biocompatibility*. Boca Raton, FL, CRC Press, 1981, vol 1, pp 159-181.

80. Shanbhag A, Yang J, Lilien J, et al: Decreased neutrophil respiratory burst on exposure to cobalt-chrome alloy and polystyrene in vitro. *J Biomed Mater Res* 1992;26:185-195.

81. Wapner KL, Morris DM, Black J: Release of corrosion products by F-75 cobalt base alloy in the rat. II. Morbidity apparently associated with chromium release in vivo: A 120-day rat study. *J Biomed Mater Res* 1986;20:219-233.

82. Hildebrand HF, Champy M: *Biocompatibility of Co-Cr-Ni Alloys*. New York, NY, Plenum Press, 1988, p 187.

83. Elves MW: Immunological aspects of biomaterials, in Williams DF (ed): *Fundamental Aspects of Biocompatibility*. Boca Raton, FL, CRC Press, 1981, vol 2, pp 159-173.

84. Lalor PA, Revell PA, Gray AB, et al: Sensitivity to titanium: A cause of implant failure? *J Bone Joint Surg* 1991;73B:25-28.

85. Gil-Albarova J, Laclériga A, Barrios C, et al: Lymphocyte response to polymethylmethacrylate in loose total hip prostheses. *J Bone Joint Surg* 1992;74B:825-830.

86. Goldblum RM, Pelly RP, O'Donnell A, et al: Antibodies to silicone elastomers and reactions to ventriculoperitoneal shunts. *Lancet* 1992;340:510-513.

87. Black J: Metallic ion release and its relationship to oncogenesis, in *The Hip: Proceedings of the 13th Open Scientific Meeting of The Hip Society*. St. Louis, MO, CV Mosby, 1986, pp 199-213.

88. Jacobs JJ, Rosenbaum DH, Hay RM, et al: Early sarcomatous degeneration near a cementless hip replacement: A case report and review. *J Bone Joint Surg* 1992;74B:740-744.

89. Gillespie WJ, Frampton CM, Henderson RJ, et al: The incidence of cancer following total hip replacement. *J Bone Joint Surg* 1988;70B:539-542.

90. Visuri T, Koskenvuo M: Cancer risk after McKee-Farrar total hip replacement. *Orthopedics* 1991;14:137-142.

91. Rock MG: Toxicity and oncogenesis, in Morrey B (ed): *Biological Material and Mechanical Considerations of Joint Replacement*. Rosemont, IL, American Academy of Orthopaedic Surgeons, 1993.

92. Black J: "And there are no data...", he said" [editorial response]. *Biomater Forum* 1990;12:9.

93. Charnley J, Follacci FM, Hammond BT: The long-term reaction of bone to self-curing acrylic cement. *J Bone Joint Surg* 1968;50B:822-829.

94. Carlsson AS, Gentz CF, Linder L: Localized bone resorption in the femur in mechanical failure of cemented total hip arthroplasties. *Acta Orthop Scand* 1983;54:396-402.

95. Huddleston HD: Femoral lysis after cemented hip arthroplasty. *J Arthroplasty* 1988;3:285-297.

96. Willert H-G, Bertram H, Buchhorn GH: Osteolysis in alloarthroplasty of the hip: The role of bone cement fragmentation. *Clin Orthop* 1990:258:108-121.

97. Jasty MJ, Floyd WE III, Schiller AL, et al: Localized osteolysis in stable, non-septic total hip replacement. *J Bone Joint Surg* 1986;68A:912-919.

98. Mulroy RD Jr, Harris WH: The effect of improved cementing techniques on component loosening in total hip replacement: An 11-year radiographic review. *J Bone Joint Surg* 1990;72B:757-760.

99. Maloney WJ, Jasty M, Rosenberg A, et al: Bone lysis in well-fixed cemented femoral components. *J Bone Joint Surg* 1990;72B:966-970.

100. Anthony PP, Gie GA, Howie CR, et al: Localised endosteal bone lysis in relation to the femoral components of cemented total hip arthroplasties. *J Bone Joint Surg.* 1990;72B:971-979.

101. Jones LC, Hungerford DS: Cement disease. *Clin Orthop* 1987;225:192-206.

102. Martell JM, Pierson RH III, Jacobs JJ, et al: Primary total hip reconstruction with a titanium-fiber coated prosthesis inserted without cement. *J Bone Joint Surg* 1993;75A:554-571.

103. Maloney WJ, Jasty M, Harris WH, et al: Endosteal erosion in association with stable uncemented femoral components. *J Bone Joint Surg* 1990;72A:1025-1034.

104. Tanzer M, Maloney WJ, Jasty M, et al: The progression of femoral cortical osteolysis in association with total hip arthroplasty without cement. *J Bone Joint Surg* 1992;74A:404-410.

105. Callaghan J, Heekin RD, Hopkinson W, et al: The uncemented porous-coated anatomic total hip prosthesis: Five to seven year results of a prospective consecutive series. *Orthop Trans* 1992;16:749.

106. Cox CV, Dorr LD: Five year results of proximal bone ingrowth fixation total hip replacement. *Orthop Trans* 1992;16:748-749.

107. Engh CA, Macalino GE: Clinical experience of the AML at 9 years. Read at the annual Harvard Hip Course, Boston, MA, Sept. 16, 1991.

108. Griffiths HJ, Burke J, Bonfiglio TA: Granulomatous pseudo-tumors in total joint replacement. *Skeletal Radiol* 1987;16:146-152.

109. Stulberg BN, Buly RL, Howard PL, et al: Porous coated anatomic acetabular failure: Incidence and modes of failure in uncemented total hip arthroplasty. Read at the annual meeting of the American Academy of Orthopaedic Surgeons, Washington, DC, Feb. 24, 1992.

110. Beauchesne RP, Kukita Y, Knezevich S, et al: Roentgenographic evaluation of the AML porous-coated acetabular component: A six-year minimum follow-up study. *Orthop Trans* 1992;16:749.

111. Schmalzried TP, Harris WH: The Harris-Galante porous-coated acetabular component with screw fixation: Radiographic analysis of eighty-three primary hip replacements at a minimum of five years. *J Bone Joint Surg* 1992;74A:1130-1139.

112. Shanbhag AS, Jacobs JJ, Glant TT, et al: Characterization of wear particles retrieved from failed uncemented total hip arthroplasty. *Trans Soc Biomater* 1992;15:29.

113. Goldring SR, Schiller AL, Roelke M, et al: The synovial-like membrane at the bone-cement interface in loose total hip replacements and its proposed role in bone lysis. *J Bone Joint Surg* 1983;65A:575-584.

114. Apple AM, Sowder WG, Hopson CN, et al: Production of mediators of bone resorption by prosthesis associated pseudomembranes. *Trans Orthop Res Soc* 1988;13:362.

115. Davis RG, Smith RL, Goodman SB, et al: Bone cement stimulates lysosomal enzyme activity of adherent mononuclear cells. *Trans Orthop Res Soc* 1990;15:234.

116. Dorr LD, Bloebaum R, Emanual J, et al: Histologic, biochemical, and ion analysis of tissue and fluids retrieved during total hip arthroplasty. *Clin Orthop* 1990;261:82-95.

117. Glant TT, Jacobs JJ, Molnár G, et al: Particulate titanium induced bone resorption in organ culture. *Orthop Trans* 1991;15:540.

118. Goldring SR, Kroop SF, Petrison KK, et al: Metal particles stimulate prostaglandin E_2 (PGE_2) release and collagen synthesis in cultured cells. *Trans Orthop Res Soc* 1990;15:444.

119. Goodman SB, Chin RC, Chiou SS, et al: Modulation of the membrane surrounding particulate polymethylmethacrylate in the rabbit tibia. *Trans Soc Biomater* 1990;13:289.

120. Goodman SB, Chin RC, Chiou SS, et al: A clinical-pathologic-biochemical study of the membrane surrounding loosened and nonloosened total hip arthroplasties. *Clin Orthop* 1989;244:182-187.

121. Horowitz SM, Frondoza CG, Lennox DW: Effects of polymethylmethacrylate exposure upon macrophages. *J Orthop Res* 1988;6:827-832.

122. Horowitz SM, Gautsch TL, Frondoza CG, et al: Macrophage exposure to polymethylmethacrylate leads to mediator release and injury. *J Orthop Res* 1991;9:406-413.

123. Kim KJ, Wilson SC, Rubash HE: Comparison study of interface tissues in cementless and cemented prostheses. *Trans Orthop Res Soc* 1990;15:236.

124. Kossovsky N, Allameh V, Campbell P, et al: Inflammatory activity of synovial macrophages retrieved from clinical arthroplasty. *Trans Orthop Res Soc* 1990;15:459.

125. Lanzer WL, Crane GK, Howard GA, et al: The effects of implant wear debris on human bone cell proliferation in vitro. *Trans Soc Biomater* 1990;13:293.

126. Mather SE, Emmanual J, Magee FP, et al: Interleukin and prostaglandin E_2 in failed total hip arthroplasty. *Trans Orthop Res Soc* 1989;14:498.

127. Murray DW, Rushton N: Macrophages stimulate bone resorption when they phacocytose particles. *J Bone Joint Surg* 1990;72B:988-992.

128. Ohlin A, Johnell O, Lerner UH: The pathogenesis of loosening of total hip arthroplasties: The production of factors by periprosthetic tissues that stimulate in vitro bone resorption. *Clin Orthop* 1990;253:287-296.

129. Perry M, Frondoza C, Jones L, et al: The response of macrophages, fibroblasts, and osteoblasts to PMMA and metal particles in tissue culture. *Trans Orthop Res Soc* 1990;15:486.

130. Spector M, Shortkroff S, Hsu H-P, et al: Tissue changes around loose prostheses: A canine model to investigate the effects of an antiinflammatory agent. *Clin Orthop* 1990;261:140-152.

131. Tanner KT, Frondoza CG, Jones L, et al: In vitro effects of polymethylmethacrylate on normal human fibroblasts. *Trans Soc Biomater* 1990;13:101.

132. Thornhill TS, Ozuna RM, Shortkroff S, et al: Biochemical and histological evaluation of the synovial-like tissue around failed (loose) total joint replacement prostheses in human subjects and a canine model. *Biomaterials* 1990;11:69-72.

133. Shanbhag AS, Jacobs JJ, Black J, et al: Pro- and anti-inflammatory mediators secreted by cells of interfacial membranes from revision total hip replacements. *Trans Orthop Res Soc* 1993;18:517.

134. Kim KJ, Greis P, Wilson SC, et al: Histological and biochemical comparison of membranes from titanium, cobalt-chromium, and non polyethylene hip prostheses. *Trans Orthop Res Soc* 1991;16:191.

135. Glant TT, Jacobs JJ, Tabith K, et al: Particulate-induced bone resorption in organ culture. *Trans Orthop Res Soc* 1992;17:44.

136. Urban RM, Sumner DR, Gilbert JL, et al: Autopsy retrieval analysis on noncircumferentially porous coated cementless femoral stems. Read at the annual meeting of The American Academy of Orthopaedic Surgeons, San Francisco,

California, Feb. 18, 1993.

137. Callaghan JJ, Fulghum CS, Glisson RR, et al: The effect of femoral stem geometry on interface motion in uncemented porous-coated hip prostheses: Comparison of straight-stem and curved-stem designs. *J Bone Joint Surg* 1992;74A:839-848.

138. Buckley CA, Gilbert JL, Urban RM, et al: Mechanically assisted corrosion of modular hip prosthesis components in mixed and similar metal combination. *Trans Soc Biomater* 1992;15:58.

139. Bauer TW, Brown SA, Jiang M, et al: Corrosion in modular hip stem. *Trans Orthop Res Soc* 1992;17:354.

140. Urban RM, Jacobs JJ, Gilbert JL, et al: Corrosion products of modular hip prostheses: Microchemical identification and histopathological significance. *Trans Orthop Res Soc* 1993;18:81.

141. Shanbhag AS, Glant TT, Jacobs JJ, et al: Macrophage stimulation of fibroblastic proliferation is affected by size composition and surface area of particulates. *Trans Orthop Res Soc* 1982;17:342.

142. Howie DW, Haynes DR, Hay S, et al: The effect of titanium alloy and cobalt chrome alloy wear particles on production of inflammatory mediators Il-1, TNF Il-6, and prostaglandin E$_2$ by rodent macrophages in vitro. *Trans Orthop Res Soc* 1992;17:344.

143. Semlitsch M, Lehmann M, Weber H, et al: New prospects for a prolonged functional life-span of artificial hip joints by using the material combination polyethylene/aluminum oxide ceramin/metal. *J Biomed Mater Res* 1977;11:537-552.

144. Huang DD, Li S: Cyclic fatigue behaviors of UHMWPE and enhanced UHMWPE. *Trans Orthop Res Soc* 1992;17:403.

145. Schmalzried TP: The metal-on-metal concept. Read at the annual Harvard Hip Course, Boston, MA, Sept. 17, 1992.

146. Engh CA, Bobyn JD, Glassman AH: Porous-coated hip replacement: The factors governing bone ingrowth, stress shielding and clinical results. *J Bone Joint Surg* 1987;69B:44-55.

147. Landon GC, Galante JO, Maley MM: Noncemented total knee arthroplasty. *Clin Orthop* 1986;205:49-57.

148. Cook SD: Hydroxyapatite-coated total hip replacement. *Dent Clin North Am* 1992;36:235-238.

149. Cook SD, Thomas KA, Haddad RJ Jr: Histologic analysis of retrieved human porous-coated total joint components. *Clin Orthop* 1988;234:90-101.

150. Jarcho M: Calcium phosphate ceramics as hard tissue prosthetics. *Clin Orthop* 1981;157:259-278.

151. Jarcho M: Biomaterial aspects of calcium phosphates: Properties and applications. *Dent Clin North Am* 1986;30:25-47.

152. Jarcho M, Kay JF, Gumaer KI, et al: Tissue, cellular, and subcellular events at a bone-ceramic hydroxyapatite interface. *J Bioeng* 1977;1:79-92.

153. Friedman RJ: Advances in biomaterials and factors affecting implant fixation, in Eilert RE (ed): *Instructional Course Lectures XIL*. Rosemont, IL, American Academy of Orthopaedic Surgeons, 1992, pp 127-136.

154. Cook SD, Thomas KA, Kay J, et al: Hydroxyapatite-coated titanium for orthopedic implant applications. *Clin Orthop* 1988;232:225-243.

155. Friedman R, Bauer T, Garg K, et al: Histologic and mechanical comparison of hydroxyapatite coated cobalt chrome and titanium implants. *Trans Soc Biomater* 1993;16:61.

156. Lacefield W: Hydroxyapatite coatings. *Ann N Y Acad Sci* 1988;523:72-80.

157. LeGeros JP, LeGeros RZ: Characterization of calcium phosphate coatings on implants. *Trans Soc Biomater* 1991;14:192.

158. Edwards B, Aberman H, Dichiara JF: In vivo performance of a hydroxylapatite coating system deposited by low pressure plasma spraying. *Trans Soc Biomater* 1991;14:173.

159. Kester MA, Manley MT, Taylor SK, et al: Influence of thickness on the mechanical properties and bond strength of HA coatings applied to orthopaedic implants. *Trans Orthop Res Soc* 1991;16:95.

160. Cook SD, Thomas KA, Dalton JE, et al: Enhancement of bone ingrowth and fixation strength by hydroxylapatite coating porous implants. *Trans Orthop Res Soc* 1991;16:550.

161. Brunski JB, Edwards JT, Cochran GVB, et al: Tensile tests of interfaces comprised of bone-titanium and bone-hydroxyapatite-coated titanium. *Trans Orthop Res Soc* 1991;16:502.

162. Berger RA, Klein AH, Rodosky MW, et al: The mechanical and histological effects of plasma sprayed hydroxyapatite coating in a canine femoral endoprosthesis model. *Trans Orthop Res Soc* 1992;17:401.

163. Thomas KA, Cook SD, Haddad RJ Jr, et al: Biologic response to hydroxyapatite-coated titanium hips: A preliminary study in dogs. *J Arthroplasty* 1989;4:43-53.

164. Soballe K, Hansen ES, Brockstedt-Rasmussen H, et al: Hydroxyapatite coating enhances fixation of porous coated implants: A comparison in dogs between press fit and non-interference fit. *Acta Orthop Scand* 1990;61:299-306.

165. Soballe K, Hansen ES, Brockstedt-Rasmussen H, et al: Tissue ingrowth into titanium and hydroxyapatite-coated implants during stable and unstable mechanical conditions. *J Orthop Res* 1992;10:285-299.

166. Soballe K, Hansen ES, Brockstedt-Rasmussen H, et al: Hydroxyapatite implant coating modifies membrane formation during unstable mechanical conditions. *Trans Orthop Res Soc* 1991;16:35.

167. Soballe K, Hansen ES, Brockstedt-Rasmussen H, et al: Hydroxyapatite coating converts fibrous anchorage to bony fixation during continuous implant loading. *Trans Orthop Res Soc* 1992;17:292.

168. Noble PC, Alexander JW, Lindahl LJ, et al: The anatomic basis of femoral component design. *Clin Orthop* 1988;235:148-165.

169. Jones LC, Kay JF, Freeburger Opishinski D, et al: Effect of hydroxylapatite coating on osteogenesis across an interface gap. *Trans Orthop Res Soc* 1991;16:549.

170. Soballe K, Hansen ES, Brockstedt-Rasmussen H, et al: Bone graft incorporation around titanium-alloy- and hydroxyapatite-coated implants in dogs. *Clin Orthop* 1992;274:282-293.

171. Stephenson PK, Freeman MA, Revell PA, et al: The effect of hydroxyapatite coating on ingrowth of bone into cavities in an implant. *J Arthroplasty* 1991;6:51-58.

172. Soballe K, Hansen ES, Brockstedt-Rasmussen H, et al: Gap healing enhanced by hydroxyapatite coating in dogs. *Clin Orthop* 1991;272:300-307.

173. Kay J, May T: HA coating for non-precision implant placements. *Trans Soc Biomater* 1991;14:12.

174. D'Antonio JA, Capello WN, Crothers OD, et al: Early clinical experience with hydroxyapatite-coated femoral implants. *J Bone Joint Surg* 1992;74A:995-1008.

175. Friedman R, Dorr L, Gustke K, et al: Two to four year results of hydroxyapatite total hip arthroplasty. Poster presented at the 9th Combined Meeting of the Orthopaedic Associations of the English-Speaking World, Toronto, Ontario, Canada, June 21-26, 1992.

176. Cook SD, Enis J, Armstrong D, et al: Early clinical results with the hydroxyapatite-coated porous LSF total hip system. *Dent Clin North Am* 1992;36:247-255.

177. Dorr L: Clinical total hip replacement with hydroxyapatite from 1984 to 1991. *Sem Arthroplasty* 1991;2:289-294.

178. Emerson R, Head W, Peters P: Comparison of the early healing course of porous titanium with hydroxyapatite-coated porous titanium hip implants. *Sem Arthroplasty* 1991;2:295-301.

179. Vaughn BK, Lombardi AV, Mallory TH: Clinical and radiographic experience with a hydroxyapatite-coated titanium plasma-sprayed porous implant. *Dent Clin North Am* 1992;36:263-272.

180. Bauer TW, Geesink RC, Zimmerman R, et al: Hydroxyapatite-coated femoral stems: Histological analysis of components retrieved at autopsy. *J Bone Joint Surg* 1991;73A:1439-1452.

181. Bloebaum RD, Merrell M, Gustke K, et al: Retrieval analysis of a hydroxyapatite-coated hip prosthesis. *Clin Orthop* 1991;267:97-102.

182. Bloebaum R, Rubman M, Bachus K, et al: Comparison of hydroxyapatite coated and porous coated femoral hip implants retrieved from the same patient. *Trans Soc Biomater* 1991;14:14.

183. Furlong RJ, Osborn JF: Fixation of hip prostheses by hydroxyapatite ceramic coatings. *J Bone Joint Surg* 1991;73B:741-745.

184. Hardy DC, Frayssinet P, Guilhem A, et al: Bonding of hydroxyapatite-coated femoral prostheses: Histopathology of specimens from four cases. *J Bone Joint Surg* 1991;73B:732-740.

185. Soballe K, Gotfredsen K, Brockstedt-Rasmussen H, et al: Histologic analysis of a retrieved hydroxyapatite-coated femoral prosthesis. *Clin Orthop* 1991;72:255-258.

186. Beeks DA, Dupont JA, Savory CG, et al: Retrieval analysis of hydroxyapatite separation and osteolysis in proximal femoral implant. *Trans Orthop Res Soc* 1993;18:465.

187. Campbell P, McKellop H, Park SH, et al: Evidence of abrasive wear by particles from a hydroxyapatite coated hip prosthesis. *Trans Orthop Res Soc* 1992;18:224.

188. Friedman R: *Arthroplasty of the Shoulder.* New York, NY, Thieme, 1993, p 299.

189. Longo JA, Poser RD, Szivek JA: HA coating enhancement of cancellous screw removal torques. *Trans Orthop Res Soc* 1991;16:521.

190. Baker JT, McKinney LA, Gunasekaran S, et al: An in vivo evaluation of artificial bone constructs. *Trans Orthop Res Soc* 1992;17:575.

191. Constantz B, Gunasekaran S, Barr B: Evaluation of bioactive cements using a rabbit femoral canal model. *Trans Orthop Res Soc* 1992;17:370.

192. Constantz B, Young S, Kienapfe H: Pilot investigations of a calcium phosphate cement in a rabbit femoral canal model and a canine humeral plug model. *Trans Soc Biomater* 1991;14:92.

193. Oonishi H: Orthopaedic applications of hydroxyapatite. *Biomaterials* 1991;12:171-178.

The Generation of Wear Debris From Cementless Hip Prostheses

John P. Collier, DE

Michael B. Mayor, MD

Victor A. Surprenant, BA

Marguerite Wrona, ME

Helene P. Surprenant

Ian R. Williams, BA

Introduction

Debris generation has been a significant concern in total hip replacement since Charnley and associates[1] first developed the concept of articulating a metal femoral head against a polymer acetabular bearing. The polytetrafluoroethylene acetabular components wore very rapidly and produced large amounts of debris. The resultant granulomatous reaction forced the revision of all patients in whom these components had been implanted. Thus began the search for a low-wear, articulating couple, which continues to this day. Charnley's replacement for polytetrafluoroethylene was ultra-high-molecular-weight polyethylene. In Charnley's clinical followups, he and others documented wear rates of this couple as varying from approximately 0.07 to 0.6 mm per year, with an average of 0.2 mm per year.[2-4] Although the total volumetric debris represented by this level of linear wear was not inconsiderable, in the vast majority of patients it did not result in a significant adverse tissue reaction. However, in some patients the generation of debris from the articular surface, combined with the generation of cement debris produced as the components loosened, resulted in an osteolytic response which became known as "cement disease."[5] The variation in patient response to the production of particulate wear in total hip replacement indicates that there is the potential for a dose/response relationship to debris, and that the response may be individual-specific.

Osteolysis in patients with cementless total hip components revealed that polyethylene debris alone could generate the same degree of bone erosion seen in the cemented components, in which the culprit was originally thought to be cement particulate debris or a combination of cement debris and polyethylene debris. In recent years, the prevalence of osteolysis in cementless components has apparently increased,[5] a phenomenon that has paralleled the increase in modularity of the cementless components. With well-fixed, one-piece femoral and acetabular prostheses, the articulating surface should be the principal source of debris generation. With the advent of more modular components, as exemplified by the development of the metal-backed acetabular prostheses described by Harris[6] in 1971, the potential sources of debris increased significantly. Recent hip components have included the use of modular heads, collars, sleeves, distal bullets, and removable pads on femoral components, and screws and removable polyethylene liners on the acetabular components. Each modular connection represents a potential site for the generation of debris. It is the goal of this paper to examine a series of retrieved modular hip prostheses to assess the potential for debris generation at the modular connections. It should be noted at the outset that because the number of specimens available is limited, it is impossible to determine the relative frequency of occurrence of any of the mechanisms of debris generation that are observed. Rather, this study provides some illumination of the potential risk of debris generation, which can be weighed against the benefits of increased modularity.

Methods

A total of 736 retrieved modular hip components (344 modular acetabular components and 392 modular femoral hip components) were examined for this study. In each case, the retrieved component was visually examined through a Nikon dissecting microscope at magnifications as high as 60X for signs of wear and corrosion. Wear was categorized on a scale of 0 to 3 using a protocol modified from the one first developed by Hood and associates.[7] The wear characteristics of scratching, burnishing, abrasion, cracking, pitting, delamination, and creep were graded individually for each polyethylene bearing received. In addition, each bearing was assessed for the degree of consolidation of the polyethylene. Acetabular components were also graded for the extent of third-body debris generated from the porous surfaces, and the degree of abrasion, scratching, and burnishing of the inside of the metal backing opposed to the polyethylene liner. Both surfaces of the polyethylene liner were graded in the same manner as tibial bearings, and each screw and screw hole was evaluated for the extent of fretting. On the femoral side, an assessment was made of the degree of loss of porous coating and the extent of proximal and distal burnishing, and fretting at all modular connections was evaluated. In addition, corrosion of the head/neck combination was evaluated for both extent and depth. Selected, corroded components were sectioned for analysis of microstructure and chemical composition.

Results

Acetabular Components

Wear of the Polyethylene Bearings Of the polyethylene liners, 92% presented evidence of debris generation from the surface opposed to the metal backing as well as the surface intended for articulation. Of these components, 14% presented evidence of considerable wearing away of the back of the polyethylene liner. Many of these components have holes in the metal backing to permit screw fixation or viewing through the apical region. Histologic examination of these components revealed that the screw holes in 32% of the components contained polyethylene debris, which had migrated through the screw holes and, therefore, was available to attack the host/implant interface (Table 1).

The evidence of micromotion leading to polyethylene wear between the bearing and the metal shell is an indication that the fixation between the two is deserving of attention as a site for considerable debris generation. Additionally and unfortunately, the debris generation from the site has direct access to the host interface (Fig. 1), unlike the debris generated at the articular surface, which has a longer and less direct path to the fixation interface. Therefore, the use of screw and apical holes in acetabular shells should be reconsidered. Screw fixation may have potential benefits, but

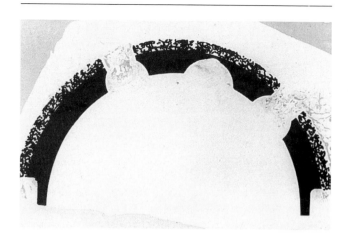

Fig. 1 The screw holes in acetabular components provide a path for migration of polyethylene debris, which was found in the fibrous tissue within the screw holes of 32% of screw-fixed components.

when no screws are used, these holes present an unnecessary risk.

Polyethylene Quality Transmitted light examination of the polyethylene bearings revealed that 60% of the retrieved components presented evidence of lack of consolidation of the polyethylene used to produce the bearings. This incomplete consolidation of the individual powder particles in the solid bar or sheet stock from which acetabular components are machined, results in fusion defects, visible as black or white spots (depending on the lighting), in the polyethylene (Fig. 2). Fusion defects may also be visible in components

Table 1
Migration of polyethylene through acetabular screw holes

	No.	% w/Poly Cold Flow Into Screw Holes	Duration
Shells w/Screw Holes	92	35	22.4
Shells w/Tissue in Screw Holes	62	44	24.4
Shells w/Poly in Screw Holes	29	59	33.6

32% of acetabula with screw holes have polyethylene migrating through those holes into the tissue.

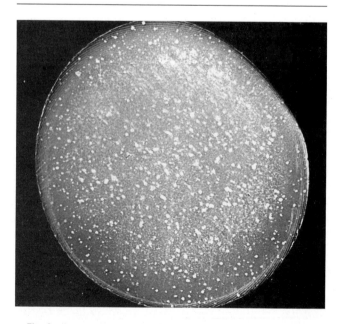

Fig. 2 Fusion defects in the polyethylene are evidence of incomplete consolidation and are visible as the white spots in this thin section, taken from an acetabular component.

molded directly from powder, if the consolidation is not complete. In knee components, poorly consolidated polyethylene has been demonstrated to be less fatigue resistant than fully consolidated polyethylene.[8] While no such correlation of wear with defects was available with acetabular components, it is likely that defects represent a material of decreased wear resistance. Therefore, it is important that surgeons become aware of the extent of variation in the polyethylene used in total hip components, and continue to urge that manufacturers strive to produce components that are completely consolidated.

Screw Fixation of Acetabular Components The majority of acetabular components affixed with screws provide evidence of fretting between the screws and the metal shell in the form of blackened tissue at the screw holes and burnishing of both the screws and the holes. In cases of loose cups affixed by screws, the motion and stresses can be so great that screws loosen and impinge against the polyethylene surface. In some cases, screws have been seen to fracture.

Fixation of the Polyethylene Liner to the Metal Shell The early designs of many modular acetabular components use small polyethylene or metal lugs, or thin rims of polyethylene to affix the bearing liner to the metal shell. In some cases, over time, these fixation mechanisms failed, leaving the polyethylene liner free to move relative to the metal component. In our retrieval series, approximately 10% of the components had lost the fixation of the bearing to the metal shell. Loss of rigid fixation can result in rapid generation of polyethylene and metal debris from the unintended articulation. Furthermore, if the polyethylene rotates out of the metal shell, direct metal-on-metal articulation can result.

Articular Cup Geometry Acetabular components should be designed to be insensitive to the angle of placement in the pelvis. Components that have hemispheric polyethylene bearings mated to hemispheric metal shells provide a uniform polyethylene thickness, and, if provided with sufficiently robust fixation of the liner to the metal shell, are relatively insensitive to orientation. However, cups that are provided with a cylindrical polyethylene liner and a cylindrical metal shell are typically provided with relatively thin polyethylene side walls and relatively thicker polyethylene in the dome regions. If an adjustment from neutral position should occur, the femoral head may articulate against the thin side walls, causing rapid creep and deformation of the liner.[9] This may result in subsequent cracking, wear through, and rotation of the liner out of the metal shell, all leading to metal-on-metal articulation (Fig. 3). Of the 92 cylindrical acetabular components, 23% were revised for failure associated with cracking and wear through of the polyethylene cup. Therefore, in general, hemispheric congruent geometries are

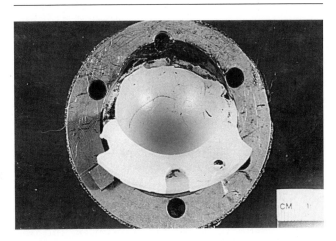

Fig. 3 Cylindrical polyethylene acetabular inserts with thin sidewalls are susceptible to early fracture, leading to the generation of large amounts of polyethylene debris and to subsequent metal-on-metal contact.

preferred over other geometries of acetabular components.

Femoral Components

The use of modular femoral heads has permitted the interoperative adjustment of leg length through various leg head/neck combinations. Additionally, it has permitted the use of ceramic and cobalt-alloy heads on titanium-alloy stems in an effort to decrease the head wear against the polyethylene bearing of the acetabular components, while decreasing the concern regarding stress shielding and bone loss. However, modular connections increase the potential for fretting and corrosion and must be designed and manufactured carefully to assure that the benefits outweigh the risks. The examination of 392 modular femoral hip prostheses has provided some insight into the possible mechanisms of debris generation on the femoral side.

Fretting There are a variety of concerns associated with the potential for fretting at modular connections. Fretting produces particulate metal debris, which can migrate to the articular surfaces, thereby increasing the wear of the polyethylene. Additionally, the generation of debris from the mating surfaces of modular connections deteriorates these connections over time, which may well result in further debris generation and a degradation in the quality of fixation at the modular connections. Perhaps of equal concern is the ensuing loss of the passive layer from fretting. All orthopaedic alloys are protected from corrosion by their passive layer. Therefore, breakdown of the layer in the crevice environment of the taper or other modular connection provides an ideal site for crevice corrosion. It is difficult to determine the extent to which fretting may be occurring at the head/neck junctions. Fretting is defined by motion, which can be as small as a micron, between two mated surfaces. Unfortunately, it is difficult to discern surface damage at this level, even with a scanning electron microscope. Evidence of gross fretting between head and neck is relatively rare, and it occurred in approximately 11% of the components which we have examined. However, retrieval and insertion/removal artifacts often make determination of fretting difficult.

Corrosion Of the 230 modular femoral hip prostheses examined for corrosion, 48 showed evidence of corrosion at the head/neck taper. In 39 of these, the corrosion was in tapers between cobalt-alloy heads and titanium-alloy stems. Eight cobalt-on-cobalt-alloy components presented corrosion of the crevice, and one modular prosthesis, comprised entirely of titanium-alloy, presented evidence of crevice corrosion (Table 2). The predominance of crevice corrosion in mixed-alloy femoral hip components in this study emphasizes the concern for proper metallurgy and tight tolerances at the head/neck taper connection. Of the 39 corroded cobalt-alloy heads affixed to titanium-alloy stems, 28 were determined to have as-cast metallurgy resulting in a very heterogeneous microstructure (Fig. 4), which is more susceptible to corrosion than either solution-annealed cobalt-alloy or machinable cobalt-alloy, both of which are more homogeneous and thus more resistant to corrosion. We have determined in the laboratory that there is nearly a 1v potential between passivated cobalt-alloy and depassivated titanium-alloy,[10] although the relative importance of this galvanic couple is yet undetermined. It is extraordinarily difficult to separate out the various factors that could lead to corrosion in the crevice environment in these clinically retrieved specimens. Fretting between the head and neck is sufficient to break down the passive film that protects the alloys from corrosion and could, alone, be sufficient to lead to crevice corrosion. However, the predominance of mixed-metal components in the series of specimens that have demonstrated corrosion continues to raise concern over the use of as-cast cobalt heads on titanium stems.[11]

Eight of 118 femoral hip components examined with cobalt-alloy heads on cobalt-alloy stems revealed

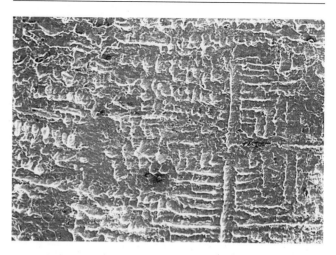

Fig. 4 Corrosion of the inside taper of the as-cast cobalt head reveals the heterogeneous nature of the dendritic structure (Magnification: 75X).

evidence of corrosion. In all eight cases, the corrosion occurred predominantly on the tapered neck of the porous-coated femoral stem. Metallurgic analysis of these corroded components indicated that the heat treatment they had been subjected to in the process of applying the porous coating resulted in a heterogeneous microstructure, in which the carbides formed along the grain boundaries. This phenomenon reduced the corrosion resistance of the grain boundaries and caused subsequent intergranular corrosion, evidenced by actual grains coming loose from the metal (Fig. 5). This corrosion is far more aggressive than the corrosion seen in the mixed-alloy components and resulted in dramatically higher penetration rates. As an example, a five-year retrieved, mixed-alloy component which presented the greatest extent and depth of corrosion was measured to have a depth of penetration of the corrosion of approximately 15 µm. In contrast, a five-year, all-cobalt-alloy prosthesis, retrieved because of femoral neck fracture caused by intergranular corrosion, revealed a depth of penetration of the corrosion of nearly 2 mm, more than an order of magnitude higher than that seen in the surface corrosion of the mixed-metal components.

One of 17 all-titanium-alloy components examined presented evidence of corrosion. The area of corrosion was small and the depth of penetration was slight, however, this specimen is evidence that any modular connection can be susceptible to crevice corrosion if there is even the slightest micromotion which can result in a breakdown of the passive film. In many instances, the benefits of modularity exceed the potential risks. However, it appears that no modular connection can be assured to be entirely risk-free. The quality of fixation at the taper is paramount, and modular connections that

Table 2
Corrosion of the head/neck taper

Head Alloy/ Stem Alloy	No. Examined	No. Corroded	% Corroded	Average Duration of Those Corroded
CC/Ti	93	39	42	37.5
Ti/Ti	17	1	6	91.5
Ti/CC	2	0	0	0
CC/CC	118	8	7	55.8

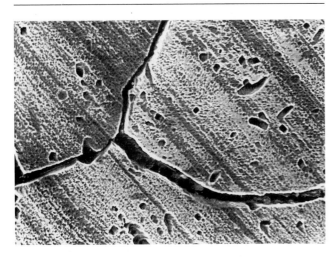

Fig. 5 The etched appearance of the grain boundaries of this sample are a result of intergranular corrosion following a sintering heat treatment, which resulted in the carbides being precipitated at the grain boundary.

permit gross micromotion will very likely result in significant debris generation and/or corrosion.

Third-Body Debris Third-body debris can be generated by any relative motion between components, such as normal articulation at the bearing surface, or by loss of any type of coating applied to the prostheses. The most severe cases of third-body debris which we have observed occurred from the shedding of loose coatings and their subsequent migration to the articular and nonarticular surfaces of the polyethylene bearing. It appears that both porous coatings and hydroxyapatite coatings are susceptible to failure, either at the time of impaction or due to fatigue in service. However, the greatest loss of coating appears to occur in components that are not bone ingrown and, therefore, are loose and able to move relative to the host bone. It is imperative that porous coatings be well adherent to the components themselves and, in the case of porous coatings, each particle must be well bonded to its neighbors. This is not always the case.[9] Of all retrieved porous coated components (both femoral and acetabular), 14% evidenced a loss of some of the porous coating particles or hydroxyapatite surface. Loss of coating occurred far less frequently in systems with well-bonded coatings than in those with less well-bonded coatings. Plasma-sprayed porous coatings appear to be at particular risk, and nearly 60% of those components presented evidence of some loss of coating. It should be noted that many of these components were loose, which tends to exacerbate the problem.

Hydroxyapatite coatings are susceptible to the same types of problems as porous metal coatings. They can be separated from the surface during impaction, while in service, or when the bond strength of the coatings

to the substrate decreases over time as the coating is resorbed. Although we have observed only two cases of particulate debris of hydroxyapatite embedded in the articular surface of the polyethylene bearing, and are aware of only one paper presented at the 1993 American Academy of Orthopaedic Surgeons Annual Meeting, which raised the concern for osteolysis as a result of hydroxyapatite debris, it is clear that there are at least some risks associated with the use of this material if it becomes third-body debris.

Conclusions

Modular hip prostheses provide a wide variety of sites for the potential generation of debris. It appears that all modular connections are at risk and therefore, components with increased modularity may be at increased risk for debris production. Tight tolerances and homogeneous metallurgy are two factors that can reduce the risk of debris generation. Other suggested design considerations follow.

Acetabular Components

(1) Ensure that the polyethylene used for the bearing is fully consolidated and defect-free. (2) Polyethylene bearings should be at least 6 mm thick to reduce the stress in the bearing and to provide sufficient material for a minimum ten-year life span (assuming a maximum 0.6 mm per year wear rate). (3) The polyethylene should be rigidly secured to the metal backing to eliminate the potential for disassociation and to minimize the potential for micromotion leading to debris generation. (4) Metal shells without holes should be provided for those surgeons who choose not to use screws. Any apical hole should be provided with tightly fitting plugs to eliminate the potential for debris migration to the host/implant interface. (5) Designs that are insensitive to cup orientation are to be preferred over those that are sensitive to cup orientation. Typically, hemispheric designs with polyethylene of uniform thickness are less sensitive to cup orientation than are cylindrical designs with thin polyethylene side walls. (6) The use of screws to affix acetabular components increases the potential for fretting debris, and the screw holes provide a pathway through which debris can migrate. Therefore, the use of screws needs further study. (7) Poorly bonded porous coatings or hydroxyapatite coatings are potential sources for third-body debris generation. Therefore, it is important to ensure that there is high-integrity bonding between the coating and the substrate and between the particles themselves.

Femoral Components

(1) Fretting between the modular connections is a paramount concern. Tight dimensional tolerances

and good design are required to minimize debris generation. (2) Corrosion of all-cobalt-alloy, mixed-alloy, and all-titanium-alloy systems has been observed, with the severity of the corrosion being largely related to the type of metallurgy. Homogeneous metal alloy systems appear to be significantly more resistant to corrosion than are heterogeneous systems. As-cast femoral heads appear to be more susceptible to corrosion than are solution annealed or wrought femoral heads. Ceramic heads are not susceptible to corrosion, although the crevice environment between a ceramic head and stem may produce corrosion of the tapered stem. (3) Porous coating heat treatments must be carefully designed and executed to assure that they result in a homogeneous microstructure of the stem. Heterogeneous stem microstructures have been associated with severe intergranular corrosion, which raises the potential for femoral neck fracture. (4) Third-body debris generation from loss of porous coating remains a concern, and the integrity of the coating/substrate bond is paramount to satisfactory long-term performance. The use of hydroxyapatite coatings should raise the same concerns. It is likely that third-body hydroxyapatite debris may produce reactions similar to those seen with bone cement, polyethylene, or metal debris.

References

1. Charnley J, Kamangar A, Longfield MD: The optimum size of prosthetic heads in relation to the wear of plastic sockets in total replacement of the hip. *Med Biol Eng* 1969;7:31-39.
2. Charnley J: Low friction principle, in *Low Friction Arthroplasty of the Hip: Theory and Practice.* Berlin, Springer-Verlag, 1979, chap 1, pp 3-15.
3. Charnley J, Cupic Z: The nine and ten year results of the low-friction arthroplasty of the hip. *Clin Orthop* 1973;95:9-25.
4. Charnley J, Halley DK: Rate of wear in total hip replacement. *Clin Orthop* 1975;112:170-179.
5. Jacobs JJ: Particulate-associated endosteal osteolysis in titanium-base alloy cementless total hip replacement, in *Symposium on Biocompatibility of Particulate Implant Materials.* San Antonio, TX, ASTM, 1990.
6. Harris WH: A new total hip implant. *Clin Orthop* 1971;81:105-113.
7. Hood RW, Wright TM, Burstein AH: Retrieval analysis of total knee prostheses: A method and its application to 48 total condylar prostheses. *J Biomed Mater Res* 1983;17:829-842.
8. Mayor MB, Jensen RE, Collier JP: The correlation between fusion defects and damage in tibial polyethylene bearings, in *The Sixth Annual Meeting of The Knee Society.* San Francisco, CA, 1993.
9. Collier JP, Mayor MB, Jensen RE, et al: Mechanisms of failure of modular prostheses. *Clin Orthop* 1992;285:129-139.
10. Collier JP, Surprenant VA, Jensen RE, et al: Corrosion between the components of modular femoral hip prostheses. *J Bone Joint Surg* 1992;74B:511-517.
11. Collier JP, Surprenant VA, Jensen RE, et al: Corrosion at the interface of cobalt-alloy heads on titanium-alloy stems. *Clin Orthop* 1991;271:305-312.

Osteolysis Caused by Polymethylmethacrylate (PMMA)

Nas S. Eftekhar, MD

Introduction

To define the reactive process that can be caused by the fragments of polymethylmethacrylate (PMMA) commonly associated with loose implants, it is first necessary to appreciate the inertness in tissue of bulk PMMA and the histologically stable interface commonly seen between the acrylic cement and skeleton. Although much of the adverse reaction found in failed prostheses has been attributed to PMMA, evidence exists that high-density polyethylene (HDP) and other debris generated in loose prostheses also contribute significantly to the process of osteolysis in cemented implants.[1] In experimental conditions, most plastics produce severe tissue reaction in their particulate forms. They also produce tumors in rats.[2,3] Any of the materials used in surgery, including autogenous bone grafts, also may produce a severe inflammatory and histiocytic reaction when used in powdered form or implanted subperiosteally.

Many surgeons have recently abandoned acrylic cement in favor of other methods of fixation of artificial joints. Although a stable cellular interface can be achieved between acrylic cement and bone, there is no agreement as to whether this stability can be maintained permanently. If it cannot, it is necessary to determine what circumstances alter a histologically stable interface, leading to bone destruction and mechanical loosening. Frequently, much of the adverse reaction found in failed prostheses has been attributed to PMMA, not to the HDP and metallic debris that are also found in most histologic specimens retrieved from failed prostheses.

Histologic Stability of Interface

According to Clarke and associates,[4] a biologically inert material is one that "does not destroy the viability of adjoining tissues and provokes no inflammatory response beyond that occasioned by trauma accompanying the insertion and by its presence as a physical and nonvital structure; and which does not impede the process of fibrous or osteogenic repair."

A histologically stable interface between the implant and the skeleton is of fundamental importance. No further development in this field is possible without first achieving a histologically stable interface following implantation of foreign materials. Charnley[5] must be credited not only with the introduction of acrylic cement and HDP as materials used in joint arthroplasty, but also with his efforts in histologic studies of response to these materials.[6] In 1968, Charnley and Crawford[7,8] described the presence of macrophages at the bone-cement interface as a direct response to PMMA particles. Among early investigators, Freeman and associates[9] interpreted the presence of macrophages at the cement-bone interface as evidence of tissue response to PMMA, whether solid or in pearls. Subsequently, Freeman and Tennant[10] concluded that "the observed difference between the metallic and PMMA interfaces may have been caused as much by their relative accessibility to high-density polyethylene debris as by any specific response to PMMA as against metal." It was concluded that the macrophages were attracted to minute particles of PMMA in the same way they are attracted to catgut and to chromium-cobalt alloy in its particulate form. Histologically, the presence of macrophages at the interface is of concern because they are precursors of osteoclasts and, thus, are instigators of bone resorption.[11] The mere presence of macrophages can be a predictor of eventual failure of fixation, because stimuli that are known to excite the macrophages include cell death, bacteria, and foreign debris (such as metals and plastics) in minute form.

Physical Form and Chemical Makeup

In addition to its chemical makeup, the physical form of the material may determine the tissue response to implants.[12,13] Teflon, which provides a classic example, does not cause any severe reaction in humans when used in bulk (plates, sheets, or rods), but when small particles are present in total hip arthroplasty, considerable tissue reaction is engendered.[14]

Surface energy and roughness of implants can influence macrophage-release mediators, which stimulate bone resorption. Murray and associates[15] demonstrated that the amount of bone resorption increased by 2.5 to 10 times when macrophages adhered to surfaces of implanted foreign materials. They concluded that bone absorption, which can cause loosening, is affected by such physical properties as surface energy and roughness of the implant, rather than by the chemical nature of the implant. As a corollary to this work, Leake and associates[16] and Rich and Harris[17] demonstrated that macrophage migration and spreading were influenced by the surface energy and the roughness of the surface on which they were cultured.

Tallroth and associates[18] postulated that loosening of implants is not an absolute prerequisite to bone lysis, which commonly occurs around a loose prosthesis. Tallroth's observation is significant because, although it is believed that acrylic cement produces little or no reaction response while it remains fixed to the bone, he indicates that occasionally a macrophage-mediated foreign body reaction can occur in the absence of cement loosening. The possible mechanism for such a reaction may be either localized fatigue of PMMA, leading to shedding of the particles, or, as suggested by Willert and associates,[19] a portion of unpolymerized acrylic may be responsible for this phenomenon. Between 14 days and 5 years after surgery, Willert observed unpolymerized acrylic polymer spherules in the cement bed of implanted histologic specimens. They believed these spherules to be incompletely polymerized polymer.

In a recent study of the nature of the "aggressive granulomatous lesions" associated with total hip arthroplasty, Santavirta and associates[20] along with others, have suggested that such lesions are a distinct entity, not only clinically, but also histopathologically and immunohistologically.[21] In their evaluation of 12 such lesions, Santavirta and associates[20] found most cells were multinucleated giant cells, C-3 bireceptors, and nonspecific esterase-positive monocyte-macrophages, which suggests the rapidly progressive lytic nature of these lesions. In their view, the process is caused by uncoupling of the normal sequence of monocyte-macrophage mediated clearance of foreign body and dead cells, normally followed by fibroblast-mediated synthesis.

The biologic response to particles of PMMA is a response to foreign material in particulate form, as evidenced by presence of histiocytic and giant cell foreign body reaction without a significant contribution by the immune system.[21]

Injury, Repair, and Remodeling

For a better understanding of tissue response following implantation, the natural response to initial injury and subsequent tissue repair also must be considered. In a classic animal study by Wiltse and associates[22] and in Willert's histologic studies after total hip arthroplasty,[23,24] immediate necrosis occurred at the interface during the first three weeks after the implantation of PMMA.[22] Necrotic tissue and fibrin up to 3 mm thick were observed and were attributed to heat of polymerization, monomeric effect, and loss of blood supply to the injured area. Larger necrotic areas observed in the trochanteric region and in the medullary cavity were indistinguishable from bone infarcts. Repair of tissue

damage at the interface began after three weeks and ended within approximately two years. This repair was manifested by peripheral hyperemia, migration of lipophages, and ingrowth of fibroblasts and capillaries.[22-24] However, the investigators observed occasional focal necrosis even at this stage; these areas were smaller than those seen during the first three weeks. The necrotic bone actually had been repaired by remodeling, reinforcement, and replacement. Repair was mainly by the mechanisms of apposition of new lamellar bone or by osteoblastic metaplasia. In these studies, the investigators found acrylic pearls in most implant beds, in foreign body giant cells, and, occasionally, in nearby connective tissue and lymphatic vessels. Rhinelander and associates,[25] using microangiography techniques, showed severe devascularization and necrosis of large areas of the cortex after reaming, followed by full recovery at six months. Repair had not occurred one year after introduction of cement after reaming.

Osteointegration of PMMA

In addition to early studies by Charnley and Crawford,[7] Charnley and associates,[6] Henrichsen and associates,[26] and Wiltse and associates,[22] direct apposition of bone formation was substantiated by electron microscopy studies of Linder and Hansson,[27] who showed that direct, viable bone, without any intervening tissue, can be found as evidence of bone remodeling after insertion of PMMA in vivo. Draenert[28] evaluated the histomorphology of the bone-cement interface. He used fully developed California rabbits to study remodeling of the cortex and revascularization of the medullary canal at the following intervals: at 1, 2, 3, 6, and 8 days; at 2, 3, 4, 6, and 8 weeks; at 3, 6, 9, and 11 months; and at 1.5, 2, and 2.5 years. The following summary is based on this animal study transposed on histology of retrieved human specimens. Bone-cement integration (osteointegration) occurred in the absence of mechanical stress. The existing gap between bone and implant was filled rapidly by newly formed bone (woven bone). Gaps up to 8 mm were filled by lamellar bone. Larger gaps were also bridged by woven bone. Regeneration of the medullary canal occurred, and the medullary canal was fully revascularized to its original state. New medullarization occurred as a second remodeling process resulting from revascularization of the cortex, replacing partially necrotic bone. The force transmission to bone optimally occurred without interruption by fibrous or molecular connection. While no tissue reaction was observed at 2.5 years after implantation, osteoblasts were deposited directly onto the bone-cement interface. This study again confirms that newly formed bone can be seen directly on the surface of the cement on the old cortex, thereby forming a new cortex.

Histology of Retrieved Human Specimens

It is important to consider the histology of bone and cement contact in the absence of infection in two separate situations: (1) in a state of rigidity, or successful arthroplasty, and (2) in a state of looseness, or failure. Charnley[5,14] was the first to report in detail the histologic findings of human specimens (37 femurs and 27 acetabulum) after patient death from natural causes; all specimens studied had a successful total hip arthroplasty. The average time after operation was 7.3 years; the longest period was 13 years, and 13 patients were evaluated more than nine years after operation. The fact that all of these cases were 100% successful arthroplasties is an essential feature in the proper interpretation of cement in contact with living tissue.

In numerous histologic reports, from both human postmortem studies and animal experimentation, investigating the necrosis of bone, periosteal new bone formation, and reaction to the implanted cement, most authors reported the presence of fibrocartilage or fibrous connective tissue in the interface between bone and cement. Some researchers believed that the implant was encapsulated by connective tissue. Others did not differentiate between materials obtained from loose prostheses and those which were rigidly fixed to the bone. Unfortunately, cellular reactions caused by metallic particles and high-density polyethylene could not be separated from those caused by PMMA particles.

Tissue Response in Rigidly Fixed Cement

Gross Appearance Close contact between cement and bone is easily recognized by close observation of a horizontal or vertical cross-section of the femur or the acetabular region. Sometimes a layer of fibrous tissue is visible to the naked eye at the cement-bone junction, especially at the areas of cancellous bone in the acetabular region. On the other hand, this fibrous layer is rarely seen at the interface between cement and femur, which is well fixed. At times however, under low-power magnification, it appears that the cement is in direct contact with bone, except close to the surface of the cement, where a normal amount of fat cells are seen. The molding of the cement injected into the cancellous bone can be appreciated after careful removal of the cement from the bone. Microradiographs obtained from this section ideally show the interface between bone and cement. The following three important histologic features of the gross specimens should be noted: (1) Negative impressions of the cement's forcible injection into the bones result from formation of a mold of the interior surface of the bone, indicating a direct bone-cement contact. This may also represent evidence of osteointegration. (2) Fibrous tissue with no preferred orientation interposed between bone and cement indicates the absence of direct contact and suggests possible loosening or inadequate

pressure injection. It may also suggest areas of bone absorption and replacement by fibrous tissue. (3) Smooth surface areas of highly organized fibrous tissue or fibrocartilage suggest possible soft tissue growth at contact and load-transmission zones.

Microscopy To recognize the histology of cement-tissue contact areas, one must be aware of the microscopic structure of acrylic cement itself when in contact with the tissue. The polymer powder is made up of spheres ranging from 20 to 80 µm. Because decalcified sections are not satisfactory for the purpose of detailed examination, the cement is usually dissolved out. The impressions left by the spherules, easily recognizable as evidence of contact between the cement and the tissue, provide evidence of osteointegration.[5,14]

Postoperative tissue damage begins at surgery and leads to bone necrosis at the site of cement insertion. The necrosis is related to metaphyseal and intramedullary interference by the trauma of broaching, devascularization of bone, and cell death by monomer or, possibly, the heat of polymerization. Therefore, it is not unusual to find segmental or zonal necrosis in the trochanteric shaft or calcar region of the femur at a later stage. One frequently observes hemispheric cement impressions in direct contact with bone trabeculae that contain living osteocytes right up to the bone-cement surface.

Within the first two or three weeks after insertion of the cement, a coagulum of connective tissue, interposed between cement and bone, is visible. The repair is manifested by local hyperemia, migration of lipophages, and ingrowth of capillaries and fibroblasts. As time progresses, the interface tissue becomes more organized and is made up of fibrous tissue, fibrocartilage, metaplasia, new bone, and fatty marrow.[14]

Femur In the femur, histologic samples from successful arthroplasty, rigidly fixed femoral components, and specimens obtained at postmortem examination show, at some points, a fibrous membrane between the acrylic cement and the bone of the femur. In specimens obtained below the level of the lesser trochanter, the interface can best be described as a delicate areolar tissue without continuity. This appearance differs somewhat from that of specimens obtained at the level of the heavily loaded femoral neck, where the interface is similar to that seen at the acetabulum. In general, in specimens obtained from the femur, the fibrous interface is usually extremely thin and never completely lines the entire endosteal surface of the femur.[5,14] Loadbearing appears to take place through caplike areas of fibrocartilage or modified bone matrix; thus, no tissue of any kind is interposed between the cement and bone. These points of contact indicated that a perfect fixation to skeleton is possible through these caps, and that load is transmitted only through selected points of the endosteal surface of the femur through the bony trabeculae. The marrow cells are separated from cement by a delicate membrane, which shows no evidence of macrophages or granulation formation.

After a successful total hip arthroplasty, absence of radiolucencies in the femur and, often, a lack of demarcation are the rule rather than the exception and can be interpreted as a positive and favorable response that is maintained in the femur over a long period of time. It is possible that at least three factors favor the use of cement in the femur: (1) the surgeon's ability to contain the cement within the femur at the time of insertion; (2) the ability to pressurize the cement in a closed cavity at surgery; and (3) the surgeon's ability to resist bleeding pressure in the femur while the cement is being polymerized. These conditions may not prevail at insertion of cement in the acetabulum.

In Malcolm's study of retrieved human specimens in patients whose operations had been performed eight to 22 years previously, he made the following observations: (1) Sixty of 78 femoral specimens showed osteointegration throughout the length of cement fixation; 18 specimens showed various amounts of fibrous tissue. (2) Viable tissue consisting of mineralized pegs of lamellar bone and a thin layer of osteoid was found in 60 specimens; scanning electron microscopy showed evidence of osteointegration. (3) A fibrous tissue, present between cement and living bone, was more prominent proximally and often disappeared distally in the femur. (4) When fibrous membrane was present, it was associated with wear particles of high-density polyethylene, metal, and evidence of macrophagic reaction (R. Malcolm, personal communication).

Acetabulum Radiologic findings after cement has been used for acetabular fixation indicate a higher incidence of radiolucencies and demarcation than are found in the femur.

Paul and Bargar[29] carried out an in vivo study in which they cemented the acetabular component in dogs using techniques for pressurization. They found that tissue response differed significantly from that in the femur. They observed new bone formation by two weeks, and bone remodeling continued to be active up to six months after operation in the femur. However, they noted little new bone formation by six weeks in the acetabulum. These differences between the acetabulum and femur were attributed to the difference in bone formation and difference in the vascularity of the bone. Certainly, micromotion and stress patterns must also play an important role in the histologic difference observed between the acetabulum and the femur.[30]

Unlike the histology of the interface in the femur, Charnley[8] noted that after 10 years, repair of the acetabulum had not reached an endpoint. The presence of histiocytes and few giant cells suggested an unstable state of repair, which he called "suspended animation," with neither positive repair nor positive destruction even after 10 to 15 years of notable clinical success. Long-term histologic specimens frequently show a fibrous membrane of various thickness present between cement and bone with plastic and metal debris.

Malcolm made a similar observation as he studied Charnley's human specimens with prostheses implanted for eight to 22 years. In contrast to evidence of osteointegration in the femur, a fibrous membrane was found between cement and bone in every acetabular specimen. The membrane contained wear particles of high-density polyethylene with evidence of macrophagic reaction (R. Malcolm, personal communication).

Tissue Reaction to Particles of PMMA

Surgical and postmortem specimens indicate that, when PMMA particles are present, loosening is the primary cause of osteolysis. Fractographic studies of retrieved cement mantles show frequent fractures at varying stages of development in the cement mantle in addition to wear of fractured surfaces of cement, adjacent prosthesis, and bone, all of which contribute significantly to tissue reaction and osteolysis caused by the release of particles of PMMA.[21] Severe macrophagic giant cell granulomatous reaction occurred at the site of fractured and fragmented cement mantles. However, occasionally a macrophage-mediated foreign body reaction also can occur in the absence of cement loosening; the possible mechanism is either a localized fatigue of PMMA, leading to shedding of particles, or particles from a portion of unpolymerized PMMA may be responsible for this phenomenon.[19]

For lack of a better term, my colleagues and I use the term prosthetic synovitis to describe the fibropseudosynovial lining of the prosthetic bed.[1] Such material is often a natural response to the debris of PMMA, HDP, metal, bone, and other materials used in arthroplasty. The interface can also be the site of bacterial infection, with or without bacteriologic proof. However, in the absence of infection and the use of HDP, the reactive tissue must be caused by the presence of PMMA.[31]

Acrylic cement can instigate the wear of high-density polyethylene by causing a three-body wear in the acetabulum. Studies of Isaac and associates[32,33] clearly indicate that PMMA and particles of barium sulfate (which is about as hard as stainless steel) used to make the cement radiopaque, may cause surface scratches on the femoral head,[34] which in turn may lead to metallic particle debris and increased high-density polyethylene wear.

In studies of synovial fluid by Salvati and associates[34] in well-fixed total hip arthroplasty, the barium level ranged from 1 mg/l to 51 mg/l. In loose prostheses, the mean synovial barium was 16-fold greater (mean, 302 mg/l; range, 30 to 8,856 mg/l). Such important observations further suggest that the impurities of PMMA, such as barium sulfate, may play an important role in production of particle-induced prosthetic synovitis. In a recent report, Isaac and associates[33] observed that only minimal wear had occurred in HDP sockets in which no cement had been used. They concluded that wear in the cemented socket was caused by fragments of cement from the acetabular side of the prosthesis.

Another source of osteolysis, and loosening of the acetabular component, may be related to the linear wear of the acetabular component, which in turn results in penetration of the head and increased mechanical stress caused by impingement and loosening. Wroblewski[35] found a significant correlation between cup wear and loosening.

From the foregoing it may be concluded that the presence of particulate PMMA can cause accelerated wear of high-density polyethylene, which can lead to loosening of the cup. Further generation of particles then results from loosening of the cement and bone. Clinical inconsistencies in the wear rate and resultant osteolysis, seen from patient to patient and between right and left hips in the same patient, may also be explained by three-body wear by particles of PMMA.

Cellular Morphology

Acute inflammatory cells are seen in the pathology material with wear debris only when infection is present. Wear debris generally provokes a chronic inflammatory response that is of no value in establishing the presence or absence of infection in pathology of joint implants. Based on 94 specimens examined by Mirra and associates,[36] using a semiquantitative grading of the materials (0, 1+, 2+, 3+), chronic inflammation of 2+ to 3- was of no value in distinguishing between infection and reaction to wear debris.

Table 1
Prosthetic Synovitis Components: (50 cases)

Components	Percent of Total
Acidophilic histiocytes	95+
Giant cells	80+
HDP	75+
Metal	16
Fibrinoid	80+
Lymphocytes/plasma cells	26
Neutrophils	8

Quantitative estimates were based on a scale of 1 to 4+ of cells and foreign body materials using microscopic examination of tissue cells sectioning, stained with hematoxylin, phloxine and saffron. (Adapted with permission from Johnston AD, Parisien MV: Pathology of reactive (prosthetic) versus septic (revisionary) synovitis, in Eftekhar NS (ed): *Infection in Joint Replacement Surgery: Prevention and Management.* St. Louis, MO, CV Mosby, 1984, chap 3, pp 97-114.)

In a similar study by Johnston and Parisien,[37] quantitative estimates were based on a scale of 1 to 4+ of cells and foreign body materials using a light microscopic examination of tissues stained with hematoxylin, as shown in Table 1. Acidophilic histiocytes were distinctive histologic hallmarks of prosthetic synovitis (95% +); giant cells, fibrinoid materials, cement, and HDP fragments (75% to 80%) comprise the bulk of the most frequently encountered remaining components, except for fragments of bone and scarred aponeurotic tissue from the articular capsule.

Acidophilic Histiocytes

The relationship established in our study between granular acidophilic histiocytes and fragments of HDP may be of significance.[1] We noted birefringent shards of HDP 2 to 5 μm long in the cytoplasm of some cells. Characteristically, particles of this size could be incorporated by mononuclear histiocytes. This association is a dominant feature of the interaction between fine particles of HDP and tissue. Tissue morphology is dominated by small fragments of birefringent material associated with sheets of histiocytes. It is not possible to identify any small fragments of acrylic cement associated with these cells. The exceptions are "foam cells," which contain minute particles of worn PMMA.[14] Acrylic cement often consists of large fragments, which are associated with multinucleated giant cells or are walled off by a connective tissue capsule. Frequently observed small acrylic polymer spherules (30 to 80 μm) are too large to be phagocytized by histiocytes, although histiocytes could be associated with the surface of individual acrylic pearls.

Multinucleated Giant Cells

Evidently, giant cells are formed in response to large fragments of acrylic cement or HDP. Fragments of cement are usually large and evidently require a syncytium of cells such as giant cells to encompass their bulk. As far as we have been able to determine, cement is not shed into the reactive tissue in the form of finely ground particles and does not appear to provoke increased numbers of mononuclear histiocytes. Whether they are formed in response to a spherule of the acrylic polymer or to large fragments of acrylic, giant cells seen in close relationship to particles of PMMA can always be distinguished from a giant cell tumor.

Radiographic Appearance of Osteolysis

Some surgeons have viewed any radiolucency between the cement and bone as evidence of osteolysis. A radiologic line of demarcation between bone and cement is often interpreted to be fibrous tissue, cartilage, or fibrocartilage. Histologies corresponding to the interface between bone and cement may also con-

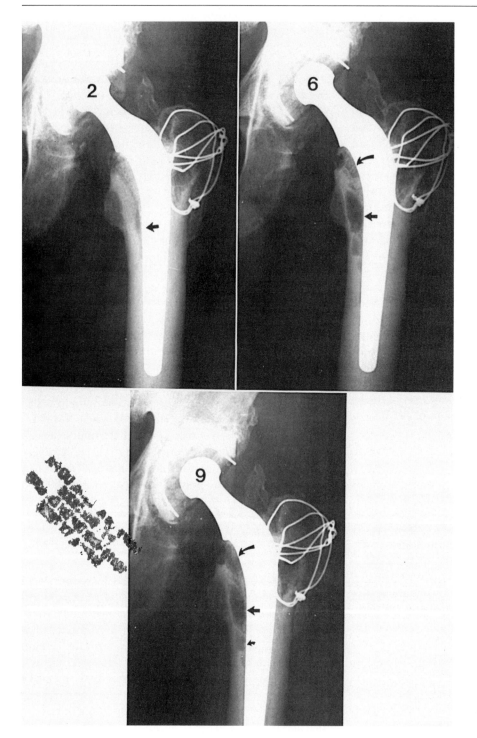

Fig. 1 **Top left**, A Charnley low friction arthroplasty was performed for a unilateral osteoarthritis in a 62-year-old man with evidence of early radiolucency at the medial aspect of the femur between cement and bone at two years postoperatively. **Top right and bottom**, Same hip at six and nine years. Progression of cystic erosion suggesting an "overstressed" medial neck and calcar region with extension to diaphysis. Note: Evidence of osteointegration of cement in femur. Patient is extremely active with weight of 95 kg and remains asymptomatic.

tain particles of HDP and small amounts of spherical acrylic cement. While the line of lucency may be a hallmark of future clinical failure, it has generally been appreciated that the incidence of loosening, that is, clinical failure, is much lower than that suggested by the radiographic lucency. Furthermore, radiolucency is especially important and can be regarded as evidence of loosening if (1) the lucency line is progressive in length, (2) the lucency line is expanding in width to more than 2 mm, and (3) the lucency line borders a line of sclerosis, which is indicative of reaction to movement. The bone lysis caused by widening of the radiolucency line appears to be erratic and expeditious, as if an associated lytic process may play a part in producing extensive bone loss. As stated, the radiologic sign alone is of no concern as long as it is not progressive or is not associated with a line of sclerosis, the latter being an indication of stress involving movement of the prosthesis and causing a reactive process.

The progressive nature of cystic erosions can be documented only by serial radiographs (Fig. 1). Most cystic erosions are asymptomatic until the implant becomes loose (Figs. 2 and 3).

Cystic resorption following loss of fixation or caused by deformation of plastic or metal or by an overly stressed bone begins either at the cement-bone interface or at the site of direct contact between metal and bone. Areas of resorption tend to expand toward the cortex and elongate up to the periosteum. The periosteum is commonly elevated, and bone remodeling may occur at the site of lysis, leading to repair and an appearance of ectasis on the radiograph. Penetration of bone by cysts is extremely uncommon, but over time

a cyst may expand into an adjacent radiographic zone (Fig. 4). Although fragments of cement particles (visible on radiograph) may gradually absorb, they resorb much more slowly than bone.[38] Although most prostheses with significant loosening may show subsidence, some may appear to be well fixed. Because prostheses tend to bend, the stem may remain fixed distally while fragmentation of cement and osteolysis occur proximally and medially. Progression of this pattern of osteolysis and loss of support may lead to stem fracture and total loss of bone proximally and medially. This mechanism of failure was frequently seen in a Charnley type prosthesis used in Huddleston's series (Fig. 4).[38] Extreme bone lysis caused by long-standing motion or particulate debris accumulation may resemble malignancy. These lesions, and even less extensive ones, are commonly progressive and do not heal spontaneously. While a biopsy of these lesions is not indicated, early

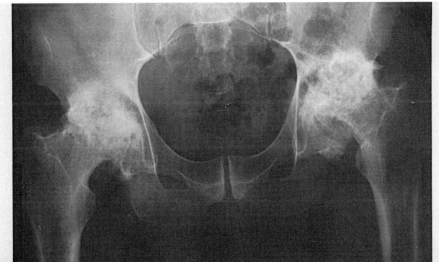

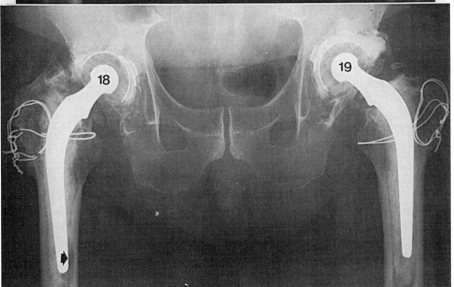

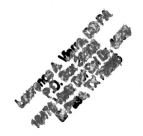

Fig. 2 **Top,** Bilateral osteo-arthritis of hip was treated by Charnley low friction arthroplasty. **Bottom,** Radiograph showing the right and left hips at 18 and 19 years after surgery. Patient's age at index operation was 48, weight 105 kg, worked as a truck driver. Patient remains asymptomatic and active.

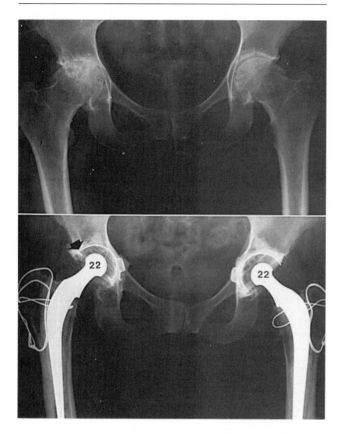

Fig. 3 **Top**, Preoperative and **bottom**, postoperative radiographs of a 50-year-old woman with degenerative osteoarthritis of the hips. At 22 years following surgery there is no evidence of osteolysis. Bone remodeling is favorably maintained. Radiographic marker is fractured presumably due to overstressed acetabular component (arrow). Patient's function remains excellent.

revision surgery offers the only chance of arresting their progression.

Histochemistry

Goldring and associates,[39] who described the histochemical characteristics of the interface membrane of loose cemented prostheses, defined a pathomechanism of bone absorption and coined the term, synovial-like membrane. They recognized three distinct zones in the membrane: (1) the synovial-like lining that forms papillary folds supported by a fibrovascular tissue at the cement-bone interface; (2) a layer containing histiocytes and giant cells, including particles of HDP and PMMA; and (3) a fibrocartilaginous layer that blends into the adjacent bone.

The first layer is lined with large polygonal cells with an eccentric nuclei. This layer (one to two cells thick) lacks a basement membrane. Occasional multinucleated giant cells are present, with a deeper lining of a loose fibrovascular stroma that contains histiocytes and mononuclear infiltrates. Occasionally, papillary folds form, with features like those of a synovial membrane.

The second (midzone) layer is predominantly made up of fibrovascular structures that contain sheets of granular histiocytes, mononuclear cells, and foreign body giant cells. The giant cells are often surrounded by large areas of dissolved PMMA, which contains the barium sulfate.

The third layer, closest to the bone and marrow, shows no evidence of acute or chronic inflammatory cells, but does have some areas of dissolved PMMA, residual granules of barium sulfate, and occasional giant cells.

The association of histiocytes and giant cells with PMMA particles at the site of bone lysis confirms that osteolysis is biologically induced by foreign body reaction in response to particulate debris. Comparison of these types of tissue reactions with tissues obtained from well-fixed prostheses suggests that none of these reactions occurs in response to well-fixed PMMA in bulk form.[39-43] In general, enzymatically active cells, such as histiocytes and monocytes, are located predominantly in the middle zone and on the cement surface of the membrane that stained positively for nonspecific esterase, lysozome, and acid esterase. These cells are consistently positive for acid phosphates. The synovial-like lining is positive only for acid phosphatase.

Based on the histochemical and cell cultures of membranes of failed total hip arthroplasty interfaces, Goldring and associates[39] deduced that the stellate cells are similar to those found in cultures of normal tissue and rheumatoid synovial tissue. The membrane has the capacity to produce large amounts of prostaglandin E_2 and collagenase, which can mediate resorption of bone and other connective tissues. Other proteolytic enzymes and cytokines, including collagenase, lactate dehydrogenase (LDH), Interleukin-1, Interleukin-6, and various growth factors and tumor necrosis factors, also have been identified. These factors are responsible for inflammation, bone resorption, and stimulation of fibrous reparative process and fibrosis.[43] It has been suggested that synovial tissue fails to develop in the absence of motion. If so, traction or motion must produce a biologic signal that causes differentiation and organization of cells into the form of synovial tissue. Edwards and associates[44] showed that repeated injection of air into subcutaneous tissue would, after a period of five to 30 days, create a lining indistinguishable from a synovial membrane.

Doty and Schofield[45] reviewed several reactive membranes from loose cemented total hip prostheses and confirmed other investigators' conclusions regarding the enzyme activities of the membrane formed between the loose prosthesis and bone.

Membranes removed during arthroplasty revisions were chemically preserved in glutaraldehyde/para-

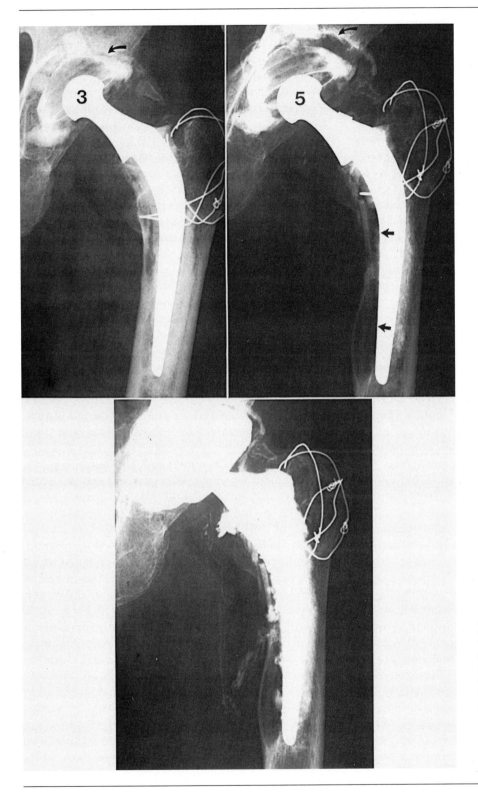

Fig. 4 Top left, A three-year postoperative radiograph of a 59-year-old man whose "Charnley-type" prosthesis had been performed for osteoarthritis at another institution. There is evidence of a radiolucent zone over the medial aspect of the femur at cement-bone interface. **Top right**, Rapid and progressive massive osteolysis is indicated (arrows) by five years, with no evidence of sepsis. **Bottom**, A spontaneous fracture of the medial cortex is being demonstrated by intra-articular injection of radiographic dye.

formaldehyde solutions and studied by light and electron microscopy. Methods were used for demonstrating acid phosphatase, alkaline phosphatase, β-galactosidase, endogenous peroxidase, and glucose oxidase.

Lysosomal enzyme activities, as indicated by acid phosphatase or naphthol esterase, were especially strong in the macrophage and giant cell populations of these membranes.[45] The connective tissue cells within the membrane were also reactive for acid phosphatase but did not appear to change in activity regardless of their location within the membrane.

The presence of PMMA or HDP particles seemed to cause activation of the macrophage or giant cell, with resulting strong lysosomal response, especially in those cells with phagocytized wear particles. β-galactosidase, an enzyme specifically synthesized by macrophages during activation, was an especially good marker for cells that had phagocytized wear products. In most cases, the presence of these particles resulted in a cellular reaction for β-galactosidase, whereas other lysosomal enzymes did not always demonstrate this effect. Thus, lysosomal enzyme activity demonstrated focal areas of cellular response within an individual membrane. This result was further complicated by the presence of very large fragments of PMMA, which appeared to be "walled off" by mononuclear connective tissue cells; these cells showed no significant increase in lysosomal enzyme activity.

Alkaline phosphatase was not demonstrable within the membrane. The enzyme would have been found in some of the leukocyte population, and endogenous peroxidase enzyme activity would have been abundant in activated leukocytes. However, these membrane samples indicated very little leukocyte activity. This also suggests that no infection was present in the specimens studied. This conclusion was supported by our microscopic studies and by cultures, in which we found no bacterial growth from these membrane samples.

Reactions for endogenous peroxidase and glucose oxidase were carried out as another indicator of macrophage activation. In general, these reactions were not uniform within samples. Macrophages or giant cells that contained phagocytized wear particles did not always show high levels of activity of these enzymes. Perhaps there is an original burst of enzyme activity when the particle is incorporated by the cell and, in time, these cells become quiescent. This would explain the "focal" localization of enzyme activities within these membranes. Goldring and associates[39] found that different areas of a single membrane displayed variable amounts of collagenase and prostaglandin activity, and that different patient samples showed a large range of these same activities. It is possible that large areas of a membrane may undergo continual active and quiescent phases during the lifetime of the prosthesis. Such a cyclic response by the membrane and the included cell populations might be mediated by mechanical stimulation between the prosthesis and the supporting bone.

Delayed Rejection

Delayed allergic reactions and rejection as the cause for osteolysis following total hip arthroplasty has been debated in the past.[46] No significant tissue lymphocytes are present in osteolytic lesions associated with loose cemented prostheses, and recent studies by Santavirta and associates[20] and Jasty and associates[43] suggest that cellular response to particle debris may not necessarily be mediated by the immune system.[20,43,47] In clinical practice, the absence of lymphocytes in some retrieved specimens from osteolytic lesions, development of unilateral lesions in patients with bilateral replacements, and absence of recurrence of the lesions after revision surgery, makes the likelihood of immune response as the cause of these lesions extremely unlikely. The fact that histiocytes and multinucleated giant cells are associated with PMMA debris suggests that osteolysis is a biologic process that is mediated by foreign-body reaction in response to PMMA particle debris.

Pathomechanics of Osteolysis

The osteolysis frequently encountered in association with loosening of femoral and acetabular components may be attributed to the presence of particles of PMMA, high-density polyethylene, and metals. However, PMMA particles may be the single causative agent in cases where no HDP was used in arthroplasty.[31] Such osteolysis was first recognized by Charnley who used the term "destructive endosteal lesion." He thought that such lesions might be due to chronic nonsuppurative infection.[5,6] Carlsson and associates[48] attributed such lesions to localized stress following loosening of the femoral component. Localized stress, abrasion, and fragmentation of cement may be the primary causes of generation of PMMA particles.

Micromotion Theory

Radiologic and histologic observations indicate that micromotion may be the cause of failure of cement fixation and osteolysis. The amplitude of such motion need not exceed 15 to 40 μm, the radius of the polymer molecule, to be sufficient to dislodge the acrylic spherules from their bed and to incorporate them into the modified bone caps.[18] These shed spherules are the small particles commonly recognizable from a mass of acrylic. In the acetabulum, the initiation of micromotion is caused by deformation of the acetabulum underload, especially if the acetabulum is made less stiff by the removal of subchondral bone.[30] Stress may then be concentrated at the exposed trabeculae, leading to bone necrosis. The necrotic bone is eventually replaced by a fibrous membrane, which may or may not turn into a strong fibrocartilaginous metaplastic weightbearing structure. If this fibrous interface results in significantly decreased stiffness, further motion will break down the acrylic and cause more looseness (micromotion).

We attribute histologic changes observed at the proximal and medial aspects of the neck of the femur (proximal to the lesser trochanter) to the same phenomenon of micromotion. The histology here differs from that found at the shaft of the femur, where a close coaptation between cement and bone is possible.

In the femur, cement fragmentation and osteolysis can occur if the cement mantle is overly stressed. For example, Huddleston[38] reported that a large number of osteolytic lesions occurred following use of a "Charnley type" prosthesis made of a deformable metal. Similarly, Jasty and associates[21] studied retrieved human specimens and found that initiation of failure was caused by overstressed cement associated with poor prosthesis design and flawed surgical technique.

During their attempt to degrade particles of PMMA and HDP, macrophages (histiocytes and multinucleated giant cells) continue to increase in number and enzyme activity level. Osteoclastic activity at the bone interface may also result from an increase in number of osteoclasts and their activities at the site. I believe that micromotion at the cement-bone interface in the acetabulum or femur in patients with late loosening, as evidenced by progressive radiolucency, results from provocation of quiescent histiocytes and macrophages at the site and the attraction and proliferation of premacrophagic stem cells. Histologically and clinically, the presence of these cells at a stable interface may eventually result in severe osteoclasis and bone loss.

Clinically, we have been able to identify categories of alteration of a stable interface, which may be related to micromotion between cement and bone: (1) defective cement techniques, such as inadequate cement mantle or varus stem; (2) young, active patients with excess elasticity of bone of the acetabulum; (3) inadequate initial fixation and the use of suboptimally designed prostheses; and (4) patients with rheumatoid disease and those with disuse atrophy. In all of these categories the common pathway may be a progressive increase in relative motion between the implant and bone, leading to particle formation and progressive osteolysis (Fig. 5).

Massive Osteolysis in Presence of Fixed Cement

Extensive osteolysis resulting from particles of cement or high-density polyethylene was also documented originally by Charnley and Crawford.[7] Bone resorption around the cemented total hip prosthesis, resulting from fragmentation of cement caused by loosening, has been documented frequently.[48] In 1976, Harris and associates[49] described an aggressive granulomatous lesion associated with a total hip prosthesis. They described four patients who had such lesions around the cemented total hip prosthesis. They defined this lesion based on the histology of four specimens removed from patients with loose prostheses as a "benign, noninflammatory tissue reaction" that caused extensive, localized, tumorlike bone resorption around the cemented femoral component.

In 1986, Jasty and associates[50] reported four cases of extensive, localized bone resorption adjacent to well-fixed total hip replacement. They found no evidence of polyethylene wear debris, but particles of PMMA were

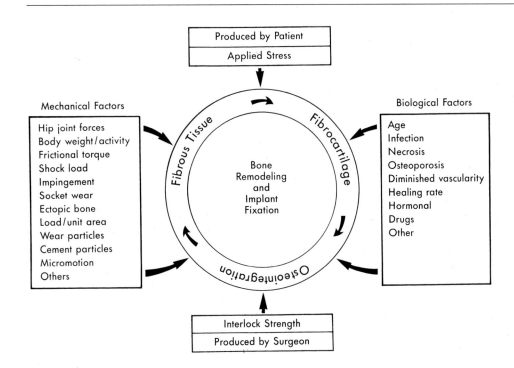

Fig. 5 The nature of the interface tissue (bone-cement junction) and its subsequent remodeling is affected by applied stress by patient (activity level, weight, etc.) and the quality of the initial fixation produced by the surgeon. Other factors, such as mechanical properties of the prosthetic device and a series of biological factors, may be equally important in maintaining the strength and function of interface tissue. (Reproduced with permission from Eftekhar N, Nercessian O: Incidence to mechanism of failure. *Ortho Clinics N Am* 1988; 19:557-566.)

abundantly present. The histologic appearance of the tissue showed sheets of macrophages and foreign-body giant cells invading the femoral cortex. However, the researchers were unable to identify the synovial-like layer at the cement surface of the membrane. They concluded that aggressive bony lysis may occur around stable, cemented stems in the absence of sepsis or malignancy.

As noted by Jasty and associates,[50] massive osteolysis in the absence of loosening is extremely rare. They were able to identify only four cases in more than 3,000 total hip arthroplasties performed at the Massachusetts General Hospital between 1972 and 1986. Most recently, Maloney and associates[51] analyzed 25 cases of severe bone lysis from the same institution, including the four previously cited cases. In three hips, postmortem specimens were also available. Data related to the histology, back-scatter scanning electron microscopy, and biochemical testing of the focal lesions confirmed a local cement fracture around an otherwise rigidly fixed implant. These researchers believed histiocytic reaction to the particulate PMMA to be the stimulus for local osteolysis. This study and other reports on localized endosteal lysis in relation to fixed cemented femoral components suggested that a focal defect in the cement mantle must exist, which enables the contents of the joint cavity to reach the bone.[52,53] Revision of arthroplasty and fixation of the components appear to arrest the progression and to prevent recurrence. Experience suggests that recurrence of osteolytic lesions following revision surgery is uncommon. For example, Eskola and associates[47] reported no recurrence of bone defects caused by osteolysis after revision of osteolytic lesions in 16 cases.

References

1. Eftekhar NS, Doty SB, Johnston AD, et al: Prosthetic synovitis, in Fitzgerald RH Jr (ed): *The Hip: Proceedings of the Thirteenth Open Scientific Meeting of the Hip Society.* St. Louis, MO, CV Mosby, 1985, chap 13, pp 169-183.
2. Oppenheimer BS, Oppenheimer ET, Danishefsky I, et al: Further studies of polymers as carcinogenic agents in animals. *Cancer Res* 1955;15:333-340.
3. Oppenheimer BS, Oppenheimer ET, Stout AP, et al: Studies of the mechanism of carcinogenesis by plastic films. *Acta Unio Internationalis Contra Cancrum* 1959;15:659-663.
4. Clarke EGC, Hickman J, Collins DH, et al: Discussion on metals and synthetic materials in relation to tissues. *Proc R Soc Med* 1953;46:641-652.
5. Charnley J: *Acrylic Cement in Orthopaedic Surgery.* Baltimore, MD, Williams & Wilkins, 1970.
6. Charnley J, Follacci FM, Hammond BT: The long-term reaction of bone to self-curing acrylic cement. *J Bone Joint Surg* 1968;50B:822-829.
7. Charnley J, Crawford WJ: Histology of bone in contact with self-curing acrylic cement, in Proceedings and reports of universities, councils and associations. British Orthopaedic Association. *J Bone Joint Surg* 1968;50B:228.
8. Charnley J: The future of total hip replacement, in Nelson JP (ed): *The Hip: Proceedings of the Tenth Open Scientific Meeting of the Hip Society.* St. Louis, MO, CV Mosby, 1982, chap 13, pp 198-210.
9. Freeman MA, Bradley GW, Revell PA: Observations upon the interface between bone and polymethylmethacrylate cement. *J Bone Joint Surg* 1982;64B:489-493.
10. Freeman MAR, Tennant RE: Cemented versus cementless hip fixation, in Tullos HS (ed): *Instructional Course Lectures XL.* Park Ridge, IL, American Academy of Orthopaedic Surgeons, 1991, chap 18, p 135.
11. Chambers TJ: The cellular basis of bone resorption. *Clin Orthop* 1980;151:283-293.
12. Goodman SB, Fornasier VL, Kei J: The effects of bulk versus particulate polymethylmethacrylate on bone. *Clin Orthop* 1988;232:255-262.
13. Stinson NE: Tissue reaction induced in guinea-pigs by particulate polymethylmethacrylate, polythene and nylon of the same size range. *Br J Exp Pathol* 1965;46:135-146.
14. Charnley J: *Low Friction Arthroplasty of the Hip: Theory and Practice.* Berlin, Springer-Verlag, 1979.
15. Murray DW, Rae T, Rushton N: The influence of the surface energy and roughness of implants on bone resorption. *J Bone Joint Surg* 1989;71B:632-637.
16. Leake ES, Wright MJ, Gristina AG: Comparative study of the adherence of alveolar and peritoneal macrophages, and of blood monocytes to methyl methacrylate, polyethylene, stainless steel, and vitallium. *J Reticuloendothel Soc* 1981;30:403-414.
17. Rich A, Harris AK: Anomalous preferences of cultured macrophages for hydrophobic and roughened substrata. *J Cell Sci* 1981;50:1-7.
18. Tallroth K, Eskola A, Santavirta S, et al: Aggressive granulomatous lesions after hip arthroplasty. *J Bone Joint Surg* 1989;71B:571-575.
19. Willert HG, Lugwig J, Semlitsch M: Reaction of bone to methacrylate after hip arthroplasty: A long-term gross, light microscopic and scanning electron microscopic study. *J Bone Joint Surg* 1974;56A:1368-1382.
20. Santavirta S, Konttinen YT, Bergroth V, et al: Aggressive granulomatous lesions associated with hip arthroplasty: Immunopathological studies. *J Bone Joint Surg* 1990;72A;252-258.
21. Jasty M, Maloney WJ, Bradgon CR, et al: The initiation of failure in cemented femoral components of hip arthroplasties. *J Bone Joint Surg* 1991;73B:551-558.
22. Wiltse LL, Hall RH, Stenehjem JC: Experimental studies regarding the possible use of self-curing acrylic in orthopaedic surgery. *J Bone Joint Surg* 1957;39A:961-972.
23. Willert HG: Reactions of the articular capsule to wear products of artificial joint prostheses. *J Biomed Mater Res* 1977;11:157-164.
24. Willert HG, Semlitsch M: Problems associated with the cement anchorage of artificial joints, in Schaldach M, Hohmann D, Thull R, et al (eds): *Advances in Artificial Hip and Knee Joint Technology.* Berlin, Springer-Verlag, 1976, pp 325-346.
25. Rhinelander FW, Nelson CL, Stewart RD, et al: Experimental reaming of the proximal femur and acrylic cement implantation: Vascular and histologic effects. *Clin Orthop* 1979;141:74-89.
26. Henrichsen E, Jansen K, Krogh-Poulsen W: Experimental investigation of the tissue reaction to acrylic plastics. *Acta Orthop Scand* 1952;22:141-146.
27. Linder L, Hansson HA: Ultrastructural aspects of the interface between bone and cement in man: Report of three cases. *J Bone Joint Surg* 1983;65B:646-649.
28. Draenert K: Histomorphology of the bone-to-cement interface: Remodeling of the cortex and revascularization of the medullary canal in animal experiments, in Salvati EA (ed): *The Hip: Proceedings of the Ninth Open Scientific Meeting of The*

Hip Society. St. Louis, MO, CV Mosby, 1981, chap 7, pp 71-110.

29. Paul HA, Bargar WL: Histologic changes in the dog acetabulum following total hip replacement with current cementing techniques. *J Arthroplasty* 1987;2:71-76.

30. Eftekhar NS, Pawluk RJ: Role of surgical preparation in acetabular cup fixation, in Riley LH Jr (ed): *The Hip: Proceedings of the Eighth Open Scientific Meeting of The Hip Society.* St. Louis, MO, CV Mosby, 1980, chap 15, pp 308-328.

31. Willert HG, Bertram H, Buckhorn GH: Osteolysis in alloarthroplasty of the hip: The role of bone cement fragmentation. *Clin Orthop* 1990;258:108-121.

32. Isaac GH, Atkinson JR, Dowson D, et al: The role of cement in the long term performance and premature failure of Charnley low friction arthroplasties. *Eng Med* 1986;15:19-22.

33. Isaac GH, Wroblewski BM, Atkinson JR, et al: Source of the cement within the Charnley hip. *J Bone Joint Surg* 1990;72B:149-150.

34. Salvati EA, Huo MH, Buly RL: Cemented total hip replacement: Long-term results and future outlook, in Tullos HS (ed): *Instructional Course Lectures XL.* Park Ridge, IL, American Academy of Orthopaedic Surgeons, 1991, chap 17, pp 121-134.

35. Wroblewski BM: Wear and loosening of the socket in the Charnley low-friction arthroplasty. *Orthop Clin North Am* 1988;19:627-630.

36. Mirra JM, Marder RA, Amstutz HC: The pathology of failed total joint arthroplasty. *Clin Orthop* 1982;170:175-183.

37. Johnston AD, Parisien MV: Pathology of reactive (prosthetic) versus septic (revisionary) synovitis, in Eftekhar NS (ed): *Infection in Joint Replacement Surgery: Prevention and Management.* St. Louis, MO, CV Mosby, 1984, chap 3, pp 97-114.

38. Huddleston HD: Femoral lysis after cemented hip arthroplasty. *J Arthroplasty.* 1988;3:285-297.

39. Goldring SR, Schiller AL, Roelke M, et al: The synovial-like membrane at the bone-cement interface in loose total hip replacements and its proposed role in bone lysis. *J Bone Joint Surg* 1983;65A:575-584.

40. Goldring SR, Jasty M, Roelke M, et al: Formation of a synovial-like membrane at the bone-cement interface: Its role in bone resorption and implant loosening after total hip replacement. *Arthritis Rheum* 1986;29:836-842.

41. Goldring SR, Jasty M, Roelke M, et al: Biological factors that influence the development of a bone-cement membrane, in Fitzgerald RH Jr (ed): *Non-Cemented Total Hip Arthroplasty.* New York, NY, Raven Press, 1988, chap 5, pp 35-39.

42. Goldring SR, Jasty M, Roelke M, et al: Factors responsible for formation of synovial-like membrane after total hip replacement (THR): Its role in prosthesis loosening. *Arthritis Rheum* 1985;28:S36.

43. Jasty M, Jiranek W, Harris WH: Acrylic fragmentation in total hip replacements and its biological consequences. *Clin Orthop* 1992;285:116-128.

44. Edwards JC, Sedgwick AD, Willoughby DA: The formation of a structure with the features of synovial lining by subcutaneous injection of air: An in-vivo tissue culture system. *J Pathol* 1981;134:147-156.

45. Doty SB, Schofield BH: Ultrahistochemistry of calcified tissues, in Dickson GR (ed): *Methods of Calcified Tissue Preparation.* Amsterdam, Elsevier, 1984, chap 4, pp 149-198.

46. Linder L, Lindberg L, Carlsson A: Aseptic loosening of hip prostheses: A histologic and enzyme histochemical study. *Clin Orthop* 1983;175:93-104.

47. Eskola A, Santavirta S, Konttinen YT, et al: Cementless revision of aggressive granulomatous lesions in hip replacements. *J Bone Joint Surg* 1990;72B:212-216.

48. Carlsson AS, Gentz CF, Linder L: Localized bone resorption in the femur in mechanical failure of cemented total hip arthroplasties. *Acta Orthop Scand* 1983;54:396-402.

49. Harris WH, Schiller AL, Scholler JM, et al: Extensive localized bone resorption in the femur following total hip replacement. *J Bone Joint Surg* 1976;58A:612-618.

50. Jasty MJ, Floyd WE III, Schiller AL, et al: Localized osteolysis in stable, non-septic total hip replacement. *J Bone Joint Surg* 1986;68A:912-919.

51. Maloney WJ, Jasty M, Rosenberg A, et al: Bone lysis in well-fixed cemented femoral components. *J Bone Joint Surg* 1990;72B:966-970.

52. Anthony PP, Gie GA, Howie CR, et al: Localised endosteal bone lysis in relation to the femoral components of cemented total hip arthroplasties. *J Bone Joint Surg* 1990;72B:971-979.

53. Fornasier VL, Cameron HU: The femoral stem/cement interface in total hip replacement. *Clin Orthop* 1976;116:248-252.

Particulate Debris in Cemented Total Hip Replacement

Eduardo A. Salvati, MD

Brian G. Evans, MD

Foster Betts, PhD

Stephen B. Doty, PhD

Introduction

Three decades have passed since Sir John Charnley's pioneering efforts introduced total hip arthroplasty (THA). Early interest focused on improving fixation of the components. However, as data become available detailing longer follow up, wear debris and the inflammatory response to this debris are becoming increasingly recognized as the significant etiologic factor associated with progressive bone loss, loosening, and failure (Fig. 1). Particulate debris is now recognized to incite a

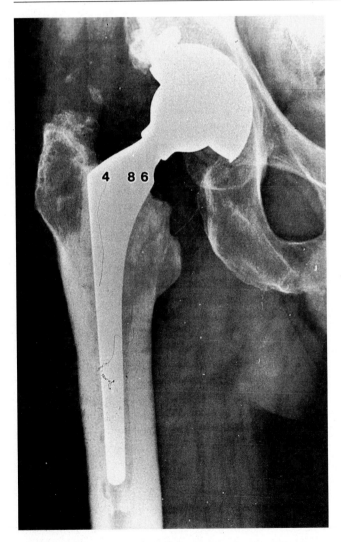
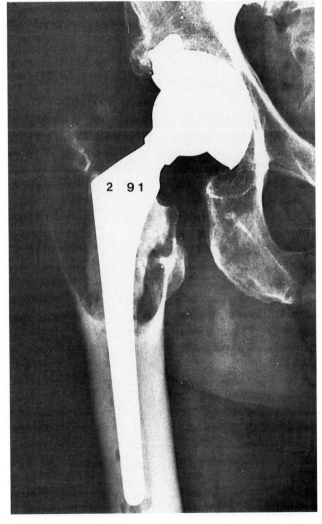

Fig. 1 **Left**, Radiograph obtained two months after a revision of a PCA femoral stem for aseptic loosening. It demonstrates an excellent cement mantle and bone cement interface in this 56-year-old male, who is 68" tall and weighs 150 lbs. **Right**, Five years post revision severe osteolysis of the proximal femur developed. Tissue obtained from the osteolytic area at the second revision revealed extensive polyethylene debris within the tissues. Note the asymmetry of the femoral head within the acetabular shell due to polyethylene wear in Zone 1.

biological response, characterized by the recruitment of macrophages, release of inflammatory mediators, and the progressive resorption of bone. This response, well recognized in cemented fixation, is now being observed in noncemented implants as well (Fig 2).[1]

In 1988 we were the first to report nine failed cemented titanium alloy total hip replacements in which severe metallosis was observed in the periprosthetic tissues.[2] Subsequent clinical observations have confirmed that titanium alloy implants have a higher rate of premature failure than those of other alloys, suggesting the possibility that titanium alloy debris may promote early loosening.[3-8]

Polyethylene debris can also incite an inflammatory response and is increasingly recognized as a significant factor in aseptic loosening.[9-11] Several studies have documented the large numbers of microscopic and submicroscopic polyethylene particles in the tissues of failed THAs.[10,12,13] Recent data have documented the production of polyethylene debris not only from the articular surface but also from the convex nonarticular surface of modular metal-backed cups and loose cemented all-polyethylene acetabular components.[14]

Bone Cement Interface

The histology of the mechanically stable bone-cement interface has been well documented.[15-17] Draenert,[15] in an animal model, demonstrated viable bone and active osteoblasts surrounding the cement mantle without intervening fibrous tissue. Jasty and associates,[16] in human retrieval studies, have demonstrated bone in intimate contact with the cement mantle with no evidence of an intervening fibrous membrane on the femoral side. Bone remodeling was noted around the well-fixed stems with the production of an osseous neocortex around the cement mantle, providing continued stable fixation even after 20 years of in vivo service. On the acetabular side, however, a fibrous membrane of variable thickness was usually present at the bone-cement interface. This membrane contained particles of polyethylene debris, particularly at the periphery.

The histologic characteristics of the fibrous membrane of failed cemented total hip components have been well defined.[12,13,18,19] Bone cement, metal, and polyethylene debris are consistently found within the fibrous tissue, and microscopic and submicroscopic particles are noted within the macrophages and giant cells. These cells are involved in the resorption of bone mediated by prostaglandins and collagenases. Increasing numbers of particles have been associated with increasing severity of the histiocytic response and tissue necrosis.[11] These wear particles may have systemic metabolic, immunologic, and oncogenic effects.[20,21]

Metallic Wear Debris

Titanium

We studied 71 all-titanium femoral stems retrieved at revision surgery.[5] Fifty patients (51 hips) underwent revision of a primary hip replacement, eight patients (eight hips) underwent rerevision surgery, and 11 patients (12 hips) underwent removal for infection. The average duration of service for the three groups was 4.5 years, 5.0 years, and 3.7 years, respectively. Radiographs were evaluated for endosteal scalloping, and bone loss was quantified. Although in most cases early postoperative radiographs revealed a well-cemented stem by current standards, the mean time to failure was only 4.5 years. Bone loss was graded as severe in 51%, moderate in 24%, and mild in 20%. Femoral endosteolysis was noted in 94% and acetabular osteolysis in 6%.

Histologic evaluation of the tissues from failed THA revealed polymethylmethacrylate debris in 75% of cases, polyethylene debris in 80%, metallic debris in 75%, and chronic inflammatory cells in all cases. Metallic debris was seen in 17% of the infected cases and in none of the eight failed revisions. Titanium debris was also observed in the regional lymph nodes, disputing the assertion of Dorr and associates,[18] that particulate debris is a local problem contained by the periprosthetic fibrous connective tissue encapsulation within the femoral canal and joint capsule.

Sixty-eight retrieved femoral components were examined for head and stem abrasion. The area of burnishing of the femoral head was mapped and quantified with a computer digitizer. The prosthetic femoral heads showed consistent abrasion and burnishing with an average involved area of 49.5% (range 2% to 96%). The stem with only 2% of the head abraded was retrieved after only a few weeks service. The extent of burnishing of the femoral head did not correlate with the duration of service.

The fact that burnishing, which was present in 70% of stems retrieved for aseptic loosening, was seen in none of the stems removed for sepsis, which were well fixed, clearly implicates motion at the stem-cement interface in the production of metallic wear debris. Several patterns of stem abrasion were noted: (1) 52% showed lateral longitudinal abrasion, primarily along the anterolateral and posteromedial edge. This pattern suggested motion against the cement in response to a posteriorly directed torque against the femoral head. (2) 13% had abrasion along the anterior and posterior shoulders as well as the medial side of the tip. This pattern was seen only with the DF-80 prosthesis and may reflect pistoning with the medial tip acting like a chisel due to its bevel. (3) 7% had diffuse areas of abrasion that did not fit any pattern, suggesting gross motion. Micromotion at the femoral metal-cement or metal-

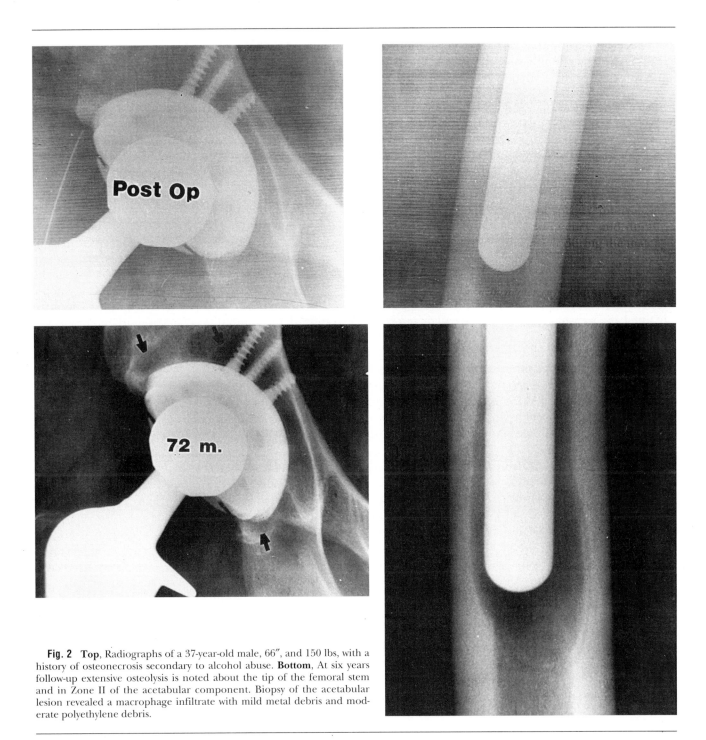

Fig. 2 Top, Radiographs of a 37-year-old male, 66″, and 150 lbs, with a history of osteonecrosis secondary to alcohol abuse. **Bottom**, At six years follow-up extensive osteolysis is noted about the tip of the femoral stem and in Zone II of the acetabular component. Biopsy of the acetabular lesion revealed a macrophage infiltrate with mild metal debris and moderate polyethylene debris.

bone interface has also been shown by Collier and associates[22] to burnish the stem and produce particulate metallic debris.

Polyethylene wear, in this group of patients, averaged 0.22 mm per year (range 0.02 to 0.60 mm per year), twice the rate of wear noted for the Charnley THA.[23-26] These findings indicate a greater amount of both polyethylene and metallic debris in patients with an all-titanium femoral prosthesis.

Intraoperatively, the periprosthetic tissues demonstrated variable degrees of gray staining and, in several cases, black staining caused by metal debris. Histologic evaluation revealed an intense histiocytic reaction at the sites of metal debris. Tissue metal levels were approximately 100 times greater in cases with failed titanium alloy stems than in a comparable series of cases with failed cobalt chromium alloy stems, as measured by atomic absorption spectrophotometry.[27]

The short duration of service and the degree of femoral osteolysis suggest accelerated loosening and failure. Bone scalloping and granuloma formation were probably caused by increased bone cement, plastic, and metallic particulate debris, which stimulated an inflammatory response and lysis.

Cobalt - Chromium

In a series of 22 patients with failed cemented cobalt chromium prostheses, metal levels were determined in the periarticular tissues.[28] In 12 hips the stem and cup were loose, in four only the cup was loose, and six were removed because of infection. The average duration of implantation was 9.5 years (range 1.0 to 17.6 years). Examination of the retrieved femoral components revealed unblemished polished surfaces and a mirror-like femoral head with rare scratches, even after 17.6 years of service. A total of 118 tissue samples were obtained (48 capsular and 70 bone-cement interface membranes).

Cobalt, chromium, and molybdenum levels varied widely from site to site within each case. Total tissue metal content (cobalt, chromium, and molybdenum averaged per case) ranged from 2.7 to 250 µg of metal per gram of tissue (mean 39 µg/g). The highest total metal levels occurred in cases revised for infection (mean 72.9 µg/g, range 5.6 to 250 µg/g), followed by cases with a loose cup and stem (mean 32 µg/g, range 6.7 to 97.8 µg/g), and those with only a loose cup, which yielded the lowest tissue metal levels (mean 8.2 µg/g, range 2.7 to 12.2 µg/g). Levels of the constituent elements generally reflected the composition of the alloy, suggesting the metal resulted from wear particles. The fact that tissues with very low metal levels did not reflect the element ratios found in the alloy suggests that corrosion may have been the source.

Histologic evaluation demonstrated fibrosis, histiocytic reaction, hemorrhage, and necrosis to be the most frequent findings. Polyethylene and cement particles were noted in approximately half the sections, and a few metal particles were seen in the tissues of infected cases. Metal levels were not found to correlate with any demographic variables or histologic findings, nor did metal content or histologic findings correlate with duration of implantation.

The low metal levels measured in the cement-bone interface and the few metal particles found histologically suggest that cobalt chromium particles may have been less important than cement or polyethylene particles in the inflammatory response and loosening. Or perhaps the large tissue metal content noted with titanium alloy stems exerts a synergistic effect with the inflammatory and lytic process initiated by cement and polyethylene particles, causing early failure. However, the accumulation of the particulate metal debris can be toxic and may have long-term implications in young patients, because cobalt, chromium, and nickel may be carcinogenic.[20,29,30]

Metal-Backed Cups

Metallic debris can also be produced from metal-backed acetabular components.[14] In noncemented components, holes are often placed in the metal shell for ancillary screw fixation. These represent a conduit for wear debris to the bone-prosthesis interface. In a recent study of 19 patients undergoing revision at The Hospital for Special Surgery, Huk and associates[14] studied the cementless titanium alloy acetabular shells and polyethylene liners. The indication for revision was recurrent dislocation in 10 cases, infection in four cases, and femoral loosening and thigh pain in five cases. Two cases were associated with osteolysis at the site of acetabular screw fixation (Fig. 2). The components were in place for an average of 21.7 months (range, 1 to 72 months). The pseudomembrane was obtained from the screw holes with and without screws and from the osteolytic lesions. This tissue was evaluated histologically for the presence of polyethylene, metal, and histiocytic reaction. Polyethylene debris was noted in 47% of the specimens and metal debris in 67% of the specimens obtained from holes containing screws. Analysis of the tissue from holes without screws revealed polyethylene debris in 88% of cases and metal debris in 31%. Material retrieved from the osteolytic lesions revealed a foreign body giant cell reaction to particulate debris, with polyethylene and metal debris identified.

Tissue from the holes with screws, of ingrowth acetabular shells, was also analyzed for metal levels. Trace metal analysis detected Ti in every specimen, regardless of the presence or absence of screws in the sampled hole. Titanium levels at the empty screw holes averaged 74 µg/g of tissue (range .72 to 331 µg/g). From the holes with screws, it averaged 959 µg/g (range 48 to 11,900 µg/g). Tissue from the two cases of osteolysis was also analyzed and the titanium level averaged 143 µg/g (138 and 147 µg/g). These high levels of titanium most likely resulted from fretting corrosion between the screws and the holes of the acetabular component and perhaps from micromotion and fretting of the wires of the fiber mesh.

Size of Particulate Debris

To investigate the possibility that higher failure rates for these prostheses might be related to significant differences in the size of metal and polyethylene debris particles, the size of the particulate debris was quantitated in tissues obtained from around 30 failed cemented femoral components—ten cobalt chromium, ten stainless steel, and ten titanium alloy femoral components.[13] Two methods of specimen preparation were used: (1) an isolation method, in which the tissue was digested leaving the metallic debris, and (2) a nonisolation method, which consisted of routine histologic preparation for light microscopy. Greater quantities of metallic debris were detected in the tissues of titanium alloy stems than in those of either cobalt chromium or stainless steel, regardless of the method of preparation. In all cases, the mean size of the particulate debris with the isolation method was 0.86 to 1.06 mm in short dimension and 1.57 to 1.79 μm in long dimension. The nonisolation method yielded significantly smaller particles, measuring 0.36 to 0.40 μm in short dimension and 0.64 to 0.69 μm in long dimension (p < 0.0001). The discrepancy between the average sizes for the two methods results from shortcomings of each of the methods: Both underestimate small particles and the nonisolation method underestimates large metal particles. However, the size of the metallic particulate debris did not differ among the alloys for either method.

Electron Microscopy

Specimens were also prepared for electron microscopy to observe the distribution of the metallic particles within the macrophage (Fig 3). In general, the metal was sequestered within phagolysosomes, vacuoles, or small transport vesicles, which appeared to fuse with larger vacuoles. This would result in large accumulations of metallic debris within some macrophages. These large vacuoles were filled with metal-containing small vesicles, which transported metal to the larger vacuole. This intracellular transport mechanism functions to carry the metal particles into the phagolysosome, a highly corrosive environment, to attempt to degrade them by enzymatic and oxidative processes. In some cases, especially with titanium particles, the metal appears to be within the cytosol, not associated with any particular organelle or structure. If this is the mechanism of sequestration used by the cell, it would explain why the intracellular deposits were often larger than the extracellular accumulations. However, in cases of rapid wear and release of metal, the extracellular accumulations were also large, suggesting a dynamic process.

A generalized phenomenon, observed with all types of metal accumulation, was the morphologic degeneration of these phagocytic cells as the metal debris accumulated. The two most apparent changes were the degeneration of the mitochondria and the development of pyknotic nuclei or nuclei with chromatin clumping. Both of these observations indicate a reduction in cell activity and an inability to maintain intracellular homeostasis. Consequently, the resulting cell death leads to an accumulation of cell debris, as the proteolytic enzymes and the metallic debris previously ingested are released.

In specimens obtained from patients with failed titanium implants, the only titanium-containing particles identified were shard-like or rectangular in shape, and usually not confined within an intracellular compartment. The dense material within lysosomes and the round-shaped dense particles in the cytoplasm did not show any sign of containing titanium within the limits of detection, using x-ray microanalysis techniques.

Wear particles and deposits of metals were found in extracellular sites as well as within the phagocytic cells. The extracellular distribution appeared random, with no obvious orientation along collagen fibrils or within the extracellular fluid. The titanium-containing specimens often demonstrated a black appearance. These large black osmiophilic deposits found adjacent to the titanium implants were observed by electron microscopy to be lamellae of lipid-like material (Fig. 4) and contained no titanium as measured by x-ray microanalysis. The appearance and distribution of these lipid-like deposits in the extracellular matrix suggested that they were the remains of cells that had degenerated within the reactive tissue.

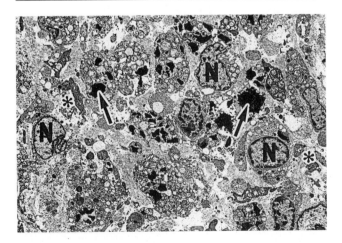

Fig. 3 This low magnification electron micrograph shows many macrophages within the soft tissue surrounding a failed prosthesis. Nuclei (N) of several macrophages are indicated, and most cells contain black deposits of metallic debris (arrows) within their cytoplasm. Cell debris (asterisks) and fragments of cells can be seen in the same area as normal cells. The fibrous extracellular matrix can be seen as light gray material between cells. [Magnification: 4,300×]

Osteolysis

In a prospective study, the metallic and cement debris were measured from tissues obtained at the site of femoral endosteolysis (FE), the bone-cement interface, and the joint pseudocapsule in 12 consecutive patients with aseptic loosening of a cemented total hip implant.[30] The mean interval between primary and revision was 9.6 years and between primary and the onset of FE 8.9 years. There were four stems each of

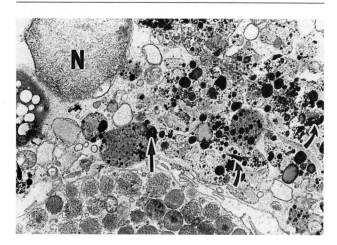

Fig. 4 This higher magnification electron micrograph shows a single macrophage found in the tissues adjacent to a failed prosthesis. The nucleus (N) is situated in a cytoplasm filled with round dense lipid deposits (straight arrow) and shards of titanium metal (curved arrows). X-ray microanalysis showed the presence of titanium within the shards, and the presence of osmium in the lipid droplets. [Magnification: 15,000×]

cases (33%). Two of the three all-titanium alloy (head and stem) femoral components had metallic debris (67%).

Detectable metal levels were found in the FE in all cases. Metal levels were 2.5 times higher in the FE than in the femoral pseudomembrane, and 4.2 times higher than levels in the joint pseudocapsule. This difference was statistically significant for the stainless steel and cobalt chromium groups but not for the titanium group, because the levels of titanium were very high in all the periprosthetic tissues.

Barium levels in areas of FE were, on average, 1.7 and 42.4 times higher than in the femoral pseudomembrane and the joint pseudocapsule, respectively. The difference between the FE and the joint pseudocapsule was significant for all three alloy groups.

Polyethylene debris was found in 65% of the joint pseudocapsule specimens and in more than 90% of the FE and femoral pseudomembranes.

Osteolysis can also be noted about the acetabular component. In a review of 71 failed cemented THA with a titanium stem, osteolysis was noted about four cups. Two had lesions noted in zone I and two in zone III.[5] Acetabular osteolysis around cemented cups, caused by metallic and polyethylene debris, has also been noted in association with stainless steel and cobalt chromium femoral implants and occurs more frequently at the periphery (Zones I and III) of the cemented acetabular component (Fig. 5). We have

stainless steel, cobalt chromium, and titanium alloy. Histologic evaluation of the tissue from the region of FE revealed a histiocytic reaction and cement debris in every case. Polyethylene debris was noted in 11 of the 12 cases (92%); metallic debris was noted in four

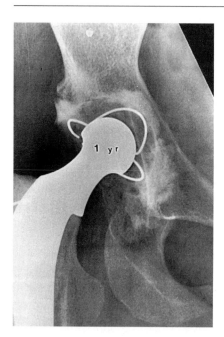
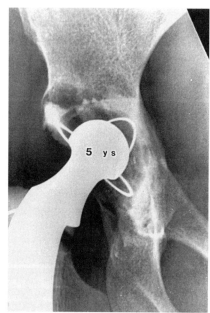
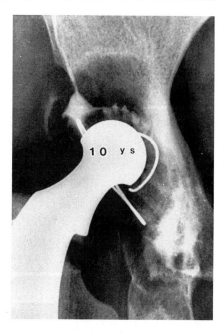

Fig. 5 **Left**, Radiograph of a cemented right total hip replacement was performed in 1980. The patient is a 36-year-old, 63″, 115-lb female with a primary diagnosis of juvenile rheumatoid arthritis. **Center**, At five-year follow-up, an asymptomatic lytic lesion was noted in Zone I of the acetabular bone cement interface and in the proximal medial femoral neck. **Right**, Ten years postoperatively the patient noted the acute onset of severe pain in the hip. The radiograph demonstrates proximal migration of the acetabular component. Also note the eccentric position of the femoral head within the acetabular cup.

also noted osteolysis in association with three noncemented acetabular components (Fig. 6). Two of these had subsequent revision surgery and biopsy of the lesions revealed metallic and polyethylene debris. All three of these lesions were in Zone II, one with extension into Zones I and III, strongly implicating the screw fixation holes as the route of access for the wear debris to the prosthesis bone interface.[14] Schmalzried and Harris,[31] in a review of 83 Harris-Galante acetabular components with average 68-month follow-up (minimum 60 months), found one case of acetabular osteolysis which was also noted in zone II.

The increased levels of polyethylene, metal debris, and particulate cement in the tissue surrounding a failed implant may act in synergy and contribute to the recruitment and activation of the macrophage infiltrate in the femoral canal.[9,12,23] This activated response may then lead to the genesis of the FE.

Synovial Fluid Metal Levels

In a prospective study, synovial fluid metal levels from stainless steel, cobalt chromium, and titanium alloy cemented total hip implants were measured by atomic absorption spectrophotometry.[32] Fluid was sampled from 37 well-fixed and 44 loose total hip arthroplasties. In addition, tissue metal levels were measured in cases that were revised.

A fivefold increase in metal levels was seen in loose compared with well-fixed stainless steel implants. However, iron, which constitutes 60% of stainless steel, is not measured, because it cannot be accurately quantitated at low levels because of contamination from hemoglobin. A sevenfold increase in metal levels was noted comparing loose to well-fixed cobalt chromium alloy implants. Titanium implants demonstrated the greatest increase, 21-fold, of loose compared to well-fixed implants. Tissue metal levels from revised cobalt chromium alloy implants averaged 45 µg/g dry tissue compared to 4,470 µg/g dry tissue from revised titanium alloy implants.

Well-fixed cemented implants had similar low synovial fluid metal levels, regardless of the alloy. However, when loosening occurred, titanium alloy implants released significantly higher levels of metal into the synovial fluid and local tissues compared to stainless steel or cobalt chromium alloy. The release occurs from the articulating surface in well-fixed implants and from abrasion of the stem against cement and bone in loose components.

Polyethylene Wear

Howie and associates[9] demonstrated in an animal model that simulated polyethylene wear particles injected intra-articularly produced bone resorption and osteolysis at the bone-cement interface, further implicating polyethylene particles in the production of osteolysis and prosthetic loosening. Ultra high molecular weight polyethylene (UHMWPE) is used as an articulating surface in most systems today for both cemented and noncemented fixation. While durable, this material is subject to wear, fatigue, oxidation, and fragmentation.[11,24,25,32-35]

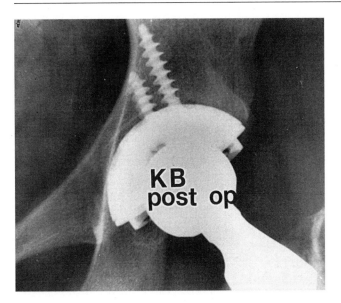 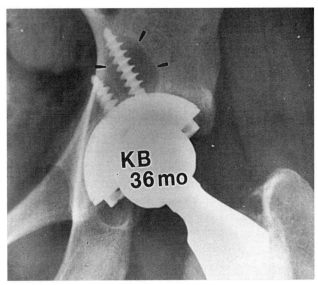

Fig. 6 **Left**, Radiograph of a right hybrid total hip prosthesis using a modular metal-backed porous ingrowth acetabular component with 4.5 mm of polyethylene thickness. The patient is a 17-year-old, 61″, 111-lb female with a primary diagnosis of juvenile rheumatoid arthritis. **Right**, At three years follow-up the patient is asymptomatic. However, a region of osteolysis has developed in Zone II about one of the acetabular fixation screws.

Charnley and Cupic[36] have estimated that polyethylene wear averaged 1.2 mm after 10 years of in vivo function. Wroblewski[25] determined the rate of wear to be 0.19 mm (range, 0.017 to 0.52 mm) per year in 22 acetabular components retrieved at the time of revision surgery. Radiographic measurements correlated well with the actual measurements in the retrieved acetabular components. In another series, Wroblewski[26] reported a wear rate of 0.096 mm per year in a radiographic review of patients with a successful result at 15 to 20 years of follow-up. McCoy and associates[37] reported a wear rate of 1.2 mm after 15 years of in vivo function in 40 hips (0.08 mm per year). The rate of wear was noted to be greater in men. Garcia-Cimbrello and Munuera[23] found the overall wear rate to be 0.13 mm per year. A significant correlation was noted between wear greater than 0.2 mm per year, age less than 50, and weight greater than 80 kg.

Livermore and associates[38] found wear to be correlated with femoral head size. Heads measuring 32 mm were associated with the greatest degree of volumetric wear, and 22-mm heads demonstrated the most linear wear. They concluded that an intermediate head size (26 to 28 mm) would provide the best compromise to minimize volumetric and linear wear (penetration of the femoral head into the polyethylene cup).

Isaac and associates[39] examined three-body wear at the femoral-head polyethylene articulation. They noted that polymethylmethacrylate, with its radiographic contrast medium barium sulfate, was able to scratch the prosthetic head, because barium sulfate has a hardness similar to that of stainless steel. We have documented by atomic absorption spectrophotometry the consistent presence of barium in the synovial fluid obtained by hip aspiration in well-fixed total hip arthroplasties (mean 19 µg/l, range 1 to 51 µg/l).[32] In loose prostheses, the mean barium level was 16-fold greater (mean 302 µg/l; range 30 to 8,856 µg/l). This observation may explain the increased wear of plastic cups in failed total hip arthroplasties.

A significant correlation between cup wear, head penetration, and acetabular loosening has been demonstrated by Wroblewski.[25,26] Garcia-Cimbrelo and Munuera,[23] in a recent study, found that 56% of patients with wear greater than 2 mm had radiographic evidence of acetabular loosening. Other possible causes of increased wear are poor tribology caused by inaccurate machining or polishing of the articular surfaces or variation in the wear characteristics of the polyethylene implanted. All of these factors can promote the production of greater numbers of wear particles, which in turn promote a greater osteolytic response and loosening.[11] Few data exist at the present time to determine which of these mechanisms is more significant, although they all contribute to the loosening.

Using light microscopy, the size of polyethylene wear debris was determined in the tissues from failed implants.[13] Tissue was obtained from failed implants of titanium, cobalt chrome, and stainless steel. The mean size of the polyethylene particles was 2.7 to 4.1 mm in short dimension and 8.1 to 12.8 mm in long dimension. The size was noted to be larger in tissues from around a titanium implant than in those from around a cobalt chromium or stainless steel implant (p < 0.001). Titanium is the alloy most susceptible to abrasion and scratching, and its roughened surface is more likely to produce large polyethylene particles than is the smooth, well-polished surface of a cobalt chromium or stainless steel prosthetic head.

Schmalzried and associates,[10] in a recent study, suggested that the particles of polyethylene debris detectable by light microscopy are only a portion of the total tissue load of plastic debris. Using polarized light, a generalized birefringence of the pseudocapsular tissue was noted, suggesting the diffuse dispersion of polyethylene particles smaller than the limits of detection by light microscopy (approximately 0.4 to 1µm).

Modularity

Acetabular

With increasing demand by clinicians for intraoperative flexibility, the use and availability of modular components are expanding. Modular acetabular components are available for both cemented and noncemented use. These designs allow replacement of a worn or damaged polyethylene liner in a well-fixed metal shell and the use or exchange of standard and extended polyethylene liners for improved stability.[40]

The introduction of the polyethylene-metal interface creates another site for wear debris production. Huk and associates[14] examined the polyethylene liners retrieved at the time of revision in 19 patients. The acetabular polyethylene liners were inspected and three modes of damage were noted: burnishing, surface deformation, and embedded metal debris. All specimens were found to have surface burnishing and deformation, the latter caused by the edges of the screw holes and prominent heads of the screws. Burnishing was documented by the loss of the machining lines from the nonarticular surface of the polyethylene liner, which represents a new source of polyethylene debris.

Several recent studies have demonstrated a marked variation between manufacturers in the metal-backed modular acetabular components.[41-43] Variability in the congruity of the polyethylene liner and the metal backing was noted with some systems that rely on rim loading and others that rely on cold flow to achieve a congruent interface. The retaining mechanisms also demonstrated marked variability in their resistance to dissociation and torsional forces. The thickness of the polyethylene liners available for each metal shell size was noted to decrease to as little as 2.5 mm in shells with the smaller outer diameter and a 32-mm inner diameter. Each surgeon must be aware not only of the range of sizes available from the manufacturer but also of the quality of the liner-retaining mechanism and the thickness of the polyethylene available for each implant selected.

Based on early studies that suggested an increasing rate of loosening with cemented cups with long-term follow-up and no improvement in long-term fixation of the cup with improved cement techniques, many clinicians now use a hybrid total hip implant consisting of a cemented femoral stem and a noncemented acetabular cup.[44-47] However, no long-term data are available to support this approach. Schmalzried and Harris[31] have published the minimum five-year results in 83 hips using the Harris-Galante fiber metal mesh acetabular component. They noted no failures for aseptic loosening, but two components were revised for liner-locking mechanism failure, one for femoral loosening with acetabular osteolysis, and one for Brooker grade IV heterotopic ossification and thigh pain. The one case of acetabular osteolysis was noted about an acetabular screw. This patient also had progressive endosteal erosion of the femur and a loose femoral component. The femur and cup were revised and, although the cup was noted to be well fixed, there was 2 mm of motion at the liner shell interface and two of three screws were found to be loose. Examination of the tissue from the acetabular lesion revealed small particles of polyethylene and a very few metal particles. Further refinement of the locking mechanism of the plastic liner with the metal shell is indicated to prevent micromotion and increased generation of debris.

Smith and associates[48] recently reported the results of wear measurements in 96 primary Harris-Galante wire mesh cups. The average follow-up was 53 months. Wear was measured from AP plain radiographs, corrected for magnification. The mean wear was noted to be .11 mm per year (range 0.0 to 0.47 mm/year). A subgroup of 18% (n=17) of these patients revealed excessive wear with a mean of 0.28 mm per year, almost three times that reported for the Charnley low friction arthroplasty.[24,26,37] These researchers were unable to find a statistically significant correlation between wear and loosening or osteolysis, perhaps because of the relatively short follow-up.[48]

As previously noted we have also identified three cases of progressive acetabular osteolysis (Figs. 2 and 6). This finding is a matter of considerable concern, because the incidence of osteolysis may increase with extended follow-up.

Femoral

Modular femoral heads offer the flexibility to adjust limb length and femoral offset and to select the femoral head size that provides optimal polyethylene thickness. The material of the femoral head can also be selected to optimize the wear properties of the articulation.[49] In the case of a revision, the modular head can be removed to improve the acetabular exposure. However, this flexibility has disadvantages as well. The femoral head can dissociate at the time of reduction of a dislocation.[50] Fractures of modular ceramic femoral heads have been reported and the long-term implications are a cause for concern.[51] The interface of the head and neck taper is a potential site for fretting, crevice, and galvanic corrosion.[22,50,51] Collier and associates[22] reported on a series of retrieved femoral stems and noted corrosion to be present on all mixed metal tapers, after only 40 months in vivo. Based on the scanning electron microscope (SEM) morphology of the corroded regions, Collier felt that galvanic corrosion was the principal mechanism. Gilbert and associates[52] also reported a series of 102 retrieved femoral stems and noted that the type of metal used in the taper did not correlate statistically with the extent of corrosion. However, there was a correlation between the time in vivo and the severity of the corrosion. This group interpreted their SEM data to implicate crevice and intergranular corrosion as the principal mechanism for degradation. They also noted crevice corrosion and cobalt depletion in several of their cobalt/chromium - cobalt/chromium tapers. While these two groups found differing forms of corrosion, the frequency of this finding is disturbing, particularly in view of the short duration of in vivo function.

Lieberman and associates,[53] at The Hospital for Special Surgery, studied 48 retrieved modular femoral stems. Twenty-six were cobalt/chromium - cobalt/chromium head neck tapers, ten were titanium alloy - cobalt/chromium tapers and 12 were titanium alloy - cobalt/chromium tapers that had been preassembled at the manufacturer with a shrink fit taper and the head-trunion interface sealed with a fine bead of silicone. No corrosion was noted in the similar metal tapers with an average time in vivo of 20 months (range, 1 to 39 months). Similarly, no corrosion was noted in the tapers of the preassembled and sealed tapers with dissimilar metals with an average time in vivo of 54 months (range 38 to 78 months). Two of the ten tapers with dissimilar metals were noted to have experienced fretting corrosion with loss of the machining marks on both the cobalt chrome head and the titanium trunion. These two implants were retrieved after 15 and 59 months in vivo, respectively. In another implant with dissimilar metals retrieved after 43 months in vivo, pitting of both the femoral head and trunion, consistent with crevice corrosion, was noted.

Thus three of ten tapers that used dissimilar metals and were not preassembled and sealed demonstrated evidence of corrosion involving the head and trunion of the modular femoral stem with an average time in vivo of only 34 months (range 13 to 59 months).

In our most recent study, synovial fluid was sampled in 33 patients, 20 with stable femoral implants (hip aspiration was performed at the time of contralateral hip surgery) and 13 at the time of revision for acetabular loosening (nine), dislocation (three), or infection (one). Nine stainless steel (SS), six monolithic cobalt-chromium (CC), ten modular CC-CC, four modular titanium-CC and four preassembled titanium-CC components were sampled. Length of implantation averaged 90 months, 110 months, 36 months, 29 months and 93 months, for the SS, monolithic CC, modular CC, modular Ti-CC and Preassembled Ti-CC components, respectively. Metal levels were determined by atomic absorption spectrophotometry.

The results revealed an average chromium level for the monolithic components of 4.20 µg/l (range, 1.4 to 10.3 µg/l) and 8.73 µg/l (range, 1 to 47.6 µg/l) for the modular components. This difference was not statistically significant. The average cobalt level was 1.1 µg/l (range, 0.2 to 2.4 µg/l) for the monolithic implants and 15.52 µg/l (range, 0.4 to 69.2 µg/l) for modular stems (p=0.017). No significant difference in metal levels was noted for mixed metal taper junctions compared to monolithic components, perhaps because of the small sample size (n=4).

The chromium/cobalt ratio is nominally 0.45 in medical grade chromium-cobalt alloy. Monolithic chromium-cobalt implants were noted to have a ratio of 4.51 (range, 2.14 to 7.00) compared with 1.05 (range, 0.32 to 2.5) for modular cobalt chromium implants (p=0.005).

These data indicate an increase in the synovial fluid metal levels of modular implants compared to monolithic implants, and there were significantly higher levels of cobalt, most likely from crevice and or intergranular corrosion at the femoral head - neck Morse taper junction. This in vivo data adds to the growing volume of data from retrieved implants demonstrating corrosion of modular implants. While few clinical problems have resulted from corrosion, careful long-term follow-up is necessary to determine the clinical significance.

Conclusions

Histologic analysis of the early failures of the titanium alloy femoral stem revealed metal particles in 75% of cases, with an average tissue titanium level of 1,047 µg/g in our first study and 4,470 µg/g in our subsequent study. The premature failure observed in the cases with the highest metal levels suggests that titanium debris may have a detrimental effect on implant fixation.

In contrast, analysis of the cobalt chromium alloy failures revealed few metal particles histologically and an average tissue metal level of 39 µg/g. Cement and polyethylene particles were observed in over 50% of cases, and these may have had a more significant role in failure. Furthermore, the average duration of implantation was 4 years for the titanium failures, compared with 9.5 years for the cobalt chromium alloy failures.

Well-fixed cemented components have low synovial fluid metal levels regardless of the alloy implanted. However, when loosening occurs, titanium alloy implants release significantly higher metal levels (x21) into the synovial fluid and local tissues, compared with cobalt chromium alloy implants (x7).

Analysis of the retrieved femoral stems consistently revealed severe burnishing of the titanium prosthetic head in comparison to the mirror-like finish of the retrieved cobalt chromium prosthetic heads, even in the component retrieved after 17.6 years of implantation. Well-fixed stems revealed no abrasion regardless of the metal. Loose stems of titanium alloy were significantly more abraded than were those of cobalt chromium alloy.

Sites of femoral endosteolysis (FE) demonstrate higher barium and metal levels than sites in the femoral pseudomembrane and pseudocapsule. In conjunction with acrylic and polyethylene debris, they contribute to the focal recruitment and activation of macrophages leading to the genesis of FE.

The sizes of the particulate metallic debris of stainless steel, cobalt chromium, and titanium alloy are similar, suggesting that debris particle size differences do not contribute significantly to the higher failure rates observed for titanium components. Polyethylene debris generated by articulation with a titanium alloy femoral head is larger, most likely because of the roughened surface of the abraded femoral head.

Electron microscopy demonstrates that the particles of metallic debris can be extremely small (a few hundredths of a micrometer). The particles are phagocytized by the macrophages and transported to the phagolysosomes. This highly corrosive environment acts on the high surface area of the metallic debris and releases metallic ions intracellularly, which may be toxic and lead to progressive cell degeneration and death, with subsequent release of intracellular enzymes, particulate, and ionic metallic debris. This cycle may repeat itself, leading to progressive tissue necrosis and osteolysis.

The results presented do not support the use of titanium alloy femoral components for cemented total hip replacement or the use of titanium alloy as an articulating surface for cemented or cementless total hip replacement. The data presented regarding modular implants is of concern. These data indicate that corrosion occurs in modular metallic interfaces of similar and dissimilar metallic interfaces. Polyethylene and titanium debris have been documented at the nonarticular surface of modular acetabular components. At the present time, few cases of implant failure resulting from modularity have been reported. However, the existing data should compel implant manufacturers to achieve and maintain high implant quality control standards. Surgeons using modular implants must optimize the interface by ensuring that the surfaces are clean, dry, and free of debris and soft tissue prior to assembly. Assembly should comply with the manufacturer's recommended techniques, and after assembly all modular interfaces must be inspected and assessed for complete seating and stability prior to closure. Clinicians must be aware of the potential problems of modular interfaces and must exercise care in the assembly of modular components at the time of surgery.

Acknowledgements

This work was supported in part by Ms. Emma A. Daniels, President of the May Ellen and Gerald Ritter Foundation.

References

1. Maloney WJ, Jasty M, Harris WH, et al: Endosteal erosion in association with stable uncemented femoral components. *J Bone Joint Surg* 1990;72A:1025-1034.
2. Agins HJ, Alcock NW, Bansal M, et al: Metallic wear in failed titanium alloy total hip replacements: A histological and quantitative analysis. *J Bone Joint Surg* 1988;70A:347-356.
3. Amstutz HC, Yao J, Dorey FJ, et al: Survival analysis of T-28 hip arthroplasty with clinical implications. *Orthop Clin North Am* 1988;19:491-503.
4. Black J, Sherk H, Bonini J, et al: Metallosis associated with a stable titanium alloy femoral component in total hip replacement: A case report. *J Bone Joint Surg* 1990;72A:126-130.
5. Buly RL, Huo MH, Salvati E, et al: Titanium wear debris in failed, cemented total hip arthroplasty: An analysis of seventy-one cases. *J Arthroplasty* 1992;7:315-323.
6. Lombardi AV Jr, Mallory TH, Vaughn BK, et al: Aseptic loosening in total hip arthroplasty secondary to osteolysis induced by wear debris from titanium alloy modular femoral heads. *J Bone Joint Surg* 1989;71A:1337-1342.
7. McKellop HA, Sarmiento A, Schwinn CP, et al: In vivo wear of titanium-alloy hip prostheses. *J Bone Joint Surg* 1990;72A:512-517.
8. Ritter MA, Stringer EA, Littrell DA, et al: Correlation of prosthetic femoral head size and/or design with longevity of total hip arthroplasty. *Clin Orthop* 1983;176:252-257.
9. Howie DW, Vernon-Roberts B, Oakeshott R, et al: A rat model of resorption of bone at the cement-bone interface in the presence of polyethylene wear particles. *J Bone Joint Surg* 1988;70A:257-263.
10. Schmalzried TP, Kwong LM, Jasty M, et al: The mechanism of loosening of cemented acetabular components in total hip arthroplasty: Analysis of specimens retrieved at autopsy. *Clin Orthop* 1992;274:60-78.
11. Willert HG, Bertram H, Buchhorn GH: Osteolysis in alloarthroplasty of the hip: The role of ultra high molecular weight polyethylene wear particles. *Clin Orthop* 1990;258:95-107.
12. Johanson NA, Bullough PG, Wilson PD Jr, et al: The microscopic anatomy of the bone cement interface in failed total hip arthroplasties. *Clin Orthop* 1987;218:123-135.
13. Lee JM, Salvati EA, Betts F, et al: Size of metallic and polyethylene debris particles in failed cemented total hip replacements. *J Bone Joint Surg* 1992;74B:380-384.
14. Huk OL, Bansal M, Betts F, et al: Generation of polyethylene and metal debris from the non-articulating surface of modular acetabular components in total hip arthroplasty. *J Bone Joint Surg*, in press.
15. Draenert K: The John Charnley Award Paper: Histomorphology of the bone-to-cement interface: Remodeling of the cortex and revascularization of the medullary canal in animal experiments. *Hip* 1981;9:71-110.
16. Jasty M, Maloney WJ, Bragdon CR, et al: Histomorphological studies of the long term skeletal responses to well fixed cemented femoral components. *J Bone Joint Surg* 1990;72A:1220-1229.
17. Linder L: Ultrastructure of the bone-cement and the bone-metal interface. *Clin Orthop* 1992;276:147-156.
18. Dorr LD, Bloebaum R, Emmanual J, et al: Histologic, biochemical, and ion analysis of tissue and fluids retrieved during total hip arthroplasty. *Clin Orthop* 1990;261:82-95.
19. Goldring SR, Schiller AL, Roelke M, et al: The synovial-like membrane at the bone-cement interface in loose total hip replacements and its proposed role in bone lysis. *J Bone Joint Surg* 1983;65A:575-584.
20. Black J: Does corrosion matter? *J Bone Joint Surg* 1988;70B:517-520.
21. Brien WW, Salvati EA, Healey JH, et al: Osteogenic sarcoma arising in the area of a total hip replacement: A case report. *J Bone Joint Surg* 1990;72A:1097-1099.
22. Collier JP, Surprenant VA, Jensen RE, et al: Corrosion between the components of modular femoral hip prostheses. *J Bone Joint Surg* 1992;74B:511-517.
23. Garcia-Cimbrelo E, Munuera L: Early and late loosening of the acetabular cup after low-friction arthroplasty. *J Bone Joint Surg* 1992;74A:1119-1129.
24. Wroblewski BM: Direction and rate of socket wear in Charnley low friction arthroplasty. *J Bone Joint Surg* 1985;67B:757-761.
25. Wroblewski BM: Wear and loosening of the socket in the Charnley low friction arthroplasty. *Orthop Clin North Am* 1988;19:627-630.
26. Wroblewski BM: 15-21-year results of the Charnley low friction arthroplasty. *Clin Orthop* 1986;211:30-35.
27. Betts F, Yau A: Graphite furnace atomic absorption spectrophotometric determination of chromium, nickel, cobalt, molybdenum and manganese in tissues containing particles of cobalt-chrome alloy. *Anal Chem* 1989;61:1235.
28. Betts F, Wright T, Salvati EA, et al: Cobalt-alloy metal debris in periarticular tissues from total hip revision arthroplasties: Metal contents and associated histologic findings. *Clin Orthop* 1992;276:75-82.
29. Lalor PA, Revell PA, Gray AB, et al: Sensitivity to titanium: A cause of implant failure? *J Bone Joint Surg* 1991;73B:25-28.
30. Huo MH, Salvati EA, Lieberman JR, et al: Metallic debris in femoral endosteolysis in failed cemented total hip arthroplasties. *Clin Orthop* 1992;276:157-168.
31. Schmalzried TP, Harris WH: The Harris-Galante porous-coated acetabular component with screw fixation: Radiographic analysis of eighty three primary hip replacements at a minimum of five years. *J Bone Joint Surg* 1992;74A:1130-1139.

32. Brien WW, Salvati EA, Betts F, et al: Metal levels in cemented total hip arthroplasty: A comparison of well fixed and loose implants. *Clin Orthop* 1992;276:66-74.

33. Bartel DL, Bicknell VL, Wright TM: The effect of conformity, thickness, and material on stresses in ultra-high molecular weight components for total joint replacement. *J Bone Joint Surg* 1986;68A:1041-1051.

34. Gabriel SM, Bartel DL: Metal backing and wear in acetabular components for total hip arthroplasty. *Trans Orthop Res Soc* 1992;17:47.

35. Isaac GH, Wroblewski GM, Atkinson JR, et al: A tribological study of retrieved hip prostheses. *Clin Orthop* 1992;276:115-125.

36. Charnley J, Cupic Z: The nine and ten year results of the low-friction arthroplasty of the hip. *Clin Orthop* 1973;95:9-25.

37. McCoy TH, Salvati EA, Ranawat CS, et al: A fifteen-year follow-up study of one hundred Charnley low-friction arthroplasties. *Orthop Clin North Am* 1988;19:467-476.

38. Livermore J, Ilstrup D, Morrey B: Effect of femoral head size on wear of the polyethylene acetabular component. *J Bone Joint Surg* 1990;72A:518-528.

39. Isaac GH, Atkinson JR, Dowson D, et al: The role of cement in the long term performance and premature failure of Charnley low friction arthroplasties. *Eng Med* 1986;15:19-22.

40. Harris WH: A new total hip implant. *Clin Orthop* 1971;81:105-113.

41. Fehring TK, Hurley PT, Braun E, et al: Modular acetabular components: Are they really metal-backed? Presented at the 59th Annual Meeting of the American Academy of Orthopaedic Surgeons, Washington, DC, Feb 21, 1992, paper no. 92.

42. Hurley PT, Fehring TK, Braun E, et al: Polyethylene liners in modular porous acetabular components: A comparative analysis. Presented at the 59th Annual Meeting of the American Academy of Orthopaedic Surgeons, Washington, DC, Feb 21, 1992, paper no. 94.

43. Parsley BS: Current concerns with modular metal-backed acetabular components. Presented at the 59th Annual Meeting of the American Academy of Orthopaedic Surgeons, Washington, DC, Feb 21, 1992, paper no. 95.

44. Beckenbaugh RD, Ilstrup DM: Total hip arthroplasty. *J Bone Joint Surg* 1978;60A:306-313.

45. Mulroy RD Jr, Harris WH: The effect of improved cementing techniques on component loosening in total hip replacement: An eleven year radiographic review. *J Bone Joint Surg* 1990;72B:757-760.

46. Stauffer RN: Ten-year follow-up study of total hip replacement. *J Bone Joint Surg* 1982;64A:983-990.

47. Sutherland CJ, Wilde AH, Borden LS, et al: A ten-year follow-up of one hundred consecutive Muller curved-stem total hip replacement arthroplasties. *J Bone Joint Surg* 1982;64A:970-982.

48. Smith EJ, Goetz D, Harris WH: Radiographic wear in the Harris-Galante porous acetabulum at 4.5 years. Presented at the 22nd Annual Hip Course, Boston, September 1992.

49. Davidson J: Surface finish of metal and ceramics. Proceedings of the Hip Society, Twentieth Open Scientific Meeting, Washington, DC, February 23, 1992.

50. Pellicci PM, Haas SB: Disassembly of a modular femoral component during closed reduction of the dislocated femoral component: A case report. *J Bone Joint Surg* 1990;72A:619-620.

51. Peiro A, Pardo J, Navarrete R, et al: Fracture of the ceramic head in total hip arthroplasty: Report of two cases. *J Arthroplasty* 1991;6:371-374.

52. Gilbert JL, Buckley CA, Jacobs JJ: Corrosion of modular head femoral components. Presented at the 22nd Annual Hip Course, Boston, September 1992.

53. Lieberman J, Rimnac C, Salvati EA: A corrosion analysis of the head-neck taper interface in hip prostheses, *Clin Orthop*, in press.

Osteolysis Due to Particle Wear Debris Following Total Hip Arthroplasty: The Role of High-Density Polyethylene

B. Michael Wroblewski, MB ChB, FRCS

Introduction

Osteolysis may be said to be present when a localized, usually clearly defined, loss of bone is observed between the implant and bone in cases of hip arthroplasty. Willert and Semlitch[1] published their observations, supported with a diagrammatic pictorial sequence of events, and suggested that the granulation tissue may act on the neighboring bone "...which is removed by extensive resorption leading to loosening of the prosthesis." Their work was done on cases where polyester was the plastic used. This theme was taken up by others[2] while Rose and associates[3] were quite categorical that "...the chief clinical question is that of biological effects of the debris and not of mechanical problems due to dimension changes." It is difficult to reconcile this statement with their suggestion that only 10% of the volumetric changes were caused by wear, whereas creep was responsible for the other 90%. More recently the terms "cement disease," "cementless disease," and "particle disease" have been used in an attempt to explain the pathology of osteolysis. The attempts to coin the phrase "cement disease" were presumably made in order not only to implicate the cement as the cause of osteolysis, but at the same time to support the use of uncemented components. When the osteolysis was described with uncemented components, the use of the term was no longer justifiable so "cementless disease" was the term used. Now, because particles of cement, polyethylene and metal have been identified in the membrane at the bone-implant interface, "particle disease" is the term most commonly used. This, however, only explains the findings, but not the cause of the osteolysis. In this chapter, the role of high-density polyethylene (HDP) wear particles as a possible cause of osteolysis will be examined. Consideration will be given to the source of the wear particles and to the incidence of osteolysis in both primary and revision surgery. Radiographic and histologic appearances will be discussed, immunohistochemical studies will be presented briefly, and, finally, the likely mechanism of these osteolytic changes will be proposed.

Source of High-Density Polyethylene (HDP) Wear Particles

Articulation

There is little doubt that most of the HDP wear particles are generated at the level of the articulation, and that wear, rather than cold flow, is the main cause of the volumetric changes. The rate of wear is primarily related to the patients' activity level[4] and the roughness of the head of the femoral component.[5] Because the head bores for itself a new, roughly cylindrical path, and the wear is mainly unidirectional, the volume of plastic shed into the tissues (T1 r^2 x d) will be roughly proportional to the depth of socket penetration (d). This fact makes it extremely difficult to distinguish between the effect of the volume of the wear particles generated (and, thus, any likely biologic effect) and the mechanical changes caused by the restriction of angular movements and impingement of the neck of the stem on the rim of the socket.[6] Two mechanisms of wear at the articulation have been identified, microscopic and macroscopic.

Microscopic Wear Asperities of the metal head remove material, in the form of relatively small wear particles, from the socket surface by abrasion and adhesion.

Macroscopic Wear is caused by buildup of subsurface fatigue strains, which lead to delamination of the plastic and larger increments of loss.[7]

Bone-Cement Interface

Histologic studies have shown that, in the cemented Charnley socket, the bone-cement interface is formed primarily of fibrous tissue; areas of true osseointegration are exceptional.[8] In studies of revised cemented HDP Charnley sockets, 32.2% showed wear on the external surface, where movement had occurred between the exposed HDP and bone.[9] Socket loosening, therefore, must occur before external socket wear can take place.

Socket-Cement Interface

More recently, radiographic evidence of the migration of the wire wear marker has been described, which suggests that movement can occur between the cement and the socket. This movement is the result of the design, the surgical technique, and the direction of the load on the socket.[10] Although no evidence has been presented that this movement generates wear particles, logic would dictate that it should.

The Incidence of Osteolysis in Revision of Failed Charnley Low-Friction Arthroplasties (LFAs)

A total of 537 consecutive Charnley LFA revisions, from various sources, have been analyzed, and the incidence of osteolysis is presented in Table 1. Although the incidence of femoral osteolysis varies, there is nothing to suggest that it is invariably present even if both components are obviously loose. Osteolysis alone, therefore, cannot be responsible for component loosening.

The Effect of Component Design and Surgical Technique on the Incidence of Osteolysis

Records of 1,342 Charnley LFAs, in patients aged 50 or younger at the time of surgery, have been analyzed to determine whether component design and surgical technique had any effect on the incidence of femoral osteolysis. The findings are shown in Tables 2 and 3. Although the groups of patients presented in Tables 2 and 3 are not strictly comparable, especially with respect to the follow-up, the evidence indicates that improvements in surgical technique of component fixation with cement reduce the likelihood of femoral osteolysis. Wear rates, and thus the volume of HDP wear debris generated, remain comparable.

Radiographic Appearance

Although osteolysis and, thus, bone destruction is the usual appearance associated with failed cases, little or no attention has been given to past experience with teflon. Therefore, it may be of interest to review some of the most destructive changes associated with the use of polytetrafluoroethylene (Teflon), and to review some of the cases in which gross bone destruction was seen at revision.

Teflon

A group of 160 cases were reviewed, of which 53 showed intrapelvic Teflon granuloma which had become calcified. In the majority of cases (79%), the calcification followed the revision to a cemented HDP socket. Calcification seen on radiographs is interpreted as a healing process.[11]

High-Density Polyethylene (HDP)

Improvement in the radiographic appearances after revision of cases with femoral osteolysis[11] is encouraging. New bone formation and even healing of the cavi-

Table 1
Incidence of femoral osteolysis in 537 cases of revision of Charnley LFAs

Indication for revision	No. of cases	No. with osteolysis	%
Loose socket	109	33	30
Fractured stem	73	23	32
Fractured stem and loose socket	33	13	40
Loose stem	125	80	64
Loose stem and loose socket	197	158	80

Table 2
The incidence of femoral osteolysis using flanged and unflanged Charnley sockets

Type of socket	No. of cases	Follow-up (years)	Osteolysis No.	%	Socket wear mm/year
Unflanged	975	10 yr 9 mth	84	8.6	0.12
Flanged	367	7 yr 1 mth	18	5.0	0.12

Table 3
The incidence of femoral osteolysis with and without intramedullary bone block

Stem fixation	No. of cases	Follow-up (years)	Osteolysis No.	%	Socket wear mm/year
No bone block	974	11 yr 9 mth	85	8.7	0.11
(1st general stem: polished)					
With bone block	368	6 yr 6 mth	17	4.6	0.13
(subsequent stem designs - round back/flanged: matt finish)					

ties would seem to counter the idea that HDP wear debris is a cause of cavitation and bone loss.

Histologic Appearance

Histology studies of intrapelvic Teflon granuloma have clearly shown calcification and even new bone formation in the presence of large masses of Teflon wear particles.[11] Similar histologic appearances are yet to be described with HDP, but the radiographic appearances suggest that this really may be the case. It is clear that the mere presence of either Teflon or HDP wear particles is not the cause of osteolysis. Some other process must be involved. A suggestion is made that it is the changes in volume and pressure within the cavity housing the implant that lead to the cavitation, and that the presence of the HDP or, in fact, any other wear debris is purely incidental. Changes in volume and pressure in the cavity containing the implant, which cause it to function as a foreign body bursa, precede the accumulation of wear particles.

Immunohistochemistry

More recently it has been suggested that initiation of the loosening of the acetabular component is biologic, and that femoral loosening is mechanical in nature.[12] It is fascinating to speculate, and begs the question, "How can nature distinguish between the two sites and where exactly is the transition from biologic to mechanical causation?"

In an attempt to shed more light on the subject, a study was undertaken to establish if there is a difference in the role of inflammatory cells in aseptic loosening of femoral and acetabular components in cemented total hip arthroplasty. This work, undertaken by Dr. S. M. Andrew and associates at Manchester University, will be published in due course (supported by The John Charnley Trust). Ten matched pairs (acetabular and femoral components and the surrounding bone-cement interface fibrous tissue) from cases of osteoarthritis were examined. The findings can be summarized as follows: (1) membranes on both sides of the arthroplasty consisted mainly of macrophages; the macrophages were "activated." (2) Quantitative results showed no difference between the cell counts positive for the various antibodies from the femoral and the acetabular sites. (3) There was a positive correlation between numbers of positive cells from the two sites of the arthroplasty. (4) The conclusion was that the inflammatory cell reactions to the loosening of the acetabular femoral components were identical. (5) The moderate number of T cells present was seen as an indication that the T cells represented a nonspecific reaction to wear debris. (6) No evidence of enhanced osteoclastic resorption of trabecular bone was found in the specimens examined. It must be emphasized that this finding was incidental, and not the objective of the study.

This important work suggests that the findings associated with cemented component loosening are more in the nature of a biologic response to a mechanical process, rather than a biologic response leading to a mechanical problem (S. M. Andrew, MD, personal communication, 1993). The findings are very encouraging. Improvements in component design, fixation with cement, and reduction in wear rates, which are within the scope of the manufacturer, designer, and the surgeon, will improve long-term results. There is no longer any justification for blaming the biologic reaction as the main cause of the problem, either on the femoral or the acetabular side.

Bone Loss and Radiographic Appearances of Femoral Osteolysis

So far no studies have been carried out to establish the extent of femoral endosteal bone loss that must occur before the changes appear on radiographs. An experimental work (unpublished) carried out by the author for this purpose is too lengthy to be quoted in detail. The summary of the findings can be outlined thus: (1) The volume of the femoral endosteal bone loss needed before it becomes obvious to the naked eye on a radiograph is not an absolute amount, but a proportion relative to the radiodensity of the femoral cortex. (2) Whether this can be distinguished from the surrounding bone will depend on whether this "bone loss" is diffuse or localized by a clearly defined edge. (3) Bone density changes are more obvious if seen in an area across the x-ray beam rather than in its plane. (4) Localized, clearly defined bone loss of 10% of the cortical density in the plane at right angles to the x-ray beam is clearly discernible.

Diffuse loss (or diffuse increase in bone density) may not be obvious until it reaches between 20% and 50% of the cortical density, and this figure may be as high as 80%. The ability to distinguish the changes probably has less to do with orthopaedic or radiologic knowledge and more to do with the ability to perceive and distinguish the shades of grey. Once radiographic changes are obvious, the loss of bone stock is already significant, and our plain radiographic assessment is clearly an underestimate.

The Mechanism of Femoral Osteolysis

Lesions indicating femoral osteolysis, when present, can be seen between the implant and the femoral cortex in the areas where a deficiency or total absence of cement can be demonstrated (Fig. 1). These areas have a scalloped, clear-cut-edge appearance, with thinning of the femoral cortex, which, at times, can lead to the fracture of the femoral shaft.

The Site

The location of the areas of femoral osteolysis can be easily explained if one considers that the total hip prosthesis, which in fact is a foreign body bursa, extends beyond the articulation and, thus, allows migration of bursal fluid and wear debris according to the changes in volume and pressure in the cavity housing the implant.

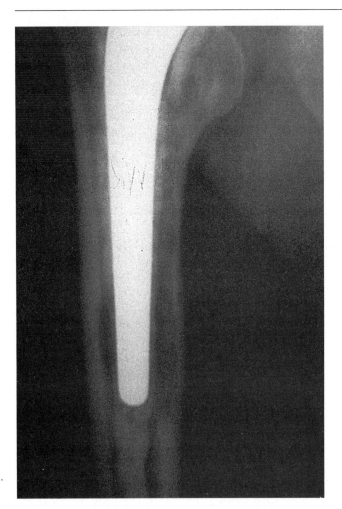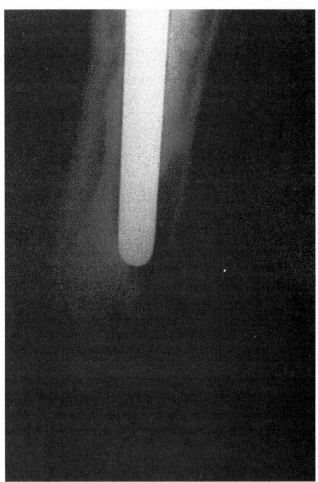

Fig. 1 Typical appearance of femoral osteolysis in an area of cement deficiency.

Shape

Uniform distribution of pressure causes a change in volume that results in a globular shape, as in a soap bubble. If such pressure changes take place within a confined space, deviations from this globular shape are determined by the surrounding structures, for example, pressure changes are unlikely to affect the hard, inert metal of the stem. Because of the pressure on the endosteal bone, the scalloped cavities of femoral osteolysis with a clearly defined edge will appear. These are by no means unique to mechanical problems attributed to loosening; they are equally obvious in cases of deep infection, where pressure and volume changes are generated locally by the infective process.

Other Areas of Endolysis

So far nothing has been said about osteolysis occurring on the acetabular side. The reason for that is probably obvious. The typical changes on the acetabu-

lar site are associated with demarcation of bone-cement interface and socket migration. Socket tilting and migration does not allow localized buildup of pressure and cavitation. This is supported by the finding of osteolysis being more than twice as common with loose stems than with loose sockets (Table 1). Loose stem-cement complex is more likely to create a one-way nonreturn value than a loose socket. If, however, such a situation can be produced, cavitation will occur. A socket that is well fixed medially but is worn thin laterally will deflect, generate pressure and volume changes at the bone-cement interface, and produce endosteal cavitation (Fig. 2).

Osteolysis Without Surgery

All the examples of osteolysis described so far have been associated with total hip arthroplasty and wear debris. However, a similar phenomenon can be seen around arthritic hips and other joints. Subchondral

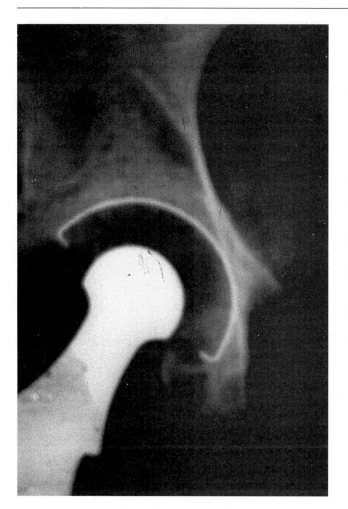 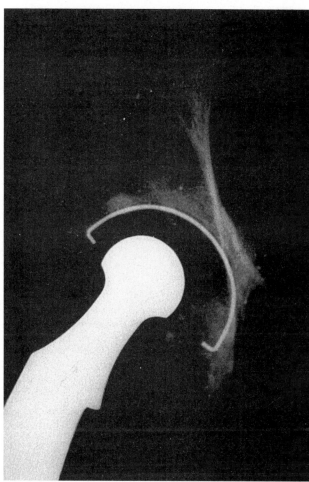

Fig. 2   Extensive cavitation at the bone-cement interface of the socket 20 years after surgery. The socket was not loose at exploration. Note the depth of socket wear.

cysts, which are common in arthritic hips, are no more than extensions of the joint cavity, which communicates with it through the defects in the subchondral plate. This communication with the joint cavity is obvious at surgery, and the enlargement and collapse of such cysts are typical of a progressive condition. Similar changes may also be seen on the femoral side, at times extending down to the neck of the femur. No wear debris, of the sort associated with artificial joints, can be implicated in the osteolysis, but fragmented bone particles may be seen. Histiocytes have been identified in such osteoarthritic cysts, but their numbers are small and they are not activated. (S. M. Andrew, MD, personal communication, 1993).

Summary

It seems likely that the osteolysis seen in total hip arthroplasty, and commonly attributed to wear debris, is actually caused by changes of volume and pressure in the cavity housing the implant. Improvements in cementing technique reduce the incidence of osteolysis. There is no evidence to suggest that this osteolysis is a biological response to wear debris or that the process is different on the femoral and the acetabular side. Similar changes can be seen on both sides of an arthritic hip joint that has not been subjected to surgery.

Acknowledgment

Supported by The Peter Kershaw Trust.

References

1. Willert HG, Semlitch M: Reaction of the articular capsule to artificial joint prosthesis, in Williams D (ed): *Biocompatibility of Implant Materials.* London, Tunbridge Wells, 1976, pp 40-48.
2. Vernon-Roberts B, Freeman MAR: The tissue response to total joint replacement prostheses, in Swanson SAV, Freeman MAR (eds): *The Scientific Basis of Joint Replacement.*

New York, NY, John Wiley and Sons, 1977, chap 4, pp 86-129.

3. Rose RM, Nusbaum HJ, Schneider H, et al: On the true wear rate of ultra high-molecular-weight polyethylene in the total hip prosthesis. *J Bone Joint Surg* 1980;62A:534-549.

4. Hodgkinson JP, Kay PR, Feler JA, et al: Activity and socket wear in the Charnley low-friction arthroplasty. Presented at the Meeting of the British Orthopaedic Association, 1992.

5. Isaac GH, Atkinson JR, Dowson D, et al: The role of cement in the long term performance and premature failure of Charnley low-friction arthroplasties. *Eng Med* 1986;15:19-22.

6. Wroblewski BM: Direction and rate of socket wear in Charnley low-friction arthroplasty. *J Bone Joint Surg* 1985;67B:757-761.

7. Fisher J, Dowson D, Cooper JR, et al: The failure and wear of UHMWPE in artificial joints. Presented at the British Orthopaedic Research Society Meeting, Leeds, March 1993.

8. Malcolm AJ: Pathology of cemented low-friction arthroplasty in autopsy specimens in Older J (ed): *Implant-Bone Interface.* London, Springer-Verlag, 1990, pp 77-82.

9. Wroblewski BM, Lynch M, Atkinson JR, et al: External wear of of the polyethylene socket in cemented total hip arthroplasty. *J Bone Joint Surg* 1987;69B:61-63.

10. Wroblewski BM: Migrating wear marker in the Charnley low friction arthroplasty. *Proc Inst Mech Eng [H]* 1992;205:125-126.

11. Wroblewski BM: *Revision Surgery in Total Hip Arthroplasty.* London, Springer-Verlag, 1990, pp 99-103.

12. Schmalzried TP, Kwong LM, Jasty M, et al: The mechanism of loosening of cemented acetabular components in total hip arthroplasty: Analysis of specimens retrieved at autopsy. *Clin Orthop* 1992;274:60-78.

Total Hip Arthroplasty

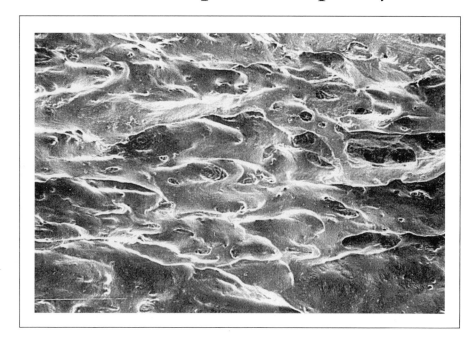

Optimizing the Outcome in Primary Hip Replacement: Continued Excellence Despite Continual Change

Clive P. Duncan, MD, FRCSC

We are at an important fork in the road on the subject of component fixation. Bone loss, caused by the inflammatory response to particular debris, has become the most significant threat to the success of joint replacement, particularly the hip. It is not a new problem. Consider for a moment Charnley's experience with the Teflon cup. But our acknowledgement of its importance and causes is new. How we use this information in the clinical and basic research settings will determine what fork in the road we will take. In the meantime we have the responsibility for continued excellence in patient care despite continual change in our understanding of the basic science of prosthetic failure. This philosophy occupies the following chapters in this section of *Instructional Course Lectures, Volume 43.*

In the academic setting, the most pressing challenge is to address osteolysis effectively, as we have done with infection. The most promising avenues would seem to include the development of a bioinert alternative to polyethylene, the minimization of volumetric wear, and the effective sealing of the host-implant junction from the ingress of debris and the ingrowth of an osteolytic membrane in response to that material. Much work remains to be done, including a reassessment of the 22-mm head and the metal-on-metal bearing.

In the community setting, the challenge is to take what information is available and choose the most appropriate fork in the road using state of the art techniques, while awaiting further information and developments.

Clearly, as outlined in the chapters by Salvati and Harris, there is every reason to be confident in cemented fixation of the stem in older patients. The intermediate and long-term results are outstanding, even in the absence of "modern" cementing techniques, if a cement-friendly stem design is used. The remaining questions, to which we may have the answers before the turn of the century, relate to the performance of the cementless cup between 10 and 20 years after implantation and the long-term results of "improved" cement use. In the meantime, the reader can be assured of continued excellence despite continual change, if the principles and practice of hip replacement in the older patient, outlined in this volume, are

carefully studied. These techniques do not represent the last or the only word on the subject; quite the opposite. But they do afford the surgeon the comfort of consistent and long-lasting success when applied to this group of patients.

What about the younger patient? It should be remembered that loosening of the stem in this group was one of the driving forces behind the development and use, in North America, of cementless stem technology. In retrospect, some of the more spectacular reports on the failure rates in young patients were stem-specific, involving the use of poor cross-sectional designs. Additionally, there is emerging evidence from some centers in the United States and the United Kingdom of very satisfactory intermediate and long-term results in patients younger than 50 years of age using other stems, such as the Charnley design. Furthermore, one of the major culprits in the osteolysis dilemma, namely polyethylene, has remained as part of most cementless systems. Did we take the wrong fork in the road?

It has to be acknowledged that cementless fixation technology is earlier in its development than we had realized, and that it will be some time before cemented and cementless fixation of the stem can be fairly compared. To abandon cementless fixation of the stem, as some did with cemented fixation, without realizing that some of our early failures may relate to poor technique and design, would be folly. It would tempt history to repeat itself and might deprive us of an opportunity for genuine advancement. After all, we did not reject the cementless socket. The early failures were due to poor manufacture and design. These were identified and corrected, and we are now enjoying, at the intermediate term, a better interface performance when compared with historical cemented controls. There have been advancements in stem design and we have new information on stem osseointegration. Thigh pain is not the major problem it was five years ago. There is emerging data which demonstrates that bone ingrowth can envelop 50% of the stem surface, a much greater percentage than was reported previously. And hydroxyapatite may promote a tight host-implant bond that will discourage interface osteolysis. There is an obligation therefore, at least in the academic setting, to continue our study of noncemented fixation. It remains to be seen whether cemented and cementless fixation, each in its third generation of development, will deliver different results at 10, 15, and 20 years in a properly designed study, particularly if we succeed in our search for an alternative to polyethylene.

Where does that leave the younger patient and the community orthopaedic surgeon? Obviously great discretion and great patience are required in the interpretation of available data while we await the outcome of the ideal study. It is not the intention of this author or the Instructional Course series to indicate which fork of the road is most appropriate for this group of patients. But it is our intention to promote continued excellence despite continual change, and the reader is encouraged to pay careful attention to the information in the following chapters, if cementless fixation is chosen, so that the outcome can be optimized. This information is far from comprehensive, and further reading is strongly recommended.

Whatever the decision of the surgeon on the vexing problem of stem fixation, there is clearly a need for improvement in how we measure, interpret, and report results. Hence the chapter by Ebramzadeh, McKellop, Dorey, and Sarmiento is a timely lesson and challenge to us all. When all is said and done, it is only by strict adherence to scientific technique that we can be sure of continued excellence despite continual change.

Noncemented Total Hip Arthroplasty in the Young Patient: Considerations for Optimizing Long-Term Implant Survival

J.D. Bobyn, PhD

Michael Tanzer, MD

C. Emerson Brooks, MD

Introduction

Over the last two decades, there has been a general tendency to extend the indication for total hip arthroplasty (THA) to younger and younger patients. One reason for this change is the overall success achieved with cemented THA in the older patient; another reason is the development of porous-coated prostheses, which may provide long-term "biologic" implant fixation by bone ingrowth. In younger, more active patients, however, there is an increased need for well-engineered and well-manufactured prostheses. The purpose of this paper is to provide details of implant design considerations as related to fixation, strength, stiffness, and wear, with focus on optimizing long-term implant survival in noncemented THA.

Basic Concepts of Noncemented Fixation

The term "biologic" fixation, originally associated with porous-coated implants designed for fixation by tissue ingrowth, is commonly used in a more general sense to refer to all joint replacement implants that are inserted without bone cement, including those with smooth surfaces, lightly textured or grit-blasted surfaces, and surfaces with calcium phosphate coatings such as hydroxyapatite. The term "press fit" is often used to refer to noncemented implants without porous coatings, although it should be used to describe tightness of fit. The extent of press fit is determined by the size of the prepared implant site relative to the size of the implant. The general recommendation for all noncemented implants is to undersize the implant site slightly in order to increase initial implant stability with an interference, or press, fit. The amount of press fit varies with the implant design and implant site. In the femur, the distal press fit may be as little as 0.2 to 0.5 mm and the proximal press fit may range from 0.5 to 1.0 mm, depending on the amount of cancellous bone left after metaphyseal preparation.[1] In the acetabulum, the press fit is typically larger, ranging from 1 to 3 mm.[2-4]

Smooth-Surfaced Implants

Smooth-surfaced implants have demonstrated reasonable longevity since the 1950s, before the advent of bone cement and porous coatings, and are still commonly used in the treatment of hip fractures in low-demand elderly patients (eg, Moore endoprosthesis). Total hip prostheses without porous coatings, often used in younger patients, particularly in Europe,[5] are primarily manufactured of both cobalt-chromium (Co-Cr) and titanium (Ti) alloy. These implants possess either smooth surfaces or micro-roughness on the order of 5 to 20 µm (created by corborundum blasting or plasma spraying) to allow increased mechanical fixation by bone apposition or ongrowth.[6] Acetabular cups typically possess threads, and femoral stems are usually tapered with proximal fins or grooves to enhance primary stability.[5] Patients are usually preselected for good bone stock and ideal femoral anatomy, thus maximizing the potential for implant stability.

In younger, more active patients, the reliability of fixation and the indications for smooth-surfaced implants are of critical importance. Although evidence of direct bone-implant contact has been demonstrated with smooth-surfaced THA prostheses,[7-9] little mechanical bonding in shear and tension can occur. As well, there is a tendency for high load-bearing, smooth-surfaced femoral prostheses to become encapsulated in fibrous tissue, especially proximally.[9,10] This may not relate so much to the surface itself as to overall implant stability, (micro) motion, and interface stress. Subsidence, typically higher in incidence and greater in extent with smooth-surfaced implants, can lead to the onset of pain and higher revision rates for mechanical loosening.[10-12] Threaded acetabular implants are more prone to migration, instability, and fibrous encapsulation than are porous-coated acetabular devices.[13-16]

Porous-Coated Implants

Experimental animal models have indicated that the optimum pore size for extent and rate of bone ingrowth is in the approximate range of 100 to 400 μm.[17-19] Most porous coatings on commercially available implants fall within this range. Human bone ingrowth, however, has been documented with pores as small as 20 to 50 μm[20] and as large as 0.5 to 2 mm.[21] As pores increase in size, the extent and likelihood of bone ingrowth decreases.[19] It has been proposed that larger pores are advantageous for bone ingrowth in the presence of implant micromotion. On a theoretical basis, however, as pores increase in size, more empty space must be filled with bone before micro-mechanical interlock is achieved—this probably increases the time required to accomplish effective biologic fixation. It is clear from several experimental animal models that immediate implant stability is crucial for bone ingrowth.[22-25] Indications are that relative motion between implant and bone in excess of 50 to 100 μm may predispose towards fibrous union.

For increased reliability in obtaining and maximizing bone ingrowth, the porous coating should be placed as close to bone as possible.[26] Although ingrowth can occur with gaps up to about 2 mm, the most consistent and the greatest extent of bone ingrowth in the femur arises from regions of cortical contact.[27-29] It is thus advantageous for the implant to possess a proximal size and shape that allows for proximity to metaphyseal cortical bone. Even implants with anatomic proximal shapes do not result in large areas of actual contact with metaphyseal cortex.[30] For implants with extensive porous coating, diaphyseal cortical contact can be reliably achieved with a straight stem and the use of rigid reamers.[17,31]

With regard to implant material, somewhat conflicting results on tissue response are reported in the dental and orthopaedic literature. In the context of animal studies, Albrektson and associates[32,33] described more favorable osseointegration with threaded implants made of commercially pure (c.p.) Ti than with those made of Ti-6Al-4V alloy or other implant metals. In contrast, Linder and associates[34,35] found a similar histologic response in rabbits to threaded implants of c.p. Ti, Ti-6Al-4V alloy, stainless steel, and Co-Cr alloy. Studies by Hoffman and associates[36] with porous-coated (sintered beads) implants placed in the distal femur of patients prior to total knee arthroplasty have shown greater bone ingrowth for Ti-6Al-4V alloy compared with Co-Cr alloy. In large series of implant retrievals, however, Collier and associates[29,38] and Cook and associates[28,37] have not observed quantitative differences between the two alloys in the amount of bone ingrowth. Any inherent difference that may exist in the bony response to titanium and cobalt-based alloys does not yet appear to be of demonstrable clinical significance. There does not appear to be a clinically significant difference in the amount of bone ingrowth that occurs between sintered beaded porous coatings and diffusion bonded fiber metal porous coatings.[39,40]

Histologic study of implants removed for pain, loosening, malposition, or infection have generally shown only a small fraction of the total porous surface area to be bone ingrown. Studies by Collier and associates[29,38] and Cook and associates[28,37] indicated the bone ingrown area to be always less than 10% and usually less than 5% of the available surface, although studies of well-functioning implants retrieved at autopsy have revealed a sharply contrasting picture. Engh and associates, in a study of eight autopsy retrievals, have demonstrated 57% of the porous surface area of AML (Depuy, Warsaw, Indiana) femoral prostheses to show bone ingrowth, both for proximally and extensively coated stems. While there was a concentration of bone ingrowth near the transition zone between porous and smooth surfaces, the bone ingrowth was distributed over most of the porous coating. Pidhorz and associates,[40] in a study of 11 autopsy-retrieved Harris-Galante-Porous (HGP, Zimmer, Warsaw, Indiana) acetabular implants, found an average of about 30% of the surface area to be bone ingrown. Compared with ingrowth around empty screw holes, there was approximately 50% more bone ingrowth adjacent to holes with screw fixation.

Data from animal studies indicate that implant shear fixation strength from cortical bone ingrowth may conservatively be estimated at about 14 MPa or 2,000 psi, approximately five times greater than that obtained by cancellous bone ingrowth.[17-19] Based on the total areas of cancellous and cortical bone ingrowth documented with autopsy-retrieved femoral prostheses, the total biologic fixation can therefore theoretically measure in the thousands of pounds.[39] At first consideration this would appear to be an exaggerated figure. However, in a canine total hip study by Brooker and associates,[41] in which proximally porous-coated femoral stems (with much less porous-coated area than on human implants) were mechanically distracted axially from the femur after one year of function, the stem removal force averaged about 4,500 Newtons or 1,000 lbs. Several studies have quantified the increased implant stability that results after bone ingrowth.[42-44] The fixation enhancement may not always be sufficient to withstand physiologic forces. Jasty and associates[45] reported that late fixation failure can occur with implants possessing very small discrete regions of porous coating. Nevertheless, porous-coated implants have the potential for an extremely high degree of fixation enhancement by bone ingrowth. In contrast to smooth-surfaced implants, porous-coated implants can also develop substantial tensile fixation by bone ingrowth.[46]

Calcium Phosphate Coatings

Artificially produced calcium phosphates such as hydroxyapatite (HA) and tricalcium phosphate (TCP) have been developed as bioactive or osteoconductive implant coatings to enhance the extent of bone development at the implant surface.[47,48] Titanium and its alloys are normally used for the implant substrate because of enhanced bond strength with calcium phosphate coatings. Hydroxyapatite, characterized by a Ca/P ratio of 1.67, is more stable and resistant to dissolution in vivo than TCP, which possesses a Ca/P ratio of 1.5.[48] Clear evidence from numerous experimental studies has shown that, compared with smooth-surfaced implants, implant fixation strength is increased both in rate and extent with the addition of calcium phosphate to the implant surface.[49,50] The addition of calcium phosphate coatings to porous-coated implants increases both the rate of development of fixation and the surface area over which bone ingrowth occurs where the implant does not initially contact bone.[51,52] For porous coated implants, the ultimate stress (fixation force per unit area) that results from bone ingrowth is similar with and without HA coating.

There are two principal approaches to the use of calcium phosphate coatings. One is to use HA on smooth-surfaced implants and rely on the physicochemical bonding properties to bone for fixation enhancement.[53-56] With this approach, the emphasis is on keeping the calcium phosphate as insoluble as possible by using HA of very high purity and crystallinity. In recognition of an inevitable and finite rate of calcium phosphate solubility, the second approach is to use HA or a mixture of HA and TCP as an additional coating on porous-coated implants and take advantage of the osteoconductive potential to enhance the mechanical interlock afforded by bone ingrowth.[51,52,57,58] In this manner, dissolution or disappearance of the calcium phosphate will have less potential long-term influence on implant fixation than it might have with a smooth-surfaced implant.

Implant Strength Considerations

Mechanical Properties of Coatings

Although they can effectively enhance implant fixation, added coatings are always at risk of debonding from the implant substrate. Debonding is more serious with implants used in young patients, because the anticipated implant life is longer and, thus, the coating-substrate fatigue behavior is apt to be more severely challenged.

The three principal types of metallic porous coatings are fiber mesh, spherical beads, and plasma spray. Coatings with metallurgic bonding to the substrate are generally more adherent than coatings that rely on mechanical bonding. Metallurgic bonding can only be achieved by the use of high temperature furnace treatments that induce atomic diffusion between the coat-

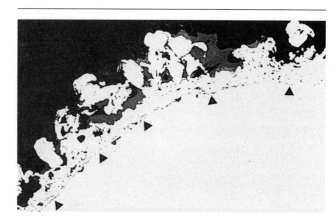

Fig. 1 Backscattered scanning electron micrograph of a plasma-sprayed titanium alloy implant used in a canine bone ingrowth study. A demarcation between the coating and the substrate is clearly evident (arrows), illustrating the absence of a metallurgic bond. Although the surface is rough, with little interconnected porosity, the ingrowth of bone is seen in some areas.

ing and the substrate. In the case of fiber metal attached to Ti-6Al-4V implants, the processing temperature is kept below the beta transus (about 1,000° C), the point that will cause a metallurgic phase change that degrades the mechanical properties of the substrate. In addition, pressure is applied to increase the rate of diffusion between fiber metal wires and the substrate. In the case of spherical beads, a high "sintering" temperature ranging from 70% to 90% of the alloy melting point is used without additional pressure to achieve the necessary bonding (gravity sintering). The manufacturing techniques used with fiber metal and sintered beaded porous coatings result in very open, interconnected porosity, with volume porosity ranging from 35% to 50%.

Plasma spraying involves the line-of-sight deposition of metallic powder onto the implant with a spray nozzle. The powder is mixed with gases in a high-energy arc and becomes molten prior to contact with the implant substrate. The plasma spray technique does not typically create a metallurgic bond with the substrate (Fig. 1), because only the powder, not the substrate, is heated. Plasma spray coatings are typically applied to a roughened implant surface in order to enhance the micro-mechanical bonding that develops after cooling of the coating. In general, plasma spray coatings have a less open or interconnected porosity than do powder-made or fiber metal-made porous coatings (Fig. 1).

The coating-substrate bond strength varies between coating type (eg, sintered beads or plasma spray) and coating material (eg, Ti-6Al-4V or Co-Cr alloy), and between different manufacturers. Manley and associates[59] compared the bond strengths of various beaded coatings and demonstrated that sintered titanium beads are substantially inferior to sintered cobalt-

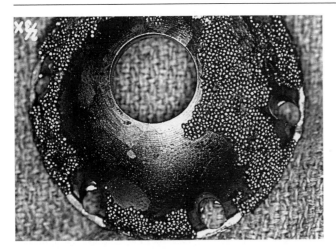
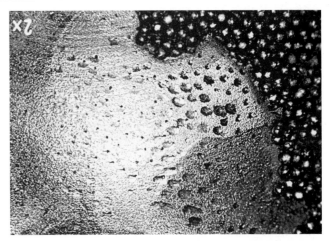

Fig. 2 Titanium alloy acetabular cup with sintered beaded porous surface removed five years after surgery for loosening. **Left,** A large portion of the porous coating had debonded from the substrate and remained embedded in the acetabulum. **Right,** Higher magnification of a debonded region shows imprinting of the individual beads into the substrate, evidence of cyclic loading of the separated interface and a probable source of metallic debris.

chrome beads unless protected by placement in a recess or pocket. Thus, titanium alloy, although advantageous from a manufacturing standpoint because of its machinability, may have a higher risk of bead debonding with certain implant designs (Fig. 2). As a rough guideline, shear strength of coatings should measure at least 30 MPa (4,400 psi) in static tests and 12 MPa (1,800 psi) in fatigue tests.[59] In clinical use, some coatings are more likely than others to dissociation from the substrate.[60-64] In addition to problems with implant fixation that could arise from a failed coating, problems with particle migration into the joint space, implant scratching, third-body wear, and osteolysis can occur (Fig. 3).

HA and TCP coatings applied to smooth implant surfaces are also susceptible to debonding, as has been shown in numerous animal studies and confirmed in analyses of retrieved human prostheses.[65-72] Bloebaum and Dupont[71] and Campbell and associates[72] have demonstrated through retrieval analyses that debonded HA particles can become embedded into the polyethylene liner of the acetabular cup. Small HA particle generation and migration have raised concerns about macrophage-mediated osteolysis and increased polyethylene debris through third-body wear mechanisms. Thinner HA coatings, on the order of 50 μm, are generally more mechanically resistant than thicker coatings.[51] In order to protect calcium phosphate coatings from shear debonding, some implants with smooth surfaces are designed with ridges or grooves that help reduce the tendency for subsidence and the development of interface shear. However, this approach does not entirely avoid the exposure of the coating to shear debonding. As mentioned earlier, an alternate approach is to apply calcium phosphate coatings to porous-coated

implants. The porous coating provides mechanical protection to as much of the calcium phosphate as possible, so as to minimize the risks associated with debonding. Although positive short-term results have been reported for various types of noncemented hip prostheses with calcium phosphate coatings,[53-55] in view of uncertainty about the long-term chemical and mechanical fate of the coatings it would seem prudent to be conservative in their application to young patients.[56]

Mechanical Properties of Implant Substrate

Implant substrate strength is degraded with heat treatments and the application of metallurgically bonded porous coatings.[73-77] Sintered Co-Cr alloy implants typically possess fatigue strength at or below that of cast Co-Cr alloy; this is about three times lower than that of forged Co-Cr alloy. Although implant fractures with porous-coated hip stems are rare, they have been reported most commonly for the smaller-sized, extensively coated AML prostheses (Fig. 4).[78] As stated earlier, fiber metal coatings are applied to Ti alloy implants at a reduced temperature, to avoid a phase change that degrades substrate fatigue strength.[76] Because the substrate of implants with plasma spray coatings is not substantially heated during processing, high fatigue strength is maintained.[77] This gain is at the expense, however, of some loss of coating bond strength.[63] It is usually not difficult to remove surface particles of plasma sprayed coatings with slight abrasive force (Fig. 1). Regardless of heat treatment parameters, metallurgic bonding of porous coatings on titanium alloy creates stress risers that lower fatigue strength by a factor of about two.[76] This resultant increased tendency for crack initiation owing to the notch sensitivity of titanium is primarily of importance to femoral prostheses because of high tensile stresses that develop during loading. Thus, for strength reasons, porous coatings on titanium alloy implants are generally restricted to the proximal stem region, with increased restriction on the lateral aspect, the region of highest tensile stresses.

Implant Design Considerations

Acetabular Implants

First-generation modular acetabular implants were generally not optimized for thickness of the polyethylene liner, conformity and support of the polyethylene liner, and liner locking strength.[63,79-83] Many problems with cold flow, motion, wear, dissociation, and fracture of the liner have recently been reported (Fig. 5).[63,84-92] There is also evidence of metallic debris generation from screw fretting against the metal shell and polyethylene debris migration through the screw holes.[40,91]

More recent acetabular implant designs have an improved locking mechanism and a more congruent fit of the liner within the metal shell. In addition, the polyethylene thickness has been increased, because experimental data show that a minimum of 6 mm is required to lower internal stresses and improve wear characteristics.[93,94] Because of concern about fretting of screws against the metal shell and particulate debris

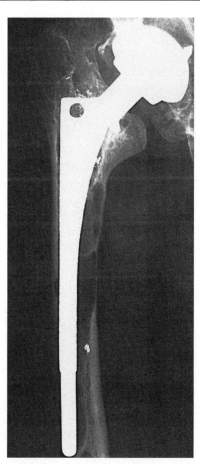

Fig. 3   This anteroposterior radiograph made five years after surgery shows an undersized fully porous-coated AML prosthesis that had progressively loosened and moved into varus. There are several clusters of porous coating that are well separated from the stem. There is a large region of osteolysis around the stem. At revision, the stem was removed easily and showed several areas of debonded porous coating. The acetabular cup liner was clearly worn and was embedded with numerous beads from the porous coating. Not evident on the radiograph is an extensive radiolucent zone behind the acetabular cup. This case illustrates the need for secure implant fixation with a well-bonded porous coating to avoid the possibility of third-body cup wear and the development of polyethylene granulomas.

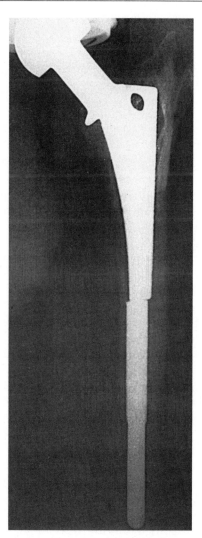

Fig. 4   This anteroposterior radiograph taken seven years after surgery shows a fractured, fully porous-coated 10.5 mm AML prosthesis. The implant had become well fixed distally and failed in cantilever loading. Debonded beads from the porous coating were also evident near the implant shoulder. This illustrates the need for implants with high fatigue properties, lacking in small diameter fully porous-coated stems subjected to high temperature heat treatments.

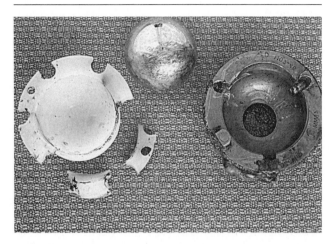

Fig. 5 Components of a 46-mm metal-backed acetabular cup that failed within two years of surgery. The polyethylene liner was less than 2 mm thick at the cup rim, and pressure from the femoral head resulted in early fracture. After liner fracture the Co-Cr femoral head came into contact with the rim of the titanium alloy metal shell, causing pronounced wear and metallosis of the joint. This failure illustrates the need for adequate polyethylene thickness, conformity, and locking mechanism, especially in the smaller cup sizes typically used in younger patients who have congenital hip dysplasia or juvenile rheumatoid arthritis.

generation and migration, there is increased emphasis on using metal shells with few or no screw holes. To minimize the potential for polyethylene debris generation from motion of the liner against the metal shell, some shells are available with a very smooth or polished concave surface.

In general, most porous-coated hemispheric acetabular cup designs have performed very well from the standpoint of fixation and stability in five- to ten-year follow-up studies.[2,15] In laboratory studies, Adler and associates[3] demonstrated the importance of proper sizing and depth of the acetabular cavity for initial cup stability. Lachiewicz and associates[95] evaluated the relative merits of screws, pegs, and spikes on acetabular stability and found advantages to screw fixation, although all three adjuvant fixation features enhanced stability compared with press fit fixation alone.[3] Concerns remain as to the longevity of noncemented acetabular cup fixation in the presence of accumulated wear debris and debris-induced osteolysis.[92] There appears to be an ever-decreasing indication for the use of cement in the acetabulum, especially in the case of younger patients, in whom preservation of bone stock is a particularly high priority.

Femoral Implants

The key to reproducibly successful noncemented femoral implant fixation—tight initial fixation—requires good metaphyseal and diaphyseal fit through careful surgery and the use of well-designed instrumentation.

In terms of primary implant stability, which is achieved through proper shape and fit, several studies have indicated that tight proximal and distal fit contribute to overall stability.[1,96,97] Markedly increased torsional stability is gained through frictional interference if the implant is either extensively porous-coated or fluted and is inserted with a slight press fit.

There has been a recent increase in femoral implants with additional sites of modularity beyond the ubiquitous head/neck taper. These have been specifically developed for noncemented fixation, and the modular components provide additional ability to match individual anatomy and increase stability through proximal and distal "fit and fill."[79] However, there is no evidence that modular femoral stems provide better clinical results than conventional one-piece implants. Moreover, concerns have been raised about particulate material generated through corrosion and fretting mechanisms at modular junctions.[63,79,98-100] With head/neck taper junctions, evidence suggests that tapers with tight tolerances work well in the long-term with both similar and mixed-metal combinations.[101] With other modular junctions, mechanical tests have shown that particulate debris is inevitably generated under physiologic loads (Fig. 6).[79] Whether the debris is sufficient to cause biologic reactions (eg, macrophage-mediated osteolysis) or to increase third-body wear of acetabular polyethylene has not been ascertained.[102] In view of the current uncertainties about long-term clinical results and mechanical and biologic issues related to multiple modular junctions, one-piece femoral implants represent a more conservative approach to THA in younger patients.

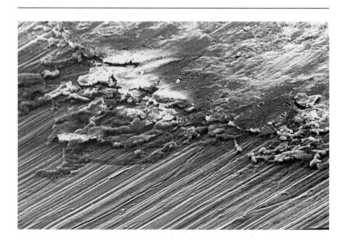

Fig. 6 Scanning electron micrograph of a titanium alloy modular hip junction subjected to 10 million loading cycles at three times body weight. Adjacent to original machining marks, there is clear evidence of surface burnishing or fretting and the creation of particulate material. (Reproduced with permission from Bobyn JD, Tanzer M, Krygier JJ, et al: Concerns with modularity in total hip arthroplasty. *Clin Orthop* 1993, in press.)

Several studies have examined the initial stability of noncemented femoral prostheses under both axial and torsional loading.[42,103-105] It is clear that micromotion measurements for noncemented stems are generally higher than for cemented stems. Also, torsional testing is a sensitive indicator of resistance to out-of-plane forces and is more revealing than axial testing in detecting differences in stability between stem designs. In a comparison of straight and anatomic stem designs, Callaghan and associates[103] showed stability characteristics to be similar for all test conditions, except that at high torsional loads the anatomic stem displayed less micromotion. It was not clear whether this difference was due to the slight bow of the anatomic stem or the increased metaphyseal filling afforded by the anatomic design. In a comparison of the initial stability of several noncemented stem designs, Schneider and associates[104] found the least torsional stability with the curved stem. In Europe and North America, straight femoral stems are strongly preferred over curved stems, perhaps because, for a straight stem, the femoral canal can be more easily and accurately machined with simple instrumentation. Depending on the degree of curvature, it is very difficult to fully insert a curved stem into the femoral canal without some oversizing of the canal distally. Thus, the fixation advantage provided by tight distal fit is more difficult to achieve with a curved stem. Also, curved distal stems do not easily accommodate the addition of flutes for enhanced torsional stability by a press fit, and extensively porous-coated and bone-ingrown curved stems present extreme challenges to removal if an implant later requires revision.

There is no convincing evidence that an implant collar or the absence of one has a positive outcome on clinical results or proximal bone remodeling. In addition to enhancing initial torsional and axial implant stability,[106] a collar also provides an obvious mechanical end point to stem insertion, transfers axial load to the proximal femur, and serves to impede implant subsidence in the presence of gross instability. However, without proper preparation of the implant site and proper use of instrumentation such as a calcar reamer, the collar can impede impaction of the stem into the tightest position and, thus, can reduce stability and proximal femoral hoop stress loading. In the presence of bone ingrowth, any benefits of the collar against subsidence are probably attenuated because of the shear resistance afforded by micromechanical interlock.

In terms of secondary implant stability, which can develop through biologic fixation or tissue ingrowth, an important design feature is the extent of porous coating of the implant. Based on data with the AML prosthesis in terms of parameters such as overall clinical scores, incidence of radiographic loosening, and revision rate for mechanical loosening, stems with extensive porous coating (defined as coating on the majority of the stem length so that the coating extends into the isthmus) are generally superior to first-generation designs, in which coating was confined to the proximal portion of the implant at the interface with the metaphysis.[17,60,107-110] Although the incidences of thigh pain and mechanical loosening are higher with the proximally coated AML prosthesis than with the extensively coated AML, this may result in part from the implant design, rather than the amount of porous coating. Proximally, the parallel-sided shape does not provide metaphyseal filling, and distally, the nonfluted smooth-surfaced stem does not provide macrointerlock. Apart from the AML, second-generation noncemented stem designs with proximal porous coating have been improved with regard to amount of porous-coated area and overall implant stability (proximal and distal); thus, some of the problems of thigh pain and early loosening experienced with first generation designs[110] will probably diminish. Considerations of bone remodeling and stem removal remain strong arguments in favor of stems with proximal porous coating.

Stem Stiffness

Stem stiffness is probably more important than a collar in its effect on proximal bone remodeling. Stem stiffness strongly influences bone remodeling, larger and stiffer stems causing increased peri-implant bone resorption.[111-116] Bending and torsional stiffness increase with the fourth power of the stem diameter, which means that an incremental change in stem size has a profound effect on stiffness. Both stem and femur stiffness are key parameters in the relationship between stiffness and bone remodeling. The same implant put into two femora of widely varying stiffnesses will cause different bone remodeling responses. Conversely, the same femur fitted with two implants of different stiffness would also be expected to remodel differently. Recent data on femur stiffness have provided the ability to identify acceptable and unacceptable stem/femur stiffness relationships.[113,117] For instance, the original stainless steel Charnley cemented stem and the 10.5 mm diameter Co-Cr AML stem are both less stiff in bending than the average femur in which they were used. After extensive (more than ten years) long-term follow-up with both implants, neither has been associated with pronounced stress-related bone resorption. In contrast, AML stems (Co-Cr) larger than 13.5 mm in diameter are increasingly stiffer than the human femur and cause a relatively high incidence of pronounced peri-implant bone resorption.[113] Clinical data indicate that with extensively coated stems peri-implant bone resorption occurs over more of the implant length.[111]

The largest stiffness difference between stem and femur is proximal.[117] As the stem flares the stiffness parameters increase exponentially and supersede the femur stiffness by factors of five to twenty or more, depending on the stem size. This disparity may help explain why peri-implant resorption tends to occur faster and is more extensive in the metaphysis. This has implications with regard to the recent generation of modular femoral prostheses designed for increased "fit and fill" of the femur. Large proximal implant segments used to fill the metaphysis will result in large proximal stiffness mismatches[118] and may increase the extent of proximal femoral stress shielding and subsequent bone resorption.

Mechanical compatibility between the femoral stem and the femur can be markedly improved with the use of Ti alloy, because it has a lower (50%) elastic modulus compared with Co-Cr alloy. Additional distal stem flexibility can be achieved through the use of simple design features such as slots or flutes. Reduction of proximal stem stiffness would probably be beneficial from a bone remodeling standpoint but is difficult to accomplish from an engineering standpoint. Composite implant technology offers the most realistic approach for achieving the large proximal stiffness reductions required for mechanical compatibility with the femur. With increased flexibility, however, comes the possibility of increased proximal micromotion.[119] Several years of development and clinical trials will be required before composite hip stems could be considered for general use in young patients.

The Problem of Wear

Although the success and progressive evolution of total hip arthroplasty were made possible by Sir John Charnley's introduction of ultrahigh molecular weight polyethylene, the last five years have witnessed a large increase in cases of rapid and excessive polyethylene wear in the hip. Recently, numerous cases of osteolytic lesions adjacent to acetabular and femoral implants have been reported in association with both cemented and noncemented prostheses.[120-122] These are believed to be caused primarily by polyethylene debris accumulation leading to macrophage activity and the release of osteoclast-activating factors.[123-129] A normally wearing hip joint will annually release approximately 50 to 200 mg of polyethylene debris. Based on the micron and submicron size range of polyethylene particles found in joint tissues, estimates of debris production range in the millions to billions of particles per year.[124-127]

Factors Influencing Polyethylene Wear on the Acetabular Side

A number of factors may contribute to increased wear and wear-related problems in the hip. The influence of various design features of modular acetabular implants on polyethylene wear has already been discussed.[79,90,129] Polyethylene wear is probably also affected by the quality of the polyethylene used.[130-132] Wide variations are known to exist between batches of polyethylene and between different polyethylene suppliers. Collier and associates[63,132] have reported evidence of voids and foci of nonconsolidated polyethylene powder in a high proportion of retrieved prostheses. Li and Howard[133] have stressed the importance of chemical stability and resistance to oxidation in order to increase mechanical resistance to such failure mechanisms as surface cracking and wear. It is important to use ultrahigh molecular weight polyethylene (UHMW-PE) with high ratings in key mechanical and physical properties (Table 1). A high level of quality control is required over parameters such as starting powder composition, extrusion processing (extruded rod generally results in better consolidation and improved properties compared with compression-molded UHMWPE sheets), postextrusion annealing (to increase crystallinity and dimensional stability), ultrasound inspection for voids and inclusions, oxidation resistance, and mechanical properties. Polyethylene that substantially exceeds minimum ASTM standards is available from several implant manufacturers.[134,135]

Factors Influencing Polyethylene Wear on the Femoral Side

Apart from material and surface finish, there are factors related to head size that influence polyethylene wear. In general, a smaller head size results in increased pressure and a higher rate of linear wear. Larger heads theoretically reduce pressure and lower the rate of linear wear. Because of surface area considerations, the higher linear rate with smaller heads results in less volumetric wear than with larger heads. Larger heads also result in higher frictional torque and this may be a significant factor in the generation of polyethylene wear debris.[136] In a large clinical follow-up of patients with 22-mm, 28-mm, and 32-mm head sizes, Livermore and associates[137] recently reported that cups with 28-mm heads were optimum for both linear and

Table 1
Properties of UHMWPE

	ASTM Standard	Commercially Available PE[134]	Commercially Available PE[135]
Molecular Weight	3×10^6	5×10^6	—
Ultimate Tensile Strength	4000 PSI	6700 PSI	6000 PSI
Tensile Yield	2800 PSI	3300 PSI	4100 PSI
Izoi Impact	20 FT-LB	No Break	No Break
Hardness	60 Shore D	69 Shore D	65 Shore D
Elongation to Failure	200%	350%	330%

volumetric wear. Kabo and associates[138] reported increasing volumetric wear of polyethylene with increasing head size. Part of the wear problem with modular acetabular implants has been attributed to the use of 32-mm heads in small cup sizes, which resulted in very thin polyethylene (Fig. 5). Increased awareness of this problem has lead to increased use of smaller head sizes, although 32-mm heads are still appropriate with larger cups having thick polyethylene (6 mm or more). Bipolar prostheses generate significantly higher amounts of polyethylene wear debris than THA prostheses, probably because of increased wear from neck impingement and the fact that there are two interfaces at which metal-polyethylene motion can occur.[139] Debris may be a serious problem in view of the wide acceptance of bipolar prostheses for treating subcapital hip fractures and avascular necrosis in the young patient.

Polyethylene wear is generally increased with the use of femoral heads made of titanium alloy because of its lower hardness and abrasion resistance. Problems with osteolysis caused by excessive head and cup wear have been reported with titanium bearing surfaces.[140-143] Attempts have been made to improve wear characteristics of titanium alloy femoral heads by surface hardening through implantation of nitrogen or oxygen into the surface or through chemical deposition of a titanium nitride surface. However, because surface affected zones are very shallow (only a fraction of a micron for ion implantation), can be damaged by three-body wear, and are probably eventually worn away, the preferred metal for femoral head bearings remains cobalt-chrome alloy because of its hardness and proven wear characteristics.

There are theoretical advantages to using ceramic heads of either alumina or zirconia for reduced polyethylene wear.[144-147] Compared with metal heads, the greater hardness of ceramics helps maintain surface finish and sphericity and increases resistance to scratching from third-body wear particles. Ceramics also possess lower coefficients of friction and greater wettability, factors that reduce adhesive wear. Finally, because of superb chemical stability, ceramics are immune to oxidative wear, the process by which oxides are continually worn away and reformed on metallic heads, which leads to progressive degradation of surface finish and increased potential for abrasive polyethylene wear. Clinical studies of polyethylene wear with ceramic heads have also reported lower wear rates than with metal heads, although the results are not as definitive as in the laboratory in view of uncontrolled variables and less than rigorous statistical analysis of the data.[148-151]

Critical factors in any studies of wear, laboratory or clinical, are surface finish and sphericity of the femoral head. A ceramic head with a rougher surface than a cobalt-chrome head will likely not perform as well in wear tests (and vice versa). Unfortunately, in most of the wear studies reported to date, information on starting surface finish is not provided, which makes it difficult to draw definitive conclusions about the superiority of one material or surface preparation over another. As the surface finish of any femoral head deteriorates, such as might be precipitated by entrapped third-body wear particles, the abrasive wear of polyethylene increases.

Finally, it should also be mentioned that there is renewed interest in metal-metal bearing combinations in total hip arthroplasty. Observations since the introduction of numerous metal-metal articulations in the 1960s and 1970s, most notably the McKee-Farrar, Sivash, and Mueller prostheses, indicate that many are still surviving, and retrieval analyses have shown wear rates one to two orders of magnitude lower than occurs with metal-polyethylene articulations.[152,153] Some of the runaway wear failures with metal-metal joints were caused by high friction and seizing secondary to deformation of thin acetabular components or by third-body wear from entrapped polymethylmethacrylate fragments.[154] With improvements in materials and fabrication techniques, metal-metal bearings may offer a reliable solution to problems with polyethylene wear. A current approach is to use non-lapped, non-paired head-cup bearing combinations with a head diameter that is about 100 microns smaller than the cup (Fig. 7).[152,155]

Migration of Polyethylene Debris

Schmalzried and associates[156] described the concept of the effective joint space and the tendency for polyethylene wear debris to migrate to remote bone-

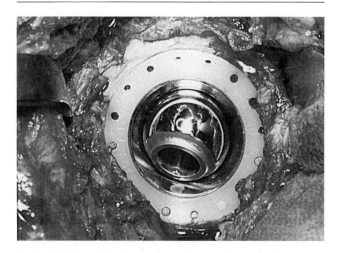

Fig. 7 Intraoperative photograph of a 28-mm diameter, metal-metal articulation made of Co-Cr alloy. The head is very slightly smaller than the cup to avoid seizing and to allow for entry and clearance of lubricating fluid.

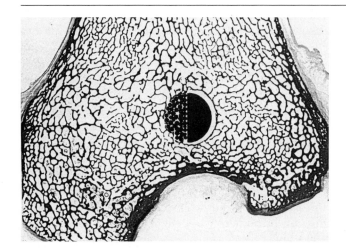 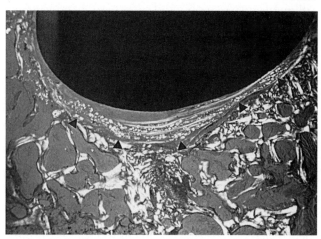

Fig. 8 Histologic sections from a canine study in which half porous-half smooth cylindrical implants in the distal femur were exposed to polyethylene particles. **Left**, Transverse section through an implant exposed to a total of 200 mg of polyethylene. There is a sharp distinction between the tissue response to the porous and smooth implant halves, a thick fibrous membrane existing only adjacent to the smooth surface. **Right**, Oblique section through an implant exposed to a total of 100 mg of polyethylene. Only the smooth implant half was surrounded by striated fibrous tissue containing clumps of polyethylene particles, highlighted under polarized light (arrows). This study supports the concept that smooth implant surfaces are more susceptible to polyethylene debris migration.

implant interfaces as a result of intra-articular joint pressure and fluid motion. With cemented THA, the propensity for polyethylene migration and erosion of the interface through osteolysis is described as being much higher on the acetabular side than on the femoral side.[157-159] Several studies have referred to the possible existence of a mechanical barrier or seal against polyethylene debris migration and that such a seal might be created through the interdigitation of cement with bone or the growth of tissue into a porous implant surface.[43,120,122]

Experimentally, Howie and associates[160] demonstrated in a rat knee model that polyethylene particles could migrate along a bone-smooth implant interface and result in peri-implant fibrosis. A subsequent study by Bobyn and associates[161] studied whether porous implant surfaces could be more resistant to polyethylene migration because of the seal that might develop through tissue ingrowth. Cylindrical implants split along the longitudinal axis into porous and smooth halves were placed into the distal end of canine femora. After a healing period the knee joints were chronically injected with simulated polyethylene wear debris (particle size = 2 to 20 µm). The total polyethylene exposure ranged from 50 to 200 mg, approximately the amount of debris produced on an annual basis in a normally wearing hip joint. The study showed that while the porous halves of the implants consistently became ingrown with bone, the majority of the smooth implant halves became surrounded by a sharply delineated fibrous membrane in association with aggregates of polyethylene particles (Fig. 8). This finding supports

the hypothesis that, compared with porous surfaces, smooth implant surfaces are more susceptible to polyethylene debris ingress and debris-mediated fibrosis. Clinical evidence also supports this hypothesis. In retrieval analyses of the original Harris-Galante-Porous (HGP, Zimmer, Warsaw, Indiana) hip stem with noncircumferential fiber metal pads, Urban and associates[162] recently showed that fibrous tissue tends to develop adjacent to the smooth regions of the implant, and that polyethylene debris accumulates within the fibrous tissue. In radiographic analyses of porous-coated femoral components used in total knee arthroplasty, Cadambi and associates[163] have shown polyethylene granulomas to develop preferentially adjacent to the smooth regions of the anterior and posterior flanges. The inference from these observations is that circumferential porous coating on noncemented femoral components can help avoid distal debris migration. On the acetabular side, preliminary radiographic evidence suggests that the tighter the press fit of the porous-coated metal shell, the lower the incidence of the peri-implant radiolucencies that develop in response to accumulated polyethylene debris.[2]

Conclusions

The ability of THA to eliminate pain and improve the quality of life of patients with hip disease is unquestionably outstanding. Successful clinical results must be tempered, however, by engineering and biological concerns, especially for younger patients who are expected to live for several decades.

In order to prevent morbidity and repetitive surgery, patient selection, prosthetic design, and surgical technique must be optimized. Only young patients with debilitating hip disease who are not candidates for an osteotomy or an arthrodesis should be considered for THA. Noncemented THA technique requires close attention to detail and careful use of instrumentation to achieve optimal implant fit and stability.[164] The key issues with implant design are reliability and reproducibility of fixation with safe, straightforward, time-proven design features. Strict emphasis should be placed on minimizing the possibility of implant mechanical failure and bone resorption caused by stress shielding. Minimizing particulate debris from wear and corrosion mechanisms and minimizing the access of debris to bone-implant interfaces is crucial to maximizing long-term implant fixation and may also be important to the patient's overall health, in view of systemic distribution of wear and corrosion products after THA and concerns about toxicity and carcinogenicity.[165]

Acknowledgments

The authors are grateful for financial assistance from the Medical Research Council of Canada and for technical assistance from Dr. R. Aribindi, Mr. A. Dujovne, and Mr. J. Krygier.

References

1. Sugiyama H, Whiteside LA, Engh CA: Torsional fixation of the femoral component in total hip replacement: The effect of surgical technique. *Trans Orthop Res Soc* 1990;15:258.
2. Hill GE: HGP press-fit at five years. *Trans 22nd Annual Hip Course* (Harris, WH, dir) Boston, MA, 1992.
3. Adler E, Stuchin SA, Kummer FJ: Stability of press-fit acetabular cups. *J Arthroplasty* 1992;7:295-301.
4. Curtis MJ, Jinnah RH, Wilson VD, et al: The initial stability of uncemented acetabular components. *J Bone Joint Surg* 1992;74B:372-376.
5. Morscher E (ed): *The Cementless Fixation of Hip Endoprostheses.* Berlin, Springer-Verlag, 1984.
6. Carlsson L, Rostlund T, Albrektsson B, et al: Removal torques for polished and rough titanium implants. *Int J Oral Maxillofac Implants* 1988;3:21-24.
7. Lintner F, Zweymuller K, Brand G: Tissue reactions to titanium endoprostheses. Autopsy studies in four cases. *J Arthroplasty* 1986;1:183-195.
8. McCutchen JW, Collier JP, Mayor MB: Osseointegration of titanium implants in total hip arthroplasty. *Clin Orthop* 1990;261:114-125.
9. Willert HG: Morphology of implant-bone interface in cemented and non-cemented endoprostheses, in Older J (ed): *Implant Bone Interface.* London, Springer-Verlag, 1990, pp 27-34.
10. Duparc J, Massin P: Results of 203 total hip replacements using a smooth, cementless femoral component. *J Bone Joint Surg* 1992;74B:251-256.
11. Simesen K: Total hip replacement ad modum Ring. *Acta Orthop Scand* 1980;51:929-935.
12. Snorrason F, Karrholm J, Lowenhielm G, et al: Poor fixation of the Mittelmeier hip prosthesis. A clinical, radiographic, and scintimetric evaluation. *Acta Orthop Scand* 1989;60:81-85.
13. Snorrason F, Karrholm J: Primary migration of fully-threaded acetabular prostheses: A roentgenstereophotogrammetric analysis. *J Bone Joint Surg* 1990;72B:647-652.
14. Huiskes R, Peeters H, Slooff TJ: Biomechanical analysis of load-transfer in acetabular-cup arthroplasty with cementless threaded sockets. *Trans Orthop Res Soc* 1987;12:507.
15. Engh CA, Griffin WL, Marx CL: Cementless acetabular components. *J Bone Joint Surg* 1990;72B:53-59.
16. More RC, Amstutz HC, Kabo JM, et al: Acetabular reconstruction with a threaded prosthesis for failed total hip arthroplasty. *Clin Orthop* 1992;282:114-122.
17. Engh CA, Bobyn JD: *Biological Fixation in Total Hip Arthroplasty.* Thorofare, NJ, Slack Inc, 1985.
18. Bobyn JD, Miller JE: Features of biologically fixed devices, in Morrey BF (ed): *Joint Replacement Arthroplasty.* New York, NY, Churchill Livingstone, 1991, chap 7, pp 61-80.
19. Bobyn JD, Pilliar RM, Cameron HU, et al: The optimum pore size for the fixation of porous-surfaced metal implants by the ingrowth of bone. *Clin Orthop* 1980;150:263-270.
20. Bobyn JD, Engh CA, Glassman AH: Histologic analysis of a retrieved microporous-coated femoral prosthesis: A seven-year case report. *Clin Orthop* 1987;224:303-310.
21. Barbos MP: Bone ingrowth into madreporic prostheses. *J Bone Joint Surg* 1988;70B:85-88.
22. Cameron HU, Pilliar RM, MacNab I: The effect of movement on the bonding of porous metal to bone. *J Biomed Mater Res* 1973;7:301-311.
23. Pilliar RM: Quantitative evaluation of the effect of movement at a porous coated implant-bone interface, in Davies JE (ed): *The Bone-Biomaterial Interface.* Toronto, University of Toronto Press, 1991, pp 380-387.
24. Pilliar RM, Lee JM, Maniatopoulos C: Observations on the effect of movement on bone ingrowth into porous-surfaced implants. *Clin Orthop* 1986;208:108-113.
25. Burke DW, Bragdon CR, Lowenstein JD: Mechanical aspects of the bone-porous surface interface under known amounts of implant motion: An in vivo canine study. *Trans Orthop Res Soc* 1993;18:470.
26. Bobyn JD, Pilliar RM, Cameron HU, et al: Osteogenic phenomena across endosteal bone-implant spaces with porous surfaced intramedullary implants. *Acta Orthop Scand* 1981;52:145-153.
27. Bobyn JD, Engh CA: Human histology of the bone-porous metal implant interface. *Orthopaedics* 1984;7:1410-1421.
28. Cook SD, Barrack RL, Thomas KA, et al: Quantitative analysis of tissue growth into human porous total hip components. *J Arthroplasty* 1988;3:249-262.
29. Collier JP, Bauer TW, Bloebaum RD, et al: Results of implant retrieval from postmortem specimens in patients with well-functioning, long-term total hip replacement. *Clin Orthop* 1992;274:97-112.
30. Robertson DD, Walker PS, Hirano SK, et al: Improving the fit of press-fit hip stems. *Clin Orthop* 1988;228:134-140.
31. Otani T, White SE, Whiteside LA: Biomechanical evaluation of reaming technique of the femoral diaphysis in cementless total hip arthroplasty. Presented at the 60th Annual Meeting of American Academy of Orthopaedic Surgeons, San Francisco, CA, 1993, p 407. (Scientific Exhibit)

32. Albrektsson T, Johansson C: Quantified bone tissue reactions to various metallic materials with reference to the so-called osseointegration concept, in Davies JE (ed): *The Bone-Biomaterial Interface.* Toronto, University of Toronto Press, 1991, pp 357-363.

33. Albrektsson T, Branemark PI, Hansson HA, et al: Osseointegrated titanium implants: Requirements for ensuring a long-lasting, direct bone-to-implant anchorage in man. *Acta Orthop Scand* 1981;52:155-170.

34. Linder L, Obrant K, Boivin G: Osseointegration of metallic implants. II. Transmission electron microscopy in the rabbit. *Acta Orthop Scand* 1989;60:135-139.

35. Linder L: Osseo-integration of metallic implants in animals and humans, in Older J (ed): *Implant Bone Interface.* London, Springer Verlag, 1990, pp 43-49.

36. Hofmann AA, Bachus KN, Bloebaum RD: In vivo implantation of identically structured and sized titanium and cobalt chrome alloy porous coated cylinders implanted into human cancellous bone. *Trans Orthop Res Soc* 1990;15:204.

37. Cook SD, Barrack RL, Thomas KA, et al: Tissue growth into porous primary and revision femoral stems. *J Arthroplasty* 1991;6(Suppl):S37-46.

38. Collier JP, Mayor MB, Chae JC, et al: Macroscopic and microscopic evidence of prosthetic fixation with porous-coated materials. *Clin Orthop* 1988;235:173-180.

39. Engh CA, Hooten JP, Zettl-Schaffer KF, et al: Evaluation of bone ingrowth with proximally and extensively porous coated AML prostheses retrieved at autopsy. *J Bone Joint Surg.* Submitted for publication.

40. Pidhorz LE, Urban RM, Jacobs JJ, et al: A quantitative study of bone and soft tissues in cementless porous-coated acetabular components retrieved at autopsy. *J Arthroplasty* 1993;8:213-225.

41. Brooker AF, Brown PR, Wenz JF, et al: Femoral ingrowth surfaces: Evaluation by whole stem pull-out testing. *J Arthroplasty* 1993, in press.

42. Engh CA, O'Connor D, Jasty M, et al: Quantification of implant micromotion, strain shielding, and bone resorption with porous-coated anatomic medullary locking femoral prostheses. *Clin Orthop* 1992;285:13-29.

43. Whiteside LA, White SE, Engh CA, et al: Mechanical evaluation of cadaver retrieval specimens of cementless bone-ingrown total hip arthroplasty femoral components. *J Arthroplasty* 1993;8:147-155.

44. Jasty M, Krushell R, Zalenski E, et al: The contribution of the nonporous distal stem to the stability of proximally porous-coated canine femoral components. *J Arthroplasty* 1993;8:33-41.

45. Jasty M, Bragdon CR, Maloney WJ, et al: Ingrowth of bone in failed fixation of porous-coated femoral components. *J Bone Joint Surg* 1991;73A:1331-1337.

46. Bobyn JD, Pilliar RM, Cameron HU, et al: The effect of porous surface configuration on the tensile strength of fixation of implants by bone ingrowth. *Clin Orthop* 1980;149:291-298.

47. Geesink RG, de Groot K, Klein CP: Chemical implant fixation using hydroxyl-apatite coatings: The development of a human total hip prosthesis for chemical fixation to bone using hydroxyl-apatite coatings on titanium substrates. *Clin Orthop* 1987;225:147-170.

48. de Groot K: Ceramics based on calcium phosphates, in Vincenzini P (ed): *Ceramics in Surgery.* Amsterdam, Elsevier Science Publishers, 1983, p 79-90.

49. de Groot K, Geesink R, Klein CP, et al: Plasma sprayed coatings of hydroxylapatite. *J Biomed Mater Res* 1987;21:1375-1381.

50. Cook SD, Thomas KA, Kay JF, et al: Hydroxyapatite-coated porous titanium for use as an orthopedic biologic attachment system. *Clin Orthop* 1988;230:303-312.

51. Soballe K, Hansen ES, Brockstedt-Rasmussen H, et al: Hydroxyapatite coating enhances fixation of porous coated implants: A comparison in dogs between press fit and non-interference fit. *Acta Orthop Scand* 1990;61:299-306.

52. Bloebaum RD, Bachus KN, Rubman MH, et al: Postmortem comparative analysis of titanium and hydroxyapatite porous-coated femoral implants retrieved from the same patient: A case study. *J Arthroplasty* 1993;8:203-211.

53. Geesink RG: Hydroxyapatite-coated total hip prostheses: Two-year clinical and roentgenographic results of 100 cases. *Clin Orthop* 1990;261:39-58.

54. D'Antonio JA, Capello WN, Jaffe WL: Hydroxylapatite-coated hip implants: Multicenter three-year clinical and roentgenographic results. *Clin Orthop* 1992;285:102-115.

55. Furlong RJ, Osborn JF: Fixation of hip prostheses by hydroxyapatite ceramic coatings. *J Bone Joint Surg* 1991;73B:741-745.

56. Morscher EW: Hydroxyapatite coating of prostheses. *J Bone Joint Surg* 1991;73B:705-706.

57. Bloebaum RD, Merrell M, Gustke K, et al: Retrieval analysis of a hydroxyapatite-coated hip prosthesis. *Clin Orthop* 1991;267:97-102.

58. Bauer TW, Stulberg BN, Ming J, et al: Uncemented acetabular components. Histologic analysis of retrieved hydroxyapatite-coated and porous implants. *J Arthroplasty* 1993;8:167-177.

59. Manley MT, Kotzar G, Stern LS, et al: Effects of repetitive loading on the integrity of porous coatings. *Clin Orthop* 1987;217:293-302.

60. Callaghan JJ, Dysart SH, Savory CG: The uncemented porous-coated anatomic total hip prosthesis: Two-year results of a prospective consecutive series. *J Bone Joint Surg* 1988;70A:337-346.

61. Davey JR, Harris WH: Loosening of cobalt chrome beads from a porous-coated acetabular component: A report of ten cases. *Clin Orthop* 1988;231:97-102.

62. Buchert PK, Vaughn BK, Mallory TH, et al: Excessive metal release due to loosening and fretting of sintered particles on porous-coated hip prostheses: Report of two cases. *J Bone Joint Surg* 1986;68A:606-609.

63. Collier JP, Mayor MB, Jensen RE, et al: Mechanisms of failure of modular prostheses. *Clin Orthop* 1992;285:129-139.

64. Rosenqvist R, Bylander B, Knutson K, et al: Loosening of the porous coating of bicompartmental prostheses in patients with rheumatoid arthritis. *J Bone Joint Surg* 1986;68A:538-542.

65. Kummer FJ, Jaffe WL: Fatigue testing of hydroxyapatite coatings: Effect of substrate material, surface preparation, and test solution. *Trans of 4th World Biomat Cong,* 1992, p 504.

66. Thomas KA, Kay JF, Cook SD, et al: The effect of surface macrotexture and hydroxylapatite coating on the mechanical strengths and histologic profiles of titanium implant materials. *J Biomed Mater Res* 1987;21:1395-1414.

67. Poser RD, Magee FP, Kay JF, et al: Biomechanical and histologic assessment of HA enhanced long-term fixation in a unique loaded canine implant. *Trans World Biomat Cong,* 1992, p 252.

68. Poser RD, May TM, Kay JF, et al: Long term performance and load sharing effects of HA coated macrotextured titanium. *Trans World Biomat Cong,* 1992, p 500.

69. May TC, Kay JF: Implant surface geometry designed for HA coating survival. *Trans World Biomat Cong,* 1992, p 506.

70. Malcolm A: Histologic analysis of hydroxyapatite coated implants, in Morrey BF (ed): *Biological, Material, and Mechanical Considerations of Joint Replacement*. New York, NY, Raven Press, 1993.

71. Bloebaum RD, Dupont JA: Osteolysis from a press-fit hydroxyapatite-coated implant: A case study. *J Arthroplasty* 1993;8:195-202.

72. Campbell P, McKellop H, Park SH, et al: Evidence of abrasive wear by particles from a hydroxyapatite coated hip prosthesis. *Trans Orthop Res Soc* 1993;18:224.

73. Pilliar RM: Powder metal-made orthopedic implants with porous surface for fixation by tissue ingrowth. *Clin Orthop* 1983;176:42-51.

74. Pilliar RM: Porous-surfaced metallic implants for orthopedic applications. *J Biomed Mater Res* 1987;21(A1 Suppl):1-33.

75. Georgette FS, Davidson JA: The effect of HIPing on the fatigue and tensile strength of a cast, porous-coated Co-Cr-Mo alloy. *J Biomed Mater Res* 1986;20:1229-1248.

76. Yue S, Pilliar RM, Weatherly GC: The fatigue strength of porous-coated Ti-6%Al-4V implant alloy. *J Biomed Mater Res* 1984;18:1043-1058.

77. Biomet, Inc: Porous coating technology: What are the issues? *J Arthroplasty* (Advertisement) 1993:8.

78. Glassman AH, Engh CA: The removal of porous-coated femoral hip stems. *Clin Orthop* 1992;285:164-180.

79. Bobyn JD, Tanzer M, Krygier JJ, et al: Concerns with modularity in total hip arthroplasty. *Clin Orthop* 1993, in press.

80. Tradonsky S, Postak PD, Froimson AI, et al: Performance characteristics of two-piece acetabular cups. Presented at the 59th Annual Meeting of American Academy of Orthopaedic Surgeons, Washington, DC, 1992.(Scientific Exhibit)

81. Fehring TK, Hurley PT, Braun E, et al: Modular acetabular components:are they really metal-backed? Presented at the 59th Annual Meeting of American Academy of Orthopaedic Surgeons, Washington, DC, 1992, p 82, Paper No. 92.

82. Hurley PT, Fehring TK, Braun E, et al: Polyethylene liners in modular porous acetabular components: A comparative analysis. Presented at the 59th Annual Meeting of American Academy of Orthopaedic Surgeons, Washington, DC, 1992, p 83, Paper No. 94.

83. Rosner B, Postak PD, Tradonsky S, et al: Cup/liner incongruity of two piece acetabular designs: Factor in clinical failure. Presented at the 60th Annual Meeting of the American Academy of Orthopaedic Surgeons, San Francisco, CA, 1993.(Scientific Exhibit)

84. Bueche MJ, Herzenberg JE, Stubbs BT: Dissociation of a metal-backed polyethylene acetabular component: A case report. *J Arthroplasty* 1989;4:39-41.

85. Ferenz CC: Polyethylene insert dislocation in a screw-in acetabular cup: A case report. *J Arthroplasty* 1988;3:201-204.

86. Kitziger KJ, DeLee JC, Evans JA: Disassembly of a modular acetabular component of a total hip-replacement arthroplasty: A case report. *J Bone Joint Surg* 1990;72A:621-623.

87. O'Brien RF, Chess D: Late disassembly of a modular acetabular component. *J Arthroplasty* 1992;7(Suppl):453-455.

88. Star MJ, Colwell CW Jr, Donaldson WF III, et al: Dissociation of modular hip arthroplasty components after dislocation: A report of three cases at differing dissociation levels. *Clin Orthop* 1992;278:111-115.

89. Kurtz SM, Gabriel SM, Bartel DL: The effect of non-conformity between metal-backing and polyethylene inserts in acetabular components for total hip arthroplasty. *Trans Orthop Res Soc* 1993;18:434.

90. Cates HE, Faris PM, Keating EM, et al: Polyethylene wear in cemented metal-backed acetabular cups. *J Bone Joint Surg* 1993;75B:249-253.

91. Huk OL, Bansal M, Betts F, et al: Generation of polyethylene and metal debris from cementless modular acetabular components in total hip arthroplasty. *Trans Orthop Res Soc* 1993;18:506.

92. Cooper RA, McAllister CM, Borden LS, et al: Polyethylene debris-induced osteolysis and loosening in uncemented total hip arthroplasty: A cause of late failure. *J Arthroplasty* 1992;7:285-290.

93. Connelly GM, Rimnac CM, Wright TM, et al: Fatigue crack propagation behavior of ultra-high molecular weight polyethylene. *J Orthop Res* 1984;2:119-125.

94. Bartel DL, Bicknell VL, Wright TM: The effect of conformity, thickness and material on stresses in ultra-high molecular weight components for total joint replacement. *J Bone Joint Surg* 1986;68A:1041-1051.

95. Lachiewicz PF, Suh PB, Gilbert JA: In vitro initial fixation of porous-coated acetabular total hip components: A biomechanical comparative study. *J Arthroplasty* 1989;4:201-205.

96. Ohl MD, Whiteside LA, McCarthy DS, et al: Torsional fixation of a modular femoral hip component. *Clin Orthop* 1993;287:135-141.

97. White SE, McCarthy DS, Whiteside LA: Effect of retaining the femoral neck on torsional stability of the femoral component in total hip arthroplasty. Presented at the 60th Annual Meeting of American Academy of Orthopaedic Surgeons, San Francisco, CA, 1993. (Scientific Exhibit)

98. Collier JP, Surprenant VA, Jensen RE, et al: Corrosion between the components of modular femoral hip prostheses. *J Bone Joint Surg* 1992;74B:511-517.

99. Mathiesen EB, Lindgren JU, Blomgren GG, et al: Corrosion of modular hip prostheses. *J Bone Joint Surg* 1991;73B:569-575.

100. Cook SD: Concerns with modular THR. *Clin Orthop* 1993, in press.

101. Bobyn JD, Dujovne AR, Krygier JJ, et al: Surface analysis of the taper junctions of retrieved and in-vitro tested modular hip prostheses, in Morrey BF (ed): *Biological, Material, and Mechanical Considerations of Joint Replacement*. New York, NY, Raven Press, 1993.

102. Urban RM, Jacobs JJ, Gilbert JL, et al: Corrosion products of modular hip prostheses: Microchemical identification and histopathological significance. *Trans Orthop Res Soc* 1993;18:81.

103. Callaghan JJ, Fulghum CS, Glisson RR, et al: The effect of femoral stem geometry on interface motion in uncemented porous-coated total hip prostheses: Comparison of straight-stem and curved-stem design. *J Bone Joint Surg* 1992;74A:839-848.

104. Schneider E, Kinast C, Eulenberger J, et al: A comparative study of the initial stability of cementless hip prostheses. *Clin Orthop* 1989;248:200-209.

105. Burke DW, O'Connor DO, Zalenski EB, et al: Micromotion of cemented and uncemented femoral components. *J Bone Joint Surg* 1991;73B:33-37.

106. Harris WH: Is it advantageous to strengthen the cement-metal interface and use a collar for cemented femoral components of total hip replacements? *Clin Orthop* 1992;285:67-72.

107. Engh CA, Bobyn JD, Glassman AH: Porous-coated hip replacement: The factors governing bone ingrowth, stress shielding, and clinical results. *J Bone Joint Surg* 1987;69B:45-55.

108. Glassman AH, Engh CA, Bobyn JD: A technique of extensile exposure for total hip arthroplasty. *Tech Orthop* 1986;1:35-46.

109. Engh CA, Glassman AH, Suthers KE: The case for porous-coated hip implants: The femoral side. *Clin Orthop* 1990;261:63-81.

110. Maric Z, Karpman RR: Early failure of noncemented porous coated anatomic total hip arthroplasty. *Clin Orthop* 1992;278:116-120.

111. Engh CA, Bobyn JD: The influence of stem size and extent of porous coating on femoral bone resorption after primary cementless hip arthroplasty. *Clin Orthop* 1988;231:7-28.

112. Bobyn JD, Glassman AH, Goto H, et al: The effect of stem stiffness on femoral bone resorption after canine porous-coated total hip arthroplasty. *Clin Orthop* 1990;261:196-213.

113. Bobyn JD, Mortimer ES, Glassman AH, et al: Producing and avoiding stress shielding: Laboratory and clinical observations of noncemented total hip arthroplasty. *Clin Orthop* 1992;274:79-96.

114. Engh CA, McGovern TF, Bobyn JD, et al: A quantitative evaluation of periprosthetic bone-remodeling after cementless total hip arthroplasty. *J Bone Joint Surg* 1992;74A:1009-1020.

115. Turner TM, Sumner DR, Urban RM, et al: A comparative study of porous coatings in a weight-bearing total hip-arthroplasty model. *J Bone Joint Surg* 1986;68A:1396-1409.

116. Sumner DR, Galante JO: Determinants of stress shielding: Design versus materials versus interface. *Clin Orthop* 1992;274:202-212.

117. Dujovne AR, Bobyn JD, Krygier JJ, et al: Mechanical compatibility of noncemented hip prostheses with the human femur. *J Arthroplasty* 1993;8:7-22.

118. Brooks CE, Bobyn JD, Burke DL, et al: Titanium modular hip prosthesis for management of arthritis. Presented at the 60th Annual Meeting of American Academy of Orthopaedic Surgeons, San Francisco, CA, 1993.(Poster Exhibit)

119. Otani T, Whiteside LA, White SE, et al: Effects of femoral component material properties on cementless fixation in total hip arthroplasty: A comparison study between carbon composite, titanium alloy, and stainless steel. *J Arthroplasty* 1993;8:67-74.

120. Anthony PP, Gie GA, Howie CR, et al: Localised endosteal bone lysis in relation to the femoral components of cemented total hip arthroplasties. *J Bone Joint Surg* 1990;72B:971-979.

121. Santavirta S, Hoikka V, Eskola A, et al: Aggressive granulomatous lesions in cementless total hip arthroplasty. *J Bone Joint Surg* 1990;72B:980-984.

122. Tanzer M, Maloney WJ, Jasty M, et al: The progression of femoral cortical osteolysis in association with total hip arthroplasty without cement. *J Bone Joint Surg* 1992;74A:404-410.

123. Willert HG, Semlitsch M: Reactions of the articular capsule to wear products of artificial joint prostheses. *J Biomed Mater Res* 1977;11:157-164.

124. Amstutz HC, Campbell P, Kossovsky N, et al: Mechanism and clinical significance of wear debris-induced osteolysis. *Clin Orthop* 1992;276:7-18.

125. Shanbhag AS, Glant TT, Gilbert JL, et al: Chemical and morphological characterization of wear debris in failed uncemented total hip replacement. *Trans Orthop Res Soc* 1993;18:296.

126. Maloney WJ, Smith RL, Huene D, et al: Particulate wear debris: Characterization and quantitation from membranes around failed cementless femoral replacements. *Trans Orthop Res Soc* 1993;18:294.

127. Lee J-M, Salvati EA, Betts F, et al: Size of metallic and polyethylene debris particles in failed cemented total hip replacements. *J Bone Joint Surg* 1992;74B:380-384.

128. Murray DW, Rushton N: Macrophages stimulate bone resorption when they phagocytose particles. *J Bone Joint Surg* 1990;72B:988-992.

129. Bobyn JD, Collier JP, Mayor MB, et al: Particulate debris in total hip arthroplasty: Problems and solutions. Presented at the 60th Annual Meeting of American Academy of Orthopaedic Surgeons, San Francisco, CA, 1993.(Scientific Exhibit)

130. Rimnac CM, Wilson PD Jr, Fuchs MD, et al: Acetabular cup wear in total hip arthroplasty. *Orthop Clin North Am* 1988;19:631-636.

131. Dumbleton JH: Wear and prosthetic joints, in Morrey BF (ed): *Joint Replacement Arthroplasty*. New York, NY, Churchill Livingstone, 1991, chap 6, pp 47-60.

132. Collier JP, Mayor MB, Surprenant VA, et al: The biomechanical problems of polyethylene as a bearing surface. *Clin Orthop* 1990;261:107-113.

133. Li S, Howard G: Characterization and description of an enhanced ultra high molecular weight polyethylene for orthopaedic bearing surfaces. *Trans Soc for Biomat*, 1990, p 190.

134. Hawkins ME: Ultra high molecular weight polyethylene. Zimmer technical report, February, 1993.

135. Depuy, Inc: A new enhanced ultra high molecular weight polyethylene for orthopaedic applications: A technical brief, 1989.

136. Ma SM, Kabo JM, Amstutz HC: Frictional torque in surface and conventional hip replacement. *J Bone Joint Surg* 1983;65A:366-370.

137. Livermore J, Ilstrup D, Morrey B: Effect of femoral head size on wear of the polyethylene acetabular component. *J Bone Joint Surg* 1990;72A:518-528.

138. Kabo JM, Gebhard JS, Loren G, et al: In vivo wear of polyethylene acetabular components. *J Bone Joint Surg* 1993;75B:254-258.

139. Kim KJ, Wilson SC, D'Antonio JA, et al: High amounts of polyethylene debris in the membranes from bipolar endoprostheses. Presented at the 59th Annual Meeting of American Academy of Orthopaedic Surgeons, Washington, DC, 1992, p 70, paper no. 68.

140. Lombardi AV Jr, Mallory TH, Vaughn BK, et al: Aseptic loosening in total hip arthroplasty secondary to osteolysis induced by wear debris from titanium-alloy modular femoral heads. *J Bone Joint Surg* 1989;71A:1337-1342.

141. Agins HJ, Alcock NW, Bansal M, et al: Metallic wear in failed titanium-alloy total hip replacements: A histological and quantitative analysis. *J Bone Joint Surg* 1988;70A:347-356.

142. Buly RL, Huo MH, Salvati E, et al: Titanium wear debris in failed cemented total hip arthroplasty. An analysis of 71 cases. *J Arthroplasty* 1992;7:315-323.

143. Witt JD, Swann M: Metal wear and tissue response in failed titanium alloy total hip replacements. *J Bone Joint Surg* 1991;73B:559-563.

144. Davidson JA: Characteristics of metal and ceramic total hip bearing surfaces and the effect on long-term UHMWPE wear. *Clin Orthop* 1993;294:361-378.

145. Poggie RA, Wert JJ, Mishra AK, et al: Friction and wear characteristics of UHMWPE in reciprocating sliding contact with Co-Cr, Ti-6Al-4V, and zirconia implant bearing surfaces, in Denton R, Keshavan MK (eds): *Wear and Friction of Elastomers, ASTM; STP 1145* Philadelphia, PA, 1992.

146. Kumar P, Oka M, Ikeuchi K, et al: Low wear rate of UHMW-PE against zirconia ceramic (Y-PSZ) in comparison to alumina ceramic and SUS 316L alloy. *J Biomed Mater Res* 1991;25:813-828.

147. McKellop H, Lu B, Benya P: Friction, lubrication and wear of cobalt-chromium, alumina, and zirconia hip prostheses compared on a joint simulator. *Trans Orthop Res Soc* 1992;17:402.

148. Weber BG: Total hip replacement: Rotating versus fixed and metal versus ceramic heads, in Salvati EA (ed): *The Hip - Proceedings of the 9th Open Scientific Meeting of the Hip Society.* St. Louis, MO, CV Mosby, 1981, pp 264-275.

149. Oonishi H, Igaki H, Takayama Y: Comparisons of wear of UHMWPE sliding against metal and alumina in total hip prosthesis. *Bioceramics* 1989;1:272-277.

150. Schuller HM, Marti RK: Ten-year socket wear in 66 hip arthroplasties: Ceramic versus metal heads. *Acta Orthop Scand* 1990;61:240-243.

151. Zichner LP, Willert HG: Comparison of alumina-polyethylene and metal-polyethylene in clinical trials. *Clin Orthop* 1992;282:86-94.

152. Semlitsch M, Streicher RM, Weber H: The wear behavior of capsules and heads of Co-Cr-Mo casts in long-term implanted all-metal hip prostheses. *Orthopade* 1989;18:377-381.

153. Jantsch S, Schwagerl W, Zenz P, et al: Long-term results after implantation of McKee-Farrar total hip prostheses. *Arch Orthop Trauma Surg* 1991;110:230-237.

154. Semlitsch M: Metallic implant materials for hip joint endoprostheses designed for cemented and cementless fixation, in Morscher E (ed): *The Cementless Fixation of Hip Endoprostheses.* Berlin, Springer-Verlag, 1984, pp 59-70.

155. Weber BG: Metal-metal total prosthesis of the hip joint: Back to the future. *Z Orthop Ihre Grenzgeb* 1992;130:306-309.

156. Schmalzried TP, Jasty M, Harris WH: Periprosthetic bone loss in total hip arthroplasty: Polyethylene wear debris and the concept of the effective joint space. *J Bone Joint Surg* 1992;74A:849-863.

157. Schmalzried TP, Kwong LM, Jasty M, et al: The mechanism of loosening of cemented acetabular components in total hip arthroplasty: Analysis of specimens retrieved at autopsy. *Clin Orthop* 1992;274:60-78.

158. Schmalzried TP, Maloney WJ, Jasty M, et al: Autopsy studies of the bone-cement interface in well-fixed cemented total hip arthroplasties. *J Arthroplasty* 1993;8:179-188.

159. Malcolm AJ: Pathology of cemented low-friction arthroplasties in autopsy specimens, in Older J (ed): *Implant Bone Interface.* London, Springer-Verlag, 1990, pp 77-84.

160. Howie DW, Vernon-Roberts B, Oakeshott R, et al: A rat model of resorption of bone at the cement-bone interface in the presence of polyethylene wear particles. *J Bone Joint Surg* 1988;70A:257-263.

161. Bobyn JD, Aribindi R, Mortimer E, et al: The effect of noncemented implant surface geometry on polyethylene debris migration and peri-implant histogenesis. *Trans Can Orthop Res Soc* 1993.

162. Urban RM, Sumner DR, Gilbert JL, et al: Autopsy retrieval analysis on noncircumferentially porous coated cementless femoral stems. Presented at the American Academy of Orthopaedic Surgeons Annual Meeting, February 1993, San Francisco, CA.

163. Cadambi A, Engh GA, Dwyer KA, et al: Osteolysis of the distal femur after total knee arthroplasty. *J Arthroplasty* 1993, in press.

164. Capello WN: Technical aspects of cementless total hip arthroplasty. *Clin Orthop* 1990;261:102-106.

165. Langkamer VG, Case CP, Heap P, et al: Systemic distribution of wear debris after hip replacement: A cause for concern? *J Bone Joint Surg* 1992;74B:831-839.

Results of Primary Total Hip Arthroplasty in Young Patients

John J. Callaghan, MD

Total hip arthroplasty should provide a durable, relatively painless hip for the lifetime of most elderly patients. The greater challenge for the orthopaedic surgeon performing total hip arthroplasty today is the treatment of younger patients, whose life expectancy is now well into the 70s and appears to be on the increase. Charnley[1] stated the problem well when he said: "The challenge comes when patients between 45 and 50 years of age are to be considered for the operation, because then every advance in technical detail must be used if there is to be a reasonable chance of 20 or more years of trouble-free activity." He also stated that "the best time to obtain a good result is the first time around."

In evaluations of the results of total hip arthroplasty in younger patients, the first question to be answered is: what is young? In order to make valid comparisons between series, the reader must be able to discern the number of patients in each decade of life. Some authors have used different age criteria, and a 10 to 15-year difference in age-grouping can make a difference in the reported results. For this lecture, in most cases, the discussion will be limited to patients who are younger than 50 years of age. However, because of the data available, some of the studies cited will include slightly older patients.

Another important consideration is the mix of diagnoses in each series of younger patients. The clinical and radiographic results in a study that includes only patients who have juvenile rheumatoid arthritis, or a high percentage of such patients, would probably differ from those in a series in which a more active group of patients had been studied. These differences must be kept in mind when comparisons are made between the series to be discussed in this paper.

Although this chapter reviews the results of total hip arthroplasty in young people, it must be remembered that the first choice of treatment for such patients should be more conservative, because the long-term durability of hip arthroplasty in younger patients is questionable. The surgeon should continue to consider alternatives, including prolonged counseling of these patients about the need to modify activity, to avoid an operation, and to use anti-inflammatory medications for as long as possible. Arthrodesis, osteotomy, and various salvage procedures for the treatment of aseptic necrosis, such as core decompression and bone-grafting, should also be considered. In addition, with the ever-increasing knowledge of the consequences related to polyethylene wear, such options as cup arthroplasty or femoral-resurfacing procedures may regain popularity as an option for this group.

Options for Treatment of Young Patients

The options for total hip replacement include insertion with cement, a hybrid technique (usually insertion of the acetabular component without cement and the femoral component with cement), and insertion without cement. The options for uncemented replacement include the use of press-fit devices, proximally porous-coated devices, extensively porous-coated devices, devices with enhancement coatings such as hydroxyapatite, and modular and custom devices.

Early Versus Later-Generation Surgical Techniques

When surgeons try to evaluate the results of total hip arthroplasty reported in the literature in order to select the best option for their patients, they must recognize that various generations of techniques and designs have evolved for both arthroplasty with cement and arthroplasty without cement. They must also keep in mind that experience (duration of follow-up) with cemented devices far exceeds that with devices inserted without cement. Hence, one is always trying to compare a shorter experience with devices inserted without cement to a longer experience with devices inserted with cement. The difficulty involved in comparison is compounded by the continuing change in technique for both types of implants and the fact that there is a learning curve with all of these procedures.[2] Hence, at any given time, readers are dealing with a later generation of techniques involving the use of cement compared with an earlier generation of techniques that do not involve cementing.

The first-generation techniques for total arthroplasty of the hip involved hand-packing of the cement in both the acetabulum and the femoral canal. The second-generation techniques included plugging of the distal aspect of the canal, the use of lavage, and the introduction of cement into the femur with a gun-injection system. The third-generation techniques added porosity reduction. The fourth-generation techniques enhanced the prosthesis-cement bond.

Modular components gained widespread use during the development of the third and fourth-generation techniques.

In the evolution of total hip arthroplasty without cement, the first generation of prostheses (the AML, Depuy, Warsaw, and Indiana prostheses) were available in only a few sizes, and only the femoral component was placed without cement. The second generation of replacements included both acetabular and femoral components of multiple sizes and modular design. The third generation included prostheses with better torsional stability, advancements in modularity, and better porous coatings (including circumferential coatings in all cases and some designs with hydroxyapatite enhancement coatings). All of these time-dependent factors introduce variables that make comparison of one technique with another less than ideal.

Results of Total Hip Arthroplasty in Young Patients

Initial Studies

Although Charnley originally recommended that cemented total hip arthroplasty be reserved for patients who are older than 60 years of age, he later expanded the indications for the procedure to include younger patients. Halley and Charnley[3] reported the results of low-friction arthroplasty in 68 hips in patients who were younger than 30 years old; most had rheumatoid arthritis or ankylosing spondylitis. At the time of follow-up six months to eight years

postoperatively, only one femoral component had failed (because the component had fractured) and no other hips had been revised for aseptic failure. These good results were substantiated by a study performed at The Hospital for Special Surgery by Bisla and associates.[4] In their series of 67 total hip arthroplasties followed for an average of 33 months, 62 hips (93%) had an excellent or good result and no hip had aseptic loosening.

These reports during the middle 1970s encouraged surgeons to undertake hip arthroplasty in younger patients. However, in 1981, Chandler and associates[5] reported that, of 33 hips in 29 patients who were younger than 30 years old, 19 (58%) had loosened components and seven (21%) had had a revision at an average of 5.5 years postoperatively. In addition, Dorr and associates[6] reported a satisfactory result in only 31 (72%) of 43 hips in patients who were younger than 45 years old, at a minimum of five years postoperatively. Only 47 (58%) of 81 hips had a satisfactory result at nine to ten years postoperatively.[6] Both in the series of Chandler and associates[5] and in those of Dorr and associates,[7] the arthroplasties were performed by various surgeons with first-generation hand-packing cementing techniques.

Long-Term Follow-up of First-Generation Cementing Techniques, Performed by One Surgeon

Collis[8,9] reported, in 1991, on 44 hips in patients who were younger than 50 years old at the time of a

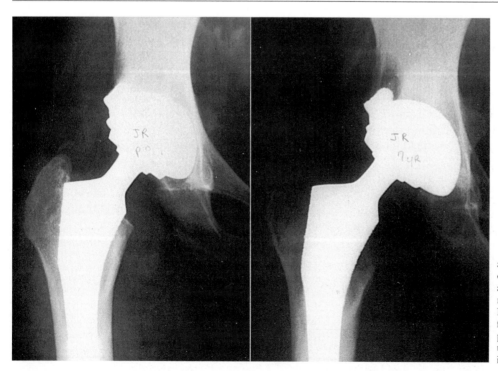

Fig. 1 Early postoperative, **left**, and seven-year follow-up radiographs, **right**, of the right hip of a woman who had a PCA total replacement at the age of 24. Note the extensive acetabular and femoral osteolysis. The eccentric placement of the femoral head in the acetabular component is indicative of polyethylene wear.

total hip arthroplasty. Twelve to 18 years postoperatively, 13 (30%) of the acetabular components and 10 (23%) of the femoral components had been revised. Thirty-three (75%) of the 44 hips were functioning well. However, 12 (39%) of the 31 unrevised acetabular components and 10 (29%) of the 34 unrevised femoral components had evidence of loosening. A number of different prostheses had been used in that series.

Sullivan and associates[10] recently reviewed the results of Johnston's series of patients who were younger than 50 years old and who had been managed with a Charnley total hip replacement with first-generation hand-packing techniques. In 84 hips followed for 16 to 21 years, 11 (13%) of the acetabular components and 2 (2%) of the femoral components had been revised for aseptic failure. However, 31 (37%) of the remaining sockets showed evidence of radiographic loosening. Only 5 (6%) of the remaining femoral components showed evidence of radiographic loosening.

Cornell and Ranawat[11] used survivorship analysis to study the hips of 100 patients who had had a cemented total hip arthroplasty before the age of 55, with all of the procedures having been performed by the same surgeon. Cornell and Ranawat reported that 90% of

the stems and 70% of the acetabular components had survived at 13 years. Solomon and associates[12] performed a survivorship analysis of cemented Charnley implants in patients who were 50 years old or younger. Of 156 hips followed for three to 16 years, with detailed results available for 130, 14 (11%) were revised, with three (2%) needing acetabular revision for aseptic loosening and eight (6%) needing femoral revision for aseptic loosening.

Results of Second-Generation Cementing Techniques, Performed by One Surgeon

Barrack and associates[13] recently reported the results of arthroplasty with the use of second-generation cementing techniques (a cement plug, jet lavage, and introduction of cement with a cement gun) in patients 50 years of age and younger. In 50 hips followed for 10 to 14 years, 11 (22%) of the acetabular components and no femoral components had been revised. Of the 50 acetabular components, 22 (44%) were radiographically loose or had been revised. Only one femoral component (2%) was radiographically loose, as assessed with stringent criteria for loosening. Ballard and associates[14] recently reviewed Johnston's series of 42 hips treated with second-generation

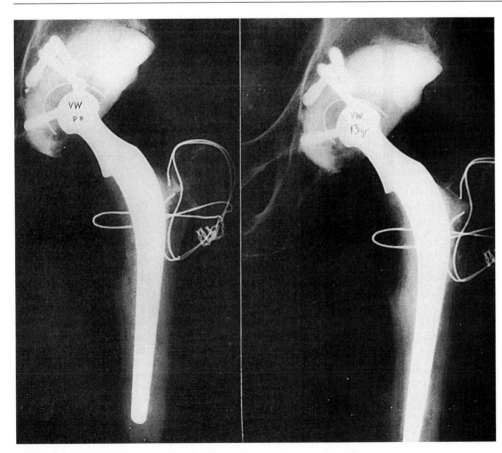

Fig. 2 Immediate postoperative, **left**, and 13-year follow-up radiographs, **right**, of the left hip of a farmer who had a Charnley total replacement with cement. There were no radiographic changes over the 13-year follow-up period, and the patient was able to continue to farm with no or slight pain.

cementing techniques. At a 10- to 12-year follow-up, 10 (24%) of the acetabular components had been revised and another four (10%) appeared loose radiographically. Two (5%) of the femoral components had been revised; however, one of the two femoral components was in a patient being treated with renal dialysis, in whom, historically, failure of total hip replacement is common.

Results of Uncemented Total Hip Arthroplasty

There have been very few reports of the results of uncemented replacement in young patients. Gustilo and associates[15] reviewed the results of the use of 69 Bias femoral components (Zimmer, Warsaw, IN) with a follow-up of five to seven years. The average Harris hip rating was 92 points, and only six (9%) of the patients had pain. Two (3%) of the femoral components had been revised, and an additional two had subsided. Heekin and associates[16] recently reported their five- to seven-year experience with the PCA total hip replacement (Howmedica, Rutherford, NJ). The average Harris hip rating was 94 points in the subset of 26 hips in patients who were younger than 50 years old. Thigh pain occurred after four (15%) of the arthroplasties. There were no femoral revisions, and there was one acetabular revision (4%). The femoral component had subsided in one hip, and the acetabular component

had migrated in one hip that had not been revised. The most alarming finding was that seven (27%) of these hips demonstrated either acetabular or femoral osteolysis, probably secondary to granuloma formation from polyethylene wear (Fig. 1).

Davies and associates[17] evaluated the results of Hedley's PCA uncemented replacements in 41 patients (48 hips) who were younger than 50 years old. At an average of three years postoperatively, 43 (90%) of these hips demonstrated an excellent or good Harrington rating. One femoral component had been revised, and three had subsided. There had been no acetabular revisions or acetabular migration.

At the 1993 Annual Meeting of The American Academy of Orthopaedic Surgeons, two papers addressed the use of uncemented hip replacements in younger patients with aseptic necrosis. Piston and associates[18] reported the results of 35 AML hip replacements, performed by Engh, in patients who were younger than 40 years old (average age, 32 years) at the time of the operation. At an average of 7.5 years postoperatively, the femoral component had been revised in one hip and was radiographically loose in another. The acetabular component had been revised in two hips (6%). Only two hips were in patients who had thigh pain. Severe or moderate stress-shielding was reported in six hips (17%) and osteolysis was

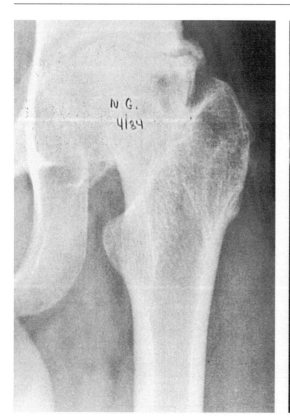
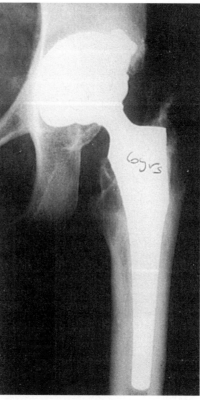

Fig. 3 Preoperative, **left**, and six-year follow-up radiographs, **right**, of the left hip of a man who had a PCA total replacement without cement at the age of 41. The follow-up radiograph demonstrates evidence of bone ingrowth. The patient functioned without pain. At present, I would not use a 32-mm head in this situation.

reported in another six. Lins and associates[19] reported the results of PCA uncemented replacement in 44 hips in patients with aseptic necrosis. The average age at the operation was 43 years. At four to six years postoperatively, there had been no femoral revisions, although one was pending, and no acetabular revisions. Six (14%) of the femoral components had subsided, and one acetabular component (2%) had migrated. In addition, two (5%) of the hips had become infected.

The early results of uncemented replacement with the use of modular and custom components are now becoming available. Cameron recently reviewed the results for 46 hips with congenital dysplasia in which a total replacement with an S-ROM modular system (Joint Medical Products Corporation, Stamford, CT) had been done (Hugh Cameron, personal communication, 1993). The average age of the patients was 44 years at the time of the operation, and there was a minimum two-year follow-up. Forty-four (96%) of the hips had a good or excellent rating, and only one (2%) was in a patient who had thigh pain. There were four minor femoral fractures (9%) during the insertion of the component. Radiographic evidence of bone ingrowth was demonstrated in 45 (98%) of the hips. Femoral subsidence occurred in only one hip, and femoral osteolysis occurred in one.

Barger and associates[20] recently reviewed the results of their first 100 primary hip replacements with custom components. The average age of the patients at the operation was 48 years, with a range of 20 to 67 years. The average duration of follow-up was three years. The average Harris hip score was 92 points. Fifteen patients had occasional thigh pain, and six had mild thigh pain. Two revisions had been performed for dissociation of the pad and two for loosening of the femoral component. Only four hips had evidence of unstable fixation. There was no noticeable stress-shielding on radiographs, and fit and fill were graded as excellent in most hips.

Enhancement Coatings

Because retrieval studies have shown bone ingrowth in only a limited proportion of each porous surface, some investigators have explored the possibility of using osteoconductive enhancement coatings to optimize the fixation of devices inserted without cement. Geesink[21] reported excellent results at two years in 100 hips in which a hydroxyapatite-coated stem had been used. Only four of these hips were in patients who had thigh pain, and there were no revisions or evidence of radiographic loosening. D'Antonio and associates[22] recently reviewed the results of replacement with a hydroxyapatite-coated stem in 148 hips in patients who

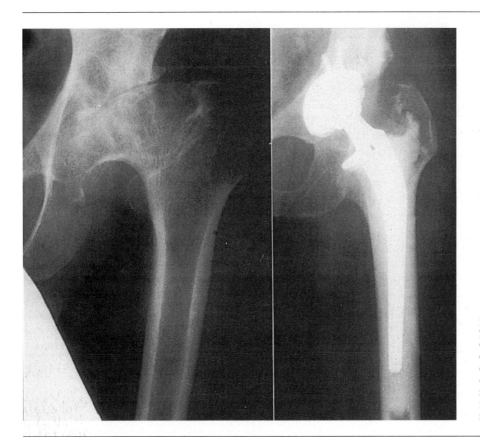

Fig. 4   Preoperative, **left**, and early postoperative radiographs, **right**, of a 44-year-old man with spondyloepiphyseal dysplasia; a total hip replacement was done with an uncemented acetabular component and a cemented femoral component. Note the use of a 22-mm femoral head. I use this construct in many young patients with abnormal femoral anatomy.

were younger than 50 years old (average age, 38 years) at the time of the operation. At an average of three to four years postoperatively, the Harris hip rating averaged 96 points. Only 2% of the hips were in patients who had thigh pain. No femoral components had been revised for aseptic loosening, and none were loose radiographically. One acetabular component demonstrated evidence of loosening radiographically. Dorr reported superior radiographic results on the femoral side when a hydroxyapatite-coated press-fit stem had been used compared with when a non-coated press-fit stem had been used; however, he reported no difference in the results of the use of a device with a porous hydroxyapatite coating compared with the use of a device of the same design with a porous non-hydroxyapatite coating (Lawrence Dorr, personal communication, 1993). Only time will tell whether any problems occur when the enhancement coating is replaced with bone or fibrous tissue and whether the enhancement coating becomes a source of particulate debris.[23,24]

In summary, because of the less durable results of total hip arthroplasty in young patients, surgeons must follow rigid indications for performance of the procedure. Alternatives to total hip arthroplasty should be considered whenever possible. Whatever form of fixation is used, it must be optimally applied (Figs. 2 through 5). The rates of loosening of cemented acetabular components have been 35% to 45% at 10 years, even when the newer techniques have been used. Although the results with uncemented devices on the acetabular side at ten years are unknown, it appears reasonable to use uncemented fixation for acetabular components in the young patient. The optimal method of femoral fixation for this population is still unknown, even after a critical review of the literature. Beyond the problems of fixation, the biologic response to particulate debris, especially the debris generated from the bearing surface, may become the most important factor in the long-term durability of the arthroplasty in this patient population. For this reason, exploration of technologies that have the potential for decreasing the problems with wear at the bearing surface must have a high priority. Currently, I use a femoral-head size that allows at least 10 mm of polyethylene thickness whenever possible. Others are using ceramic heads in this active patient population to address the issue of polyethylene wear.

References

1. Charnley J: *Low Friction Arthroplasty of the Hip. Theory and Practice.* New York, Springer, 1979, p 1.

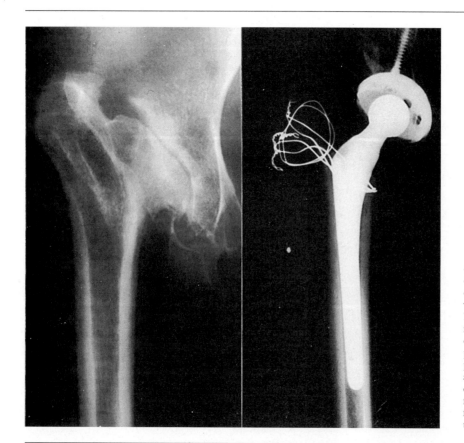

Fig. 5 Preoperative, **left**, and early postoperative radiographs, **right**, of the right hip of a 31-year-old woman with developmental dysplasia; a total hip arthroplasty was done with an uncemented porous-coated acetabular component and a hydroxyapatite-coated femoral component. I use hydroxyapatite-coated femoral components in young patients with small femoral canals in which press-fit fixation is possible but that require a stem that is too small for safe application of porous surfaces, which weakens the femoral-stem construct. Note the 22-mm femoral head, which allows the use of a thicker polyethylene cup.

2. Callaghan JJ, Heekin RD, Savory CG, et al: Evaluation of the learning curve associated with uncemented primary porous-coated anatomic total hip arthroplasty. *Clin Orthop* 1992;282:132-144.

3. Halley DK, Charnley J: Results of low friction arthroplasty in patients thirty years of age or younger. *Clin Orthop* 1975;112:180-191.

4. Bisla RS, Inglis AE, Ranawat CS: Joint replacement surgery in patients under thirty. *J Bone Joint Surg* 1976;58-A:1098-1104.

5. Chandler HP, Reineck FT, Wixson RL, et al: Total hip replacement in patients younger than thirty years old: A five-year follow-up study. *J Bone Joint Surg* 1981;63-A:1426-1434.

6. Dorr LD, Takei GK, Conaty JP: Total hip arthroplasties in patients less than forty-five year old. *J Bone Joint Surg* 1983;65A:474-479.

7. Dorr LD, Luckett M, Conaty JP: Total hip arthroplasties in patients younger than 45 years: A nine- to ten-year follow-up study. *Clin Orthop* 1990;260:215-219.

8. Collis DK: Cemented total hip replacement in patients who are less than fifty years old. *J Bone Joint Surg* 1984;66A:353-359.

9. Collis DK: Long-term (twelve to eighteen-year) follow-up of cemented total hip replacements in patients who were less than fifty years old: A follow-up note. *J Bone Joint Surg* 1991;73A:593-597.

10. Sullivan P, MacKenzie J, Callaghan J, et al: Long-term follow-up of cemented total hips in patients under fifty. Unpublished data.

11. Cornell CN, Ranawat CS: Survivorship analysis of total hip replacements: Results in a series of active patients who were less than fifty-five years old. *J Bone Joint Surg* 1986;68A:1430-1434.

12. Solomon MI, Dall DM, Learmonth ID, et al: Survivorship of cemented total hip arthroplasty in patients 50 years of age or younger. *J Arthroplasty* 1992;7:347-352.

13. Barrack R L, Mulroy RD Jr, Harris WH: Improved cementing techniques and femoral component loosening in young patients with hip arthroplasty: A 12-year radiographic review. *J Bone Joint Surg* 1992; 74-B(3):385-389.

14. Ballard T, Callaghan J, Johnston R: Total hip arthroplasty in patients under age 50 using contemporary techniques. Unpublished data.

15. Gustilo RB, Bechtold JE, Giacchetto J, et al: Rationale, experience, and results of long-stem femoral prosthesis. *Clin Orthop* 1989;249: 159-168.

16. Heekin RD, Callaghan JJ, Hopkinson WJ, et al: The porous-coated anatomic total hip prosthesis, inserted without cement: Results after five to seven years in a prospective study. *J Bone Joint Surg* 1993;75-A:77-91.

17. Davies JF: Uncemented total hip replacement in the young patient. *Orthop Trans* 1991;15:750.

18. Piston RW, de Carvalho PI, Suthers KE: Treatment for femoral head osteonecrosis by noncemented total hip replacement. Read at the Annual Meeting of The American Academy of Orthopaedic Surgeons, San Francisco, California, Feb. 23, 1993.

19. Lins R, Barnes B, Callaghan J, et al: Evaluation of uncemented total hip arthroplasty in patients with avascular necrosis of the femoral head. Unpublished data.

20. Barger W, Taylor J, Newman M: Custom femoral components: report of the first 100 primary total hip replacements. Unpublished data.

21. Geesink RG: Hydroxyapatite-coated total hip prostheses: Two-year clinical and roentgenographic results of 100 cases. *Clin Orthop* 1990;261: 39-58.

22. D'Antonio JA, Capello WN, Crothers OD, et al: Early clinical experience with hydroxyapatite-coated femoral implants. *J Bone Joint Surg* 1992;74A:995-1008.

23. Bauer TW, Geesink RC, Zimmerman R, et al: Hydroxyapatite-coated femoral stems. Histological analysis of components retrieved at autopsy. *J Bone Joint Surg* 1991;73A:1439-1452.

24. Lemons JE: Bioceramics: Is there a difference? *Clin Orthop* 1990;261:153-158.

Cementless Fixation in the Young Patient

William N. Capello, MD

Introduction

The management of disabling hip disease in the young patient continues to be a challenge for today's orthopaedic surgeon. Dissatisfaction with conventional cemented total hip arthroplasty in this patient population has led to the introduction of a number of alternative treatments over the years. Surface replacement arthroplasty was one such attempt which, although conceptually a reasonable idea, was discontinued because of its inability to provide a durable arthroplasty in the treatment of young adults. More recently, cementless implants were introduced with the thought that they could provide a more durable and longer-lasting arthroplasty than conventional cemented total hips. Whether or not these new implants will fulfill their promise remains to be determined. This chapter will focus on the use of these cementless implants in this very difficult patient group. Guidelines for their use will be discussed and alternatives in certain situations will be provided.

I believe that there are three goals in cementless total hip replacement. The first goal is the establishment of immediate rigid fixation of the implant to the femur. The second goal is conversion of this immediate fixation into a long-lasting and, ideally, permanent bond between the prosthesis and the femur. Finally, the third goal of cementless fixation is to achieve the first two goals with minimal stress shielding of the femur in the process.

Immediate Fixation

Proximal

The proximal femur is capable of providing immediate stabilization of a cementless implant in a significant number of the patients we encounter. There are two requirements that are necessary for this to occur. First, the bone of the proximal femur must be of good quality, ie, the cortical bone must be of relatively normal thickness and the cancellous bone must have structural integrity. The second requirement is that the surgeon must use precise and exacting methods of inserting the implant. Most current implants designed for proximal fixation have a double wedge configuration (Fig. 1). This geometric design allows for the immediate lock of the prosthesis into the bone. To take advantage of this design feature the preparation in the bone should be as close to the cortex as is physically possible, ie, be slightly undersized relative to the implant to be inserted. This undersizing provides an interference fit that will resist normal forces on the hip until the implant is secondarily stabilized. It has been my experience that placing a prophylactic cable or a cerclage wire around the proximal femur before inserting the implant allows the surgeon to insert the largest possible implant while at the same time minimizing the risk of fracture of the proximal femur. I have also found it useful to test the implant with a torque wrench once it is in place, delivering 150 inch-pounds of rotational torque to the implant. Occasion-

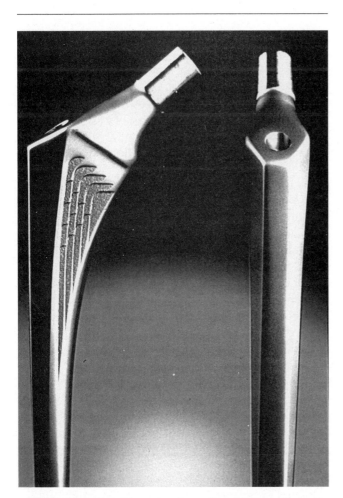

Fig. 1 Example of cementless femoral component with double wedge configuration for proximal fixation.

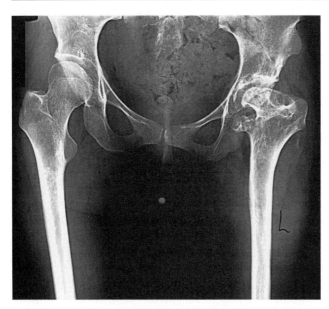 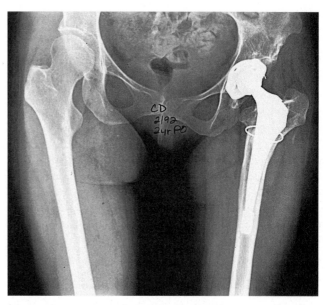

Fig. 2   Left, Preoperative radiograph of left hip of a 28-year-old female with dysplasia and post-valgus osteotomy now showing secondary degenerative joint disease. **Right,** Two-year postoperative radiograph of 28-year-old female with custom implant.

ally, although the surgeon may be confident that the implant is well-fixed as evidenced by the amount of force necessary to insert it, torquing it will reveal that it is actually not as stable as one hoped. I believe that this testing reduces the likelihood of early loosening of implants.

In some situations, the femur is slightly approportional, which means that the standard geometries available for proximally fixed implants will not adequately fill both the proximal and distal femur as well as the surgeon would like. There is some work to suggest that the percent fill of the distal femur is related to the onset of thigh pain (R.G. Averill, personal communication, 1986). There is good experimental work to show that adequate filling of the distal canal minimizes proximal micromotion.[1] Therefore, if there is a major mismatch proximal to distal, it is recommended that the surgeon consider using one of the many modular implants currently on the market. These implants, which provide for independent filling of the proximal and distal femur, enhance proximal fixation.

Diaphyseal

In situations in which the proximal bone is of very poor quality or is simply not available, as in revision settings, a proximally fixed implant is not a reasonable choice. In these situations, I believe that a more extensively fixed, diaphyseal-filling implant is an appropriate alternative. These implants require basically a cylindri-

cal preparation of the diaphysis that leaves it slightly undersized relative to the final implant. This undersizing provides both the axial and rotatory stability necessary to secure the implant until the secondary stabilizing events occur.

Although the main emphasis of this chapter is cementless fixation in the young adult, I believe that in settings in which proximal fixation is not possible or is questionable, and in which the alternative diaphyseal fixation would require a massive implant, cement should be considered as an alternative form of fixation. This situation is frequently seen in metabolically impaired patients, such as those who are undergoing chronic renal dialysis. In these patients there is a generalized osteopenia and frequently a widened diaphysis. Other settings in which cement should be considered are in such unusual circumstances as complete congenital dislocation of the hip, which requires a low resection level, one that is at or slightly below the level of the lesser trochanter. In those instances, the proximal femur is surgically removed and hence is not available for fixation purposes. In these settings I often use cement to secure the implant, although cementless distally fixed implants are a possible alternative.

The final implant choice to be discussed is the custom implant. In my practice, these are reserved for those unique abnormalities in geometry, either developmental or acquired, that preclude the use of off-the-shelf prostheses (Fig. 2). In my own practice, I rarely have occasion to use custom implants.

Secondary Fixation

I believe that a biologic event is necessary to stabilize cementless implants permanently to the skeleton. Such biologic events include bone growth into a three-dimensional surface such as porous coating or wire mesh, bone growth onto a roughened surface such as plasma spraying or arc depositing or, finally, bone growth onto a bioactive surface such as hydroxyapatite. Although some data support the use of press-fit implants without any means for secondary biological stabilization,[2] I believe that it is currently insufficient to recommend this as a routine procedure. Our own experience with a smooth press fit implant was not favorable,[3] nor was that of Geesink and associates.[4] In their experimental work with dogs where one femur had a hydroxyapatite-coated implant and the other had an identical implant of titanium alloy without the coating, it was apparent upon retrieval of these implants that the non-coated implants did not show any evidence of integration. They were routinely demarcated from the femur by a fibrous membrane and had little or no mechanical integrity with regard to their ability to stay fixed to the femur. The uncoated implants were radiographically and histologically loose.

The design of the implant can augment secondary fixation or stabilization. I believe that this is particularly true in proximally fixed implants in which the double wedged configuration continues to augment the secondary biologic fixation. In addition, I believe that the remodeling changes that occur around these implants, specifically the endosteal condensation of bone that seems to occur with some regularity in cementless proximally fixed implants, also helps to stabilize the prosthesis secondarily (Fig. 3).

Stress Shielding

Stress shielding or adverse remodeling of the proximal femur is inevitable with any intramedullary implant. The degree to which it is seen, I believe, depends on at least three factors. The first of these factors is the quality of the bone into which the implant is placed. Thinned osteoporotic bone, such as that seen in revision settings, is more likely to undergo further deterioration than is thick healthy cortical bone. This may be due simply to the larger size implant needed to accommodate these thinned femora, or it may, in fact, be related to the biologic activity of the bone.

The second factor that influences stress shielding is the level of fixation. It is generally agreed that the more proximal the fixation of the prosthesis to the femur the less stress shielding that is seen.[5]

The final determinant is the stiffness of the implant. This may well be the most significant of the three factors. Engh and Bobyn[6] have clearly shown that extensively integrated implants produce varying amounts of subsequent stress shielding as a function of the diameter of the implant. The thinner the implant and hence

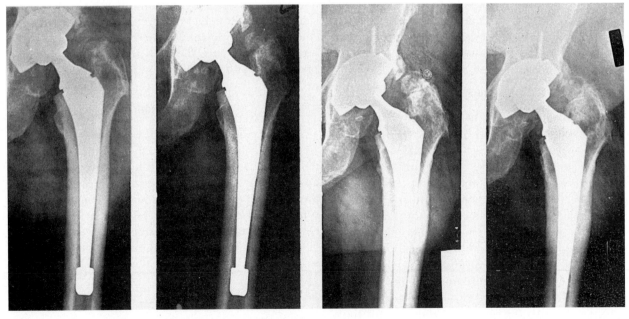

Fig. 3 Serial radiographs (immediately postoperative, one year, three years, and five years postoperative) of a 60-year-old male with cementless total hip arthroplasty demonstrating remodeling changes of cortical hypertrophy and endosteal condensation.

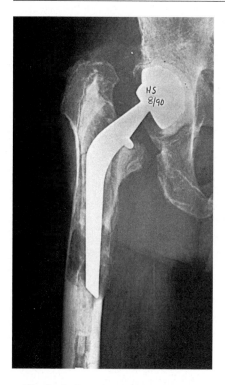
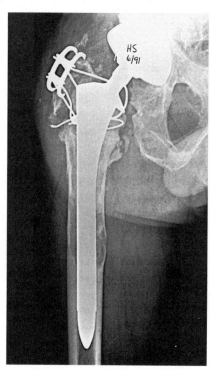
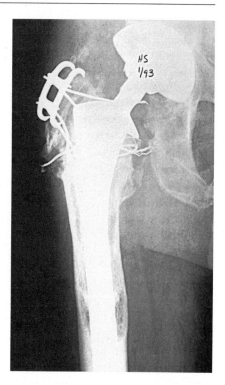

Fig. 4   Left, Radiograph preoperative to revision total hip replacement in 77-year-old male. **Center,** One-year postoperative radiograph showing revision to extensively coated implant in 77-year-old male. **Right,** Two-year postoperative radiograph showing no obvious stress shielding and healing of pre-existing osteolytic lesions in 77-year-old male.

the more flexible the implant, the less stress shielding that is noted independent of the extensiveness of the fixation (Fig. 4). This factor has influenced my thinking on the use of massive implants in thinned bone situations. I am reluctant to place large canal-filling implants in these settings for fear that the resultant stress shielding may be dramatic and could lead to long-term problems should revision become necessary or even threaten the integrity of the implant itself.

Optimum Implant

I believe that the optimum cementless implant should be fixed extensively to the femur and should have some capacity to fill at least the proximal and distal femur. It should also be flexible to minimize stress shielding. Unfortunately, no implant with this combination of qualities exists at present in our current array of cementless prostheses. Therefore, until such an implant is developed, my recommendations for the management of significant hip disease in the young individual are as follows. In individuals with Dorr Type A bone,[7] I suggest using a non-modular, proximally fixed implant. If there is a significant mismatch proximally to distally with regard to the ability to fill the canal with a non-modular implant, then I suggest that a modular implant be considered. If the proximal

femur is of poor bone quality or has significant deficiencies, so that a proximally fixed implant would have little likelihood of remaining fixed, then a more distally fixed diaphyseal filling implant is appropriate. However, in settings where this might entail the use of a massive implant, I recommend that the surgeon consider the use of cement as an alternative. Finally, the role of custom implants, I believe, is small and reserved for situations where the anatomy is so distorted that off-the-shelf implants are not practical.

Conclusion

I believe that the surgeon has an obligation to individualize as much as possible the prosthetic choice to the patient. I would advise against trying to force one prosthetic system to work in each and every case that the surgeon encounters. In my experience there currently exists no prosthetic system that is complete enough to handle all the situations that we encounter in dealing with the young adult with disabling hip disease.

References

1. Manley MT, Capello WN, Averill RG, et al: Effect of stem design parameters, stem fit and bone quality on the torsional stability of femoral stems. Presented at the 57th annual meet-

ing of the American Academy of Orthopaedic Surgeons, New Orleans, February 8-13, 1990, paper No. 355.

2. Blaha JD, Grappiolo G, Gruen TA, et al: Five to eight-year follow-up of a cementless, press-fit, non-bone ingrowth total hip stem. Presented at the 60th annual meeting of the American Academy of Orthopaedic Surgeons, San Francisco, February 18, 1993, paper No. 56.

3. Hupfer TA, Capello WN, Hile LE: Comparison of identical geometry press-fit and ingrowth femoral prostheses. Presented at the 56th annual meeting of the American Academy of Orthopaedic Surgeons, Las Vegas, February 10, 1989, paper No. 97.

4. Geesink RG, de Groot K, Klein CP: Chemical implant fixation using hydroxyl-apatite coatings: The development of a human total hip prosthesis for chemical fixation to bone using hydroxyl-apatite coatings on titanium substrates. *Clin Orthop* 1987;225:147-170.

5. Bobyn JD, Mortimer ES, Glassman AH, et al: Producing and avoiding stress shielding: Laboratory and clinical observations of noncemented total hip arthroplasty. *Clin Orthop* 1992;274:79-96.

6. Engh CA, Bobyn JD: The influence of stem size and extent of porous coating on femoral bone resorption after primary cementless hip arthroplasty. *Clin Orthop* 1988;231:7-28.

7. Dorr LD, Absatz M, Gruen TA, et al: Anatomic porous replacement hip arthroplasty: First 100 consecutive cases. *Semin Arthroplasty* 1990;1:77-86.

Cementless Fixation of the Femur: Pros and Cons

Cecil H. Rorabeck, MD, FRCS(C)

Robert B. Bourne, MD, FRCS(C)

Peter Devane, MBChB, FRACS, MSc

Gordon A. Veale, MBChB, FRACS

Introduction

Cemented total hip replacement has been extremely effective in affording pain relief and improvement of function. Complications from cemented stems have been reduced by improvements in design and materials, as well as improvements in the cementing and insertional techniques. Thus, the incidence of revision for a failed cemented femoral stem using contemporary techniques is reported to be as low as 5% at 10 years.[1] Although it is generally agreed that a well-done cemented total hip replacement remains the gold standard in the older age group, attempts have been made to improve the results of total hip replacement in the younger age group using cementless technique. The reason for this stems from the pessimistic reports of the results of cemented total hip replacements in patients younger than 50 years of age. Chandler and associates[2] report a 40% revision rate in patients undergoing cemented total hip replacement under the age of 40. Other studies have not been as pessimistic[3,4]; but all authors are in agreement that a cemented hip replacement in a younger patient with osteoarthritis is less likely than a cemented hip replacement done in the older age group to withstand the test of time.

To conclude that cementless hip replacement was developed purely to address the problems of total hip replacement in the younger patient is to oversimplify the situation. In order to fully understand cementless fixation, and define its role in total hip replacement (THR), it is necessary to trace its development back in time.

The Development of Cementless Fixation

In 1940, Moore and Bohlman[5] fabricated a stainless steel prosthesis used as a replacement for a proximal femur which was resected because of a giant cell tumor. This device has been credited as the forerunner of a prosthesis which still bears its originators name and is implanted today. In 1950 J. E. M. Thompson developed a short-stemmed metallic device that came to be known as the "light-bulb" prosthesis.

Starting in 1973 and working independently, Gilberty and Bateman developed the prototypes of the present bipolar endoprosthesis, which employed metallic cups lined with ultra-high density polyethylene locked securely onto the head of a femoral component. All of these femoral components had a smoothly coated stem and none attempted to obtain bony ingrowth, because at that time fixation at the prosthesis/bone interface was not recognized as a major problem.

Failure of the femoral endoprosthesis on the acetabular side of the joint led to the acceptance of the need for an acetabular component. In 1951, McKee and Watson-Farrar of Norwich, England, developed their prosthesis, which, by the time it became available in the mid 1950s, had been modified to incorporate acrylic cement.[6]

In 1958 Sir John Charnley began the classic work that was to earn him a place in history as the father of the present-day THR. With his reporting of the long-term results in 1972,[7] THR gained world-wide acceptance as a therapeutic rather than experimental procedure for hip disease. Acrylic bone cement had initially been developed by Charnley to obtain stable early fixation of total hip arthroplasty. However, by the mid 1970s, with careful long-term follow-up, several problems with cemented implants had become evident. The most important of these was aseptic loosening, and a large portion of the blame for this (whether rightly or wrongly is still being debated today) was attributed to the acrylic cement. This concern, which led many to try to develop a better method of fixation at the bone/prosthesis interface, was the true beginning of cementless fixation as we know it today.

A variety of total hips were developed in Europe for use without cement, including those designed by Lord, Judet, and Mittlemeier. These had large surface irregularities and were known as macrointerlock, but they also had a high late failure rate.

The concept of biologic ingrowth was modified by Engh, Hungerford, and others in the United States in the late 1970s and early 1980s. The AML™ (DePuy, Warsaw, IN) and PCA™ (Howmedica, Rutherford, NJ) devices were initially quite successful, and they remain in use at this time with only minor modifications.

During the mid and late 1980s a large number of additional press-fit microinterlock components became commercially available. Although the short-term results with most press-fit femoral components are quite good, a new group of problems began to appear. These can be categorized as: (1) thigh pain and limp and (2) stress shielding.

These problems made the indications for uncemented femoral fixation less well defined, and led, in the late 1980s and early 1990s, to the development of hybrid THRs (cemented femoral components and press-fit acetabular cups). There has also been a recent swing back to fully cemented components. This leaves the surgeons in the difficult position of deciding which type of femoral fixation is the best for a particular patient. It is the purpose of this paper to review these concerns and, in so doing, to define what the authors believe to be the role of cementless femoral stems in patients with osteoarthritis of the hip.

Clinical Study

In an effort to determine the incidence and the significance of thigh pain in a population of patients undergoing cementless total hip replacement in a single institution, a study was initiated comparing two implants, namely the PCA and the Mallory-Head™ (Biomet, Warsaw, IN) (Fig. 1). All patients who underwent cementless total hip replacement at the University Hospital between the years 1975 to 1981 were included in this study. The study population was made up of 432 patients who received the cementless PCA hip replacement and 864 patients who received a cementless Mallory-Head replacement. The patients are consecutive with no exclusions. The preoperative diagnosis included osteonecrosis, rheumatoid arthritis, and post-traumatic arthritis. Ninety percent of the procedures were done, however, for osteoarthritis.

The PCA femoral stem is a modular proximally beaded cobalt chrome anatomic implant designed to obtain a tight interference fit both in the metaphysis and at the level of the isthmus. The canal was reamed and then rasped in sequential fashion, following which the appropriate sized femoral component was inserted. Attempts were made in all cases to obtain a tight interference fit. The Mallory-Head cementless femoral com-

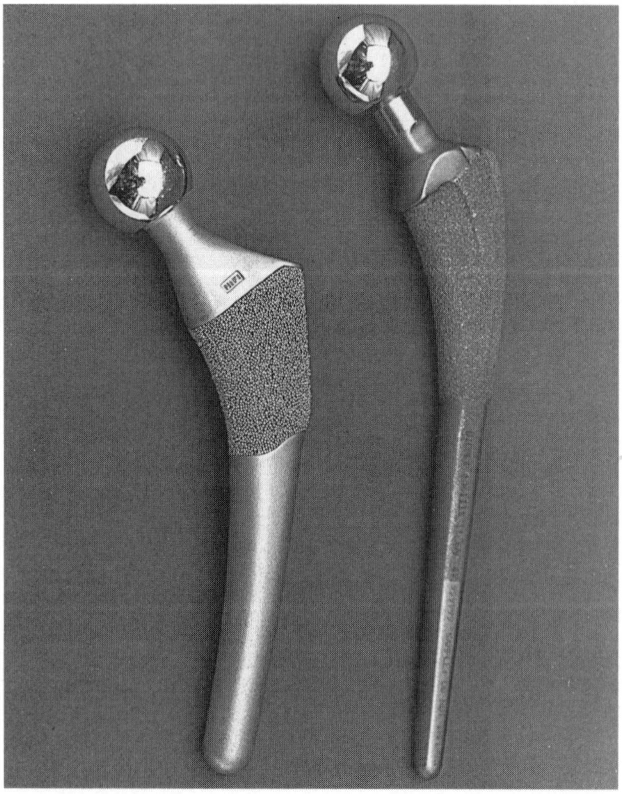

Fig. 1 **Left** Porous Coated Anatomic (Co Cr Mb) femoral component. **Right**, Mallory-Head (Titanium) femoral component.

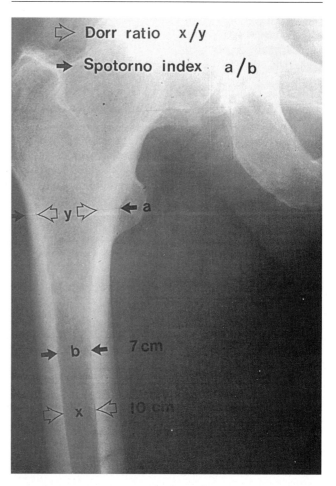

Fig. 2 Radiograph demonstrating the Dorr ratio and the Spotorno index.

ponent is a straight stem, titanium alloy implant, with plasma spray applied proximally to act as a surface for bony ingrowth. It differs from the PCA in that the stem is not anatomic, is longer, and is made of a different material. It also has a proximal fin to give it torsion resistance.

Preoperatively, all patients were examined both clinically and radiographically using standardized techniques. The preoperative radiographic assessment included the canal calcar isthmus ratio (Dorr) as well as a Spotorno Index (Fig. 2).[8] The former is a ratio of the canal diameter at a point 10 cm distal to the calcar isthmus. The smaller the ratio (x/y) the better the potential for a tight interference fit with a cementless implant. As the ratio approaches 1, the possibility of a good proximal and distal match decreases. Using this ratio, femurs were classified into Type A, B, or C according to Dorr (Fig. 3).[9]

Postoperatively, the patients were seen at three months, six months, one year, and yearly thereafter. Clinical assessment was done using a Harris Hip Score. In addition a Visual Analogue scale was used to record thigh pain (Fig. 4). The patient was asked to mark the Visual Analogue graph at some point between zero and ten with zero being no thigh pain and ten being severe thigh pain. The Harris Hip score, as well as all follow-up data, was done by a nurse.

Postoperative radiographic assessment included the presence or absence of spot welds, subsidence, sclerotic or radiolucent lines, loose beads, cortical hypertro-

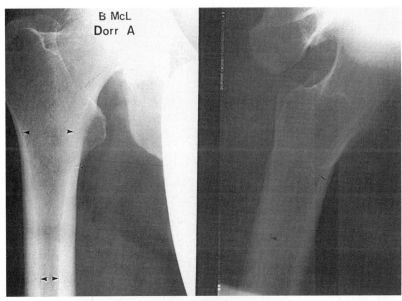

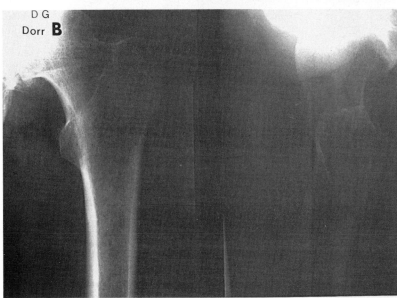

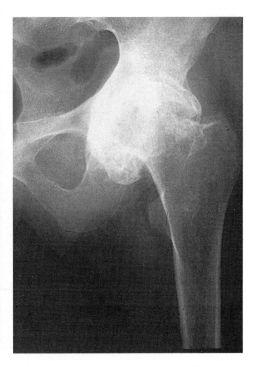

Fig. 3 **Top left** and **top right**, Radiographic examples of a Dorr type A femur, AP and lateral views. **Bottom left** and **center**, Radiographic example of a Dorr type B femur, AP and lateral views. **Bottom right**, Radiographic example of a Dorr type C femur, AP view.

How much "thigh pain" do you experience during your daily activities?

Please put a mark on the following line:

No   Severe
Thigh |——————————————————————| Thigh
Pain   Pain

Fig. 4 Visual Analogue Scale for thigh pain.

Clinical Results

The incidence of thigh pain in the PCA group was 13% at two years and 23% at four years.[10] Conversely, the incidence of thigh pain in the Mallory-Head group was 7% at one year and 3% at two years. An analysis of the incidence of thigh pain in patients younger than 50 years of age demonstrated no difference in the incidence.[11]

Comparison of the severity of thigh pain between the two implants showed no difference at two years. More than 80% of patients with thigh pain in both groups graded their pain as mild (less than 3). The remaining patients in the Mallory-Head group graded their thigh pain as moderate (4-7) with none in the severe category. Similarly, 15% of the PCA patients graded their pain as moderate with 5% rating it as severe (8-10). An analysis of those patients coming to revision for thigh pain alone demonstrated that, although the symptom was relatively common, it was not of sufficient severity in either hip system to compel either the surgeon or the patient to recommend or ask for exploratory surgery. Four percent of the PCA and none of the Mallory-Head underwent exploratory surgery and revision for thigh pain within the first four years.

phy or pedestal formation. For purposes of this review, a stem was considered stable (ingrown) if one could demonstrate a spot weld and/or the absence of any reactive lines around the stem (Fig. 5). Conversely, a stem was considered to be unstable and, hence, lacking bony ingrowth if any of the following parameters were present: recent migration greater than 2.0 mm; widening of radiolucent lines; a global sclerotic line, especially in Zone 7; progressive particle shedding; pedestal formation.

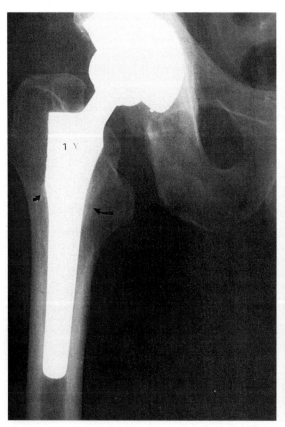
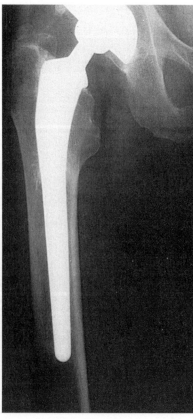

Fig. 5 Left, Spot welds seen on the AP radiograph of a PCA femoral component. **Right,** Spot welds seen on the AP radiograph of a Mallory-Head femoral component.

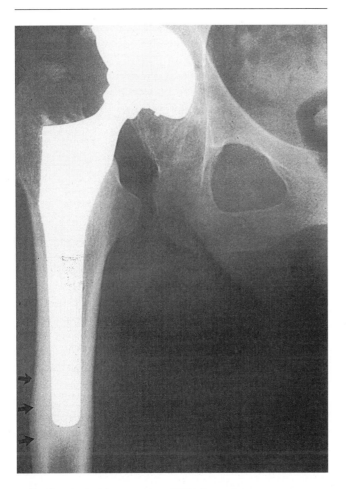

Fig. 6 Cortical hypertrophy of PCA femoral component as seen on the AP radiograph.

Radiographic Results

Careful radiographic analysis was done to determine if thigh pain could be predicted on the basis of either preoperative radiographs or postoperative radiographic appearance. While it was clear from this study that a patient with a clear diagnosis of stem loosening would have thigh pain, nevertheless, a solidly bony ingrown stem did not insure the absence of thigh pain. In addition to stem migration, factors found to correlate with thigh pain included the appearance of a pedestal distally, subsidence in excess of 4 mm, and radiolucent or radiosclerotic lines globally in the zone of porous coating. Bone quality was not a factor in the incidence of thigh pain. The presence or absence of good metaphyseal fill or distal fit did not seem to be of any predictive value in the etiology of thigh pain.

In the PCA group, radiographic features pertaining to the femoral component that positively correlated with thigh pain included a tight diaphyseal fit through the isthmus, subsidence greater than 2 mm, periosteal cortical hypertrophy at the stem tip, cancellous hypertrophy, and platform sclerosis of the tip stem (Gruen Zone 4) (Fig. 6). Conversely, in the Mallory-Head group, no positive correlation could be made between preoperative bone quality or postoperative femoral component fill and thigh pain. Similarly, after statistical analysis, no positive correlation could be made with any of the radiographic features examined for the small group of patients in the Mallory-Head group who had thigh pain (Fig. 7).

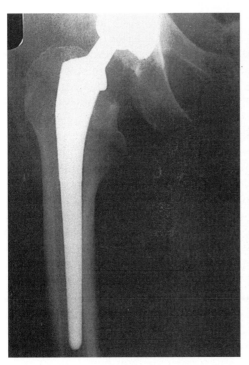
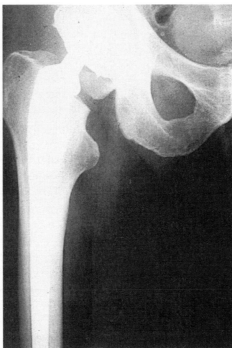

Fig. 7 Left, An example of good metaphyseal fit and fill with the Mallory-Head femoral component. **Right**, An example of poor metaphyseal fit and fill with the Mallory-Head femoral component.

Discussion

Thigh Pain

Virtually all reported studies of cementless total hip replacement report a "new" early symptom of thigh pain in patients receiving cementless femoral stems.[12-23] The percentage of patients experiencing this symptom varies according to the surgeons performing the operation and the type of implant used. The reported incidence of thigh pain after insertion of the PCA prosthesis varies from 4%[18] to 41%.[22] Callaghan and associates[13] reported a 16% incidence of thigh pain with the PCA prosthesis in two years, while Campbell and associates[12] reported a 17% incidence of thigh pain at two years using the same prosthesis. Other authors have suggested the incidence of thigh pain decreases with time.

Hedley and associates,[24] using the PCA prosthesis, reported a 40% incidence of thigh pain three months postoperatively, which by two years had reduced to a 4% incidence.[24] Katz and associates,[25] in a comparison of total hip arthroplasty in younger patients with osteonecrosis of the hip, noted an incidence of thigh pain of 29% at two-year follow-up in patients who received a cementless femoral stem. Hedley's observations of a decreasing incidence of thigh pain with time were substantiated by Plotz and associates.[26] Their study of 106 consecutive cementless total hip replacements demonstrated a steadily decreasing incidence of thigh pain, from 53% at three months to 6.6% at 15 months following surgery. Other authors, using different implants (tri-lock femoral component), have also commented on a decreasing incidence of thigh pain between one year and two years.[21]

Thigh pain is not a symptom unique to the PCA implant. At an average follow-up of 36 months, Haddad and associates[16] noted an incidence of isolated thigh pain with the AML prosthesis of 13%. The comparable figure for a group of patients who received PCA prostheses was 10%. Engh and associates,[14] who used defined radiographic criteria of bony or fibrous ingrowth, reported a different incidence of thigh pain with the AML prosthesis. At two-year follow-up with the prosthesis defined as demonstrating bony ingrowth, a 7.8% incidence of mild thigh pain was noted. At the same follow-up period, 20.6% of patients defined radiographically as having fibrous ingrowth complained of some thigh pain. Other researchers have been unable to correlate radiographic findings with the incidence of severity of thigh pain. Bands and associates,[27] in a study of 68 cementless PCA implants, noted that there was no correlation between thigh pain and the degree of bone prosthesis radiolucency or the fit of the femoral stem. Similar observations have been noted by Ghazal and associates.[10]

The phenomenon of thigh pain following a cementless femoral stem is not new. Ring[28] stated that the most common complaint of patients with symptoms after insertion of a cementless prosthesis was thigh pain. He did not report the incidence but rather talked anecdotally. Andrew and associates,[29] in follow-up data on the Ring prosthesis, noted that almost all of 116 patients complained of thigh pain, especially start-up pain. It must be remembered, however, that the Ring prosthesis is a Moore's (press fit) type stem, and it does not have a porous coating to encourage ingrowth of new bone.

Theories on the Etiology of Thigh Pain

While it is clear that thigh pain had a positive correlation with a radiographically loose stem, nevertheless, there are a group of patients whose solid bony ingrowth can be demonstrated radiographically, but who continue to have thigh pain. The question arises as to the etiology of thigh pain in this group of individuals. When considering thigh pain, one must ask the question, "Is it avoidable?" In order to answer the question, it is necessary to understand the etiology of thigh pain and its relationship to cementless implants. While a loose femoral stem, whether cemented or cementless, will cause thigh pain necessitating revision, there is a unique symptom of mild thigh pain, reported with all cementless implants, that does not normally require revision. Many theories regarding the etiology of thigh pain associated with cementless femoral stems have been suggested. The majority of these relate to factors that directly affect the fixation of the implant. The underlying premise is that the implant will cause thigh pain.

Thigh pain in cemented total hip replacement is rarely seen immediately postoperatively, and its appearance is usually considered an indication that the cemented femoral stem has loosened. Bourne and associates,[30] who compared a series of patients receiving cementless PCA prostheses with another group who received a cemented Harris Design-2 (HD2TM, Howmedica, Rutherford, NJ), noted a 17% incidence of thigh pain at two years with a cementless PCA and no thigh pain at two years using the cemented HD2 prosthesis. Phillips and Messieh,[20] who used a cementless bipolar prosthesis, considered thigh pain on weightbearing to be the major problem and attributed this pain to loosening of the femoral component.

In addition to the above, a number of other factors have been implicated in the etiology of thigh pain. Many of these are also cited as causes of loosening or as reasons for failure to obtain early adequate fixation of a cementless stem. These factors include (1) inadequate diaphyseal fit, (2) inadequate metaphyseal fit, (3) extent of porous coating, (4) location of porous coating, (5) quality of patient's bone stock, (6) weight of the patient, (7) insufficient femoral stem length, (8) too stiff a femoral stem, and (9) presence or absence of radiologic signs confirming bony ingrowth.

All of these factors can be construed to have a direct or indirect effect on the fixation of a cementless femoral component of a total hip replacement. The literature, however, is confusing when one attempts to determine the relative importance of each of these factors.

In a study of the AML prosthesis, Engh and associates,[14] in a review of 195 patients with a press fit AML stem, found that patients with radiographic hallmarks of a femoral stem with bony ingrowth had a lower incidence of thigh pain than patients with radiographic signs of fibrous ingrowth. In their opinion, a good press fit at the isthmus of the femoral canal leads to a better chance of bony ingrowth into the porous coating of the prosthesis, better fixation, and, hence, less chance of thigh pain.

Whiteside[23] also emphasized the important of a "tight distal fit" to prevent toggle of the stem in the medullary canal. Testing this hypothesis, he found that 53% of patients with a loose distal fit had some degree of thigh pain at one year postoperatively where only 3% of those with a tight distal fit had pain at the same follow-up period. Although no porous ingrowth occurred in the distal part of the prosthesis used by Whiteside, in contrast to that used by Engh and associates, Whiteside did note a positive correlation between thigh pain and loose distal fit.

Other reports, however, have not noted the same correlation between the distal fit and thigh pain. Skinner and Curlin[31] measured the gap at a point 5 cm above the distal tip of the femoral stem using PCA, AML, and Harris-Galante™ (Zimmer, Warsaw, IN) prostheses and found no relationship between thigh pain and the gap between the bone and the prosthesis. Similarly, in a retrospective study of 110 PCA hips, Campbell and associates[12] noted that a good "isthmal fit" was no guarantee of elimination of thigh pain. His study demonstrated an equal incidence of thigh pain between those patients with good and those with poor isthmal fit.

Bone quality has been suggested as a factor in predicting whether a patient is likely to experience postoperative thigh pain, but here, too, a review of the literature generates confusion. Engh and associates[14] found that patients with poor bone quality, as defined by their own 10-point scale, were more likely to experience postoperative thigh pain (26% versus 11%) than those with good bone quality. It should be noted, however, that the authors also found that bone quality did not have a statistically measurable influence on the radiographic likelihood of bone ingrowth or on the incidence of postoperative limp. Conversely, Campbell and associates[12] failed to find any correlation between bone quality and thigh pain.

Several conclusions are drawn from the literature: (1) No report has yet given a reliable predictor (either clinical or radiologic) of thigh pain. (2) Radiologic indicators of bony ingrowth and thigh pain are prosthesis specific. (3) The relationship between thigh pain and radiologic loosening is not clear.

We believe that the reason that thigh pain is still a symptom and not a diagnosis is because thigh pain is prosthesis specific. The causes of thigh pain in a PCA and in an AML may be completely different. This difference explains many of the anomalies in the literature, such as the association of the painful PCA implant and loosening, compared to the painful AML implant, which has not been associated with loosening. We have noted that PCAs that show tip sclerosis on the lateral radiograph have a higher incidence of thigh pain. This pain may occur because the tip of the prosthesis irritates the anterior femoral cortex from within, despite the presence of radiologic bony ingrowth.

The radiologic signs of bony ingrowth are also prosthesis specific. Radiologic signs of ingrowth for the AML, which have been extensively documented (spot welds, tip sclerosis, etc.), are not seen with the Mallory-Head implant.

Running through all reports is an almost unconscious attempt to relate cementless femoral problems to fixation. Undoubtedly, a loose implant will always cause problems, but the converse does not necessarily apply. Most hip surgeons will recall cases of having revised solidly fixed femoral stems because of pain.

Stress Shielding

Another criticism of cementless fixation relates to the issue of stress shielding, which is defined as the loss of proximal femoral bone stock because of solid distal fixation (Fig. 8). Again this is prosthesis specific, and depends on the design, material, and pattern of porous coating of the femoral prosthesis. Because other factors can mimic this condition (infection, polyethylene debris), the importance of stress shielding has been mainly theoretical.

With the introduction of the isoelastic implant it has been suggested that it is important to match implant stiffness to the stiffness of the bone.[19,32,33] By so doing, movement is reduced at the bone implant interface, which provides a more ideal climate for bone ingrowth into the prosthesis. Theoretically, at least, if one could match the modulus of the implant with that of bone, the issue of thigh pain might be reduced. Skinner and Curlin[31] attempted to correlate the ratio of the flexural rigidity of the bone to the flexural rigidity of the femoral stem with the presence or absence of thigh pain. In their study they examined the Harris-Galante, the PCA, and the AML hips and found that determining the flexure rigidity ratio of the painful hips and the non-painful hips revealed no significant difference. They did, however, demonstrate that there was a mildly positive correlation with the pain score to the flex-

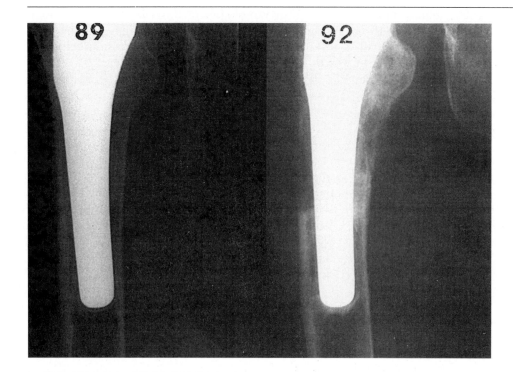

Fig. 8 AP radiograph demonstrating stress shielding at 3 years with a Porous Coated Anatomic femoral component.

ure rigidity of the implant, which demonstrated a trend toward lower pain with more flexible stems. They then attempted to correlate the pain score to flexural rigidity ratio divided by patient weight, and achieved a statistically significant correlation (p=0.0222). The flexural rigidities for a standard chromium cobalt implant ranging in thickness from 9 to 16.5 mm is 72 to 804 N•m². On the other hand, for titanium prostheses of the same size, the corresponding range would be half this—36 to 402 N•m². It is possible, therefore, to compare the flexural rigidity of bone to the flexural rigidity of the implant for differing bone-prostheses constructs. While the importance of the flexural rigidity ratio is yet to be determined in the etiology of thigh pain, our clinical and radiographic findings would tend to support those of Skinner and Curlin; namely, that the incidence of thigh pain is somewhat higher when this ratio is compared to patient's weight.

What is the Place of Cementless Femoral Fixation Today?

The case for cementless femoral fixation remains unproven. Acrylic cement has given good long-term results in low demand patients.[1] Total hip arthroplasties using biologic ingrowth, have been implanted only since the mid 1970s, and, although some studies suggest they may be as good, there are none that clearly demonstrate cementless femoral fixation to be superior to cemented stems. One would hope that the incidence of late aseptic loosening would be lower than for cemented implants but this has yet to be proven. The two basic questions that must be answered are, "Which patients should have a cementless femoral stem, and how can one minimize the problems of thigh pain and stress shielding?"

Patient Factors

Cementless arthroplasty was developed to address the problem of aseptic loosening of cemented prostheses, which in turn affects the longevity of an implant. For this reason we consider it the fixation of choice in patients who are younger than 65 years of age and who have adequate bone stock.

Dorr, Spotorno, and others have suggested that bone quality is the most important factor in determining clinical success of a cementless total hip replacement. They have defined several femoral morphologic indices in an attempt to act as a guide for surgeons performing cementless total hip replacement. Our studies would suggest that their value has yet to be proven, for we have been unable to correlate femoral morphology with clinical outcome in an early (four-year) follow-up, and that other factors, such as interference fit, need to be considered.[10,11]

Surgeon-Related Factors

Cementless arthroplasty of the hip is technically demanding. Despite the fact that all surgery in both group of patients was performed by the same two surgeons using the same approach, it is important to note that virtually all of the PCA implants were done before the Mallory Head series was started. Thus, the authors had gained more experience and a new appreciation for the role of initial stem stability in osseous integration in porous ingrowth implants. Undoubtedly this has played a role in the improvement in short-term clinical success with cementless implant using the Mallory-Head system.

We believe there is a definite relationship between initial stability of the implant in the operating room and the chances, pattern, and amount of bony ingrowth. It is essential that initial stem stability be achieved at the time of implantation in order to achieve later bony ingrowth.

References

1. Kavanagh BF, Dewitz MA, Ilstrup DM, et al: Charnley total hip arthroplasty with cement: Fifteen-year results. *J Bone Joint Surg* 1989;71A:1496-1503.
2. Chandler HP, Reineck FT, Wixson RL. et al: Total hip replacement in patients younger than thirty years old: A five-year follow-up study. *J Bone Joint Surg* 1981;63A:1426-1434.
3. Dorr LD, Luckett M, Conaty JP: Total hip arthroplasties in patients younger than 45 years: A nine to ten year follow-up study. *Clin Orthop* 1990;260:215-219.
4. Dorr LD, Takei GK, Conaty JP: Total hip arthroplasties in patients less than forty-five years old. *J Bone Joint Surg* 1983;65A:474-479.
5. Moore AT, Bohlman HR: Metal hip joint: A case report. *J Bone Joint Surg* 1943;25A:688-692.
6. McKee GK, Watson-Farrar J: Replacement of arthritic hips by the McKee-Farrar prosthesis. *J Bone Joint Surg* 1966;48B:245-259.
7. Charnley J: The long-term results of low-friction arthroplasty of the hip performed as a primary intervention. *J Bone Joint Surg* 1972;54B:61-76.
8. Spotorno L, Schenk RK, Dietschi C, et al: Personal experiences with uncemented prostheses. *Orthopade* 1987;16:225-238.
9. Dorr LD: Optimizing results of total joint arthroplasty, in Stauffer ES (ed): *American Academy of Orthopaedic Surgeons Instructional Course Lecture XXXIV.* St. Louis, MO, CV Mosby, 1985, p 401-404.
10. Ghazal ME, Bourne RB, Rorabeck CH, et al: Thigh pain in osteoarthritic patients with uncemented Porous Coated Anatomic hip replacements: A five year study. *J Bone Joint Surg*, in press.
11. Burkart BC, Bourne RB, Rorabeck CH, et al: Thigh pain in cementless total hip arthroplasty: A comparison of two systems at two years follow-up. *Clin Orthop* 1993;24:645-653.
12. Campbell AC, Rorabeck CH, Bourne RB, et al: Thigh pain after cementless total hip arthroplasty: Annoyance or illomen. *J Bone Joint Surg* 1992;74B:63-66.
13. Callaghan JJ, Dysart SH, Savory CG: The uncemented porous-coated anatomic total hip prosthesis: Two-year results of a prospective consecutive series. *J Bone Joint Surg* 1988;70A:337-346.
14. Engh CA, Bobyn JD, Glassman AH: Porous-coated hip replacement: The factors governing bone ingrowth, stress shielding, and clinical results. *J Bone Joint Surg* 1987;69B:45-55.
15. Engh CA, Massin P: Cementless total hip arthroplasty using the anatomic medullary locking stem: Results using a survivorship analysis. *Clin Orthop* 1989;249:141-158.
16. Haddad RJ Jr, Skalley TC, Cook SD, et al: Clinical and roentgenographic evaluation of noncemented porous-coated anatomic medullary locking (AML) and porous-coated anatomic (PCA) total hip arthroplasties. *Clin Orthop* 1990;258:176-182.
17. Harris WH, Maloney WJ: Hybrid total hip arthroplasty. *Clin Orthop* 1989;249:21-29.
18. Hedley AK, Gruen TAW, Borden LS, et al: The Hip, in Brand RA (ed.): Proceedings of the Fourteenth Open Scientific Meeting of the Hip Society. St. Louis, MO, CV Mosby, 1987.
19. Morscher EW, Dick W: Cementless fixation of "isoelastic" hip endoprostheses manufactured from plastic materials. *Clin Orthop* 1983;176:77-87.
20. Phillips TW, Messieh SS: Cementless hip replacement for arthritis: Problems with a smooth surface Moore stem. *J Bone Joint Surg* 1988;70B:750-755.
21. Smith SE, Garvin KL, Jardon OM, et al: Uncemented total hip arthroplasty: Prospective analysis of the tri-lock femoral component. *Clin Orthop* 1991;269:43-50.
22. Vaughan BK, Mallory TH, Buchert PK, et al: Porous coated anatomic cementless total hip replacement: Clinical and radiographic results with minimum two-year follow-up. Presented at the Fifty-fifth Annual Meeting of the American Academy of Orthopaedic Surgeons. Atlanta: Feb. 4-9, 1988.
23. Whiteside LA: The effect of stem fit on bone hypertrophy and pain relief in cementless total hip arthroplasty. *Clin Orthop* 1989;247:138-147.
24. Hedley AK, Gruen TA, Borden LS, et al: Two-year follow-up of the PCA noncemented total hip replacement. *Hip* 1987;225-250.
25. Katz RL, Bourne RB, Rorabeck CH, et al: Total hip arthroplasty in patients with avascular necrosis of the hip: Follow-up observations on cementless and cemented operations. *Clin Orthop* 1992;281:145-151.
26. Plotz W, Gradinger R, Rechl H, et al: Cementless prosthesis of the hip joint with "spongy metal" surface: A prospective study. *Arch Orthop Trauma Surg* 1992;111:102-109.
27. Bands R, Pelker RR, Shine J, et al: The noncemented porous-coated hip prosthesis: A three-year clinical follow-up study and roentgenographic analysis. *Clin Orthop* 1991;269:209-219.
28. Ring PA: Five to fourteen year interim results of uncemented total hip arthroplasty. *Clin Orthop* 1978;137:87-95.
29. Andrew TA, Berridge D, Thomas A, et al: Long-term review of ring total hip arthroplasty. *Clin Orthop* 1985;201:111-122.
30. Bourne RB, Rorabeck CH, Chess DG, et al: A prospective two year comparison of total hip replacements. *Compl Orthop* 1991;30:108.
31. Skinner HB, Curlin FJ: Decreased pain with lower flexural rigidity of uncemented femoral prostheses. *Orthopedics* 1990;13:1223-1228.
32. Andrew TA, Flanagan JP, Gerundini M, et al: The isoelastic, noncemented total hip arthroplasty: Preliminary experience with 400 cases. *Clin Orthop* 1986;206:127-138.
33. Jakim I, Barlin C, Sweet MB: RM isoelastic total hip arthroplasty: A review of 34 cases. *J Arthroplasty* 1988;3:191-199.

Preoperative Templating and Choosing the Implant for Primary THA in the Young Patient

James A. D'Antonio, MD

Introduction

Two decades of total hip arthroplasty (THA) have shown the importance of preoperative planning. No single prosthesis is suitable for all patients, young and old. Variations in bone quality, bone shape, physiologic age, activity level, and patient expectations exist. The goals with hip reconstruction are to achieve pain relief, restoration of function, and long-term fixation, and to minimize wear. To optimize the results in the young adult and reach these goals, it is essential to select the most appropriate prosthesis, one that will obtain immediate implant stability and restore hip biomechanics. For young adults the emphasis is on cementless fixation, but both cemented and cementless systems require accurate preoperative planning and templating.

In the past, preoperative templating was performed to equalize leg length and select implant size. In my experience, traditional techniques, which used intraoperative pins and rulers, calipers, and measured resections, yielded inconsistent results. Today we template accurately to restore normal hip biomechanics, and to select an implant system that best fits the patient's anatomy.[1-3] In order to restore normal hip mechanics, the surgeon must locate the anatomic center of the acetabulum and then simultaneously restore, to as close to normal as possible, the relationship of the femur to the pelvis (both horizontal and vertical offsets). Some alteration in the hip center can be tolerated as long as it is not extreme and the appropriate hip abductor moment-arm is restored. While superior elevation of the hip center may not be detrimental to joint loading, lateral socket placement results in higher joint reactive forces and, therefore, higher implant loads.[4-6] Reconstruction of the normal femoral offsets is essential if restoration of the abductor moment-arm and optimization of leg length, stability, and implant loads is to be achieved. Valgus positioning of the femoral component (decreased horizontal offset) shortens the abductor moment-arm, increases joint reactive force and implant loads, and can increase wear at the bearing surface (Fig. 1). Varus position (increased horizontal femoral offset) decreases joint reactive force, but it increases the bending moment, shear stress, and rotational stresses on the femoral stem (Fig. 1). An increase in the vertical offset will result in excessive leg lengthening; a decrease may

result in soft tissue laxity and possible instability.

Over the past decade a variety of proportional implant systems have been developed to satisfy the needs of the majority of patients undergoing THA. The instruments used to insert these proportional implants have been improved to the point where the bones on both sides of the hip joint can be accurately shaped to accept off-the-shelf implants. Variations in the patient's anatomy, such as head-neck angle and offset, can be managed with appropriate planning and reconstructive maneuvers. For example, the femoral neck-shaft angle can vary from the average 127° in both varus and valgus directions. By combining neck resection levels with a range of available head-neck lengths, accurate templating makes it possible to match the majority of these variations. To do this it is necessary for implant manufacturers to supply the surgeon with accurately magnified templates that match the acetabular and femoral implant sizes and clearly indicate the femoral head-neck offset possibilities. In addition, it is essential that plain radiographs of both hips and both proximal femurs be obtained. The radiographs must be reproducible and must have magnification markers in place. In those patients where the anatomy is severely altered by congenital or acquired disease, off-the-shelf implant systems may not meet the patient's needs. In such cases, if cementless reconstruction is most desirable, planning to include CT scan reconstruction of the

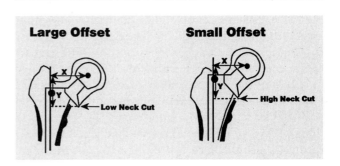

Fig. 1 This illustration of low and high neck resection levels shows how they affect abductor moment-arm while maintaining leg length. Low neck resection and the use of a longer neck (+10) creates a more varus reconstruction with increase in abductor moment-arm. The high resection illustrated, which uses a short neck (+0 head) creates a more valgus orientation and shortens the abductor moment-arm.

bony anatomy and custom implant design may be necessary. Finally, where these bony abnormalities exist, cemented total hip arthroplasty can be used, even in the young, to satisfy the goals of total hip arthroplasty.

Prosthetic Selection

Prosthetic selection in the young adult is an important part of planning and templating if long-term success is to be achieved. For the acetabulum, the state-of-the-art is a press-fit, uncemented spherical or complex geometry acetabular shell. This shell is press-fit into an undersize acetabular cavity of good bone with immediate stability. From a technical standpoint, it is most desirable to template the acetabular shell from a point just lateral to the teardrop to the lateral superior edge of the opening of the acetabulum at 40° to 45° inclination, and to prepare a slightly undersized acetabular bed (1 to 3 mm) to achieve the highest level of peripheral rim interference. We believe that this concept will prove longer lasting than our previous experiences with cemented acetabular components, but long-term studies are not yet available to prove conclusively the value of this technique. During the past ten years, extensive experience with press-fit porous-coated sockets has, in general, been excellent. However, reports of prosthetic migration and of accelerated polyethylene wear and associated bone lysis indicate that some press-fit modular cup designs of the 1980s may have been flawed.[5]

The first choice for prosthetic selection on the femoral side is one that is designed for proximal biologic fixation and that can be press-fit with a high degree of initial stability in quality bone. Experience with both straight and curved stems indicates that a high degree of success can be achieved with proximally fixed implants. With either stem shape, templating in two planes is crucial to determine size and offset possibilities at a given neck resection level. The use of curved implants allows a more anatomic positioning of the femoral stem in most femurs, but has the disadvantage of limiting the ability to machine the femur in cases in which the implant does not fit. With straight stems, accurate cutting instruments can be used safely to machine the intramedullary canal of the proximal femur to fit the off-the-shelf implants and to achieve a predictable, high level of interference fit. The use of distally fixed or more extensively coated femoral implants should be a last choice for the younger patient because these implants increase the risk of proximal stress shielding and proximal bone loss. These implants should be reserved for unusual problems, such as for fixation of a subtrochanteric osteotomy for correction of rotational or angular deformities, or perhaps where poor proximal bone precludes the use of a proximally coated stem. Distally fixed femoral

implants do offer ease of adjustment of femoral offsets with variations in neck resection level, and they are easy to machine for distal interference. Custom femoral implants are indicated when the size and fit of the femur preclude the use of stock implants to achieve the goals of total hip arthroplasty. Finally, cemented femoral stems are still occasionally necessary or useful in young adults with shortened life expectancy, poor bone quality (large diameter canal), or distorted femoral anatomy (developmental dysplasia of the hip).

Materials: Radiographs and Templates

For routine cases, an anteroposterior projection of both hips that includes the proximal femurs and a lateral radiograph of the diseased proximal femur are obtained with magnification markers. For the anteroposterior projection, both hips are included, with the proximal 8 inches of both femurs, and with the femurs internally rotated to a maximum of 15° to 20° (Fig. 2).[1,3] Internal rotation of the diseased hip is usually not possible, but in the majority of cases the opposite, or normal, hip can be internally rotated to achieve an anteroposterior appearance of the femoral neck and head as close to the zero plane as possible. It is in this plane that the true head-neck offset and femoral neck-shaft angle can best be evaluated with designed anteroposterior templates. For this reason, templating must by necessity begin with the hip that is appropriately internally rotated (usually the normal side). The templated calculations will then be transposed to the pathologic side, making the assumption that prior to the disease process the anatomy of the pathologic proximal femur matched that of the normal side, an

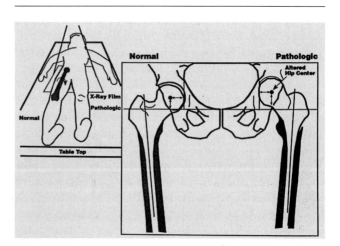

Fig. 2 Anteroposterior view of hips and proximal femurs with magnification markers on inner thigh and hips internally rotated 15° to 20° when possible.

assumption that is usually correct. In cases where bilateral hip disease exists and neither hip can be adequately internally rotated, or in those cases where there is distorted anatomy of one or both of the proximal femurs, alternative radiographs may be necessary. An anteroposterior view of the proximal femur can be obtained by elevating the pelvis to effectively internally rotate the femur, but this technique distorts the proximal femur and further alters magnification. A second technique is to obtain a posterolateral radiograph of the proximal femur and hip with the patient prone and the foot externally rotated 15° to 20°, with the opposite hip elevated to allow proper rotation of the pathologic hip.[3] The preferred lateral radiograph is a table-down lateral view (Lowenstein) of the proximal femur. With the patient in a nearly lateral position, the affected side is turned down on the x-ray table with the knee and thigh flexed towards 90°. The opposite limb is extended and the x-ray is directed perpendicular to the proximal femur and table. This technique for the lateral radiograph is easily reproducible and gives a standardized radiograph that can be used safely to gauge the maximum proximal anteroposterior dimension and overall length of the femoral stem. All radiographs are obtained using a 40-inch focal film distance with a reciprocating grid between the patient and the film.

Templates supplied by the manufacturer of the implants should be magnified to 115% and 120%. These templates should be representative of all acetabular component sizes in the anteroposterior plane and of all femoral components, illustrating both the size and offset possibilities in both the anteroposterior and lateral planes, again magnified at both 115% and 120%.

Radiographic Evaluation

Before templating, the radiographs are studied to identify normal anatomic landmarks as well as acetabular bone stock deformities or proximal femoral bone abnormalities. The following landmarks on the anteroposterior hip radiograph are marked for future reference: teardrops, ischial tuberosities, bottom of obturator foramen, top of the lesser trochanter, top of the greater trochanter, lateral superior edge of the acetabulum, and normal center of rotation of the normal hip when available. Deficiencies in the acetabular bone stock are identified, and their biomechanical significance is studied. The acetabular implant will be positioned from just lateral to the teardrop, which represents the unicortical plate at the depth of the acetabular fossa, and the lateral superior edge of the acetabulum at 40° to 45°. A line drawn beneath the ischial tuberosities or at the bottom of the obturator foramina will intersect the femurs and give a measurement of leg-length inequality. The tops of the lesser and greater trochanters, one or the other, can be used as a reference in templating to gauge the femoral offsets to optimize the reconstruction.

Templating Technique: Five Steps

Having established the magnification of the radiographs from the magnification markers for both the anteroposterior and lateral radiographs, the appropriately magnified templates are selected for use.

Step One: Leg-length determination on anteroposterior radiograph of hips Using a line connecting the bottom of the obturator foramen or the bottom of the ischial tuberosities, the intersection of that line on both femurs will be gauged from the top of the lesser trochanter to measure the leg-length inequality with the magnified template (Fig. 3).

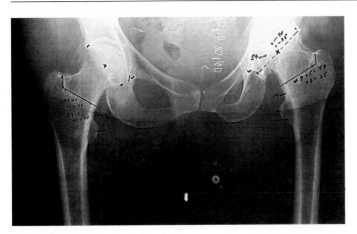
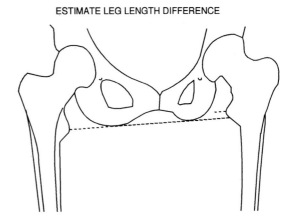

ESTIMATE LEG LENGTH DIFFERENCE

Fig. 3   This anteroposterior view of hips with lines drawn beneath ischial tuberosities where they intersect the femurs at the level of the lesser trochanter illustrates approximate leg-length difference.

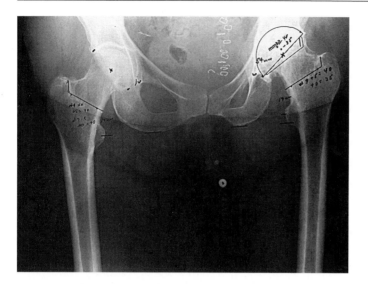

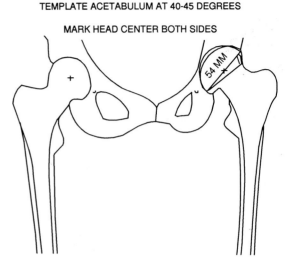

TEMPLATE ACETABULUM AT 40-45 DEGREES

MARK HEAD CENTER BOTH SIDES

54 MM

Fig. 4   Anteroposterior hips with normal acetabular center of rotation marked through template on the normal and pathologic hips placing the template just lateral to the teardrop at an inclination of 40° to 45° to the superolateral acetabular rim.

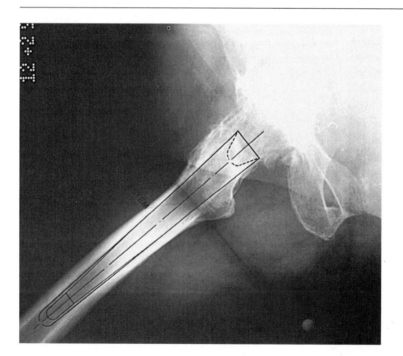

FEMORAL FIT ON PATHOLOGIC HIP

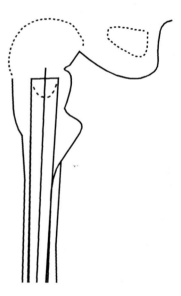

Fig. 5   Step Three: This lateral proximal femur is templated to illustrate proximal fill and overall stem length for maximum size allowable.

Step Two: Acetabular size and position on anteroposterior radiograph of hips Beginning on the normal hip, the center of rotation is marked through the template overlaying the femur and acetabulum. The socket is sized to remove the minimal amount of peripheral rim with the template positioned from just lateral to the teardrop to the superolateral edge of the acetabulum at an inclination of 40° to 45°. The center of that templated socket on the normal side should correlate closely to the anatomic center of the normal

hip. This process is then repeated on the pathologic side, again from the same position lateral to the teardrop to the pathologic lateral superior acetabular edge. Frequently, because of the disease progress and superior erosion of the acetabulum, the socket diameter size may differ from the templated normal size and result in some slight elevation of the center of rotation (Fig. 4).

Step Three: Femoral component size and length on lateral radiograph of the proximal femur The appropriately magnified lateral templates are now placed over the lateral radiograph to determine the maximum proximal femoral size and length that the femur will accommodate, whether that be for a press-fit, metaphyseal, and canal-filling prosthesis or for cemented implants that allow for an adequate cement mantle (Fig. 5).

Step Four: Femoral component sizing using anteroposterior hip radiograph Anteroposterior templates of proper magnification are placed over the normal proximal femur (most often) unless the pathologic hip can be internally rotated 20° (unusual). When templating for proximally coat-

ed implants, the proximal (metaphyseal) fill, distal diaphyseal fit, and length of stem are all appropriately noted. The implant size that fits best both proximally and distally and is within the maximum allowable size on the lateral film is selected. When using cement, an implant several sizes smaller must be used to permit an adequate cement mantle without destruction of the cancellous bone. When using extensively coated implants designed for diaphyseal fixation, an accurate estimate in both planes with regards to diameter of stem can be determined (Fig. 6).

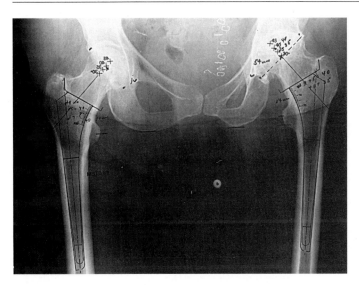
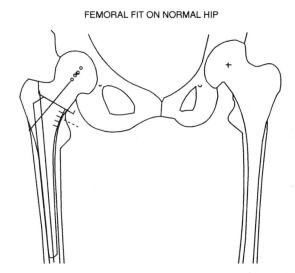

FEMORAL FIT ON NORMAL HIP

Fig. 6 Step Four: Anteroposterior hips templating normal femur for proximal fill, distal fit, and stem length to correlate with Step Three.

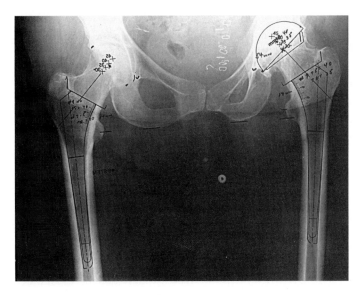
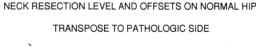
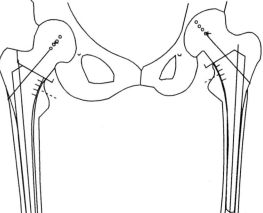

NECK RESECTION LEVEL AND OFFSETS ON NORMAL HIP

TRANSPOSE TO PATHOLOGIC SIDE

Fig. 7 Templating on anteroposterior hips beginning on the normal side to reproduce the normal femoral offsets. Neck resection level is measured from the top of the lesser trochanter, and the plan is transposed to the pathologic hip at the same neck resection level. Correlating the new head center on the pathologic hip with the new socket center will yield a leg-lengthening estimate that should approximate the leg-length discrepancy determined in Step One.

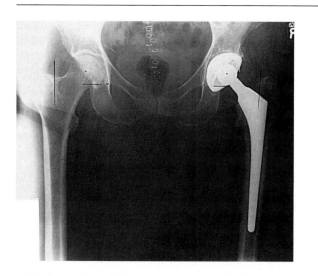 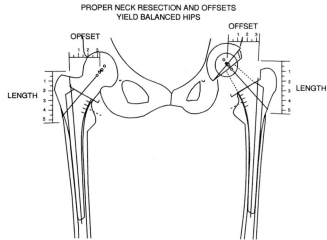

Fig. 8 A balanced hip reconstruction results from restoration of the normal socket center and femoral offsets.

Step Five: Femoral neck resection level and offset reconstruction on anteroposterior radiograph of hips Using the selected femoral size (Step Three and Step Four), the overlay templates on the normal hip are now used to determine the neck resection level that best permits reproduction of the normal neck-shaft angle and offsets for the patient. By moving the neck resection level in a proximal and distal direction, and combining this with the offset possibilities of the hip system being evaluated, the vertical and horizontal offsets can usually be duplicated closely. Once this is accomplished, the level of this neck resection is marked on the femoral neck and measured either from the tip of the greater trochanter or, preferably, from the top of the lesser trochanter. This planned resection is then transposed to the pathologic hip at the same femoral neck resection measured from the top of the lesser trochanter. If no leg-length discrepancy is present, superimposition of the center of the prosthetic head to the planned acetabular center will maintain existing leg length. However, when a discrepancy in leg length is present (Fig. 7), the new planned prosthetic head center templated and marked on the pathologic hip will not correspond to the templated planned acetabular center of rotation. The distance measured between those two centers should closely approximate the previously measured leg-length discrepancy obtained in Step One. During this important fifth templating step, when possible, templating for a midrange head-neck length (+5) will facilitate intraoperative adjustment (+0 or +10) if prosthetic seating intraoperatively is finalized at a level above or below the planned femoral neck resection level (Fig. 7). Evaluation of postoperative radiographs (Fig. 8) shows hip reconstruction that has restored the normal acetabular center of rotation and both femoral

offsets. This results in a balanced hip reconstruction with restoration of normal biomechanics. A second illustration of the templating technique is demonstrated in Figure 9. In this 46-year-old male, with slipped capital femoral epiphysis, significant alterations in hip mechanics are present. The preoperative planning process resulted in a reconstruction that not only restored his leg length equality but also insured a close approximation to the patient's normal femoral offsets and hip center of rotation.

An alternate plan for that unusual patient with distorted anatomy may be necessary where off-the-shelf stock implants do not template to a solution. Where acetabular bony abnormalities exist, the true anatomic center of rotation of the hip may be far removed from the pathologic center, as in high-riding developmental dysplasia of the hip. In this situation, accurate templating must be performed to determine the available bone for reconstruction, the possible need for structural graft, and the need for unusual socket sizes and shapes, whether they be very small, very large, or of a custom shape and size. Where femoral bony abnormalities exist, rotational deformities, such as excessive anteversion, may require a planned subtrochanteric derotational osteotomy. Angular femoral deformities are best handled by osteotomies through the level of deformity. Femoral shortening, as is seen in high-riding developmental dysplasia of the hip, may be necessary through the subtrochanteric region to complete the reconstruction. In these difficult situations, CT scanning with or without foam models can be extremely useful in planning for a reconstruction with or without custom prostheses. Finally, in these situations where a lower femoral neck resection level, poor bone quality, or appropriate fit-and-fill cannot be achieved, cement-

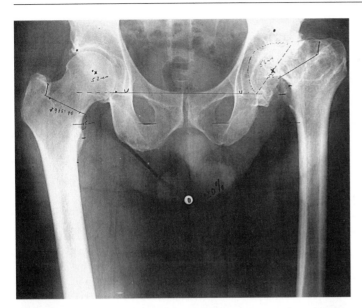

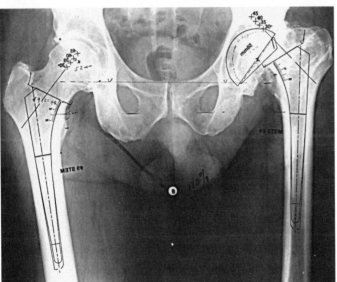

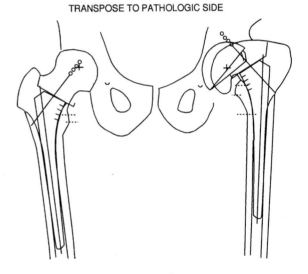

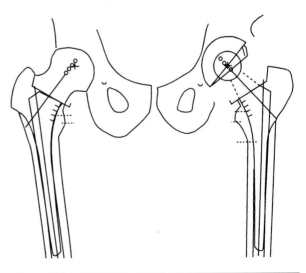

Fig. 9 Top , This anteroposterior view demonstrates significant alteration in biomechanics in a pathologic left hip. **Center left** and **right,** Preoperative templating and planning illustrates on the normal right hip a reconstructive plan, which, when transposed to the pathologic left side, restores near-normal leg length and offsets. **Bottom left** and **right,** Postoperative radiograph and illustration of reconstruction.

NECK RESECTION LEVEL AND OFFSETS ON NORMAL HIP

TRANSPOSE TO PATHOLOGIC SIDE

PROPER NECK RESECTION AND OFFSETS
YIELD BALANCED HIPS

ed, custom, or extensively coated implants may be the procedure of choice when templating to a satisfactory solution.

Postoperative radiographs must be evaluated to compare the reconstruction to the preoperative templated plan. This exercise will sharpen the surgeons' templating and planning skills

Conclusion

Preoperative templating is essential to achieve consistently good, long-term results with total hip arthroplasty. Accurate templating can help the surgeon restore proper hip biomechanics and optimize implant function and loading. Good quality radiographs of known magnification, used in combination with magnified templates, can assist the surgeon in prosthetic selection and positioning to best duplicate the patient's normal hip anatomy.

References

1. Capello WN: Preoperative planning of total hip arthroplasty, in Anderson LD (ed): American Academy of Orthopaedic Surgeons *Instructional Course Lectures Volume XXXV.* St. Louis, MO, CV Mosby, 1986, chap 26, pp 249-257.
2. DeOrio JK, Blasser KE: Indications and patient selection, in Morrey BF (ed): *Joint Replacement Arthroplasty.* New York, NY, Churchill-Livingstone, 1991, chap 39, pp 547-559.
3. Engh CA: Recent advances in cementless total hip arthroplasty using the AML prosthesis. *Techniques Orthop* 1991;6:3.
4. Johnston RC, Brand RA, Crowninshield RD: Reconstruction of the hip: A mathematical approach to determine optimum geometric relationships. *J Bone Joint Surg* 1979;61A:639-652.
5. Stulberg BN, Buly RL, Howard PL, et al: Porous coated anatomic acetabular failure: Incidence and modes of failure in uncemented total hip arthroplasty. Presented at the 59th Annual Meeting of the American Academy of Orthopaedic Surgeons, Washington, DC, 1992, p 168.
6. Yoder SA, Brand RA, Petersen DR, et al: Total hip acetabular component position affects component loosening rates. *Clin Orthop* 1988;228:79-87.

Primary Total Hip Arthroplasty in the Older Patient: Optimizing the Results

David D. Dore, MD

Harry E. Rubash, MD

Basic Templating Skills and Choosing the Implant

Preoperative planning for total hip arthroplasty (THA) is an integral part of reconstructive surgery on the adult hip. The choice of implant and method of fixation must take into account the patient's age, weight, activity level, and bone quality, as well as the presence of bone disease, tumor, or other medical problems. Preoperative templating enables the surgical team to determine the approximate size needed for the acetabular and femoral components, the prosthetic neck length required, the appropriate level of neck resection, and the leg-length difference. Having this knowledge preoperatively aids the team in avoiding intraoperative complications, reduces operative time, and identifies special needs for a particular case (eg, somatosensory evoked potentials, iliac crest bone grafting, allograft, specific type of prosthesis, or custom prosthesis). Such information also enables the formulation of alternative plans, shortens the learning curve for a new implant system, improves technical skills, and ultimately can improve the clinical results.[1-4]

Proper Radiographs for Preoperative Planning

Accurate preoperative planning requires an anteroposterior (AP) radiograph of the pelvis (Fig. 1), and an AP radiograph of the proximal half of the femur

(Fig. 2) (in both AP radiographs the hips should be internally rotated approximately 15°), and a lateral radiograph of the proximal half of the femur (Fig. 3), all of known magnification. Internal rotation of the hip is required on the AP radiograph to eliminate the normal anteversion of the hip (15° of internal rotation places the head and neck parallel to the cassette). The

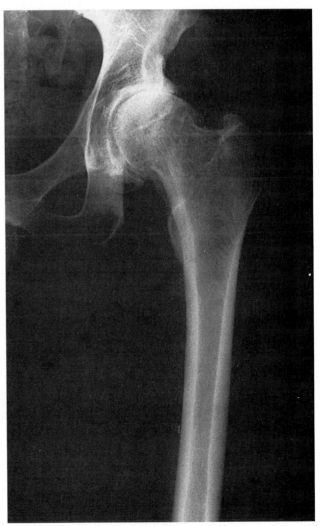

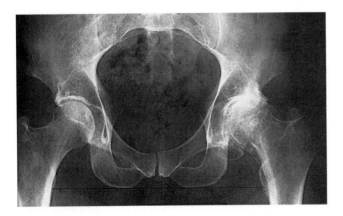

Fig. 1 Anteroposterior radiograph of the pelvis with the hips internally rotated approximately 15° to eliminate the normal anteversion of the hips. The acetabulum may be sized and the new acetabular center of rotation determined on this radiograph.

Fig. 2 Anteroposterior radiograph of the proximal half of the femur with the hip internally rotated approximately 15°. The femur may be sized and the neck resection level determined on this radiograph.

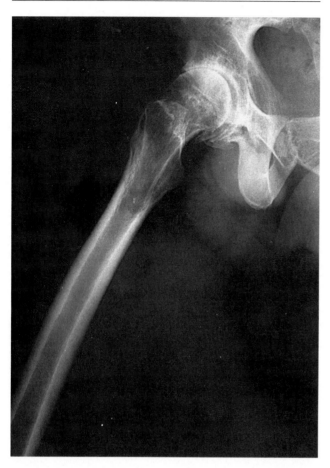

Fig. 3 Lowenstein lateral radiograph of the proximal half of the femur. Sizing of the femoral component must be performed in this plane.

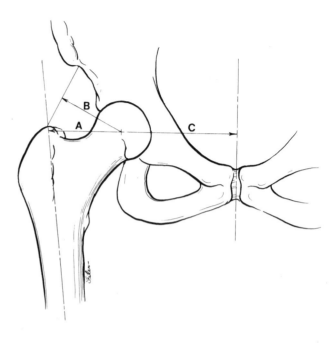

Fig. 4 Line A is the offset: the distance from the center of the femoral head to the long axis of the femur. Line B is the abductor moment arm: the distance from the femoral head to the abductor muscles. Line C is the body weight lever arm: the distance from the center of the body to the center of the femoral head.

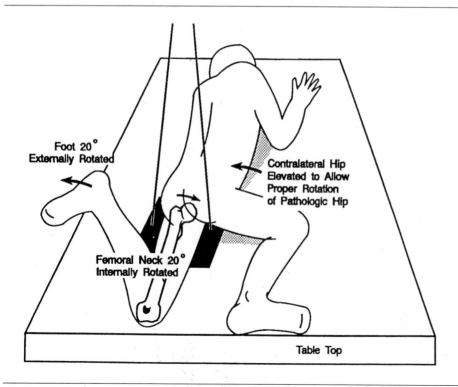

Fig. 5 The alternative technique for positioning a patient to obtain a radiograph of the proximal femur in the desired amount of internal rotation. When the hip is stiff, this is the only method that can be used to determine the internal shape of the femur in the plane of 0° of femoral neck anteversion. (Reproduced with permission from Engh CA: Recent advances in cementless total hip arthroplasty using the AML prosthesis. *Techniques Orthop* 1991;6(3):59-72, Figure 3.)

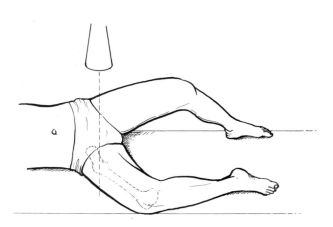

Fig. 6 Lowenstein lateral of hip and proximal femur: The patient's hip, knee, and ankle are placed on the table and the x-ray beam is centered over the lesser trochanter at a 90° angle to the proximal femur.

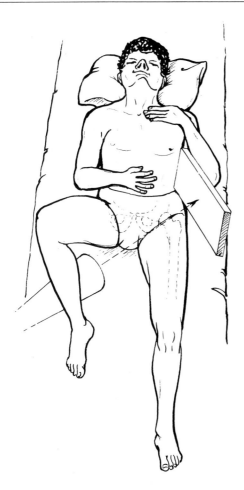

Fig. 7 Modified surgical lateral: The patient's leg is extended and internally rotated 15° to 20°. The contralateral leg is suspended above the patient. The x-ray cassette is placed parallel to the neck; the beam is perpendicular to the neck and centered over the femoral head and neck.

templates are manufactured for use in this plane; thus, the true neck-shaft angle and offset (distance from center of femoral head to long axis of the femur) can be measured (Fig. 4). Patients with advanced arthritis of the hip often have an external rotation contracture and cannot internally rotate the hip 15° to 20°. In most such cases, one can assume that before disease onset the diseased hip was identical to the contralateral normal hip. Therefore, femoral templating can be performed on an AP radiograph of the normal hip in the appropriate amount of internal rotation. Occasionally, this assumption may not be valid or both hips may be diseased, and instead, an AP radiograph of the involved hip with the femoral neck in neutral version must be obtained in the manner described by Engh (Fig. 5).[2] Magnification of the radiograph is determined by placing a marker of known dimensions (such as a plexiglass rod with lead spheres embedded in both ends exactly 100 mm apart) at the level of the greater trochanter and parallel to the x-ray cassette. This known distance then is measured on the radiograph to determine the magnification.

The Lowenstein lateral view is our lateral radiograph of choice for preoperative templating (Fig. 6). This view is obtained by placing the patient's hip, knee, and ankle on the table and centering the x-ray beam over the lesser trochanter at a 90° angle to the proximal femur. The magnification marker is placed on the anterior thigh, halfway between the medial and lateral borders, with the superior edge at the level of the crease of the leg. This view does not distort the femoral canal shape and shows the maximum amount of anterior femoral bow. Other lateral radiographs may be used for preoperative templating. The modified surgical lateral view is obtained by fully extending the involved

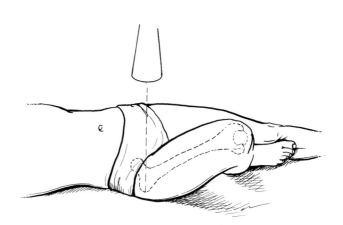

Fig. 8 The unilateral frog-leg lateral: the hip and knee are flexed, and the hip is abducted 40°. The beam is perpendicular to the table and centered over the femoral head and neck.

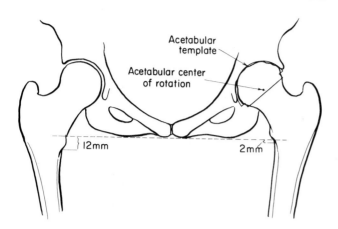

Fig. 9 Templating begins on the anteroposterior radiograph of the pelvis. A line is drawn across the ischial tuberosities, and leg-length differences due to hip disease are calculated by measuring from this line to a fixed point on the lesser trochanters. In this example, the left leg is 10 mm shorter as a result of hip disease. The acetabulum is sized and the acetabular center of rotation marked.

straight (to eliminate any contraction at the hip and/or knee) or a computerized tomographic scanogram (if the contraction cannot be eliminated) can be helpful in preoperative planning. If a fixed hip flexion contracture goes undetected, the clinical measurement of the involved leg will be too short; consequently, release of the flexion contracture during THA may over-lengthen the leg.

Next, the acetabular templates are used to determine the size of the acetabular component needed (Fig. 9). The template should contact the lateral margin of the teardrop; its inferior edge should extend just below the teardrop, and it should span the distance from the teardrop to the acetabular lateral rim at approximately 45°. The center of rotation of the acetabular component then can be marked on the radiograph.

The size of the femoral component to be used is determined by templating on the AP radiograph of the involved hip and proximal femur (Fig. 10). For femoral components that will be cemented, one should allow at least 2 mm circumferentially about the

leg, internally rotating the foot 15° to 20°, and suspending the contralateral leg above the patient. The cassette is placed parallel to the long axis of the femoral neck. The central ray is directed perpendicular to the long axis of the femoral neck and centered over the femoral head and neck (Fig. 7). The unilateral frog-leg lateral is obtained by having the patient flex the affected hip and knee as far as possible. The foot is then turned inward to brace against the opposite knee, and the hip is abducted approximately 40°; the central ray is directed perpendicular to the table and centered on the femoral head and neck (Fig. 8).

Templating Skills

Planning begins with the AP pelvic radiograph, on which a line is drawn across the most inferior aspect of the ischial tuberosities (Fig. 9). The distance between this line and a fixed point on the lesser trochanters accurately indicates any leg-length discrepancy due to hip disease. This difference in leg lengths must be compared to measurements obtained clinically.[5] These clinical measurements must be obtained with both lower extremities in a symmetrical position to determine the true leg-length difference. Failure to do this when an extremity has a fixed contracture can lead to erroneous clinical measurements. A patient may have unequal leg lengths for reasons not associated with the current hip disease, such as a prior fracture, growth plate disturbance, or congenital disorder. In such cases, a scanogram performed with the legs

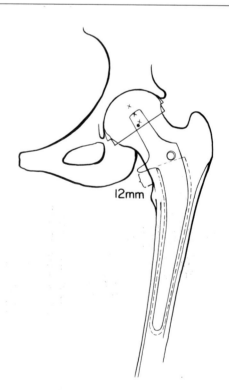

Fig. 10 The anteroposterior radiograph of the involved hip is used for selecting the size of the femoral component and the level of neck resection. By performing a neck cut approximately 12 mm above the lesser trochanter and using a medium length neck, the involved leg will be lengthened 10 mm (the vertical distance from the femoral center of rotation is 10 mm above the acetabular center of rotation), thereby equalizing the leg lengths.

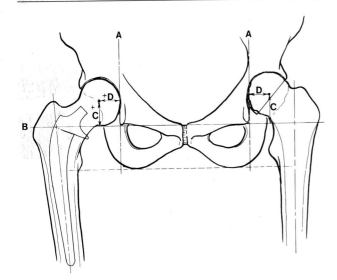

Fig. 11 When a radiograph of the involved hip with appropriate internal rotation cannot be obtained, femoral templating can be performed on the contralateral normal hip. The acetabulum is templated on the involved (left) side in the routine fashion. The distance from the new acetabular center of rotation to vertical (A) and horizontal (B) lines through the teardrop are measured (distances D and C, respectively). The new acetabular center of rotation is then transferred to the normal (right) hip and templating of the proximal femur is performed in the routine fashion. The prosthetic neck length (medium) and neck resection level (12 mm above the lesser trochanter) that most closely reproduce the biomechanics of the normal hip should be selected.

implant for the cement mantle; most current templates have this margin built in. A femoral template that best fits the femoral canal is chosen. For proximally porous-coated press-fit implants, a femoral template that best fits the porous-coated section of the prosthesis is chosen. The diaphyseal portion of the femur is assessed to ensure the amount of bone is adequate to withstand machining of the canal for intimate contact of the cylindrical portion of the prosthesis. For stems that have porous-coating distally, the femoral component is sized based on diaphyseal fill. Often, it is necessary to drill the intramedullary canal until the medial and lateral endosteal surfaces are parallel for at least 3 cm. The next step is to measure the diameter of the prosthesis that will contact the endosteal surfaces over the surgically created isthmus and the length of the prosthesis over which porous coating must be applied in order to reach through the isthmus.

The neck resection level and prosthetic neck length then are determined. This can be performed on the involved side if significant distortion of the hip joint and change in the offset have not occurred. If they have, or if a film with appropriate rotation of the

involved side is not obtainable, the contralateral normal side of the pelvis can be used. Templating of the normal rather than the severely distorted hip will more reliably produce normal hip biomechanics postoperatively. Templating on the involved side: if no leg-length discrepancy exists, superimposing the centers of rotation of the prosthetic head and acetabulum will maintain the existing leg length and offset. If leg lengths differ, then the vertical distance from the acetabular center to the femoral center should equal this difference. With the femoral component in the desired position, the neck resection level can be measured from the superior aspect of the lesser trochanter; a neck length then is chosen that will equalize the leg lengths.

Templating on the noninvolved hip, the prosthetic acetabular center of rotation of the involved hip must be transferred to the normal side. To accomplish this, the distance is measured from the planned acetabular center of rotation to horizontal and vertical reference lines through the teardrop (Fig. 11), and this position is transferred to the normal side.[2] This position will be different from the center of the normal femoral head. Then the previously determined femoral template is adjusted vertically within the canal to approximate the acetabular center to one of the prosthetic femoral head centers. The femoral neck resection level and prosthetic neck length are recorded. Placement of the acetabular and femoral components in these positions, with the neck resection made at the appropriate level and use of the predetermined prosthetic neck length will place the diseased femur the same distance from the pelvis as the contralateral femur (offset and leg-length difference caused by hip disease will be equalized).

The femoral neck osteotomy level will affect the size of the femoral component needed to fill the proximal femur. A higher neck cut will necessitate a larger proximal implant; a lower cut, a smaller implant (Fig. 12). Several press fit implant systems offer various-sized proximal components to maximize the proximal fit. Based on the osteotomy level, the appropriate size of the proximal component is chosen.

The lateral femoral template then is placed on the lateral radiograph to ensure that the stem diameter and stem length are appropriate in this plane and to check for femoral anatomical variations (Fig. 13). This view is especially important in planning for the longer-stem implants used primarily in revision surgery, in which particular attention must be paid to the amount of anterior bow. In selecting the size and length of a specific implant, one major consideration is the avoidance of intraoperative perforation of the cortex. With the femoral template at the desired vertical level, the press fit stem should achieve three point contact with the endosteal surface.

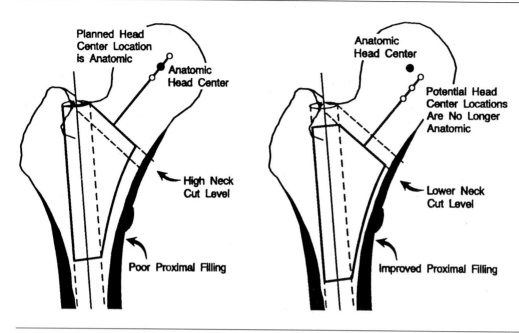

Planned Head Center Location is Anatomic

Anatomic Head Center

High Neck Cut Level

Poor Proximal Filling

Anatomic Head Center

Potential Head Center Locations Are No Longer Anatomic

Lower Neck Cut Level

Improved Proximal Filling

Fig. 12 Adjustments in the vertical position of the prosthesis within the femur will affect both the proximal canal fill and the prosthetic head center location. In the case example illustrated, a prosthesis with larger medial-to-lateral dimension would be required to fill the canal at the best possible neck resection level. (Reproduced with permission from Engh CA: Recent advances in cementless total hip arthroplasty using the AML prosthesis. *Techniques Orthop* 1991;6 (3):59-72, Figure 11.)

Changes in the Acetabular Position

Medialization of the Cup

Though Charnley originally advocated medialization of the acetabular component to decrease the body weight lever arm (Fig. 4) and, thereby, decrease joint reactive forces; the ability to do so is limited by the medial wall of the acetabulum. Excessive medial placement of the socket will result in weakening or penetration of the medial wall, which may necessitate bone grafting. Component placement in an overly medial position also causes increased stresses in the peripheral rim, decreased offset, abductor muscle laxity, and less hip stability. Moreover, the patient will be more likely to suffer impingement on both the anterior and posterior column, fracture of the acetabulum, development of progressive acetabular protrusio, and loosening of the implant. A clinical situation in which medialization of the femoral head has occurred is seen in patients with acetabular protrusio. Acetabular protrusio has been observed in 5.2% of patients with rheumatoid arthritis and is associated with several other conditions including ankylosing spondylitis, osteomalacia, osteoporosis, rickets, Paget's disease, and traumatic injury.[6] Radiographically, acetabular protrusio is diagnosed and progression followed by the relationship of the femoral head to Köhler's line (ilioischial line, a line drawn from the medial border of the ilium to the medial border of the ischium) and the center-edge (CE) angle of Wiberg[7] (the angle formed by a vertical line drawn through the center of the femoral head and a line from the center of the femoral head to the lateral border of

the acetabulum) (Fig. 14). Acetabular protrusio is present if the femoral head has migrated medial to Köhler's line or the CE angle is greater than 35°.

Preoperative templating should place the cup so that it assumes its true anatomic position, thereby restoring proper joint biomechanics.[8] The cup should

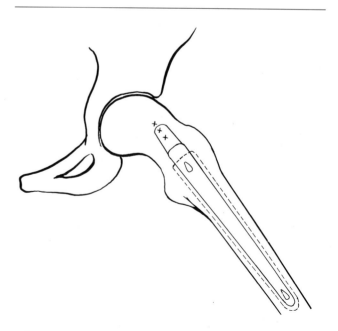

Fig. 13 The Lowenstein lateral radiograph is used for lateral templating. The chosen implant template is placed at the planned neck resection level, and the stem diameter and length are assessed in this plane.

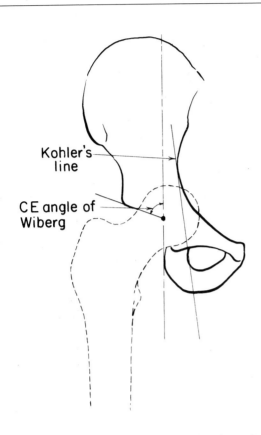

Fig. 14 Köhler's line (ilioischial line) is a line drawn from the medial border of the ilium to the medial border of the ischium. The center-edge (CE) angle of Wiberg is the angle formed by a vertical line through the center of the femoral head and a line from the center of the femoral head to the lateral border of the acetabulum. Acetabular protrusio is present if the femoral head migrates medial to Köhler's line or the CE angle of Wiberg is greater than 35°.

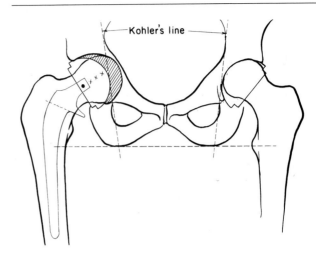

Fig. 15 Acetabular protrusio: The acetabular cup is placed as close as possible to its anatomic location. The goal is to obtain a stable hip through good peripheral rim contact. Medial bone grafting is then performed. The femur is then sized in the routine fashion. The neck resection level and prosthetic neck length that will most closely equalize leg lengths and restore normal offset is chosen.

be placed just lateral to the teardrop, and should span the distance from the teardrop to the lateral edge of the acetabulum; the cup's inferior margin should be just below the teardrop (Fig. 15). The goal is to achieve good peripheral rim contact, and then bone graft the defect in the medial wall. Medial displacement of the cup can be further resisted in severe acetabular protrusio with the use of heavy wire mesh, metal rings, or custom cups.

The prosthetic acetabulum is typically larger than the natural socket and the center of rotation is more superior than on the normal side because of the axial and superior migration of the femoral head associated with protrusio acetabuli. In addition, the involved leg preoperatively is shorter and has less offset than on the normal side. Templating the contralateral normal hip, as previously described, can indicate the true amount of offset and the femoral neck resection level required to equalize leg length in patients with hip disease.

However, if the protrusio acetabulum is longstanding, soft tissue tightness may prevent the full restoration of offset and leg length. Often, a lower neck cut, a shorter prosthetic neck, or a prosthesis with less offset can be used to maximize leg length, joint biomechanics, and stability of the hip.

Lateralization of the Cup

Many patients with advanced degenerative joint disease of the hip have a large medial osteophyte that requires considerable reaming in order to reach the old medial wall of the acetabulum (unicortical plate) (Fig. 16). Intraoperatively, the transverse acetabular ligament can be seen crossing the acetabular notch. The notch leads into the acetabular fossa, which is at the center of the articular surface of the acetabulum. The inferior edge of the acetabular fossa corresponds to the bottom of the radiographic teardrop (Fig. 17). The lateral aspect of the teardrop represents the unicortical plate at the depth of the acetabular fossa. Reaming of the medial osteophyte is most easily accomplished with a small reamer and should be carried back to, but not through, the unicortical plate. Then, progressively larger, but not more medial, reaming should continue until peripheral contact is made. Failure to reach to the depth of the acetabular fossa will cause lateralization of the cup, which, in turn, can result in less bony coverage of the cup, less-than-ideal acetabular bed bleeding, and consequently decreased ingrowth. Lateralization of the cup will also increase the abductor lever arm and the offset.

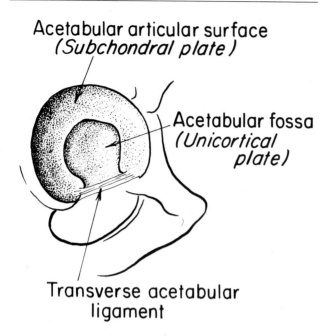

Acetabular articular surface
(Subchondral plate)

Acetabular fossa
(Unicortical plate)

Transverse acetabular ligament

Fig. 16 The anatomic landmarks of the acetabulum should be located intraoperatively.

Superior Placement of the Cup

Superior positioning of the cup may cause shortening of the leg unless a longer prosthetic neck is used or a higher neck cut made. If the cup is made to span down to the bottom of the acetabular fossa, then a larger-than-normal cup will be required, which will necessitate greater reaming of the anterior and posterior columns to obtain a hemispherical shape.

Patients with developmental dysplasia of the hip (DDH) who develop significant arthritis requiring THA can present a challenging problem to the orthopaedic surgeon. Crowe and associates[9] classified dysplastic hips according to the amount of subluxation: group I, less than 50%; group II, 50-75%; group III, 75-100%; and group IV, more than 100%. Many surgeons place the cup in a superior and lateral position in the area of the false acetabulum. However, several studies have shown that this practice increases forces in the hip and subsequently promotes the risk of loosening for both the femoral and acetabular components.[9-15] Ideally, the center of the hip is placed at the anatomic position. This site can be identified intraoperatively by locating the anterior inferior iliac spine, ischial tuberosity, and the obturator foramen and then reaming at the junction of these three anatomical landmarks.[9] However, patients with DDH often do not have adequate bone stock in the region of the true acetabulum, and superior placement of the component (without lateralization) or bone grafting superiorly may be

required.[9,13,16] Because of the bone deficiency in DDH, the prosthetic acetabular component is smaller than normal and often a component that is not routinely available may be needed.[9,17]

In DDH, the proximal femur is also dysplastic, causing increased anteversion and posterior migration of the greater trochanter. This condition may require a femoral component with a straighter stem and a smaller diameter than normal, a component system with variable version, or a proximal osteotomy.[9,17,18] If a high hip center has been chosen for acetabular placement, the leg will be shortened; a high neck cut or a longer prosthetic neck may partially compensate for this. The use of a high hip center also increases the likelihood of impingement on the anterior column with flexion, adduction, and internal rotation and on the posterior column with extension and external rotation. Often, the anterior inferior iliac spine, a portion of the ischium, or a portion of the greater trochanter must be resected to improve stability.

Lengthening of the leg is often a desirable event in patients with DDH. If the preoperative plan is to gain more than 2 cm of length, somatosensory evoked potentials (SSEP) can be used intraoperatively to help monitor peroneal and posterior tibial nerve function.[19] We currently use SSEP on all patients we plan to lengthen 2 cm or more. Intraoperatively, leg lengths can be monitored by placing a pin in the ilium and measuring to a mark on the proximal femur, distal to the planned femoral neck osteotomy site before hip dislocation.[20,21] After placement of the trial femoral components, this distance can be measured again and com-

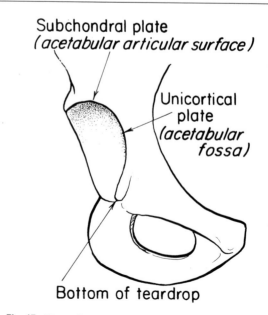

Subchondral plate
(acetabular articular surface)

Unicortical plate
(acetabular fossa)

Bottom of teardrop

Fig. 17 The radiographic landmarks of the acetabulum.

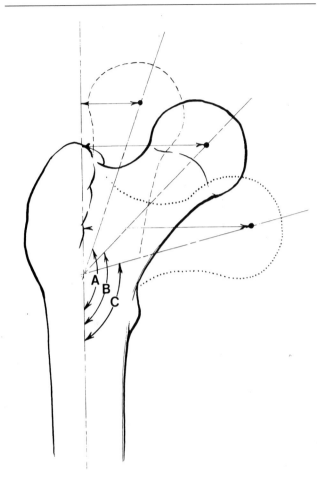

Fig. 18 The neck shaft angle will affect the vertical height of the neck and the offset. Coxa valga (A=160°) increases the vertical neck length and decreases the offset, whereas a normal neck shaft angle (B=135°) results in an intermediate vertical neck length and offset. Coxa vara (C=115°) causes a decrease in the vertical neck height and an increase in offset.

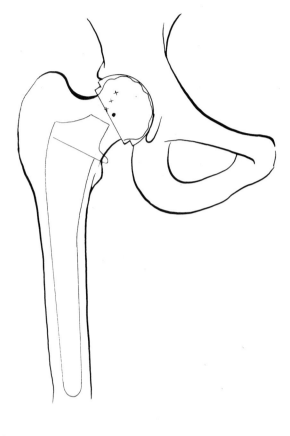

Fig. 19 Patients with coxa vara have apparent greater trochanteric overgrowth, increased offset, and decreased vertical neck length. Consequently, the neck resection level must be lower and/or a shorter prosthetic neck length must be used to avoid over-lengthening of the leg. The increased offset in patients with coxa vara is best handled by using a prosthesis with built-in increased off-set in order to avoid abductor muscle laxity and instability. Abductor musculature may also be tightened by lengthening the leg or performing a greater trochanteric advancement.

pared to the initial reading. We use this simple means of monitoring leg length in all total hip arthroplasties.

Inferior Placement of the Cup

When the cup is placed too inferiorly, the bone will be of poor quality and superior coverage of the cup will be decreased, thereby sacrificing cup stability. In addition, the center of the cup will be lower than normal, thus lengthening the leg unless a shorter prosthetic neck and/or lower neck cut is used.

Changes in Femoral Neck-Shaft Angle

Coxa Vara

Patients with coxa vara have a shortened leg and a hip with increased offset (Fig. 18). Failure to take this into consideration can lead to an over-lengthened leg and/or instability. The acetabulum is templated in the normal fashion. A lower-than-normal femoral neck cut is needed to avoid over-lengthening. In addition, the increased offset requires the use of a prosthesis with increased offset. If not, trochanteric advancement may be needed intraoperatively to help stabilize the hip. Use of a longer prosthetic neck or higher femoral neck cut will lengthen the hip, which, by increasing the tension in the abductor musculature will increase hip stability; however, limb lengthening may not be the desired result (Fig. 19).

A patient with coxa vara and a femoral neck fracture is particularly prone to adverse clinical results when treated with prosthetic replacement. Failure to recognize and adapt the procedure in patients with coxa vara, for example, performing a standard neck cut, using a low-offset prosthesis, and adjusting prosthetic neck length to maximize stability, can result in significant clinical lengthening and nerve palsy (Fig. 20).

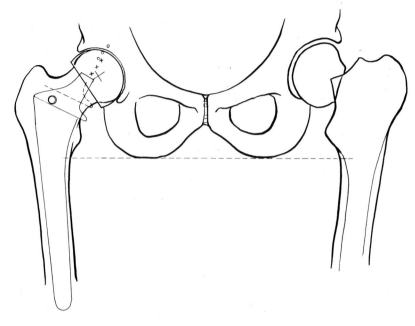

Fig. 20 Displaced femoral neck fractures which require prosthetic replacement are best templated on the contralateral normal side. In patients with coxa vara, a low-neck osteotomy and placement of a shorter-neck prosthesis will more closely reproduce the normal anatomy ("____" represents the neck resection level and "+" represents the femoral head center of rotation). A more normal neck osteotomy level ("----" represents the neck resection level and "o" represents the femoral head center of rotation) and placement of a longer-neck prosthesis will significantly lengthen the leg.

Coxa Valga

Patients with coxa valga have a relatively long leg and decreased offset (Fig. 18). On radiographs taken with the hips externally rotated, the neck shaft angle appears to be higher than normal. Therefore, if the patient cannot internally rotate the hip enough to achieve neutral neck version, femoral templating should be performed on the contralateral normal hip, or the alternative AP radiograph described above (Fig. 5) should be obtained for the involved hip to allow proper templating. In patients with true coxa valga, the acetabulum is templated in the normal fashion. The femur requires a higher-than-normal neck cut to maintain length and the femoral component should not have an increased offset (Fig. 21). If a normal neck cut and a graduated offset prosthesis are used, the radiographic findings appear more normal, but, the extremity may be too short, the abductor muscles may be tight, and adduction may be limited.

Offset

Femoral offset is one of the most effective and accessible mechanical variables that the surgeon can manipulate to optimize the biomechanics in THA.[22] A decrease in offset compared to a patient's normal anatomic offset can lead to instability, limp, and increased joint reactive force. The decrease in the abductor lever arm raises the energy requirements for gait. Stability is diminished by both bony impinge-ment and soft tissue laxity, and the increase in joint reactive force potentially hastens the failure of one or both components. Conversely, an increase in the off-set increases the abductor lever arm and causes a decrease in the abductor force required for gait, in joint reactive force, and in overall energy require-ments for gait (Fig. 4). In addition, the risk of both bony impingement and soft tissue laxity are reduced. Although increased offset increases the bending moment of the prosthesis, the resultant strain in the prosthesis is still well below the fatigue strain of the superalloys. Intraoperatively, if the patient's anatomic offset is found to exceed the prosthetic offset, three remedies are available. The first is to transfer the greater trochanter distally, thus reducing the instabil-ity and decreasing the likelihood of limping. Second, a longer prosthetic neck can be used, thus lengthen-ing the leg, increasing the offset, reducing abductor laxity, and increasing stability. Finally, a prosthesis with greater offset can be used. This is the best solu-tion, but the implant may not be available intraopera-tively, especially if preoperative planning did not allow for this possibility.

Summary

Preoperative planning is the first step in adult reconstructive surgery of the hip. When executed properly, it provides a template of the procedure for the whole surgical team. Thorough planning also

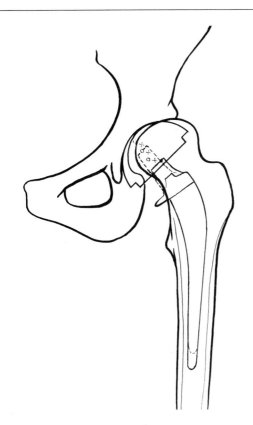

Fig. 21 In patients with coxa valga, a higher-than-normal femoral neck resection level and a femoral component without increased offset should be used ("x" represents the femoral head center of rotation of the femoral component without increased offset, "o" represents the femoral head center of rotation of the femoral component with increased offset).

helps the team anticipate intraoperative problems and avert complications. It reduces surgical trial and error, thus reducing operative time. Planning shortens the learning curve for a new implant system, improves technical skills for performing THA, and ultimately can improve the clinical results.

References

1. Capello WN: Preoperative planning of total hip arthroplasty, in Anderson LD (ed): American Academy of Orthopaedic Surgeons *Instructional Course Lectures, XXXV.* St. Louis, MO, CV Mosby, 1986, chap 26, pp 249-257.
2. Engh CA: Recent advances in cementless total hip arthroplasty using the AML prosthesis. *Techniques Orthop* 1991;6:59-72.
3. Fitzgerald RH Jr, Brindley GW, Kavanagh BF: The uncemented total hip arthroplasty: Intraoperative femoral fractures. *Clin Orthop* 1988;235:61-66.
4. Knight JL, Atwater RD: Preoperative planning for total hip arthroplasty: Quantitating its utility and precision. *J Arthroplasty* 1992;7(Suppl):403-409.
5. Abraham WD, Dimon JH III: Leg length discrepancy in total hip arthroplasty. *Orthop Clin North Am* 1992;23:201-209.
6. Hastings DE, Parker SM: Protrusio acetabuli in rheumatoid arthritis. *Clin Orthop* 1975;108:76-83.
7. McCollum DE, Nunley JA, Harrelson JM: Bone-grafting in total hip replacement for acetabular protrusion. *J Bone Joint Surg* 1980;62A:1065-1073.
8. Ranawat CS, Dorr LD, Inglis AE: Total hip arthroplasty in protrusio acetabuli of rheumatoid arthritis. *J Bone Joint Surg* 1980;62A:1059-1065.
9. Crowe JF, Mani VJ, Ranawat CS: Total hip replacement in congenital dislocation and dysplasia of the hip. *J Bone Joint Surg* 1979;61A:15-23.
10. Dunn HK, Hess WE: Total hip reconstruction in chronically dislocated hips. *J Bone Joint Surg* 1976;58A:838-845.
11. Johnston RC, Brand RA, Crowninshield RD: Reconstruction of the hip: A mathematical approach to determine optimum geometric relationships. *J Bone Joint Surg* 1979;61A:639-652.
12. Linde F, Jensen J, Pilgaard S: Charnley arthroplasty in osteoarthritis secondary to congenital dislocation or subluxation of the hip. *Clin Orthop* 1988;227:164-171.
13. Russotti GM, Harris WH: Proximal placement of the acetabular component in total hip arthroplasty: A long-term follow-up study. *J Bone Joint Surg* 1991;73A:587-592.
14. Tronzo RG, Okin EM: Anatomic restoration of congenital hip dysplasia in adulthood by total hip displacement. *Clin Orthop* 1975;106:94-98.
15. Yoder SA, Brand RA, Pedersen DR, et al: Total hip acetabular component position affects component loosening rates. *Clin Orthop* 1988;228:79-87.
16. Harris WH, Crothers O, Oh I: Total hip replacement and femoral-head bone-grafting for severe acetabular deficiency in adults. *J Bone Joint Surg* 1977;59A:752-759.
17. Woolson ST, Harris WH: Complex total hip replacement for dysplastic or hypoplastic hips using miniature or microminiature components. *J Bone Joint Surg* 1983;65A:1099-1108.
18. McQueary FG, Johnston RC: Coxarthrosis after congenital dysplasia: Treatment by total hip arthroplasty without acetabular bone-grafting. *J Bone Joint Surg* 1988;70A:1140-1144.
19. Wasielewski RC, Crossett LS, Rubash HE: Neural and vascular injury in total hip arthroplasty. *Orthop Clin North Am* 1992;23:219-235.
20. McGee HM, Scott JH: A simple method of obtaining equal leg length in total hip arthroplasty. *Clin Orthop* 1985;194:269-270.
21. Woolson ST, Harris WH: A method of intraoperative limb length measurement in total hip arthroplasty. *Clin Orthop* 1985;194:207-210.
22. Steinberg B, Harris WH: The "offset" problem in total hip arthroplasty. *Contemp Orthop* 1992;24:556-562.

Total Hip Replacement in the Elderly: Cost-Effective Alternatives

Brian G. Evans, MD

Eduardo A. Salvati, MD

Introduction

Total hip arthroplasty (THA) is a common elective procedure in orthopaedic surgery today, particularly in the elderly. During the last few decades, this segment of the population has demonstrated the largest increase in numbers, a trend that is expected to continue into the next century. In view of escalating health-care costs, pressure is being applied to hospitals and physicians to reduce expenditures and the length of stay (LOS) of patients in the hospital. The cost of orthopaedic implants is also being reviewed in a critical fashion, and an increasing number of institutions are including cost in the selection process. For this paper elderly was defined arbitrarily as age greater than 80 years. The authors recognize that many factors in addition to chronologic age contribute to the physiologic age of an individual patient.

Hospital Cost and Length of Stay

The average hospital cost at The Hospital for Special Surgery (HSS) for the 890 primary THAs performed during 1991, in patients younger than 80 years of age, was $14,465 (range $6,376 to $72,510). During that same period, the average cost for the 87 primary THAs in patients 80 years of age and older was $17,074 (range $7,455 to $32,703). The increased cost of $2,609 (18%) for the elderly group was statistically significant (p<0.001) as well as fiscally significant. The average hospital cost for all patients receiving a primary THA in 1991 was $14,697. In 1992, the average cost for primary THA increased to $16,255, an increase of $1,558 (11%).

The LOS for all patients admitted for a primary THA was 10.9 days; for those 80 years of age or older it was 13.2 days. Thus, hospitalization for patients in the older group was approximately 18% more expensive, and their hospital stay was two days longer than for the general population.

The average hospital cost of a one-stage bilateral THA performed during 1991 was $24,459 (range $13,421 to $63,673). That year, one-stage bilateral THA was performed in only three patients older than 80 years of age. The average cost was $38,094 (range $30,687 to $44,747), or $14,445 (59%) more expensive. Comparing the data for single THA and one-stage bilateral THA for the patients younger than 80, the bilateral procedure is $9,762 (66%) more expensive. However, in patients over the age of 80 the procedure is $21,020 (123%) more expensive.

The average LOS of 98 patients with a one-stage bilateral THA was 14.52 days, 3.58 days longer than a single primary THA. In patients 80 years of age or older the average LOS was 24.67 days, 11 days longer than a primary single THA in the same age group.

While the number of patients 80 years of age or older who had a bilateral THA was small, their length of stay was almost twice as long as that required for a single primary THA (24.67 versus 13.67 days), and their hospitalization cost was an additional $21,020, more than twice the cost of a unilateral THA in the same age group. While many medical and social factors must be considered prior to one-stage bilateral THA, this procedure is also more costly for the elderly than for the general population.

Results of THA in the Elderly

Several studies have investigated the results of THA in elderly patients. Holmberg[1] compared the six-year survival of 646 patients undergoing THA, with a mean age of 74 years, to an age- and sex-matched control group from the general population (all individuals in both groups were at least 40 years of age). At six years, the cumulative mortality rate was 15% for elective THA in patients with rheumatoid or osteoarthritis, significantly lower than the control rate of 36%. The highest cumulative mortality (50% at six years) was noted in patients who had a femoral neck fracture and who were 80 years of age or older.

Pettine and associates[2] compared the results of elective THA in patients 80 years of age or older with a control group of patients aged 64 to 67, chosen to represent the average THA patient. The mean length of stay was 18 days in the elderly group and 16 days in the control group. In the elderly group, 51% had minor and 8% had major complications, compared with 26% and 2% within the control group. One patient in the control group and none in the elderly population died while hospitalized. At five year follow-up, 20 of the 91 elderly patients had died (22%); in the control group 7 of 87 patients died (8%). Clinical evaluation at follow-up revealed 66% of the elderly patients to be ambulating well without complaints related to the THA. Twelve patients, 13%, were noted to be confined to a wheelchair for reasons unrelated to their arthroplasty.

Ekelund and associates[3] also studied the outcome of THA in a group of patients 80 years of age or older. They followed 157 patients with 162 arthroplasties for one year after THA. The patients were divided into two groups based on preoperative diagnosis. Seventy-nine patients, 84 hips, were classified in the degenerative joint disease (DJD) group with a preoperative diagnosis of osteoarthritis, rheumatoid arthritis, or atraumatic osteonecrosis of the femoral head. The fracture group included 78 patients (78 arthroplasties) who were treated primarily with a THA for a proximal fracture, after failure of primary fixation, or for posttraumatic arthritis. Four patients died in the first three months following surgery; an additional three patients died between three and 12 months following surgery. The cumulative mortality at one year was 7 patients (4.5%).

Eighty percent of patients had no complications within the first year. Four patients had a deep venous thrombosis, three a nonfatal myocardial infarction, three had transient renal insufficiency, and one patient developed pneumonia in the early postoperative period. One patient developed a colonic ileus, required a colostomy, and was later found to have a primary colon tumor, requiring resection. Two patients were found to have a deep infection and were treated successfully with two-stage reimplantation and intravenous antibiotics. Fifteen hips dislocated (9.2%), four in the DJD group and 11 (14%) in the fracture group. Nine (82%) of these, all in the fracture group, became recurrent. The dislocation rate was 11% with the lateral approach without trochanteric osteotomy and 4% with the posterior approach. No dislocations occurred in 13 patients who had a lateral approach with a trochanteric osteotomy. Asymptomatic aseptic loosening was noted in five patients at one year. One additional patient had a revision at one year for symptomatic aseptic loosening.

The mean LOS was 13 days. After surgery, 97% of patients in the DJD group and 83% in the fracture group returned to their previous living situation. At one-year follow-up, good to excellent results were found in 94.5% of the DJD group and in 80% of the fracture group.

Boettcher[4] also studied a group of 42 patients 80 years of age and older who were treated with a THA. Of these patients, 75% experienced a complication. The most common complications were excessive bleeding (31 patients), postoperative confusion (12 patients), urinary tract infection (4 patients) and dislocation (4 patients). The average LOS was 16 days, compared to 12 days for the younger patients. One in-hospital death occurred. Of the remaining 41 patients, 50% were alive at five-year follow-up. The cost for surgery was $12,250 per patient or $514,500 for 42 patients. The comparable cost for one year of nursing

home care was $30,000 per patient or $1,260,000 for the group. The author calculated an overall savings of $3,885,000 for the care for the remaining 41 patients. However, this savings calculation assumes that all those patients without THA surgery will require nursing home care, an assumption that may not be accurate. Also, some patients who have THA may require nursing home care postoperatively. However, disabled patients who do not have THA often require additional help with activities of daily living, which can be expensive. THA provides additional benefit in terms of pain relief, ambulation, function, reducing the need for medications, and improving the quality of life. The author concluded that THA surgery was a cost-effective procedure in the elderly patient.

Wiklund and Romanus[5] evaluated the quality of life using the Nottingham Health Profile preoperatively and one year after THA. Significant improvements were noted in pain relief, energy, sleeping, and social isolation. A significant decrease was found in the frequency of health-related problems that affected housework, holidays, hobbies, social and family life, and sexual function. When the postoperative group was compared to a normal control group, matched for age and sex, no significant differences were noted. Thus, THA is very effective in providing pain relief and improving the quality of life.

Age Distribution and Mortality of THA

Peterson and associates[6] analyzed the rates of total hip and knee arthroplasties, during 1988, among Medicare beneficiaries in the United States. Coverage by Medicare usually starts at the age of 65, and only patients 65 and older were considered. THA was performed in 52,062 patients covered by Medicare, 65 years of age and over in 1988. The largest number were performed in patients 70 to 74 years of age (Fig. 1). Bilateral THA, either one-stage or during one hospitalization, was performed in 1.6% of the patients. THA was performed in 9,912 patients 80 years of age or older, representing 19% of the total number 65 years of age and over.

The overall mortality rate was 72/10,000 (0.72%) after THA. Increasing age correlated with increasing mortality (Fig. 2). The mortality rate almost doubles from the 75 to 79-year age group to the 80 to 84-year age group (60 to 110/10,000) and triples after the age of 90 years (370/10,000).

Recent data collected at The Hospital for Special Surgery found a significant decrease in postoperative (in-hospital) mortality with changes in the anesthesia techniques over a ten-year period.[7] From 1981 to 1985, general anesthesia was used for most patients who received joint replacement arthroplasty at HSS. During that time, 23 of 5,874 (0.39%) patients receiving a total hip or knee replacement died during their hospitaliza-

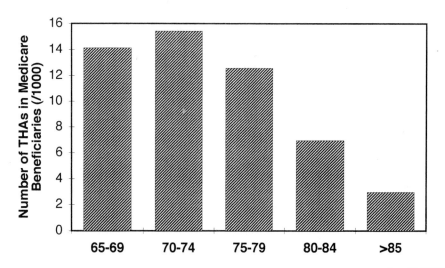

Age Distribution of Medicare Beneficiaries 65 years and Older Receiving THA in 1988 (N=52,062)

Fig. 1 The total number of patients having a THA covered by Medicare was 52,062. The age distribution of Medicare beneficiaries 65 years of age and over receiving a THA reveals that 19% are older than 80 years of age. The largest age group is between 70 and 74 years of age. Data from 1988. (Derived from Peterson MGE, Hollenberg JP, Szatrowski TP, et al: Geographic variations in the rates of elective total hip and knee arthroplasties among Medicare beneficiaries in the United States. *J Bone Joint Surg* 1992;74A:1530-1539.)[6]

tion. After 1985, a transition was made to the use of epidural anesthesia, radial artery monitoring, pulse oximetry, and ECG on a routine basis. High-risk patients and those receiving a one-stage bilateral joint replacement or a revision arthroplasty received pulmonary artery catheters. High-risk patients were also kept in the recovery room for at least 24 hours with nursing and anesthesia surveillance. From 1987 to 1991, only 10 of 9,685 (0.10%) joint replacement patients died during their hospitalization. The reduction from 0.39% to 0.10% was statistically significant (p=0.0003). When THA was considered separately, the

reduction in mortality, from 0.36% to 0.10%, was also significant (p=0.0277) and substantially less than the rate of 0.72% for Medicare beneficiaries throughout the United States.[6] These data support the use of regional anesthesia for joint replacement, the increased use of invasive monitoring, and close postoperative surveillance in high-risk patients or those undergoing long or complex procedures.

Considerations in Cost Containment

As previously noted, the average life expectancy for patients after a THA is greater than that for the general

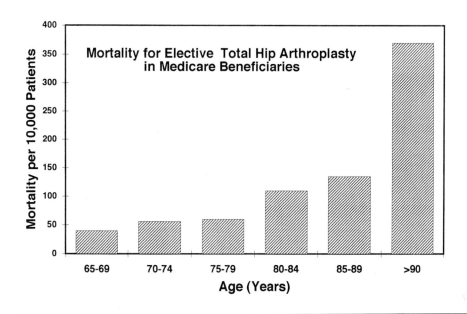

Mortality for Elective Total Hip Arthroplasty in Medicare Beneficiaries

Fig. 2 The mortality rate for elective THA in Medicare beneficiaries doubles from the 75- to 79-year age group to the 80- to 84-year age group. The rate doubles again from the 85- to 89-year age group to those older than 90 years. The overall mortality rate for elective THA in Medicare beneficiaries was 72/10,000. (Derived from Peterson MGE, Hollenberg JP, Szatrowski TP, et al: Geographic variations in the rates of elective total hip and knee arthroplasties among Medicare beneficiaries in the United States. *J Bone Joint Surg* 1992;74A:1530-1539.)[6]

population.[1] In part, this is the result of patient selection for major elective surgery. Severe medical problems or cognitive impairment are potential contraindications to THA. Longer life expectancy will increase the demands placed upon the arthroplasty. Cost containment cannot compromise the quality or longevity of the joint replacement, but is placing increased pressure on manufacturers to produce less expensive implants and on institutions and surgeons to select cheaper prostheses.

As the hospital reimbursement for THA decreases, the relative cost of the implant becomes even more significant.[8] Cemented implants (acetabulum, femoral stem and head) cost 25% to 48% less than cementless implants from the same manufacturer. This can result in a difference of $1,000 to $2,000 in implant costs alone, resulting in savings of 7% to 14% of the total hospital cost per patient.[8] The existing literature demonstrates excellent long-term results in elderly patients with cemented THA, with a survivorship of 78% to 90% at 11 to 20 years follow-up.[9-11]

The Acetabular Side

Early radiographic data suggested there would be an increase in the failure of cemented acetabular cups.[12-15] However, long-term studies have not supported this prediction.[9-11] McCoy and associates[10] found the survivorship of cemented acetabular components to be superior to that of cemented femoral components, with survivorship of 98% for the cups and 93% for the stems at 15 years. No acetabular revisions were required between the 10-year and 15-year follow-up periods.

Kavanagh and associates,[9] in a report of the 15-year results of Charnley THA, noted that the probability of radiographic loosening of the acetabular component was 8.5%, and the probability of femoral loosening was 26%. The probability of revision at 15 years was 10.9%.

Schulte and associates[11] recently reported the minimum 20-year follow-up of 330 Charnley THA (264 patients) implanted between 1970 and 1972. In this study, 83 patients (98 hips) were found to be living, and only five patients were lost to follow-up. The revision rate for the entire series was 9.4%, with 6.1% being revised for aseptic loosening. Including only those patients who lived for 20 years following their THA, 15.2% were revised, 11.1% for aseptic loosening. The acetabular component was revised for aseptic loosening in 5.7% of all patients and in 10.6% of those living for a minimum of 20 years. These excellent results with cemented acetabular components were obtained with early component design and cementing techniques.

Several biomechanical analyses predicted that metal backing would decrease stress concentration at the prosthesis-cement and cement-bone interface.[16-19]

These theoretical advantages, however, have not translated into improved clinical results.[20,21] Ritter and associates[21] noted a significantly increased rate of failure of the metal-backed cup compared to the all-polyethylene acetabular components. In a group of 238 cemented THAs, 138 with a metal-backed cup and 100 with an all-polyethylene cup, 8 metal-backed cups and only 2 all-polyethylene cups (p<0.0034) required revision at an average follow-up of 5.2 years. Significant differences in radiographic loosening and migration were also noted, with a complete lucent line around 54 metal-backed and 23 all-polyethylene cups (p<0.0001) and migration in 6 metal-backed cups and only 2 all-polyethylene cups (p<0.0001). Recent studies using finite element analysis have shown that thin polyethylene and metal backing increase the stresses within the polyethylene, which may result in increased wear.[22] Metal backing increases the cost of the implant and introduces an additional interface, for wear and possible disassociation, at the metal-polyethylene nonarticular interface.[15,16]

Data regarding cementless acetabular components do not have comparable long-term follow up. Schmalzried and Harris[23] recently reported the minimum five-year follow-up of a series of 83 consecutive Harris-Galante Fiber Metal Mesh acetabular components. None of the cups was revised for loosening; however, two had failure of the liner locking mechanism with dissociation of the liner from the shell. Lysis about the acetabular screw holes was seen at the time of revision in one patient whose acetabular prosthesis was revised for femoral loosening. The appearance of new radiolucent lines about the acetabular component was also noted in 49 of the 83 cups. The significance of these lines is unclear at this time and further follow-up is necessary. While these results are encouraging, they do not represent a substantial improvement in acetabular fixation.

In a recent study of 19 patients undergoing revision at The Hospital for Special Surgery, Huk and associates[24] studied the cementless titanium alloy acetabular shells and polyethylene liners obtained at revision. Two cases were associated with osteolysis at the site of acetabular screw fixation. The 19 components were in place for an average of 21.7 months (1 to 72 months). The pseudomembrane obtained from the empty screw holes revealed acellular necrotic tissue in one half of the specimens and dense fibro-connective tissue and foreign body giant cell reaction in the other half. The pseudomembrane obtained from the holes with screws revealed polyethylene debris in 47% of the specimens and metal debris in 67%. Material retrieved from the osteolytic lesions revealed a foreign body giant cell reaction to particulate debris, with polyethylene and metal debris identified. When the convex nonarticular surfaces of the acetabular polyethylene liners were inspected, three modes of damage were noted: burnishing, surface deformation, and embedded metal debris. All specimens were found to have surface burnishing and deformation caused by micromotion and by the edges of the screw holes and prominent heads of the screws, which represent a new source of polyethylene debris.

Tissue from the screw holes of ingrowth acetabular shells was also analyzed for metal levels. Trace metal analysis detected Ti in every specimen, regardless of the presence or absence of screws in the sampled hole. Titanium levels at the empty screw holes averaged 74 µg/g of tissue (range 0.72 to 331 µg/g). At the holes with screws the levels averaged 959 µg/g (range 48 to 11,900 µg/g). Titanium tissue levels from tissues obtained from the two osteolytic lesions averaged 143 µg/g (138 and 147 µg/g). These high levels of titanium most likely resulted from fretting corrosion between the screws and the holes of the metallic shell and, perhaps, from micromotion and fretting of the wires of the fiber mesh.

Metal backing and porous coating increase the cost of the implant. All-polyethylene acetabular cups cost $300 to $500, metal-backed cemented cups cost $720 to $960, and a porous-coated metal-backed shell and liner cost $1,000 to $1,500, an increase of approximately 300%. The elevated cost for metal-backed cemented and cementless components is difficult to justify based upon clinical outcome, particularly in the elderly patient.

The Femoral Side

Economic forces have stimulated implant manufacturers to produce a series of inexpensive femoral implants. The adequacy of these implants must be carefully evaluated based on more than 30 years of clinical experience and study of the biomaterials, design, and biomechanics of THA. The femoral stem must be made of a biomaterial capable of tolerating long-term cyclic loading and in a geometry that minimizes peak stresses within the cement mantle. Modern stem design and materials have virtually eliminated the 2% to 5% incidence of stem fracture of early femoral components.[12] Recent data have also clearly demonstrated that untreated titanium is not an acceptable articulating surface.[25-28] The results of ion impregnation to harden the surface of the titanium and improve wear resistance have not been in use long enough to determine any clinical improvement.

As shown in Table 1, stainless steel, cobalt-chromium, and titanium alloys demonstrate substantial variation in grain size and material properties with different manufacturing techniques (casting, forging, hot isostatic pressing, or cold working).[29,30] For the simple geometry of most cemented femoral stems, the additional cost of these treatments is minimal. In The Dana Center for Orthopaedic Implants at HSS, an unfinished cobalt-chromium cast stem is approximately equal in cost to a forged cobalt-chromium alloy stem, with slight variation related to the size of the implant.

Addressing cemented versus cementless fixation for femoral implants, the long-term clinical data demonstrate a clear advantage for cemented fixation, particularly in elderly patients. Kavanagh and associates[9] reported the probability of radiographic femoral loosening with the Charnley THA to be 12.1% at five years, 16.6% at ten years, and 26% at 15 years. The corresponding figures for femoral revision were 3.5%, 7.6%, and 10.9%, respectively.

Table 1
Mechanical Properties of Hip Implant Biomaterials:

Alloy	Yield Strength	Ultimate Tensile Strength	Fatigue Strength
Cobalt Chrome			
Cast	≥450 MPa	≥655 MPa	245-280 MPa
Annealed	241-448 MPa	793-1000 MPa	340 MPa
Cold-Worked	≥1586 MPa	≥1793 MPa	405 MPa
Elgiloy	1900 MPa	2500 MPa	617 MPa
*PM	840	1270	725 MPa
Stainless Steel			
Annealed	≥170 MPa	≥480 MPa	190-230 MPa
Cold Worked	310-690 MPa	655-860 MPa	530-700 MPa
Ortron	333 MPa	1150 MPa	583 MPa
Titanium Alloy:			
Ti-6Al-4V			
α-β worked, annealed	1000 MPa	1100 MPa	670 MPa

*Powder metallurgic processed cobalt chromium alloys.
(Adapted with permission from Ducheyne P. Cohen CS: Biomaterials: Structure, processing, and mechanical properties, in Steinberg ME (ed): *The Hip and Its Disorders.* Philadelphia, PA, WB Saunders, 1991, pp 905-928.)

McCoy and associates[10] reported a 15-year survival rate of 91% for the Charnley femoral component (failure defined by removal). Schulte and associates[11] found the 20-year revision rate of the femoral component to be 2.5% for all patients and 3.2% for patients surviving a minimum of 20 years after the arthroplasty. Of their patients, 90% either had died with the primary implant still in place or were functioning well 20 years after surgery. The long-term follow-up data clearly indicate that, even with early techniques, a primary cemented total hip arthroplasty should survive the lifetime of the elderly patient. It is likely that improvements introduced in biomaterials, design, and cementing techniques may improve the survivorship in the future.[31-33]

Maloney and Harris[34] studied a group of 50 patients, 25 with a cementless total hip arthroplasty and 25 matched patients with a hybrid arthroplasty (cemented stem and cementless cup). The average follow-up was 32 months for the hybrid group and 37 months for the noncemented group, with a minimum two-year follow-up in both groups. Mild to severe thigh pain was noted in 24% of the cementless THR. Four of 25 (16%) cementless arthroplasties required reoperation. In the hybrid group no reoperations were required. Callaghan[35] reported a 1.1% rate of femoral revision, a 5.5% rate of femoral loosening and a 10% rate of femoral lysis at five- to seven-year follow-up of the noncemented PCA THA. These data compare unfavorably with the 20-year follow-up of the cemented Charnley THA with femoral revision, loosening, and lysis rates of 3.0%, 7.5%, and 3.3%, respectively.[10] The clinical data do not justify the use of noncemented implants in the elderly, particularly in light of the excellent results with cemented fixation.

The price for cementless femoral and acetabular components ranges from $3,800 to $4,300, compared to a range of $2,060 to $3,205 for a cemented system.[7] This can result in a $1,000 to $2,000 (30% to 40%) cost savings per patient. Because it is difficult to machine a smooth, round femoral head attached to a femoral stem, modularity of the femoral component does not increase the cost of the femoral stem and metal head unit. However, the modular interface does provide a potential site for disassembly in vivo.[36] The potential for crevice corrosion exists at the head-neck interface, and galvanic corrosion can occur if dissimilar metals are used for the stem and head.[37,38] However, in patients 80 years of age and older, it is not likely that corrosion will be a significant problem leading to clinical failure. The cost of a modular implant can be dramatically increased if a ceramic femoral head is used. A ceramic femoral head costs approximately $950, compared with approximately $350 for a metal femoral head, a difference of approximately 270%. Limited clinical data exist to support the hypothesis that ceramic femoral heads reduce polyethylene wear; however, recent reports documenting fracture of the ceramic heads have raised questions of their safety in clinical application.[39,40] At present, there is no reason to use a ceramic femoral head in an elderly patient. In summary, the clinical data and the cost of the implants favor cemented THA for both acetabular and femoral fixation in the elderly.

The Implant Distributors and Manufacturers

Implant costs are also affected by the volume of cases done at a hospital and by the competition between various distributors and manufacturers. Significant discounts can be negotiated if the hospital has a consistent volume of arthroplasties. The volume discount, which can be as high as 50%, may encourage hospitals and surgeons to select one manufacturer to provide most of the implants.

Summary

The cost of the prosthetic components can represent approximately 15% to 25% of the total cost of hospitalization, depending upon whether cemented or cementless fixation is selected. The excellent long-term clinical data of cemented fixation and the cost of the implants clearly favor cemented fixation for total hip arthroplasty in the elderly patient.

Acknowledgments

Olga Huk, MD, Assistant Clinical Professor, Hotel-Dieu DeMontreal, University of Montreal, provided the data on polyethylene and titanium wear debris production with modular acetabular components. Margaret G. E. Peterson, PhD, Cornell Musculoskeletal Disease Center, The Hospital for Special Surgery, provided data on the age distribution and mortality in Medicare patients and performed the statistical analysis of the cost data. John R. Reynolds, BA, Vice President for Financial Affairs, Stacey Malakoff, BS, CPA, Controller, and Timothy Brown, BS, Reimbursement Analyst, Department of Finance, The Hospital for Special Surgery, provided the data on the hospital costs and length of stay for patients at The Hospital for Special Surgery. Supported in part by Ms. Emma Daniels, President of The May Ellen and Gerald Ritter Foundation and by Dr. and Mrs. Alberto Foglia.

References

1. Holmberg S: Life expectancy after total hip arthroplasty. *J Arthroplasty* 1992;7:183-186.
2. Pettine KA, Aamlid BC, Cabanela ME: Elective total hip arthroplasty in patients older than 80 years of age. *Clin Orthop* 1991;266:127-132.

3. Ekelund A, Rydell N, Nilsson OS: Total hip arthroplasty in patients 80 years of age and older. *Clin Orthop* 1992;281:101-106.

4. Boettcher WG: Total hip arthroplasties in the elderly: Morbidity, mortality, and cost effectiveness. *Clin Orthop* 1992;274:30-34.

5. Wiklund I, Romanus, B: A comparison of quality of life before and after arthroplasty in patients who had arthrosis of the hip joint. *J Bone Joint Surg* 1991;73A:765-769.

6. Peterson MGE, Hollenberg JP, Szatrowski TP, et al: Geographic variations in the rates of elective total hip and knee arthroplasties among Medicare beneficiaries in the United States. *J Bone Joint Surg* 1992;74A:1530-1539.

7. Sharrock NE, Cazan MG, Hargett MJL, et al: Mortality following total hip and knee arthroplasty: Changes in anesthesia techniques over a ten year period. *Anesth Analg*, in press.

8. Levine DB, Killen AR, Keenen M, et al: Cost awareness and containment for the 1990's: Recycling orthopaedic implants. *Contemp Orthop* 1992;25:376-381.

9. Kavanagh BF, Dewitz MA, Ilstrup DM, et al: Charnley total hip arthroplasty with cement: Fifteen-year results. *J Bone Joint Surg* 1989;71A:1496-1503.

10. McCoy TH, Salvati EA, Ranawat CS, et al: A fifteen-year follow-up study of one hundred Charnley low-friction arthroplasties. *Orthop Clin North Am* 1988;19:467-476.

11. Schulte KR, Callaghan JJ, Kelley SS, et al: The outcome of Charnley total hip arthroplasty with cement after a minimum twenty-year follow-up: The results of one surgeon. *J Bone Joint Surg* 1993;75:961-975.

12. Beckenbaugh RD, Ilstrup DM: Total hip arthroplasty. *J Bone Joint Surg* 1978;60A:306-313.

13. Stauffer RN: Ten-year follow-up study of total hip replacement. *J Bone Joint Surg* 1982;64A:983-990.

14. Sutherland CJ, Wilde AH, Borden LS, et al: A ten-year follow-up of one hundred consecutive Möller curved-stem total hip-replacement arthroplasties. *J Bone Joint Surg* 1982;64A:970-982.

15. Hurley PT, Fehring TK, Braun E, et al: Polyethylene liners in modular porous acetabular components: A comparative analysis. Presented at the 59th annual meeting of the American Academy of Orthopaedic Surgeons, Washington DC, February 21, 1992, paper No. 94, p 83.

16. Parsley BS: Current concerns with modular metal-backed acetabular components. Presented at the 59th annual meeting of the American Academy of Orthopaedic Surgeons, Washington DC, February 21, 1992, paper No. 95, p 83.

17. Bartel DL, Wright TM, Edwards D: The effect of metal backing on stresses in polyethylene acetabular components, in *The Hip: Proceedings of the 11th Open Scientific Meeting for The Hip Society*. St. Louis, MO, CV Mosby, 1983, chap 13, pp 229-239.

18. Crowninshield RD, Pedersen DR, Brand RA, et al: Analytical support for acetabular component metal backing, in *The Hip: Proceedings of the 11th Open Scientific Meeting for The Hip Society*. St. Louis, MO, CV Mosby, 1983, chap 11, pp 207-215.

19. Carter DR: Finite element analysis of a metal-backed acetabular component, in *The Hip: Proceedings of the 11th Open Meeting for The Hip Society*. St. Louis, MO, CV Mosby, 1983, chap 12, pp 216-228.

20. Harris WH, Penenberg BL: Further follow-up on socket fixation using a metal-backed acetabular component for total hip replacement: A minimum ten-year follow-up study. *J Bone Joint Surg* 1987;69A:1140-1143.

21. Ritter MA, Keating EM, Faris PM, et al: Metal-backed acetabular cups in total hip arthroplasty. *J Bone Joint Surg* 1990;72A:672-677.

22. Gabriel SM, Bartel DL: Metal backing and wear in acetabular components for total hip arthroplasty. Presented at the Orthopaedic Research Society, February 17-20, 1992, Washington, DC.

23. Schmalzried TP, Harris WH: The Harris-Galante porous-coated acetabular component with screw fixation: Radiographic analysis of eighty-three primary hip replacements at a minimum of five years. *J Bone Joint Surg* 1992;74A:1130-1139.

24. Huk OL, Bansal M, Betts F, et al: Generation of polyethylene and metal debris from the non-articulating surface of modular acetabular components in total hip arthroplasty. Accepted for publication, *Br J Bone Joint Surg*, 1993.

25. Agins HJ, Alcock NW, Bansal M, et al: Metallic wear in failed titanium-alloy total hip replacements: A histological and quantitative analysis. *J Bone Joint Surg* 1988;70A:347-356.

26. Lombardi AV Jr, Mallory TH, Vaughn BK, et al: Aseptic loosening in total hip arthroplasty secondary to osteolysis induced by wear debris from titanium-alloy modular femoral heads. *J Bone Joint Surg* 1989;71A:1337-1342.

27. Robinson RP, Lovell TP, Green TM, et al: Early femoral component loosening in DF-80 total hip arthroplasty. *J Arthroplasty* 1989;4:55-64.

28. Amstutz HC, Yao J, Dorey FJ, et al: Survival analysis of T-28 hip arthroplasty with clinical implications. *Orthop Clin North Am* 1988;19:491-503.

29. Ducheyne P, Cohen CS: Biomaterials: Structure, processing, and mechanical properties, in Steinberg ME (ed): *The Hip and Its Disorders*. Philadelphia, PA, WB Saunders, 1991, chap 43, pp 905-928.

30. Black J: Metals, in Black J (ed): *Orthopaedic Biomaterials in Research and Practice*. New York, NY, Churchill Livingstone, 1988, pp 163-189.

31. Barrack RL, Mulroy RD Jr, Harris WH: Improved cementing techniques and femoral component loosening in young patients with hip arthroplasty: A 12-year radiographic review. *J Bone Joint Surg* 1992;74B:385-389.

32. Mulroy RD Jr, Harris WH: The effect of improved cementing techniques on component loosening in total hip replacement: An 11-year radiographic review. *J Bone Joint Surg* 1990;72B:757-760.

33. Russotti GM, Coventry MB, Stauffer RN: Cemented total hip arthroplasty with contemporary techniques: A five-year minimum follow-up study. *Clin Orthop* 1988;235:141-147.

34. Maloney WJ, Harris, WH: Comparison of a hybrid with an uncemented total hip replacement: A retrospective matched-pair study. *J Bone Joint Surg* 1990;72A:1349-1352.

35. Callaghan JJ: Primary cementless femoral components PCA at five to seven years. Presented at the 22nd Annual Hip Course, Boston, September 16-19, 1992.

36. Pellicci PM, Haas SB: Disassembly of a modular femoral component during closed reduction of the dislocated femoral component: A case report. *J Bone Joint Surg* 1990;72A:619-620.

37. Collier JP, Surprenant VA, Jensen RE, et al: Corrosion between the components of modular femoral hip prostheses. *J Bone Joint Surg* 1992;74B:511-517.

38. Lieberman J, Rimnac C, Salvati EA: A corrosion analysis of the head-neck taper interface in hip prostheses. *Clin Orthop*, in press.

39. Oonishi H, Takayaka Y, Clarke IC, et al: Comparative wear studies of 28-mm ceramic and stainless steel total hip joints over 2 to 7 year period. *J Long Term Effects of Medical Implants* 1992;2:37-47.

40. Peiro A, Pardo J, Navarrete R, et al: Fracture of the ceramic head in total hip arthroplasty: Report of two cases. *J Arthroplasty* 1991;6:371-374.

The Case for Cemented Fixation of the Femur in Every Patient

William H. Harris, MD

After the dismay of the mid 1970s in total hip replacement, characterized by the widespread recognition of the stark figures for a very high incidence of loosening of cemented femoral components[1,2] and lysis[3-6] of the femur using first-generation femoral cementing techniques, and after the strident, conflicting claims of the 1980s, characterized as "cement versus cementless," the 1990s have brought resolution of these concerns and conflicts. The experience of the 1980s has provided the data needed to make rational and important decisions concerning fixation of the femoral component. Speculation about which system, cement or cementless, is better for which group of patients can only, in reality, be resolved by long-term clinical data. Those data now exist.[7-11] All femoral components should be cemented. The data strongly support this conclusion, independent of age, weight, sex, diagnosis, and primary or revision operation.

What are the data that support such a strong statement? Two observations dominate this decision. The first is the excellent long-term results that occur with improved femoral cementing.[7-11] The second is the high and increasing incidence of lysis in association with cementless femoral components. Lysis of the femur around cementless femoral components is progressive, earlier in onset, higher in incidence, and more aggressive in extent, compared to the use of improved femoral cementing techniques.[12-17] Each of these two factors is important. Both are dominating. And both strongly favor the use of cement. The decision about using cement fixation for the femur in every patient becomes an easy decision.

Examine first the data on results of improved femoral cementing. The well-known reports from the Mayo Clinic[1] and the Cleveland Clinic[2] characterized the long-term results of large series of patients who underwent first-generation femoral cementing. The features that defined first-generation femoral cementing were the absence of a medullary plug, finger packing the cement, no pressurization, the use of femoral components made of cast materials, femoral stem designs that often had a narrow medial border with sharp corners, commonly the absence of a collar, and in many instances a banana-shaped stem. Even in the use of Charnley's technique with Charnley's stem, representative 10-year figures[1] showed that 29.5% of the femora were loose by radiographic criteria at 10 years. With the Muller stem, this figure was even higher.[2]

After our report on lysis in the femur in association with loose cemented femoral components,[3] in which we demonstrated the intense macrophage response, the recognition of this process increased substantially in North America.

The high rates of loosening of the femoral component and lysis of the femur prompted the introduction of three avenues of progress—the surface replacement, improved cementing techniques, and elimination of cement. The surface replacement proved to be a short-lived phenomenon. The decade of the 1980s represented the contest between improved cementing techniques and the use of cementless femoral components.

Improved cementing techniques have dramatically and extensively reversed the incidence of both loosening of femoral components and lysis of the femur. At 11 years, the total femoral loosening rate reported from the Massachusetts General Hospital was 3% (total) including the revision rate for femoral loosening of 2%.[7] At the Mayo Clinic, the figures for loosening were 7% total and 3% revision for loosening (Richard Stauffer, personal communication). At the Brigham and Women's, the figure for loose femoral component at eight years using improved cemented techniques was zero. (Clement Sledge, personal communication).

Moreover, in the report from Massachusetts General, the incidence of major femoral lysis was zero. There were 7% of the femurs that showed small focal areas of lysis in femoral components that were rigidly fixed. This process, which we reported under the designation of "lysis without looseness,"[6] has been shown to be secondary to defects in the cement mantle or areas of very thin cement[18] and generally is nonprogressive. All of these figures were in older patients (average age 57) and, in short, indicate that in patients aged 55 and older, approximately 95% of the femoral components remain rigidly fixed over ten years and only approximately 3% require revision for loosening of the femoral component.[7]

These figures are in sharp contrast with reports of cementless femoral fixation after a minimum five-year follow-up (Table 1). The minimum five-year follow-up is essential for two reasons. First, it is now clear that two-year data on cementless femoral components is nondiscriminatory. All cementless femoral components look about the same after two years. Second, lysis

Table 1
Lysis around uncemented femoral components

Prosthesis	Author/Source	Lysis Incidence	Average Followup
AML	Oh et al[13]	56%	6.5 yrs
	Beauchesne et al[12]	22%	6.0 yrs
APR	Cox et al[16]	16%	5.0 yrs
HGP	Smith & Harris[39]	31%	4.5 yrs
	Martel et al[40]	7.5%*	5.5 yrs
PCA	Oh et al[13]	37%	5.5 yrs
	Crutcher et al[14]	26%	5.9 yrs
	Stulberg et al[17]	19%	5.7 yrs
	Callaghan et al[41]	8%	5.0 yrs

* Stable implant

generally does not begin until three years or more after insertion. Therefore, five-year follow-up data are essential for understanding the real incidence of lysis around cementless femoral components.

These figures are stark. The details of these reports show that the lysis in association with cementless femoral components comes on earlier, is more extensive, is progressive,[19] and increases in incidence (E.J. Smith and William Harris, unpublished data). It is more extensive and more common than with the use of cement. Keep in mind that the 7% figures for the small focal lysis without looseness in the cementless series with improved cementing techniques was reported at 11 years,[7] not at five or six years. The corresponding figure from the same series with improved cementing at six years was only 2%, and, once again, represented lysis that was all focal. The femoral components were all tight. It is inevitable that the lysis figures for these various groups of cementless femoral components, when restudied at 11 years, will be substantially worse than those given at five years.

In addition to the lysis issue, which clearly is the dominant issue regarding cementless femoral components, it is also clear that the incidence of thigh pain, limp, loosening, and revision for loosening is higher in cementless femoral components than in those cemented using improved cementing techniques. Some series also report a higher incidence of heterotopic ossification.[20]

Thus, it is quite clear that improved cementing techniques have dramatically reduced femoral loosening at 11 years and have also dramatically reduced femoral lysis. It is also clear that the concept that the lysis was secondary to "cement disease" has proved false. The expectation that eliminating the cement would eliminate the lysis has proven equally false and, moreover, it is now clear that the incidence of lysis in association with cementless femoral components, independent of

design, independent of proximal versus extensive coating, independent of chromium cobalt versus titanium, and independent of modular versus monoblock, is substantially and importantly worse with cementless femoral components. These data strongly support the use of improved cementing techniques for primary operations in older patients, regardless of sex, age, or diagnosis.

Improved cementing techniques can be divided into two subsets: second-generation and third-generation cementing techniques. The second-generation techniques, adopted about the mid 1970s, include the use of a medullary plug, the use of a cement gun, and the beginning of pressurization of the cement. The femoral components were changed to the use of super alloys, and almost all femoral components adopted a contour with a broad medial border, a rounded medial border, no sharp corners, and, in many cases, a collar.

Subsequent to that, in the third-generation, a number of additional important advances were made, including porosity reduction, which increases the fatigue life of bone cement by at least a factor of five (and compared with the weakest cements, 50 to 75 times).[21,22] This porosity reduction is achieved by centrifugation or vacuum mixing.[21,23] Pressurization has also been improved.[24-26] In another important development, the role of debonding as the leading initiating cause of loosening of cemented femoral components became established and led to an improved understanding of the need to strengthen the cement-metal interface. This can be done both by precoating the surface with a thin layer of polymethylmethacrylate[27,28] and by creating a rough surface on the metal.[28] Finally, centralization of the component has helped eliminate the lysis without looseness.[29]

From these new insights into the understanding of the mechanism of failure of fixation of cemented femoral components and these techniques for overcoming the weak areas in the cementing process has come a startling revelation. In a matched pair retrospective study, we compared a series of patients who were identical in every way except for having a cemented or a cementless femoral component. Patients were matched for age, gender, diagnosis, weight, duration of follow-up, surgeon, surgical approach, postoperative rehabilitation, acetabular component, femoral head size, femoral head metal (chromium cobalt), and radiographic interpretation. The only distinction was that in one group the femoral component was a cemented component and in the other group it was a cementless component. The specific differences were that the femoral component in one group was cementless, made of titanium alloy with a proximal porous surface and a titanium/chromium cobalt combination at the head/neck junction. In the other group the femoral component was designed for use with cement and made of chromium cobalt, and the Morse taper was a chromium cobalt/chromium cobalt junction.

The astonishing finding is that the incidence of femoral lysis in the cementless group was 31% and in the third generation femoral cementing group was zero. This is a statistically significant difference (p = 0.002). It states simply and eloquently that cement prevents femoral lysis.

Consider what an astonishing statement that is. Fifteen years ago it was widely believed that cement caused femoral lysis. We now know that lysis is not so-called "cement disease." There is no such thing as "cement disease." There is fragmented cement disease just as there is particulate polyethylene disease and particulate metal disease. But if the cement does not fragment, there is no lysis from cement.[18] It is a remarkable reversal of our understanding of the nature of total hip replacement to come to the realization that third-generation femoral cementing actually protects against femoral lysis.

When cementless total hip replacements began, they were widely used preferentially in the two groups of patients in which the record with cement was particularly poor, namely the young and in revisions. What effect has improving the femoral cementing techniques had on these two groups? Consider first the question of cement versus cementless in younger patients.

We have recently published our 12-year results with improved cementing techniques on the femoral side in patients age 50 and under (average age 41).[10] At 12 years, 100% of the femoral components were in place and 98% of the femoral components remained solidly fixed. The incidence of lysis was zero. No cementless series has approached those figures. Similar excellent long-term results of good cementing have been reported in young patients by Johnston (R. J. Johnston, personal communication).

Many of the reports of extremely poor results of cemented femoral components in younger patients were examples of the poor results of first-generation femoral cementing.[30-32] The improvement in durability and prevention of lysis with improved cementing techniques on the femoral side in the young is even more dramatic than it is in the elderly. The justification for using cementless femoral components in the young has vanished.

Consider next the issue of femoral revision surgery. For obvious reasons, the results of fixation of cemented femoral revision operations were even poorer than the primary results. Using first-generation femoral cementing techniques, Kavanagh and associates,[33] Pellici and associates,[34,35] and Callahan and associates[36] have all reported a high incidence of failure of fixation at relatively short periods of time, with average figures showing 30% to 40% of the components loose at three

to five years and 20% or more of the femoral components having been rerevised by eight years or so, when first-generation femoral cementing techniques were used.

To assess the impact of second-generation femoral cementing on revision surgery, we studied two groups of patients, those with follow-ups of five to ten years and those with ten to 15 years. In the ten- to 15-year group the average follow-up was nearly 12 years. At that time 90% of the femoral components were still in place and 80% were solidly fixed by radiographic criteria.[11] This represents a remarkable improvement in stability with second-generation femoral cementing. The figures for the five- to ten-year group show that only 7% were revised for loosening at an average of nine years, and 87% were still solidly fixed.[37]

The figures for the combined group show that of the 86 femoral revisions done with modern cementing with an average follow-up of ten years, about 90% are still in place and 80% are solidly fixed. Only 10% of the femoral stems were revised and only 7% were revised for femoral loosening.

We have also addressed the issue of whether or not a patient who has major lysis in association with a loose cemented femoral component is likely to get lysis again after a revision with cement. Among the issues involved in this is the question of whether or not there is an idiosyncratic response to the use of bone cement in that patient in that femur. In fact, at a follow-up of nine years in a group of femurs with major lysis in the femur, which were revised using modern cementing, only one in seven showed a lytic response following revision.[38]

No 10-year data exist for cementless femoral components used in revision. However, all of the short-term data that have been reported clearly show a substantially higher incidence of complications, including thigh pain, limp, loosening, the need for support, and revision. These data strongly support the use of cement in femoral revision surgery. No cementless series has matched the figures reported above with the use of improved cementing.

An additional important point deals with the issue of cementing in cases in which there is a defect in the femur. Many surgeons consider that in such cases the use of cement is impossible. In point of fact, it is easy to close the defect temporarily by using a stent. The stent is made of a layer of rubber dam, followed by a layer of sterile felt, followed by the application of a layer of malleable lead sheet. The lead sheet is cerclaged tightly to the femur. This stent provides a hermetic seal for the defect and allows excellent cement pressurization. When the cement has hardened, the stent is removed and a bone graft is then added across the defect. This has proven to be an excellent method of dealing with these complex problems.

In summary, improved cementing techniques provide by far the best long-term survival of the femoral component in primary total hip replacements in older patients. They also provide by far the best fixation in the young and in femoral revision surgery. Lysis in association with cementless femoral components occurs at an earlier time, in higher incidence, in greater severity, in increasing incidence, and is progressive.

All of these data strongly support the conclusion that cement is the optimum form of fixation of femoral components for total hip replacement regardless of age, sex, diagnosis, and primary versus revision surgery. In fact, the data strongly show that modern cementing protects against femoral lysis.

References

1. Stauffer RN: Ten-year follow-up study of total hip replacement. *J Bone Joint Surg* 1982;64A:983-990.
2. Sutherland CJ, Wilde AH, Borden LS, et al: A ten-year follow-up of one hundred consecutive Müller curved-stem total hip-replacement arthroplasties. *J Bone Joint Surg* 1982;64A:970-982.
3. Harris WH, Schiller AL, Scholler JM, et al: Extensive localized bone resorption in the femur following total hip replacement. *J Bone Joint Surg* 1976;58A:612-618.
4. Willert HG, Bertram H, Buchhorn GH: Osteolysis in alloarthroplasty of the hip: The role of ultra-high molecular weight polyethylene wear particles. *Clin Orthop* 1990;258:95-107.
5. Huddleston HD: Femoral lysis after cemented hip arthroplasty. *J Arthroplasty* 1988;3:285-297.
6. Jasty MJ, Floyd WE III, Schiller AL, et al: Localized osteolysis in stable, non-septic total hip replacement. *J Bone Joint Surg* 1986;68A:912-919.
7. Mulroy RD Jr, Harris WH: The effect of improved cementing techniques on component loosening in total hip replacement: An 11-year radiographic review. *J Bone Joint Surg* 1990;72B:757-760.
8. Roberts DW, Poss R, Kelley K: Radiographic comparison of cementing techniques in total hip arthroplasty. *J Arthroplasty* 1986;1:241-247.
9. Russotti GM, Coventry MB, Stauffer RN: Cemented total hip arthroplasty with contemporary techniques: A five-year minimum follow-up study. *Clin Orthop* 1988;235:141-147.
10. Barrack RL, Mulroy RD Jr, Harris WH: Improved cementing techniques and femoral component loosening in young patients with hip arthroplasty: A 12-year radiographic review. *J Bone Joint Surg* 1992;74B:385-389.
11. Estok DM, Harris WH: Long-term results of cemented femoral revision surgery using second generation techniques: Average 11.7 year follow-up. *Clin Orthop*, in press.
12. Beauchesne RP, Kukita Y, Knezevich S, et al: Roentgenographic evaluation of the AML porous coated acetabular component: A six year minimum follow-up study. Presented at the 59th Annual Meeting of the American Academy of Orthopaedic Surgeons, Washington, DC, Feb. 25, 1992, paper no. 416.
13. Oh J-H, Kim Y-H, Kim VEM: Endosteal osteolysis in cementless porous coated femoral components. Presented at the 59th Annual Meeting of the American Academy of Orthopaedic Surgeons, Washington, DC, Feb. 25, 1992, paper no. 407.
14. Crutcher JP Jr, Borden LS, Hedley AK, et al: Minimum five year follow-up of uncemented total hip arthroplasty for primary osteoarthritis. Presented at the 58th Annual Meeting of the American Academy of Orthopaedic Surgeons, Anaheim, CA, March 9, 1991, paper no. 198.
15. Jasty M, Haire T, Tanzer M: Femoral osteolysis: A generic problem with cementless and cemented components. Presented at the 58th Annual Meeting of the American Academy of Orthopaedic Surgeons, Anaheim, CA, March 9, 1991, paper no. 222.
16. Cox CV, Dorr LD: Five-year results of proximal bone ingrowth fixation total hip replacement. Presented at the 59th Annual Meeting of the American Academy of Orthopaedic Surgeons, Washington, DC, Feb. 25, 1992, paper no. 415.
17. Stulberg BN, Buly RL, Howard PL, et al: Porous coated anatomic acetabular failure: Incidence and modes of failure in uncemented total hip arthroplasty. Presented at the 59th Annual Meeting of the American Academy of Orthopaedic Surgeons, Washington, DC, Feb. 24, 1992, paper no. 282.
18. Maloney WJ, Jasty M, Burke DW, et al: Biomechanical and histologic investigation of cemented total hip arthoplasties: A study of autopsy-retrieved femurs after in vivo cycling. *Clin Orthop* 1989;249:129-140.
19. Tanzer M, Maloney WJ, Jasty M, et al: The progression of femoral cortical osteolysis in association with total hip arthroplasty without cement. *J Bone Joint Surg* 1992;74A:404-410.
20. Maloney WJ, Krushell RJ, Jasty M, et al: Incidence of heterotopic ossification after total hip replacement: Effect of the type of fixation of the femoral component. *J Bone Joint Surg* 1991;73A:191-193.
21. Burke DW, Gates EI, Harris WH: Centrifugation as a method of improving tensile and fatigue properties of acrylic bone cement. *J Bone Joint Surg* 1984;66A:1265-1273.
22. Davies JP, O'Connor DO, Greer JA, et al: Comparison of the mechanical properties of Simplex P, Zimmer Regular, and LVC bone cements. *J Biomed Mater Res* 1987;21:719-730.
23. Wixson RL, Lautenschlager EP, Novak MA: Vacuum mixing of acrylic bone cement. *J Arthroplasty* 1987;2:141-149.
24. Oh I, Carlson CE, Tomford WW, et al: Improved fixation of the femoral component after total hip replacement using a methacrylate intramedullary plug. *J Bone Joint Surg* 1978;6A:608-613.
25. Oh I, Bourne RB, Harris WH: The femoral cement compactor. An improvement in cementing technique in total hip replacement. *J Bone Joint Surg* 1983;65A:1335-1338.
26. Bourne RB, Oh I, Harris WH: Femoral cement pressurization during total hip arthroplasty: The role of different femoral stems with reference to stem size and shape. *Clin Orthop* 1984;183:12-16.
27. Ahmed AM, Raab S, Miller JE: Metal/cement interface strength in cemented stem fixation. *J Orthop Res* 1984;2:105-118.
28. Davies JP, Singer G, Harris WH: The effect of a thin coating of polymethylmethacrylate on the torsional fatigue strength of the cement-metal interface. *J Appl Biomater* 1992;3:45-50.
29. Noble PC, Jay JL, Lindahl CJ, et al: Methods of enhancing acrylic bone cement.Transaction of Society for Biomaterials 13th Annual Meeting, New York, June 3-7, 1987; paper no. 169.
30. Chandler HP, Reineck FT, Wixson RL, et al: Total hip replacement in patients younger than thirty years old: A five-year follow-up study. *J Bone Joint Surg* 1981;63A:1426-1434.
31. Dorr LD, Luckett M, Conaty JP: Total hip arthroplasties in patients younger than 45 years: A nine- to ten-year follow-up study. *Clin Orthop* 1990;260:215-219.

32. Dorr LD, Takei GK, Conaty JP: Total hip arthroplasties in patients less than forty-five years old. *J Bone Joint Surg* 1983;65A:474-479.

33. Kavanagh BF, Ilstrup DM, Fitzgerald RH Jr: Revision total hip arthroplasty. *J Bone Joint Surg* 1985;67A:474-479.

34. Pellicci PM, Callaghan JJ, Wilson PD Jr, et al: Results of revision total hip replacement, in Welch RB (ed): *The Hip: Proceedings of the Twelfth Open Scientific Meeting of the Hip Society.* 1984, chap 14, pp 247-253.

35. Pellicci PM, Wilson PD Jr, Sledge CB, et al: Revision total hip arthroplasty. *Clin Orthop* 1982;170:34-41.

36. Callaghan JJ, Salvati EA, Pellicci PM, et al: Results of revision for mechanical failure after cemented total hip replacement, 1979 to 1982: A two to five-year follow-up. *J Bone Joint Surg* 1985;67A:1074-1085.

37. Pierson JL, Harris WH: Comparisons of first and second generation femoral cementing for revision surgery. Presented at the 60th Annual Meeting of the American Academy of Orthopaedic Surgeons, San Francisco, CA, February 1993, paper no. 64.

38. Jasty M, Pierson JL: What is the fate of recementing into femoral osteolysis? Average nine year follow-up. Presented at the 60th Annual Meeting of the American Academy of Orthopaedic Surgeons, San Francisco, CA, February 1993, paper no. 236.

39. Smith EJ, Harris WH: The increasing incidence of femoral osteolysis after cementless total hip arthroplasty. Presented at the 60th Annual Meeting of the American Academy of Orthopaedic Surgeons, San Francisco, CA, February 1993.

40. Martell JM, Galante JO, Pierson R III, et al: Results of primary total hip reconstruction with the cementless Harris-Galante prosthesis: Minimum five-year results. Presented at the 58th Annual Meeting of the American Academy of Orthopaedic Surgeons, Anaheim, CA, March 9, 1991, paper no. 192.

41. Callaghan JJ, Heekin RD, Hopkinson WJ, et al: Porous coated anatomic primary total hip arthroplasty: Five to seven year results in a prospective consecutive series. Presented at the 59th Annual Meeting of the American Academy of Orthopaedic Surgeons, Washington, DC, Feb. 25, 1992, paper no. 417.

Cemented Fixation of the Femur

Murali Jasty, MD

Total joint replacement surgery has provided dramatic relief of pain and improvement in function for millions of patients with end-stage arthritis. Long-term follow-up results from procedures done in the 1970s, however, have shown unacceptably high rates of failures (20% to 50% at ten years) in part because of inadequate designs of some of the first-generation components and cementing techniques.[1-4] Prosthetic components made of suboptimal materials and designs were used, and these either fractured or created fractures in the cement mantle by virtue of stress concentration created by sharp corners. Adequate cement intrusion probably was not obtained, because the cement was mixed by hand and packed with finger pressure into the canal without occluding the medullary canal.

In the past two decades, major advances have taken place in improving the long-term success rates of cemented femoral component fixation. Knowledge of the complex biomechanics of the hip and the stress transfer around cemented femoral components has been considerably expanded by several in vitro mechanical studies and analytical modeling techniques.[5-8] Newer materials have been developed that can withstand the weightbearing stresses with larger safety margins. As a result, newer prosthetic designs and surgical techniques became available,[9-12] and these have improved long-term success rates of cemented total hip replacements. For example, femoral component fractures have been virtually eliminated by the introduction of superalloy materials. Techniques to optimize the penetration of cement into cancellous bone by medullary canal plugging and by the use of cement delivery and pressurizing systems introduced in the 1970s have been responsible for the more favorable results from the second half of the decade. Several investigators have been able to reduce the rates of femoral component loosening remarkably (to less than 3% at ten years) using these techniques.[11,12] The combined information from these studies established that technical improvements in material and design do in fact extend the longevity of cemented total joint arthroplasty.

Recent morphologic studies, on femurs retrieved at autopsy from patients who underwent total hip arthroplasty many years earlier, have provided additional valuable information on the mechanisms involved in the initiation of femoral component loosening.[13] These studies have shown that in the absence of cement fractures and fragmentation, the cement is tolerated very well by the skeleton over the long term. Osseointegration of the cement with minimal fibrous tissue formation at the cement-bone interface is noted in many cases. The studies have also shown that loosening of the components is most commonly initiated by cement fragmentation. Local or generalized cement fractures were associated with the disruption of the cement-bone interface and periprosthetic osteolysis. Sharp corners of the prostheses, thin or incomplete cement mantles, debonding at the cement-metal interface, and voids in the cement were the factors responsible for fracturing cement. The two sites of the cement mantle where most cement fractures occurred were at the most proximal and most distal ends of the femoral components, precisely the two regions where high stresses in the cement mantle would be expected to occur based on finite element and experimental models. These studies have improved the understanding of the mechanisms involved in the initiation of femoral component loosening and have provided new avenues to pursue in further improving the long-term reliability of cemented femoral components.

Cemented femoral arthroplasty involves creation of a composite structure, the members of which are the prosthesis, cement, and the bone, anchored to each other through the cement-metal and cement-bone interfaces. Long-term success of such a construct is dependent on maximizing and maintaining the mechanical interlock of the interfaces, and on preventing mechanical failure of the three members of the composite over time. The weakest member or members of the composite determine the likelihood of failure of the whole structure. Furthermore, the mechanical and physical properties of each of these members and their interfaces can alter the load transfer across the whole composite structure and affect the stresses within the adjacent members.

Optimizing the Outcome: Primary Cemented Femoral Components

The Optimum Prosthetic Component

The femoral components selected should be made of superalloy metals, such as cobalt chromium-based alloys (Fig. 1). Femoral components with rounded corners and broad lateral surfaces are preferred to those

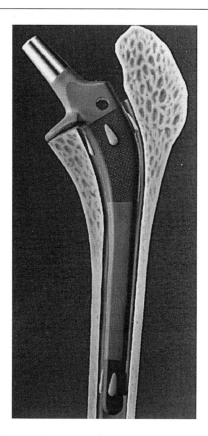

Fig. 1 Contemporary femoral stem made of high-strength cobalt chromium-based superalloy material, with smooth borders, methylmethacrylate precoating over the proximal and distal segments, and with preformed centralizers.

with sharp corners. A broad medial collar on the femoral component is recommended, because it maximizes load transfer to the calcar and reduces the stresses in the proximal femoral cement mantle. The largest stem that will fit the canal, yet leave room for a cement mantle 2 to 3 mm thick all around the prosthesis should be chosen to avoid defects in the cement mantle. Preformed centralizers on the femoral components greatly assist in centering the components in the femoral canal to provide a cement mantle of uniform thickness. Design features that enhance the bond strength between the metal and the cement, such as precoating or texturing, should be used, particularly at the proximal and distal ends of the prostheses. The rationale for choosing such a femoral component is discussed below.

Since the introduction of total hip replacements with stainless steel femoral components by Charnley,[14] femoral components of various designs have been introduced in Europe and North America. Engineering analyses have shown that certain design configurations produce unfavorable stresses in the stem and cement mantle, by virtue of their load trans-

fer mechanisms.[5,6,8] Cast metals used for the first-generation femoral components occasionally contained inclusions and impurities in the material. Cracks that arose in these areas led to prosthetic fractures. The fabrication methods have since been substantially modified by such techniques as forging and hot isostatic pressing, which markedly improved the strength of the metals by giving the microstructure a finer grain and eliminating the voids. The introduction of superalloy materials such as the cobalt chromium-based alloys also has led to significant improvements in the fatigue strengths of the femoral components and has promoted their widespread use in joint replacement surgery. Availability of materials and techniques to optimize the geometry now makes it possible to design a femoral component with high fatigue strength. With these designs and modern cementing techniques, it is hoped that the serious complication of fatigue fracture of the femoral component will largely be a problem of the past.

Several features in the design of femoral components are critically important in protecting the cement mantle from fracturing. The cross-sectional shape, geometric configuration, length, and material properties profoundly influence the distribution of load transfer around the hip. Using finite element techniques, Crowninshield and associates[5] found that increasing femoral stem length from 100 mm to 130 mm reduced the predicted maximum compressive stresses in the cement by 26%. Increasing the cross-sectional stem size by 20% produced a 5% reduction in predicted maximal compressive cement stresses and a 12% reduction in maximal tensile stresses within the stem. Femoral components with broad medial borders and large area moments of inertia help to lower the stresses within the cement mantle. In addition, for implants with a broad lateral surface, proportionately more of the surrounding cement mantle is subjected to compressive rather than tensile loads, which is an advantage, because the compressive strength of polymethylmethacrylate (PMMA) is higher than its tensile strength. Femoral components made of cobalt-based alloys are preferable to those made of titanium alloys, because their higher elastic modulus and, therefore, higher proximal bending stiffness helps reduce the proximal cement stresses. Lower bending stiffness at the distal end of the prosthesis is beneficial in that it lowers the distal cement stresses, and tapering the components at the distal end lowers their bending stiffness.[7]

Femoral components with narrow, sharp corners will create substantial stress risers in the cement. Components such as the Mueller and Aufranc-Turner, therefore, may be at risk for creating fractures in the cement mantle, especially on the medial side. Support for avoiding sharp medial borders on the femoral components also comes from the long-term clinical experience with these implants in which there has been a substantially higher incidence of loosening than with other designs from the same era. Proper stem design, therefore, plays an important role in minimizing cement stresses.

The next issue in the selection of the femoral component involves the metal-cement interface. Cement does not possess good adhesive properties, and the strength of the cement-metal interface is usually lower than that of the bulk cement. Ahmed and associates[15] found that the cement-metal interface prepared in the standard fashion fails at loads of only 200 psi under pull-out testing. Separation at the cement-metal interface may adversely affect the adjacent cement mantle. Hampton and associates,[6] using finite element analysis, showed that loosening the bond between the metal and cement substantially increases the axial stresses in the proximal-medial cement mantle, a finding that has been verified by experimental studies with embedded strain gauges.[16] Evidence for the importance of the cement-metal interface in initiating femoral component loosening is provided by follow-up clinical radiographic studies and pathologic studies.[2,13] These studies show that radiolucencies at the proximal lateral cement interface often are associated with femoral component loosening, and that debonding at the metal-cement interface is one of the features associated with initiation of femoral component loosening.

Various methods for strengthening the metal-cement interface have been explored, including the use of components with porous or textured surfaces, and components with PMMA precoating.[17] Porous surfaces, however, may trap air, blood, or fat particles in vivo and weaken the cement. Textured surfaces enhance interfacial shear strength but do not resist tensile forces at the interfaces well. In precoating, an industrial process, the surface of the prosthesis is cleaned meticulously, and the PMMA coating is electrostatically deposited onto the prosthesis. In this process, intermolecular adhesion forms between the cement and metal, thus improving both tensile and shear strength. Ahmed and associates[15] found that precoating improves the interfacial shear strength on push-out tests by an order of magnitude, and that failure of the precoated specimens usually occurred within the cement and not at the interface. The improvement in strength is even more pronounced in a saline environment, which drastically reduces the interface strength of nonprecoated specimens but does not affect the precoated specimens.

Centering the stem within the femoral canal to obtain a cement mantle of uniform thickness is an important issue that is being addressed currently. Experimental and finite element studies have shown that a uniform cement mantle thickness is desirable in maintaining the stresses within a safe level.[7,8,13] Mantles less than 2 mm thick are at risk for fracture, particularly at the proximal and distal ends of the prostheses, where the stresses are highest. Studies of femurs retrieved at autopsy provide direct evidence that thin and incomplete mantles are associated with cement fractures and fragmentation, prosthetic loosening, and periprosthetic osteolysis.[13]

Manual centering of the femoral component is tedious and unreliable. Metal fins and ribs on the femoral components effectively center the component, but may be undesirable because they can also produce defects in the mantle. Preformed PMMA spacers, which are attached to the prosthetic components just before femoral component insertion, are also effective in centering, but they are cumbersome and have the additional disadvantages of trapping air and blood within the cement. For these reasons, preformed PMMA spacers attached to the prosthesis during the manufacturing are now preferred. The shapes of these spacers are optimized to allow the cement to flow freely, which eliminates the problems of air and blood entrapment. It is important to centralize both the proximal and distal ends of the components, because these are the two regions where most cement fractures occur.

Optimizing the Cement

Charnley's application of polymethylmethacrylate bone cement to artificial joint fixation in 1959 was a milestone achievement in the development of joint replacement surgery.[18] Almost 30 years later, PMMA is still the standard material for anchoring total joint implants to the skeleton. Despite its enormous success, however, PMMA has several recognized shortcomings as a structural material. Several studies have shown that in the vast majority of cases nonseptic prosthetic loosening of cemented total joint replacements can be attributed to disruption of the integrity of the cement mantle or its interfaces.[2,3,13] Identification of the causes of the poor strength of bone cements and attempts to improve the fatigue life of bone cements are of major importance in cemented joint replacement surgery.

Several different formulations of methylmethacrylate bone cements are available for total joint replacement surgery. All of them contain a powder phase, which consists of prepolymerized particles of polymethylmethacrylate, and a liquid phase, which consists of methylmethacrylate monomer. However, subtle differences in the chemical and physical characteristics of the powder and liquid constituents among the commercially available bone cement formulations can lead to differences in the mechanical properties of the cements.[19] Zimmer Regular, LVC, and CMW bone cement powders contain PMMA polymer. Palacos R cement powder contains a methylmethacrylate-methacrylate copolymer, and Simplex P cement powder contains a mixture of polymethylmethacrylate and methyl methacrylate-Styrene Copolymer, in a one-to-five ratio. Zimmer Regular, LVC, CMW, and Simplex P cements contain barium sulphate to make them radiopaque. Palacos R uses zirconium oxide to make the cement radiopaque. Furthermore, chlorophyll is used in Palacos R to provide a green tint. The particle sizes of the powder are also varied in some formulations to obtain different viscosities and working and setting times. These subtle differences in the chemical and physical characteristics of the different commercial formulations of the bone cements can affect their mechanical properties and fatigue strengths.

Porosity in cured surgical bone cements can adversely effect their mechanical properties.[13,20-24] Plexiglass, the commercial preparation of basically the same acrylic material, is cured industrially under high temperature and pressure, and it exhibits substantially better fatigue strength than surgical bone cement. In contrast, hand mixing the surgical bone cement leads to the formation of numerous voids, which act as stress risers and compromise its mechanical strength, particularly if the voids are located in regions where the cement is exposed to high stresses.

Efforts to improve the fatigue strengths of bone cements have included attempts to increase the degree of polymerization and the use of reinforcing fiber additives,[24,25] such as carbon, graphite, Kevlar, or metal fibers. The high developmental costs and changes in the viscosity, elastic modulus, and creep behavior of the cement have limited the clinical utility of these techniques.

A more practical approach involves reducing the porosity of the bone cement by techniques such as vacuum mixing and centrifugation after mixing. Wixson and associates[26] reported that vacuum mixing significantly reduces the porosity of Simplex P (7.1% vs 0.1%), increases in its fatigue life by tenfold and improves its toughness. Burke and associates[20] have shown that centrifugation after mixing markedly improves the fatigue strength of Simplex P bone cement by reducing its porosity. Centrifugation of Simplex P for only thirty seconds after mixing increased its fatigue life by 136%. More striking are the results of the subsequent studies by this group. Using optimized centrifugation techniques, they were able to increase the fatigue life of centrifuged Simplex P five-fold.[22]

O'Connor and associates[27] related the increase in fatigue strength to the mechanical requirements of the surgical bone cement around the femoral components by using embedded strain gauges to measure the strains in the femoral cement mantle under simulated physiologic loads. They found that, at physiologic strain levels, 70% of uncentrifuged PMMA samples will fail before 10 million cycles (approximately ten years

of normal walking). In sharp contrast, under the same loads, none of the centrifuged specimens failed at 10 million cycles, a dramatic increase in the endurance of otherwise traditional Simplex P, without significantly altering the setting time or peak setting temperature of PMMA.

In order to choose the optimum cement and preparation technique, Davies and associates[21,22] investigated the amount of porosity and the fatigue strengths of various commercial bone cements prepared by standard mixing, mixing with chilled monomer, and centrifugation. They found that the best fatigue strength was obtained with Simplex P prepared by centrifugation. Centrifugation of Simplex P for 30 seconds after mixing with room temperature monomer resulted in a cement that was easy to use and had excellent fatigue strength. Simplex P centrifuged for 2 minutes after mixing with monomer at room temperature exhibited higher fatigue strength, but the cement became too viscous and was difficult to inject from the syringe. Simplex P, when mixed with monomer at 0°C and centrifuged for 60 seconds, provided an excellent low viscosity state and high fatigue strength. In contrast, LVC bone cement, which had the lowest porosity as mixed by standard techniques, remained significantly weaker than Simplex P even after centrifugation. Palacos R had a slightly higher fatigue strength than Simplex P when mixed in standard fashion, but centrifugation of Palacos R was not very effective in either reducing the porosity or further improving the fatigue strength. Thus, Simplex P, mixed with chilled monomer and centrifuged for 30 to 60 seconds or vacuum mixed appears to be optimal for use in total hip arthroplasty.

It is clear from these studies that substantial improvements in the fatigue strengths of bone cements can be realized by porosity reductions. Davies and associates[23] have also shown that porosity reduction of surgical cement improves its fatigue strength even in the presence of the significant asperities on the surface seen in vivo because of trabecular bone interdigitations. Tests of centrifuged specimens with sharp notches and trabecular bone on the surface have confirmed the importance of porosity reduction to improve the fatigue strength of bone cement in conditions that simulate the in vivo environments.

Optimizing the Cement and Prostheses Insertion

The poor results of early studies on cemented total hip replacements have led to the speculation that cement is not a biocompatible material, and that loosening is initiated primarily by biologic reactions to the cement. This theory is based on the finding of periprosthetic osteolysis around some of the failed prostheses. Histologic studies of tissues from the regions of osteolysis usually show numerous macrophages and foreign body giant cells along with particulate debris of methylmethacrylate.[28] Biochemical studies have shown that this tissue produces large amounts of prostaglandin E_2 and collagenase—known mediators of pathologic bone resorption.

The adverse tissue response that occurs at the cement-bone interface, however, is related to fragmented cement and not to bulk cement. In contrast to the granulomatous tissue that forms around failed prostheses, very little soft tissue forms if the prosthetic components are fixed well to the skeleton,[28] and, when present, it contains relatively little particulate debris and does not produce high levels of prostaglandins. Data from the femurs retrieved at autopsy from patients with well-functioning prostheses also support the view that cemented femoral components are tolerated very well by the skeleton over a long term, if the cement is intruded well into the bone and has not fragmented.[13]

The poor results reported with first-generation cemented femoral components may therefore reflect the suboptimal cement techniques used at the time. Adequate cement intrusion probably was not achieved consistently in those days, because the cement was inserted into the canal with digital pressure only, without employing special techniques to enhance cement intrusion into bone. The results of clinical studies showing low long-term loosening rates with improved cementing techniques and the data from autopsy material indicate that adequate intrusion of cement into the endosteal surface of the femur is of paramount importance in minimizing the failures of cemented femoral arthroplasty.

The two critical features that determine the intrusion of cement into the bone are the viscosity of the cement and the pressure used to deliver the cement.[29-31] Meticulous cleaning and drying of the femoral canal, plugging the canal, delivering the cement in a less viscous (more fluid) form with cement syringes and pressuring the delivered cement are surgical techniques that improve cement intrusion.

The viscosity of the cement depends on the formulation of the cement and the techniques used to mix it. The CMW and Palacos cements become very stiff soon after mixing. In contrast, LVC retains its low viscosity for more than five minutes after mixing. Simplex P cement has an intermediate viscosity, which steadily increases during the usual working period of three to five minutes after mixing. Chilling the monomer can also prolong the low viscosity state of certain cements.

Rey and associates[31] studied the intrusion characteristics of Simplex P, LVC and Palacos R cements into bovine cancellous bone at different ambient temperatures and with injection pressures of 20, 40, and 60 psi. The intrusion depth of cement was directly related to the intrusion pressure and inversely related to the cement viscosity. For Simplex P mixed in the standard fashion for 60 seconds under operating room environmental conditions, and injected with a commercially available gun at 20 psi, a minimum cement intrusion depth of 5 mm was obtained even into dense bovine cancellous bone. They found that intrusion can be improved using either low viscosity cement (LVC) and low pressure or higher viscosity cement (Simplex P) and higher pressure. Thus, use of a low viscosity cement is not an absolute requirement for optimal cement intrusion, because even the higher viscosity cements can intruded by higher pressures. Furthermore, it may not be desirable to use cements with very low (LVC) or very high viscosities (Palacos), because their fatigue strength after centrifuging or vacuum mixing is lower than that of Simplex P.

Plugging the distal medullary canal to contain the cement in the medullary canal during pressurization adds greatly to cement intrusion. By occluding the femoral canal 2 cm to 4 cm beyond the tip of the stem, the distal flow of cement is prevented and the cement is confined to the proximal canal. Various devices, such as bone plugs and polyethylene plugs, have been used to occlude the medullary canal. Although improved cement-bone interface pressures can be achieved with bone or plastic plugs, in practice it is difficult to completely seal the distal canal in all cases, particularly if the femoral canal at the level of the plug is wider than the femoral canal immediately distal to it. Bourne and associates[29] demonstrated that substantially greater pressurization can be obtained reliably with the use of a cement plug than with bone or plastic plugs. Special calibrated medullary plug syringes[10] markedly simplify the insertion of the cement plug. One half pack of Simplex (20 g of polymer, 10 cc of monomer) is mixed to make the plug and loaded into the plug syringe. After the cement reaches the dough state, 4 cc of it is inserted 3 cm below the planned level of the tip of the stem using the calibrated syringe. After the cement has been injected, the nozzle should be rotated several times in a clockwise and counterclockwise direction to separate the plug from the tip of the syringe. No further manipulation inside the femoral canal should be done until the plug is completely hardened.

Once the methacrylate plug has hardened, the medullary canal should be meticulously cleaned, to remove blood, marrow fat, and residual bone debris, and dried. This enhances cement intrusion and prevents laminations in the cement, caused by inclusions of blood and fat, which can have a deleterious effect on the strength of PMMA.[17] The cleaning can be effectively accomplished using pulsatile (radially directed) jet saline lavage and suction. Special polyethylene intramedullary brushes can also be used to mechanically remove medullary debris. After cleaning, the canal is thoroughly dried by packing with sponges.

Sponges soaked in dilute adrenalin solution (0.5 cc of 1:1000 adrenaline in 250 cc of saline) and packed into the femoral canal are used to reduce bleeding from the endosteal surface. Hypotensive anesthesia will also decrease the bleeding and is recommended if there are no medical contraindications. A final dry sponge is passed down the canal just before the cement is inserted, and the distal end of the canal near the plug is suctioned to remove any pooled blood. The combination of these techniques should leave the interstices of the cancellous bone clean and dry, which will promote maximal cement interdigitation and achieve a superior cement-bone interface.

The various commercial cement guns are invaluable for delivering the cement deep into the femoral canal and for pressurizing the cement. The cement gun offers the major advantages of improving the mechanical properties of the cement, by pressurizing it, of diminishing the likelihood of entrapping blood and air, as commonly occurs during finger packing.[32] To prevent air entrapment during delivery, the nozzle on the gun should be passed to the level of the plug and the cement should be injected into the femoral canal in a retrograde fashion. The cement should be inserted just prior to the "doughy" phase, or at the moment the cement will not stick to the surgeon's glove. In this state, excellent cement intrusion can be achieved and the risk of erratic movement of the stem during insertion and during polymerization is substantially reduced.

After delivering the cement into the femoral canal, it should be pressurized by using a femoral canal seal[29,33] and continued compaction of the cement. Pressurizing the cement by finger packing does not produce high enough pressures, because some of the cement can escape out of the femoral neck. By virtue of the intermittent nature of finger packing, the pressure rise is repeatedly interrupted and is of very short duration. Slow and continuous injection of the cement into the femoral canal occluded distally by the plug and proximally by the seal is much more effective in creating sustained pressures and improving cement intrusion. A larger volume of PMMA will be needed when the cement is pressurized in this manner, because the trabecular spaces are filled more completely. It is wise to plan on mixing one extra pack of cement than is customarily used without pressurization.

The femoral component should then be placed into the pressurized cement in neutral orientation to the long axis of the medullary canal, avoiding varus or valgus positioning and defects in the cement mantle. The preformed centralizers attached to the proximal and distal ends of the prosthesis are a great help in centering the femoral component within the medullary canal. The surgeon should also anticipate greater resistance to passing the stem because of the more com-

plete filling of the available space with PMMA. The additional pressure generated during the femoral component insertion improves the intrusion of the cement into the endosteal surface of the femoral diaphysis. It is important to hold the femoral component steady until the cement hardens completely, because movement of the femoral component when the cement is in the dough phase will produce separation of the cement-metal interface.

The combination of techniques discussed above will insure void-free cement of high fatigue strength with excellent interdigitation with the endosteal trabecular bone (Fig. 2). Ideally there should be a uniform, void-free cement mantle, 2 mm to 3 mm in thickness around the entire circumference of the femoral component, with no radiolucencies at the cement-bone interface on the radiographs.

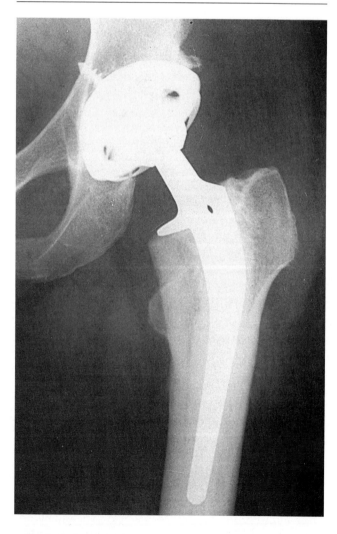

Fig. 2 Radiograph of a well-cemented total hip arthroplasty. Note excellent intrusion of the cement into bone, and void-free cement.

References

1. Beckenbaugh RD, Ilstrup DM: Total hip arthroplasty. *J Bone Joint Surg* 1978;60A:306-313.

2. Stauffer RN: Ten-year follow-up study of total hip replacement. *J Bone Joint Surg* 1982;64A:983-990.

3. Sutherland CJ, Wilde AH, Borden LS: A ten-year follow-up of one hundred consecutive Müller curved-stem total hip-replacement arthroplasties. *J Bone Joint Surg* 1982;64A:970-982.

4. Wroblewski BM: Fractured stem in total hip replacement: A clinical review of 120 cases. *Acta Orthop Scand* 1982;53:279-284.

5. Crowninshield RD, Brand RA, Johnston RC, et al: An analysis of femoral component stem design in total hip arthroplasty. *J Bone Joint Surg* 1980;62A:68-78.

6. Hampton SJ, Andriacchi TP, Galante JO: Three dimensional stress analysis of the femoral stem of a total hip prosthesis. *J Biomech* 1980;13:443-448.

7. Huiskes R, Chao EY: A survey of finite element analysis in orthopedic biomechanics: The first decade. *J Biomech* 1983;16:385-409.

8. Lewis JL, Askew MJ, Wixson RL, et al: The influence of prosthetic stem stiffness and of a calcar collar on stresses in the proximal end of the femur with a cemented femoral component. *J Bone Joint Surg* 1984;66A:280-286.

9. Amstutz HC, Markolf KL, McNeice GM, et al: Loosening of total hip components: Cause and prevention, in *The Hip, Proceedings of the Fourth Open Scientific Meeting of The Hip Society.* St. Louis, MO, CV Mosby, 1976, chap 10, pp 102-116.

10. Harris WH (ed): *Advanced Concepts in Total Hip Replacement.* Thorofare, NJ, SLACK Inc, 1985.

11. Mulroy RD Jr, Harris WH: The effect of improved cementing techniques on component loosening in total hip replacement: An 11-year radiographic review. *J Bone Joint Surg* 1990;72B:757-760.

12. Russotti GM, Coventry MB, Stauffer RN: Cemented total hip arthroplasty with contemporary techniques: A five-year minimum follow-up study. *Clin Orthop* 1988;235:141-147.

13. Jasty M, Maloney WJ, Bragdon CR, et al: The initiation of failure in cemented femoral components of hip arthroplasties. *J Bone Joint Surg* 1991;73B:551-558.

14. Charnley J: *Low Friction Arthroplasty of the Hip: Theory and Practice.* New York, NY, Springer-Verlag, 1979.

15. Ahmed AM, Raab S, Miller JE: Metal/cement interface strength in cemented stem fixation. *J Orthop Res* 1984;2:105-118.

16. Crowninshield RD, Tolbert JR: Cement strain measurement surrounding loose and well fixed femoral component stems. *J Biomed Mater Res* 1983;17:819-828.

17. Park JB, von Recum AF, Gratzick GE: Pre-coated orthopedic implants with bone cement. *Biomater Med Devices Artif Organs* 1979;7:41-53.

18. Charnley J: The bonding of prostheses to bone by cement. *J Bone Joint Surg* 1964;46B:518-529.

19. Lautenschlager EP, Stupp SI, Keller JC: Structure and properties of acrylic bone cement, in Ducheyne P, Hastings GW (eds): *Functional Behavior of Orthopaedic Biomaterials.* Boca Raton, FL, CRC Press, 1984, chap 4, vol 2, pp 87-119.

20. Burke DW, Gates EI, Harris WH: Centrifugation as a method of improving tensile and fatigue properties of acrylic bone cement. *J Bone Joint Surg* 1984;66A:1265-1273.

21. Davies JP, O'Connor DO, Greer JA, et al: Comparison of the mechanical properties of Simplex P, Zimmer Regular, and LVC bone cements. *J Biomed Mater Res* 1987;21:719-730.

22. Davies JP, Jasty M, O'Connor DO, et al: The effect of centrifuging bone cement. *J Bone Joint Surg* 1989;71B:39-42.

23. Davies JP, O'Connor DO, Burke DW, et al: The effect of centrifugation on the fatigue life of bone cement in the presence of surface irregularities. *Clin Orthop* 1988;229:156-161.

24. Saha S, Pal S: Mechanical properties of bone cement: A review. *J Biomed Mater Res* 1984;18:435-462.

25. Knoell A, Maxwell H, Bechtol C: Graphite fiber reinforced bone cement: An experimental feasibility investigation. *Ann Biomed Eng* 1975;3:225-229.

26. Wixson RL, Lautenschlager EP, Novak M: Vacuum mixing of methylmethacrylate bone cement. *Trans Orthop Res Soc* 1985;10:327.

27. O'Connor DO, Burke DW, Davies JP, et al: SN curve for centrifuged and uncentrifuged PMMA. *Trans Orthop Res Soc* 1985;10:325.

28. Goldring SR, Jasty M, Roelke M, et al: Biological factors that influence the development of a bone-cement membrane, in Fitzgerald RH Jr (ed): *Non-Cemented Total Hip Arthroplasty.* New York, NY, Raven Press, 1988, chap 5, pp 35-39.

29. Bourne RB, Oh I, Harris WH: Femoral cement pressurization during total hip arthroplasty: The role of different femoral stems with reference to stem size and shape. *Clin Orthop* 1984;183:12-16.

30. Krause WR, Miller J, Ng P: The viscosity of acrylic bone cements. *J Biomed Mater Res* 1982;16:219-243.

31. Rey R, Paiement G, McGann W, et al: A study of intrusion characteristics of LVC, Simplex P and Palacos cements in a bovine cancellous bone model. *Clin Orthop* 1987;215:272-278.

32. Gruen TA, Markolf KL, Amstutz HC: Effects of laminations and blood entrapment on the strength of acrylic bone cement. *Clin Orthop* 1976;119:250-255.

33. Oh I, Bourne RB, Harris WH: The femoral cement compactor: An improvement in cementing technique in total hip replacement. *J Bone Joint Surg* 1983;65A:1335-1338.

Contributions of Basic and Applied Sciences to Hip Replacement in the Older Patient

Philip C. Noble, MS

Introduction

The essential goal of total hip replacement is restoration of normal function to the diseased, painful hip joint. This is achieved by exchanging the femoral head and the articulating surface of the acetabulum for a mechanical facsimile of metal and plastic. In practice, the long-term outcome of this procedure depends on both the accuracy of replication of the original position of the joint center and the durability of the bond formed between each of the prosthetic components and the skeleton. The present success of total hip replacement has been due to many advances in scientific knowledge, including our understanding of the biomechanics of the hip joint and of the effect of mechanical and biologic factors on the longevity of the interfaces formed between polymer, metal, cement, and bone.

In the younger patient, debate has raged over the relative merits of cemented and cementless modes of implant fixation of femoral prostheses, but few authorities dispute the virtues of cemented fixation in the elderly. Within the acetabulum, however, widespread clinical practice has affirmed the use of cementless fixation independent of age, although a place still remains for cement. In this chapter, we will focus on the biomechanical aspects of total hip replacement and their influence on the outcome of this procedure in the older patient.

Restoration of the Hip Joint

The femoral and acetabular components are designed to restore the normal anatomic relationship of the pelvis and femur. In the coronal plane, the center of rotation of the femoral head is fixed by two variables: (1) its offset, medially, from the axis of the femoral shaft and (2) its height, cephalad, with respect to the greater and the lesser trochanters (Fig. 1). In the normal population, the medial offset of the femoral head varies by approximately 37 mm, from 24 to 61 mm (Fig. 2). The offset of the head is affected principally by the inclination of the femoral neck with respect to the femoral axis, which ranges from 106° to 155° in the normal population.[1] The anterior position of the femoral head also varies considerably, corresponding to a range of anteversion of ±18 degrees.[1]

Restoration of the correct medial offset during hip replacement is important because it recreates the cor-

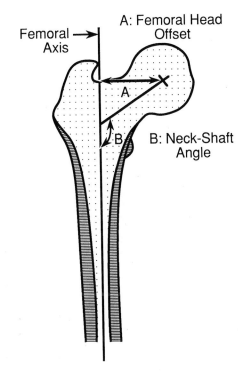

Fig. 1 Diagrammatic representation of the position of the femoral head with respect to the axis of the medullary canal. (Reproduced with permission from Noble PC: Biomechanical advances in total hip replacement, in Niwa S, Hattori T (eds): *Biomechanics in Orthopedics.* Berlin, Springer-Verlag, 1992, pp 46-75.)

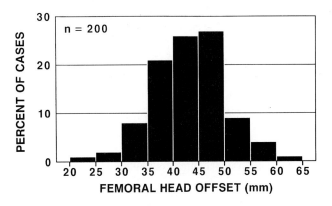

Fig. 2 Distribution of values of the medial offset of the femoral head from a cadaveric population of 200 femora. (Reproduced with permission from Noble PC: Biomechanical advances in total hip replacement, in Niwa S, Hattori T (eds): *Biomechanics in Orthopedics.* Berlin, Springer-Verlag, 1992, pp 46-75.)

rect mechanical balance between two factors: the abductor forces, which act lateral to the hip joint, and the body weight, which is applied medially. Too small an offset of the femoral shaft from the femoral head (or too valgus a prosthesis) will cause shortening of the abductors in addition to a reduction in the abductor moment arm. As the force of contraction of the abductor muscles must balance the adducting effect of the weight of the body, any reduction in the medial offset of the femur must cause the force of contraction of the abductors to increase, leading to an even greater resultant force across the artificial joint. Alternately, too long an offset (or too varus a prosthesis) will lateralize the proximal femur; this can lead to increased bending moments on the femoral shaft and the femoral component. Although this reduces the joint reaction force, increased stresses within the cement mantle and the cement-bone interface may eventually lead to failure of fixation and loosening of the prosthesis. In addition, some patients may complain of an asymmetric appearance of their hips if the greater trochanter is excessively lateralized.

The success of any procedure that attempts to restore normal joint anatomy depends upon the availability of prosthetic devices with sufficient flexibility to match the normal anatomic variability of the human femur. In total hip replacement, modular femoral heads allow the surgeon to vary the neck length of the prosthesis over a range of up to 20 mm, corresponding to a variation of 14 mm in medial head offset. This is less than half of the normal anatomic range of all femora and only 70% of the range of head offsets observed in femora of any one canal size[2,3] Greater coverage of the anatomic range can be provided if the head offset of the prosthesis is varied with its medial-lateral width and medial curvature (Fig. 3). This approach is based on the observation that femoral canals with a varus curvature have large medial head offsets whereas those having a valgus configuration have a head offset that is significantly smaller. This strategy results in a set of implants having two basic shapes, one with a valgus (straighter) medial profile and the other with a varus (more curved) medial profile with corresponding variations in neck/shaft angle and head offset. This enables much of the anatomic variation present within the normal bone population to be accommodated within a single system of prostheses.

The Biomechanics of Cemented Fixation

In cemented hip replacements, loads are transmitted from the femoral stem to the femur via three key mechanical elements: (1) the stem-cement interface; (2) the mantle of acrylic bone-cement; and (3) the cement-bone interface. The long-term durability of the prosthesis depends upon the ability of each of these three mechanical elements to transmit load without

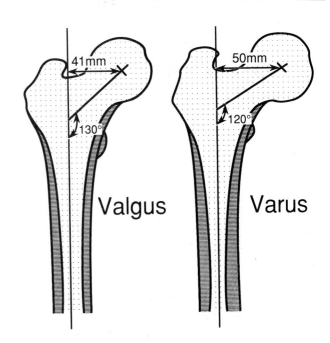

Fig. 3   The shape of the medial cortex is observed to be related to the neck/shaft angle of the femur and the medial offset of the femoral head. (Reproduced with permission from Noble PC: Biomechanical advances in total hip replacement, in Niwa S, Hattori T (eds): *Biomechanics in Orthopedics.* Berlin, Springer-Verlag, 1992, pp 46-75.)

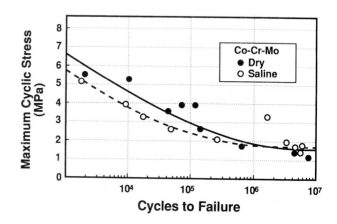

Fig. 4   The observed variation of the fatigue strength of the cement-stem interface in dry and saline environments. (Reproduced with permission from Raab S: Endoprosthetic fixation and the implant/bone-cement interface. Montreal, Canada, University of McGill, 1980, Dissertation.)

failure, as overload of any one element could ultimately compromise the entire fixation system. Though often weaker than the cement itself, the interfaces play a vital role in allowing the prosthesis and the femur to protect the cement mantle from excessive loading. Thus, any attempt to increase the durability of cemented fixation must address the strength of the interfaces formed by the cement mantle with the adjacent bone and prosthesis.

The Stem-Cement Interface

Recent investigations of cemented stems retrieved at postmortem have shown that the occurrence of fractures within the cement mantle is frequently preceded by separation of the stem-cement interface.[4] Previous computer studies predicted that debonding would increase the strain within the cement mantle by 100% to 200% and so it may be argued that failure of the stem-cement interface might ultimately lead to aseptic loosening of cemented components, especially if additional sources

of weakness exist within the cement.[5,6] A number of finite element models have predicted that the stresses developed at the stem-cement interface can be quite high. This is especially true during stair-climbing, when it is predicted that peak stresses of 4 to 8 MPa are developed within the interface at the level of the femoral neck osteotomy and the distal tip of the implant.[7,8] In contrast, the fatigue strength of a typical interface formed between cement and satin-finished Co-Cr is only 1 to 2 MPa in physiologic conditions (Fig. 4).[9,10]

The relative weakness of the stem-cement interface may be attributed to a number of factors.[11] Porous, boundary layers often form over the surface of the prosthesis during its implantation into the femur (Figs. 5

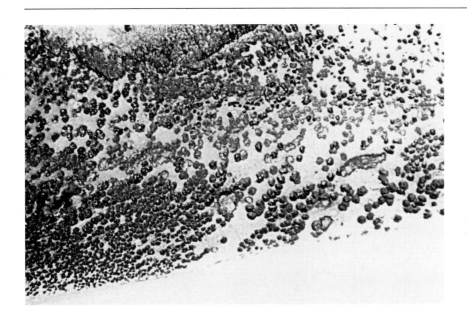

Fig. 5 A section of a cement mantle removed from the surface of a retrieved femoral stem and stained with India ink. Areas of extreme cement porosity are seen in direct contact with the femoral stem. (Reproduced with permission from Noble PC, Ward KS: Factors affecting the strength of cemented interfaces, in *The Implant/Bone Interface.* Berlin, Germany, Springer-Verlag, 1992.)

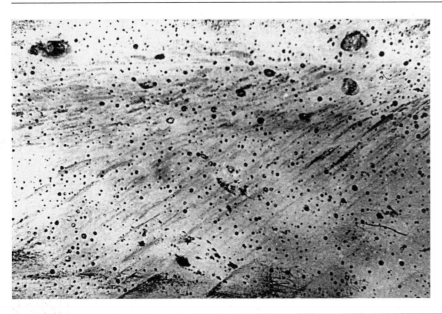

Fig. 6 Typical surface features of the cement mantle formed in direct contact with the femoral stem and loaded in vivo. Pores of varying size are seen intermingled with scratches caused by relative motion of the mantle and the metal.

and 6), leading to interfaces that are considerably weaker than the acrylic cement, especially in tension. The low fracture toughness of these interfaces, especially under repetitive loading, can lead to failure of adhesive bonding. Several enhancements to the surface of the femoral stem have been proposed to increase the durability of its bonding with the cement mantle, including: use of stems with porous coatings, similar to those designed to support tissue ingrowth[12]; application of a thin film of methylmethacrylate (pre-coating)[13]; and fabrication of implants with macrostructured, high-roughness surface textures, designed to maximize load transfer in shear.[14] Although, under clinical conditions, the relative efficacy of these alternate methods is unknown, laboratory studies have shown that reliable bonding can be achieved only by mechanical interlock, because adhesive bonds between the implant and acrylic cement are weak in the presence of physiologic fluids.[15]

Although porous metal coatings provide the stem-cement interface with the greatest resistance to shear stresses, the bonds formed between cement and beaded coatings are weak in tension because a relatively small area of cement is present between adjacent beads within the porous surface. Nonetheless, the bond developed with these surfaces is still stronger and more durable than the interfaces formed with precoated or surface textured prostheses.

Theoretically, PMMA precoating appears to be an ideal method of maximizing the strength of the cement-metal interface.[16,17] A thin film of PMMA is applied to the femoral component under industrial conditions by a process designed to remove weak surface layers from the metal to provide the best possible interface with acrylic cement. Then, in the operating room, wet cement is bonded to the precoated layer rather than to the metal implant surface, which is normally covered with an adherent oxide layer that forms weak interfaces with cement. Despite these measures, the fatigue performance of pre-coated interfaces under physiologic conditions has been disappointing (Fig. 7). In the presence of saline, these interfaces lose 70% to 80% of their initial strength with repetitive loading, so that coatings with initial bond strengths of 8 to 10 MPa in tension fail at stresses only 2 to 3 MPa (Fig. 8).[10,15] This progressive weakening is expected to result in a service life of only one million cycles or approximately one year within the body. The cause of this degradation is unknown, but may be related to diffusion of water vapor through the very thin precoated layer or the presence of pores within the interface between the precoated surface and the cement mantle. The bond strength of precoated surfaces is also highly variable, even when the acrylic coating is applied to the metal substrate under seemingly constant conditions.[15] This may cause the integrity of the bond between the

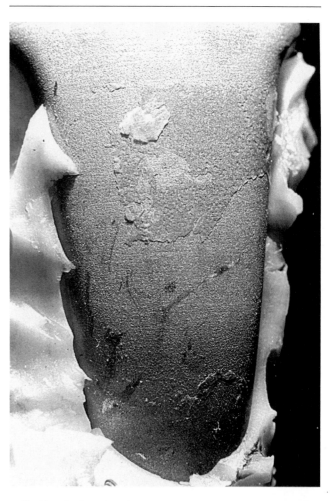

Fig. 7 The lateral surface of a PMMA pre-coated prosthesis that failed by aseptic loosening after three years in the body. The cement mantle is seen to be separated from the stem, which is now predominantly uncoated, indicating failure of the stem-pre-coat interface. In other areas a PMMA film remains attached to the prosthesis suggesting failure of initial adhesion between the cement mantle and the acrylic pre-coating.

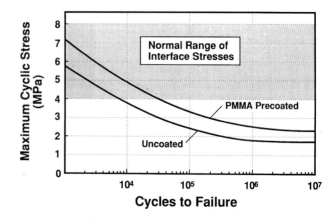

Fig. 8 The fatigue strength of uncoated and PMMA pre-coated surfaces (Co-Cr alloy) compared to the range of interface stresses that are predicted to be generated during normal activities. Both interfaces appear to be too weak to maintain their integrity in the long term.

stem and the cement mantle to vary unpredictably from implant to implant.

The third option for enhancement of stem-cement bonding is to roughen the surface of the prosthesis, especially in areas of the stem that are exposed to large interface stresses. Suitable surface textures may be formed by forging, plasma spray coating, machining, or arc deposition, and provide interfaces with initial strengths of 9 to 24 MPa in shear and 6 to 7 MPa in tension.[18,19] However, interfaces formed between acrylic cement and nonporous, textured surfaces weaken dramatically with repetitive loading, failure often occurring at stresses of less than 2 MPa in saline under fatigue conditions.[10] Nonetheless, these surfaces have the advantage that shear stresses are transferred between the stem and the cement by mechanical interlock, even in the absence of adhesive bonding.

An additional consideration is the ease of removal of cemented prostheses from the femur, as even well-fixed femoral stems occasionally require early revision for malposition and other causes. Revision of cemented stems is often extremely difficult if measures have been adopted to enhance bonding at the stem-cement interface. In such cases, it is essential that some means be available to allow the stem-cement bond to be broken in a controlled manner without trauma to the patient or the need to split the femur. The most effective method presently available for removal of cemented prostheses involves disruption of the stem-cement interface using a handheld ultrasonic probe; however, the cost of this equipment limits its widespread availability.

The Cement-Bone Interface

In many cases of prosthetic loosening, failure is initiated at the cement-bone interface. This may occur if structurally inadequate bone is left prior to cementing or if the penetration of cement into the endosteal surface is shallow because of poor pressurization or ineffective bone preparation.[20] Intraoperatively, an effective mechanical interlock can be obtained at the cement-bone interface if the strongest available porous bone is exposed prior to cementing; if blood, fat, and debris are removed from trabecular spaces to make room for cement interdigitation; and if the cement is kept under sustained pressure after its delivery to the femur.[21,22]

Preparation of the Implantation Site Bone preparation plays a critical role in the development of a strong cement-bone interface. As the loadbearing capacity of metaphyseal cancellous bone is highly variable, all weak trabeculae must be removed to leave a structure that is capable of supporting the cemented prosthesis. In addition, the prepared surface of the implantation site must be porous to allow interdigitation of cement. Unfortunately, the porosity of the cancellous structure of the femoral metaphysis varies considerably because of the orientation of the trabeculae. Posteriorly, within the femoral canal, the calcar femoral has almost no inherent porosity and forms a physical barrier that is relatively impenetrable to pressurized cement (Fig. 9). Laterally, the trabeculae form concentric arcades that are parallel to the cement-bone interface and resist

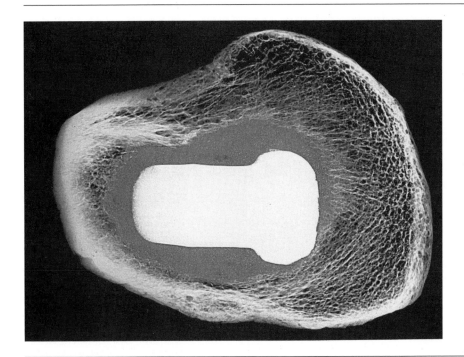

Fig. 9 A contact radiograph of a proximal slice taken through a cemented femoral stem within the femur. Some cement penetration is visible medially, anteriorly, and laterally; however, on the posterior surface, the trabeculae run parallel to the interface and have only superficial contact with the cement mantle.

penetration of cement in a radial direction. To overcome these obstacles, a series of holes may be drilled into the cancellous bed to provide access to the trabecular spaces of the proximal femur (Klaus Draenert, personal communication, May 1992). These holes allow the pressurized cement to flow circumferentially around the implantation site, thereby increasing the strength and uniformity of mechanical interlock.

Significant reinforcement of the stem-cement interface is also provided by the endosteal surface within the medullary canal, although little cancellous bone is often present below the level of the lesser trochanter. Nonetheless, the cortical wall does have a rough, irregular surface, which can develop significant bond strength, even in elderly and postmenopausal patients with poor quality bone stock (Fig. 10). Although metaphyseal cement penetration has been emphasized by previous authors, the diaphyseal interface may serve as a secondary line of defense when cement fixation within the metaphysis is inadequate. In this situation, endosteal interlock can provide resistance to micromotion and can enhance the stiffness of the interface in torsion, especially in femora where the medullary canal is relatively circular.

Because of the potential importance of the diaphyseal cement/bone interface, reaming instruments should be used carefully within the femur in order to preserve the porous intramedullary surface. If a cylindrical reamer is used in the isthmus, it is recommended that enlargement of the canal be limited to 2 mm whenever possible. Conical reaming instruments should also be used cautiously; the reamer should be directed laterally and not distally to ensure neutral alignment of the implantation site.[23]

Cementing Technique Effective pressurization of bone cement is also essential for durable implant fixation. However, the proximal femur can be difficult to pressurize, because the irregular metaphyseal cavity is hard to seal effectively. Anatomically contoured sealing devices are now available that conform to the shape of the implantation site in the proximal femur. These devices minimize leakage of cement, thus maximizing the pressure that can be developed during cement delivery (Fig. 11).[24] Using these devices, pressures to 55 to 60 psi can be developed using a cement gun in conjunction with a distal intramedullary plug. This is in contrast to conventional manual cementing techniques, which typically produce intermittent pressurization of the interface to pressures of less than 10 psi (Fig. 12).

In order to contain the cement within the implantation site, the intramedullary plug must be able to withstand considerable pressure, typically from 50 to 100 psi, without distal displacement. In practice, few contemporary plug designs have this capability. In fact, our experimental studies have shown that the intramedullary plugs in common use will only withstand pressures up to about 50 psi without distal migration in 22% to 80% of femora, depending upon the individual plug design and the size of the canal (Fig. 13). This problem becomes marked in canals larger than 12 to 14 mm, in which most commercial devices will resist pressures of only 30 to 40 psi (Fig. 14).

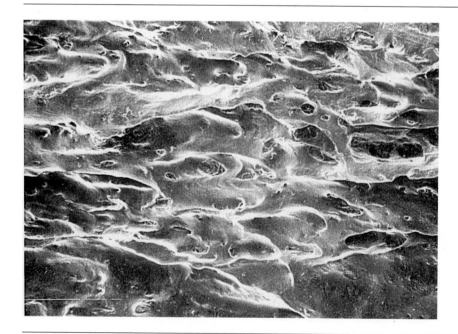

Fig. 10 A scanning electron micrograph of the endosteal surface of the unreamed diaphysis of the femur.

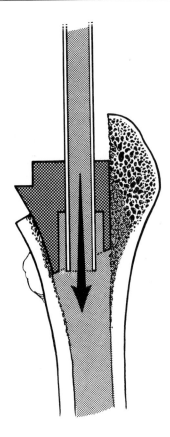

Fig. 11 Schematic representation of an anatomically contoured flexible pressurizing seal occluding the mouth of the medullary canal during pressurization of bone cement with a cement gun. (Reproduced with permission from Noble PC: Biomechanical advances in total hip replacement, in Niwa S, Hattori T (eds): *Biomechanics in Orthopedics.* Berlin, Springer-Verlag, 1992, pp 46-75.)

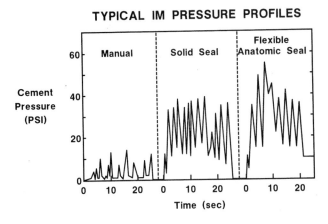

Fig. 12 Typical performance of three methods of pressurizing the proximal cement/bone interface. The manual (two thumbs) technique provides relatively low cement pressures, which decay rapidly with release of the force against the doughy cement. The alternate methods are used with lower viscosity cement delivered with a cement syringe. The solid and flexible proximal seals allow a minimum level of cement pressure to be maintained between clicks of the cement gun, thus minimizing back-bleeding. (Reproduced with permission from Noble PC, Ward KS: Factors affecting the strength of cemented interfaces, in *The Implant/Bone Interface.* Berlin, Germany, Springer-Verlag, 1992.)

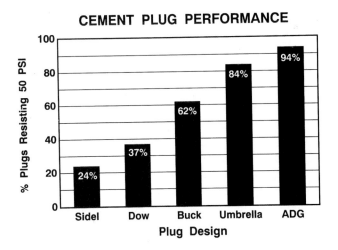

Fig. 13 The relative performance of five commercial designs of polymeric intramedullary plugs, assessed in terms of the percentage of devices resisting cement pressures of 50 psi without migration in the canal. All tests were performed in identical femoral specimens ranging in diameter from 8 to 18 mm.

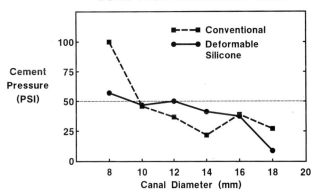

Fig. 14 The average cement pressure required to cause 5 mm of migration of two designs of intramedullary plugs, a conventional design (Seidel plug, Howmedica Inc.) and a deformable silicone plug (Dow Corning Inc.), expressed as a function of the diameter of the medullary canal.

The Cement Mantle

The durability of the cement mantle may be enhanced by increasing the fatigue strength of the cement itself[25] and by reducing the stresses developed during weight-bearing.[14] Although most intraoperative methods of enhancing acrylic cement increase its average strength by 20% to 30%, optimization of the shape of the mantle can reduce peak stresses by 50% to 90%.[6,14,26]

Various computer models have been employed to study the relationship between the mantle geometry and cement stresses.[6] These studies have shown that the strongest cement mantle is not of uniform thickness but ranges from a minimum of 2 mm distally to 3 to 7 mm proximally.[27] During normal activities, the stresses borne by the mantle are very uneven and tend to concentrate in the areas of greatest discontinuity of stiffness. Proximally, maximum cement stresses are present at the level of the femoral neck osteotomy; distally, the peak stress occurs at the level of the tip of the prosthesis. Within the distal cement, the peak stress increases dramatically with the bulk of the implant within the canal (Fig. 15). Thus, the thinner the mantle, the higher the cement stress and the greater the risk of fracture and fragmentation of the cement column. In practice, because any reduction in the distal diameter of the femoral stem is limited by the strength of the stem itself, a compromise must be reached where both the cement mantle and the implant are bulky enough to function without eventual failure. This generally corresponds to 70% to 80% filling of the medullary canal by the prosthesis, leaving a distal mantle of at least 1 to 2 mm in thickness.

Proximal cement stresses follow different guidelines (Fig. 15). In the proximal-medial area of the cement mantle, minimum cement stresses occur when the stem fills 80% to 90% of the canal, which corresponds to a medial cement thickness of 3 to 7 mm. As the mantle becomes thicker, peak stresses increase gradually; however, if the mantle becomes thinner, stresses can rise to catastrophic levels and lead to failure of the mantle with weightbearing.

Some clinical support for these predictions is found in a number of series of cemented hip replacements.[28-30] Sarmiento and Green[28] looked at the effect of the thickness of the proximal medial cement on the incidence of significant calcar resorption, a phenomenon that appears to be a response to the generation of particulate debris. These investigators found that significant resorption became alarmingly prevalent once the thickness of the proximal cement was less than 2 mm.

On the basis of a long-term review of 864 primary cemented cases they recommended an optimum proximal cement thickness of 2 to 5 mm.[30]

Thin and inadequate cement mantles are a common source of particulate debris, which can lead to osteolysis at the cement-bone interface. To eliminate the formation of defective mantles, prostheses are needed that allow sufficient space with respect to the femoral canal for formation of a mantle of adequate thickness. The implant must also be centered within the cement mantle so that it will not impinge against the endosteal surface. The most common form of malfitting arises when the femoral canal has a less pronounced medial curvature than the implant. In these cases, thin areas of cement are observed medially at the level of the femoral neck osteotomy and the distal tip of the stem, exactly the two positions where peak cement stresses are greatest. Ironically, canals with a straighter, stovepipe shape are more common in older patients, the age group in whom cement is used most frequently. Consequently, inadequate cement mantles resulting from mismatches between the implant and the canal tend to occur most frequently in older patients. This problem can be overcome if cemented prostheses have a straighter, more valgus medial contour than their cementless counterparts. This means that implants of one fixed geometry cannot be used for cemented and cementless hip replacement without compromising the minimum thickness of the cement mantle, leading to increased risk of aseptic loosening and osteolysis.

Centralization

The benefits of an optimum cement mantle remain theoretical unless the stem can be positioned centrally within the medullary canal. The recent emergence of centralizing devices now makes this possible (Fig. 16). Detailed study of the mantles of femurs harvested from cadavers shows that areas of fissuring and perforation

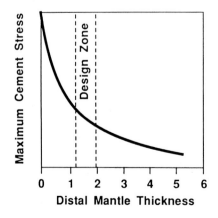

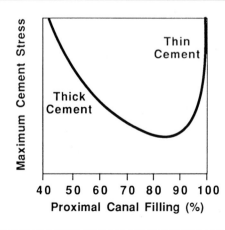

Fig. 15 Variation of the maximum stress within the cement mantle, distally (**left**), adjacent to the distal tip of the prosthesis, and proximally (**right**) near the level of the femoral neck osteotomy. Stresses are plotted as a function of the thickness of the distal cement mantle and the percentage of the proximal canal occupied by the femoral stem. (Reproduced with permission from Huiskes R: Some fundamental aspects of human joint replacement: Analysis of stresses and heat. *Acta Orthop Scand* 1992;63:250.)

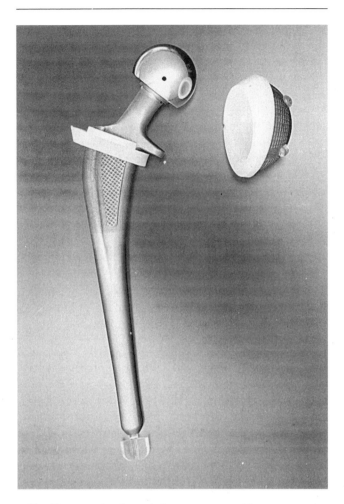

Fig. 16 Femoral and acetabular components with cement spacing and centralizing devices. (Reproduced with permission from Noble PC: Biomechanical advances in total hip replacement, in Niwa S, Hattori T (eds): *Biomechanics in Orthopedics*. Berlin, Springer-Verlag, 1992, pp 46-75.)

of the cement mantle are extremely common in cemented hip replacement.[27] This is not surprising, given that the position of the stem in the canal is difficult to control by feel alone and that prostheses are often implanted in increased anteversion to maximize joint stability and in some degree of valgus to avoid a varus stem position. However, both these deviations almost inevitably cause impingement of the stem against bone in some area of the canal, a situation that often goes unnoticed during implantation.

Centralizing devices are now commonly used to prevent stem impingement by fixing the minimum possible thickness of the cement mantle in key areas, generally proximally and distally.[31] Although various designs are available, most centralizing devices are fabricated from polymethylmethacrylate, which bonds with the wet cement, thus avoiding the formation of stress concentrations through mechanical or structural disconti-

nuities. Both proximal and distal centralizers must be used to guarantee the integrity of the cement mantle, because centralization of the distal stem within the medullary canal has little influence on the proximal position of the implant within the metaphysis.

Acetabular Replacement

A finding common to many series of cemented hip replacements is development of progressive radiolucent lines between the cement and the bone within the acetabulum. Although these radiographic indications of biologic incompatibility are not always associated with frank loosening of acetabular components, cementless acetabular fixation has been adopted by many surgeons for use in patients of all ages, including those who would routinely receive a cemented femoral component. At present, the best results are obtained using hemispherical cementless cups with porous-coated outer surfaces and with modular polyethylene liners. This design allows the surgeon the greatest flexibility in obtaining secure intraoperative fixation within the pelvis while retaining the ability to maximize coverage of the femoral head by positioning the bearing liner within the cup.

Despite the early clinical success of cementless acetabular cups, several issues appear to compromise the long-term durability of these components. These include the integrity of mechanisms providing liner-shell attachment, the fit and method of fixation of the shell to the bony acetabulum, and the occurence of osteolysis in response to polyethylene wear debris.

Late loosening of cemented acetabular cups is not generally caused by inadequate initial fixation, but rather by progressive osteolysis secondary to the accumulation of polymeric wear debris at the cement-bone interface.[32] Typically, localized areas of fibrous membrane at the interface serve as sites for osteoclastic resorption of bone. This process undermines the fixation of the cement and leads to increased micromotion and eventual loosening of the cemented component. Histologic examination of retrieved implants suggests that this process is not related to the presence of acrylic cement but to the accumulation of particles of polyethylene generated by abrasive wear of the bearing surface. If this is indeed true, the longevity of all acetabular components, including cementless prostheses fixed without acrylic cement, is threatened by the effects of wear debris. Indeed, several clinical reviews have demonstrated that osteolysis can be a disturbing complication of cementless acetabular fixation with an incidence of 9% to 15% at five to nine years postimplantation.[33-35]

Several measures can be adopted to minimize the prevalence of osteolysis following cementless acetabular replacement. Materials are becoming available that may reduce the rate of wear of the acetabular cup and the volume of fine debris entering the joint. These include metal-on-metal bearings, ceramic femoral heads, and new forms of ultra-high-molecular-weight polyethylene. However, the efficacy of each of these options in reducing osteolysis remains unproven.

Osteolysis may also be eliminated if the area of bony ingrowth into the acetabular cup is maximized and all gaps between the shell and the acetabulum are removed that could allow ingress of wear debris. Retrieval studies of cementless cups have demonstrated that most of the surface of the prosthesis is ingrown with fibrous tissue and that the area of bony attachment is highly variable.[36-38] Moreover, it is uncommon for a complete, circumferential band of bony ingrowth to be present between the cup and the acetabular margin. These observations are not surprising, given the flexibility of the acetabulum, which can undergo deformations of up to 200 mm during normal weightbearing. An additional factor is the ellipsoidal shape of the socket, which often cannot be made truly hemispherical without excessive reaming at surgery.

One popular method of increasing the stability of cementless cups, adjunctive screw fixation, is often used with a slightly oversized shells, typically 1 to 2 mm larger than the reamed acetabulum. Screw fixation provides a number of benefits to the surgeon, because screws enhance the stability of cup fixation and increase the area of direct contact between the implant and the underlying bone. However, transacetabular placement of screws and drills is also associated with some hazard to the patient and can result in serious neurovascular injuries, or even death. These tragic complications typically occur secondary to perforation of vital structures within the pelvis by screws that have been passed through the inner pelvic wall in an attempt to obtain bicortical thread purchase. As the only way to avoid neurovascular injuries and still use screw fixation is to avoid bicortical fixation entirely, we have examined in some detail the optimal placement of unicortical screws within the pelvis.

In a cadaveric study, we measured the intracortical thickness of the pelvis as a function of the position of screw placement on the acetabular surface.[1] Eight specimens spanning the anatomic range of the acetabular diameter were embedded in foam and divided into 16 pie-shaped slices. On an outline of each transected slice, we measured the distance between the inner and outer cortices measured at right angles to the surface of the acetabular shell. From these measurements, we determined the maximum length of a screw that would engage cancellous bone without penetrating of the inner wall of the pelvis. By repeating the process for all bone slices, a three-dimensional map of the surface of the acetabulum was developed

to guide the length and placement of screws used for acetabular fixation (Fig. 17).

The zones of safe screw placement varied with the length of the screw. When the length of the screw equalled 40% of the acetabular diameter (16 to 24 mm), positions for "safe" screw placement were restricted to approximately one quarter of the available acetabular surface, almost entirely within the posterior half of the socket (Fig. 18). Based on this observation, it is recommended that screws should be positioned with considerable care, avoiding the anterior half of the acetabular surface and the rim and dome on the posterior side. In addition, whenever possible, the length of screws should be restricted to only 40% of the diameter of the reamed acetabulum. As this generally corresponds to short screws providing limited fixation, the primary stability of the acetabular shell should be obtained through accurate reaming of the acetabulum and placement of an oversized prosthetic component.

One objection to the use of screws to augment acetabular fixation is that the holes present in the shell allow ingress of wear debris to the cementless interface. Although this is true, laboratory experiments have shown that even in the absence of screw holes, almost all of the cup-bone interface is accessible to small particles. Given that polyethylene wear debris ranges in size from approximately 0.2 to 5 mm, gaps of 0.5 to 1 mm (500 to 1,000 mm), which are present between some part of the shell and the acetabulum,

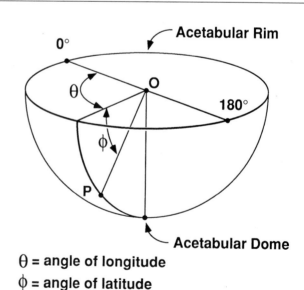

θ = angle of longitude
φ = angle of latitude

Fig. 17 The position of screw placement within the acetabulum may be defined in terms of two angular coordinates that are analogous to the angles of latitude and longitude used to describe the locations of geographic landmarks.

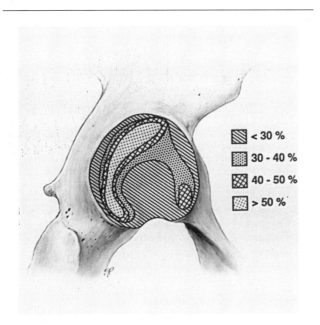

Fig. 18 Distribution of intracortical thickness of the pelvis for screws passing perpendicular to the acetabular surface. All thicknesses are normalized with respect to the diameter of the acetabulum. (Reproduced with permission from Noble PC: Biomechanical advances in total hip replacement, in Niwa S, Hattori T (eds): *Biomechanics in Orthopedics.* Berlin, Springer-Verlag, 1992, pp 46-75.)

provide an easy portal for infiltration of particles to any area of the interface where direct contact is not present between the ingrowth coating and the underlying bone.

Conclusion

While the short history of total hip replacement is firmly grounded in the inspiration and dedication of many farsighted surgeons tempered with an understanding of basic scientific principles, the future of this endeavor will be increasingly within the realm of the basic sciences. It is hoped that in the years ahead new developments in surgical techniques and biomaterials will provide even greater longevity to total hip replacement. However, today most of the issues that face us in extending the durability of this procedure can only be truly resolved through greater insight into the mechanisms of implant loosening, prosthetic wear, and the biologic response to foreign materials.

References

1. Noble PC: Biomechanical advances in total hip replacement, in Niwa S, Hattori T (eds): *Biomechanics in Orthopedics.* Tokyo, Springer-Verlag, 1992, pp 46-75.
2. Noble PC, Alexander JW, Lindahl LJ, et al: The anatomic basis of femoral component design. *Clin Orthop* 1988;235:148-165.
3. Noble PC: Proximal femoral geometry and the design of cementless hip replacements. *Orthop Rel Sci* 1990;1:86-92.
4. Maloney WJ, Jasty M, Burke DW, et al: Biomechanical and histologic investigation of cemented total hip arthroplasties: A study of autopsy-retrieved femurs after in vivo cycling. *Clin Orthop* 1989;249:129-140.
5. McNiece GM, Amstutz HC: Finite element studies in hip reconstruction, in Komi PV (ed): *Biomechanics V: Proceedings of the 5th International Congress on Biomechanics.* Baltimore, MD, University Park Press, 1976, pp 339-405.
6. Huiskes R: Some fundamental aspects of human joint replacement: Analyses of stresses and heat conduction in bone-prosthesis structures. *Acta Orthop Scand* 1980;185(suppl):1-208.
7. Lu Z, Ebramzadeh E, McKellop H, et al: The influence of the stem-cement bonding strength on the cement stresses in total hip arthroplasty. *Trans Orthop Res Soc* 1992;17:377.
8. Estok DM, Orr TE: The strain gradient across the cement mantle in a cemented femoral component: A detailed mapping. *Trans Orthop Res Soc* 1992;17:371.
9. Raab S, Ahmed AM, Provan JW: The quasistatic and fatigue performance of the implant/bone-cement interface. *J Biomed Mater Res* 1981;15:159-182.
10. Davies JP, Harris WH: Fatigue strength of cement-metal interface: Comparison of metal, metal with precoating and metal with rough surface and precoating, in *Proceedings of the 16th Annual Meeting of the Society for Biomaterials.* Minneapolis, MN, Society for Biomaterials, 1990, p 34.
11. Raab S: *Endoprosthetic Fixation and the Implant/Bone-Cement Interface.* Montreal, University of McGill, 1980. Dissertation.
12. Welsh RP, Pilliar RM, Macnab I: Surgical implants: The role of surface porosity in fixation to bone and acrylics. *J Bone Joint Surg* 1971;53A:963-977.
13. Ahmed AM, Raab S, Miller JE: Metal cement interface strength in cemented stem fixation. *J Orthop Res* 1984;2:105-118.
14. Levy RN, Noble PC, Scheller A, et al: Prolonged fixation of cemented total hip replacement. *Surgical Rounds For Orthopaedics* 1988;April:15-22.
15. Raab S, Ahmed AM, Provan JW: Thin film PMMA precoating for improved implant bone cement fixation. *J Biomed Mater Res* 1982;16:679-704.
16. Park JB, Malstrom CS, von Recum AF: Intramedullary fixation of implants pre-coated with bone cement: A preliminary study. *Biomater Med Devices Artif Organs* 1978;6:361-373.
17. Raab S: Bone connective prostheses adapted to maximize strength and durability of prostheses: Bone cement interface and methods of forming same. 1982 U.S. Patent Number 4,336,618.
18. Arroyo NA, Stark CF: The effect of textures, surface finish and precoating on the strength of bone cement-stem interfaces, in the *Proceedings of the 13th Annual Meeting of the Society for Biomaterials.* Minneapolis, MN, Society for Biomaterials, 1987, p 218.
19. Noble PC, Scheller AD Jr, Tullos HS, et al: Applied design criteria for total hip prosthesis, in Stillwell WT (ed): *The Art of Total Hip Arthroplasty.* Orlando, FL, Grune and Stratton, 1987, chap 5, pp 51-68.
20. Krause WR, Krug W, Miller J: Strength of the cement-bone interface. *Clin Orthop* 1982;163:290-299.
21. Ling RSM: Prevention of loosening of total hip components, in Riley LH Jr (ed): *The Hip: Proceedings of the Eighth Open Scientific Meeting of the Hip Society.* St Louis, MO, CV Mosby, 1980, chap 14, pp 292-307.
22. Miller J, Johnson JA: Advances in cementing techniques in total hip arthroplasty, in Stillwell T, Chandler JL (eds): *The Art of Total Hip Arthroplasty.* Orlando, FL, Grune and Stratton, 1987, chap 19, pp 277-291.
23. Balu RG, Noble PC: Effect of canal reaming on

cement/bone interface. Presented at the 60th Annual Meeting of the American Academy of Orthopaedic Surgeons, San Francisco, CA, February 1993, paper no. 72.

24. Noble PC, Alexander JW, Hammerman SM, et al: Innovations in cementing techniques in total hip replacement. Presented at the 54th Annual Meeting of the American Academy of Orthopaedic Surgeons, San Francisco, CA, January 1987, scientific exhibit no. 3142.

25. Burke DW, Gates EI, Harris WH: Centrifugation as a method of improving tensile and fatigue properties of acrylic bone cement. *J Bone Joint Surg* 1984;66A:1265-1273.

26. Davies JP, Jasty M, O'Connor DO, et al: The effect of centrifuging bone cement. *J Bone Joint Surg* 1989;71B:39-42

27. Noble PC, Tullos HS, Landon GC: The optimum cement mantle for total hip replacement: Theory and practice, in Hugh S. Tullos (ed): *Instructional Course Lecture, XL*. Park Ridge, IL, American Academy of Orthopaedic Surgeons, 1991, chap 20, pp 145-150.

28. Sarmiento A, Gruen TA: Radiographic analysis of a low-modulus titanium-alloy femoral total hip component: Two to six-year follow-up. *J Bone Joint Surg* 1985;67A:48-56.

29. Huddleston HD: Femoral lysis after cemented hip arthroplasty. *J Arthroplasty* 1988;3:285-297

30. Madsen NS, Brick GW, Poss R, et al: Minimum five year follow-up of modern cement technique and single femoral stem design. Presented at the 58th Annual Meeting of the American Academy of Orthopaedic Surgeons, Anaheim, CA, March 7-12, 1991, paper no. 89.

31. Scheller A, Levy RN, Noble PC, et al: A comparative analysis of total hip component position and cement technique. Presented at the 56th Annual Meeting of the American Academy of Orthopaedic Surgeons, Las Vegas, NV, February 9-14, 1989, paper no. 386.

32. Schmalzried TP, Kwong LM, Jasty M, et al: The mechanism of loosening of cemented acetabular components in total hip arthroplasty: Analysis of specimens retrieved at autopsy. *Clin Orthop* 1992;274:60-78.

33. Beauchesne RP, Kukita Y, Knezevich S, et al: Roentgenographic evaluation of the AML porous coated acetabular component: A six year minimum follow-up study, Presented at the 59th Annual Meeting of the American Academy of Orthopaedic Surgeons, Washington, DC, February 18-23, 1992, paper no. 416.

34. Stulberg BN, Buly RL, Howard PL, et al: Porous coated anatomic acetabular failure: Incidence and modes of failure in uncemented total hip arthroplasty. Presented at the 59th Annual Meeting of the American Academy of Orthopaedic Surgeons, Washington, DC, February 18-23, 1992, paper no. 168.

35. Lavernia C, Tsao AK, Hungerford DS: Silent osteolysis: Polyethylene debris in cementless total hip replacement. Presented at the 60th Annual Meeting of the American Academy of Orthopaedic Surgeons, San Francisco, CA, February 18-23, 1993, paper no. 230.

36. Schwartz JT, Engh CA, Forte MR, et al: Evaluation of initial surface apposition in porous coated acetabular components. *Trans Orthop Res Soc* 1991;16:243.

37. Zettl-Schaffer KF, Engh CA, Sweet D, et al: Histologic and roentgenographic assessment of well functioning porous coated acetabular components: A human postmortem retrieval analysis, in *Proceedings of the Implant Retrieval Symposium of the Society for Biomaterials*. Minneapolis, MN, Society for Biomaterials, 1992, p 43.

38. Pidhorz LE, Urban RM, Sumner DR, et al: Autopsy retrieval analysis of cementless porous coated acetabular components. Presented at the 60th Annual Meeting of the American Academy of Orthopaedic Surgeons, San Francisco, CA, February 18-23, 1993, paper no. 244.

Fixing the Cup

Pasquale Petrera, MD

Harry E. Rubash, MD

Historical Issues

Charnley's original concept of low-friction arthroplasty was of paramount importance in the development of the total hip replacement. His intention was to find two materials that when used together would approximate the low coefficient of friction of human cartilage. His first attempts mated a stainless steel femoral component that had a 42-mm head with a socket made of polytetrafluorethylene (PTFE), otherwise known as Teflon. PTFE was being used in engineering and aerospace industries for its low coefficient of friction. Although its characteristics in the human body were not known, Charnley believed it ideal for the socket of the low-friction arthroplasty. With time, Charnley reduced the head size of the femoral component to 22.5 mm to allow for a thicker PTFE cup. More than 300 total hip replacements were implanted using these materials before Charnley began to see the poor results caused by low wear resistance and the body's reaction to PTFE debris. The cups wore quite quickly, producing a large amount of PTFE particles. These particles formed large periprosthetic granulomas and this reaction caused severe bony destruction and implant loosening. Attempts at reinforcing the PTFE by filling it with fiberglass ended dismally, because the new socket wore just as quickly and the filler acted as an abrasive.[1] Revision was required, with removal of the cup, in all of these PTFE arthroplasties to halt the progress of wear-debris generated particle disease.

In 1962, Charnley discovered that high-molecular-weight polyethylene made an effective bearing surface for the acetabular component. Laboratory studies using this new material had shown that its coefficient of friction, though higher than that of PTFE, decreased when it was subjected to high stress.[2]

Charnley fixed the polyethylene cups in the acetabular bone using polymethylmethacrylate (PMMA), which was then being used as a dental repair material. Six months after implantation, radiographs showed the disturbing occurrence of demarcation between cement and bone. These radiolucencies around the cup were not progressive, but were of concern to Charnley because they were not evident around the femoral stem. Charnley felt that these radiolucencies were a sure sign of loosening and ultimate failure of the cup. Instead of using bone cement he began to implant a press-fit socket.

More than 300 press-fit sockets were implanted between 1962 and 1965 before they, too, were abandoned. Charnley observed that the acetabular radiolucencies around cemented cups did not progress beyond the amount visible at one year and the patient's clinical results were excellent regardless of the radiologic findings. Moreover, patients who had bilateral low-friction implants and both types of sockets invariably preferred the cemented side. Convinced of the success of polyethylene components fixed with PMMA, Charnley directed his attention toward improving the design and the implantation of polyethylene sockets. For the next 15 years total hip arthroplasty was performed using a cemented socket.

Cement remained the standard of socket fixation until the mid 1980s, when concerns about radiographic loosening and "cement disease" prompted the initiation of press-fit implants and the use of techniques to promote bone ingrowth; these methods were applied to both the femoral and acetabular components. Today, we see a growing trend toward the use of uncemented sockets in total hip replacement. Is this trend justified, or have we abandoned a proven technique in the face of a new technology?

Cemented Components

To compare cemented and uncemented acetabular components, it is first necessary to delineate the clinical and radiographic determinants of failure. All studies define revision as failure of the implant, but loosening also must be considered. Furthermore, the fact that the definition of loosening varies with different studies makes comparisons difficult. Cemented sockets can show radiographic signs of loosening without clinical signs of failure. Migration or change in position of the socket indicates gross loosening. A socket surrounded by a continuous 2-mm radiolucency in all three zones is *probably loose* as described by DeLee and Charnley.[3] Hodgkinson and associates[4] found that acetabular components with any continuous radiolucent line, irrespective of width, had a 94% probability of being found loose intraoperatively.

Plain radiographs are frequently inadequate for determining whether an acetabular component is loose. Sensitivities ranging from 37% to 63% and specificities ranging from 63% to 89% have been reported in diagnosing loose cups by plain radiographs.[5,6]

Arthrograms are more helpful, having a sensitivity of 89% to 100% and a specificity of 75% to 98%.[5-7] The seepage of injected dye along the bone-cement interface is indicative of loosening (Fig. 1). Lyons and associates[5] reviewed 34 loose cups and found arthrographic signs of loosening for 33, whereas plain radiographs showed loosening in only 24. Among 35 loose cups, O'Neill and Harris[6] found arthrograms accurate for 66%, while plain radiographs were diagnostic for 37%. Thus, arthrograms are better than plain radiographs in diagnosing a loose acetabular component and are useful in the evaluation of a painful or suspected loose socket.

A review of the short-term results for Charnley components, as reported during the late 1970s and early 1980s, reveals similar results with respect to loosening as defined by revision or migration. At four years, Charnley found revision necessary in 1% of 582 cemented acetabular components. Concurrent review of 169 press-fit sockets in this same paper revealed that 6.5% required revision.[8] This study vindicated his abandonment of the press-fit socket after limited evaluation. Cupic[9] noted a 0.7% loosening rate among 409 implants at five years, and Eftekhar[10] reported a 1.5% acetabular revision rate at seven to eight years. In another series, Eftekhar[11] found that 0.8% of acetabular components were revised by five to 15 years.[11] In addition, Griffith and associates[12] reviewed 547 cemented implants at 8.3 years and found 18 loose cups, only five of which required revision. Among 2,012 total hip arthroplasties, Coventry and associates[13] noted a 0.1% rate of acetabular loosening at up to five years.

Although the results of cemented Charnley sockets are certainly acceptable, the incidence of radiolucencies has been disturbing. The recently described progressive nature of these radiolucencies, coupled with the inaccuracy of plain radiographs in diagnosing loosening, is significant. Given the high association between radiolucencies and loosening described by Hodgkinson and associates,[4] the actual number of

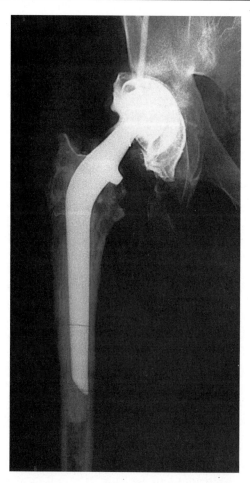

Fig. 1 Arthrogram of a loose metal-backed cemented cup ten years after implantation using modern cementing techniques.

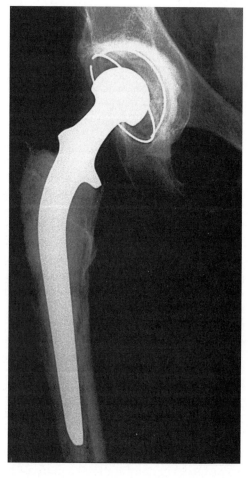

Fig. 2 Anteroposterior radiograph of a cemented all-polyethylene cup placed 13 years earlier shows no evidence of loosening.

loose sockets is probably much higher than the values stated in early reports.

The presence and progression of acetabular radiolucencies must be viewed in light of the fact that a radiographically loose cemented component may continue to function well clinically for a number of years.[4,14,15] The upper limits of this dichotomy need to be defined in order to determine the realistic longevity of cemented sockets (Figs. 2 and 3).

Charnley cemented acetabular components evaluated at five to seven years have been found to do well. Various studies have found that the failure rate at ten years is higher. For example, Stauffer[16] characterized 26 of 231 components as loose, with 17 of these showing progression of radiolucent lines or migration. Three percent had been revised. Of 1,041 components studied by Hozack and associates,[17] 150 cups were radiographically loose, but only 15 had been revised. Survivorship for the socket at ten years was 99%. At 11 years, Older[18] found radiographic loosening in 15% of 153 Charnley components; one-half of which had migrated without clinical symptoms, and 2% of which required acetabular revision.

Comparing the five- and ten-year results for cemented Charnley sockets reveals, in general, a higher revision rate at longer follow up (Table 1). Of more concern than revision rates alone are the proportionately much larger increases in loosening rates. Given the high probability that most of these radiographically loose cups will require revision, dependent on patient longevity, the actual failure rate is much higher than the stated revision rates. The relatively small numbers of revisions can be misleading in light of the much larger group of patients with impending failure. This has been one of the driving forces behind finding a new technique for acetabular implantation.

The large patient attrition rate over the course of long-term studies also must be considered. Survivorship analysis has been used to compensate for these

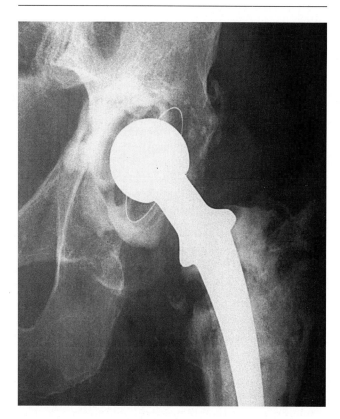

Fig. 3   Anteroposterior radiograph of a cemented all-polyethylene cup placed 12 years previously. Evidence of severe loosening and migration are seen.

deficiencies and is based on the assumption that patients who are lost to follow-up are no more or less likely to have had failed implants as described by the investigators.[19] Also, the fact that a patient still has the implant does not always equate with good clinical results, and herein lies the weakness of survivorship analysis. Despite these shortcomings, survivorship

Table 1
Intermediate and long-term results of Charnley cemented all-polyethylene cups

Investigator	Number of Patients	Follow-up (yrs)	Revisions	Loose
Charnley (1972)[8]	582	4	1 %	—
Cupic (1979)[9]	409	5	0.7 %	—
Eftekhar (1971)[10]	138	7-8	1.5 %	0
Eftekhar (1987)[11]	449	5-15	0.8 %	—
Griffith et al (1978)[12]	547	8.3	0.91%	3.3 %
Coventry et al (1974)[13]	2,012	0-5	0.1 %	—
Stauffer (1982)[16]	231	10	3.0 %	11.3 %
Hozack et al (1990)[17]	1,041	10	1.65%	25 %
Older (1986)[18]	153	10-12	2.0 %	15 %
García-Cimbrelo and Munuera (1992)[20]	680	12.7	4.3 %	9.0 %
McCoy et al (1988)[21]	100	15	1.0 %	6.0 %
Kavanagh et al (1989)[22]	166	15	7.2 %	14 %
Welch et al (1988)[24]	100	15-17	6 %	—

analysis enables direct comparison between results of different studies and, for this reason, is a useful tool.

The results of longer follow-up have been analyzed recently using survivorship analysis. At an average of almost 13 years, Garcia-Cimbrelo and Munuera[20] found that 9% of 680 Charnley prostheses were radiographically loose; the revision rate was 4.3%. Survivorship analysis showed a 19% total cumulative probability of loosening at 18 years. They also categorized these sockets as having early loosening (within ten years of surgery) or late loosening (after ten years of surgery). Early loosening was associated with deficiencies in the acetabular bone, whereas late loosening was associated with linear acetabular polyethylene wear of more than 2 mm. Although the process of wear debris is slower with the polyethylene cup than the PTFE cup, polyethylene debris has been implicated in the late loosening of cemented acetabular components. This is supported by the rates of late loosening in Garcia-Cimbrelo and Munuera's study.[20]

McCoy and associates[21] studied the results of 100 Charnley prostheses at 16 years, finding that 6% had migrated and 1% had required revision. Survival analysis for mechanical failure showed 98% survival of the socket at 15 years. At 15 years, among 166 Charnley implants, Kavanagh and associates[22] found that 9% had migrated and 14% were probably loose. The probability of loosening of the socket was 8.5% at 15 years. After a 15- to 17-year follow-up of patients with a Charnley prosthesis, Welch and associates[24] reported that 6% of the acetabular components had required revision without radiographic follow-up.

Cemented all-polyethylene sockets reviewed in long-term investigations have continued to function well with low revision rates, despite a relatively higher incidence of radiographic loosening. Other early attempts at acetabular component fixation have not been as successful. The Ring prosthesis consisted of a metal cup with a threaded stem that was screwed into the iliopubic bar of bone of the pelvis. This articulated, metal-on-metal, with a modified Austin-Moore prosthesis having a 40-mm head. Acetabular revisions averaged 16%, with survivorship at ten years being 70.6%.[25] Buchholz and Heinert[23] calculated a 72% acetabular survivorship for the St. George 38-mm head size prosthesis at 15 years. Uncemented ceramic components have also been implanted with little success.[26] Early work with threaded acetabular cups showed no advantage over cemented cups.[27] Another review showed disturbingly high rates of failure, especially in revision situations, and "discretionary use was advised" (Fig. 4)[28] Pegged, uncemented polyethylene components have been implanted with no revisions at the relatively short follow-up of 18 months.[29] Long-term follow-up has yet to be reported. Charnley's initial experience with press fit showed loosening rates

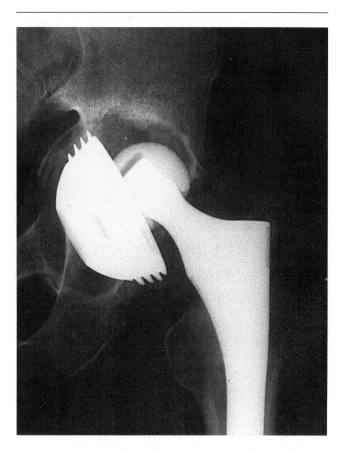

Fig. 4 Anteroposterior radiograph of a threaded acetabular component placed seven years prior to this catastrophic failure.

of 15% at seven to eight years and 35% at 12 to 15 years.[30]

Attempts at Improving Cemented Fixation

Efforts to improve cementing technique and thereby decrease both radiographic and clinical signs of loosening have had mixed results. Pressurization of cement, along with centrifugation, has been used for femoral components and has led to longer component survival as well as a lower rate of loosening. Improvement in acetabular component survival was hypothesized with these same modern cementing techniques. Oh and associates[31] believed that a major cause of cup loosening was poor interdigitation of the cement with the bone and cup. He recommended a flanged polyethylene component to aid in pressurizing acetabular cement. He also thought that cement equalizing pods, positioned around the outside perimeter of the cup, would provide a uniform periprosthetic cement mantle and avoid eccentric cup seating (bottoming out).

The objective of a cemented all-polyethylene cup is to transfer stress to bone via an acrylic layer, that is,

PMMA, which serves as a low-modulus energy absorber.[32] Deficiencies in this layer of cement, evidenced by bottoming out of the acetabular component, will result in suboptimal fixation and performance of the cup in the long term.

Other factors have been thought to influence fixation of the cemented acetabular component. The blood pressure of bone, approximately 25 mm Hg, has been found to be sufficient to force blood between bone and cement during cup insertion and cement curing. Shelley and Wroblewski[33] found that a flanged cup will produce cement pressures high enough to overcome this back pressure of blood. They also believed that a flanged component seats concentrically without bottoming out, and that it helps to provide an equal cement mantle surrounding the cup.

In the initial technique of cemented total hip arthroplasty recommended by Charnley, the socket was reamed into the cancellous bone of the pelvis. This method sacrificed the important subchondral bone of the acetabulum, which is stronger than the deeper cancellous bone. Preservation of subchondral bone, combined with the drilling of multiple 6-mm anchor holes, has resulted in significantly fewer late radiologic findings of socket demarcation, according to the criteria of DeLee and Charnley, and has decreased linear polyethylene wear.[34] This improvement is attributed to the subchondral bone's ability to tolerate higher stresses and to transmit loads more evenly to the underlying cancellous areas. In spite of these improvements, however, revision rates for cemented polyethylene cups have not changed significantly.

Mulroy and Harris[35] found that using modern cementing techniques for both components did not prolong the life of the acetabular side, despite the proven benefit on the femoral side. Using modern cement techniques and an all-polyethylene cup with a 26-mm head, Berry had a rate of 7.5% acetabular revisions for aseptic loosening at eight to ten years (D Berry, Mayo Clinic, personal communication). Callaghan and Johnston, using the same techniques, found 31% probably or definitely loose at ten years (JJ Callaghan and RC Johnston, personal communication, 1993). Thus, although modern cementing techniques may benefit the femoral side, the acetabular results are the same as the initial results of Charnley and his colleagues, if not worse.

In contradistinction, Ranawat and associates[36] compared conventionally cemented sockets with sockets cemented using modern technique. This study was done retrospectively in a matched population. At ten years, 14% of the conventionally cemented sockets had migrated, and 2.7% had been revised. At five years, no revisions had been performed in the sockets cemented by modern technique, and this group had significantly fewer radiolucencies. Ten-year follow-up of the newer technique is anxiously awaited to determine whether these better results will be maintained. Ten-year follow-up of uncemented sockets will also be available at this time, allowing direct comparison of both methods.

Metal-backed cemented cups have been developed in an attempt to increase longevity of acetabular implants. Use of these components initially was studied with finite element analysis, which indicated that a metal-backed cup could reduce bone stress in the acetabulum. This theoretical benefit was then studied in vivo (Table 2). Along with its ability to maintain a near-normal stress pattern in the innominate bone, the metal backing also allowed for replacement of the polyethylene liner in cases of severe wear; a potential clinical advantage.[37,38] Ten-year follow-up revealed that 21% of these metal-backed acetabuli had required revision and another 21% were radiographically loose.[14] As with cemented all-polyethylene cups, the radiographic findings did not always correlate with the clinical findings. Ritter and associates[39] found inferior results at 5.2 years with metal backing and recommended that it not be used for cemented acetabular components (Fig. 5). In short, a potential improvement in cemented acetabular technique once again has offered no long-term benefit over initial attempts with all-polyethylene cups. Other causes of the relatively consistent loosening rate of cemented acetabuli need to be examined.

Polyethylene Wear

Polyethylene wear has been a cause of great concern since the advent of total hip arthroplasty. Acetabular components rarely "wear out," but polyethylene wear debris has been implicated as a cause of component loosening.

A review of the literature reveals a mean linear rate of wear in Charnley acetabular components of 0.07 to 0.21 mm per year, with the average being 0.1 mm per

Table 2
Results with metal-backed cemented acetabular sockets

Investigator	Number of Patients	Follow-up (yrs)	Revisions	Loose
Harris and White (1982)[37]	51	6.5	39%	2.0%
Harris and Penenberg (1987)[14]	48	11.3	21%	21%
Ritter et al (1990)[39]	138	5.2	6%	43%

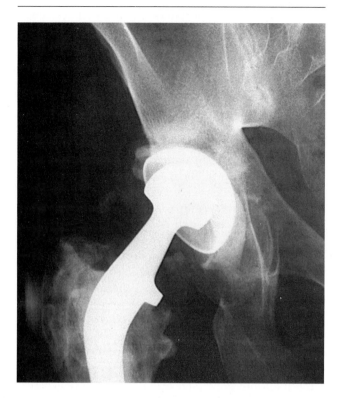

Fig. 5 Gross loosening and eccentric polyethylene wear is evident in this anteroposterior radiograph of a metal-backed cemented cup placed ten years earlier.

year. The 32-mm-head size Muller and Aufranc-Turner components wore an average of 0.1 mm–0.2 mm annually.[40,41]

Although these linear wear rates are relatively similar, volumetric wear must be considered. Livermore and associates[40] estimated the volume of wear debris by the formula $v = \pi r^2 w$, where v is volume of debris, w is the linear wear, and r is the radius of the femoral head. Thus, whereas linear wear rates for different femoral head sizes are similar, the volume of wear debris is proportional to the square of the radius of the femoral head. Consequently, larger heads will produce more polyethylene debris, making loosening more likely. Livermore and associates[40] confirmed this in a study of 22-, 28-, and 32-mm head sizes. The acetabular components used were all-polyethylene cemented components obtained from a single supplier. The wear rate of 28-mm heads (0.08 mm per year) was less than for the other two and the difference was statistically significant. The volumetric wear of 32-mm heads was almost double that of 22- and 28-mm heads; this difference was also statistically significant.[40] Furthermore, Morrey and Ilstrup,[41] who reviewed 6,128 total hip arthroplasties that used a variety of implants, found that at any given year, the probability of acetabular revision was greater for patients who

had a 32-mm component than for those with a 22- or 28-mm component. In a smaller series, Ritter and associates[42] found similar results, with 32-mm components showing a significantly higher rate of revision (Fig. 6).

A detailed postmortem histologic study of cemented acetabular components by Schmalzried and associates[43] demonstrated that loosening of cemented sockets is biologic rather than mechanical in nature. Polyethylene wear debris plays a critical role in the initiation of this biologic process. These investigators observed that a membrane between the bone-cement interface of sockets was invariably present at the intra-articular margin and in continuity with the pseudocapsule. Away from the intra-articular margin, they saw direct apposition of bone and cement. They theorized that a "cutting wedge" of bone resorption is responsible for the progressive disruption of the bone-cement interface. This theory is consistent with the location of radiolucencies and their progressive nature. Such disruptive membranes are full of polyethylene wear debris particles, both extracellularly and within macrophages. The local macrophage response to polyethylene debris leads to bone resorption (Fig. 7). The process begins at the periphery of the cup and extends toward the dome, resulting in loosening. These researchers believed the high rate of metal-backed acetabular component loosening to be associated with the reported 37% increase in the rate of polyethylene wear from these components.[43,44] The greater amount of wear most likely results from the

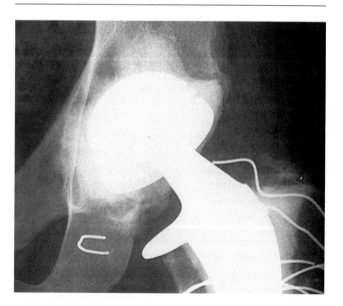

Fig. 6 Anteroposterior radiograph of a cemented metal-backed cup with extreme polyethylene wear as manifested by eccentricity of the head in the socket.

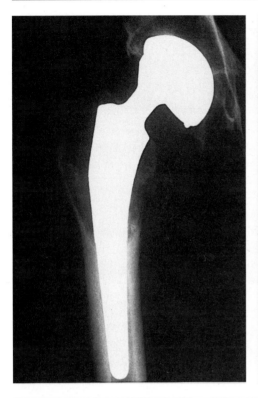 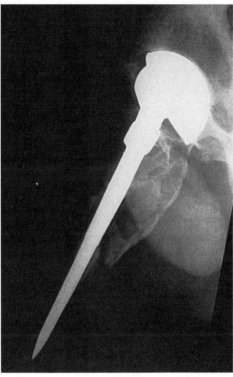

Fig. 7 **Left**, Anteroposterior, and **right**, lateral radiographs of the hip of a 42-year-old man who had arthroplasty 12 years before. Severe polyethylene wear and massive pelvic and femoral osteolysis are evident.

altered stress transfer of metal-backed cups, caused by the interposition of a stiff metallic shell between polyethylene and cement.

Acetabular Deficiencies

Another variable in cemented acetabular sockets is the pelvic anatomy. Patients undergoing primary total hip replacement sometimes have altered socket anatomy. Acetabular deficiencies, especially of the superior weightbearing area, are frequently associated with congenital hip dysplasia. Protrusio acetabuli is often associated with rheumatoid arthritis and ankylosing spondylitis. Such anatomic variations can make acetabular reconstruction difficult. Arthroplasty techniques have been modified to deal with these defects. For acetabuli with congenital dysplasia, studies showed success with bulk femoral head autografting. In 47 patients at seven years, Gerber and Harris[45] found all grafts united radiographically. However, in another series of patients reconstructed with the same technique, 32% of the components had loosened at 5.9 years follow-up, and 16% of the hips required revision.[46] This technique is not recommended at this time.

Another approach to the problem of congenital dysplasia is to place a small acetabular component in the anatomic position and to fill the superior gap with cement. McQueary and Johnston[15] used this technique

in 61 patients. At an average follow-up of 8.5 years, 10% of the acetabular components showed radiographic evidence of loosening, but none had been revised. The authors believed that this method of fixation was superior and recommended its use. Although their results are better than those obtained with bulk autografting, concern remains. Given the mechanism of cemented acetabular loosening and the radiographic signs of loosening in 10% of patients who underwent this technique, it is likely that, with time, those 10% plus additional patients eventually will require revision.

Protrusion remains a problem, especially in patients with rheumatoid arthritis. For such patients encouraging results have been obtained with bone grafts, which have united and halted the protrusion.[47,48] The fate of bone grafts in patients with protrusio is quite different from that of bulk autografts used to withstand weightbearing, most likely because of the contained nature of the bone graft in protrusio acetabuli and the decreased stresses therein (Figs. 8 and 9). After a 10.9-year follow-up of patients with cemented acetabular components, Gates and associates[49] found that autografting had arrested progression of the protrusion in 90%. Ten percent of the patients had required revision, and another 5% were radiographically loose. These researchers recommended this technique for reconstruction of protrusio acetabuli with a cemented component.

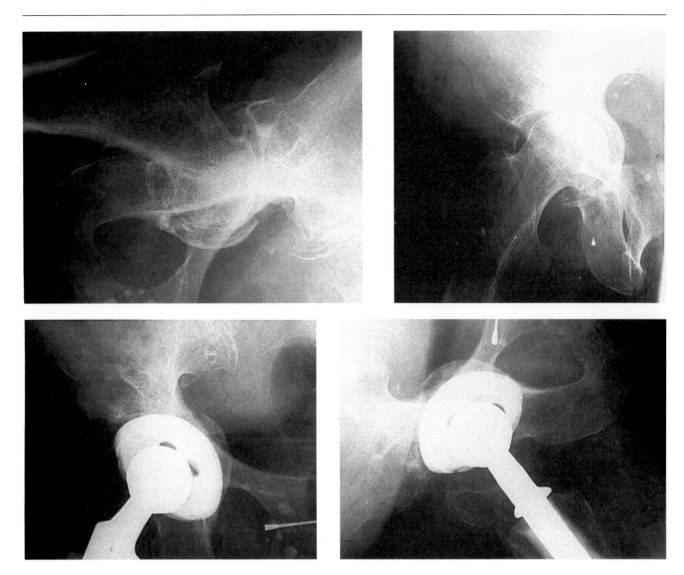

Fig. 8 **Top left,** Anteroposterior, and **top right,** lateral radiographs of a 79-year-old patient with protrusio acetabuli and a central acetabular fracture that was reconstructed using press-fit technique. **Bottom left** and **right,** Incorporation of the contained bone graft is evident.

Positioning of the acetabular component is important in total hip arthroplasty and affects the long-term survival of both the acetabular and femoral components. Yoder and associates[50] demonstrated that nonanatomic superior and lateral placement of the acetabular component resulted in significantly high rates of femoral loosening. Investigation by Russotti and Harris[51] implicated lateral displacement of the acetabular component in early loosening. McQueary and Johnston[15] agreed. In their study of coxarthrosis after congenital dysplasia, the only variable that correlated significantly with acetabular loosening was lateral displacement of the cup in excess of 25 mm. A biomechanical study by Doehring and associates[52] confirmed that joint forces are increased with hip center lateralization. These elevations in joint force can be attrib-

uted to an increase in the adduction moment. Superior-only hip center relocation did not significantly alter the joint force. Reconstruction of acetabular deficiencies can be accomplished by moving the center of hip rotation superiorly. Lateralization of the component should be avoided (Fig. 10).

Uncemented Components

Attempts to achieve biologic fixation of total hip components by tissue ingrowth have continued to increase in popularity over the last decade. In a human postmortem retrieval study of well-functioning implants, Engh and associates[53] found an average of 32.3% bony ingrowth after 12 to 99 months. They concluded that cementless acetabular reconstruction can "consistently achieve durable fixation by bone ingrowth into a porous surface." Sumner and associates[54] examined 19 titanium fiber-metal acetabular components and found ingrowth in up to 80% of the metal surface. They concluded that fixation occurs by both bony and fibrous fixation. Finally, Thomas and associates[55] reported from 5% to 70% surface ingrowth into titanium sockets.

These postmortem and retrieval studies have consistently demonstrated bony ingrowth with interspersed fibrous tissue. The implants studied had been functioning well clinically and were removed for reasons other than loosening. The remaining question is whether this fibrous tissue is an integral part of the metal-cement interface or a variation of the macrophage-laden membrane of a loosening cemented socket. If this membrane is similar to the destructive membrane described by Schmalzried and associates,[43] once again socket fixation may be compromised in the long term.

Reported studies of various cementless implants have described differences in function both radiographically and clinically (Table 3). This may be due to differences in materials, manufacturing, prosthetic head size, or implantation method. One study of the porous-coated anatomic (PCA) component, one of the first widely available uncemented systems, found 18% loosening of beads from the acetabular component at two years. Also, progressive acetabular lucencies, seen in 8% of patients, were of concern to the investigators.[56] Longer follow-up of PCA components found 6% to be loose, revision rate was 3% at five to seven years. Of more concern is the 4% incidence of acetabular lysis noted with the 32-mm head.[57] Among 91 cases

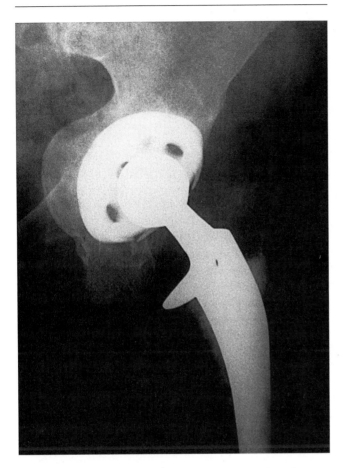

Fig. 9 Anteroposterior radiograph after reconstruction of protrusio acetabuli in a 69-year-old patient reveals excellent incorporation of the bone graft.

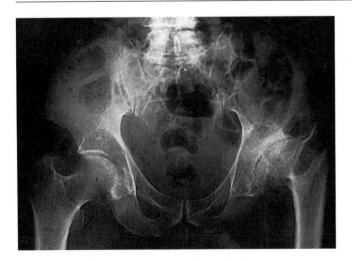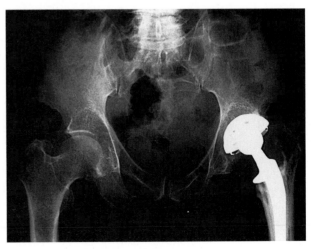

Fig. 10 **Left**, Preoperative, and **right**, postoperative anteroposterior pelvic radiographs of a 64-year-old patient with an untreated slipped capital femoral epiphysis. Reconstruction was achieved using a high hip center without lateralization. Note the medialization of the press-fit uncemented cup to the anatomic tear drop.

Table 3
Intermediate results of uncemented sockets

Investigator	Implant	Number of Patients	Follow-up (yrs)	Revisions	Loose
Callaghan et al (1988)[56]	PCA+	50	2	0%	2%
Heekin et al (1993)[57]	PCA+	91	5-7	3%	6%
Capello (1992)	Dual Geometry	91	5.5	0%	1.1%
Schmalzried (1992)[58]	HGP* w/screws	83	5-7	0%	0%
Pierson (1991)[59]	HGP* w/screws	199	5 (minimum)	0%	0%
Lachiewicz (1992)[60]	HGP* w/screws	100	2-5	0%	2%
Jordan (1993)	HGP* w/screws	92	7	0%	0%
Schmalzried et al (1993)[62]	HGP* no screws	122	4.7	0%	0%

+PCA - Porous Coated Anatomic
*HGP - Harris-Galante Porous

with the dual geometry cup without screws, Capello found that no revisions had been performed and only one cup had loosened at 5.5 years. Clinical results were excellent (W Capello, personal communication, 1992).

Schmalzried and Harris[58] studied the six-year outcome in 83 patients who had a titanium fiber metal cup with screws; no loosening had occurred and no revisions were necessitated by mechanical loosening. However, the authors were troubled by progressive radiolucent lines seen in 27% of the acetabular components. These were equally common in the three acetabular zones; no component was surrounded by a continuous radiolucent line. No migration was noted in this series. Results at minimum 5-year follow-up with the same component fixed with screws at another institution in 199 cases found no revisions and no migration. Acetabular radiolucencies less than 1 mm were observed in one third of all cases in the peripheral zones, and seven cups showed complete radiolucencies.[59] The authors in both of these studies found excellent clinical results with well-functioning implants and no revisions at five to six years. The presence of radi-

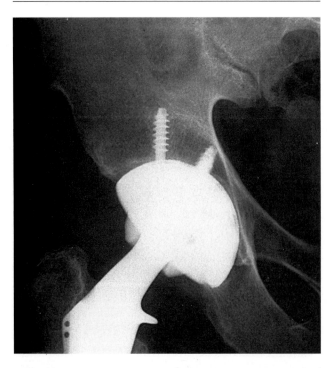

Fig. 11 In this anteroposterior radiograph of an uncemented cup with screws, placed six years earlier, peripheral radiolucency is evident in zone 1.

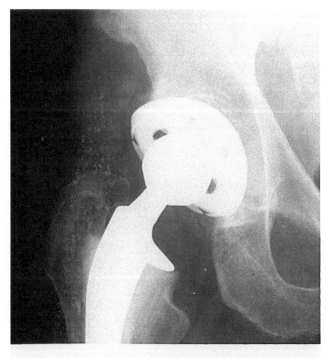

Fig. 12 Anteroposterior radiograph of a press fit uncemented component with no radiolucencies.

olucencies was concerning, but their ultimate significance remains unknown.

At two to five years, Lachiewicz and associates[60] found that no revisions were needed and clinical results were excellent in patients with 100 titanium metal cups. Two percent of the patients had nonprogressive radiolucent lines 1 mm wide in all three zones. Acetabular radiolucencies were also noted in all three zones, with the most (21%) noted in zone 3. Jordan, reporting average 7-year follow-up in 92 titanium metal cups, found 0% acetabular loosening and excellent clinical functioning (Louis Jordan, Norfolk, VA, personal communication, 1993).

The meaning of the lucencies noted in these studies is unclear, but their presence may bode poorly for the long-term stability of uncemented cups implanted with screw fixation. The cups in these studies were placed after reaming line to line using a component the same size as the final reamer. This method does not allow the cup to fit tightly. Fixation of the cup to the acetabular bone relies on transfixing screws, which are usually placed in the polar regions. Cook and associates[61] reported that ingrowth mainly occurs around these screws. Because ingrowth and close apposition of the metal-bone interface occurs in the polar region, the peripheral zones have less congruence, and radiolucencies can occur (Fig. 11). Their presence is worrisome because, as in cemented components, they will allow polyethylene debris and macrophages to enter the critical fixation interface. This problem is the impetus for press fitting ingrowth cups.

Press fitting involves implanting a cup that is 1 to 4 mm larger than the size of the last reamer. This results in a tight and exact fit around the periphery of the socket. Theoretically, a successful press fit will prevent access to the critical implant-bone interface at the periphery and will avoid the biologic initiation of membrane formation and cup loosening modulated by polyethylene wear debris (Fig. 12). Of critical importance in this technique is full concentric seating of the implant throughout its entirety. Lack of seating in the polar region with a tight peripheral fit may allow the ingress of polyethylene wear debris through the unfilled screw holes of the component. Theoretically, the same mechanism of loosening can occur, but from a different point of initiation and direction. The technique of placing bone graft in screw holes or using ingrowth cups without screw holes may then have some relevance in the future of ingrowth acetabular components.

Among 122 press-fit implants without screws, Schmalzried[62] found no revisions had been needed at 56 months. No fractures were noted from impacting an oversized cup into the acetabular bed and no component changed position postoperatively. More importantly, the incidence of progressive peripheral radiolu-

cencies was much less than with screw fixation, and the difference was statistically significant. Most of the gaps they saw in the metal-bone interface were at the dome of the implant (Fig. 13). Many of these gaps resolved, but the occurrence of progressive radiolucencies also occurred in this same zone. This supports the concept of a tight peripheral press fit, along with bottoming out of the cup.

Comparison of Cemented and Uncemented Results

The intermediate results of uncemented and cemented acetabular components should be compared. In all but two of the studies reviewed here, the uncemented sockets have performed vastly better than cemented all-polyethylene cups after an average of five years. Although revision rates for cemented cups are 1% or less, their much higher rate of radiographic loosening cannot be ignored. Under critical scrutiny all of these cups must be considered impending failures irrespective of their clinical function. In contrast, uncemented cups have a 0% average revision rate save for one study. These numbers are the benchmark for which future five-year studies need to strive.

One report quotes a 0% revision rate for cemented components, and a 3% revision rate is mentioned in a review of an uncemented component.[36,57] We believe that these results are the exception rather than the

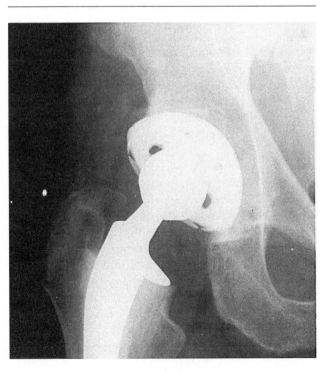

Fig. 13 On this anteroposterior radiograph, radiolucencies at the dome (zone 2) reveal incomplete seating of a press-fit uncemented component.

norm. The promising results for the cemented component may be related to the technical abilities of the surgeons or to meticulous adherence to strict technique. Unfortunately, other investigators have been unable to duplicate these results. The poor results for the uncemented technique may be due to a number of factors, including the use of a 32-mm-head prosthesis and the large amount of polyethylene wear generated with such large components, as described by Livermore and associates.[40] Wixson and associates'[63] direct comparison of cemented and uncemented acetabular components at two to four years revealed fewer loose components and radiolucent lines in the uncemented group. Twelve percent of cemented acetabular components were loose, while only 3% of the uncemented cups showed a change in position. These were both statistically significant differences.

Current Recommendations

The realization that the cause of cemented acetabular loosening was not mechanical in nature, but rather biologic and related to polyethylene wear debris, has led to changes in uncemented component design and technique. The present use of press-fit uncemented components is intended to achieve a tight peripheral fit, thus preventing polyethylene-debris-laden macrophages from gaining access to the critical bone-implant interface. Hopefully, the lessons learned from postmortem studies of cemented cups will increase the survivorship rates of ingrowth components in the long term.

Our recommendations for acetabular component fixation and technique are as follows. The patient is placed on the operating room table in the lateral decubitus position and a modified lateral approach to the hip joint is made. After leg length has been assessed and appropriate markings made, the hip is dislocated and the femoral neck cut is completed at the appropriate level. Excellent acetabular exposure is obtained with the use of two self-retaining retractors. Uterine tenacula are used to grasp the acetabular capsule and labrum. This is removed using electrocautery, taking small, sharp, well-defined bites and being careful not to stray into surrounding muscle or fat.

Once the periphery of the acetabulum is cleared of all soft tissue, the floor of the acetabulum is located using an osteotome to remove the central osteophyte, if present, or a curette to scrape away soft tissue and cartilage. When the floor of the acetabulum has been identified, all cartilage is removed from it using a large, long-handled curette. Reaming commences with a reamer approximately 44 to 46 mm in diameter. Reaming increases in 2-mm increments, and the first three to four reamers are used to medialize to the floor of the natural acetabulum. The acetabulum is

then reamed wider until good bony contact is achieved with the final reamer. This reamer is then placed free in the acetabulum to ensure that good bony contact is present throughout the acetabular bed. Maintenance of full contact between the reamer and bed at this time is of the utmost importance.

Any defects in the subchondral bone are now packed with cancellous reamings, and a porous-coated component that is 2 mm larger than the last reamer is impacted in 40° to 45° of abduction and 10° to 15° of anteversion using the socket-positioning device. The positioner is then removed, and final impaction is performed with the metal impactor. Full seating of the component is ascertained by examining the screw holes and looking for intimate bone-implant contact. If full contact is not present, further reaming to obtain concentricity or bone grafting is necessary. Stability of the acetabular component is then tested by manual distraction using pliers. If screws are necessary, they are now placed using the quadrant system of Wasielewski and Rubash, placing screws in the posterosuperior or posteroinferior quadrants.[64] Two screws of length no greater than 25 mm usually are sufficient for cup stability. Next, a non-lipped liner is impacted into the acetabulum after turning in one of the acetabular tines. We prefer to use a polyethylene liner that is at least 8 mm thick. The head size used is chosen taking this into consideration (Table 4). Postoperatively, our patients, whether undergoing uncemented or hybrid total hip arthroplasty, are limited to touch-down weightbearing for six weeks using a walker, are then advanced to full weightbearing with a walker for two weeks, and then use a cane with full weightbearing for another six weeks.

Cemented cups have performed admirably, but shortcomings remain. Tight fixation between the bone and cement is difficult to achieve at insertion, allowing the entrance of polyethylene wear debris implicated in acetabular socket loosening. Such debris is present in all total hip replacements that have polyethylene acetabular bearing surfaces. The amount of polyethylene wear debris varies depending on femoral head size, polyethylene thickness, and cup position. Linear wear rates of polyethylene sockets are relatively similar, but large differences in volumetric wear have been

Table 4
HGP-II cup size necessary to achieve at least 8 mm polyethylene thickness

Head Size	Cup Size
22 mm	50 mm
26 mm	54 mm
28 mm	56 mm
32 mm	60 mm

reported. Thirty-two-mm heads, metal-backed acetabular components, and uncemented metal-backed cups with a thin polyethylene bearing surface all have been associated with high revision rates. The failure of these components is thought to be related to the larger volume of polyethylene wear debris generated by these designs.

The exact mechanism of failure of cemented acetabuli was recognized after uncemented sockets were popularized. Efforts are now underway to prevent similar failure mechanisms in the uncemented socket. This is the rationale behind press fitting acetabular components. Under-reaming the acetabulum enables a tight press fit, especially at the periphery. This circumferential "peripheral block" to the entry of polyethylene wear debris is critical. It is hoped that by preventing the debris' access to the metal-bone interface, it will be possible to avoid the initiation of biologic loosening, as described by Schmalzried.[43]

In the technique of press fitting a cup, it is also important to seat the component fully to avoid any gaps in the interface at the dome of the implant, because it is possible that these gaps may also be a source of biologic loosening. Investigation of the uncemented cup with screws reveals that radiolucencies are present and may be progressive. This is a cause for concern and is the driving force behind press fitting components instead of using line-to-line sizing. Long-term review of both press fitting and line-to-line sizing with screws will be necessary to determine if the theoretical concerns and benefits have a basis in reality.

Indications for using cemented acetabuli still exist. Neoplasms or metastatic disease of the acetabulum should be reconstructed using cement. Cement also can be helpful for the patient with severe osteoporosis of the acetabular bed. Elderly patients, for whom revision surgery will not be needed based on life expectancy, may benefit from the decreased blood loss and immediate mobilization offered by cementing a cup. Reconstruction of the acetabulum in patients with Paget's disease may also require cement to obtain firm fixation in the sclerotic acetabular bony bed and to stop the increased intraoperative and postoperative bleeding associated with this disease.

Comparison of uncemented and cemented sockets reveals the superiority of ingrowth cups. Revisions for aseptic loosening are much less common and the radiographic results are better in the uncemented sockets. Certain uncemented sockets have not fared well under critical scrutiny, but these negative results are most likely the result of defects in design or implementation, not theory.

In 1993, we recommend the use of uncemented press-fit acetabular sockets for total hip reconstruction in almost all patients. The procedure is much easier with uncemented sockets and, based on their performance to date, we believe they will outdistance all types of cemented cups in both performance and longevity.

References

1. Charnley J: Low friction principle, in *Low Friction Arthroplasty of the Hip: Theory and Practice*. New York, Springer-Verlag, 1979, chap 1, pp 3-15.
2. Waugh W: The plan fulfilled: Wrightington, in *John Charnley: The Man and the Hip*. New York, Springer-Verlag, 1990, chap 10, pp 113-138.
3. DeLee JG, Charnley J: Radiological demarcation of cemented sockets in total hip replacement. *Clin Orthop* 1976;121:20-32.
4. Hodgkinson JP, Shelley P, Wroblewski BM: The correlation between the roentgenographic appearance and operative findings at the bone-cement junction of the socket in Charnley low friction arthroplasties. *Clin Orthop* 1988;228:105-109.
5. Lyons CW, Berquist TH, Lyons JC, et al: Evaluation of radiographic findings in painful hip arthroplasties. *Clin Orthop* 1985;195:239-251.
6. O'Neill DA, Harris WH: Failed total hip replacement: Assessment by plain radiographs, arthrograms, and aspiration of the hip joint. *J Bone Joint Surg* 1984;66A:540-546.
7. Murray WR, Rodrigo JJ: Arthrography for the assessment of pain after total hip replacement: A comparison of arthrographic findings in patients with and without pain. *J Bone Joint Surg* 1975;57A:1060-1065.
8. Charnley J: The long-term results of low-friction arthroplasty of the hip performed as a primary intervention. *J Bone Joint Surg* 1972;54B:61-76.
9. Cupic Z: Long-term follow-up of Charnley arthroplasty of the hip. *Clin Orthop* 1979;141:28-43.
10. Eftekhar N: Charnley "low friction torque" arthroplasty: A study of long-term results. *Clin Orthop* 1971;81:93-104.
11. Eftekhar NS: Long-term results of cemented total hip arthroplasty. *Clin Orthop* 1987;225:207-217.
12. Griffith MJ, Seidenstein MK, Williams D, et al: Eight year results of Charnley arthroplasties of the hip with special reference to the behavior of cement. *Clin Orthop* 1978;137:24-36.
13. Coventry MB, Beckenbaugh RD, Nolan DR, et al: 2,012 total hip arthroplasties: A study of postoperative course and early complications. *J Bone Joint Surg* 1974;56A:273-284.
14. Harris WH, Penenberg BL: Further follow-up on socket fixation using a metal-backed acetabular component for total hip replacement: A minimum ten-year follow-up study. *J Bone Joint Surg* 1987;69A:1140-1143.
15. McQueary FG, Johnston RC: Coxarthrosis after congenital dysplasia: Treatment by total hip arthroplasty without acetabular bone-grafting. *J Bone Joint Surg* 1988;70A:1140-1144.
16. Stauffer RN: Ten-year follow-up study of total hip replacement. *J Bone Joint Surg* 1982;64A:983-990.
17. Hozack WJ, Rothman RH, Booth RE, et al: Survivorship analysis of 1,041 Charnley total hip arthroplasties. *J Arthroplasty* 1990;5:41-47.
18. Older J: Low-friction arthroplasty of the hip: A 10-12-year follow-up study. *Clin Orthop* 1986;211:36-42.
19. Dorey F, Amstutz HC: The validity of survivorship analysis in total joint arthroplasty. *J Bone Joint Surg* 1989;71A:544-548.
20. García-Cimbrelo E, Munuera L: Early and late loosening of the acetabular cup after low-friction arthroplasty. *J Bone Joint Surg* 1992;74A:1119-1129.

21. McCoy TH, Salvati EA, Ranawat CS, et al: A fifteen-year follow-up study of one hundred Charnley low-friction arthroplasties. *Orthop Clin North Am* 1988;19:467-476.

22. Kavanagh BF, Dewitz MA, Ilstrup DM, et al: Charnley total hip arthroplasty with cement: Fifteen-year results. *J Bone Joint Surg* 1989;71A:1496-1503.

23. Buchholz HW, Heinert K: Long-term results of cemented arthroplasty: Analysis of complications fifteen years after operation. *Orthop Clin North Am* 1988;19:531-540.

24. Welch RB, McGann WA, Picetti GD III: Charnley low-friction arthroplasty: A fifteen- to seventeen-year follow-up study. *Orthop Clin North Am* 1988;19:551-555.

25. Bryant MJ, Mollan RA, Nixon JR: Survivorship analysis of the Ring hip arthroplasty. *J Arthroplasty* 1991;6(Suppl):S5-S10.

26. Kummer FJ, Stuchin SA, Frankel VH: Analysis of removed autophor ceramic-on-ceramic components. *J Arthroplasty* 1990;5:28-33.

27. Apel DM, Smith DG, Schwartz CM, et al: Threaded cup acetabuloplasty: Early clinical experience. *Clin Orthop* 1989;241:183-189.

28. Shaw JA, Bailey JH, Bruno A, et al: Threaded acetabular components for primary and revision total hip arthroplasty. *J Arthroplasty* 1990;5:201-215.

29. Knahr K, Salzer M, Frank P: Experience with uncemented polyethylene acetabular prostheses, in Morscher E (ed): *The Cementless Fixation of Hip Endoprosthesis.* Berlin, Springer-Verlag, pp 205-210.

30. Charnley J: Long-term radiological results, in *Low Friction Arthroplasty of the Hip: Theory and Practice.* New York, Springer-Verlag, 1979, chap 6, pp 66-90.

31. Oh I, Sander TW, Treharne RW: Total hip acetabular cup flange design and its effect on cement fixation. *Clin Orthop* 1985;195:304-309.

32. Amstutz HC, Yao J, Dorey FJ, et al: Acrylic fixation—stem and socket replacement: Results, principles, and technique, in Amstutz HC (ed): *Hip Arthroplasty.* New York, Churchill Livingstone, 1991, chap 19, pp 239-260.

33. Shelley P, Wroblewski BM: Socket design and cement pressurisation in the Charnley low-friction arthroplasty. *J Bone Joint Surg* 1988;70B:358-363.

34. Kobayashi S, Terayama K: Radiology of low-friction arthroplasty of the hip: A comparison of socket fixation techniques. *J Bone Joint Surg* 1990;72B:439-443.

35. Mulroy RD Jr, Harris WH: The effect of improved cementing techniques on component loosening in total hip replacement: An 11-year radiographic review. *J Bone Joint Surg* 1990;72B:757-760.

36. Ranawat CS, Rawlins BA, Harju VT: Effect of modern cement technique on acetabular fixation total hip arthroplasty: A retrospective study in matched pairs. *Orthop Clin North Am* 1988;19:599-603.

37. Harris WH, White RE Jr: Socket fixation using a metal-backed acetabular component for total hip replacement: A minimum five-year follow-up. *J Bone Joint Surg* 1982;64A:745-748.

38. Harris WH: A new total hip implant. *Clin Orthop* 1971;81:105-113.

39. Ritter MA, Keating EM, Faris PM, et al: Metal-backed acetabular cups in total hip arthroplasty. *J Bone Joint Surg* 1990;72A:672-677.

40. Livermore J, Ilstrup D, Morrey B: Effect of femoral head size on wear of the polyethylene acetabular component. *J Bone Joint Surg* 1990;72A:518-528.

41. Morrey BF, Ilstrup D: Size of the femoral head and acetabular revision in total hip-replacement arthroplasty. *J Bone Joint Surg* 1989;71A:50-55.

42. Ritter MA, Stringer EA, Littrell DA, et al: Correlation of prosthetic femoral head size and/or design with longevity of total hip arthroplasty. *Clin Orthop* 1983;176:252-257.

43. Schmalzried TP, Jasty M, Harris WH: Periprosthetic bone loss in total hip arthroplasty: Polyethylene wear debris and the concept of the effective joint space. *J Bone Joint Surg* 1992;74A:849-863.

44. Cates HE Jr, Faris PM, Keating EM, et al: Polyethylene wear with cemented metal-backed acetabular cups in total hip arthroplasty. Presented at the 59th Annual Meeting of the American Academy of Orthopaedic Surgeons, Washington, DC, February, 1992.

45. Gerber SD, Harris WH: Femoral head autografting to augment acetabular deficiency in patients requiring total hip replacement: A minimum five-year and an average seven-year follow-up study. *J Bone Joint Surg* 1986;68A:1241-1248.

46. Jasty M, Harris WH: Salvage total hip reconstruction in patients with major acetabular bone deficiency using structural femoral head allografts. *J Bone Joint Surg* 1990;72B:63-67.

47. Ranawat CS, Dorr LD, Inglis AE: Total hip arthroplasty in protrusio acetabuli of rheumatoid arthritis. *J Bone Joint Surg* 1980;62A:1059-1065.

48. Mendes DG, Roffman M, Silbermann M: Reconstruction of the acetabular wall with bone graft in arthroplasty of the hip. *Clin Orthop* 1984;186:29-37.

49. Gates HS III, McCollum DE, Poletti SC, et al: Bone-grafting in total hip arthroplasty for protrusio acetabuli: A follow-up note. *J Bone Joint Surg* 1990;72A:248-251.

50. Yoder SA, Brand RA, Pedersen DR, et al: Total hip acetabular component position affects component loosening rates. *Clin Orthop* 1988;228:79-87.

51. Russotti GM, Harris WH: Proximal placement of the acetabular component in total hip arthroplasty: A long-term follow-up study. *J Bone Joint Surg* 1991;73A:587-592.

52. Doehring TC, Rubash HE, Shelley FJ, et al: High hip center: Experimental measurements of joint force magnitude and direction in normal, superior, and superolateral hip-center positions. Presented at the 39th Annual Meeting of Orthopaedic Surgeons, San Francisco, CA, 1992.

53. Engh CA, Zettl-Schaffer KF, Kukita Y, et al: Histological and radiographic assessment of well functioning porous-coated acetabular components: A human postmortem retrieval study. *J Bone Joint Surg* 1993;75A:814-824.

54. Sumner DR, Jasty M, Turner TM, et al: Bone ingrowth in porous-coated cementless acetabular components retrieved from human patients. *Trans Orthop Res Soc* 1987;12:509.

55. Thomas BJ, Amstutz HC, Campbell P: Cementless acetabular reconstruction, in Amstutz HC (ed): *Hip Arthroplasty.* New York, Churchill Livingstone, 1991, chap 21, pp 279.

56. Callaghan JJ, Dysart SH, Savory CG: The uncemented porous-coated anatomic total hip prosthesis: Two-year results of a prospective consecutive series. *J Bone Joint Surg* 1988;70A:337-346.

57. Heekin RD, Callaghan JJ, Hopkinson WJ, et al: The porous-coated anatomic total hip prosthesis, inserted without cement: Results after five to seven years in a prospective study. *J Bone Joint Surg* 1993;75A:11-91.

58. Schmalzried TP, Harris WH: The Harris-Galante porous-coated acetabular component with screw fixation: Radiographic analysis of eighty-three primary hip replacements at a minimum of five years. *J Bone Joint Surg* 1992;74A:1130-1139.

59. Pierson RH III, Martell JM, Padgett DE, et al: Cementless acetabular reconstruction in primary total hip arthroplasty: Minimum five year results. Presented at the 58th Annual Meeting of the American Academy of Orthopaedic Surgeons, Anaheim, CA, March, 1991, p 213.

60. Lachiewicz PF, Anspach WE III, DeMasi R: A prospective study of 100 consecutive Harris-Galante porous total hip arthroplasties: 2-5-year results. *J Arthroplasty* 1992;7:519-526.

61. Cook SD, Thomas KA, Haddad RJ Jr: Histologic analysis of retrieved human porous-coated total joint components. *Clin Orthop* 1988;234:90-101.

62. Schmalzried TP, Hill GE, Wessinger SJ, et al: Harris-Galante Porous (HGP) acetabular component press-fit without screw fixation: Five-year radiographic analysis of primary cases. Presented at the 60th Annual Meeting of the American Academy of Orthopaedic Surgeons, San Francisco, CA, February, 1993.

63. Wixson RL, Stulberg SD, Mehlhoff M: Total hip replacement with cemented, uncemented, and hybrid prostheses: A comparison of clinical and radiographic results at two to four years. *J Bone Joint Surg* 1991;73A:257-270.

64. Wasielewski RC, Cooperstein LA, Kruger MP, et al: Acetabular anatomy and the transacetabular fixation of screws in total hip arthroplasty. *J Bone Joint Surg* 1990;72A:501-508.

Spine

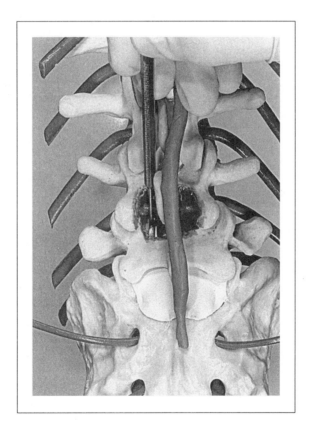

CHAPTER 40

Spinal Stenosis: Indications for Laminectomy

Steven R. Garfin, MD

Srdjan Mirkovic, MD

Harry N. Herkowitz, MD

The indications for surgery for symptoms related to spinal stenosis are often less clear than for sciatica related to acute disk herniations. This is because, as previously noted, the history may be nonspecific, and the physical findings equivocal or, perhaps, nonexistent. Complicating the decision to operate, and the type of procedure to perform, is the fact that the "abnormalities" seen on imaging studies in spinal stenosis may be the same as those found in the normal aging spine. Once, however, it is decided that surgery will be performed, the surgeon must decide the type of operation and the length or extent of the operation (cephalad to caudal).

The timing of surgery is usually based on the patient's decision that his or her quality of life, related to back and leg complaints, is unsatisfactory. This frequently occurs in an aged patient, who may have concomitant medical problems (cardiovascular, pulmonary, or other diseases).[1,2] This is particularly significant when the treatment for a cardiac condition may be controlled exercise, but the leg symptoms from the stenosis limit the patient's ability to exercise. The medical condition may also complicate the surgery, because cardiac or pulmonary disease can significantly increase the risks to the patient from anesthetics, blood loss, etc. We have found a close affiliation with a gerontologist, who is aware of the importance of ambulation and exercise in the elderly, knows the limitations created by spinal stenosis, and appreciates the benefits of surgery, frequently allows us to operate successfully on patients who otherwise might have been denied surgery by a general internist or family physician. Age, by itself, should not be used as a criteria to avoid surgery and deprive patients of possible benefits.[2-4] Articles by Deyo and associates[1] and Turner and associates[2] demonstrate the success of decompressive surgery for elderly patients with spinal stenosis, although in individuals older than 75 to 80 years of age the complications were increased. Mortality increased after age 75 for patients undergoing decompression and fusion, and after age 80 if only a decompression was performed. Interestingly, the percentages cited are similar to the expected mortality for this age group.[1,2]

The surgical decision, as noted, is based on the patient's complaints of limited ability to ambulate because of hip and/or leg pain, weakness, and/or dysesthesias. Additionally, there are frequently low back complaints, but this should not be the driving force towards surgery. The primary indication is gradual onset of leg pain, associated with activities. Pain, weakness with ambulation, dysesthesias, numbness, or other vague proprioceptive type complaints may prevent patients from ambulating or participating in sports activities (treadmill, swimming) at a level they feel to be adequate for their mental and physical well-being. Clinically, the examination may show focal or disparate, noncontiguous, neurologic deficits, or it may, as it is in most cases, be normal. If the patient's symptoms are characteristic of spinal stenosis, the fact that an examination is normal should not dissuade the surgeon from considering surgery.

Imaging studies may show a focal deficit, consistent with unilateral leg complaints, or diffuse, more generalized, compressive pathology related to the disk(s), facets, vertebral body subluxations (degenerative spondylolisthesis), degenerative or pre-existing scoliosis, ligamentous intrusions into the canal, or some combination of the above. These studies may depict a number of lesions, involving one or more levels, with predominant central compression, lateral stenosis, and/or foraminal stenosis. Additionally, the radiographic findings may involve more levels than the subjective complaints or objective deficits initially suggest.

Indications

There is no evidence of predictable definite progression in symptoms or neurologic deterioration in patients who present with spinal stenosis and who do not undergo surgery. Johnsson and associates,[5] in a limited follow-up study, evaluated 64 patients who had myelographically confirmed symptoms and signs of spinal stenosis. Of these patients, 44 elected surgery and 20 did not. Ten of the 20 nonoperated patients were followed by the authors for nearly three years. Of these ten, 58% improved over the three year period of follow-up, 37% reported no change, and only one worsened symptomatically. Of the 44 who chose surgery, 17 were followed for an average of 3.5 years. In the group of patients who had surgery, 63% felt they improved, 32% felt they did not, and one patient worsened. Functionally, walking capacity improved in 42% of patients who did not undergo any surgical procedure, 32% noted no change, and only 26% worsened. In patients who underwent surgical decompression and had an incomplete myelographic block, 55%

noted improvement in their walking capacity following surgery, 27% noted no change, and 23% worsened. In those patients who had a complete myelographic block, 79% noted improvement in lower extremity function following surgery, and 21% felt they lost some functional capacity.

These findings are consistent with our experience. There does not appear to be an urgent need to operate on patients who are clinically stable and functioning well. Despite this, many patients, in an effort to return to an active, healthy lifestyle, choose surgery rather than delay. In general, therefore, we have established the following three guidelines for recommending surgical decompression for patients presenting with symptoms of spinal stenosis. The first is persistent leg pain that interferes with the patient's quality of life. (This is related to the patient's activity level, not a proscribed limitation mandated for the entire group.) Second is the failure of nonoperative care to relieve symptoms over a period of at least two to three months. This care includes some combination of modalities such as time, anti-inflammatories, alterations in exercise pattern under physical therapy guidance, and/or epidural steroids. Mild, functional incapacitation or neurologic deficits are useful confirmatory symptoms and signs of spinal stenosis, but by themselves do not necessitate urgent decompression. Certainly, however, if there is a fairly rapid neurologic loss or a diminution in bowel or bladder function (both are rare), then following a workup, more urgent decompression may be indicated. Third is documented spinal stenosis confirmed on either myelogram/computed tomographic scan and/or a magnetic resonance scan.

In the majority of patients, surgery can provide relief for leg pain complaints related to spinal stenosis and can be rewarding for both the patient and the surgeon. However, strict criteria should be followed when selecting a patient for surgery. The workup, as noted, should include: (1) a trial of nonoperative care; (2) medical evaluation; (3) laboratory tests, including a complete blood count, a chemistry panel with renal and liver function tests, and a urinalysis; (4) plain radiographs, including flexion-extension lateral films; (5) a magnetic resonance imaging scan; (6) possibly a myelogram with a flexion-extension lateral, followed by a computed tomographic scan; and, if there is any inconsistency in the history, physical examination, and radiographic studies (7) an electromyogram (EMG) or more detailed neurologic evaluation (Outline 1).[6]

At this time, the mainstay of the surgical approach to the symptoms related to spinal stenosis is lumbar laminectomy. The surgeon operating on the lumbar spine for spinal stenosis should approach the procedure in a fairly standardized fashion. Loupe magnification and headlight illumination, to enhance visualiza-

tion of the dura, nerve roots, and epidural veins, are important aids in the decompression process. Hemostasis, obtained at every level to avoid pooling of blood along the neural elements, will also help in visualization and will make the procedure less frustrating for the surgeon. Frequently, central decompression is not enough, and lateral recess stenosis must also be addressed. Central canal stenosis is occasionally related to inferior facet hypertrophy; more lateral stenosis, along the nerve root, is related to impingement from the superior facet.[7-11] To decompress a nerve root, it may be necessary to remove up to one half of the superior facet.[12] Frequently, removal of the medial one half, or less, of the facet joints on both sides of one motion segment allows adequate decompression centrally and laterally, without creating spinal instability.[13] However, the nerve root must be adequately decompressed. More of the facet joint may be removed if necessary, but in such cases fusion should be considered at the time of surgery. Details of the procedure are listed in the chapter on techniques. In the properly selected patient, with appropriate radiographic findings and adequate surgical decompression (and possibly instrumentation with stabilization as necessary), one can anticipate an 85% to 90% success rate in the relief (diminution) of leg symptoms and improvement in the quality of life.[3,14]

Laminectomy

The goals of surgery should be the adequate (relatively complete) decompression of all areas of the lumbar spine that on imaging studies (radiographs,

---

Outline 1
Protocol for patients undergoing decompressive laminectomy

1. Preoperative History and Physical Examination
2. Plain Radiographs with Flexion-Extension Lateral
3. MR Scan
4. Myelogram followed by CT Scan
5. EMG, if symptoms and signs are not consistent with the radiographic findings. This study helps rule out polyneuropathy or other neuromuscular diseases.
6. Medical Evaluation
7. Routine Blood Work (CBC, chemistry panel, urinalysis)
8. Coagulation Studies including prothrombin time, partial thromboplastin time, and platelet count
9. Discontinuation of all Anti-Inflammatory Medications at least 10 days before surgery
10. Consideration of autologous blood donation

Intraoperative
1. IV antibiotics prior to surgery and for 24 hours post-operative
2. Thromboembolic disease support hose and/or alternating venous compression stockings
3. Proper positioning on a surgical frame
4. Standardized approach to the lumbar spine
5. Decompress all areas compressed on preoperative studies

MRI, or enhanced CT) demonstrate stenosis. The operation should include a central laminectomy, usually from the lowest to the most proximal involved levels. The majority of patients with spinal stenosis have compression at the L4-5 level and L5 root symptoms. Though the S1 root may not be involved, surgically it is often technically easier and, perhaps, safer to enter at the L5-S1 interlaminar space and then proceed proximally, even though this lowest level may not necessarily require decompression. The laminectomy should decompress all roots in the areas operated on, with the most attention paid to one side, if there is primarily unilateral symptomatology. However, all lumbar roots involved in the surgical decompression should be explored, re-evaluated for compression, and foraminotomies performed as necessary, to allow a small nerve probe (such as a DeBakey #3 dilator or a Frazier dural elevator) to be passed out the neuroforamen. One should attempt, if possible, to preserve as much of each facet joint as possible, while adequately decompressing the foramina and the lateral recess. To do this, the foraminotomies can be performed with curettes, burrs, undercutting Kerrison punches, and/or small, fine spinal osteotomes (see the chapter on technique).

The decision to fuse the spine may be made preoperatively or decided on intraoperatively, based on creation of "instability" at the time of decompression.[15-17] The possibility of fusion should be considered preoperatively and discussed with the patient to ensure that the success of an adequately performed decompression of the spinal nerve roots laterally is not compromised by a lack of such requirements for surgical fusion as appropriate consent, autologous blood, and cell savers.

The laminectomy, to provide immediate relief of leg pain, is probably the most significant portion of the procedure. Some patients will also obtain relief from back pain, particularly as they become more mobile and stand more erect. Relief of back pain is related to the lack of leg pain complaints when the spine is extended, as well as removal of the thickened posterior elements and ligaments. If the decompression is complete, the short-term results are exceedingly rewarding to the patient and the surgeon. It is the long-term results that lead to the concern for fusion, with or without instrumentation, and these are addressed in a later chapter.[15,18,19]

As distinct from herniated disks, which present as asymmetric focal defects, frequently with a single radicular pattern, the symptoms of spinal stenosis are related to a more diffuse and generalized degenerative process. Therefore, surgical treatment must be directed at both central canal and lateral recess pathology, as well as foraminal encroachment. The results of surgery for spinal stenosis are best when the goal is to relieve symptoms of leg pain related to the spinal stenosis and to halt, if not reverse, progression in lower extremity weakness and dysfunction. With these goals, leg pain relief can be expected nearly 85% of the time. However, with regard to the relief of back pain, the results are rarely as good.[3,14-18,20]

Results

Our experience in decompressive surgery for spinal stenosis and our reported results allow us to anticipate a nearly 85% improvement in leg pain complaints in patients undergoing surgery for spinal stenosis. The results of surgery in other series vary widely, however, with satisfactory results ranging from 60% to 95%.[3,5-23] Johnsson and associates[16] noted good to excellent results in 60% of patients who underwent decompressive surgery for spinal stenosis. In their series, factors leading to a good result were: (1) a myelogram showing significant compression of the dural sac (patients with high degree blocks did better than those with incomplete blocks); (2) adequate decompression of the lateral recesses; and (3) duration of preoperative symptoms less than two years. Our data agree with the above. Surin and associates[24] noted 86% good to excellent results following decompressive laminectomy for spinal stenosis. As opposed to Johnsson's study, however, the patients in Surin's group did better if there was only moderate, as opposed to severe, compression of the thecal sac. They agreed, however, with Johnsson's findings that the results were better if the stenotic symptoms had been present for less than two years before surgery. Paine[21] reported 91% of his patients improved following decompression. In his series, results were better when only one or two levels were decompressed. He observed that when more levels were decompressed, low back pain complaints increased. Of 170 patients undergoing laminectomy for spinal stenosis, Garfin and associates[3] reported a 94% patient satisfaction rate postoperatively. Of this group of patients, 87% had complete or partial relief of low back pain, while leg pain complaints were improved over 90% of the time.

Herkowitz and Garfin[15] and Herkowitz and Kurz[18] reviewed 125 patients who underwent decompression for myelographically confirmed spinal stenosis. The follow-up for this study ranged from two to seven years with a mean of 3.9. Of patients with degenerative stenosis, without spondylolisthesis, 84% reported good to excellent results in terms of leg pain relief. If there was concomitant degenerative spondylolisthesis, 78% noted good to excellent results. The percentage of patients in the latter group improved significantly if fusion had been added at the level of the degenerative spondylolisthesis.[15,18] The primary reason for poor results in most series is related to multi-level decompression and the development of postoperative instabilities.

In general, spinal stenosis surgery in properly selected patients is usually successful in relieving leg pain. The risks of operating on elderly patients are not insignificant; the benefits from the procedure and improvement in quality of life generally exceed the risks.

References

1. Deyo RA, Cherkin DC, Loeser JD, et al: Morbidity and mortality in association with operations on the lumbar spine: The influence of age, diagnosis, and procedure. *J Bone Joint Surg* 1992;74A:536-543.
2. Turner JA, Ersek M, Herron L, et al: Surgery for lumbar spinal stenosis: Attempted meta-analysis of the literature. *Spine* 1992;17:1-8.
3. Garfin SR, Glover M, Booth RE, et al: Laminectomy: A review of the Pennsylvania hospital experience. *J Spinal Disord* 1988;1:116-133.
4. Parrish TF: Lumbar disk surgery in patients over 50 years of age. *South Med J* 1962;55:667-669.
5. Johnsson KE, Rosen I, Uden A: The natural course of lumbar spinal stenosis. *Acta Orthop Scand (Suppl)* 1993;251:67-68.
6. Amundson G, Garfin SR: Minimizing blood loss during spine surgery, in Garfin SR(ed): *Complications of Spine Surgery.* Baltimore, MD, Williams & Wilkins, 1989, chap 2, pp 29-52.
7. Kirkaldy-Willis WH: The relationship of structural pathology to the nerve root. *Spine* 1984;9:49-52.
8. Kirkaldy-Willis WH, Wedge JH, Yong-Hing K, et al: Lumbar spinal nerve lateral entrapment. *Clin Orthop* 1982;169:171-178.
9. Schatzker J, Pennal GP: Spinal stenosis, a cause of cauda equina compression. *J Bone Joint Surg* 1968;50B:606-618.
10. McIvor GWD, Kirkaldy-Willis WH: Pathological and myelographic changes in the major types of lumbar spinal stenosis. *Clin Orthop* 1976;115:72-76.
11. Wiltse LL, Kirkaldy-Willis WH, McIvor GWD: The treatment of spinal stenosis. *Clin Orthop* 1976;115:83-91.
12. Verbiest H: A radicular syndrome from developmental narrowing of the lumbar vertebral canal. *J Bone Joint Surg* 1954;36B:230-237.
13. Booth RE Jr: Spinal stenosis, in Anderson LD (ed): *American Academy of Orthopaedic Surgeons Instructional Course Lectures XXXV.* St. Louis, MO, CV Mosby, 1986, pp 420-435.
14. Tile M, McNeil SR, Zarins RK, et al: Spinal stenosis: Results of treatment. *Clin Orthop* 1976;115:104-108.
15. Herkowitz HN, Garfin SR: Decompressive surgery for spinal stenosis. *Semin Spine Surg* 1989;1:163-167.
16. Johnsson KE, Willner S, Johnsson K: Postoperative instability after decompression for lumbar spinal stenosis. *Spine* 1986;11:107-110.
17. Kirkaldy-Willis WH, Paine KWE, Cauchoix J, et al: Lumbar spinal stenosis. *Clin Orthop* 1974;99:30-50.
18. Herkowitz HN, Kurz LT: Degenerative lumbar spondylolisthesis with spinal stenosis: A prospective study comparing decompression with decompression and intertransverse process arthrodesis. *J Bone Joint Surg* 1991;73A:802-808.
19. Johnsson KE, Willner S, Pettersson H: Analysis of operated cases with lumbar spinal stenosis. *Acta Orthop Scand* 1981;52:427-433.
20. Spengler DM: Degenerative stenosis of the lumbar spine. *J Bone Joint Surg* 1987;69A:305-308.
21. Paine KWE: Results of decompression for lumbar spinal stenosis. *Clin Orthop* 1976;115:96-100.
22. Verbiest H: Results of surgical treatment of idiopathic developmental stenosis of the lumbar vertebral canal: A review of twenty-seven years' experience. *J Bone Joint Surg* 1977;59B:181-188.
23. Garfin SR, Rydevik BL, Lipson SJ, et al: Spinal stenosis, in Rothman RH, Simeone FA, Herkowitz HN, et al (eds): *The Spine.* Philadelphia, PA, WB Saunders, 1992, pp 791-875.
24. Surin V, Hedelin E, Smith L: Degenerative lumbar spinal stenosis: Results of operative treatment. *Acta Orthop Scand* 1982;53:79-85.

Controversies in Low Back Pain: The Surgical Approach

Edward N. Hanley, Jr, MD

Daniel M. Spengler, MD

Sam Wiesel, MD

James N. Weinstein, DO

Introduction

The following chapter is a description of four controversial topics that face spine surgeons on a daily basis. The first topic discussed is recurrent disk herniation. The question asked of the course presenters is: "Should I fuse a patient who has had a recurrent disk herniation at the same level?" The second topic discussed is dark disk disease, and in this case the question asked of the panel was: "Should I operate on a 45-year-old laborer with unrelenting low back pain and a dark disk on MRI at the L4-5 level?" The third topic discussed is degenerative scoliosis. In this case the question asked of the panel was: "How should I approach a 55-year-old female with back and increasing right leg pain of six months duration who has a degenerative lumbar scoliosis?" The fourth and final topic discussed is spinal stenosis with instability. In this case the panel was asked: "When should I fuse a patient in whom I am planning to do a spinal decompression for stenosis?"

In each case the panel was asked to approach these questions and to consider whether or not spinal instrumentation should be considered. This chapter provides both sides of each controversy and attempts to present the reader with the appropriate decision-making literature for each of these difficult patient problems.

Recurrent Disk Herniation: Excision With Fusion

The once controversial issue of whether or not to perform a spinal arthrodesis with primary disk excision for radicular symptoms appears to be a settled issue.[1-8] Results of multiple studies indicate successful relief of radicular pain in approximately 90% of cases when surgical indications are appropriate (predominant radicular pain, tension signs, correlative imaging study, stable psychometrics).[9,10] Fragment excision through a limited exposure approach without extensive disk extirpation is the favored current method.[11] With this technique, a 5% to 10% incidence of recurrent disk herniation and 10% to 15% incidence of major postoperative low back pain is accepted.[9] With this approach, however, comes the acknowledgment that certain patients

will later experience radicular lower extremity pain, with or without concomitant low back pain, and may be candidates for further interventional treatment.[12-15] The form of such further treatment is the topic of this discussion.

The correct approach to use for patients with recurrent disk herniation depends on the characteristics of the complaints, the physical findings, results of imaging studies, and the period of time elapsed and pain-free interval, if any, since the primary procedure. Those patients whose minor residual lower extremity pain and/or low back pain is bothersome but not incapacitating are best managed by accepted nonsurgical measures—nonsteroidal anti-inflammatory medication, brief periods of rest, instruction on the various manifestations of the problem, and physical and psychological measures to deal with it. For individuals with persistent and severe dermatomal-sclerotomal radicular pain, further evaluation and, possibly, more aggressive intervention is indicated. An algorithmic approach may be beneficial in such circumstances.[14] The two broad categories into which such patients can be divided (Fig. 1) are those with radiculopathy only and those with a combination of radiculopathy and low back pain.

Because the vast majority of symptomatic lumbar disk herniations occur at L4-5 and L5-S1, our discussion will be limited to problems at these levels, although the principles for L4-5 disease can be applied to upper lumbar problems.[16]

Radiculopathy Only

Most patients with recurrent disk herniation have recurrent symptoms referable to the same anatomic level and side. The absence of at least some period of pain relief after the primary operation is cause for concern and usually indicates improper patient selection for surgery, failure to operate at the proper level, or failure to achieve nerve root relief. For those patients who have experienced a pain-free interval, the major diagnostic possibilities are recurrent disk herniation at the same level or, less likely, nerve root entrapment caused by epidural scar formation.[10,12-14]

Plain radiographs, which help to confirm that

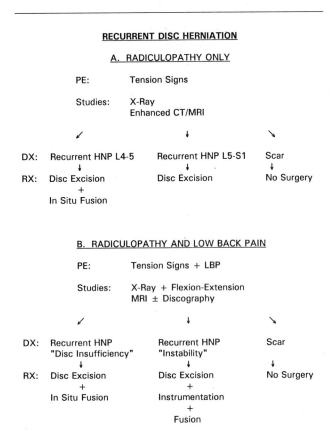

RECURRENT DISC HERNIATION

A. RADICULOPATHY ONLY

PE:　　　Tension Signs

Studies:　X-Ray
　　　　　Enhanced CT/MRI

DX:　Recurrent HNP L4-5　　Recurrent HNP L5-S1　　Scar

RX:　Disc Excision　　　　　Disc Excision　　　　　No Surgery
　　　+
　　　In Situ Fusion

B. RADICULOPATHY AND LOW BACK PAIN

PE:　　　Tension Signs + LBP

Studies:　X-Ray + Flexion-Extension
　　　　　MRI ± Discography

DX:　Recurrent HNP　　　Recurrent HNP　　　Scar
　　　"Disc Insufficiency"　"Instability"

RX:　Disc Excision　　　Disc Excision　　　No Surgery
　　　+　　　　　　　　+
　　　In Situ Fusion　　Instrumentation
　　　　　　　　　　　　+
　　　　　　　　　　　　Fusion

Fig. 1 Algorithmic approach to recurrent disk hernation. Patients can be divided into those with radiculopathy only (A) and those with radiculopathy and low back pain (B).

surgery was indeed performed at the appropriate site and that there has been no unrecognized or acquired hypermobility, may also help to rule out the possibility of post-operative diskitis. Disk-space narrowing, although difficult to assess, is most often present after disk excision but because it has been shown to bear no relationship to symptoms, it should not be used as a criterion for therapeutic decision making.[9] Computed tomography, with and without intravenous contrast, is a reliable and proven study, which in the majority of instances will differentiate a recurrent herniation from scar formation. Magnetic resonance imaging is extremely sensitive but not very specific for such purposes and may show major and confusing postoperative changes even in the face of no symptoms.

If a recurrent disk herniation is unequivocally identified and an appropriate conservative treatment regimen has failed, consideration of a second surgical procedure may be appropriate. In such circumstances, the level of involvement influences the choice of procedure (Fig. 1). If the involvement is at L5-S1, problems related to abnormal mechanical stress, recurrences, or bad back pain are minimal. It is thought that this is

true because this segment is protected by the restraining influences of the iliotransverse ligaments and the fact that it is recessed within the pelvis. At L4-5, however, these protective influences are not present. Some authorities believe that the L4-5 level is exposed to accentuated rotational forces because of the fulcrum effect of the upper spine (believed to be a factor in degenerative spondylolisthesis) and hence is predisposed to higher rates of re-recurrent disk herniation and/or back pain. In fact, some authors note that improved surgical results are exhibited (decreased recurrence rate, less back pain, lower re-operation rate) when primary L4-5 disk excision is combined with a spinal arthrodesis.[17] A similar approach has been advocated for young patients undergoing primary surgery.[18] Because no gross instability pattern is present in such patients (radicular pain only), instrumentation, which adds no advantage and will increase operative time, blood loss, and complications, is not appropriate. In general, a traditional posterolateral intertransverse one-level fusion will suffice. Successful surgical results should exceed 80%.

Patients whose recurrent symptoms are found to be related to epidural scar formation should be managed without surgery.

Radiculopathy and Low Back Pain

Patients with recurrent radiculopathy and low back pain present more of a challenge. Here the major debate is whether or not back pain symptoms are related to mechanical insufficiency of the disk or to definable instability (Fig. 1). Again, appropriate symptoms and findings are imperative prior to considering surgery. Plain radiographs and lateral flexion-extension views may reveal instability caused by degenerative change or iatrogenic spinal destabilization from facet removal, pars interarticularis excision, or fracture. MRI may show disk degeneration/dehydration but is viewed by some as insufficient to assess discogenic pain from insufficiency. Provocative diskography, although controversial, may be useful in such circumstances.[15]

What is instability or hypermobility? Although numerous criteria have been proposed, most are either vague or incomprehensible. Probably the most reasonable objective measure of hypermobility is greater than 4 mm of translation and/or more than 10° of angular change on lateral motion radiographs.[15]

If no gross hypermobility pattern is present, repeat surgery with disk excision and posterolateral fusion is appropriate. Although it has been suggested that the addition of instrumentation or combined anterior disk excision and fusion may be indicated here, surgery of this magnitude is rarely necessary. The expected outcome in more than 75% of cases should be relief of radicular pain and mild residual low back pain. If, by the previously mentioned criteria, the level of recurrence demonstrates frank translational or angular instability then supplementary fixation-instrumentation may help hold the spine in a stable anatomic position while fusion consolidation occurs. Although not objectively proven in clinical series, the rate of arthrodesis consolidation may be slightly improved with such techniques. Success with such measures should be in the 75% range.

Again, patients in this group with a diagnosis of epidural scar should not be operated upon with the possible exception of stabilization of those with gross instability patterns, and then with limited expectations. For patients with compensable work-related situations, expected success rates should diminish by 10% for disk excision alone and by 30% for disk excision combined with fusion.[19]

Summary

Patients who do in fact have recurrent lumbar disk herniations can be expected to enjoy surgical outcomes nearly as good as the initial diskectomy procedure without the need for fusion. Recurrent herniations in patients who have experienced a pain-free interval of greater than one year offer the best outcome. Recurrence at a new level offers results nearly as good as an index diskectomy. Although surgical stabilization seems appropriate in patients with recurrent disk herniation at L4-5, recurrence of radiculopathy with back pain and/or instability or more than two recurrences at the same level, this opinion is not supported by hard data.

Dark Disk Disease

The term "dark disk disease" has been largely derived from the appearance of the intervertebral disk on magnetic resonance imaging (MRI). On T2 weighted images, the normal hydrated disk should appear white. Conversely, the less hydrated disk will appear dark. Recently, authors and paper presenters have suggested that a dark disk represents a disease process and, furthermore, that this disease process can be improved with various spinal fusion procedures. A dark disk on an MRI usually reflects a normal physiologic process of aging which, in general, has nothing to do with any disease process. The disease, if there is one, remains ill-defined.

The indications for surgical intervention for a process affecting the disk would need to establish neural compression, segmental instability, or both.[20,21] Short of this, the treating physician is dealing with a patient who has idiopathic lower back pain and evidence of a normal aging process on MRI. Clearly, a thorough assessment of the patient is warranted to exclude the multiple possible causes for the symptom of lower back pain. In particular, various causes for referred pain, such as tumor, aortic aneurysm, peptic ulcer disease, or endometriosis, must be excluded.

Assuming there is no evidence of any serious pathologic process, the most appropriate treatment for idiopathic lower back pain must be initiated.[22-24] Such measures include symptom control methods using salicylates or nonsteroidal anti-inflammatory drugs. Exercise programs, using aerobic conditioning and trunk strengthening, also appear to have merit.[25-27] In patients with a chronic symptom complex (one that has continued for longer than six months), a more comprehensive assessment and carefully considered treatment approach must be implemented.[24,28] Psychological assessment and consultation with a clinical psychologist and/or psychiatrist, one interested in patients with chronic benign pain problems, are essential. Identification of environmental issues that reinforce pain behaviors, such as ongoing litigation, must be identified and addressed appropriately. One cannot expect any patient to "feel better" or to exhibit "well behavior" when lowered financial recovery may result from "diminished illness." For the motivated individual who has become deconditioned, work transition programs do appear to have potential benefit.[25-27]

In summary, dark disk disease, when not associated with either neural compression or segmental spinal instability, represents physiologic aging, not a disease. For patients who have symptoms and who have only dark disks on MRI, treatment should be the same as for any other patient with idiopathic lower back pain.

On the other hand, in the investigation of patients with mechanical back pain and/or those under consideration for spinal fusion, the use of MRI and/or diskography has been investigated to determine whether or not an intervertebral disk is normal or not. In one of the only prospective studies, Calhoun and associates[29] attempted to define the role of diskography in the investigation of patients with low back pain with and without nondermatomal pain in the lower limb. In this study, 195 patients were followed for a minimum of two years. Of 137 patients in whom diskography revealed morphologically abnormal disks, 89% had significant concordant pain. This group derived measurable and sustained clinical benefit from spinal fusion. In 25 patients whose disks were morphologically abnormal but for whom the provocation of symptoms on diskography was not present, only 52% had clinical success. These authors therefore advocate lumbar diskography for the further investigation of a particular group of patients with back and leg pain. Similar results were reported by Blumenthal and associates.[30] They treated patients whose diagnosis was internal disk disruption, a syndrome of traumatically induced low back pain arising from the intervertebral disk.[31] They feel the diagnosis is confirmed by an abnormal diskogram with concordant pain reproduction at the affected level or levels. Thirty-four patients with internal disk disruption at one level were reviewed and followed an average of 29 months. Of these, 53% underwent anterior lumbar fusion at L4-5, 32% at L5-S1, and the remainder at L2-3, L3-4. Treatment was considered successful if the patient returned to work or normal activities and required either no medications or only anti-inflammatories. By the above criteria, 25 of these 34 patients (74%) with internal disk disruption had a successful outcome. The average time to return to work or normal activities in this group was 6.1 months. The overall union rate was reported to be 73% with an average time to union of one year. They did report graft extrusion requiring revision and retrograde ejaculation as being complications. However, these occurred in only one patient.

However, diskography remains controversial despite nearly 50 years of study. Diskography was first alluded to by Steindler in 1938 and popularized by Lindbloom in 1944. In 1968 Holt performed the classic study in which a 37% false-positive rate was reported.[32] The problems of Holt's study have been well documented.[33] In fact, recalculating Holt's data from his original paper would suggest a false-positive rate of only 25.7%, and if herniated disk patients were excluded from his study, that rate would be even less.[33] In the paper by Walsh and Weinstein,[33] which used currently acceptable techniques, the number of subjects with abnormal disk images was similar to that seen in Holt's study (50%). This study, as opposed to Holt's, used current techniques, valid diskograms, independent observers,

pain intensity three or more on a scale of five, concordance of the pain, and two or more pain behaviors. The false-positive rate was reported to by 0%.[33] However, this study does not raise a flag to diskography and does not answer the question of what to do with a positive study.

The advocates of diskography support the following indications: (1) to diagnose internal derangement or disruption; (2) as a last resort in patients with lower pack pain and in whom results of standard diagnostic procedures are normal; and (3) to determine the disk level causing symptoms when multi-level disk degeneration is present.

Many questions are still left unanswered. For example, "Is pain associated with diskography related to the patient's symptoms?" and "Can diskography be used to predict outcome of spinal surgery, such as fusion?" Answers to these two questions require prospective randomized studies. Provided that dark disk disease exists as a clinical entity and appropriate studies can be performed, an algorithm to treatment might be as follows (Fig. 2): If this algorithm is true, what is the best treatment approach? There are obviously many options (Fig. 3) but few answers.

Degenerative Scoliosis

Degenerative scoliosis can be defined as scoliosis in the thoracolumbar spine developing after the age of 60. It is associated with disk degeneration and facet joint arthrosis. The curve is generally no greater than 400. Depending on the orientation of the facet joints,

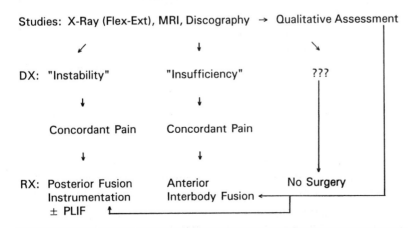

Fig. 2 Algorithmic approach to "Dark Disk Disease." If the diagnosis is unclear, no surgical treatment is indicated.

Treatment Options
(Controversial)

Fusion Surgeries

● Anterior Interbody Fusion (ALIF)
- No Hardware
- With Hardware

● Circumferential 360° Fusion

● Posterior Lumbar Interbody Fusion (PLIF)
- No Hardware
- With Hardware

Fig. 3 Surgical treatment options for patients with degenerative "Dark Disk Disease." These procedures are controversial and not yet scientifically validated.

there can be an associated lateral shift in the antero-posterior plane of one vertebral body on another as well as spondylolisthesis in the lateral plane. The overall result of the scoliosis and the degenerative processes is to reduce the volume of the spinal canal. Depending on the degree of canal size reduction, symptomatic spinal stenosis can occur.

A More Aggressive Surgical Approach

The evaluation and treatment of adult scoliosis patients is challenging and controversial. Expectations of treatment outcome should not mirror those reported for younger patients. Adult scoliosis can be divided into two major categories; that which is present before skeletal maturity (pre-existent scoliosis) and that which arises de novo later in life as a result of degenerative change and osteoporosis (degenerative scoliosis). Pre-existent scoliosis follows the patterns of that seen in adolescent patients and may be associated with pain, curve progression, cosmetic concerns, and, on occasion, pulmonary decompensation or neurologic compromise. Degenerative scoliosis primarily affects the lumbar spine, and presentation is related to mechanical insufficiency of the spine (low back pain) with or without neurologic symptoms (claudication/radiculopathy).[15,34,35] For both groups, nonsurgical treatment (NSAIDs, bracing, exercise, dietary and smoking measures, psychological support) is always indicated before consideration of surgery.

Degenerative scoliosis may develop de novo without any pre-existent deformity. Grubb and associates[36] analyzed a group of adults who developed scoliosis of the lumbar spine with an associated loss of lumbar lordosis. In contrast to patients with a pre-existent idiopathic scoliosis, these individuals were noted to be older at the time of the symptom onset, to have an equal female-male ratio, to exhibit an absence of structural

changes, and to be more osteoporotic.

The presenting symptoms of patients with degenerative scoliosis may be nonspecific. In general, these patients present a combination of lower back pain and spinal stenosis. As opposed to most groups with spinal stenosis, however, these patients often fail to obtain relief of their stenosis symptoms with sitting.[34] The major problem is that of spinal collapse caused by disk degeneration, osteoporosis, facet degenerative change, and rotational abnormality. These abnormalities result in both absolute stenosis, from decrease in spinal canal volume, and relative stenosis, caused by collapse and translational and rotational shift of the spine. Although it is commonly believed that radicular symptoms will predominate on the side of collapse (concavity),[37-39] neural symptoms may occur as a result of traction and shift on the convexity of the curve.[40]

The symptoms and signs may be very nonspecific. Pain is generally of gradual onset and can be located in the back, the legs, or more commonly a combination of the two. Ambulation may increase the leg pain. Physical findings range from objective neurologic findings of the involved nerve roots to vague tenderness in the lumbosacral area. The straight-leg-raising test is usually negative in the sense that it reproduces the leg pain.

Plain radiographs are quite diagnostic and will demonstrate the level of scoliosis as well as the degenerative pathology. No other test is really necessary unless one wants to rule out other pathology (tumor), or unless surgery is being considered. Should surgery be contemplated, a myelogram followed by a CAT scan is preferred because it is a dynamic study in the sense that one can observe the water soluble dye traveling up and down the spinal canal.

Conservative treatment, consisting of the measures previously mentioned, may be beneficial on occasion. A trial of nonsteroidal anti-inflammatory medication, education, rest, and epidural steroids may be tried. Soft lumbar supports or corsets may provide some support, but these usually will not provide sufficient immobilization to relieve symptoms. More rigid braces, even custom-fabricated TLSOs, are often poorly tolerated by this elderly patient population. A gentle exercise program is instituted at any time during the course of therapy if it provides the patient with symptomatic relief. Over 80% of patients will respond favorably.

The vast majority of these patients can be managed by nonsurgical means. If significant symptoms continue, surgery can be considered.

Proponents of decompression procedures alone include Epstein and associates,[37] Nachemson,[41] and San Martino and associates,[38] but decompression can lead to failure of back pain relief, to progressive spinal collapse, and to exacerbation of neural symptoms,[15,42] making secondary surgical treatment even more difficult.

Recent experiences have emphasized the benefits of a more comprehensive surgical approach, in which aggressive decompression is combined with deformity correction and stabilization with segmental pedicle screw fixation constructs. Simmons and Simmons[39] recently reported a series of 42 patients treated by this technique, with satisfactory outcomes in 93% of patients and minimal medical or device-related complications. They emphasized the difference between this type of problem and those of pre-existent scoliosis patients and the benefits of indirect decompression provided by segmental adjustment of the involved levels. Similar results have been reported by Marchesi and Aebi[44] in 27 patients with an apparent pseudarthrosis rate of only 4%.

Surgical experience with this condition, with secondary treatment of patients previously decompressed, showed some initial relief of radicular symptoms but worsened back pain followed by progressive neural deterioration. These patients have been treated with secondary stabilization with pedicle fixation (usually T12 or L1 to L5) with moderately good pain relief and functional improvement. Recent experience in 30 patients with primary surgical treatment of this condition with extensive bilateral decompression followed by correction-stabilization-arthrodesis with pedicle screw fixation had results which mirrored those of Simmons and Simmons[39] and Marchesi and Aebi.[44]

For the above reasons decompression with or without a combination of segmental correction and fusion with instrumentation is recommended for patients whose incapacitating spinal stenosis symptoms and back pain are caused by degenerative scoliosis and who have failed nonsurgical treatment measures.[15] For the occasional patient with single nerve root involvement and no major back pain, unilateral root decompression may be indicated. For the rare presentation of painful collapsing degenerative scoliosis with back pain only, there may be a role for corrective instrumentation and fusion alone. Despite reports of the apparent success of such approaches, one must keep in mind that other health factors may preclude surgical treatment in some elderly patients, regardless of the severity of their symptoms and the functional disability caused by them. Judicious therapeutic decision-making is imperative in this disorder. An algorithmic approach to this condition is presented in Figure 4.

Stenosis and Instability

Degenerative Spondylolisthesis—Fusion?: To Instrument or Not

Spinal stenosis may be defined as an absolute or relative narrowing of the spinal canal and/or foramen to

DEGENERATIVE SCOLIOSIS

A. LBP

PE: Deformity, Imbalance, LBP
↓
Studies: X-Ray, Bend X-Ray, Hip X-Ray
Myelo/CT
↓
DX: Degenerative Scoliosis

Sx: mild-moderate ↙   ↘ Sx: severe

Nonop Rx   Surgical Rx
Brace   Segmental Instrumentation
NSAI   Fusion
± Anterior Surgery
Brace

B. LBP + CLAUDICATION/RADICULOPATHY

PE: Deformity, Imbalance, LBP, Neuro
↓
Studies: X-Ray, Bend X-Ray, Hip X-ray
Myelo/CT, EMG
↓
DX: Degenerative Scoliosis + Stenosis

Sx: mild-moderate ↙   ↘ Sx: severe

Nonop Rx: Surgical Rx:
Brace   Decompression
NSAI   Segmental Instr.
± Epidural Steroids   Fusion
Brace

Fig. 4 Algorithmic approach to degenerative scoliosis. Patients with this condition are best divided into those with low back pain (LBP) only (A) and those with low back pain with claudication and/or radiculopathy (B).

produce compression of the neural elements. An additional instability component may occur depending on the tropism (sagittal orientation) of the facet joints. The more vertical the facets are in the anterior-posterior plane the more likely instability is to occur. Instability may be defined as dynamic when one vertebral body moves 4 mm or more relative to another on weight-bearing, lateral flexion-extension radiographs. It is static when there is a fixed slip. This latter situation is the most common and is generally referred to as degenerative spondylolisthesis.

The complaint of back pain, leg pain, or both is common. Leg pain may significantly increase with ambulation to the point where the patient has to stop walking. This is referred to as neurogenic claudication and needs to be carefully differentiated from vascular pathology. Back pain can be a major component especially if instability is present.

Degenerative spondylolisthesis is an acquired condition thought to be caused by chronic disk degeneration and long-standing segmental instability.[45] Facet changes and rotational instability characterize the pathologic process.[46] Slippage occurs most often at L4-5, although it may be present at adjacent levels. It rarely progresses to more than 25% to 30% of vertebral body width. As the olisthesis progresses, patients may present with sciatica or claudication. Back pain is a frequent complaint but usually equal to or less than the neural symptomatology. This problem is common in the elderly population. The average age at presentation is approximately 60 years.

The physical examination may not be very rewarding. The neurologic examination and tension signs are usually negative. In some cases where the patient is asked to reproduce his leg pain by walking, a specific neurologic deficit may be obtained. This is termed a stress test.

Plain radiographs will demonstrate the pathology. Weightbearing lateral flexion-extension films should be included. Disk degeneration, facet joint arthrosis and static/dynamic slips will be easily identified. One must constantly be aware that other pathology, such as metastatic tumor, must be ruled out because many patients can have the radiographic picture of spinal stenosis and be asymptomatic. No other diagnostic studies are necessary unless surgery is being contemplated, in which case a myelogram followed by a CAT scan is preferred because of its dynamic quality.

The majority of these patients can be treated in a nonoperative manner. The most important aspect is patient education. If the patient understands the process and what can be accomplished from treatment, unrealistic goals will not be expected. Actual treatment consists of controlled physical activity, anti-inflammatory medication and braces/corsets. For those patients who continue to have symptoms, epidural steroids may be an appropriate next step.

Surgical treatment may be indicated when the disease becomes functionally incapacitating or neurologic dysfunction is progressive (rare). Again, patient education as to the realistic goals for surgery is necessary if both the patient and surgeon wish to be satisfied with the outcome.

The surgical treatments advocated have consisted of decompression, arthrodesis, or a combination of both. Until recently, reports have not shown objective data to support one approach or the other.[47,48] Lombardi and associates[49] concluded that the group treated by decompression with fusion "continued to feel better and stronger with time." Feffer and associates[47] also reported that those who had decompression with fusion appeared to have more favorable outcomes. Rosenberg[46] and, more recently, Herron and Trippi[50] concluded that routine fusion was not necessary if preoperative radiographs did not show instability and if the decompression procedure did not compromise structural integrity of the spine. Reynolds and Wiltse[48]

looked at results of surgical treatment in patients of different ages. They concluded that fusion is beneficial in patients under the age of 65 but is not necessarily indicated in older patients. Some surgeons have tended to selectively fuse only younger patients or those who required extensive decompressive procedures.[45] Others have suggested an initial decompressive procedure, followed by selective arthrodesis if the initial procedure fails.[46,51] More recent uncontrolled surgical reports suggest that arthrodesis provides long-term stability, resists torsional and translational forces, and results in successful outcomes in approximately 85% of patients.[52-55]

The best and most objective information on this disease subset was reported in 1991 by Herkowitz and Kurz.[56] They provide invaluable information, which may serve to settle the issue of whether or not to combine fusion with decompression in the treatment of degenerative spondylolisthesis. They prospectively studied 50 patients with spinal stenosis in conjunction with degenerative spondylolisthesis, performing decompression alone in 25 patients and decompression and intertransverse fusion in the other 25. The patients in the two groups were similar in character and mimicked those reported previously. At a follow-up of three years (range 2.4 to 4 years), results were significantly better with respect to pain in the back and lower extremities in those patients who had a concomitant arthrodesis (96% versus 44% satisfactory, p = 0.0001). Spondylolisthesis increased postoperatively in 96% of patients without an arthrodesis and in only 28% of those who had an arthrodesis performed. Although the radiographic pseudarthrosis rate was 36% in patients who had undergone fusion, this did not appear to affect the clinical result.

While this report seems to settle the issue of whether or not to fuse patients with degenerative spondylolisthesis, it does not provide insight into whether or not to stabilize the spine with instrumentation during the procedure. Although claims have been made to support the instrumentation concept, there is no objective evidence to support or denigrate it. While we await the outcome of a prospective multicenter study on this issue, our approach has been to apply known principles. For the typical patient with degenerative spondylolisthesis with spinal stenosis and no evidence of gross instability on flexion-extension radiographs, a decompressive procedure is performed in conjunction with a lateral arthrodesis as advocated above. For patients with objective instability, defined as translational excursion of more than 4 mm or angular change of more than 10° on motion radiographs, segmental instrumentation is advocated. A similar approach is proposed for patients with the other disease entities within this category of lumbar spinal stenosis with instability (isthmic spondylolisthesis and

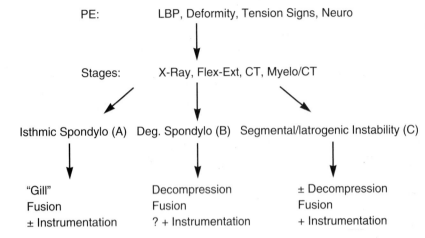

STENOSIS AND INSTABILITY

CLAUDICATION/RADICULOPATHY ± LBP

PE: LBP, Deformity, Tension Signs, Neuro

Stages: X-Ray, Flex-Ext, CT, Myelo/CT

Isthmic Spondylo (A)   Deg. Spondylo (B)   Segmental/Iatrogenic Instability (C)

"Gill"   Decompression   ± Decompression
Fusion   Fusion   Fusion
± Instrumentation   ? + Instrumentation   + Instrumentation

Fig. 5   Algorithmic approach for stenosis with instability. Most patients with this will have some component of back pain, but lower extremity and neural symptoms usually predominate. Surgical success appears best in the degenerative spondylolisthesis group (B).

A. HISTORY   -   Back and/or leg pain with increased leg pain on ambulation.

B. PHYSICAL   -   +/– neurological deficit or tension sign. Positive stress test.

C. DIAGNOSTIC STUDY   -   Dynamic lateral weightbearing plain x-rays. Myelogram/CT scan before surgery.

D. TREATMENT   -   a. Initially anti-inflammatory medication, controlled physical activity and a corset.
b. Epidural steroids.
c. Surgery
    (1) Decompression with adequate removal of ligamentum flavum - open foramen.
    (2) Bilateral lateral fusion.
    (3) Only time to consider instrumentation is with motion greater than 4 mm.
    (4) Do not remove disk or this will lead to progression and increased symptoms.

Fig. 6   Outline of the standardized diagnostic and treatment approach to patients with stenosis and instability.

segmental/iatrogenic instability) (Fig. 5). As always, all therapeutic decision-making must take into consideration the age and general health of the patient, previous results of nonsurgical treatment measures, and applicable psychosocial and/or compensation issues. A relatively standardized and objective approach to these patients may ultimately help in improving outcome results (Fig. 6).

References

1. Adkins EWO: Lumbo-sacral arthrodesis after laminectomy. *J Bone Joint Surg* 1955;37B:208-223.

2. Frymoyer JW, Hanley E, Howe J, et al: Disc excision and spine fusion in the management of lumbar disc disease: A minimum ten-year follow-up. *Spine* 1978;3:1-6.

3. Frymoyer JW, Matteri RE, Hanley EN, et al: Failed lumbar disc surgery requiring second operation: A long-term follow-up study. *Spine* 1978;3:7-11.

4. Hoover NW: Indications for fusion at the time of removal of the intervertebral disc. *J Bone Joint Surg* 1968;50A:189-193.

5. LaRocca H: Failed lumbar surgery. *The Lumbar Spine (ISSLS)*. Philadelphia, PA, WB Saunders, 1990, pp 872-881.

6. Lehmann T, LaRocca H: Repeat lumbar surgery. *Spine* 1981;6:615-619.

7. Nachlas IW: End-result study of the treatment of herniated nucleus pulposus by excision with fusion and without fusion. *J Bone Joint Surg* 1952;34A:981-988.

8. Turner JA, Ersek M, Herron L, et al: Patient outcomes after lumbar spinal fusions. *JAMA* 1992;268:907-911.

9. Hanley EN Jr, Shapiro DE: The development of low-back pain after excision of a lumbar disc. *J Bone Joint Surg* 1989;71A:719-721.

10. Ruggieri F, Specchia L, Sabalat S, et al: Lumbar disc herniation: Diagnosis, surgical treatment, recurrence: A review of 872 operated cases. *Ital J Orthop Traumatol* 1988;14:15-22.

11. Sprangfort EV: The lumbar disc herniation. *Acta Orthop Scand* 1972;(Suppl):142.

12. Cauchoix J, Ficat C, Girard B: Repeat surgery after disc excision. *Spine* 1978;3:256-259.

13. Fager CA, Freidberg SR: Analysis of failures and poor results of lumbar spine surgery. *Spine* 1980;5:87-94.

14. Federowicz SG, Wiesel SW: An algorithm for the multiply operated low back patient and treatment of operative complications. *Semin Spine Surg* 1991;3:175-183.

15. Hanley EN Jr, Phillips ED, Kostuik JP: Who should be fused?, in Frymoyer JW, Ducker TB, Hadler NM, et al (eds): *The Adult Spine: Principles and Practice*. New York, Raven Press, 1991, vol 2, chap 91, pp 1893-1917.

16. Spengler DM, Ouellette EA, Battié M, et al: Elective discectomy for herniation of a lumbar disc. *J Bone Joint Surg* 1990;72A:230-237.

17. Vaughan PA, Malcolm BW, Maistrelli GL: Results of L4-L5 disc excision alone versus disc excision and fusion. *Spine* 1988;13:690-695.

18. DeOrio JK, Bianco AJ Jr: Lumbar disc excision in children and adolescents. *J Bone Joint Surg* 1982;64A:991-996.

19. Waddell G, Kummel EG, Lotto WN, et al: Failed lumbar disc surgery and repeat surgery following industrial injuries. *J Bone Joint Surg* 1979;61A:201-207.

20. Frymoyer J: Are we performing too much spinal surgery? *Iowa Orthop J* 1989;9:32-36.

21. Turner JA, Ersek M, Herron L, et al: Patient outcomes after lumbar spinal fusions. *JAMA* 1992;268:907-911.

22. Deyo RA: Conservative treatment for low back pain: Distinguishing useful from useless therapy. *JAMA* 1983;250:1057-1062.

23. Fordyce WE, Brockway JA, Bergman JA, et al: Acute back pain: A control-group comparison of behavioral vs traditional management methods. *J Behav Med* 1986;9:127-140.

24. Scientific approach to the assessment and management of activity-related spinal disorders: A monograph for clinicians: Report of the Quebec Task Force on Spinal Disorders. *Spine* 1987;12:S1-S59.

25. Kellett KM, Kellett DA, Nordholm LA: Effects of an exercise program on sick leave due to back pain. *Phys Ther* 1991;71:283-293.

26. Mayer TG, Gatchel RJ, Kishino N, et al: Objective assessment of spine function following industrial injury: A prospective study with comparison group and one-year follow-up. *Spine* 1985;10:482-493.

27. Mayer TG, Barnes D, Kishino ND, et al: Progressive isoinertial lifting evaluation I & II: A standardized protocol and normative database. *Spine* 1988;13:993-1002.

28. Jensen MP, Turner JA, Romano JM, et al: Coping with chronic pain: A critical review of the literature. *Pain* 1991;47:249-283.

29. Calhoun E, McCall IW, Williams L, et al: Provocation discography as a guide to planning operations on the spine. *J Bone Joint Surg* 1988;70B:267-271.

30. Blumenthal S, Baker J, Dossett A, et al: The role of anterior lumbar fusion for internal disc disruption. *Spine* 1988;13:566-569.

31. Crock HV: A reappraisal of intervertebral disc lesions. *Med J Aust* 1970;1:983-988.

32. Holt EP: The question of lumbar discography. *J Bone Joint Surg* 1968;50A:720-726.

33. Walsh T, Weinstein J, Spratt K, et al: Lumbar discography in normal subjects: A controlled prospective study. *J Bone Joint Surg* 1990;72A:1081-1088.

34. Grubb SA, Lipscomb JH: Diagnostic findings in painful adult scoliosis. *Spine* 1992;17:518-527.

35. Jackson RP, Simmons EH, Stripinis D: Incidence and severity of back pain in adult idiopathic scoliosis. *Spine* 1983;8:749-756.

36. Grubb SA, Lipscomb HJ, Coonrad RW: Degenerative adult onset scoliosis. *Spine* 1988;13:241-245.

37. Epstein BS, Epstein JA, Jones MD: Symptomatic lumbar scoliosis with degenerative changes in the elderly. *Tex Med* 1978;74:56-64.

38. San Martino A, D'Andria FM, San Martino C: The surgical treatment of nerve root compression caused by scoliosis of the lumbar spine. *Spine* 1983;8:261-265.

39. Simmons ED Jr, Simmons EH: Spinal stenosis with scoliosis. *Spine* 1992;17(6 Suppl):S117-S120.

40. Hanley EN Jr, Eskay ML: Degenerative lumbar spinal stenosis. *Adv Orthop Surg* 1985;8:396-403.

41. Nachemson A: Adult scoliosis and back pain. *Spine* 1979;4:513-517.

42. Benner B, Ehni G: Degenerative lumbar scoliosis. *Spine* 1979;4:548-552.

43. Lonstein JE: Adult scoliosis, in Bradford DS, Lonstein JE, Ogilvie JW, et al (eds): *Moe's Textbook of Scoliosis and Other Spinal Deformities*, ed 2. Philadelphia, WB Saunders, 1987, chap 17, pp 369-390.

44. Marchesi DG, Aebi M: Pedicle fixation devices in the treatment of adult lumbar scoliosis. *Spine* 1992;17(8 suppl):S304-S309.

45. Fitzgerald JA, Newman PH: Degenerative spondylolisthesis. *J Bone Joint Surg* 1976;58B:184-192.

46. Rosenberg NJ: Degenerative spondylolisthesis: Surgical treatment. *Clin Orthop* 1976;117:112-120.

47. Feffer HL, Wiesel SW, Cuckler JM, et al: Degenerative spondylolisthesis: To fuse or not to fuse. *Spine* 1985;10:287-289.

48. Reynolds JB, Wiltse LL: Surgical treatment of degenerative spondylolisthesis. *Spine* 1979;4:148-149 (abstract).

49. Lombardi JS, Wiltse LL, Reynolds J, et al: Treatment of degenerative spondylolisthesis. *Spine* 1985;10:821-827.

50. Herron LD, Trippi AC: L4-5 degenerative spondylolisthesis: The results of treatment by decompressive laminectomy without fusion. *Spine* 1989;14:534-538.

51. Cauchoix J, Benoist M, Chassaing V: Degenerative spondylolisthesis. *Clin Orthop* 1976;115:122-129.

52. Hanley EN Jr: Decompression and distraction-derotation arthrodesis for degenerative spondylolisthesis. *Spine* 1986;11:269-276.

53. Kaneda K, Kazama H, Satoh S, et al: Follow-up study of medial facetectomies and posterolateral fusion with instrumentation in unstable degenerative spondylolisthesis. *Clin Orthop* 1986;203:159-167.

54. Knox BD, Harvell JC Jr, Nelson PB, et al: Decompression and luque rectangle fusion for degenerative spondylolisthesis. *J Spinal Disord* 1989;2:223-228.

55. Wiltse LL, Kirkaldy-Willis WH, McIvor GW: The treatment of spinal stenosis. *Clin Orthop* 1976;115:83-91.

56. Herkowitz HN, Kurz LT: Degenerative lumbar spondylolisthesis with spinal stenosis: A prospective study comparing decompression with decompression and intertransverse process arthrodesis. *J Bone Joint Surg* 1991;73A:802-808.

Lumbar Spinal Stenosis: Indications for Arthrodesis and Spinal Instrumentation

Harry N. Herkowitz, MD

Introduction

The previous chapters outlined the indications and techniques for decompressive laminectomy. There appears to be a clear-cut consensus that patients who present with clinical symptoms of spinal stenosis and a confirming imaging study should undergo decompression of the involved segment(s) when nonsurgical treatment fails. The expected success rate is 75% to 90%.[1-6]

Deciding which patents would benefit from a concomitant arthrodesis is more difficult. At the time of the decompressive laminectomy the decision to fuse is based on two factors. The first is the preoperative structural integrity of the lumbar spine. The second takes into account any structural changes that occur during the decompressive laminectomy itself.

The significant preoperative structural alterations are: (1) presence of degenerative spondylolisthesis along with spinal stenosis, (2) scoliosis and/or kyphosis along with spinal stenosis, and (3) recurrent spinal stenosis at a previously decompressed spinal level with or without iatrogenic spondylolisthesis.

The significant intraoperative changes are: (1) excessive removal of lumbar facet(s) and (2) "radical" excision of the intervertebral disk at the level of decompression. Each of these structural alterations will be discussed in depth and the rationale for the addition of a concomitant arthrodesis will be presented.

Preoperative Structural Alterations

Degenerative Spondylolisthesis

Until recently, controversy centered on the role of arthrodesis in patients undergoing decompressive laminectomy when an associated spondylolisthesis was present (Fig. 1). Numerous articles have appeared in the literature advocating no arthrodesis; others have supported arthrodesis at the time of the decompressive laminectomy.[6-15] Herkowitz and Kurz[15] published a prospective study that compared decompressive laminectomy alone and decompressive laminectomy with intertransverse arthrodesis in 50 patients with single level spinal stenosis associated with degenerative spondylolisthesis. That study demonstrated statistically significant better results in those patients who underwent a concomitant arthrodesis. Based on that data,

the authors recommended arthrodesis for all patients undergoing decompressive laminectomy with an associated degenerative spondylolisthesis (Fig. 2). Several articles published since then have supported the addition of an arthrodesis when the stenotic segment is associated with a degenerative spondylolisthesis.[16-18]

Postacchini and Cinotti[16] reported on the occurrence of laminar regrowth following decompressive laminectomy for spinal stenosis. They reviewed 40 patients with an average follow-up of 8.6 years. Of the 40 patients, degenerative spondylolisthesis was present

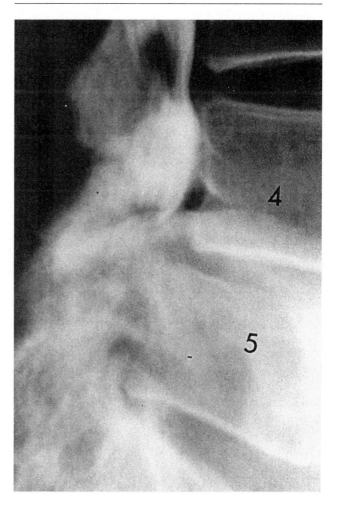

Fig. 1 Lateral lumbar myelogram indicating complete block at L4-L5 in patients with spinal stenosis and degenerative lumbar spondylolisthesis.

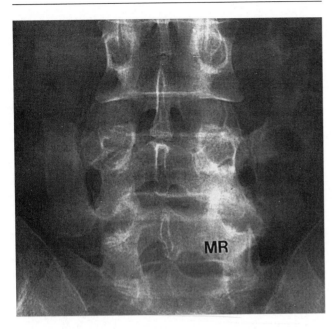

Fig. 2 Postoperative AP radiograph demonstrating solid postero-lateral arthrodesis at L4-L5.

addition of a posterolateral arthrodesis at the time of the decompressive laminectomy.

Scoliosis-Kyphosis

The surgical management of spinal stenosis in association with pre-existing idiopathic or degenerative lumbar scoliosis does not present as clear-cut a picture as that of degenerative spondylolisthesis (Fig. 3). Prior studies have focused on retrospective analysis of surgical technique without comparative reviews of various surgical options.[19-22]

It is clear that not all patients with surgically significant spinal stenosis within a lumbar scoliosis and/or kyphosis require a concomitant arthrodesis. Therefore, the following five factors need to be considered in making a surgical decision for a concomitant arthrodesis. The first of these is curve flexibility. On side-bending films the curve demonstrates at least 50% correction (Fig. 4). A decompressive laminectomy alone would most likely increase the risk of curve progression unless arthrodesis is added when a flexible curve exists. The second factor is a documented preoperative

preoperatively in 16 patients. Six of these 16 had a decompression alone; ten had an added arthrodesis. Those patients without an arthrodesis had more bone regrowth and a significantly poorer clinical outcome than the group with the arthrodesis.

Further support for the addition of an arthrodesis when spinal stenosis is associated with a degenerative spondylolisthesis was reported by Satomi and associates.[17] In a series of 41 surgical patents, 27 patients underwent anterior lumbar interbody fusion and 14 patients had a posterior decompression only. Good to excellent results were 93% and 72%, respectively, in the two groups. Although the arthrodesis group was fused anteriorly rather than by the traditional postero-lateral approach, superior results with an arthrodesis were still demonstrated.

Caputy and Luessenhop[18] reported on 96 patients who underwent decompression alone for spinal stenosis. At five years postoperatively, 26 patients were considered failures. Of these 26 patients, 16 had recurrent leg pain, and five of the 16 had a pre-existing degenerative spondylolisthesis. Ten of the 26 patients were considered failures because of recurrent low back pain. Five of these ten had a pre-existing degenerative spondylolisthesis at the stenotic level. Based on the findings of their study, the authors recommended the addition of an arthrodesis for all patients undergoing surgery with degenerative spondylolisthesis associated with spinal stenosis.

In summary, the data regarding spondylolisthesis in association with spinal stenosis strongly support the

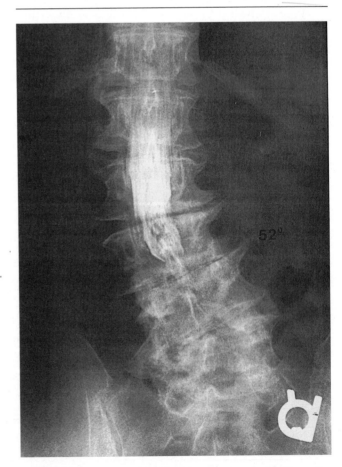

Fig. 3 AP radiograph demonstrating degenerative lumbar scoliosis with a myelographic block at L3 in a patient with spinal stenosis.

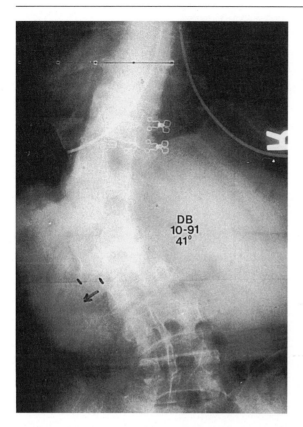
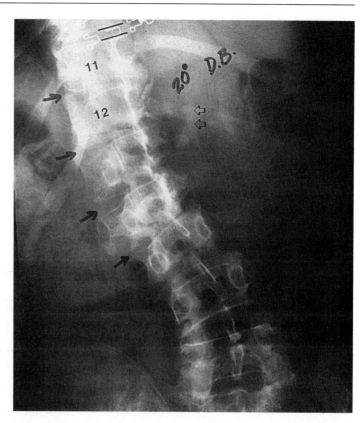

Fig. 4 **Left**, AP lumbar radiograph depicting a 41° left lumbar scoliosis with an associated lateral listhesis of L2 on L3. **Right**, Left lateral bending radiograph showing correction of the lumbar curve from 41° to 20°.

history of curve progression. This, alone, would be an indication for arthrodesis. Third is scoliosis with a predominant radiculopathy within the concavity of the curve (Fig. 5, *top*). In this case, a decompressive laminectomy with partial facetectomy may not be sufficient to alleviate nerve root compression in the concavity. Because the root may be compressed between the pedicles of the concavity, partial correction of the deformity is indicated to reduce pedicular kinking (Fig. 5, *bottom*). Fourth, loss of lumbar lordosis, such that the patient is in sagittal imbalance, is defined by a standing lateral radiograph including the entire spine, from the base of the skull to the sacrum. On this radiograph, a plumb line is draw inferiorly from the odontoid process. Normally, this line should pass through the posterior half of the vertebral body of L5. In a patient with sagittal imbalance, this line will pass anterior to this point (Fig. 6, *left*). Because persistence of a "flat back" can lead to increasing back pain postoperatively, improving this sagittal imbalance is necessary at the time of decompressive surgery (Fig. 6, *right*). The fifth factor is lateral spondylolisthesis. Lateral listhesis that demonstrates correction on side-bending films is an indication of a hypermobile segment, which may become more unstable following a decompressive

laminectomy (Fig. 7, *left*). Therefore, arthrodesis is indicated to prevent further shifting of the vertebrae (Fig. 7, *right*).

The magnitude of the scoliotic curve itself is not a sufficient reason, in itself, to recommend arthrodesis, if none of the other pre-existing factors outlined above is present. As an example, a 60° rigid lumbar curve with satisfactory sagittal balance and three-level spinal stenosis would require only a decompressive laminectomy.

Recurrent Spinal Stenosis at the Same Segment

Patients who require a second decompressive laminectomy at the same segment are candidates for an arthrodesis. Further compromise of the facet joints is usually necessary in order to accomplish decompression of the central canal and lateral recesses in these cases. Sacrificing more than 50% of each facet joint renders that motion segment unstable, especially when the facet joints lie in the usual sagittal orientation above L5-S1.[23,24] Segmental instability may be detected when adequate flexion-extension radiographs can be obtained. Excessive translational and angular movement of the motion segment is defined as greater than 4 mm of translational movement (Fig. 8) or greater

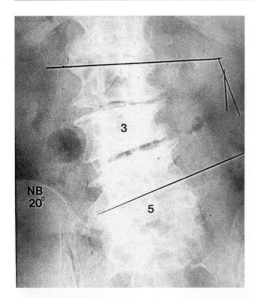

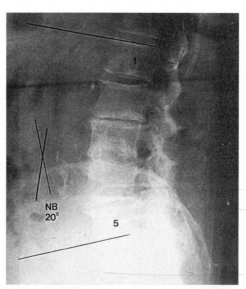

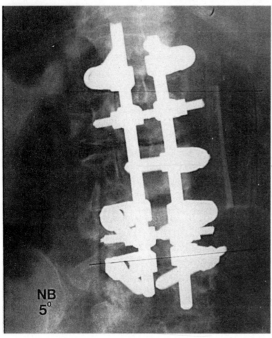

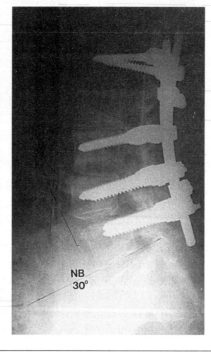

Fig. 5 Top left, AP lumbar radiograph showing a 20° lumbar scoliosis. This patient had predominant left lumbar radiculopathy which was within the curve's concavity. **Top right**, This lateral lumbar radiograph depicts the loss of lumbar lordosis. **Bottom left**, This anteroposterior postoperative radiograph shows reduction of the scoliosis and distraction of the pedicles on the concave side of the curve (Isola instrumentation). **Bottom right**, This lateral postoperative radiograph shows restoration of lumbar lordosis (Isola instrumentation).

than 10° of angular change measured at the endplate (Fig. 9). Patients who develop a recurrent stenosis in conjunction with an iatrogenic spondylolisthesis also require concomitant arthrodesis, because further instability will be produced following the second decompression.[25-28] Patients who develop stenosis above a previous posterior fusion require only decompression unless excessive resection of the facet joints occurs.

Intraoperative Structure Alterations

Excessive Removal of the Facet Joints

Abumi and associates[23] have demonstrated in cadaveric specimens the importance of the lumbar facet joints for the structural stability of the motion segment. Upon performing progressive facetectomies of the lumbar motion segment and subjecting the specimens to cyclical loading in an Instron machine, they concluded that removal of greater than 50% of each facet joint led to unacceptable movement of that motion segment (defined as greater than 50% of each facet joint). Therefore, when excessive facet excision occurs during surgery, posterolateral arthrodesis should be added to prevent postoperative instability.

Disk Excision

The incidence of disk herniation in conjunction with spinal stenosis has been reported as from 5% to

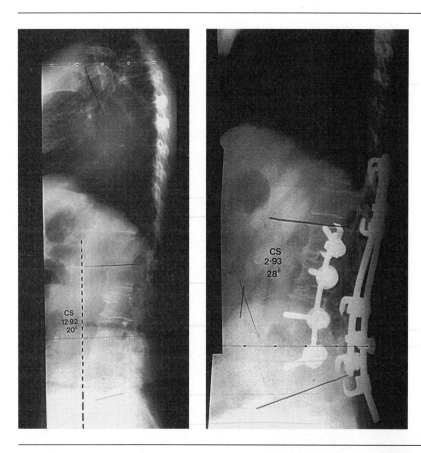

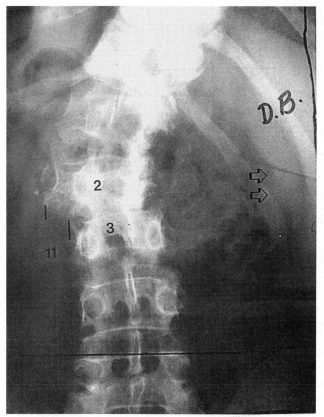

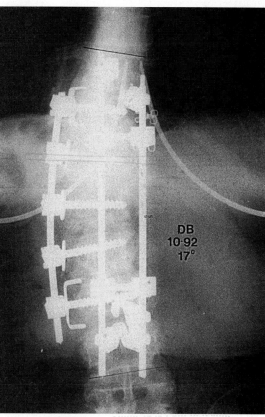

Fig. 6   Left, Lateral lumbar radiograph in patient CS with history of lumbar scoliosis and spinal stenosis. Note plumb line passes anterior to the vertebral body L5 (20° kyphosis). **Right,** Postoperative lateral lumbar radiograph demonstrating restoration of lumbar lordosis. Note plumb line now passes through the L5 vertebral body (28° lordosis) (TSRH instrumentation).

Fig. 7   Left, Lateral listhesis L2-L3 in patient DB with associated scoliosis. Partial correction noted on right side bending. **Right,** AP postoperative radiograph depicts correction of the scoliosis (41° to 17°) and correction of the lateral listhesis.

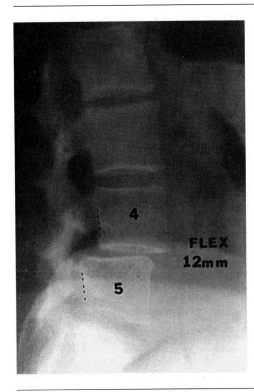

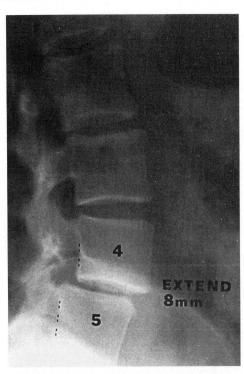

Fig. 8 Flexion and extension lateral radiographs demonstrating excessive translational motion at L4-L5 in a patient who had undergone a previous decompressive laminectomy.

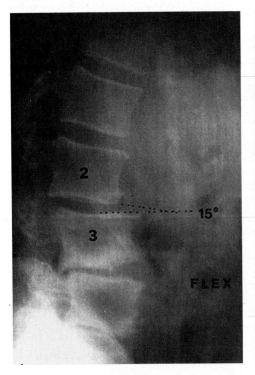

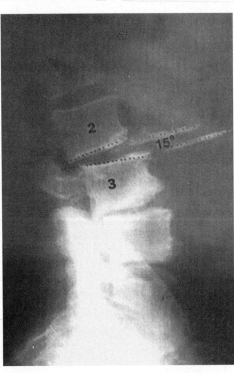

Fig. 9 Flexion and extension lateral radiographs demonstrating excessive angular motion at L2-L3 in a patient who had undergone a previous decompressive laminectomy.

25%.[1,2] Most disk herniations that occur in this group represent extrusions or free fragments of disk at the level of the foramen. In those cases simple removal of the disk fragment at the time of decompressive laminectomy is all that is required. "Radical" disk excision, removal of as much disk material as possible, may lead to an iatrogenic spondylolisthesis, because it destabilizes the anterior column after the posterior column has been compromised by the decompressive laminectomy.[10] If a "radical" diskectomy was felt to be necessary, then a posterolateral arthrodesis should be added.

Spinal Instrumentation

The goals of internal fixation are to correct deformity, to stabilize the spine, to protect the neural elements, to improve the rate of fusion, to reduce the number of segments requiring arthrodesis, and to reduce rehabilitation time.

Fixation into the lumbar and lumbosacral spine presents special problems, especially when dealing with an aged population. Lumbar spinal instrumentation in older patients must address osteoporosis and the lack of lamina available for fixation that occurs following the decompressive laminectomy. Traditional posterior distraction systems such as Harrington rods or Knodt rods often lead to a loss of lumbar lordosis. The maintenance of lumbar lordosis is a critical factor in long-term surgical success, because failure to maintain lumbar lordosis is a significant cause of recurrent back and/or leg pain.

Pedicle fixation appears to solve the technical problems of the traditional implant systems when a spinal instrumentation system is indicated following a decompressive lumbar laminectomy. Pedicle fixation places the fixation points through the lumbar pedicle—the strongest part of the osteopenic vertebrae.[29] It allows segmental fixation, which improves torsional stability and aids in maintaining lumbar lordosis (Fig. 5). In addition, segmental fixation may reduce the number of motion segments that require arthrodesis, thus preserving distal lumbar segments, which is a significant factor for reducing the incidence of low back pain. Pedicle screw systems are also better able than conventional hook and rod systems to achieve adequate sacral fixation.[30] Finally, reduction of spinal deformity is accomplished more efficiently with pedicle segmental fixation (Fig. 10).

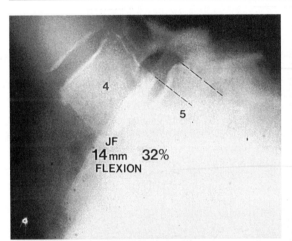

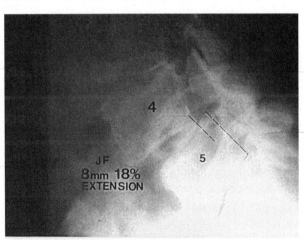

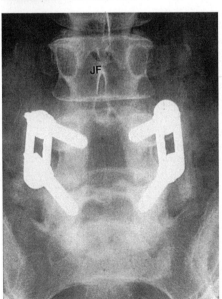

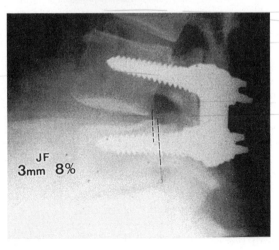

Fig. 10 **Top**, Preoperative lateral flexion extension radiographs in a patient with recurrent spinal stenosis and translational instability. **Bottom**, Postoperative AP and lateral radiographs demonstrating partial reduction of the spondylolisthesis with pedicle screw fixation at L4-L5.

Pedicle fixation also has disadvantages. First, a significant learning curve exists even for experienced spine surgeons.[31,32] Failure to place the pedicle screw in the correct location may lead to neurologic deficit and loss of fixation.[33] In addition, the longevity of pedicle fixation systems can now be evaluated. Boos and associates[34] evaluated the AO internal fixator and the Cotrel-DuBousset system following their implantation for degenerative disorders of the lumbar spine. At two plus years post surgery, only 70% of the implants remained "intact."

The disadvantages of pedicle fixation must be weighed against the advantages to allow the surgeon to decide whether an implant system is necessary at the time of arthrodesis. With the increasing efforts surgeons must make to control costs, this consideration becomes even more important.

The surgeon contemplating the addition of a spinal implant to the arthrodesis in patients with spinal stenosis is faced with the fact that hard scientific data are lacking to assist the surgeon in making an informed decision. In most cases, instrumentation is added following decompression and arthrodesis (1) to improve the chance for a solid arthrodesis and (2) to correct a pre-existing deformity.

The incidence of pseudarthrosis following posterolateral fusion increases with the number of levels being fused. The rates of pseudarthrosis for one-, two-, and three-level fusions are 3.5% to 10%, 15% to 20%, and 25% to 33%, respectively.[35] In addition, the pseudarthrosis rate increases if segmental instability is present at that motion segment, for example, when a prior decompressive laminectomy with translational or angular instability is present. Therefore, when these conditions are present, instrumenting the arthrodesis may aid in obtaining a successful fusion.

The indications for the addition of instrumentation following spinal stenosis decompression and arthrodesis are: (1) correction of scoliosis and/or kyphosis, (2) arthrodesis of two or more motion segments with an associated decompressive laminectomy, (3) recurrent spinal stenosis with iatrogenic spondylolisthesis, (4) translational motion greater than 4 mm in flexion and extension, and (5) angular motion greater than 10° in flexion and extension. Is the addition of instrumentation indicated for a one-level arthrodesis in degenerative spondylolisthesis following decompressive laminectomy or if excessive facet excision has occurred at the time of the one-level laminectomy? The answers to these questions are not presently available.

In summary, this section has outlined the indications for arthrodesis and spinal instrumentation in degenerative lumbar spinal stenosis. It has not attempted to detail surgical technique. Analysis of the various implant systems, along with their advantages and disad-vantages, has been omitted because it is beyond the scope of this discussion.

Much needs to be clarified regarding arthrodesis and instrumentation for lumbar degenerative disorders. Only prospective controlled studies will answer these questions so that we can provide our patients with the most effective and longest lasting surgical treatment.

References

1. Garfin SR, Glover M, Booth RE, et al: Laminectomy: A review of the Pennsylvania hospital experience. *J Spinal Disord* 1988;1:116-133.
2. Herkowitz HN, Garfin SR: Decompressive surgery for spinal stenosis. *Semin Spine Surg* 1989;1;163-167.
3. Herron LD, Mangelsdorf C: Lumbar spinal stenosis: Results of surgical treatment. *J Spinal Disord* 1991;4:26-33.
4. Katz JN, Lipson SJ, Larson MG, et al: The outcome of decompressive laminectomy for degeneratve lumbar stenosis. *J Bone Joint Surg* 1991;73A:809-816.
5. Spengler DM: Current concepts review: Degenerative stenosis of the lumbar spine. *J Bone Joint Surg* 1987;69A:305-308.
6. Tile M, McNeil SR, Zarins RK, et al: Spinal stenosis: Results of treatment. *Clin Orthop* 1976;115:104-108.
7. Bolesta MJ, Bohlman HH: Degenerative spondylolisthesis: The role of arthrodesis. Presented at the 56th Annual Meeting of the American Academy of Orthopaedic Surgeons. Las Vegas, NV, February 1989, paper No. 374, p 193.
8. Brown MD, Lockwood JM: Degenerative spondylolisthesis, in Evarts CM (ed): *American Academy of Orthopaedic Surgeons Instructional Course Lectures XXXII.* St. Louis, MO, CV Mosby, 1983, pp 162-169.
9. Chang KW, McAfee PC: Degenerative spondylolisthesis and degenerative scoliosis treated with a combination segmental rod-plate and transpedicular screw instrumentation system: A preliminary report. *J Spinal Disord* 1988;1:247-256.
10. Dall BE, Rowe DE: Degenerative spondylolisthesis: Its surgical management. *Spine* 1985;10:668-672.
11. Feffer HL, Wiesel SW, Cuckler JM, et al: Degenerative spondylolisthesis: To fuse or not to fuse. *Spine* 1985;10:287-289.
12. Fitzgerald JAW, Newman PH: Degenerative spondylolisthesis. *J Bone Joint Surg* 1976;58B:184-192.
13. Herkowitz HN, Kurz LT: Degenerative lumbar spondylolisthesis with spinal stenosis: A prospective study comparing decompression with decompression and intertransverse process arthrodesis. *J Bone Joint Surg* 1991;73A:802-808.
14. Herron LD, Trippi AC: L4-5 degenerative spondylolisthesis: The results of treatment by decompressive laminectomy without fusion. *Spine* 1989;14:534-538.
15. Lombardi JS, Wiltse LL, Reynolds J, et al: Treatment of degenerative spondylolisthesis. *Spine* 1985;10:821-827.
16. Postacchini F, Cinotti G: Bone regrowth after surgical decompression for lumbar spinal stenosis. *J Bone Joint Surg* 1992;74B:862-869.
17. Satomi K, Hirabayashi K, Toyama Y, et al: A clinical study of degenerative spondylolisthesis: Radiographic analysis and choice of treatment. *Spine* 1992;17:1329-1336.
18. Caputy AJ, Luessenhop AJ: Long-term evaluation of decompressive surgery for degenerative lumbar stenosis. *J Neurosurg* 1992;77:669-676.
19. Kostuik JP, Errico TJ, Gleason TF: Luque instrumentation in degenerative conditions of the lumbar spine. *Spine* 1990;15:318-321.
20. Nasca RJ: Rationale for spinal fusion in lumbar spinal steno-

sis. *Spine* 1989;14:451-454.

21. Marchesi DG, Aebi M: Pedicle fixation devices in the treatment of adult lumbar scoliosis. *Spine* 1992;17(8 Suppl):S304-S309.

22. Simmons ED Jr, Simmons EH: Spinal stenosis with scoliosis. *Spine* 1992;17(6 Suppl):S117-S120.

23. Abumi K, Panjabi MM, Kramer KM, et al: Biomechanical evaluation of lumbar spinal stability after graded facetectomies. *Spine* 1990;15:1142-1147.

24. Grobler LJ, Robertson PA, Novotony JE, et al: Etiology of spondylolisthesis: Assessment of the role played by lumbar facet joint morphology. *Spine* 1993;18:80-91.

25. Hopp E, Tsou PM: Postdecompression lumbar instability. *Clin Orthop* 1988;227:143-151.

26. Johnsson KE, Willner S, Johnsson K: Postoperative instability after decompression for lumbar spinal stenosis. *Spine* 1986;11:107-110.

27. Lee CK: Lumbar spinal instability (olisthesis) after extensive posterior spinal decompression. *Spine* 1983;8:429-433.

28. Ruge D, Wiltse L: Postoperative spondylolisthesis in lumbar spondylosis, in *Spinal Disorders: Diagnosis and Treatment.* Philadelphia, PA, Lea & Febiger, 1977, pp 184-194.

29. Zindrick MR, Wiltse LL, Widell EH, et al: A biomechanical study of intrapeduncular screw fixation in the lumbosacral spine. *Clin Orthop* 1986;203:99-112.

30. Carlson GD, Abitbol JJ, Anderson DR, et al: Screw fixation in the human sacrum: An in vitro study of the biomechanics of fixation. *Spine* 1992;17(6 Suppl):S196-S203.

31. Weinstein JN, Spratt KF, Spengler D, et al: Spinal pedicle fixation: Reliability and validity of roentgenogram-based assessment and surgical factors on successful screw placement. *Spine* 1988;13:1012-1018.

32. Whitecloud TS, Skalley TC, Cook SD, et al: Roentgenographic measurement of pedicle screw penetration. *Clin Orthop* 1989;245:57-68.

33. Davne SH, Myers DL: Complications of lumbar spinal fusion with transpedicular instrumentation. *Spine* 1992;17(6 Suppl):S184-S189.

34. Boos N, Marchesi D, Aebi M: Survivorship analysis of pedicular fixation systems in the treatment of degenerative disorders of the lumbar spine: A comparison of Cotrel-Dubousset instrumentation and the AO internal fixator. *J Spinal Disord* 1992;5:403-409.

35. Jackson RK, Boston DA, Edge AJ: Lateral mass fusion: A prospective study of a consecutive series with long-term follow-up. *Spine* 1985;10:828-832.

Spinal Stenosis: History and Physical Examination

Srdjan Mirkovic, MD

Steven R. Garfin, MD

Introduction

With progressive neural compression spinal stenosis may become clinically significant, although the severity of symptoms does not necessarily correlate with the magnitude of compression seen on spinal imaging studies. An accurate diagnosis rests on a combination of clinical symptoms and signs. Imaging evidence of spinal stenosis, although it is essential in confirming the diagnosis, cannot be relied on exclusively, because of the high incidence of positive radiographic findings in asymptomatic patients.[1]

Types

Spinal stenosis can be classified into several categories (Outline 1). Congenital or developmental stenosis[2,3] may be seen in individuals of normal stature with congenitally short pedicles, or in patients, such as achondroplastic dwarfs, who have epiphyseal disorders.[4] In these individuals, short pedicles decrease the anteroposterior diameter of the characteristically trefoil canal, thus largely contributing to central stenosis. Patients in this category first experience symptoms in their 30s and 40s,[5] an age when early degenerative changes lead to subsequent spinal canal narrowing and progressive neural compromise.

Acquired, most commonly degenerative, stenosis begins later, in the mid- to late-50s, or early 60s.[6-9] The average age of presentation of the female patient is 73; male patients tend to be younger. Earlier studies[6,10-12] noted a male predominance of three-to-one to 12-to-one; however, recent reports[13,14] suggest a female predominance, which more closely reflects that seen in our practice. In addition to central stenosis, lateral recess,[15] as well as foraminal stenosis, are common findings. Degenerative spondylolisthesis,[16-18] typically at L4-5, is often seen in association with degenerative stenosis, and is frequently a contributing factor in neurogenic claudication.[19]

Further narrowing of the spinal canal may also be a consequence of a traumatic event or a metabolic process affecting the spine,[20-25] while iatrogenic stenosis can occur following spinal surgery.

History

Because spinal stenosis most commonly occurs as a sequela of degenerative changes, it is not surprising that early symptoms are insidious in onset,[26] resembling those seen in lumbar spondylosis. Vague complaints of low back ache and stiffness, often aggravated by humid and cold weather and relieved with heat, as well as mechanical-type symptoms exacerbated with activity and relieved with rest, are typical. These indispositions can persist for a prolonged period of time, perhaps depending on cultural background, overall previous experience, and one's perception of pain. When they become worse, some patients seek an explanation from a doctor, often their primary care physician or other allied health professional. The majority, however, learn to accept their discomfort as an integral part of the aging process, along with the moderate limitations in activities of daily living that their symptoms may impose.

Orthopaedic consultation is generally sought when symptoms become increasingly frequent and severe, particularly when they interfere with such everyday activities as self-care, shopping, and walking (Table 1). By the time this stage is reached, symptoms become more consistent with neurogenic claudication as described by Van Gelderen[26] and Ehni,[27] characterized

---

Outline 1 Classification of spinal canal stenosis

I. CONGENITAL/DEVELOPMENTAL
   A. Idiopathic
   B. Achondroplastic
   C. Osteopetrosis

II. ACQUIRED
   A. Degenerative
      1. Central
      2. Lateral Recess and Foraminal
      3. Degenerative Spondylolisthesis
   B. Iatrogenic
      1. Post Laminectomy
      2. Post Fusion
      3. Post Discectomy
   C. Miscellaneous Disorders
      1. Acromegaly
      2. Paget's
      3. Fluorosis
      4. Ankylosing Spondylitis
   D. Traumatic

III. COMBINED
   Any Combination of Congenital, Developmental, or Acquired Stenosis

Table 1
Differential diagnosis of symptoms

Findings	Neurogenic Claudication	Vascular Claudication	Lumbar Spondylosis
Pain			
Type	Vague Cramping, Aches, Sharp, Burning in Legs	Tightness, Cramping (Usually in Calf)	Dull, Ache (In the Low Back)
Location	Back, Buttocks, Legs	Leg Muscles	Back
Radiation	Common Proximal to Distal	Localized in Legs	Localized Back
Exacerbation	Standing (Particularly with Trunk Extended) Walking - Less Bicycling - None, Unless Trunk Extended	Walking, Bicycling (Lower Extremity Activities)	General Activities, Bending, Standing, Twisting, Lifting
Improvement	Sitting, Flexing, Squatting	Standing, Cessation of Muscular Activity	Decreased Activity, Rest
Time to Relief	Slow	Quick	Slow
Walking Uphill	No Pain	Pain	± Pain
Walking Downhill	Pain (Lumbar Hyperextension)	Pain	± Pain
Back Pain	Common	Uncommon	Common
Limitation of Spinal Movement	Common	Uncommon	Common

by leg pain, achiness, numbness, and tingling, as well as cramping and weakness. In the first author's series, as in the series previously reported by Garfin and associates,[28] 85% of patients experienced a dull aching pain, paresthesias was noted in 57%, and 47% complained of subjective lower extremity weaknesses. Only 15% experienced a cramping sensation. Onset of symptoms tends to be proximal in the low back and buttocks,[29,30] with subsequent propagation distally to the knees, often in a not characteristically dermatomal pattern. Though asymmetrical involvement of the lower extremities is common, generally both extremities are involved.[10,29,31,32]

Unilateral involvement in a dermatomal distribution, typical of a radiculopathy,[33] is more often seen with severe foraminal and lateral recess stenosis. A sudden onset of sciatica, or worsening of previous symptoms, must alert the physician to the possibility of a concomitant disc herniation, in addition to a preexisting spinal stenosis.[1]

The sine qua non of spinal stenosis is exacerbation of symptoms with extension, and improvement with flexion,[26] because the capacity of the spinal canal varies with posture.[11,26] Patients experience limitations with simple activities of daily living, such as prolonged standing, often more so than walking up an incline, repetitive overhead reaching, and sleeping in the prone position. It is important to realize that the constellation of symptoms, and the subsequent limitations in activities of daily living, compromise the basic requirements for independent living. In the elderly patient, whose overall function may already be jeopardized, these limitations, aside from the symptoms, often cause concern and anxiety. Patients should be reassured that the possibility of a progressive and permanent disability, particularly a paralytic condition, is highly unlikely.

Lumbar flexion with the patient sitting, in contrast to standing and/or extending, alleviates symptoms in 80% of cases, and more than 75% note improvement with forward bending. Although patients have difficulty explaining their symptoms, relief often occurs with squatting or leaning on a shopping cart, bench, lawn mower, or against a wall. The majority of patients (92%) relay a history of progressively decreased walking distance over a period of months. The flexed posture may allow patients to bicycle without difficulty, although walking may be limited to a few blocks (Table 2).[26] The stooped, so-called simian, posture may be easily observed in the elderly individual with spinal stenosis who presents for evaluation.

Neurogenic claudication should be distinguished from vascular claudication[26,34,35] secondary to vascular insufficiency. In patients with vascular insufficiency, walking distance before the onset of symptoms tends to be relatively constant, and cramping occurs in a distal to proximal direction. Commonly, patients experience fairly prompt resolution of symptoms if they continue to stand, which is associated with decreased muscular activity. In contradistinction, pain in patients

Table 2
Differential diagnosis of signs

Findings	Neurogenic Claudication	Vascular Claudication	Lumbar Spondylosis
Neurologic Examination	Occasional Findings, Usually Asymmetric	Rare Findings, Symmetric if Present	No Findings Negative
Straight Leg Raise	Negative, Rarely Positive	Negative	Negative
Femoral Stretch Test	Negative, Rarely Positive	Negative	Negative
Pulses	Present, or Symmetrically Diminished	Diminished or Absent, Often Asymmetric	Symmetric
Skin	Normal	Hair Loss	Normal
Bicycle Test	Negative/Positive with Lumbar Hyperextension	Positive	Negative

with neurogenic claudication resolves more gradually, and does not improve with standing. They must often sit or bend forward in order to obtain relief of their symptoms.

Patients with vascular claudication rarely complain of regular low back pain or have significant limitations in their lumbar range of motion, though it may occur concomitantly with neurogenic claudication in this aged population. Because vascular claudication relates to increased muscular exertion and is independent of truncal position, patients are unable to ride a bicycle for prolonged periods of time.[36]

Peripheral neuropathy[37,38] must also be differentiated from neurogenic claudication secondary to spinal stenosis. Clinically, peripheral neuropathy manifests itself as a bilaterally symmetrical areflexia, with sensory neuropathy and little or late-developing motor loss. A distal "glove and stocking" distribution is characteristic, with an irregular upper border of sensory loss. Both ankle jerks are frequently absent, and vibratory sensation is commonly diminished. Symptoms may consist of burning feet, paresthesias, and pain, typically at night and unrelated to activity. A history of diabetes, drug use, exposure to toxins, and alcoholism should be sought. The possibility of an occult malignancy or compromised renal function should also be investigated. If the diagnosis is in doubt, electromyographic and nerve conduction studies should be performed.[39]

Physical Examination

Neurologic examination is often normal unless spinal stenosis has been present for an extended period of time and is well advanced. Although many patients complain of leg weakness, a specific motor deficit is rarely noted on manual examination or hand-held dynamometer testing, especially if performed after the patient has rested for a period of time.

Deconditioning, as well as activity restrictions secondary to pain, may be an explanation for the perceived weakness. However, in cases of severe stenosis, and particularly with degenerative spondylolisthesis, motor dysfunction is a more frequent finding. Generally, patients have little difficulty with toe and heel walking, or with repetitive unilateral toe raises. The majority of elderly patients have difficulty squatting, secondary to degenerative changes in the hips and knees, which, in addition to disuse weakness, makes this a poor test for motor strength. Weakness of the extensor hallucis longus muscle (L-5 nerve root) is the most frequently noted motor deficit, characteristically seen in the presence of degenerative changes, such as spondylolisthesis, at L4-5. At times, a paramedian disk herniation at L4-5, associated with central or lateral recess stenosis, may also lead to an acute L-5 motor deficit. Although paresthetic discomfort is a common complaint, loss of pin prick and light touch sensation is unusual. Sensory changes, if present, should raise suspicion of a coexistent peripheral neuropathy. Commonly, reflexes tend to be symmetrically decreased in the elderly. Asymmetric reflexes suggest stenosis, as opposed to degenerative age-related alterations. We have found the post ambulation stress neurologic reexamination to be helpful in demonstrating objective findings, such as a change in reflexes or motor examination compared to the resting state. We routinely retest patients after brisk walking in the office hallway, once their symptoms have been reproduced.

The straight leg raise test (Table 2) is characteristically negative, despite complaints of radicular-type pain distribution; this can be explained on the basis of slow circumferential root entrapment restricting nerve root motion, unlike that seen with a herniated nucleus pulposus, which leads to a sudden asymmetric compression. Similarly, the crossover straight leg raise test tends to be negative. Unless a concurrent disc herniation is present at the upper lumbar levels, the femoral stretch test is most often negative.

Long tract involvement secondary to cervical or thoracic spinal canal stenosis should be sought by assessing for upgoing toes (Babinski response), hyperreflexia, and clonus. The presence of these signs should make one wary of coexistent cervical and lumbar stenosis. With spinal stenosis of long duration, thigh and calf atrophy may be noted, particularly if lateral recess or foraminal stenosis predominates.[10] Commonly, the only positive neurologic finding may be diminished vibratory sensation.

Signs associated with vascular claudication, such as diminished or absent distal pulses and absence of skin hair, should also be recorded. Similarly, a brief abdominal examination with the legs flexed, to rule out a pulsatile abdominal mass associated with an abdominal aortic aneurysm, should be performed.

Examination of the back, more often than not, reveals a loss of lumbar lordosis with no tenderness to palpation or percussion, and no evidence of trigger points. Range of motion is generally good in flexion with notable limitation in extension,[32] which correlates with the history. A positive extension test, with reproduction of the patient's symptoms, can often be elicited by asking patients to lie prone and hyperextend their backs by pushing their upper body off the examining table with their arms. Frequently patients obtain prompt symptomatic relief by sitting in a forward stooped position on the examining table after the extension test. The complete examination should also entail evaluation of both hips to rule out degenerative joint disease, as well as palpation of the greater trochanters for greater trochanteric bursitis, to assure that a minor, easily treatable condition is not missed.

Pain drawings[40] have become a useful adjunct in the evaluation of low back pain; therefore, one should be familiar with the typical pain drawing in patients with spinal stenosis (Fig. 1). Because there are a wide spectrum of symptoms in patients with lumbar spinal stenosis, a graphic representation may vary and may not be characteristic or "classic" (Fig. 2). The pain diagram may be misclassified as lumbar spondylosis, a benign condition (Fig. 3).

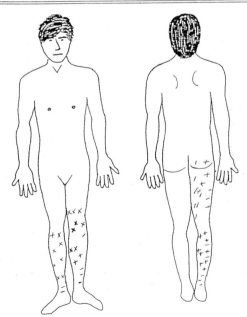

Fig. 1 Typical spinal stenosis.

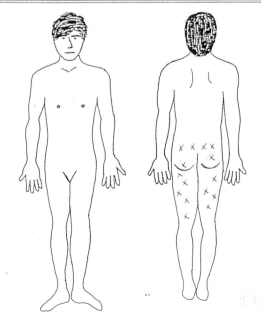

Fig. 2 Atypical spinal stenosis.

MARK ALL AFFECTED AREAS WITH APPROPRIATE SYMBOLS

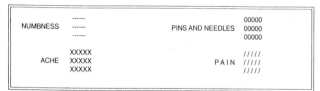

NUMBNESS	------ ------ ------	PINS AND NEEDLES	00000 00000 00000
ACHE	XXXXX XXXXX XXXXX	PAIN	///// ///// /////

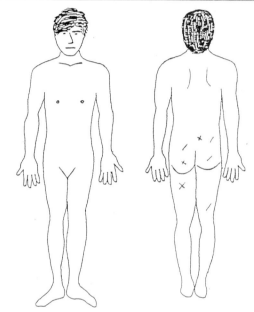

Fig. 3 Spondylosis.

Conclusion

Careful history taking is paramount because, due to overall vague symptoms and a paucity of findings on physical examination, an accurate diagnosis can be difficult. Imaging studies may be extremely helpful in making a diagnosis, but their evaluation must be correlated with the history and physical examination. Attempts have been made to quantify the magnitude of spinal stenosis,[41] but correlation with the severity of clinical symptoms is rarely accurate. Often, differentiating lumbar spondylosis from a surgically treatable spinal stenosis may be more arduous than the differentiation from vascular claudication or peripheral neuropathy (Table 2). In such cases, a period of nonoperative care is perhaps the best diagnostic tool.

We have found that patients gain a significantly better understanding of the etiology of their symptoms if compression of the neural structures, seen with extension of the lumbar spine, is demonstrated on a spine model and correlated with the radiographic findings.

References

1. Wiesel SW, Tsourmas N, Feffer HL, et al: 1984 Volvo Award in Clinical Sciences: A study of computer-assisted tomography: I. The incidence of positive CAT scans in an asymptomatic group of patients. *Spine* 1984;9:549-551.
2. Postacchini F: *Lumbar Spinal Stenosis.* Wien, Springer-Verlag, 1989, chap 3, chap 4, pp 49-74.
3. Verbiest H: A radicular syndrome from developmental narrowing of the lumbar vertebral canal. *J Bone Joint Surg* 1954;36B:230-237.
4. Bethem D, Winter RB, Lutter L, et al: Spinal disorders of dwarfism: Review of the literature and report of eighty cases. *J Bone Joint Surg* 1981;63A:1412-1425.
5. Surin V, Hedelin E, Smith L: Degenerative lumbar spinal stenosis: Results of operative treatment. *Acta Orthop Scand* 1982;53:79-85.
6. Jones RAC, Thomson JLG: The narrow lumbar canal: A clinical and radiological review. *J Bone Joint Surg* 1968;50B:595-605.
7. Kirkaldy-Willis WH, Paine KWE, Cauchoix J, et al: Lumbar spinal stenosis. *Clin Orthop* 1974;99:30-50.
8. Moreland LW, Lopez-Mendez A, Alarcon GS: Spinal stenosis: A comprehensive review of the literature. *Semin Arthritis Rheum* 1989;19:127-149.
9. Epstein JA, Epstein BS, Lavine LS, et al: Degenerative lumbar spondylolisthesis with an intact neural arch (pseudospondylolisthesis). *J Neurosurg* 1976;44:139-147.
10. Hall S, Bartleson JD, Onofrio BM, et al: Lumbar spinal stenosis: Clinical features, diagnostic procedures, and results of surgical treatment in 68 patients. *Ann Intern Med* 1985;103:271-275.
11. Schonstrom NSR, Bolender NF, Spengler DM: The pathomorphology of spinal stenosis as seen on CT scans of the lumbar spine. *Spine* 1985;10:806-811.
12. Roberson GH, Llewellyn HJ, Taveras JM: The narrow lumbar spinal canal syndrome. *Radiology* 1973;107:89-97.
13. Lipson S: Clinical diagnosis of spinal stenosis. *Semin Spine Surg* 1989;1:143-144.
14. Iida H, Shikata J, Yamamuro T, et al: A pedigree of cervical stenosis, brachydactyly, syndactyly, and hyperopia. *Clin Orthop* 1989;247:80-86.
15. Ciric I, Mikhael MA, Tarkington JA, et al: The lateral recess syndrome: A variant of spinal stenosis. *J Neurosurg* 1980;53:433-443.
16. Macnab I: Spondylolisthesis with an intact neural arch: The so-called pseudo-spondylolisthesis. *J Bone Joint Surg* 1950;32B:325-333.
17. Newman PH: Stenosis of the lumbar spine in spondylolisthesis. *Clin Orthop* 1976;115:116-121.
18. Getty CJM: Lumbar spinal stenosis: The clinical spectrum and the results of operation. *J Bone Joint Surg* 1980;62B:481-485.
19. Mirkovic S, Garfin SR, Rydevik B, et al: Pathophysiology of spinal stenosis, in Eilert RE (ed): *Instructional Course Lectures XLI.* Park Ridge, IL, American Academy of Orthopaedic Surgeons, 1992, pp 165-177.
20. Weisz GM: Lumbar spinal canal stenosis in Paget's disease. *Spine* 1983;8:192-198.
21. Weisz GM: Stenosis of the lumbar spinal canal in Forestier's disease. *Int Orthop* 1983;7:61-64.
22. Weisz GM: Lumbar spinal canal stenosis in osteopoikilosis. *Clin Orthop* 1982;166:89-92.
23. Epstein N, Whelan M, Benjamin V: Acromegaly and spinal stenosis: Case report. *J Neurosurg* 1982;56:145-147.
24. Yoshikawa S, Shiba M, Suzuki A: Spinal-cord compression in untreated adult cases of vitamin-D resistant rickets. *J Bone Joint Surg* 1968;50A:743-752.

25. Singh A, Dass R, Hayreh SS, et al: Skeletal changes in endemic fluorosis. *J Bone Joint Surg* 1962;44B:806-815.

26. Van Gelderen CH: Ein Orthotisches (Lordotisches) Kauda-syndrome. *Acta Psychiatr Neurol* 1948;23:57-68.

27. Ehni G: Spondylotic cauda equina radiculopathy. *Tex J Med* 1965;61:746-752.

28. Garfin SR, Glover M, Booth RE, et al: Laminectomy: A review of the Pennsylvania hospital experience. *J Spinal Disord* 1988;1:116-133.

29. Schatzker J, Pennal GF: Spinal stenosis: A cause of cauda equina compression. *J Bone Joint Surg* 1968;50B:606-618.

30. Wilson CB: Significance of the small lumbar spinal canal: Cauda equina compression syndromes due to spondylosis: Part III. Intermittent claudication. *J Neurosurg* 1969;31:499-506.

31. Grabias S: Current concepts review: The treatment of spinal stenosis. *J Bone Joint Surg* 1980;62A:308-313.

32. Spengler DM: Degenerative stenosis of the lumbar spine. *J Bone Joint Surg* 1987;69A:305-308.

33. Joffe R, Appleby A, Arjona V: "Intermittent ischaemia" of the cauda equina due to stenosis of the lumbar canal. *J Neurol Neurosurg Psychiatr* 1966;29:315-318.

34. Hawkes CH, Roberts GM: Neurogenic and vascular claudication. *J Neurol Sci* 1978;38:337-345.

35. Dodge LD, Bohlman HH, Rhodes RS: Concurrent lumbar spinal stenosis and peripheral vascular disease: A report of nine patients. *Clin Orthop* 1988;230:141-148.

36. Dyck P, Doyle JB Jr: "Bicycle test" of Van Gelderen in diagnosis of intermittent cauda equina compression syndrome: Case report. *J Neurosurg* 1977;46:667-670.

37. Thomas PK: Clinical features and differential diagnosis, in Dyck PJ, Thomas PK, Lambert EH, et al (eds): *Peripheral Neuropathy*, ed 2. Philadelphia, PA, WB Saunders, 1984, vol 2, chap 51, pp 1169-1190.

38. Brown MT: Neuropathy. *Semin Neurol* 1987;7:1.

39. Jacobson RE: Lumbar stenosis: An electromyographic evaluation. *Clin Orthop* 1976;115:68-71.

40. Mann NH III, Brown MD, Enger I: Expert performance in low-back disorder recognition using patient pain drawings. *J Spinal Disord* 1992;5:254-259.

41. Ullrich CG, Binet EF, Sanecki MG, et al: Quantitative assessment of the lumbar spinal canal by computed tomography. *Radiology* 1980;134:137-143.

The Surgery of Spinal Stenosis

Robert E. Booth, Jr, MD

Jeffrey Spivak, MD

Introduction

When performed adroitly and for the proper indications, the surgery of spinal stenosis should yield the same excellent results as simple disk excisions, even though the symptoms may be of greater longevity and the patients of significantly greater age. Unlike disk surgery, however, the surgery of spinal stenosis presents some unique conceptual and technical challenges. An organized and anatomic approach is mandatory, because the penalty for an incomplete or unsuccessful procedure is greater in the spine than in other surgical arenas. A decompressive laminectomy that is unsuccessful—often the result of poor hemostasis, loss of intraoperative orientation, incomplete understanding of the surgical pathology, or inadequate decompression and stabilization—creates a "failed back" and a pain problem for which there is frequently no solution.

Procedure

Preparation

Little controversy remains about patient positioning. The kneeling posture on a laminectomy frame produces a dependent abdomen and minimizes both operative hemorrhage and the change of epidural hematoma. Elastic stockings to support venous pressure in the lower extremities, spinal anesthesia to provide a pharmacologic phlebotomy, and ocular magnification for the surgeon are operative mechanics with which almost every surgeon would agree. The greatest disincentive to the kneeling position is the obligatory hyperextension of the spinal column, making laminotomy and facet joint decompression technically more difficult (Fig. 1). Conversely, the position of spinal hyperextension reproduces the appendicular and axial compression of the neural elements. Thus if a spine is effectively decompressed in this hyperextended posture, complete relief of pain when the patient is erect and active should be expected.

Localization of the appropriate level for spinal incision begins with examination of the anteroposterior radiograph. Spinal abnormalities such as transitional vertebrae, bifid spinous processes, asymmetric transverse processes, and other structural abnormalities are excellent clues to identify a specific spinal level. Palpation of the bony spine can be accomplished in even the most obese patient. Not only does the surgeon palpate for the presence of the spinous processes at the level of the lumbosacral junction, but also for the level of the iliac crest relative to the bony spine, as it is the most common landmark. It is important to remember to discount the supplemental thickness of skin, fat, and muscle, which will falsely elevate the apparent level of the iliac crest. Once the dissection is carried below the skin and fat, one can usually identify the almost constant anatomic decussation of the fascial fibers of the lumbodorsal fascia at the L5-S1 innerspace, which provides an anatomic clue to the site of the lumbosacral junction.

Exposure of the sacrum itself at the bottom of the skin incision provides further certainty of the L5-S1 level. Palpation of the termination of the interlaminar spaces, the hollow sound created by scraping of the sacral periosteum, the palpation of the alar prominences laterally, and the demonstration of motion by grasping the spinous processes with towel clips all provide further confirmation of the lumbosacral junction.

An additional advantage of the kneeling position is the facility in obtaining a lateral lumbosacral intraoperative radiograph, using pins or clips to confirm the appropriate spinal level. The penalty for exposing an incorrect level is so high that one should have a very low threshold for obtaining this radiograph. It should be remembered that when an incorrect spinal level has

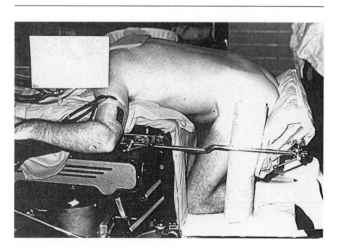

Fig. 1 Kneeling position on a laminectomy frame.

been decompressed, the general error is to be too high in the spine, rarely too low. Thus, the subsequent exploration for the correct level should proceed distally rather than proximally, after further attempts to identify the lumbosacral junction and obtain proper orientation.

Incision and Dissection

The initial skin incision is made in the midline, directly over the spinous processes, which are palpable just beneath the skin. Dissection is carried down through the subcutaneous fat to the lumbodorsal fascia, which is a very thick structure seen clearly in the anatomic specimen in Figure 2. The lumbodorsal fascia forms a thick envelope that encompasses the erector spiny muscle and coalesces with the psoas fascia anterior and the periosteum of the lamina and spinous process medially. It is crucial to preserve this envelope of fascia and periosteum by performing a subperiosteal dissection of the bony elements of the spine. This avoids violation of the intramuscular vessels, allows for tamponade of the paraspinous veins by postsurgical muscle swelling, and prevents the surgical field from becoming obscured with blood. Hemostasis is crucial at every level of the dissection in order to prevent the welling of blood in the depth of the wound from concealing critical anatomic structures. Skin and fascial vessels must be meticulously coagulated before deeper levels of dissection may be begun.

When the subperiosteal dissection of the spinous processes and lamina is begun, it is performed in a distal to proximal direction. This is because the paraspinous musculature has an oblique insertion onto the bony elements of the spine. Instruments passed from caudad to cephalad will stay in the subperiosteal plane, avoiding further muscle hemorrhage. Instruments such as an electrocautery or periosteal elevator should be angled away from the midline to account for the bulbous enlargement of the tip of the spinous process, which is part of the pathophysiology of spondyloarthrosis.

Once the subperiosteal dissection has been carried laterally to the margin of the facet joints, self-retaining retractors should be placed to enlarge the operative field and to compress the intramuscular vasculature and reduce hemorrhage. Some additional bleeding may now be encountered from the small facetal arteries, which course around the medial aspect of each facet joint and provide the primary source of intraoperative bleeding outside of the spinal canal itself (Fig. 3). These arteries can be safely controlled with electrocautery because the neural elements are still protected by the bone above them. Meticulous hemostasis should again be achieved.

At this juncture, many surgeons prefer to remove the spinous processes with a large bone biter, occasionally exposing venous lakes within the soft bone of the elderly patient. Even though these bony structures may subsequently be removed, the use of bone wax to preclude hemorrhage will keep the wound dry during the impending laminectomy.

With the spine now dry and exposed, the surgeon should review the surgical anatomy and planned dissection before opening the spinal canal itself. In particular, one must identify and articulate the location of

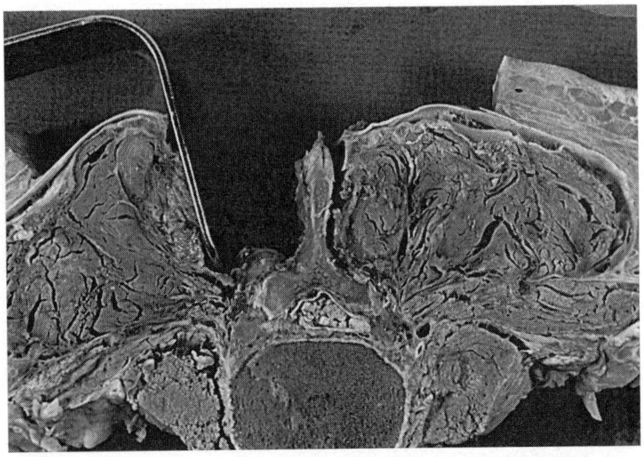

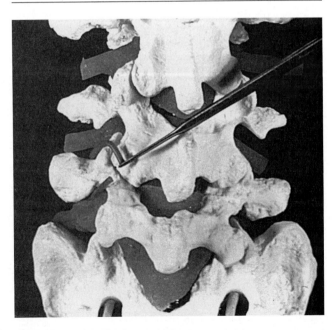

Fig. 2   Anatomic specimen showing the lumbodorsal fascia and paravertebral muscles.

Fig. 3   Most intraoperative bleeding outside the spinal canal comes from the small facetal arteries.

the pedicles, which are the key to any subsequent anatomic dissection (Fig. 4). It is around the pedicles that the neural elements will be found, by which the nerve roots will be numbered, and which will remain even after the rest of the dorsal spinal elements have been excised and the spinal canal is completely open. It is surprisingly easy to become disoriented when the usual posterior bony landmarks have been excised and the spinal canal is completely open.

Decompression

Preoperative planning will identify the specific nerve roots to be decompressed. Although the spinal stenosis syndrome encompasses a wide variety of anatomic variations, each individual nerve root is generally at risk in two areas—in the lateral recess and in the neural foramen. It is very helpful to articulate to oneself the location of these areas before proceeding with further dissection (Fig. 5).

Even the most effective subperiosteal dissection will leave some short muscle fibers attached to the laminae and ligamentum flavum, and these can be excised with a large curette. This is done with a gentle scraping motion, preferably moving from the lateral area of the facet joint towards the midline of the spinous process, so that the final excursion of the instrument does not violate the parafacetal arteries or paraspinous muscle envelope.

When the ligamentum flavum has been cleanly exposed, a small curette may then be gently used to dissect the insertion of the ligament from the undersurface of the superior vertebra. Curettes are quite

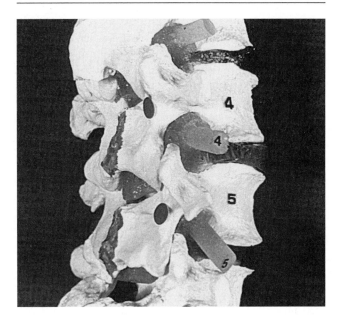

Fig. 5 Model showing nerve roots and relationship to neuroforamen and posterior aspect of pedicle (circles).

effective at this task, and they enjoy the additional safety of presenting a blunt ball to the delicate neural elements beneath. This step, and all subsequent steps to remove the laminae, should be initiated in the midline and then proceed laterally. This is because even in the most narrow spinal canal, the midline is the last area to become stenotic and the safest area in which to begin a dissection.

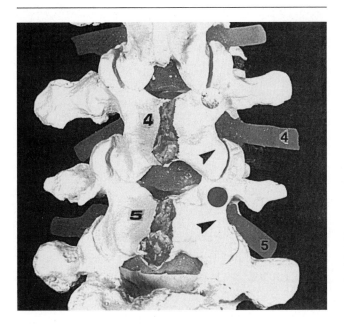

Fig. 4 The vertebral pedicles are the key to subsequent dissection.

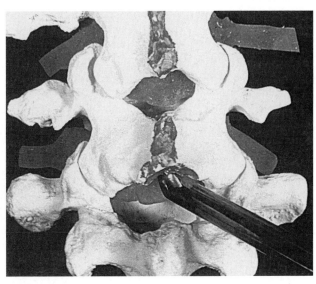

Fig. 6 Dissection of laminar bone using a Kerrison punch.

When the inferior edge of the lamina has been exposed, a rongeur or Schlesinger punch is used to begin dissecting the bone of the lamina itself (Fig. 6). Again, this step should be initiated in the midline and then carried smoothly to the lateral sides of the spinal canal. The round bowl of the Schlesinger punch protects the neural elements, particularly if pressure is directed dorsally.

The dura in patients with severe spinal stenosis may be quite thin, and the typical dorsal fat may be absent. In inflammatory spondylopathies, such as ankylosing spondylitis, the dura may even be adherent to the anterior surface of the lamina, and extreme care must be taken in the dissection. As the laminar dissection proceeds cephalad, curettes or Frazier palpator scan be used to ensure that the path ahead is free of adhesions. The ligamentum flavum of succeeding interspaces can then be dissected using the same technique.

The result of this midline dissection will be a central trough extending proximally and distally over the appropriate levels to be decompressed. This central gutter may then be extended laterally to the medial edge of the facet joints. The dura will be readily visible, and any bleeding encountered at this point from the epidural vessels should be controlled with bipolar electrocautery, topical coagulants, or sponges. The surgical field again should be completely dried before attempting any further examination of the neural elements.

Patients with a pure central spinal stenosis make up a very small proportion of those seen in daily practice. In these patients, this dissection alone will alleviate neurologic symptoms. These patients are typically young and possess a congenitally narrow spinal canal, usually by virtue of short pedicles.

In the vast majority of patients, however, the area of stenosis is in the lateral recess or foramen, and further dissection will be necessary. It is mandatory that every nerve root at jeopardy be examined in the lateral recess and its neural foramen. An appreciation for stenosis in these areas is first gained by placing a probe along the path of the nerve root in question (Fig. 7). This maneuver, as well as the insertion of all subsequent dissecting instruments, should be performed from proximal to distal with the instrument parallel to the nerve root. This minimizes the chance of damaging the neural fascicles. The most common offending element will be the overgrown superior facet, and this can be readily palpated and removed using an obliquely oriented Schlesinger punch (Fig. 8). Undercutting the overgrown and hypertrophic superior facet will decompress the lateral recess but will not destabilize the facet joint itself. This maneuver can be performed throughout the length of the exposed spinal levels, providing a complete release of the lateral recess. This dissection alone will eliminate the symptoms of spinal stenosis in the vast majority of surgical patients.

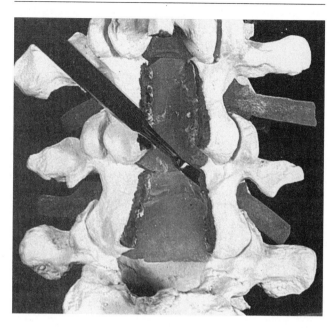

Fig. 7 A dequate root decompression is determined by probing along the path of the nerve root.

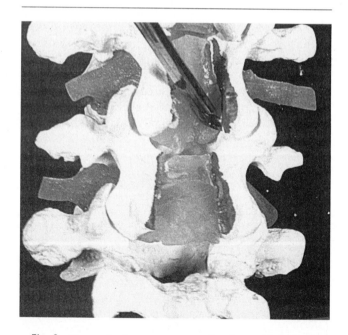

Fig. 8 Removal of overgrown superior facet with a Kerrison punch.

At this juncture it is appropriate to consider the adequacy of spinal decompression. Lamentably, this is an area where the surgeon can rely only on judgment, experience, and the "feel" of a decompressed nerve root. Although the importance of preoperative planning must never be underestimated, in the operating theater it is necessary to avoid clinging to preconceived and presurgical notions of where the pathology may lie. Instead, one must rely on one's tactile and visual senses at the time of surgery to be sure that each nerve root is free from compression in the central canal, the lateral recess, the neural foramen, and, if necessary, beyond. There is no test or objective criterion by which to quantify this situation, and the surgeon must constantly bear in mind the occasionally delicate balance between complete neural freedom and spinal stability. Nonetheless, no surgical dissection for spinal stenosis should be terminated until the nerve roots at jeopardy are no longer under pressure. Once the central spinal canal and the lateral recess have already been decompressed, the handling of the foraminal and extraforaminal sources of nerve compression is crucial in the successful treatment of spinal stenosis.

Common Problems

Although any of a wide variety of anatomic variants can cause foraminal or extraforaminal stenosis, there are four common problems that should always be considered when a nerve root, decompressed to the extent of its lateral recess, fails to move appropriately under direct palpation. The first of these patterns involves the entrapment of the spinal nerve between the superior facet of one vertebra and the posterolateral aspect of the vertebral body of the suprajacent vertebra (Fig. 9). To resolve this problem, the surgeon need only undermine further the superior facet or perhaps excise the facet joint itself.

A related problem is seen when the nerve root is caught between the superior facet of one vertebra and the descending pedicle of the vertebra above (Fig. 10). Again, the nerve can be freed by excising the tip of the

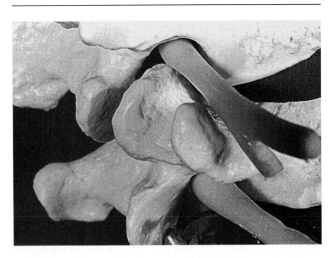

Fig. 10 Nerve entrapped between the superior facet of one vertebra and the descending pedicle of the vertebra above.

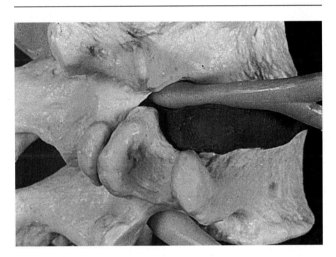

Fig. 11 Nerve entrapped between the bulging annulus of a degenerated disk and the vertebral body of the suprajacent vertebra.

superior facet or the entire facet joint if necessary. The third, and perhaps most common, of these lateral syndromes is seen when the nerve root is entrapped between the bulging annulus of the degenerated disk and the vertebral body of the suprajacent vertebra (Fig. 11). This is more of a soft-tissue problem than the two preceding stenosis patterns, and it is sometimes difficult to appreciate. It is usually the result of a subannular herniation or the severe degeneration and collapse of the intervertebral disk. This problem can be resolved in two ways. The easiest approach is to excise the lateral annulus, either with a pituitary rongeur or small knife. A small knife is preferable because it minimizes the fibrosis that may promote recurrence of the problem. A second approach is to take down the inferomedial aspect of the vertebral pedicle, either with a curette or an osteotome. Certainly, both of these techniques are

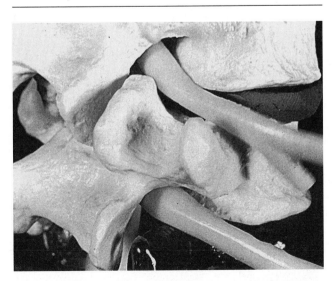

Fig. 9 Nerve entrapped between the superior facet of one vertebra and the posterolateral aspect of the vertebral body of the suprajacent vertebra.

quite delicate, and adequate protection of the neural elements must be provided.

The fourth pattern of neural decompression at the foraminal level occurs in degenerative spondylolisthesis (Fig. 12). It is most common at the L4-L5 level, producing symptoms when the L5 nerve root is caught between the vertebral body of L5 itself and the advancing inferior facet of L4, which has eroded through the superior facet of the subjacent vertebra. Although these degenerative spondylolistheses will produce a dramatic myelographic defect, often a complete block at L4 to L5, the vertebral body of L4 almost never advances more than one third of the width of the L5 vertebral body. At this point, the L4 inferior facets impinge on the body of L5 and halt the progressive spondylolisthesis. One is obliged to free the entrapped nerve root by sacrificing the offending part of the facet joint.

Instability

It is obvious from the discussion of these "lateral syndromes" that some compromise of the facet joints is often necessary to provide neural decompression. At some point, it is necessary to address the resultant spinal instability. Preoperatively, one can to some degree predict instability when 4 mm of translation, 10° of angulation, degenerative lateral listheses, or gross motion are seen on spinal radiographs. Less objective factors such as a low intercrestal line, disk space preservation, physiologic youth, high activity, or a significant proportion of low back pain may mitigate towards spinal stabilization. The simplest rule of thumb available to spinal surgeons is merely to retain the total of one facet joint at each spinal level. That is, a unilateral hemifascetectomy or even complete fascitectomy can be performed without significantly compromising the stability of the lumbar spine. A bilateral hemifacetectomy will likewise leave enough facet joint to prevent spondylolisthesis (Fig.13). Bilateral complete facetectomies however, render the spine unstable and must be treated with a lumbar fusion.

In order to avoid iatrogenic instability, alternative techniques of lumbar decompression are widely practiced. When specific isolated areas of neural entrapment have been clearly identified preoperatively, a localized dissection involving the medial pars interarticularis and adjoining lamina may be sufficient to expose the nerve root in question (Fig. 14). Partial dissection of this facet joint will only minimally compromise stability if the residual spinal structures remain intact.

In the technique of multiple subarticular fenestrations, a burr is used first to remove the medial third of the facet joint, often with the aid of an operative microscope. The burr is then turned obliquely to undercut the lateral two thirds of the facet joint overlying the ligamentum flavum removing the bony compression in the lateral recess (Fig. 15).

Another limited and focal technique uses a Wiltse muscle-splitting incision, exposure of the transverse processes, and careful removal of the intertransverse ligament to expose the most lateral margins of the neural foramen (Fig. 16). This approach does not allow any investigation of the spinal canal or lateral recess, and focal pathology beyond the neural foramen must clearly be the source of the patient's symptoms.

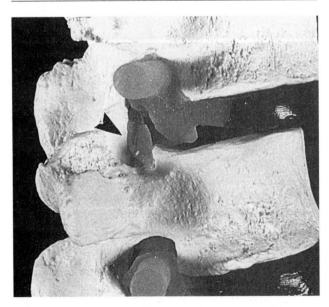

Fig. 12 L5 nerve root caught between the vertebral body of L5 and the inferior facet of L4.

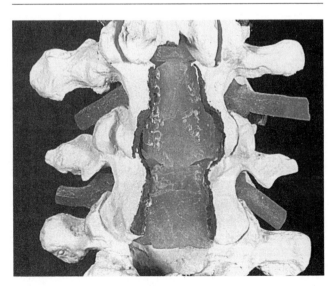

Fig. 13 Bilateral hemifacetectomies.

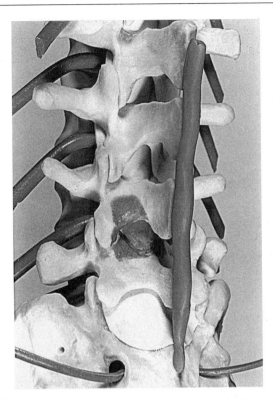

Fig. 14 Shaded area (center) denotes portion of medial pars interarticularis and adjoining lamina which should be removed.

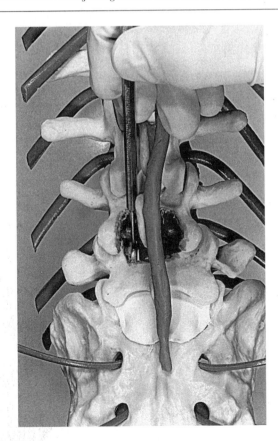

Fig. 15 Technique used to remove bony compression in the lateral recess.

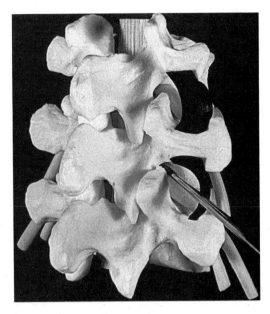

Fig. 16 Technique used to expose the lateral margin of the neural foramen using the Wiltse approach.

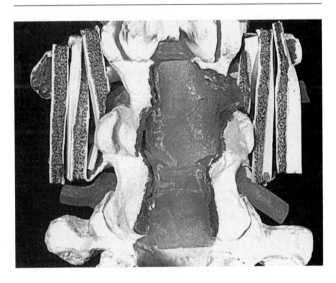

Fig. 17 Bilateral lateral fusion.

Bilateral lateral fusions remain the vogue for most forms of spinal instability, both perceived and predicted. Midline fusions are to be discouraged, lest overgrowth of the graft create a new central stenosis (Fig. 17).

Pedicle screw fixation techniques have gained significant popularity in recent years, enhancing the rates of lumbar fusion and expediting patient recuperation. Higher morbidity, increased infection rates, and greater technical complications have been the price for this advance. Most surgeons favor the "anteromedial approach" to pedicle screw fixation, in which the screw

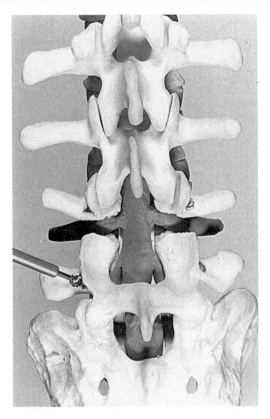

Fig. 18   Pedicle screw fixation via the "anteromedial approach".

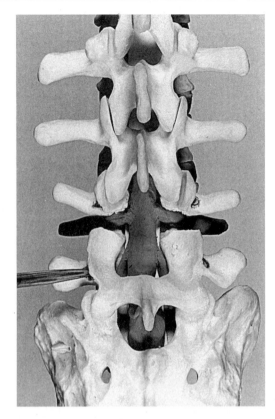

Fig. 20   Use of probe to palpate the pedicle.

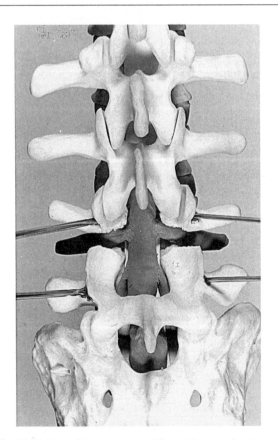

Fig. 19   Radiographic markers used in pedicle screw fixation.

entry point is at the intersection of a transverse line through the transverse processes and a vertical line through the center of the facet joints (Fig. 18). A burr applied to this point will expose the pedicle. Screws are directed medially and parallel to the superior vertebral endplate, preceded by radiographic markers. Steinmann pins on one side and drill bits on the other facilitate radiographic identification (Fig. 19). A gearshift pedicle probe, followed by a Penfield probe, ensures protection from the screws by the bony cortices of the pedicle walls (Fig. 20). Decortication of the lateral gutters and transverse processes should then be performed, before rod insertion is begun. Rods, crosslinking bars, and graft material can then be placed to secure the fusion (Fig. 21). It is important to avoid the creation of a kyphosis in the attempt to open the foramina or to reverse a degenerative scoliosis.

Conclusion

Although supplemental techniques such as autogenous fat grafting, electrical stimulation of fusions, and internal and external supports have been used, the real success of spinal stenosis surgery lies in the control of hemorrhage, the treatment of the appropriate

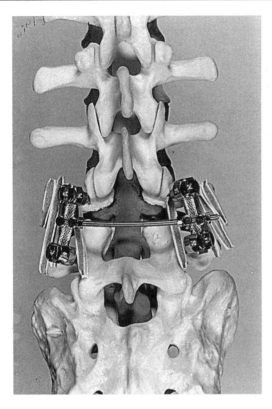

Fig. 21 Application of rods, crosslinking bars, and graft material.

spinal levels, and the adequacy of decompression and stabilization. If these techniques and principles are kept in mind, the high level of success achieved in simple disk surgery can be approximated and a happy result will ensure for both the surgeon and the patient.[1-31]

References

1. Aebi M, Etter C, Kehl T, et al: Stabilization of the lower thoracic and lumbar spine with the internal spinal skeletal fixation system: Indications, techniques, and first results of treatment. *Spine* 1987;12:544-551.
2. Booth RE: Spinal stenosis, in Anderson LD (ed): *American Academy of Orthopaedic Surgeons Instructional Course Lecture XXXV*. St. Louis, MO, CV Mosby, 1986, pp 420-435.
3. Burton CV: Successful surgical management of lateral spinal stenosis, in ES Stauffer (ed): *American Academy of Orthopaedic Surgeons Instructional Course Lecture XXXV*. St. Louis, MO, CV Mosby, 1985.
4. Caputy AJ, Luessenhop AJ: Long-term evaluation of decompressive surgery for degenerative lumbar stenosis. *J Neurosurg* 1992;77:669-676.
5. Deyo RA, Cherkin DC, Loeser JD, et al: Morbidity and mortality in association with operations on the lumbar spine. *J Bone Joint Surg* 1992;74A:536-543.
6. Garfin SR, Glover M, Booth RE, et al: Laminectomy: A review of the Pennsylvania Hospital experience. *J Spinal Disord* 1988;1:116-133.
7. Getty CJ, Johnson JR, Kirwan EO, et al: Partial undercutting fasciectomy for bony entrapment of the lumbar nerve root. *J Bone Joint Surg* 1981;63B:330-335.
8. Herron LD, Mangelsdorf C: Lumbar spinal stenosis: Results of surgical treatment. *J Spinal Disord* 1991;4:26-33.
9. Herkowitz HN, Kurz LT: Degenerative lumbar spondylolisthesis with spinal stenosis. *J Bone Joint Surg* 1991;73A:802-808.
10. Hopp E, Tsou PM: Postdecompression lumbar instability. *Clin Orthop* 1988;227:143-151.
11. Johnsson KE, Willner S, Johnsson K: Postoperative instability after decompression for lumbar spinal stenosis. *Spine* 1986;11:107-110.
12. Johnsson KE, Willner S, Pettersson H: Analysis of operated cases with lumbar spinal stenosis. *Acta Orthop Scand* 1981;52:427-433.
13. Johnsson KE, Wilner S, Petterson H: Analysis of instability after decompression for lumbar spine stenosis. *Spine* 1986;11:107-110.
14. Kabins MB, Weinstein JN: Pedicle screw fixation: Indications, techniques, and systems, in Andersson GBJ, McNeill TW (eds): *Lumbar Spinal Stenosis*. St. Louis, MO, CV Mosby, 1992, pp 349-371.
15. Katz JN, Lipson SJ, Larson MG, et al: The outcome of decompressive laminectomy for degenerative lumbar stenosis. *J Bone Joint Surg* 1991;73A:809-816.
16. Kirkaldy-Willis WH, McIvor GWD: Spinal stenosis. *Clin Orthop* 1976;115:2-144.
17. Kirkaldy-Willis WH, Wedge JH, Yong-Hing K, et al: Pathology and pathogenesis of lumbar spondylosis and stenosis. *Spine* 1978;3:319-328.
18. Kirkaldy-Willis WH: The relationship of structural pathology to the nerve root. *Spine* 1984;9:49-52.
19. Kirkaldy-Willis WH, Wedge JH, Yong-Hing K, et al: Lumbar spinal nerve lateral entrapment. *Clin Orthop* 1982;169:171-178.
20. Krag MH, Frederickson BE, Yuan HA: Spinal instrumentation, in Weinstein JN, Wiesel SW (eds): *The Lumbar Spine*. Philadelphia, PA, WB Saunders, 1990, pp 916-955.
21. Magerl FP: Stabilization of the lower thoracic and lumbar spine with external skeletal fixation. *Clin Orthop* 1984;189:125-141.
22. McNeill TW: Decompressive laminectomy, in Andersson GBJ, McNeill TW (eds): *Lumbar Spinal Stenosis*. St. Louis, MO, Mosby Year Book, 1992, pp 339-347.
23. Nixon JE: Surgical management, in Nixon JE (ed): *Spinal Stenosis*. London, Edward Arnold, 1991, pp 309-322.
24. Paine K: Results of decompression for lumbar spinal stenosis. *Clin Orthop* 1976;115:96-100.
25. Rothman RH, Simeone FA: *The Spine*, ed 2. Philadelphia, PA, WB Saunders, 1982, vol 1.
26. Roy-Camille R, Saillant G, Mazel C: Internal fixation of the lumbar spine with pedicle screw plating. *Clin Orthop* 1986;203:7-17.
27. Tarlov IM: The knee-chest tion for lower spinal operations. *J Bone Joint Surg* 1967;49A:1193-1194.
28. Verbiest H: A radicular syndrome from developmental narrowing of the lumbar vertebral canal. *J Bone Joint Surg* 1954;36B:230-237.
29. Verbiest H: Results of surgical treatment of idiopathic developmental stenosis of the lumbar vertebral canal: A review of twenty-seven years' experience. *J Bone Joint Surg* 1977;59B:181-188.
30. Wiltse LL, Hutchinson RH: Surgical treatment of spondylolisthesis. *Clin Orthop* 1964;35:116-135.
31. Young S, Veerapen R, O'Laoire SA: Relief of lumbar canal stenosis using multilevel subarticular fenestrations as an alternative to wide laminectomy: Preliminary report. *Neurosurgery* 1988;23:628-633.

Diagnostic Imaging

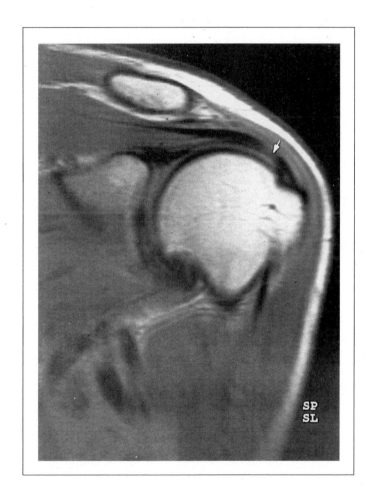

The Use of Scintigraphy to Detect Increased Osseous Metabolic Activity About the Knee

Scott F. Dye, MD

Mailine H. Chew, MD

Scintigraphy of human joints with techniques such as technetium imaging can provide a direct assessment of periarticular osseous physiology. Of the imaging modalities currently used to evaluate human joints, only scintigraphy requires a living, metabolically functioning organism. Radiography, computed tomography, magnetic resonance imaging (MRI), and ultrasound yield images that reflect primarily structural, rather than physiologic, characteristics. As orthopaedic surgeons, our perceptions of injury and disease have been profoundly influenced by the predominance of structural information provided by such anatomic imaging modalities. Our orthopaedic lexicon contains structurally oriented terminology (for example, fracture, ligament rupture, meniscal tear, and disc herniation) that has changed little during this century.[1-3] Even our conceptualization of degenerative osteoarthrosis is replete with structurally descriptive words. Osteophytes, osteosclerosis, subchondral cysts, osteopenia, and joint-space narrowing are characteristics easily seen on plain radiographs, and they reflect macrostructural change that has already occurred. This language does not describe the active pathophysiology of this disease.[4,5]

Over the past 12 years, many independent research efforts in the United States and Europe have concentrated on the use of technetium scintigraphy to assess normal and abnormal joints—primarily, the knee. These studies have indicated that a heretofore unrecognized and unappreciated process of increased bone remodeling and turnover is occurring about the joints of many patients. This osseous remodeling often occurs despite the demonstration of normal findings by current diagnostic methods, including radiography, computed tomography, and even MRI.[6] The purpose of this paper is to summarize these findings and to delineate the uses of radionuclide imaging in the assessment and treatment of periarticular symptoms of the knee. We will describe some factors that may initiate and sustain increased osseous metabolic activity, and we will discuss how scintigraphic findings have altered our concepts of musculoskeletal injury and the body's adaptation to injury.

Scintigraphy With Technetium-99m Methylene Diphosphonate

Historically, use of scintigraphic information about the knee and other joints has been limited. Aside from the occasional use for the patient with a tumor,[7] an infection,[8] osteonecrosis,[9] osteolysis,[10] metabolic[11] or metastatic bone disease,[12] or reflex sympathetic dystrophy,[13] the most accepted use for periarticular bone scintigraphy seems to be the delineation of sites of increased stress or degenerative changes, or both, in older patients who are being considered for arthroplasty[5] (Fig. 1). However, similar patterns of periarticular uptake have been demonstrated in knees with injuries previously thought to be confined to soft-tissue damage at a time before radiographically identifiable osseous changes have occurred. For example, a scintigraphic pattern of subchondral three-compartment uptake may be seen in a patient for whom radiographic findings were normal and in whom the only structural damage is an unstable bucket-handle tear of the lateral meniscus (Fig. 2).

The scintigraphic marker that is commonly used to show metabolic characteristics of periarticular bone is

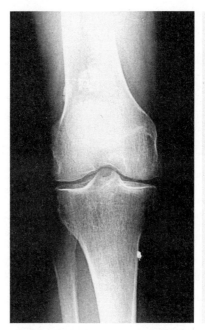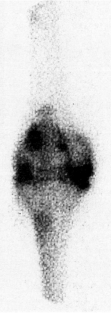

Fig. 1 A patient with osteoarthrosis of the right knee involving three compartments. **Left**, Radiograph revealing overt degenerative changes of the knee, including osteophytes and osteopenia. **Right**, Technetium scintiscan showing increased uptake in all three compartments.

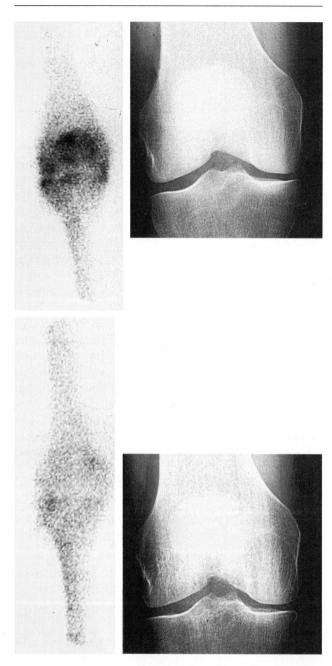

Fig. 2 A patient in whom a large bucket-handle tear of the lateral meniscus in the right knee was the only documented structural abnormality. This patient was initially thought to have an injury confined to soft tissues (a meniscal tear) but showed increased scintigraphic activity in bone before the appearance of radiographic changes. **Top left**, Technetium scintiscan showing three-compartment uptake. **Top right**, Normal preoperative radiograph. **Bottom left**, Technetium scintiscan, made 23 months after the repair of the lateral meniscus,[73] showing nearly complete resolution of the increased scintigraphic activity that had been seen preoperatively. **Bottom right**, Radiograph made at 23 months, showing mild osteopenia.

technetium-99m (metastable). Technetium-99m, a reliable emitter of gamma radiation (a photon with an energy of 140 kiloelectronvolts) with a short (six-hour) half-life, is produced in a generator by transmutation

from molybdenum 99.[14] It is administered in a liquid aliquot chemically attached to a methylene diphosphonate moiety, which is readily adsorbed to the hydration shell of living bone (the metabolically active region of mineral turnover).[15] A typical study involves the intravenous injection of 20 mCi of technetium-99m methylene diphosphonate (Tc 99m-MDP). Whole-body radiation exposure roughly equals that of a series of radiographs of the lumbosacral spine, with the bladder receiving the highest dose because of urinary clearance of the agent. A gamma camera detects the gamma photon rays emitted by the target organ by means of a sodium iodide crystal, which produces a visible wavelength photon on absorption of a high-energy gamma photon. Beneath the crystal is a set of photomultiplier tubes connected to a computer, which produces an image manifesting geographic distribution and location of the Tc 99m-MDP complex. The regions of gamma photon production are represented as dark spots on a clear background.

Typical studies consist of either a three-phase or a delayed static study. The first of the three phases, the blood-flow phase, reflects arterial blood passage through, or perfusion of, a region and is obtained on initial injection of the technetium aliquot. The second phase, the blood pool, which is acquired several minutes later, shows the relative vascularity of the region of interest.[15] In our experience with major joints, such as the knee and the ankle, acquisition of the first two phases is rarely indicated unless the clinical finding suggests the possibility of reflex sympathetic dystrophy, infection, or tumor. We think that the study of greatest interest and value is the third phase, the delayed static images acquired three hours after the injection. These delayed images show the differential distribution of the Tc 99m-MDP within physiologically active bone. This differentiation is a function of the coupled processes of blood supply and tracer extraction by metabolically active bone.[16]

At our institution, a Siemens 750S-ZLC gamma camera (Erlangen, Germany) with an 18-inch (45.7-centimeter) diameter, 3/8-inch (0.96-centimeter) thick sodium-iodide crystal is used. We use a low-energy all-purpose collimator and acquire 500,000 counts per image. Anterior and posterior views of a normal adult knee show activity in the femur and tibia, with an indistinct joint line (Fig. 3, *left*). The activity in the patella does not differ perceptibly from that of the femur. The activity in the proximal-lateral region of the tibia is typically slightly increased compared with that of the medial region. The femoral and tibial physeal regions often show more activity than do the condyles or plateaus in individuals who are younger than 35 years old. On lateral and medial projections of a normal knee (Fig. 3, *right*), the activity in the femur fades imperceptibly into that of the tibia, and the patello-

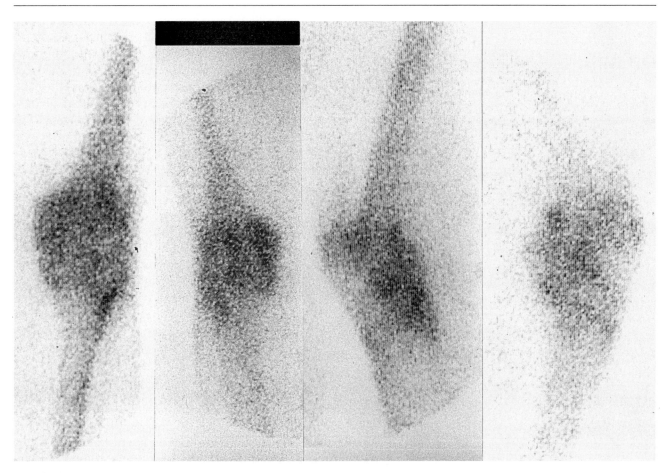

Fig. 3 Typical technetium scintigraphic images of the left knee of an asymptomatic individual. **Left**, Anterior scintiscan showing characteristics of osseous homeostasis. There is uniform femoral activity fading into the tibial region without an identifiable joint line. The patellar activity is indistinct. The activity in the proximal-lateral region of the tibia is typically slightly increased. **Left center**, Posterior scintiscan revealing uniform femoral activity fading into the tibial region. **Right center**, Lateral scintiscan showing femoral activity fading imperceptibly into the tibial region. The patellar activity is roughly equal to that of the distal aspect of the femoral diaphysis. **Right**, Medial scintiscan of a control knee, showing femoral activity fading into the tibial region.

femoral joint line is likewise indistinct. The activity in the patella roughly equals that of the distal aspect of the femoral diaphysis.[17]

Single-photon-emission computed tomography provides more accurate localization of tracer accumulation, because the tomographic method separates overlying structures.[18] We have not found this technique to be necessary for the assessment of joints such as the knee and ankle, for which we routinely acquire four views on the delayed static image. The use of single-photon-emission computed tomography is considered to be more valuable for imaging of deep osseous structures, such as the spine or hips.

Quantitative Assessment of Scintigraphic Activity

In an earlier study, in order to assess more accurately the qualitative readings for the patella, one of us (SFD), along with Boll, developed a quantitative method of comparing computer-generated ratios of regions of interest; this was called the percent patellar activity (Fig. 4).[17,19] The ratio of the scintigraphic counts of the patella to those of the patella and the femoral diaphysis, combined, within specified pixels should indicate the percentage of the total activity contributed by the patella alone. Typical control values ranged from 49% to 60%, with values of more than 65% being considered abnormal. At present, however, we rarely use quantitative techniques in the typical clinical setting because whenever the scintigraphic activity was determined to be qualitatively increased, the quantitative data were also in the abnormal range.[19] A simple, yet effective, alternative semiquantitative method for the classification of periarticular activity in different regions (for example, the medial femoral condyle or the medial tibial plateau) involves assignment of numbers from 0 (normal) to 4 (intense activity).[20]

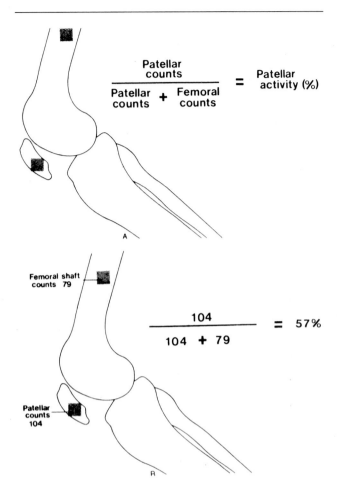

$$\frac{Patellar\ counts}{Patellar\ counts + Femoral\ counts} = Patellar\ activity\ (\%)$$

Femoral shaft counts 79

$$\frac{104}{104 + 79} = 57\%$$

Patellar counts 104

Fig. 4 **Top,** Schematic representation of the quantitative technique of determining the percent patellar activity. **Bottom,** The actual scintigraphic counts of a control individual with 57% patellar activity. (Reproduced with permission from Dye SF, Boll DA: Radionuclide imaging of the patellofemoral joint in young adults with anterior knee pain. *Orthop Clin North Am* 1986;17:252.)

Osseous Lesions

By the early 1980's, our group at Letterman Army Medical Center, Presidio of San Francisco, California, had established that a heretofore unappreciated osseous process, shown by technetium scintigraphy, was occurring in the region of the patella in many patients who had anterior pain in the knee but normal radiographic findings and, often, grossly normal articular cartilage. Knowing that a wide variety of clinical conditions, including tumors and infections, are associated with increased scintigraphic activity, we were interested in establishing the actual histologic nature of the osseous process detected in our patients. While treating the patients, we obtained (with the patients' knowledge and permission and with the approval of the Institutional Review Board) sagittally oriented bone samples, 3 mm in diameter, from the patellae of 15 individuals with normal radiographic findings, positive

findings on patellar scans, and persistent symptoms. Six age-matched cadaveric patellae, obtained from a tissue-transplant bank, served as control specimens.[21]

The typical histologic appearance of the subchondral region of the control patellae under polarized light consisted of articular cartilage, calcified cartilage, and a thin subchondral layer of bone with projecting spicules of patellar trabeculae (Fig. 5, *top left*).[22] The sections revealed even lamellations of the trabeculae, which we consider to be a histologic indicator of osseous homeostasis. A whorled lamellar pattern in the area, deep to the zone of calcified cartilage, was seen; it represented a normal region of slightly increased metabolic activity. Biopsy of a similar region of the patella of a symptomatic patient with positive scintigraphic findings revealed thickened trabeculae; more reversal lines; a generalized whorled, burled-walnut appearance of the lamellar pattern on polarized light, indicative of remodeling activity (Fig. 5, *top right*); and vascular invasion across the tidemark zone. On occasion, we found evidence of classic cutting-cone activity (Fig. 5, *bottom left*) and Howship lacunae (Fig. 5, *bottom right*), with multinucleated osteoclastic giant cells as well as metabolically active woven bone.

None of the 15 biopsies revealed any evidence of a tumor, an infection, a bone cyst, or necrosis. In no patient was the sedimentation rate or white blood cell count elevated. We now believe that the osseous process detected by the bone scans in these patients was a spectrum of increased bone turnover and remodeling not associated with a tumor or an infection. We believe that this process represents increased osseous metabolic activity.

Bone is an ancient tissue that has evolved a characteristically delimited ability to respond to stimuli and that typically follows a pattern of osteoclastic resorption and osteoblastic remodeling with remineralization of newly formed osteoid (Fig. 6).[23] A positive bone scan demonstrates regions of metabolically active bone where this biologic spectrum of increased remodeling has been activated. Biopsies on patients with more discomfort and intense scintigraphic findings have demonstrated more osteoclastic activity.

Factors Leading to Increased Osseous Metabolic Activity

There are three clinical phenomena associated with increased osseous scintigraphic activity that may provide insight into the nature and cause of this process: mechanical osseous trauma, neurovascular dysfunction, and production of humoral factors.

Mechanical Osseous Trauma

Bone overload, either through a single event such as an overt fracture or through the supraphysiologic stresses of repetitive submaximum loading, can initiate

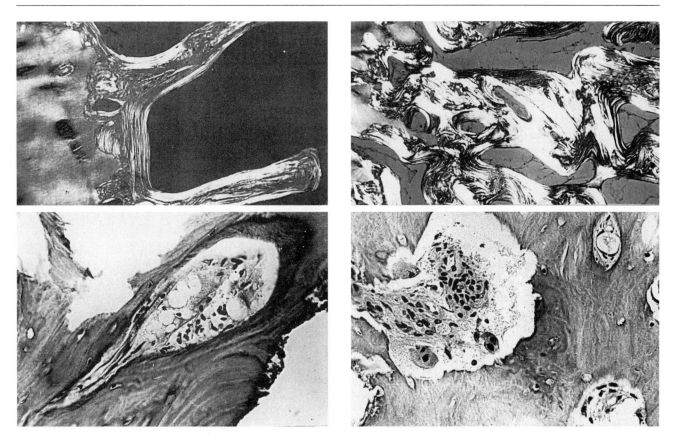

Fig. 5 **Top left**, Histologic section of the subchondral region of a normal patella, showing thin trabeculae and even lamellations with polarized light (hematoxylin and eosin, x 250). **Top right**, Histologic section of the subchondral region of a symptomatic patella with increased scintigraphic activity, demonstrating thickened trabeculae, an increased number of reversal lines, and a whorled lamellar pattern on polarized light (hematoxylin and eosin, x 250). (Reproduced with permission from Dye SF: Radionuclide imaging of the knee, in Aichroth P, Cannon WD (eds): *Knee Surgery, Current Practice*, London, Martin Dunitz, 1992, p 41.) **Bottom left**, Histologic section of a symptomatic patella with increased scintigraphic activity, showing a classic cutting cone (hematoxylin and eosin, x 300). **Bottom right**, Histologic section of a symptomatic patella with increased scintigraphic activity, showing a Howship lacuna (hematoxylin and eosin, x 350).

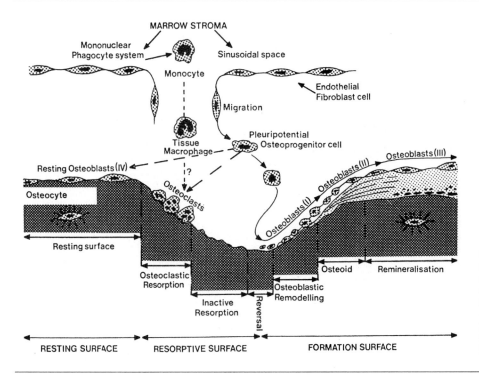

Fig. 6 Schematic representation of the biologic process of osteoclastic resorption and osteoblastic remodeling and remineralization of newly formed osteoid. Osteoblasts (I through IV) represent cells of increasing maturity. (Reproduced with permission from Parsons V: *Color Atlas of Bone Disease*, Chicago, IL, Year Book Medical Publishers, 1980, p 36.)

the increased osseous metabolic activity of bone that is detectable with scintigraphic methods.[24-26] We define these supraphysiologic stress loads as loads that are less than that required to cause an immediate fracture, but that will, with repetition, stimulate and initiate the biologic cascade of increased osseous metabolic activity that is detectable with technetium scintigraphy. These stresses are enough to induce increased bone-remodeling and may, with time, cause overt structural changes in the bone. These changes may be seen in the early stages of a stress fracture, when osteoclastic activity has begun but osteoblastic activity has not. We believe that the pathokinematics created by a tear of intra-articular soft tissues (for example, a rupture of the anterior cruciate ligament or a meniscal tear) also can result in supraphysiologic osseous loading, triggering the biologic cascade of increased remodeling.

McBride and associates,[27] using a rabbit model, showed that technetium scintigraphy detects regions of physiologically active bone in which increased remodeling resulted in degenerative changes prior to the appearance of radiographic abnormalities. In their study, post-traumatic osteoarthrosis was induced by sectioning of the anterior cruciate ligament in 38 rabbits. At two weeks, scintigraphy with Tc 99m-MDP revealed positive findings in 100% of the knees in which the anterior cruciate ligament had been sectioned; radiographic findings remained negative until the eighth postoperative week.

In order to study controlled trauma to the patella of an asymptomatic individual, one of us (SFD) allowed his patella to be penetrated, under local anesthesia, with a 15-gauge needle for an intraosseous pressure measurement. The pre-study control bone scan showed a classically normal image indicative of osseous homeostasis (Fig. 7, *left*). Seven weeks after the osseous injury, increased uptake was noted at the site of the needle penetration within the medial facet of the patella (Fig. 7, *center*). We interpret the increased scintigraphic activity following the controlled trauma as representing osseous remodeling in response to direct trabecular injury. Fourteen months later, after clinical healing, a third technetium bone scan revealed resolution of the abnormal patellar uptake (Fig. 7, *right*), indicating restoration to osseous homeostasis. We know of no other study that has documented, in a human model, osseous homeostasis followed by a known degree of trauma, subsequent scintigraphic evidence of increased remodeling activity, and eventual restoration of homeostasis.

Neurovascular Dysfunction

As exemplified by the clinical syndrome of reflex sympathetic dystrophy, neurovascular dysfunction is also recognized as a cause of intense osseous remodeling activity detectable with scintigraphic techniques.[17,28] We believe that, in many individuals with a history of only mild or moderate retinacular strain, subsequent demonstration of intense activity in the patella on bone-scanning represents a process in the bone similar to that seen with reflex sympathetic dystrophy—that is, alteration of the normal neurovascular osseous supply

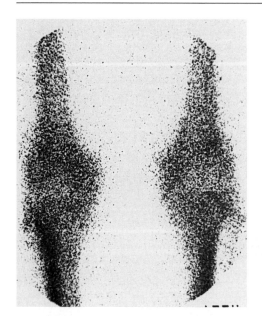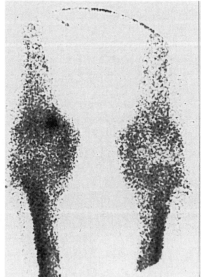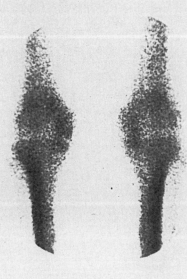

Fig. 7 Anterior technetium scintiscans made before and after penetration trauma to the medial facet of the right patella with a 15-gauge needle. **Left,** Osseous homeostasis was seen before the procedure. **Center,** Markedly increased uptake in the region of the medial facet seven weeks after the penetration trauma. **Right,** Restoration of osseous homeostasis 14 months after the penetration trauma.

resulting in increased osseous turnover.[29,30] There is also evidence that intraosseous hypertension can stimulate increased osseous metabolic activity and remodeling, resulting in formation of new cancellous bone.[31-33]

Humoral Factors

Various locally produced cytokines (for example, prostaglandins,[34,35] interleukin-1,[36,37] tumor necrosis factor,[38] interferon gamma,[36] and colony-stimulating factors[39]) can have a potent stimulating effect, increasing bone metabolic activity to levels detectable by scintigraphy. MacKinnon and Holder[40] reported experimental evidence that prostaglandin E, for example, is a potent stimulator of bone resorption. There has been speculation that the powerful action of cytokines on bone metabolism may be a process common to many etiologies of increased bone-remodeling, with prostaglandins and other factors released from sites of osteocyte injury or soft-tissue inflammation inducing the biologic cascade resulting in increased bone turnover.[41]

Combining the available basic-science information with clinical experience, we developed a theoretical model of osseous homeostasis (Fig. 8). Beginning with the initial premorbid condition of osseous homeostasis, one or more factors (triggers) may induce the biologic cascade of increased remodeling activity of bone that is detectable with scintigraphy with Tc 99m-MDP. Once initiated, the increased metabolic activity of bone resorption and formation can continue indefinitely because of the persistence of the triggering factors. Many activities of daily living, such as stair-climbing, that are well tolerated under normal conditions may result in supraphysiologic loads to the metabolically activated bone after initiation of remodeling—that is, the threshold for continued activation of remodeling is lowered.

Eventual restoration of osseous homeostasis, as documented by normal findings on a technetium scan, is possible without any net change in bone morphology.[42] Restoration of osseous homeostasis is the desired clinical outcome. If persistent osteoclastic resorption predominates, net loss of bone (osteolysis), such as seen with reflex sympathetic dystrophy, can occur. Restoration of osseous homeostasis with stable osteopenia, documented by normal scintigraphic findings, is possible (Fig. 2, *bottom*). If chronic osteoblastic activity predominates, osteophytes and osteosclerosis could develop and eventually become metabolically dormant. As Radin and Rose[43-45] indicated, the loss of bone compliance associated with osteosclerosis could negatively affect the viability of articular cartilage, resulting in clinical osteoarthrosis. Stressed biologic tissues are complex systems, and regions of increased bone density and osteopenia can develop within the same joint. Intermittent periods of metabolic activation and dormancy (punctuated equilibrium) also may occur. We believe that osteoarthrosis is commonly such an intermittently activated process.

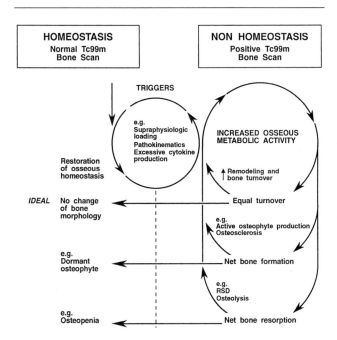

Fig. 8 Theoretical model of osseous homeostasis with multiple triggers inducing increased remodeling activity detectable by technetium scintigraphy. The increased osseous metabolic activity can continue for an indefinite period because of the effects of recurrent triggers. If bone turnover is equal, no change of bone morphology occurs; if osteoblastic activity predominates, osteopenia can develop; and, if osteoblastic activity predominates, osteosclerosis and osteophytes can develop. Restoration of osseous homeostasis, documentable by normal findings on a technetium scan, is possible with or without osseous morphologic changes. RSD = reflex sympathetic dystrophy.

Scintigraphy in Patients With Symptoms in the Anterior Aspect of the Knee

An early, non-traditional use of technetium scintigraphy of the knee was the evaluation of patients with anterior pain in the knee. Many research groups have established the presence of increased patellar scintigraphic activity in such patients, often in the absence of other objective abnormalities.[17,42,46-50]

An initial clinical study from Letterman Army Medical Center involved the use of technetium scintigraphy for 113 patients, between the ages of 18 and 45, who had anterior discomfort in 167 knees.[17] Technetium bone scans were obtained and evaluated in relation to various radiographic and physical findings. Patients were excluded from the study if they had radiographically identifiable abnormalities (such as a fracture, osteophytes, or osteopenia) or a history of a previous operation. Of the 167 symptomatic patellae, 81 (49%) had qualitatively increased scintigraphic activity as compared with only three (4%) of 70 age-matched and activity-matched control knees for which bone scintigraphy had been done. Although many theoretical indicators of malalignment were examined, no difference could be detected between the alignment of the patella in the symptomatic patients and the alignment of 158 control knees (79 individuals).[47] The rate of increased scintigraphic activity in the patella (four of 25) in the patients who had symptoms that were primarily parapatellar in nature, such as those associated with an inflamed plica or with retinacular or patellar-ligament pain, was not statistically different from that of the control patellae (three of 70). However, 77 (54%) of the 142 patients with pain that was primarily patellar demonstrated an abnormally increased scintigraphic uptake. Five of 12 individuals with positive patellar scans who eventually had an arthroscopic examination were found to have grossly normal articular cartilage, an observation confirmed by Butler-Manuel and associates.[46] Grossly normal synovial tissue

was also documented in many patients. Thus, osseous abnormalities detected scintigraphically are not necessarily related to overt cartilaginous failure or synovitis but can be a consequence of other factors.

After following several patients with anterior pain in the knee with sequential bone scans before and after conservative treatment, it became clear that the detected abnormal osseous activity was a dynamic process that could, with time, return to normal (Fig. 9). We documented the patterns and possible dynamics of the osseous process in 78 patients with 114 symptomatic knees that had been treated conservatively.[42] Patients with abnormal findings on initial patellar scans had a significantly greater chance of persistence of symptoms compared with the patients with normal findings on the initial patellar scans (Student t test, $p < 0.001$). We also noted four recurrent patterns of initial patellofemoral uptake. Two, focal and diffuse, were often associated with resolution of symptoms and a return to normal activity on the scan (Fig. 10, *left*). The other two,

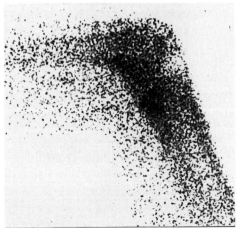
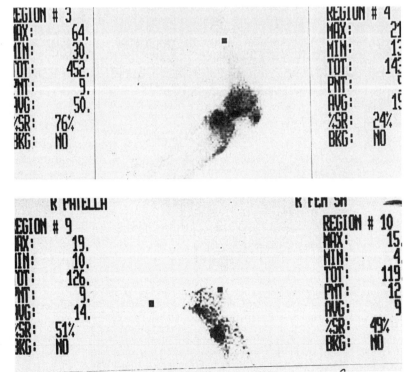
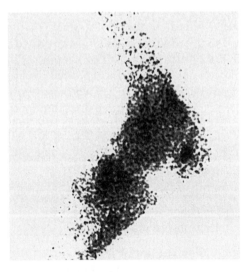

Fig. 9 Technetium scintiscans demonstrating comparative qualitative and quantitative readings in an individual who had a three-month history of retropatellar discomfort. **Top left**, Qualitative scintiscan showing focal patellar uptake. **Top right**, Quantitative scintiscan showing patellar activity of 76%, which is well into the abnormal range. **Bottom left**, Qualitative technetium scintiscan made three months later, after resolution of the symptoms with a conservative treatment program, showing restoration of osseous homeostasis. **Bottom right**, Quantitative technetium scintiscan, made at three months, documenting restoration of the percent patellar activity to within the normal range (51%).

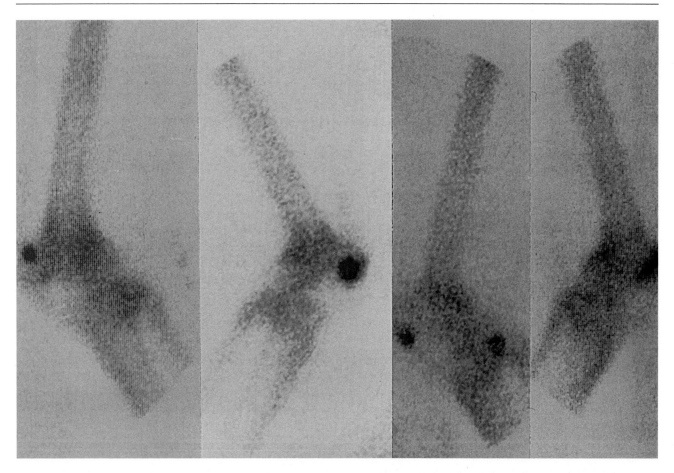

Fig. 10 Patterns of increased patellar scintigraphic activity. **Left**, The focal pattern, which is associated with likely resolution of symptoms. **Left center**, The diffuse pattern, which is associated with likely resolution of symptoms. **Right center**, The focal inferior-pole pattern, which is associated with persistence of symptoms. **Right**, The trochlear and patellar pattern, which is associated with persistence of symptoms.

inferior pole as well as femoral trochlear and patellar, were associated with persistence of symptoms and continued increased activity (Fig. 10, *right*). The mean duration of symptoms for the patients with initially positive findings on the scan was 11 months (range, 3 to 18 months), suggesting that once the scintigraphically detected patellar osseous process is initiated, a return to homeostasis is often prolonged. Thus, the determination that conservative therapy has failed, as a rationale for surgical intervention, in patients with patellofemoral pain who do not have mechanical symptoms but who have a positive result on technetium study, should not be made too soon (for example, after only six weeks of treatment). In patients with negative findings on a bone scan, a diagnosis of parapatellar soft-tissue strain and inflammation was most often made. One patient in this group had an eventual diagnosis of symptoms referred to the patellar region from saphenous nerve entrapment. This diagnosis was documented by electrodiagnostic studies.

Scintigraphy in Patients With a Tear of the Anterior Cruciate Ligament or a Meniscal Lesion

Increased osseous metabolic activity also has been seen with other knee disorders previously considered to involve only soft-tissue failure, including symptomatic tears of the anterior cruciate ligament[51-54] and meniscal tears.[55-58] In our experience[22] with 86 patients with a chronically symptomatic tear of the anterior cruciate ligament, 73 (85%) exhibited increased subchondral scintigraphic activity (Fig. 11, *left*), often in the presence of normal osseous findings on radiographs and MRI scans.[6] We have also documented that restoration of osseous homeostasis is possible after reconstruction of a torn anterior cruciate ligament (Fig. 11, *right*).

In recent studies[53,54] involving MRI of acute injuries of the anterior cruciate ligament, regions of "edema," presumably excess extracellular fluid, or bone "infraction," presumably trabecular fractures, have been demonstrated most often in the lateral compartment.

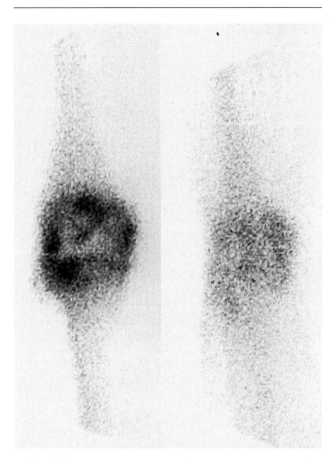

Fig. 11 Anterior technetium scintiscans of the right knee of a patient with a chronic symptomatic tear of the anterior cruciate ligament. **Left,** Three-compartment uptake is seen. Radiographs revealed normal findings. **Right,** Eighteen months after reconstruction with an autogenous graft consisting of the central third of the patellar ligament, there was restoration of osseous homeostasis. The findings on the postoperative radiograph remained normal.

In a study of 13 patients, Marks and associates[53] reported that bone scintigraphy detected all of the regions of osseous injury indicated by MRI scans and detected additional areas that had been missed in two patients. In knees with a chronic tear of the anterior cruciate ligament, imaged by technetium scintigraphy, the medial compartment is most often involved, followed by the lateral and then the patellofemoral compartment.[51,52] Mooar and associates[58] described four patterns of uptake in knees with internal derangement; one pattern was three-compartment uptake associated with rotatory instability of the knee without overt radiographic changes. We have found that a wide spectrum of increased subchondral uptake can occur in knees with internal derangement or instability associated with a torn anterior cruciate ligament.

The knees of individuals with symptomatic tears of the anterior cruciate ligament may be likened, in essence, to a transmission system with linkage failure. The knee with a biologic linkage failure can demon-strate a spectrum of abnormal scintigraphic activity that reflects regions of supraphysiologically stressed bone, either as a function of the initial trauma or, as is more likely in the chronic setting, activation of the remodeling cascade due to the pathokinematics secondary to the loss of the anterior cruciate ligament and to possible meniscal injury.

In a recent study, Fritschy and associates[20] reported an unexpectedly high percentage of abnormal findings on bone scans and degenerative changes in patients following reconstruction of the anterior cruciate ligament, despite restoration of normal laxity parameters. The authors used a semiquantitative scoring system for bone-scan activity and radiographic degenerative changes. Twenty-two patients had had reconstruction of the anterior cruciate ligament, and there were 75 patients in the control group. The mean score for the activity on the technetium bone scan was 12.1 of a possible 24 points for the reconstructed knees and 4.7 points for the control knees. The mean score for radiographic evidence of degeneration was 6.2 of a possible 18 points for the reconstructed knees and 0.7 point for the control knees. The results of this study emphasize the importance of physiologic as well as structural criteria in the assessment of such patients.

Studies by Marymont and associates,[57] Bauer and associates[55] Mooar and associates,[58] Lohmann and associates,[56] and us[59,60] have documented the association of meniscal tears with increased osseous metabolic activity. The typical scintigraphic finding in patients with a symptomatic meniscal tear is increased subchondral activity in the involved compartment (Fig. 2, top left). Bauer and associates[55] and Mooar and associates[58] described this activity as being located exclusively in the tibia, but our experience has differed. Frequently, we have identified increased activity in the adjacent femoral subchondral bone as well as in other compartments without an overt meniscal lesion.

In a recent study,[59] 28 (82%) of 34 knees with documented meniscal abnormalities, normal findings on preoperative radiographs, and no overt ligamentous damage demonstrated abnormally increased scintigraphic activity in at least the involved compartment. On postoperative follow-up examination (at an average of 18 months), 20 (59%) showed normal or nearly normal scintigraphic activity. Fairbank[61] changes (radiographic narrowing, osseous-ridge formation, and flattening of the femoral condyles) developed in six of the 14 patients for whom the postoperative bone scans either had not shown improvement or had shown worsening. In contrast, such changes developed in only one of the 20 patients for whom the scans had shown resolution of the lesion (Student t test, $p < 0.001$). Persistent, increased osseous metabolic activity in these patients was thus a prelude to eventual radiographically identifiable degenerative changes.

Atypical Scintigraphic Patterns

The reproducibility of the abnormal scintigraphic patterns has been so consistent that an atypical bone scan should be immediately apparent and should often lead to a revised diagnosis. As an example, a woman was referred from an internist with a presumptive diagnosis of a torn lateral meniscus. A technetium bone scan revealed normal activity in the lateral compartment and intensely abnormal uptake at the proximal tibiofibular joint (Fig. 12). This study led to the correct diagnosis of active rheumatoid arthritis affecting the proximal tibiofibular joint. Another patient in whom an atypical scintigraphic study led to a different diagnosis than had been initially suspected was a middle-aged man who had noted increasing pain at the medial joint line soon after he had started jogging. Clinically, the symptoms were consistent with a diagnosis of a symptomatic degenerative tear of the medial meniscus. The scan revealed atypical, intense pancondylar uptake in the medial femoral condyle (Fig. 13). Radiographs and high-resolution computed tomography revealed normal findings, as did arthroscopic examina-

tion. The diagnosis of transient osteolysis was made following biopsy of the medial femoral condyle.

Scintigraphic Findings in the Contralateral Knee

When a patient with unilateral symptoms has a technetium study of the knees, some increased uptake may be noted in the contralateral knee. It is rare to find intense activity in these instances. This activity in the contralateral knee may be a result of increased loading to protect the symptomatic joint or may be a reflection of normal regions of clinically silent bone adaptation. In some patients, a careful history and physical examination can reveal a subjective component, such as intermittent slight aching and tenderness to palpation of the active region.

Scintigraphy of Joints Other Than the Knee

Scintigraphic imaging data of other joints has convinced us that similar dynamic osseous metabolic characteristics are probably common and fundamental to all joints. We are performing an ongoing study in which bone scans are obtained for patients with normal radiographic findings and persistent pain in the

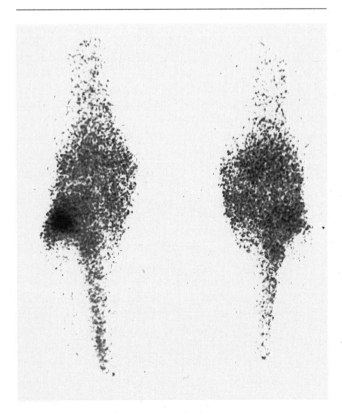

Fig. 12 Anterior technetium scintiscan of a patient with active rheumatoid arthritis affecting the proximal tibiofibular joint that had been suspected of being a tear of the lateral meniscus. The study shows increased activity in the proximal tibiofibular joint, with normal findings in the lateral compartment.

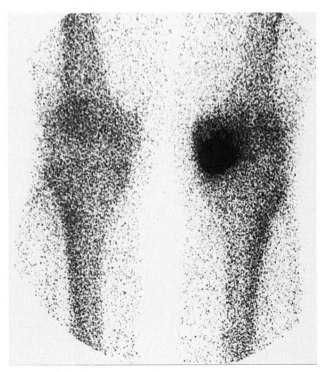

Fig. 13 Anterior technetium scintiscan of a patient with transient osteolysis of the medial femoral condyle that was suspected of being a tear of the medial meniscus. The study shows intense pancondylar activity in the medial femoral condyle.

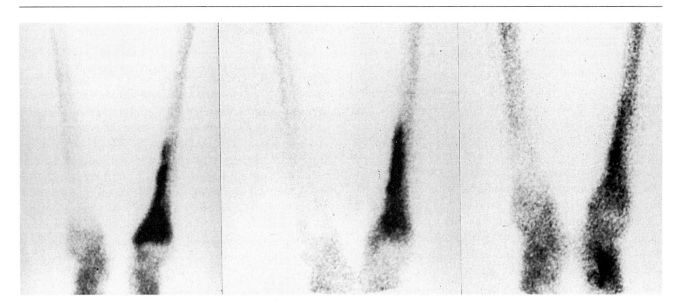

Fig. 14 Anterior technetium scintiscans of the ankle of a patient with a history of a sprain two months prior to the study. Radiographs revealed normal findings. **Left,** Initial scintiscan showing intense activity in the distal one-fourth of the tibia. **Center,** Four months after the initial study and institution of conservative therapy, there was a moderate decrease in the abnormal tibial activity. **Right,** Nine months after the initial study, there was a marked decrease in the abnormal distal tibial activity.

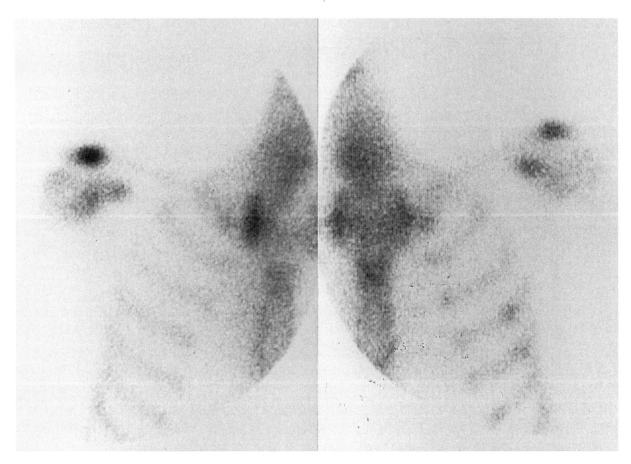

Fig. 15 **Left,** Anterior technetium scintiscan of the right shoulder of a patient with acromioclavicular symptoms, showing increased activity in the acromioclavicular joint. Radiographs revealed normal findings. **Right,** Anterior technetium scintiscan of the asymptomatic left shoulder, showing normal activity in the acromioclavicular joint.

ankle following a sprain. Of the more than 20 patients imaged so far, all have exhibited abnormal uptake about the ankle despite normal radiographs. Our early sequential data also indicate that once the increased osseous metabolic activity has been established, the process tends to persist, as we have seen in the knee (Fig. 14). In independent work that included MRI and arthrography, Pavlov and associates[62,63] noted a similar variety of abnormal patterns of scintigraphic uptake about the foot and ankle. According to these observations, technetium scintigraphy is invaluable for the determination of which osseous component is the source of symptoms.

Recently, we have begun to use scintigraphy for patients with symptoms in the upper extremities. Symptomatic acromioclavicular joints often reveal similar patterns of increased osseous metabolic activity, even when radiographic findings are normal (Fig. 15). Johnson[64] described scintigraphic information as being useful for the determination of which symptomatic acromioclavicular joints may be best treated surgically. We also have found that technetium scintigraphy can show periarticular activity in inflamed facet joints of the spine (Fig. 16).

Recently, investigation of the temporomandibular joint[65,66] has shown the value of technetium scintigraphy for the demonstration of osseous stresses despite normal findings on radiographs. As a result, many practitioners now routinely use scintigraphic information to aid in their therapeutic decision-making when treating symptomatic temporomandibular joints (L. Kaban, personal communication, 1991).

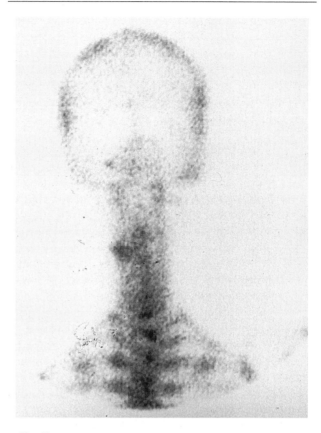

Fig. 16 Posterior technetium scintiscan of the cervical spine of a symptomatic patient, showing increased activity in the left fourth and fifth cervical facets.

Clinical Recommendations

Scintigraphy with Tc 99m-MDP can provide valuable adjunctive physiologic information to aid in the diagnosis of selected periarticular symptoms, when the results of therapy are being assessed, and when medicolegal cases are being evaluated.

Diagnosis of Periarticular Symptoms

Technetium scintigraphy is an excellent adjunctive imaging modality in the evaluation of patients in whom the source and clinical importance of periarticular symptoms remain in doubt. For example, it can help to clarify the diagnosis in patients with a vague history of symptoms in the knee and MRI findings suggestive of structural damage, such as a torn meniscus. When a bone scan reveals increased subchondral activity in the involved compartment, independently confirming that the periarticular bone has been physiologically overstressed, it is more likely that a lesion demonstrated by MRI is clinically important. In contrast, if the bone scan indicates osseous homeostasis of the suspected compartment, one should be cautious

before attributing clinical importance to the finding of possible structural damage on the MRI scans.

Middle-aged athletes with symptoms of chronic, intermittent periarticular pain following participation in high-impact sports, such as jogging or racquetball, are ideal candidates for technetium scintigraphic evaluation. If the findings on the technetium scan are normal, indicating osseous homeostasis, the patient can be reassured that the joint is withstanding the loads being placed across it without evidence of osseous overload. If, however, the scan shows a substantial increase in scintigraphic activity, there is objective evidence that the joint is being overloaded and therapeutic intervention is indicated. Patients with an untreated chronic tear of the anterior or posterior cruciate ligament and persistent intermittent symptoms are also good candidates for evaluation with a technetium scan.

Assessment of Therapeutic Results

Another clinical role for the use of technetium scintigraphy is the assessment of results of meniscal or ligamentous procedures. We recommend a follow-up bone scan between 18 and 24 months after the operation, in order to determine whether osseous homeostasis has been restored in the involved joint. When symptoms persist after the operation, the scan should be considered sooner. If there is a substantial loss of osseous homeostasis, the physician should counsel the patient about being at risk for possible degenerative changes and should provide appropriate therapeutic recommendations.

Medicolegal Assessment

Technetium scintigraphy also can be of great value for the assessment of medicolegal cases. A bone scan provides a direct reflection of the physiologic characteristics of a joint. It is independent of joint position or loading at the time of the study. For instance, a normal technetium bone scan in a patient who claims to have persistent, profound pain following a knee injury rules out active reflex sympathetic dystrophy or osteolysis and suggests that the diagnosis of active degenerative changes is inappropriate. On the other hand, a technetium bone scan can confirm the existence of increased osseous metabolic activity not shown by other imaging modalities and can support the patient's claim. For example, severe patellofemoral symptoms developed in both knees of a man who repaired telephone power lines. The findings of an extensive workup, which included radiography, MRI, and arthroscopy, were interpreted as being within normal limits, and the patient was about to return to his normal occupation of climbing telephone poles. Then, a technetium bone scan revealed intense activity in the patellofemoral joints bilaterally and provided an objective reason for him to continue restriction of that type of activity.

Therapeutic Recommendations

If the technetium bone scan of a symptomatic patient reveals regions of increased osseous metabolic activity, the clinician can assume that the joint is being physiologically overstressed. Our treatment approach involves three areas: addressing of any existing pathomechanics, administration of appropriate anti-inflammatory therapy, and rehabilitation.

Pathomechanics

The physician must identify any external or internal source of recurrent mechanical or traumatic triggers. External factors include supraphysiologic loading resulting from participation in high-impact activities (for example, racquetball or basketball) and aggravating activities of daily living (for example, excessive stair-climbing). Such supraphysiologic loading often leads to continued increased osseous metabolic activity and must be restricted at least temporarily. Often, minimum changes in activity can reduce loads to levels that are within the joint's physiologic capacity for load acceptance. Patients with severe malalignment, such as a varus configuration, as well as persistently increased physiologic stress in the medial compartment should be considered for surgical correction of the malalignment.

Treatment should also address any internal pathomechanical factors, such as a torn meniscus or a torn or attenuated ligament. A correlative positive bone scan supports a decision for surgical intervention. However, no single technetium study alone should be used to determine whether surgical intervention should be undertaken. For example, some patterns of patellar pain are associated with resolution of symptoms over time, if appropriate conservative therapy has been instituted.

Anti-Inflammatory Therapy

We believe that regions of increased osseous metabolic activity represent zones of continued activation by excessive local cytokine production. We therefore recommend an ongoing anti-inflammatory program. This should include achievement of therapeutic blood levels of an anti-inflammatory non-steroidal medication of the clinician's choice and application of ice for 20 minutes two or three times daily for several weeks or until the symptoms have fully resolved. Two technetium studies of the ankle performed a week apart on one of our patients documented that application of ice for a single 20-minute period decreased a zone of increased osseous metabolic activity by 80% (Fig. 17).

Rehabilitation

Patients should maintain muscle tone and active function of the cerebellar-proprioceptive control mechanisms[67-69] through the use of appropriate exercises that do not result in supraphysiologic loading of periarticular structures. For example, bicycling with low or no resistance and swimming are ideal forms of exercise for most injured knees.

Conclusions

Often, within periarticular bone, there are regions of dynamic metabolic adaptations characterized by increased turnover and remodeling. These dynamic osseous events have been generally unrecognized because most current imaging modalities reveal anatomic and structural instead of physiologic characteristics of tissues. The addition of osseous metabolic information is complementary to other diagnostic information, including that derived from a thorough history, physical examination, and anatomic imaging studies.

Multiple triggers, including mechanical, neurovascular, and hormonal factors, may initiate increased

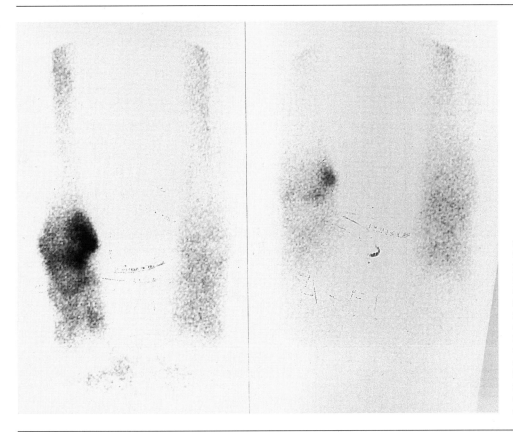

Fig. 17 Left, Anterior technetium scintiscan of a patient with a three-month history of pain in the ankle that had been diagnosed as a sprain. The study shows a marked increase in the activity in the medial malleolar region. Radiographs revealed normal findings. **Right**, Anterior technetium scintiscan made one week later. Ice was applied to the right ankle for 20 minutes before injection of the technetium-99m methylene diphosphonate. The study shows marked diminution of osseous metabolic activity.

osseous metabolic activity that is detectable with technetium scintigraphy. We think that chronic, supraphysiologic loading or abnormal joint mechanics (pathokinematics) combine with chronic, excessive periarticular cytokine production to produce the persistently increased remodeling in most patients. The presence of regions of increased osseous metabolic activity, therefore, can help the clinician to determine the extent to which such persistent factors have affected the joint. We have noted that persistently increased osseous metabolic activity of periarticular bone identifies a subgroup at risk for early structural changes.

We have found that the simplicity and starkness of a positive bone scan is comprehensible to patients. Their awareness of physiologic overload often leads them to cooperate with a program of appropriate restriction of activity, anti-inflammatory therapy, rehabilitation, and possibly surgical intervention that eventually results in restoration of homeostasis. Our goal is that homeostasis be restored before structural changes occur.

The achievement of cellular homeostasis is a broad fundamental principle of therapy throughout the field of medicine.[70] It should be no less a goal for orthopaedists, who have traditionally sought evidence of structural restoration instead of documentation of physiologic normalcy. Scintigraphic techniques provide the clinician with a simple, safe, and available method of visualizing these characteristics of periarticular bone. An improved understanding of metabolic adaptations of musculoskeletal systems can be expected as subsequent scintigraphic investigations include the use of positron-emission tomography.[71,72]

Acknowledgements

The authors thank the many individuals who have assisted in this work over the years, including Lottie Applewhite; Juanita Chase; Anne Shew; Gill Gardener; Frances Neagley; Percival Dunigan, MD; Paul Peartree, MD; Michael Stowell, MD; Jack McBride, MD; Gilberto Sostre, MD; Robert Lull, MD; Daniel Boll, MD; George Westin, MD; Mark Via, MD; Christian Andersen, MD; Donald Campbell, MD; Michael Fry, MD; Paul Fry, MD; Gene Galvin, MD; Harry Jergesen, MD; Douglas Mason, MD; Steve Shifflett, MD; W. Dilworth Cannon, Jr, MD; Kenneth DeHaven, MD; and Geoffrey Vaupel, MD.

References

1. Hutchins WC: Miscellaneous affections of joints, in Crenshaw AK (eds): *Campbell's Operative Orthopaedics*, ed 5. St. Louis, MO, CV Mosby, 1971, pp 987-1029.
2. Rockwood CA Jr, Green DP (eds): *Fractures in Adults*, ed 2. Philadelphia, PA, JB Lippincott, 1984, p 17.

3. Thomas CL (ed): *Taber's Cyclopedic Medical Dictionary*, ed 16. Philadelphia, PA, FA Davis, 1989.

4. Egund N, Frost S, Brismar J, et al: Radiography and scintigraphy in the assessment of early gonarthrosis. *Acta Radiol* 1988;29:451-455.

5. Thomas RH, Resnick D, Alazraki NP, et al: Compartmental evaluation of osteoarthritis of the knee: A comparative study of available diagnostic modalities. *Radiology* 1975;116:585-594.

6. Dye S, Bessolo R, Chew M, et al: Comparison of magnetic resonance imaging and technetium scintigraphy in the detection of increased osseous metabolic activity about the knee. Read at the Annual Meeting of The American Academy of Orthopaedic Surgeons, San Francisco, California, Feb. 22, 1993.

7. McNeil BJ: Value of bone scanning in neoplastic disease. *Semin Nucl Med* 1984;14:277-286.

8. Handmaker H, Leonards R: The bone scan in inflammatory osseous disease. *Semin Nucl Med* 1976;6:95-105.

9. Lotke PA, Ecker ML: Osteonecrosis of the knee. *Orthop Clin North Am* 1985;16:797-808.

10. Strashun A, Chayes Z: Migratory osteolysis. *J Nucl Med* 1979;20:129-132.

11. Fogelman I, Mckillop JH, Gray HW: The "hot patella" sign: Is it of any clinical significance? *J Nucl Med* 1983;24:312-315.

12. Kipper MS, Alazraki NP, Feiglin DH: The "hot" patella. *Clin Nucl Med* 1982;7:28-32.

13. Simon H, Carlson DH: The use of bone scanning in the diagnosis of reflex sympathetic dystrophy. *Clin Nucl Med* 1980;5:116-121.

14. Rollo FD (ed): *Nuclear Medicine Physics, Instrumentation, and Agents.* St. Louis, MO, CV Mosby, 1977, pp 398-399.

15. Holder LE: Current concepts review: Radionuclide bone-imaging in the evaluation of bone pain. *J Bone Joint Surg* 1982;64A:1391-1396.

16. Siegel BA, Donovan RL, Alderson P, et al: Skeletal uptake of 99mTc-diphosphonate in relation to local bone blood flow. *Radiology* 1976;120:121-123.

17. Dye SF, Boll DA: Radionuclide imaging of the patellofemoral joint in young adults with anterior knee pain. *Orthop Clin North Am* 1986;17:249-262.

18. Collier BD, Johnson RP, Carrera GF, et al: Chronic knee pain assessed by SPECT: Comparison with other modalities. *Radiology* 1985;157:795-802.

19. Dye SF, Boll DH, Westin GW, et al: Assessing patellar scintigraphic activity: A new quantitative method. *Orthop Trans* 1985;9:459.

20. Fritschy D, Daniel DM, Rossman D, et al: Bone imaging after acute knee hemarthrosis. *Knee Surgery, Sports Traumatology, Arthroscopy: Official Journal of the ESSKA.* 1993;1:20-27.

21. Dye SF, Daniel DM, et al: The correlation of increased scintigraphic activity and patellar osseous pathology in young patients with patellofemoral pain. *Orthop Trans* 1986;10:480.

22. Dye SF: Radionuclide imaging of the knee, in Aichroth P, Cannon WD (eds): *Knee Surgery, Current Practice.* London, Martom Dunitz, 1992, pp 38-44.

23. Parsons V: *Color Atlas of Bone Disease.* Chicago, IL, Year Book Medical Publishers, 1980, pp 36-37.

24. Brill DR: Sports nuclear medicine: Bone imaging for lower extremity pain in athletes. *Clin Nucl Med* 1983;8:101-116.

25. Matin P: Bone-scanning of trauma and benign conditions, in Freeman LM, Weissman HS (eds): *Nuclear Medicine Annual 1982.* New York, NY, Raven Press, 1982, pp 81-118.

26. Rosenthall L, Hill RO, Chuang S: Observation on the use of 99mTc-phosphate imaging in peripheral bone trauma. *Radiology* 1976;119:637-641.

27. McBride JT, Rodkey WG, Brooks DE, et al: Early detection of osteoarthritis using technetium 99m MDP imaging, radiographs, histology and gross pathology in an experimental rabbit model. *Orthop Trans* 1991;15:348-349.

28. Kozin F, Ryan LM, Carrera GF, et al: The reflex sympathetic dystrophy syndrome (RSDS): III. Scintigraphic studies, further evidence of the therapeutic efficacy with systemic corticosteroids, and proposed diagnostic criteria. *Am J Med* 1981;70:23-30.

29. Hokfelt T, Kellerth JO, Nilsson G, et al: Experimental immunohistochemical studies on the localization and distribution of substance P in cat primary sensory neurons. *Brain Res* 1975;100:235-252.

30. Kimball E: Involvement of cytokines in neurogenic inflammation, in Kimball S (ed): *Cytokines and Inflammation*, Boca Raton, FL, CRC Press, 1991, pp 169-189.

31. Arnoldi CC, Linderholm H, Mussbichler H: Venous engorgement and intraosseous hypertension in osteoarthritis of the hip. *J Bone Joint Surg* 1972;54B:409-421.

32. Kelly PJ, Bronk JT: Venous pressure and bone formation. *Microvasc Res* 1990;39:364-375.

33. Welch RD, Johnston CE II, Waldron NJ, et al: Bone changes associated with intraosseous hypertension in the caprine tibia. *J Bone Joint Surg* 1993;75A:53-60.

34. Klein DC, Raisz LG: Prostaglandins: Stimulation of bone resorption in tissue culture. *Endocrinology* 1970;86:1436-1440.

35. Sato K, Fujii Y, Kasono K, et al: Stimulation of prostaglandin E2 and bone resorption by recombinant human interleukin 1 alpha in fetal mouse bones. *Biochem Biophys Res Commun* 1986;138:618-624.

36. Gowen M, Mundy GR: Actions of recombinant interleukin-1, interleukin-2, and interferon-gamma on bone resorption in vitro. *J Immunol* 1986;136:2478-2482.

37. Lorenzo J: Cytokines and bone metabolism: Resorption and formation, in Kimball S (ed): *Cytokines and Inflammation.* Boca Raton, FL, CRC Press, 1991, pp 145-168.

38. Bertolini DR, Nedwin GE, Bringman TS, et al: Stimulation of bone resorption and inhibition of bone formation in vitro by human tumour necrosis factors. *Nature* 1986;319:516-518.

39. Evans DB, Bunning RA, Russell RG: The effects of recombinant human granulocyte-macrophage colony-stimulating factor (rhGM-CSF) on human osteoblast-like cells. *Biochem Biophys Res Commun* 1989;160:588-595.

40. MacKinnon SE, Holder LE: The use of three-phase radionuclide bone scanning in the diagnosis of reflex sympathetic dystrophy. *J Hand Surg* 1984;9:556-563.

41. Mundy GR: Cytokines and local factors which affect osteoclast function. *Int J Cell Cloning* 1992;10:215-222.

42. Dye SF, Peartree PK: Sequential radionuclide imaging of the patellofemoral joint in symptomatic young adults. *Am J Sports Med* 1989;17:727.

43. Radin EL: Aetiology of osteoarthrosis. *Clin Rheumatol* 1976;2:509-522.

44. Radin EL: The relationship between biological and mechanical factors in the aetiology of osteoarthrosis. *J Rheumatol Suppl* 1983;9:20-21.

45. Radin EL, Rose RM: Role of subchondral bone in the initiation and progression of cartilage damage. *Clin Orthop* 1986;213:34-40.

46. Butler-Manuel PA, Guy RL, Heatley FW, et al: Scintigraphy in the assessment of anterior knee pain. *Acta Orthop Scand* 1990;6:438-442.

47. Dye SF, Boll DA: An analysis of objective measurements including radionuclide imaging in young patients with patellofemoral pain. *Am J Sports Med* 1985;13:432.

48. Hejgaard N, Diemer H: Bone scan in the patellofemoral pain syndrome. *Int Orthop* 1987;11:29-33.

49. Kahn D, Wilson MA: Bone scintigraphic findings in patellar tendonitis. *J Nucl Med* 1987;28:1768-1770.

50. Kohn HS, Guten GN, Collier BD, et al: Chondromalacia of the patella: Bone imaging correlated with arthroscopic findings. *Clin Nucl Med* 1988;13:96-98.

51. Alexander A, Barrach R, Dorchak J, et al: Radionuclide imaging of the chronic ACL-deficient knee. Read at the First World Congress of Sports Trauma, Majorca, Spain, May 25, 1992.

52. Dye SF, Andersen CT, Stowell MT: Unrecognized abnormal osseous metabolic activity about the knee of patients with symptomatic anterior cruciate ligament deficiency. *Orthop Trans* 1987;11:492.

53. Marks PH, Goldenberg JA, Vezina WC, et al: Subchondral bone infractions in acute ligamentous knee injuries demonstrated on bone scintigraphy and magnetic resonance imaging. *J Nucl Med* 1992;33:516-520.

54. Vellet AD, Marks PH, Fowler PJ, et al: Occult posttraumatic osteochondral lesions of the knee: Prevalence, classification, and short-term sequelae evaluated with MR imaging. *Radiology* 1991;178:271-276.

55. Bauer KC, Persson PE, Nilsson OS: Tears of the medial meniscus associated with increased radionuclide activity of the proximal tibia: Report of three cases. *Int Orthop* 1989;13:153-155.

56. Lohmann M, Kanstrup IL, Gergvary I, et al: Bone scintigraphy in patients suspected of having meniscus tears. *Scand J Med Sci Sports* 1991;1:123-127.

57. Marymont JV, Lynch MA, Henning CE: Evaluation of meniscus tears of the knee by radionuclide imaging. *Am J Sports Med* 1983;11:432-435.

58. Mooar P, Gregg J, Jacobstein J: Radionuclide imaging in internal derangements of the knee. *Am J Sports Med* 1987;15:132-137.

59. Dye SF, Chew M, McBride JT, et al: Restoration of osseous homeostasis of the knee following meniscal surgery. *Orthop Trans* 1992;16:725.

60. Dye SF, McBride JT, Chew M, et al: Unrecognized abnormal osseous metabolic activity in patients with documented meniscal pathology. *Am J Sports Med* 1989;17:723-724.

61. Fairbank TJ: Knee joint changes after meniscectomy. *J Bone Joint Surg* 1948;30B:664-670.

62. Pavlov H: Imaging of the foot and ankle. *Radiol Clin North Am* 1990;28:991-1018.

63. Pavlov H, Torg JS, Freiberger RH: Tarsal navicular stress fractures: Radiographic evaluation. *Radiology* 1983;148:641-645.

64. Johnson LL: Diagnostic and Surgical Arthroscopy of the Shoulder. St. Louis, MO, CV Mosby, 1993, pp 406-408.

65. Blankestijn J, Panders AK, Vermey A, et al: Synovial chondromatosis of the temporo-mandibular joint: Report of three cases and a review of the literature. *Cancer* 1985;55:479-485.

66. Epstein DH, Graves RW, Higgins WL: Clinical significance of increased temporomandibular joint uptake by planar isotope bone scan. *Clin Nucl Med* 1987;12:705-707.

67. Marr D: A theory of cerebellar cortex. *J Physiol* 1969;202:437-470.

68. Sanes JS: A theory of cerebellar function. *Math Biosci* 1971;10:25-51.

69. Schmahmann JD: An emerging concept: The cerebellar contribution to higher function. *Arch Neurol* 1991;48:1178-1187.

70. Guyton AC (ed): *Textbook of Medical Physiology*, ed 7. Philadelphia, PA, WB Saunders, 1986, p 3.

71. Muehllehner G, Karp JS: A positron camera using positron-sensitive detectors: PENN-PET. *J Nucl Med* 1986;27:90-98.

72. Muehllehner G, Karp JS: Positron emission tomography imaging—technical considerations. *Semin Nucl Med* 1986;16:35-50.

73. Henning CE: Arthroscopic repair of meniscus tears. *Orthopedics* 1983;6:1130-1132.

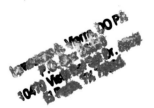

Magnetic Resonance Imaging of the Postoperative Spine

Harry K. Genant, MD

Magnetic resonance imaging is being increasingly used for studies of the lumbar spine and has become the modality of choice in assessment of patients with symptoms following spinal surgery—the failed back surgery syndrome (FBSS).[1-5] FBSS includes a heterogeneous group of disorders whose hallmark is back pain, sciatica, and functional impairment. Few other disease entities represent such a tangled complexity of organic, psychologic, and social factors. The failed back represents a major clinical problem for both the patient and the health care system, because the worldwide failure rate of initial spinal surgery ranges from 25% to 40%, with subsequent spinal exploration failure rate even higher, at 70% to 90%. An estimated 25,000 to 50,000 new cases of FBSS occur in the United States each year. The severity of FBSS and its resulting disability varies, but it is often sufficiently severe to necessitate either occupational change or early retirement.[6-8]

The diagnostic evaluation of patients presenting with FBSS is a major challenge to both radiologists and surgeons. Clinical assessment is difficult, and the physical signs and sensory symptoms are frequently bizarre. Today MRI has established itself as the diagnostic modality of choice for imaging of the postoperative spine. The multiplanar imaging capability, superior contrast resolution, and excellent tissue characterization are its major advantages. Most recently, Gadolinium-DTPA-enhanced MRI of the spine, combined with noncontrast MRI, has shown heretofore unparalleled sensitivity and accuracy.[4,5,9]

The most important causes of FBSS are recurrent disk herniation, postoperative fibrosis with scar formation, lateral spinal stenosis, archnoiditis, pseudarthrosis, and postoperative infection.

Postoperative Scar

Postoperative scar usually presents as an extradural mass of irregular configuration, with unsharp margination and, typically, without any contiguity to the disk. Located along the path of surgery, it presumably arises as a result of tissue insult. Absence of mass effect displacing neural structures away from the scar is fairly characteristic for scar tissue. Sometimes, however, there is retraction of neural structures towards the scar tissue.[2,5,10]

The signal intensity characteristics of nonenhanced scar tissue depend on many factors: scar morphology, fat content, age of the scar, vascularity, its specific location, inflammation, and technical factors. Newly formed scar, or scar in the immediate postoperative period, consists of budding granulation tissue, which has high signal intensity on T2-weighted images. As scar tissue ages with time, it develops a relative preponderance of fibrous elements. As this occurs, the scar acquires signal intensity characteristics similar to those of other fibrous tissue in the body, and it becomes hypointense on both T1- and T2-weighted images. Scar morphology and volume seem to affect its signal intensity. When scar appears mostly in strands of tissue, it tends to have low signal intensity on both T1- and T2-weighted images. However, mass or band-like scars more often demonstrate intermediate signal intensity on T1- and T2-weighted images. Some investigators, who believe that the location of scar influences its signal intensity, have stated that there is a difference between anterior scar and posterior scar, with laterally placed scar somewhere in between the two. Anterior scar, for unknown reasons, maintains high signal intensity on T2-weighted images over a long time period, while posterior scar becomes fibrotic as it ages, as described above.[3,10,11]

The administration of Gd-DTPA shows characteristic enhancement of this abnormal epidural soft tissue on early images, those made six to ten minutes postinjection.[4,5,9] This presence of early enhancement is one of the major criteria used to distinguish scar from recurrent disk herniation. It is postulated that scar enhances early because of its abundant vascularity. Histologically, in the immediate postoperative period, scars consists of an abundance of small capillaries interspersed between a stroma of collagen and fibroblasts. For 30 to 45 minutes postinjection, this enhancement continues, with the high signal intensity of scar becoming more homogeneous, presumably as a result of equal filling of the extravascular spaces within the fibrous tissue.

Recurrent Disk Herniation

The intervertebral disk consists of three distinct parts—the cartilaginous endplate, the annulus fibrosus, and the nucleus pulposus. On T1-weighted images, the normal intervertebral disk has a central portion of intermediate signal intensity and a peripheral portion of decreased signal intensity. On T2-weighted images, the central portion becomes hyperintense while the peripheral portion remains of low signal intensity.

Differentiation of epidural fibrosis from herniated disk is crucial, because reoperation on scar unaccompanied by disk material often leads to a poor surgical result.[2,4,7,9] Disk herniations are characterized by a focal extension of the disk beyond the margins of adjacent endplates, and may be central, lateral, or both. The criteria used to identify abnormal disks are the same as for scar—morphologic, epidural location, and the presence or absence of mass effect. Morphologically, the diagnosis of recurrent disk herniation is made when there is a discrete, focal, globular, smooth, and sharply marginated posterior protrusion of aberrant soft tissue contiguous with the parent disk. Recurrent herniated disk typically appears as isointense on T1-weighted images, and hyperintense on T1- or T2*-weighted images when compared to the parent disk. On T1-weighted images, the disk is contrasted sharply with hyperintense extradural fat and the hypointense thecal sac. On T2-weighted images, it is contrasted with the hyperintense thecal sac. Presence of mass effect with displacement of normal tissues is considered to be typical of disk. The sagittal imaging plane is more sensitive for defining deformities of the thecal sac at the disk-thecal sac interface. Axial images are used to evaluate neural foramina and nerve root compression in cases of lateral or posterolateral disk herniation. Sometimes, the path of extruded nuclear material is outlined on axial T2-weighted images, the so-called diskogram effect.

Following Gd-DTPA injection, there is no enhancement of the intervertebral disk on early T1-weighted images, in contrast to the early enhancement of scar tissue. However, signal enhancement is the rule in delayed, 30- to 45-minute postinjection imaging. The signal intensity of gadolinium-enhanced disk generally does not become as high as that of enhanced scar, and tends to remain inhomogeneous. However, to avoid any confusion, early imaging is performed to differentiate scar from disk on the basis of enhancement. The lack of early enhancement of the intervertebral disk is attributed to its relative avascularity. As disk has a voluminous extracellular space and an almost negligible intravascular space, late enhancement is presumed to result from the diffusion of contrast into the disk from surrounding vascular tissues.[4,5,9,10] The characteristics of early Gd-DTPA enhancement, in conjunction with the other characteristics—morphological features, presence of mass effect, and its epidural location—should be used as the major criteria in distinguishing recurrent disk herniation from postoperative scar.

Fusion Complications

The place of spinal fusion in the treatment of intervertebral joint disease remains controversial. Still, many spinal fusions are performed each year for mechanical or segmental instability, and, of these patients, about 30% to 40% experience recurrent or persistent pain.[6-8] Spinal fusion, a surgical procedure, consists of placing a bone graft across a spinal segment in order to eliminate motion across that spinal segment. As the graft is incorporated, the spinal motion decreases and finally ceases.

The appearance of bone grafts on MRI depends partly on the initial status of their bone marrow.[2,12] They have a variable appearance. Iliac autografts usually show high signal intensity on T1-weighted images because of the presence of fatty bone marrow. Allografts will usually show low signal intensity on T1- and T2-weighted images. The margins of the bone grafts are well-defined, linear areas of low signal intensity on both T1- and T2-weighted images, representing cortical bone. Other factors that influence graft appearance are the extent of trauma involved in the surgical procedure, the postoperative stress placed on the fusion mass, and the amount of revascularization.

Persistent lumbar instability is a frequent cause of recurrent postoperative back pain in patients who have undergone lumbar fusion. Segmental instability is difficult to detect clinically, especially in patients with multiple back surgeries, where symptoms might be related to other common causes of FBSS. While conventional radiography and computed tomography are excellent tools for evaluation of structural integrity, that is, they confirm the presence of a firm attachment of an unbroken bone graft, they cannot be used to evaluate functional integrity. Functional integrity means that levels intended to be fused move as a one unit, not as separate segments. One of the major advantages of MRI of the postoperative spine is that it makes it possible to differentiate stable from unstable fusions and, thus, makes repair possible.[2,12] These MRI changes appear as a result of events related to the amount of stress placed on vertebrae above and below the fusion. They typically require 12 months or more to develop fully. In clinical instability, the spine, under physiologic loads, is no longer able to maintain the relationships between vertebrae. This instability leads to irritation of the spinal cord or roots, or to the development of incapacitating deformities. The vertebral bodies at the level of stable spinal fusions have increased signal intensity on T1-weighted images, as result of fatty marrow conversion of the subchondral bone at the corresponding levels. These changes reflect decreased vertebral biomechanical stress. Fusion instability is demonstrated by a band of low signal intensity on T1-weighted images adjacent to the endplates, and an increase in signal intensity with progressive T2-weighting. These changes are presumed to result from reparative granulation tissue, inflammation, edema, and hyperemic changes in the unstable fusion.[12]

MRI appears to be unique in its assessment of functional fusion stability. It is probably most useful in symptomatic patients with post-fusion pseudarthrosis, in whom both CT and conventional radiography fail to demonstrate any anatomic disruption.

References

1. Bobman SA, Atlas SW, Listerud J, et al: Postoperative lumbar spine: Contrast-enhanced chemical shift MR imaging. *Radiology* 1991;179:557-562.
2. Chafetz N, Lang P, Genant HK: Assessment of the postoperative spine by magnetic resonance, in Genant HK (ed): *Spine Update*. Radiology Research and Education Foundation, University Press, 1987, pp 273-283.
3. Hochhauser L, Kieffer SA, Cacayorin ED, et al: Recurrent postdiskectomy low back pain: MR-surgical correlation. *Am J Roentgenol* 1988;151:755-760.
4. Hueftle MG, Modic MT, Ross JS, et al: Lumbar spine: Postoperative MR imaging with Gd-DTPA. *Radiology* 1988;167:817-824.
5. Ross JS, Delamarter R, Hueftle MG, et al: Gadolinium-DTPA-enhanced MR imaging of the postoperative lumbar spine: Time course and mechanism of enhancement. *AJR Am J Roentgenol* 1989;152:825-834.
6. Burton CV: Causes of failure of surgery on the lumbar spine: Ten-year follow-up. *Mt Sinai J Med* 1991;58:183-187.
7. Burton CV: Clinical review of the failed back surgery syndrome, in Genant HK (ed): *Spine Update*. Radiology Research and Education Foundation, University Press, 1987, pp 247-252.
8. Burton CV, Kirkaldy-Willis WH, Yong-Hing, et al: Causes of failure of surgery on the lumbar spine. *Clin Orthop* 1981;157:191-199.
9. Glickstein MF, Sussman SK: Time-dependent scar enhancement in magnetic resonance imaging of the postoperative lumbar spine. *Skeletal Radiol* 1991;20:333-337.
10. Sotiropoulos S, Chafetz NI, Lang P, et al: Differentiation between postoperative scar and recurrent disc herniation: Prospective comparison of MR, CT, and contrast-enhanced CT. *AJNR* 1989;10:639-643.
11. Stoller DW, Genant HK, Lang P: The spine, in Stoller DW, Genant HK, Helms CA, et al (eds): *Magnetic Resonance Imaging in Orthopaedics and Rheumatology*. Philadelphia, JB Lippincott, 1989, pp 322-375.
12. Lang P, Chafetz N, Genant HK, et al: Lumbar spinal fusion: Assessment of functional stability with magnetic resonance imaging. *Spine* 1990;15:581-588.

Sonography of Tendons: Patterns of Disease

Marnix van Holsbeeck, MD

Joseph H. Introcaso, MD, DMD

Patricia A. Kolowich, MD

Introduction

Until recently the diagnosis of tendon disease has been based solely on clinical examination. The superficial location of many tendons, such as those of the hand and wrist, facilitates clinical diagnosis. Techniques such as xeroradiography and computed tomography (CT) have had little impact on the diagnosis of tendon abnormalities.[1] Invasive techniques, such as arthrography and tendonography, are able to address a limited number of very specific problems, but cannot be applied to all tendons. Arthroscopy is clearly the gold standard for articular evaluation, but, because of their extra-articular location, almost all tendons are inaccessible to the arthroscope. The notable exceptions to this are the tendons of the rotator cuff of the shoulder.

Recently, magnetic resonance imaging (MRI) and ultrasound have emerged as powerful tools in the evaluation of tendon pathology.[1-7] Improvements in ultrasound transducer technology and digital signal processing have greatly enhanced resolution of ultrasound images. At the same time MRI surface coils have been developed to facilitate imaging of joints and periarticular structures of the extremities. Significant differences exist between MRI and ultrasound with regard to image characteristics and method of examination. MRI is a static examination in many ways. It requires large stationary magnets weighing up to 9 tons, greatly limiting access. In addition, the fact that the patient must remain motionless during the examination precludes examination of a joint or extremity throughout its normal range of motion.[8] MRI generates images based on the chemical composition of tissues, largely relying on the mobile protons of water molecules to obtain its signal. Images produced using MRI have excellent soft tissue contrast, but are of limited use in the evaluation of compact bone and tendon structure.

Ultrasound produces images of anatomic structures based on reflectivity and acoustic impedance. This provides excellent imaging of soft tissue structures and the surface of cortical bone, but will not demonstrate medullary bone or cortical bone thickness. When applied to evaluation of soft tissue structures, such as tendons, ultrasound has many advantages over MRI.[8] The small size of the equipment makes it more accessible. Ultrasound machines are inexpensive, easily transportable, and do not have special power requirements.

The relatively small cost of ultrasound examinations increases access in several ways. Ultrasound examinations are one third to one tenth the cost of MRI. Also, the ease of transport of ultrasound equipment permits the machine to be moved to the outpatient clinic, where imaging examinations may be performed at the time of the initial clinical evaluation. Examination time is much shorter for ultrasound than for MRI. Most ultrasound examinations can be completed within 10 minutes. In addition, ultrasound is a real-time imaging modality that allows visualization of structures throughout their range of motion during both active and passive mobilization. In many cases this reveals lesions that are occult on static MRI images. Rapid comparison with the contralateral extremity is also possible, without sacrificing image resolution or greatly increasing the length of the examination. Unlike MRI, patients with cardiac pacemakers may be examined without risk, and orthopaedic implants do not degrade images. These factors make ultrasound ideal for the evaluation of tendon pathology.

Examination of the musculoskeletal system is best performed with high frequency transducers (7.5, 10, 15, or 25 MHz).[9] Image resolution is proportional to transducer frequency; that is, image resolution increases as transducer frequency is increased. However, the ability of the sound beam to penetrate the tissues decreases as transducer frequency is increased. Therefore, the best transducer for imaging a tendon will have the highest frequency that is able to penetrate to the desired depth. Superficial tendons of the hand and the Achilles tendon may be examined using 15 or 25 MHz transducers.

Tendons are composed of regularly arranged collagen fibers. The ultrasound beam is reflected at interfaces of these collagen bundles, producing a striated pattern (Fig. 1) of alternating bright echogenic and dark hypoechoic bands. A greater number of striations are evident with higher frequency transducers.[9] MRI is unable to demonstrate the internal architecture of tendons with the detail provided by ultrasound. Because of their highly regular architectural pattern of collagen bundles, tendons exhibit a property referred to as anisotropy.[10] Anisotropic tissues display different properties, depending on the angle from which they are observed. Therefore, proper sonographic evaluation of tendons must be performed with the path of the incident sound beam perpendicular to the long axis of the

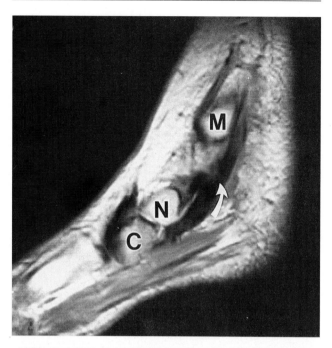

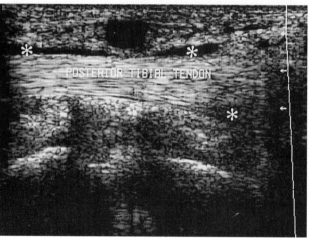

Fig. 1 **Top,** MRI image of the normal posterior tibial tendon. Tendons are of low signal intensity on MRI images. Internal tissue structure cannot be recognized. Posterior tibial tendon (curved arrow); Cuneiform (C); Navicular (N); Medial malleolus (M). **Bottom,** Ultrasound image of the normal posterior tibial tendon. Ultrasound produces images of anatomic structures based on reflectivity and acoustic impedance. The tendon sheath appears as a hypoechoic sac surrounding the tendon (asterisks). The image of the tendon consists of alternating bright echogenic and dark hypoechoic bands. These bands are created by reflection of the ultrasound beam at the interfaces of the collagen bundles. Changes in this striated pattern in pathologic tendons correlate well with microscopic damage in the tendon substance.

tendon. Oblique imaging will result in a falsely hypoechoic appearance of the tendon, leading to an incorrect diagnosis.

Shoulder

Normal tendons of the rotator cuff appear as a hyperechoic band covering the humeral head, deep to the deltoid. Beginning at the age of 20 years, slowly progressing degenerative changes occur in the rotator cuff, and these changes can be observed sonographically. The tendons demonstrate a diffuse decrease in echogenicity. These changes progress gradually, and by the age of 50 years the cuff is isoechoic or possibly hypoechoic relative to the deltoid muscle. Thickening of the subacromial-subdeltoid bursa, biceps tendon, and sheath are also frequent findings in aging shoulders. The incidence of rotator cuff tears also increases with age.[6,7] Of patients who come in for evaluation of cuff tears, 50% have tears larger than 4 cm in greatest dimension with the tendons fully retracted beneath the acromion. Sonographically, these lesions appear as nonvisualization of the rotator cuff beneath the deltoid, a finding well documented in the literature.[6,8,11] Herniation of the deltoid muscle into the tendon defect may also be observed.[8] Classic criteria for diagnosis of rotator cuff tears are complete absence of the cuff and focal defects that involve the entire cross section of the tendon.[6] These defects are noted during transverse and longitudinal scanning of the cuff tendons.

The introduction of ultrasound as an accurate noninvasive screening test for the detection of rotator cuff pathology is intended to reduce the number of patients who present for treatment with the findings of severe end-stage disease. For this reason, we feel that the classic criteria for sonographic diagnosis of rotator cuff tears must be refined. These new criteria will be discussed below. In 1991, 72 of our shoulder ultrasound patients were evaluated surgically. Using our new criteria, we diagnosed full-thickness tears with a sensitivity of 100% and specificity of 97%. In this same group, 18 partial-thickness tears confirmed at surgery were diagnosed with a sensitivity and specificity of 94%. These numbers have not been equaled by MRI. Recent MRI studies[12] have reverted to introducing gadolinium into the joint in an attempt to improve their statistics in detection of partial tears. However, this MR arthrogram appears counterproductive, in that it turns a noninvasive diagnostic test into a longer, more expensive, invasive test.

Small full-thickness tears of the rotator cuff may be smaller than the beam width of the transducer, therefore making them visible in only one imaging plane. This is analogous to a transverse type II fracture of the odontoid process of C2, which is very often occult on transverse axial CT imaging. Figure 2 illustrates this principle. A horizontal tear—by far the most common type of small full-thickness tear of the rotator cuff—is the earliest phase of an impingement tear. The tendon fibers are separated from the greater tuberosity and withdrawn, uncovering the tuberosity. We refer to this as the "naked tuberosity sign" (Fig. 3). The tendon ends abruptly, terminating short of the lateral-most extent of the greater tuberosity, unlike the normal

HORIZONTAL TEAR

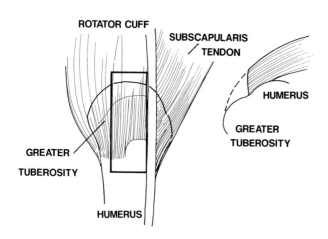

Fig. 2 Small horizontal full-thickness tear (diagram). The diagram on the left shows the most common type of small full-thickness tear as seen by the surgeon. It is a lateral view on the supraspinatus after the deltoid has been removed. The rectangle shows the transducer positioned longitudinally over the supraspinatus tendon. The drawing on the right illustrates the sonographic appearance of this tear during longitudinal scanning. The tendon fibers are separated from the greater tuberosity and withdrawn, uncovering the tuberosity.

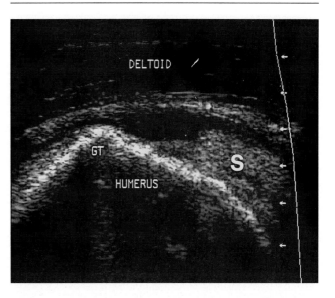

Fig. 3 Small horizontal full-thickness tear. The supraspinatus tendon (S) withdraws from the greater tuberosity (GT) and leaves the bone uncovered ("naked tuberosity sign").

insertion of the tendon, which tapers smoothly to meet the lateral-most extent of the greater tuberosity. Coronal scanning often demonstrates this subtle abnormality; transverse imaging fails to demonstrate the lesion. The degree of medial retraction of the torn

end of the tendon can accurately be assessed sonographically to the level of the acromion and is an important factor in determining the operability and surgical approach.

The less common type of small, full-thickness tears are those that extend vertically (Fig. 4), parallel to the fibers of the supraspinatus tendon. As expected, these lesions are most easily detected on transverse imaging.

VERTICAL TEAR

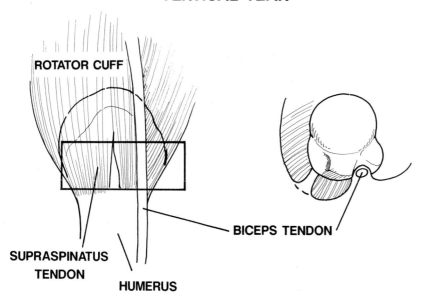

Fig. 4 Small vertical full-thickness tear (diagram). Some traumatic tears extend vertically in the supraspinatus along the collagen bundles of the tendon. The diagram on the left shows the surgeon's view of a vertical tear. The figure on the right is the sonographic appearance of this abnormality. These tears are best seen during transverse scanning and may be overlooked on longitudinal images. The transducer position is indicated by the rectangle.

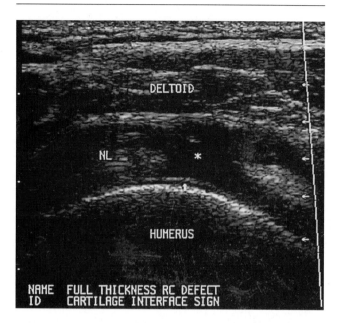

Fig. 5 Small vertical full-thickness tear. The tendon defect of small vertical tears often fill with fluid (asterisk). The articular cartilage surface of the humeral head (small arrow) is then very clearly demonstrated. Normal (NL) supraspinatus tendon is seen at the margins of the tear.

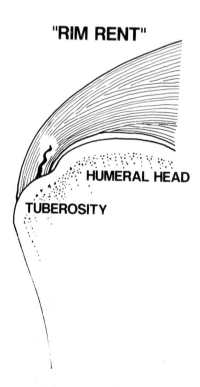

Fig. 6 Partial-thickness tear of the rotator cuff (diagram). Partial-thickness tears are typically located at the undersurface of the supraspinatus. A hyperechoic retracted bundle of fibers is surrounded by a hypoechoic segment in the tendon. This decreased echogenicity likely represents edema within the tendon.

Patients with vertical tears often give a history of a single traumatic event resulting in symptoms. Fluid usually fills the defect and provides an excellent sonographic window for demonstration of the articular cartilage of the humeral head. This results in very sharp delineation of the cartilage surface. We refer to this as the "cartilage interface sign" (Fig. 5). The fluid that fills the defect is often hemorrhagic in nature, attributable to the inciting trauma.

Partial-thickness tears of the rotator cuff are frequently identified at the medial aspect of the greater tuberosity, along the undersurface of the cuff.[13] A small amount of hypoechoic or anechoic fluid is usually seen within the tendon defect. Retracted torn tendon fibers form hyperechoic bundles along the margins of the lesion. We apply the term "rim rent" (Figs. 6 and 7) to describe these lesions, which correspond to the original pathologic description of Codman.[14] Typical patients having this type of tear are in their late 20s or early 30s. Their symptoms, localized pain and tenderness at the site of the lesion, may continue for weeks or even months.

Knee

Tendinitis involving the knee is a common affliction of athletes. Anterior knee pain may be the result of either quadriceps or patellar tendinitis. Medial knee pain in runners may be the result of pes anserine tendinitis. Biceps femoris tendinitis will cause pain at the posterolateral aspect of the knee. Patients with tendinitis of the knee present with localized pain and tenderness. Depending on the location, the pain syndrome may mimic patellofemoral or meniscal disease. Thus,

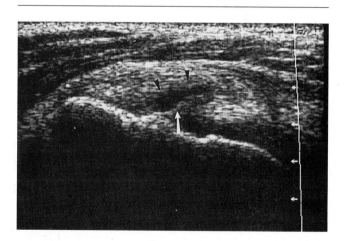

Fig. 7 Partial-thickness tear of the supraspinatus. The hyperechoic lesion (arrow) in the deep aspect of the tendon is suggestive of a retracted collagen fiber bundle. Surrounding decreased echogenicity (arrowheads) corresponds to synovial fluid.

the clinical picture may be misleading. These lesions are often missed on MRI because of the "Magic Angle Phenomenon"[15] and the lack of optimal left-right comparison. Tendinitis cannot be confirmed by arthroscopic examination because it is extra-articular.

Tendinitis is diagnosed sonographically by increased dimension and decreased echogenicity of the tendon. The diameter of the tendon may more than double. Unlike tenosynovitis of the hand and wrist, these lesions represent microscopic damage to tendon fibers and should be regarded as small intrasubstance tears. The best known example is patellar tendinitis, jumper's knee.[16] Patients present with pain and swelling over the anterior knee.[5] Classic sonographic findings[11] are swelling of the patellar tendon adjacent to the patellar apex, best demonstrated on longitudinal images. This proximal location coincides with the most common site of patellar tendon rupture (Fig. 8). Transverse images reveal the swelling to be nodular, involving the central portion of the tendon.[8,11] Distal patellar tendinitis and quadriceps tendinitis may also result in anterior knee pain, but are much less common. When present, they are usually the result of trauma or a sports-related injury. However, quadriceps tendinitis and rupture[8] are increasingly seen in patients who have undergone knee replacement surgery. Two other types of tendinitis—distal biceps and pes anserine tendinitis—are noteworthy because of difficulty in diagnosing these entities clinically.[8,11] These entities are rare but are often misdiagnosed. Athletes are most often affected,

but these lesions may also be found in obese patients. Biceps tendinitis occurs focally at the insertion of the biceps tendon on the fibular head. The distal 1 to 2 cm of the tendon are swollen and decreased in echogenicity, signs best appreciated by comparison with the contralateral extremity. Similarly, pes anserine tendinitis is characterized by swelling and decreased echogenicity of the insertion on the anteromedial aspect of the tibia. The semitendinosus insertion often shows the greatest degree of involvement. When treated with local injection of steroids, these lesions often progress to rupture.

Ankle

Chronic ankle pain most frequently originates from extra-articular structures. Pain is often caused by inflammation of tendons, tendon sheaths, or bursae. The Achilles tendon lacks a synovial tendon sheath. Pain localized over the Achilles tendon is usually accompanied by local swelling. Two distinct types of Achilles tendinitis can be identified—proximal and distal.[11] Proximal tendinitis is characterized by segmental swelling of the tendon approximately 6 cm proximal to its insertion on the calcaneus. This is a degenerative type of tendinitis, which tends to become symptomatic during the fourth decade of life. The location of this proximal lesion coincides precisely with the most common site of Achilles tendon rupture.[3,11] Distal tendinitis is seen in younger patients, some of whom report a remote trauma as the inciting factor. These lesions are observed sonographically to involve the distal-most extent of the Achilles tendon. Retrocalcaneal bursitis is often an associated sonographic finding.[11]

Traumatic injury of the tendons at the medial and lateral aspects of the ankle is less commonly encountered. Inversion and eversion injuries usually tear the collateral ligaments of the ankle, but on rare occasions tendons may also be involved. The posterior tibial and peroneus tendons are most commonly involved.[8,11] Prolonged ankle pain following inversion or eversion injury with medial or lateral point tenderness raises suspicion of tendon injury.[17-19] Predisposing factors include rheumatoid arthritis, diabetes, obesity, and steroid use.

Tears of the peroneus and posterior tibial tendons typically follow the long axis of the tendon.[11] These lesions are well demonstrated sonographically. Different cleavage planes are often identified (Fig. 9).[20] Tears may follow the course of the tendon and split the tendon apart, resulting in a frayed appearance. This is often seen in obese women (Fig. 10). Transverse tears, which are usually the result of more severe trauma, may be seen isolated or after closed ankle fracture (Fig. 11). Supramalleolar and inframalleolar ruptures occur with equal frequency.[20]

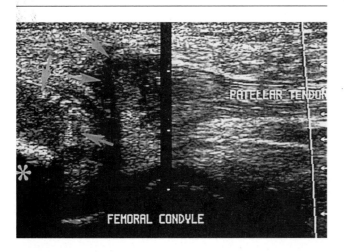

Fig. 8 Patellar tendon rupture. Split-screen image of a ruptured patellar tendon. The patient was a basketball player with recurrent episodes of patellar tendinitis and sudden onset of knee pain prior to admission. The intact distal patellar tendon is seen at the right. The left side of the split screen shows the retracted end of the ruptured tendon (arrows). The rupture occurred just distal to the patellar apex (asterisk). This is the most common location for patellar tendon rupture.

POSTERIOR TIBIAL TENDON

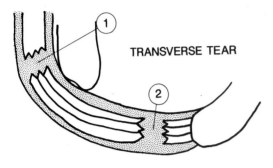

TRANSVERSE TEAR

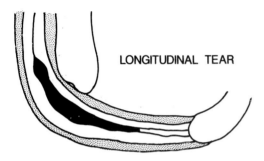

LONGITUDINAL TEAR

Fig. 9 Patterns of posterior tibial tendon rupture (diagram). Tears of the ankle tendons may be transverse or longitudinal. Acute traumatic posterior tibial tendon tears are often transverse. In our patient population these tears occur in supramalleolar and infra-malleolar locations with equal frequency (Sites 1 and 2). Degenerative type tears are common in the posterior tibial tendon. The orientation of these tears is most frequently longitudinal.

Conservative treatment fails in these patients. These lesions are often well treated surgically, sometimes requiring tendoplasty with the flexor digitorum tendon. If the tendon is greatly retracted, triple arthrodesis of the foot may be the only surgical correction possible. If unrecognized, these lesions will lead to a painful flatfoot deformity. Abnormal stress placed on the subtalar joint will result in joint destruction resembling a neuropathic joint. Ultrasound is not only useful in diagnosis of these tendon tears, but is also accurate in measuring the degree of retraction, allowing better preoperative planning.

In addition to rupture, tendinitis and tenosynovitis may affect the peroneus and posterior tibial tendons.[8,11,20] Increased fluid may be detected within the synovial sheath of the tendon. This can be treated effectively by simple casting. However, swelling and decreased echogenicity of these tendons is histologically similar to the intrasubstance tears demonstrated in the patellar tendon. Conservative treatment of these lesions often fails. Sonography accurately distinguishes between these two entities.

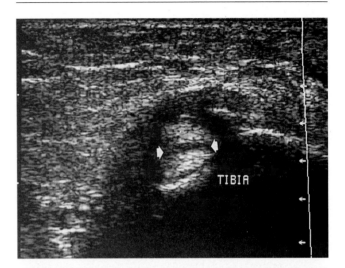

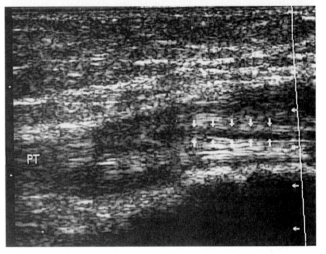

Fig. 10 **Top**, Longitudinal tear of the posterior tibial tendon. This transverse image shows that the tendon is split down the middle. The tear appears hypoechoic (arrows). **Bottom**, Longitudinal tear of the posterior tibial tendon. This longitudinal image shows a split (arrows) in the tendon (PT). The tear extends along the long axis of the tendon.

Conclusion

Tendon disease is among the most common causes of chronic pain in athletes. A large number of individuals are increasing their level of physical activity to improve their overall health. As a result, the incidence of tendon disease is increasing markedly. Ultrasound provides an accurate, noninvasive, cost-effective method of diagnosis. It affords better treatment planning and can be used for follow-up to determine when a patient may safely return to a normal level of activity.

References

1. Cheung Y, Rosenberg ZS, Magee T, et al: Normal anatomy and pathologic conditions of ankle tendons: Current imag-

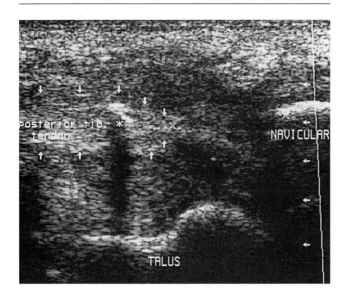

Fig. 11 Transverse tear of the posterior tibial tendon. A hypoechoic gap is noted in the distal aspect of the inframalleolar posterior tibial tendon. The proximal tendon is separated from the navicular attachment (x) along with an osseous fragment (asterisk).

ing techniques. *Radiographics* 1992;12:429-444.

2. Fornage BD, Rifkin MD, Touche DH, et al: Sonography of the patellar tendon: Preliminary observations. *AJR* 1984;143:179-182.

3. Fornage BD: Achilles tendon: US examination. *Radiology* 1986;159:759-764.

4. Kalebo P, Allenmark C, Peterson L, et al: Diagnostic value of ultrasonography in partial ruptures of the Achilles tendon. *Am J Sports Med* 1992;20:378-381.

5. Karlsson J, Kalebo P, Goksor LA, et al: Partial rupture of the patellar ligament. *Am J Sports Med* 1992;20:390-395.

6. Mack LA, Nyberg DA, Matsen FA III: Sonographic evalua-tion of the rotator cuff. *Radiol Clin North Am* 1988;26:161-177.

7. Middleton WD, Reinus WR, Totty WG, et al: Ultra-sonographic evaluation of the rotator cuff and biceps ten-don. *J Bone Joint Surg* 1986;68A:440-450.

8. van Holsbeeck M, Introcaso JH: Musculoskeletal ultrasonog-raphy. *Radiol Clin North Am* 1992;30:907-925.

9. Martinoli C, Cittadini G Jr, Pastorino C, et al: High-resolu-tion US of tendon echostructure: Normal findings and pathologic changes. *Radiology* 1992;185(suppl):144.

10. Rubin JM, Carson PL, Meyer CR: Anisotropic ultrasonic backscatter from the renal cortex. *Ultrasound Med Biol* 1988;14:507-511.

11. van Holsbeeck M, Introcaso JH: Sonography of tendons, in van Holsbeeck M: *Musculoskeletal Ultrasound*. St. Louis, Mosby Year Book, 1991.

12. Hodler J, Kursunoglu-Brahme S, Snyder SJ, et al: Rotator cuff disease: Assessment with MR arthrography versus stan-dard MR imaging in 36 patients with arthroscopic confirma-tion. *Radiology* 1992;182:431-436.

13. van Holsbeeck M, Kolowich PA, Introcaso JH: Sonographic appearance of partial-thickness tears of the rotator cuff. *Radiology* 1992;185(suppl):144.

14. Codman EA: *The Shoulder: Rupture of the Supraspinatus Tendon and Other Lesions in or About the Subacromial Bursa*. Boston, Thomas Todd, 1934.

15. Erickson SJ, Cox IH, Hyde JS, et al: Effect of tendon orienta-tion on MR imaging signal intensity: A manifestation of the "magic angle" phenomenon. *Radiology* 1991;181:389-392.

16. Martens M, Wouters P, Burssens A, et al: Patellar tendinitis: Pathology and results of treatment. *Acta Orthop Scand* 1982;53:445-450.

17. Downey DJ, Simkin PA, Mack LA, et al: Tibialis posterior tendon rupture: A cause of rheumatoid flat foot. *Arthritis Rheum* 1988;31:441-446.

18. Kerry HD: Posterior tibial tendon rupture. *Ann Emerg Med* 1988;17:649-650.

19. Mueller TJ: Rupture and lacerations of the tibialis posterior tendon. *J Am Podiatr Assoc* 1984;74:109-119.

20. van Holsbeeck M, Katcherian D, Wu KK, et al: Patterns of posterior tibial tendon abnormality. *Radiology* 1992;185 (suppl):143-144.

Magnetic Resonance Imaging Studies of the Shoulder: Diagnosis of Lesions of the Rotator Cuff

Michael P. Recht, MD

Donald Resnick, MD

Shoulder pain can result from instability, abnormalities involving the bicipital tendon, ischemic necrosis of bone, degenerative osteoarthrosis, calcific tendinitis, and rotator cuff disorders. Shoulder pain is one of the more frequent medical complaints, and a disorder of the rotator cuff is one of the more common etiologies.[1]

Roentgenograms are useful for the diagnosis of osseous abnormalities and soft-tissue calcification; for identification of the shape of the acromion[2-4]; and for the diagnosis of osseous changes associated with impingement syndrome, such as subacromial enthesophytes (spurs) and flattening and sclerosis of the greater tuberosity of the humerus. In addition, osseous changes believed to be associated with chronic rotator cuff tears, such as a concave depression on the inferior surface of the acromion,[5] an acromiohumeral distance of less than 7 mm, and superior migration of the humeral head, can be visualized on radiographs. However, the rotator cuff cannot be evaluated with the use of radiographs.

Arthrography, which is used most frequently to evaluate rotator cuff tears, has a reported accuracy of 94% to 99%.[6,7] Arthrography is of little value for the detection of partial tears involving the superior (bursal) surface of the rotator cuff, intratendinous tears, or tendinopathy or tendinitis of the rotator cuff.[8] Furthermore, arthrography is an invasive procedure.

Ultrasonography, a non-invasive method, has been used to assess problems related to the rotator cuff; however, clinical studies have demonstrated conflicting results about its accuracy in the diagnosis of rotator cuff tears.[9-11] The quality of the results closely parallels the expertise of the ultrasonographer.[12]

Magnetic resonance imaging (MRI), by virtue of its superior soft-tissue contrast, lack of ionizing radiation, non-invasive nature, and ability to outline structures in multiple planes, has become the primary diagnostic method in the evaluation of joints such as the knee and the temporomandibular joint.[13,14] The role of MRI studies in the evaluation of lesions of the shoulder has not been well defined. This is due in part to controversy and uncertainty regarding the appearance of the normal shoulder on the imaging studies and in part to the technical difficulties of imaging of the shoulder. Recent improvements in the hardware and software, as well as an increased understanding of the normal anatomy of the shoulder, have decreased some of the problems. This should make it possible to conduct clinical studies to further define the role of MRI studies in the evaluation of a patient who has shoulder pain.

This paper includes a review of the technique for obtaining MR images of the shoulder; a discussion of the normal anatomy of the shoulder, as seen on the imaging studies; a description of the images that are representative of lesions of the rotator cuff; and comments on future developments in shoulder imaging.

Technical Considerations

There are three technical problems with regard to MRI of the shoulder. First, the geometry of the magnet bore does not allow the shoulder to be placed in the isocenter of the magnet. This necessitates the use of an off-center field of view, a feature that is standard on the newest scanners. However, because of decreased magnetic-field homogeneity in the periphery of the magnet compared with the magnetic isocenter, specialized sequences that require high magnetic-field homogeneity, such as fat-saturation images, are more difficult to obtain in shoulder imaging than in imaging of areas of the body that can be placed in the magnetic isocenter.

Second, the need for high-resolution images to distinguish adequately between a normal and an abnormal rotator cuff makes use of thin imaging sections with small fields of view (14 to 16 cm) mandatory. The resultant small voxel size leads to a decreased signal-to-noise ratio. In order to maintain an adequate signal-to-noise ratio with such small voxel sizes, it is necessary to use a dedicated shoulder surface coil. The two most commonly used surface-coil designs include paired coils, one placed anterior and one placed posterior to the shoulder in a Helmholtz configuration (Fig. 1, *left*), and a single anterior looped coil configured to fit the shape of the shoulder (Fig. 1, *right*).[15-17]

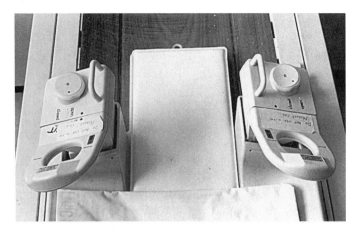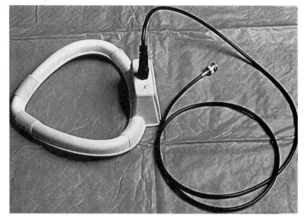

Fig. 1   Surface coil designs. **Left,** Bilateral Helmholtz-type coils (one anterior and one posterior). **Right,** Form-fitted anterior looped coil.

Third, the optimum planes for visualization of the rotator cuff are oblique, not orthogonal. This oblique imaging capability is a standard feature of the new scanners.

Imaging Technique

The patient is placed supine in the coil with the arm at the side. An internally rotated position of the arm, although often the most comfortable for the patient, tends to lead to an overlap of the images of the supraspinatus and infraspinatus tendons, making it difficult to image these tendons in continuity.[18] Because this can simulate a lesion of the rotator cuff, imaging with the humerus in internal rotation should be avoided. External rotation allows the tendons to be more easily visualized in continuity, but this position is often more uncomfortable to the patient, leading to the increased possibility of motion artifacts. Therefore, the arm should be placed with the shoulder in a neutral or slightly externally rotated position. To evaluate the anatomy of the shoulder adequately, it is necessary to image the shoulder in three planes: transaxial, coronal oblique, and sagittal oblique.

The first imaging sequence, in the evaluation of rotator cuff lesions, is a coronal localizer and uses a large field of view (40 cm), which makes it possible to choose the optimum location for the off-center field of view. The second sequence, a gradient-echo sequence obtained in the transaxial plane from the level of the acromion superiorly to the level of the inferior glenoid margin caudally, uses a small field of view (14 to 16 cm) and a 4-mm slice thickness. These images are useful as a screening method in the diagnosis of lesions of the labrum and capsule, for identification of the subscapularis muscle and tendon, for detection of Hill-Sachs deformities, and for assessment of the tendon of

the long head of the biceps in the intertubercular groove. Additionally, the axis of the supraspinatus muscle and tendon is visualized on the transaxial images, and this permits proper positioning of the coronal oblique and sagittal oblique imaging planes.

The coronal oblique imaging plane is chosen to extend parallel to the axis of the supraspinatus muscle and tendon. This is the most important plane for identification of a lesion of the rotator cuff, as the supraspinatus and infraspinatus muscles and tendons are imaged in continuity with their insertion on the greater tuberosity. It also allows for the assessment of the relationship between the supraspinatus tendon and the overlying acromion and acromioclavicular joint. The protocol for evaluation of the rotator cuff includes both T1- and T2-weighted coronal oblique spin-echo sequences with use of a 14-cm field of view and a 4-mm slice thickness.

The final weighting sequence is a sagittal oblique T1- or T2-weighted spin-echo sequence that affords the best view of the supraspinatus outlet, which is the opening between the coracoacromial arch and the glenoid through which the supraspinatus passes to its insertion.[19] It also allows assessment of the shape of the acromion, which has been postulated to play a role in the development of rotator cuff lesions.[20-22]

Anatomy of the Shoulder on MRI

This section delineates some of the basic principles involved in the interpretation of MRI studies. On spin-echo T1-weighted images that have a short repetition time and a short echo time, fat has a high signal intensity, muscle and hyaline cartilage have an intermediate signal intensity, and fluid has a low signal intensity. Conversely, on T2-weighted images, fluid has the highest signal intensity and fat and muscle have an intermediate signal intensity. Structures that lack mobile proteins, such as cortical bone, the fibrous glenoid labrum, and tendons, have a low signal intensity on all of the images.

The transaxial plane is used to evaluate the capsule of the shoulder, including the glenoid labrum, the subscapularis muscle and tendon, the tendon of the long head of the biceps, and the humeral head (Fig. 2). The glenoid labrum is a fibrous structure[23] and it produces a low signal intensity. There is great variability in the shape and configuration of the anterior and posterior aspects of the labrum, although both are most commonly triangular or round.[24] The sites of insertion of the posterior and anterior aspects of the capsule usually are well visualized on the transaxial images. Although the glenohumeral ligaments can occasionally be identified, they are not visualized consistently unless a joint effusion is present.

The insertion of the subscapularis tendon into the lesser tuberosity, and the signal void of the bicipital tendon within the intertubercular groove, can also be identified on transaxial images. A Hill-Sachs lesion, identified as a notched defect of flattening of the humeral head, should be considered to be present only when the flattening is at or proximal to the level of the coracoid process because there is a normal area of flattening on the posterolateral aspect of the humer-

al head at the point of transition to the humeral shaft.[25]

The coronal oblique plane (Fig. 3) is best for identification of the supraspinatus muscle and tendon in their entirety. The infraspinatus and teres minor muscles and tendons are visualized on posterior coronal oblique images. Although the subscapularis muscle and the tendon of the long head of the biceps may be visualized on anterior coronal oblique images, they are more easily visualized on transaxial images. The coracoclavicular, coracohumeral, and coracoacromial ligaments can be visualized in the coronal oblique plane although they cannot always be identified. The coronal oblique plane affords the best visualization of the subacromial-subdeltoid fat plane and bursa.

Anterior coronal oblique images may be used to study the acromioclavicular joint and the relationship of the supraspinatus muscle and tendon to the acromioclavicular joint and the anterior aspect of the acromion. The sagittal oblique plane (Fig. 4), however, allows optimum visualization of the supraspinatus outlet and of the shape of the acromion.

Knowledge of the appearance of the normal anatomy of the shoulder on the images can help to prevent misinterpretation of two areas — the anterior interval and the articular cartilage.[17] An area of increased signal may be seen in the space between the superior bor-

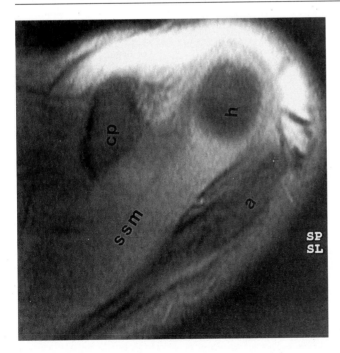

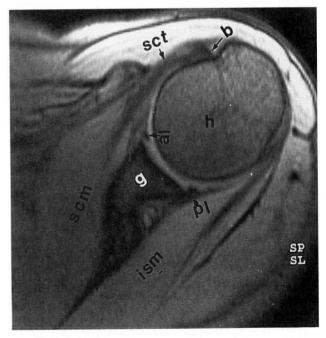

Fig. 2 MRI in the transaxial plane (repetition time, 500 ms; echo time, 13 ms; flip angle, 25°). The images are from cranial to caudal. cp = coracoid process, h = humerus, ssm = supraspinatus muscle, a = acromion, al = anterior aspect of the labrum, b = biceps tendon, g = glenoid, ism = infraspinatus muscle, pl = posterior aspect of the labrum, scm = subscapularis muscle, sct = subscapularis tendon, SP = slice position, and SL = slice thickness.

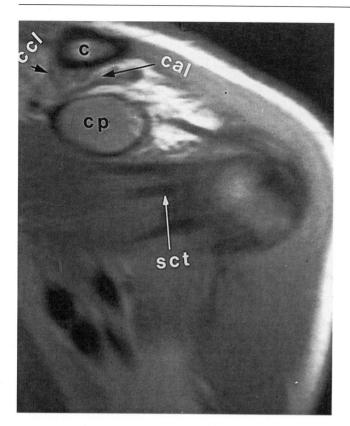
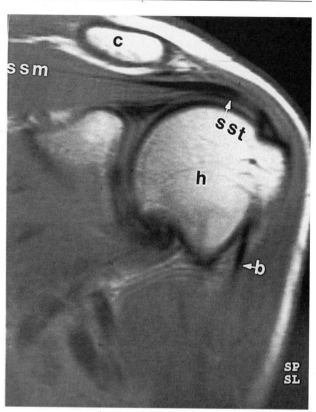

Fig. 3 MRI in the coronal oblique plane (repetition time, 2,000 ms; echo time, 20 ms). The images are from anterior to posterior. c = clavicle, cal = coracoacromial ligament, sct = subscapularis tendon, ccl = coracoclavicular ligament, cp = coracoid process, b = biceps tendon, h = humerus, ssm = supraspinatus muscle, sst = supraspinatus tendon, SP = slice position, and SL = slice thickness.

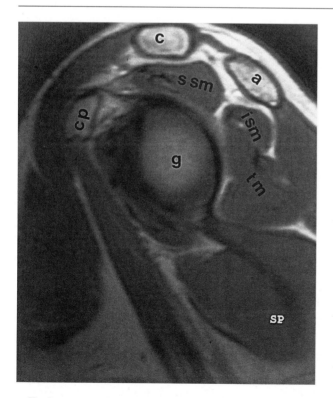
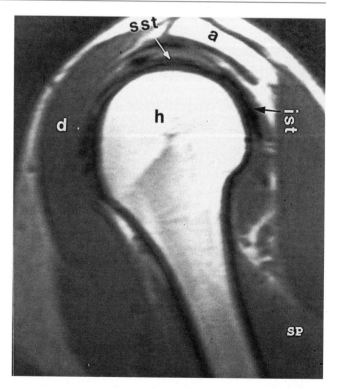

Fig. 4 MRI in the sagittal oblique plane (repetition time, 600 ms; echo time, 20 ms). The images are from medial to lateral. a = acromion, c = clavicle, cp = coracoid process, tm = teres minor muscle, ssm = supraspinatus muscle, g = glenoid, ism= infraspinatus muscle; d = deltoid, h = humerus, ist = infraspinatus tendon, sst = supraspinatus tendon, and SP = slice position.

der of the subscapularis muscle and tendon and the supraspinatus muscle and tendon, and it may be misinterpreted as focally increased signal within the supraspinatus tendon.[26] This area is identified on an anterior coronal oblique slice that includes the supraspinatus tendon, the subscapularis tendon, and the tendon of the long head of the biceps. This appearance is due to the fact that the supraspinatus tendon often curves anteriorly at this site, which may cause it to be partially averaged on the image with membranous tissues that are present in the anterior rotator interval, leading to an increased signal intensity compared with the normal signal intensity of the tendon. This pitfall can be avoided by recognition of the characteristic location of this increased signal; the fact that it is usually confined to one slice; and the fact that, on the T2-weighted images, this signal is of lower intensity than the fluid-like signal intensity seen in most rotator-cuff tears.

Another possible error is the interpretation of the intermediate signal intensity of the articular cartilage of the humeral head as an increased signal within the rotator cuff. Knowledge of the expected location and intensity of the signal within the rotator cuff, and the expected location and intensity of the signal of the articular cartilage, aid in the recognition of this signal as being separate from, and just inferior to, the supraspinatus tendon.

Lesions of the Rotator Cuff

The pathophysiology of disorders of the rotator cuff is controversial. Neer[4,27] popularized the theory that impingement of the supraspinatus tendon, when the arm is raised, between the greater tuberosity of the humerus and the unyielding coracoacromial arch (composed of the acromion, the coracoacromial ligament, the coracoid process, and the acromioclavicular joint) leads to disorders of the rotator cuff. Neer stated that 95% of rotator cuff tears are initiated by impingement.[4] Some authors have believed that the impingement theory is valid because of the association of supraspinatus tendon ruptures with distally pointing osteophytes of the acromioclavicular joint[28] and with variations in acromial shape and slope.[22] Morrison and Bigliani[22] described three distinct acromial shapes: type 1, a flat acromion; type 2, a curved acromion; and type 3, a hooked acromion; they found that the majority (90% to 100%) of rotator cuff tears were seen in patients with a type-2 or a type-3 acromion.[20]

Neer[4] suggested that there were three progressive stages of the impingement syndrome. Stage I consists of edema and hemorrhage, which may result from excessive overhead use in sports or work activities. This stage typically is seen in patients who are younger than 25 years of age and is reversible with conservative ther-

apy. Stage II is characterized by fibrosis and thickening of the supraspinatus tendon, biceps tendon, and subacromial bursa and is a result of chronic inflammation or repeated episodes of impingement.[4,29] This stage is usually seen between the ages of 25 and 40 years and may necessitate surgical intervention if conservative therapy fails. Stage III is marked by a partial or complete tear of the rotator cuff; degeneration or a tear, or both, of the tendon of the long head of the biceps; and secondary osseous changes on the undersurface of the anterior portion of the acromion and greater tuberosity.

Another theory is that rotator cuff disease is the result of degenerative tendinopathy, which presumably develops as a result of ischemia. This theory, initially proposed by Codman,[30-32] was supported by Rathbun and Macnab,[33] who described an area that was relatively avascular where tendon degeneration was first seen and was most extensive. In recent studies, Ozaki and associates[34] and Ogata and Uhthoff[35] also concluded that most rotator cuff tears were a result of an intrinsic degenerative process of the rotator cuff rather than of impingement. They believed this to be the case because of the lack of changes of the undersurface of the acromion in the face of a partial tear of the undersurface of the cuff, the correlation between aging and cuff tears, and the lack of correlation between aging and degenerative changes of the undersurface of the acromion. Ogata and Uhthoff,[35] however, suggested that partial tears, once present, may permit proximal migration of the humeral head, leading to secondary impingement with progression to a full-thickness tear.

It is probable that both impingement and intrinsic tendon degeneration and ischemia contribute to the development of rotator cuff disease.[17] The challenge for MRI studies is the demonstration, not only of complete rotator cuff tears, but also of the earlier changes of rotator cuff tendinopathy and partial tears.

Description of MRI Findings

The normal supraspinatus tendon was described, in early reports, as possessing little or no signal intensity on all imaging sequences.[36-38] Intratendinous signal was therefore considered abnormal and indicative of pathological changes in the rotator cuff. A number of recent studies, however, have demonstrated intermediate signal intensity within the supraspinatus tendon of normal, asymptomatic volunteers (Fig. 5).[39-41] Various explanations for this increased signal have been proposed. They include partial volume-averaging if the tendon is not imaged in continuity[18]; the presence of multiple slips of the supraspinatus tendon, with muscle or soft tissue, or both, interposed between the tendinous slips[40,41]; and the so-called angle phenomenon.[42] The angle phenomenon is observed due to the collagen fibers having a T2 relaxation time dependent on

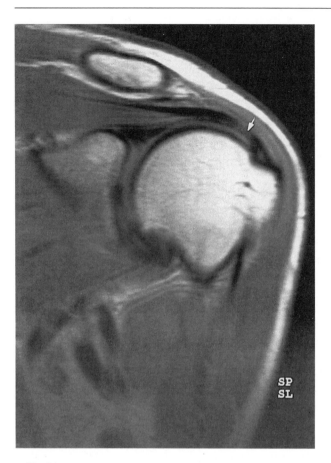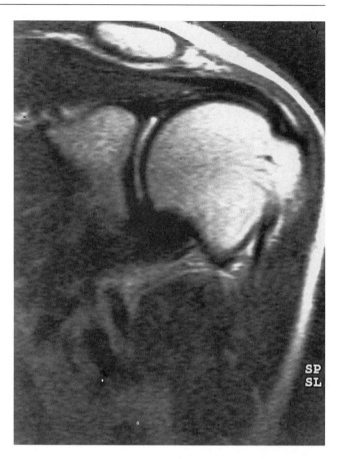

Fig. 5 Signal intensity (arrow) within the supraspinatus tendon of a normal volunteer as seen on a proton density-weighted image, **left** (repetition time, 2,000 ms; echo time, 20 ms) and a T2-weighted image, **right** (repetition time, 2,000 ms; echo time, 80 ms). The intermediate signal intensity on the proton density-weighted image is decreased on the T2-weighted image. The morphology of the supraspinatus tendon is normal. SP = slice position and SL = slice thickness.

their orientation with respect to the main magnetic field. When short echo-time sequences are used to image tendons that are at the angle, defined on the condition $(3 \cos^2\Theta - 1) = 0$, where Θ (55°) is the angle between the static field and the tendon being studied, the tendons demonstrate increased signal. Another explanation for the increased signal intensity in the supraspinatus tendon is the presence of asymptomatic degenerative changes of the tendon.[40] It is clear that the intermediate signal intensity commonly seen within the normal supraspinatus tendon should not be considered pathological unless it is associated with altered tendon morphology, such as thinning or irregularity, or when the intratendinous signal intensity is greater than that of muscle on T2-weighted images.[39,41]

Tendinopathy or tendon degeneration is characterized by abnormal tendon morphology associated with intermediate signal intensity on T1-weighted images and proton-density-weighted images (a long repetition time and a short echo time). On T2-weighted images, this signal can be of intermediate intensity or of decreased intensity, but it should not be of markedly increased intensity (Fig. 6).[36,38,43]

A partial tear of the rotator cuff is seen as a focal area of intermediate signal intensity on T1 and proton-density-weighted images, and as a moderate or marked increase in signal intensity that does not extend through the entire thickness of the tendon on T2-weighted images (Fig. 7).[15-17] Partial tears can involve the articular or bursal surface or they can be intratendinous. Intratendinous tears are difficult to distinguish from tendinitis with active inflammation. The signal abnormality associated with tendinitis is more diffuse than that associated with partial tears.[15] In addition, the increased signal intensity associated with tendinitis is usually oriented horizontally within the tendon, while the increased signal intensity associated with partial tears is usually oriented vertically within the tendon.

Complete tears of the rotator cuff are seen as areas of discontinuity that extend through the entire thickness of the tendon. The defect has increased signal

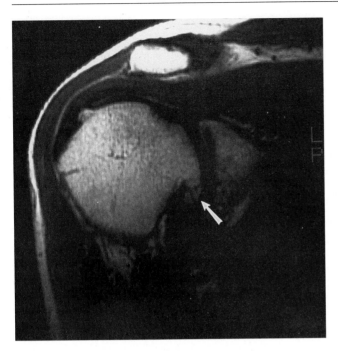 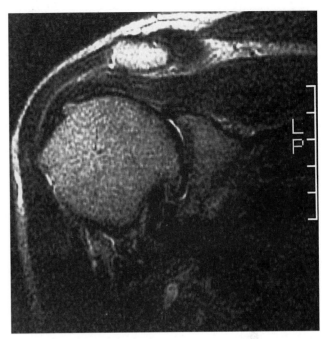

Fig. 6   T1-weighted image, **left** (repetition time, 600 ms; echo time, 20 ms) and T2-weighted image, **right** (repetition time, 2,000 ms; echo time, 90 ms) demonstrating tendinopathy of the supraspinatus tendon. There is intermediate signal intensity within the tendon on the T1-weighted image, associated with thinning of the tendon. The relative signal intensity is decreased on the T2-weighted image. Note the osteophytes arising from the humeral head (arrow).

intensity on T1 and proton-density-weighted images and usually shows a marked increase in signal intensity on T2-weighted images (Fig. 8).[36,38,43] A few complete tears may be visualized as an attenuation and irregularity of the tendon with moderate or low signal intensity on T2-weighted images.[43] The lack of high signal intensity on T2-weighted images may be secondary to scar or granulation tissue having filled the tendon defect. Diagnosis of these tears is made on the basis of marked abnormality of the tendon contour associated with secondary signs, such as retraction of the musculotendinous junction and atrophy of the supraspinatus muscle.[43]

A number of secondary signs, such as fluid in the subacromial-subdeltoid bursa and loss of continuity of the peribursal fat stripe, have been used to differentiate tendon degeneration from partial and small complete tears of the rotator cuff.[38] These signs have been shown to be sensitive but non-specific for rotator cuff tears.

A number of clinical studies have documented the accuracy of magnetic resonance-imaging studies in the diagnosis of rotator cuff lesions.[5,6,36,38,43-47] The sensitivity for the detection of rotator cuff tears has ranged from 69% to 100%, and the specificity has ranged from 88% to 100%.[6,36,44] These studies have also shown excellent correlation for the size of the tears (r = 0.95) and the quality of the torn edges, as confirmed at the time of the operation.[36,43] The usefulness of imaging studies in the assessment of a shoulder after surgery has not been well assessed.

Osseous and soft-tissue changes that are associated with the impingement syndrome, such as subacromial osteophytes, osteophytes on the acromioclavicular joint, and capsular hypertrophy, as well as the shape of the acromion can be assessed with magnetic resonance-imaging studies.[5,17] It is important to remember, however, that shoulder impingement is a clinical diagnosis and the imaging studies cannot be obtained with the shoulder in positions that produce signs of impingement. Therefore, although these studies can be used to diagnose the changes that are associated with impingement syndrome, they cannot be used to make the clinical diagnosis of a shoulder impingement syndrome.

Future Developments

A number of new pulse-sequence designs that may be used in imaging of the shoulder are being tested. These include fat-suppressed and hybrid-RARE (rapid acquisition relaxation-enhancement) images. Fat-suppressed images have been advocated[40] because the suppression of subcutaneous fat helps to decrease respiratory artifacts. In addition, the expansion of the dynamic range that is possible when the high signal of fat is

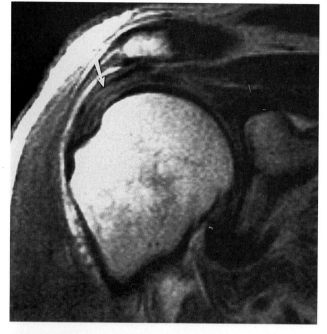

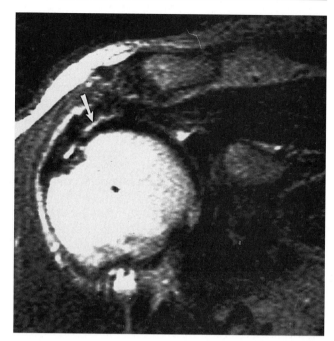

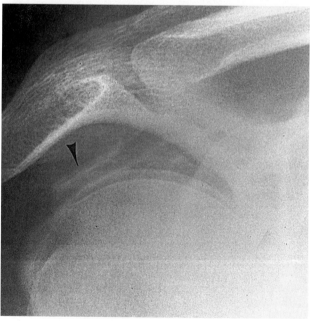

Fig. 7 Partial tear (arrow) of the supraspinatus tendon as seen on a T1-weighted image, **top left** (repetition time, 600 ms; echo time, 20 ms) and a T2-weighted image, **top right** (repetition time, 2,000 ms; echo time, 20 ms). The relative intensity of the signal within the supraspinatus tendon (arrow) is increased on the T2-weighted image. **Bottom,** The partial tear (arrow) seen in the T1- and T2-weighted images was confirmed on double-contrast arthrography.

suppressed improves soft-tissue contrast, making the lesion of the rotator cuff more obvious on the images.

Hybrid-RARE sequences[48] provide T2 weighting in a fraction of the time that is necessary for acquisition of routine spin-echo T2-weighted images. This allows for faster scan times and an increased number of signal acquisitions, thereby decreasing motion artifacts and providing an increased signal-to-noise ratio. Clinical studies comparing both hybrid-RARE and fat-suppressed sequences with standard spin-echo and gradi-

ent-echo sequences are necessary to determine their usefulness in the evaluation of rotator cuff disease.

Magnetic resonance arthrography, accomplished with the intra-articular injection of Gadopentate dimeglumine (gadolinium-diethylenetriamine-acetic acid) is being studied in the evaluation of abnormalities of the rotator cuff, the labrum, and the capsule. Two recent studies[49,50] have demonstrated improvement in the detection of rotator cuff tears, especially partial tears of the articular surface, with this method.

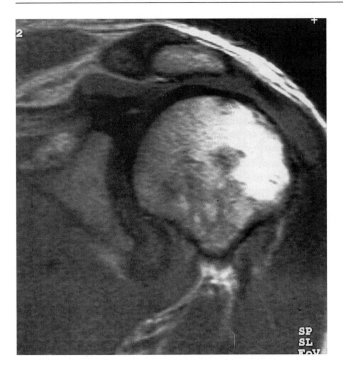 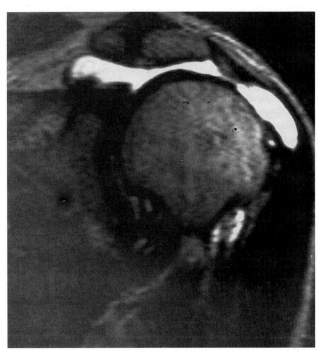

Fig. 8 A large, complete tear of the supraspinatus tendon with muscle atrophy. The T1-weighted image, **left** (repetition time, 550 ms; echo time, 20 ms) and T2-weighted image, **right** (repetition time, 2,000 ms; echo time, 20 ms) demonstrate fluid filling the large gap in the tendon and extending into the subacromial-subdeltoid bursa. There is retraction of the tendon with fatty atrophy of the supraspinatus muscle. SP = slice position and SL = slice thickness.

The disadvantages are that it is an invasive procedure, and the duration of the examination is increased. Additional clinical studies are necessary to determine the role of this method in the evaluation of rotator cuff disease.

References

1. Bonafede RP, Bennet RM: Shoulder pain: Guidelines to diagnosis and management. *Postgrad Med* 1987;82:185-189,192-193.
2. Cone RO III, Resnick D, Danzig L: Shoulder impingement syndrome: Radiographic evaluation. *Radiology* 1984;150:29-33.
3. Kilcoyne RF, Reddy PK, Lyons F, et al: Optimal plain film imaging of the shoulder impingement syndrome. *AJR Am J Roentgenol* 1989;153:795-797.
4. Neer CS II: Impingement lesions. *Clin Orthop* 1983;173:70-77.
5. Seeger LL, Gold RH, Bassett LW, et al: Shoulder impingement syndrome: MR findings in 53 shoulders. *AJR Am J Roentgenol* 1988;150:343-347.
6. Burk DL Jr, Karasick D, Kurtz AB, et al: Rotator cuff tears: Prospective comparison of MR imaging with arthrography, sonography, and surgery. *AJR Am J Roentgenol* 1989;153:87-92.
7. Mink JH, Harris E, Rappaport M: Rotator cuff tears: Evaluation using double-contrast shoulder arthrography. *Radiology* 1985;157:621-623.
8. Resnick D: Shoulder arthrography. *Radiol Clin North Am* 1981;19:243-253.
9. Brandt TD, Cardone BW, Grant TH, et al: Rotator cuff sonography: A reassessment. *Radiology* 1989;173:323-327.
10. Soble MG, Kaye AD, Guay RC: Rotator cuff tear: clinical experience with sonographic detection. *Radiology* 1989;173:319-321.
11. Wiener SN, Seitz WH Jr: Sonography of the shoulder in patients with tears of the rotator cuff: Accuracy and value for selecting surgical options. *AJR Am J Roentgenol* 1993;160:103-107.
12. Mack LA, Matsen FA III, Kilcoyne RF, et al: US evaluation of the rotator cuff. *Radiology* 195;157:205-209.
13. Kursunoglu-Brahme S, Resnick D: Magnetic resonance imaging of the knee. *Orthop Clin North Am* 1990;21:561-572.
14. Rao VM, Farole A, Karasick D: Temporomandibular joint dysfunction: correlation of MR imaging, arthrography, and arthroscopy. *Radiology* 1990;174:663-667.
15. Boorstein JM, Kneeland JB, Dalinka MK, et al: Magnetic resonance imaging of the shoulder. *Curr Probl Diagn Radiol* 1992;21:3-27.
16. Kursunoglu-Brahme S, Resnick D: Magnetic resonance imaging of the shoulder. *Radiol Clin North Am* 1990;28:941-954.
17. Zlatkin MB: *MRI of the Shoulder*, New York, Raven Press, 1991, pp 21-97.
18. Davis SJ, Teresi LM, Bradley WG, et al: Effects of arm rotation on MR imaging of the rotator cuff. *Radiology* 1991;181:265-268.
19. Neer CS II, Poppen NK: Supraspinatus outlet. *Orthop Trans* 1987;11:234.
20. Bigliani LU, Morrison DS, April EW: The morphology of the acromion and its relationship to rotator cuff tears. *Orthop Trans* 1986;10:216.
21. Epstein RE, Schweitzer ME, Frieman BG, et al: Hooked acromion: Prevalence on MR images of painful shoulders. *Radiology* 1993;187:479-481.

22. Morrison DS, Bigliani LU: The clinical significance of variations in acromial morphology. *Orthop Trans* 1987;11:234.

23. Moseley HF, övergaard B: The anterior capsular mechanism in recurrent anterior dislocation of the shoulder. *J Bone Joint Surg* 1962;44B:913-927.

24. Neumann CH, Petersen SA, Jahnke AH: MR imaging of the labral-capsular complex: Normal variations. *AJR Am J Roentgenol* 1991;157:1015-1021.

25. Workman TL, Burkhard TK, Resnick D, et al: Hill-Sachs lesion: Comparison of detection with MR imaging, radiography and arthrography. *Radiology* 1992;185:847-852.

26. Nobuhara K, Ikeda H: Rotator interval lesion. *Clin Orthop* 1987;223:44-50.

27. Neer CS II: Anterior acromioplasty for the chronic impingement syndrome in the shoulder: A preliminary report. *J Bone Joint Surg* 1972;54A:41-50.

28. Petersson CJ, Gentz CF: Ruptures of the supraspinatus tendon: The significance of distally pointing acromioclavicular osteophytes. *Clin Orthop* 1983;174:143-148.

29. Hawkins RJ, Abrams JS: Impingement syndrome in the absence of rotator cuff tear (stages 1 and 2). *Orthop Clin North Am* 197;18:373-382.

30. Codman EA: *The Shoulder: Rupture of the Supraspinatus Tendon and Other Lesions In or About the Subacromial Bursa.* Boston, MA, Thomas Todd, 1934.

31. Codman EA: Rupture of the supraspinatus 1834 to 1934. *J Bone Joint Surg* 1937;19:643-652.

32. Codman EA, Akerson IB: The pathology associated with rupture of the supraspinatus tendon. *Ann Surg* 1931;93:348-359.

33. Rathbun JB, Macnab I: The microvascular pattern of the rotator cuff. *J Bone Joint Surg* 1970;52B:540-553.

34. Ozaki J, Fujimoto S, Nakagawa Y, et al: Tears of the rotator cuff of the shoulder associated with pathological changes in the acromion: A study in cadavera. *J Bone Joint Surg* 1988;70A:1224-1230.

35. Ogata S, Uhthoff HK: Acromial enthesopathy and rotator cuff tear: A radiologic and histologic postmortem investigation of the coracoacromial arch. *Clin Orthop* 1990;254:39-48.

36. Iannotti JP, Zlatkin MB, Esterhai JL, et al: Magnetic resonance imaging of the shoulder: Sensitivity, specificity, and predictive value. *J Bone Joint Surg* 1991;73A:17-29.

37. Kieft GJ, Bloem JL, Obermann WR, et al: Normal shoulder: MR imaging. *Radiology* 1986;159:741-745.

38. Zlatkin MB, Iannotti JP, Roberts MC, et al: Rotator cuff tears: Diagnostic performance of MR imaging. *Radiology* 1989;172:223-229.

39. Kaplan PA, Bryans KC, Davick JP, et al: MR imaging of the normal shoulder: variants and pitfalls. *Radiology* 1992;184:519-524.

40. Mirowitz SA: Normal rotator cuff: MR imaging with conventional and fat-suppression techniques. *Radiology* 1991;180:735-740.

41. Neumann CH, Holt RG, Steinbach LS, et al: MR imaging of the shoulder: appearance of the supraspinatus tendon in asymptomatic volunteers. *AJR Am J Roentgenol* 1992;158:1281-1287.

42. Erickson SJ, Cox IH, Hyde JS, et al: Effect of tendon orientation of MR imaging signal intensity: A manifestation of the "magic angle" phenomenon. *Radiology* 1991;181:389-392.

43. Rafii M, Firooznia H, Sherman O, et al: Rotator cuff lesions: Signal patterns at MR imaging. *Radiology* 1990;177:817-823.

44. Evancho AM, Stiles RG, Fajman WA, et al: MR imaging diagnosis of rotator cuff tears. *AJR Am J Roentgenol* 1988;151:751-754.

45. Farley TE, Neumann CH, Steinbach LS, et al: Full-thickness tears of the rotator cuff of the shoulder: Diagnosis with MR imaging. *AJR Am J Roentgenol* 1992:158:347-351.

46. Kieft GJ, Bloem JL, Rozing PM, et al: Rotator cuff impingement syndrome: MR imaging. *Radiology* 1988;166:211-214.

47. Kneeland JB, Middleton WD, Carrera GF, et al: MR imaging of the shoulder: Diagnosis of rotator cuff tears. *AJR Am J Roentgenol* 1987;149:333-337.

48. Haacke EM, Tkach JA: Fast MR imaging: techniques and clinical applications. *AJR Am J Roentgenol* 1990;155:951-964.

49. Flannigan B, Kursunoglu-Brahme S, Snyder S, et al: MR arthrography of the shoulder: Comparison with conventional MR imaging. *AJR Am J Roentgenol* 1990;155:829-832.

50. Hodler J, Kursunoglu-Brahme S, Snyder SJ, et al: Rotator cuff disease: Assessment with MR arthrography versus standard MR imaging in 36 patients with arthroscopic confirmation. *Radiology* 1992;182:431-436.

Osteonecrosis

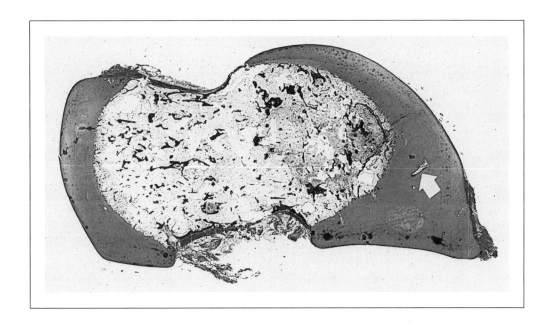

Treatment of Osteonecrosis of the Femoral Head With Electrical Stimulation

Roy K. Aaron, MD

Several clinical studies of the conservative management of osteonecrosis of the femoral head (ONFH) have indicated that, in the adult, once radiographic changes are apparent, this is a progressive disease that leads to femoral head collapse and osteoarthritis.[1-5] These studies, with an average follow-up of 31 months, demonstrated that clinical progression occurs in approximately 86% and radiographic progression in approximately 78% of hips. Other studies indicate that 80% to 100% of patients who have ONFH experience clinical progression within 18 months, and that more than 50% undergo arthroplasty within three years (D.W. Lennox, T. Ebert-Smith, personal communication).[6] Most studies suggest that progression occurs within two to three years after the onset of symptoms regardless of underlying cause. An exception is osteonecrosis in elderly patients with displaced intracapsular fractures of the hip, of whom about 50% exhibit progression.

A number of surgical procedures have been developed to preserve the femoral head. While each of these procedures has achieved some success, each procedure has major limitations in its application. The need for major surgical intervention, substantial incidence of failure, and application limited to early stages of the disease have stimulated the development of noninvasive or minimally invasive methods of treatment. Because of its success in augmenting bone repair, electric stimulation has generated interest as a potential treatment for ONFH.

Rationale for the Use of Electric Fields in the Treatment of ONFH

The pathophysiology of ONFH has been described as a coupled process of resorption and repair.[7,8] The repair process in cancellous bone is limited in that the replacement of dead with living bone is not complete. In subchondral bone, the rate of resorption exceeds that of bone formation, resulting in a loss of structural integrity, subchondral fracture, and collapse. It is not the presence of dead bone itself but rather the resorption of the bone that leads to the loss of mechanical integrity and collapse of the femoral head. Exposure to electric stimulation may alter the balance between resorption of dead bone by osteoclasts and osteoblastic production of new bone so as to retard the net loss of bone substance, preserve the strength of subchondral

bone, and prevent collapse.

Electric fields have been recorded in bone as a function of mechanical loading (strain-related potentials) or injury and repair (bioelectric potentials). Strain-related potentials arise from mechanical deformation of bone, are dependent on the intrinsic material properties of the tissue, and are quantitatively related to the magnitude and frequency of the applied load. While the exact physiologic role of strain-related potentials is not fully known, they have been implicated in information transfer to the osteocyte regarding the nature of its extracellular matrix and its biophysical environment. Electric currents of appropriate frequency and amplitude may signal bone cells to synthesize or resorb bone matrix and, thereby, to adapt or remodel in response to applied mechanical loads. The application of exogenous electric and electromagnetic fields has been shown to have a favorable effect on several biologic processes pertinent to the pathophysiology of ONFH.

Bone formation can be stimulated by electric fields of appropriate configurations. This has been shown in multiple in vitro and in vivo models, including cell and organ culture and whole bone repair and bone graft incorporation.[9] In an experimental model of endochondral ossification, exposure to an electromagnetic field used clinically for bone repair has produced significant increases in calcification and maturation of trabecular bone.[10] Clinical studies with similar signals have suggested an enhancement of repair of fractures and osteotomies.[11,12] Clinical studies have demonstrated healing in 87% of delayed or ununited tibial fractures.[13] Enhancement of bone repair has been achieved with direct current stimulation as well. Nonunions have been subjected to a 60 kHz capacitively coupled electric signal. Of 22 well-established nonunions treated for an average of six months, 77% achieved healing.[14]

Bone resorption can be suppressed by appropriately configured electric fields. Inductively coupled, or pulsed, electromagnetic fields have been used experimentally to prevent disuse osteoporosis.[15] Pulsed fields of 1.5 Hz frequency have produced increases in bone mass associated with suppression of endosteal bone resorption. The pulse configuration used in the treatment of ONFH has been shown also to decrease parathyroid hormone receptor activity on osteoblast cell membranes and to decrease osteoclast content of lysosomal enzymes.[16,17] Other studies have confirmed the ability of this signal to suppress bone resorption.[18] The suppression of bone resorption may be of particular significance in altering the balance of resorption and synthesis of bone in ONFH. Electrical stimulation may, by decreasing bone resorption in ONFH, maintain bone mass in the osteonecrotic femoral head, retard the loss of structural integrity associated with bone resorption, and prevent femoral head collapse.

Clinical Techniques for the Electric Stimulation of ONFH

Three methods have been used to expose the femoral head to electric fields. Electric fields have been applied to the hip invasively by the placement of electrodes within the femoral head or noninvasively by capacitive or inductive coupling. In the invasive, or D.C. techniques, electric current is applied through surgically implanted electrodes, with the cathode placed into the site of bone repair and the anode in nearby soft tissues. The current generating unit is either implantable or external and supplies a constant direct current (D.C.) of 2 to 20 µA. These devices usually require surgical removal at the end of the stimulation period. In the hip, the cathode has typically been inserted into a core decompression track together with bone graft.[19] Electric fields may also be produced noninvasively by capacitive or inductive coupling. In the capacitive coupling technique, skin electrodes are centered anteriorly and posteriorly over the femoral head.[20] Electric fields can also be induced into the femoral head by inductive coupling with a time-varying, or pulsed, electromagnetic field.[21,22] This technique uses a current-carrying coil driven by an external generator. The electric current from the generator establishes a proportional magnetic field in the coil, and the femoral head is exposed to this field. The induced current in the femoral head is related to characteristics of the applied magnetic field and to the biologic properties of the bone.

Clinical Studies

Electric stimulation with an invasive D.C. technique has been reported by Steinberg and associates[19] as an adjunct to core decompression and grafting and has been compared with core decompression and grafting alone (Table 1). This study used a surgically implantable power source, which delivered a constant direct current of 20 µA for 24 hours per day for six months. Seventy-four hips were treated with core decompression, grafting, and electric stimulation, and the results were compared to those of 42 hips treated with core decompression and grafting alone. The minimum follow-up time was two years. The mean follow-up time was 33 months without electric stimulation

Table 1
Hips requiring arthroplasty

	Nonoperative	Core Decompression and Graft	Core Decompression Graft and D.C.
Precollapse (II, III)	74%	43%	25%
Collapse (IV, V)	90%	43%	47%

(Reproduced with permission from Steinberg ME, Brighton CT, Corces A, et al: Osteonecrosis of the femoral head: Results of core decompression and grafting with and without electrical stimulation. *Clin Orthop* 1989; 249:199-208.)

and 44 months with electric stimulation. Results were evaluated clinically by Harris hip scores. Hips treated with electric stimulation and core decompression had better clinical outcomes than those treated with core decompression alone. Of hips treated with electric stimulation, 64% were rated as improved or unchanged compared with 43% without electric stimulation. Considering those hips which did not go on to arthroplasty, 83% treated with electric stimulation were improved or unchanged compared to 58% without electric stimulation. The mean Harris hip scores improved from 65 to 70 in the electrically stimulated group; those without electric stimulation declined from 65 to 62. Results were evaluated radiographically by the method of Steinberg. No significant difference in radiographic progression was seen between the two groups. Examining hip survival, 43% of hips with precollapse lesions treated with core decompression and grafting alone required total hip replacement; 25% of those treated with core decompression, grafting, and electric stimulation went to arthroplasty. In a comparison group of hips with precollapse lesions treated nonoperatively, 74% required total hip replacement. In this study, the addition of electric stimulation improved clinical results and hip survival but did not affect radiographic outcome.

Electric stimulation has also been reported as an adjunct to core decompression and grafting using a noninvasive capacitive coupling technique for the administration of the electric field.[20] All patients underwent core decompression and grafting. Patients were randomized to additional treatment groups with either active or inactive electric stimulation devices. Twenty hips were followed in each of the active and inactive stimulation groups for two to four years follow-up with a mean follow-up of 31 months. The outcome was evaluated clinically by Harris hip scores and radiographically by the method of Steinberg. As reported in the previous study, hips treated with core decompression and grafting had better clinical and radiographic outcome than hips treated nonoperatively. The adjunctive use of capacitively coupled electrical

Table 2
Results with pulsed fields

	Radiographic Progression	Arthroplasty
Precollapse (II, III)	0%	0%
Collapse (IV, V)	18%	25%

(Reproduced with permission from Bassett CA, Schink-Ascani M, Lewis SM: Effects of pulsed electromagnetic fields on Steinberg ratings of femoral head osteonecrosis. *Clin Orthop* 1989; 246:172-185.)

stimulation did not result in significant improvement clinically or radiographically compared with hips with inactive units. This study did not evaluate the role of capacitively coupled electric stimulation alone, without core decompression and grafting.

Results with a series of patients with ONFH treated with a pulsed, or time-varying, inductively coupled field have been reported (Table 2).[22] In this study, 118 hips were followed for an average of four years. Clinical results were reported with the d'Aubigne scoring system and radiographs were described by the method of Steinberg. No comparison group was included. In all stages of ONFH, 78% of the femoral heads were preserved. No arthroplasties were performed in 15 hips with precollapse lesions. Of hips with collapse on radiograph, 25% underwent arthroplasty. None of the 15 hips with precollapse lesions progressed radiographically. Of the hips with collapse on radiograph at the start of treatment, 18% progressed further over the study. Direct comparison of these data with other studies of the natural history of ONFH is difficult but the rates of clinical and radiographic progression appear to be less than those reported in several studies of the conservative management of this disease.

Electric stimulation for the treatment of ONFH has been compared with the results of core decompression

Table 3
Results with pulsed fields

		Clinical Success	Radiographic Success	Combined Success
Pulsed Field	II	76%	67%	67%
	III	35%	45%	23%
Core	II	36%	24%	20%
Decompression	III	4%	33%	4%

(Reproduced with permission from Aaron RK, Cimobor DM, McK D: Electrical stimulation of bone induction and grafting, in Habal MB, Reddi AH (eds): *Bone Grafts and Bone Substitutes*. Philadelphia, PA, WB Saunders, 1992, pp 192-205.)

(Table 3).[21] In this study, an electric field was induced noninvasively in the femoral head by exposure to an externally applied pulsed, or time-varying, electromagnetic field. The device was worn for 8 hours a day for 12 to 18 months. Hips were evaluated clinically with a modified d'Aubigne hip scoring system and by a quantitative method of radiographic progression.

Radiographic progression was defined as either an advance of one Ficat stage or progressive collapse of 2 mm or more. Treatment was considered a success if patients improved clinically, retained their femoral head, and demonstrated the absence of radiographic progression. Fifty-six hips treated with the pulsed field were compared to 50 hips treated with core decompression, with a mean follow-up time of 36 months. Of patients with Ficat II lesions, 62% treated with core decompression were considered by clinical criteria to be successfully treated, compared with 87% treated with pulsed fields. Of Ficat II hips treated with core decompression, 38% showed no radiographic progression, whereas 74% treated with pulsed fields were radiographically stable. By combined clinical and radiographic criteria, 70% treated with pulsed fields and 35% treated with core decompression were successfully treated. Both treatments were less successful in the presence of subchondral collapse. In Ficat III lesions, 55% of those treated with pulsed fields were successfully treated by clinical assessment compared to 25% of those treated with core decompression. A significant number of hips in both groups exhibited radiographic collapse. This study concluded that exposure to pulsed fields produced results superior to those seen with core decompression in both Ficat stages II and III.

This patient population has now been followed for six years, and the results of hips treated with pulsed fields appear to be more durable than those seen with core decompression, particularly in stage II hips. Of Ficat II hips treated with pulsed fields, 81% have been clinically successful and 71% exhibited stability radiographically with no progression. By comparison, in Ficat II hips treated with core decompression, 44% were clinically successful and 32% exhibited the absence of radiographic progression. Eighty-one percent of the hips treated with pulsed fields and 52% of those treated with core decompression were preserved. Of Ficat III hips treated with pulsed fields, 35% were considered to be clinically successful and 32% exhibited stable radiographs. Of these hips, 45% were preserved. None of the Ficat stage III hips treated with core decompression were clinically successful, and only one hip did not progress radiographically. Hip survival, defined as the percentage of hips preserved by treatment (not undergoing total hip arthroplasty), was compared among three groups—those undergoing treatment with pulsed fields or core decompression and a third group of hips treated with partial weightbearing. Survival in those hips treated with partial weightbearing exhibited a roughly logarithmic decay over five years of follow-up. Of the nonoperatively treated Ficat II hips, 28% were preserved during this period. By comparison, 52% of hips treated with core decompression were preserved.

Hip survival in Ficat II hips treated with pulsed fields demonstrated stability over the five-year follow-up period, with 81% of the hips being retained. Of Ficat stage III hips treated nonoperatively, only 15% were retained at five years follow-up. Treatment with core decompression did not appear to provide any benefit. In this group, the hip survival curve was essentially identical to that of nonoperatively treated hips. Of Ficat III hips treated with pulsed fields, 45% were preserved at five years follow-up.

Conclusion

Exposure to a time-varying, pulsed electromagnetic field appears to produce results superior to those of conservative nonoperative management or core decompression. These results appear to be durable over a six-year follow-up period. The results indicate that this technique is applicable to both Ficat stage II and Stage III lesions, with considerably better results being observed in precollapse hips. The adjunctive use of direct current stimulation with the surgical implantation of an electrode appears to give better results when used with core decompression and grafting than those observed with the surgical procedure alone. The clinical studies presented should be regarded as promising but preliminary, because the optimal signal characteristics, method of application, and alterations in pathophysiology are not yet known. More efficacious stimulation techniques can perhaps be devised once the specific effects on the pathophysiology of ONFH are determined.

References

1. Patterson RJ, Bickel WH, Dahlin DC: Idiopathic avascular necrosis of the head of the femur: A study of fifty-two cases. *J Bone Joint Surg* 1964;46A:267-282.

2. Merle D'Aubigné R, Postel M, Mazabraud A, et al: Idiopathic necrosis of the femoral head in adults. *J Bone Joint Surg* 1964;47B:612-633.

3. Musso ES, Mitchell SN, Schink-Ascani M, et al: Results of conservative management of osteonecrosis of the femoral head: A retrospective review. *Clin Orthop* 1986;207:209-215.

4. Steinberg ME, Hayken GD, Steinberg DR: A new method for evaluation and staging of avascular necrosis of the femoral head, in Arlet J, Ficat RP, Hungerford DS (eds): *Bone Circulation.* Baltimore, MD, Williams & Wilkins, 1984, pp 398-403.

5. Zizic TM, Hungerford DS: Avascular necrosis of bone, in Kelley WN, Harris EO, Ruddy S, et al (eds): *Textbook of Rheumatology,* Vol 2, 2nd edition. Philadelphia, PA, WB Saunders, 1985, pp 1689-1710.

6. David AW, Stulberg BN, Bauer TW, et al: Osteonecrosis of the femoral head: A prospective randomized treatment protocol. *Trans Orthop Res Soc* 1989;14:77.

7. Aaron RK, Lennox D, Bunce GE, et al: Durability of outcome in osteonecrosis of the femoral head treated with PEMF or core decompression, in Brighton CT, Pollack SR (eds): *Electromagnetics in Medicine and Biology.* San Francisco, CA, San Francisco Press, 1991, p 309.

8. Glimcher MJ, Kenzora JE: Nicolas Andry Award. The biology of osteonecrosis of the human femoral head and its clinical implications: I. Tissue biology. *Clin Orthop* 1979;138:284-309.

9. Aaron RK, Coimbor DM: Electrical stimulation of bone induction and grafting, in Habal MB, Reddi AH (eds): *Bone Grafts and Bone Substitutes.* Philadelphia, PA, WB Saunders, 1992, pp 192-205.

10. Aaron RK, Coimbor DM, Jolly G: Stimulation of experimental endochondral ossification with low-energy pulsing electromagnetic fields. *J Bone Miner Res* 1989;4:227-233.

11. Bassett CA, Valdes MG, Hernandez E: Modification of fracture repair with selected pulsing electromagnetic fields. *J Bone Joint Surg* 1982;64A:888-895.

12. Borsalino G, Bagnacani M, Bettati E, et al: Electrical stimulation of human femoral intertrochanteric osteotomies: Double-blind study. *Clin Orthop* 1988;237:256-263.

13. Bassett CA, Mitchell SN, Gaston SR: Treatment of ununited tibial diaphyseal fractures with pulsing electromagnetic fields. *J Bone Joint Surg* 1981;63A:511-523.

14. Brighton CT, Pollack SR: Treatment of recalcitrant nonunion with a capacitively coupled electrical field: A preliminary report. *J Bone Joint Surg* 1985;67A:577-585.

15. Rubin CT, McLeod KJ, Lanyon LE: Prevention of osteoporosis by pulsed electromagnetic fields. *J Bone Joint Surg* 1989;71A:411-417.

16. Luben RA, Cain CD, Chen MC, et al: Effects of electromagnetic stimuli on bone and bone cells in vitro: Inhibition of responses to parathyroid hormone by low-frequency fields. *Proc Nat Acad Sci USA* 1982;70:4180-4184.

17. Ryaby J, Doty S: Electromagnetic field effects on skeletal tissues in vitro. *J Electron Chem Soc* 1982;129:133-140.

18. Skerry TM, Pead MJ, Lanyon LE: Modulation of bone loss during disuse by pulsed electromagnetic fields. *J Orthop Res* 1991;9:600-608.

19. Steinberg ME, Brighton CT, Corces A, et al: Osteonecrosis of the femoral head: Results of core decompression and grafting with and without electrical stimulation. *Clin Orthop* 1989;249:199-208.

20. Steinberg ME, Brighton CT, Bands RE, et al: Capacitive coupling as an adjunctive treatment for avascular necrosis. *Clin Orthop* 1990;261:11-18.

21. Aaron RK, Lennox D, Bunce GE, et al: The conservative treatment of osteonecrosis of the femoral head: A comparison of core decompression and pulsing electromagnetic fields. *Clin Orthop* 1989;249:209-218.

22. Bassett CA, Schink-Ascani M, Lewis SM: Effects of pulsed electromagnetic fields on Steinberg ratings of femoral head osteonecrosis. *Clin Orthop* 1989;246:172-185.

Concepts of Etiology and Early Pathogenesis of Osteonecrosis

John Paul Jones, Jr, MD

Current pathophysiologic evidence suggests that traumatic osteonecrosis (ON) is the result of a sudden ischemic event, rather than some gradual or chronic process. However, the etiology and early evolution of nontraumatic ON are poorly understood in terms of cause and effect. Exposure to several seemingly unrelated risk factors and confounding variables is explored, using the talus as an example, in an attempt to determine if a single final common pathway can consistently cause ON in various disorders.

The body of the talus, articulating with both the ankle joint and subtalar joint, is similar to the femoral head in being virtually surrounded by articular cartilage with relatively few vascular foramina. Blood supply to the talar body predominantly enters retrograde through the subtalar neck region[1,2] as the anastomotic artery of the tarsal canal, originating from the posterior tibial artery. Secondary supply is derived from deltoid branches of the posterior tibial artery, which enter the talar body on its medial periosteal surface. The artery of the tarsal canal has extraosseous anastomoses with the artery of the tarsal sinus, and there is tertiary, anterolateral supply to the talar body through anastomoses with the dorsalis pedis artery.

Posttraumatic Correlations

The superolateral two thirds of the femoral head is especially susceptible to ON following displaced intracapsular fractures,[3] because its blood supply comes primarily from the lateral epiphyseal branches of the medial femoral circumflex artery. Likewise, the reported incidence of ON of the humeral head after four-part fractures is about 37%,[4] and the intraosseous arcuate branch of the anterior circumflex artery is the most important vessel. In contrast, ON is relatively rare with nondisplaced talar neck fractures, because adequate intraosseous anastomoses remain intact within the talar body. However, displaced fractures of the talar neck with dislocation of the subtalar joint have an increased incidence of ON. In this injury, two of the three main sources of blood are interrupted. ON was identified in 40% to 50% of these fracture-dislocations.[5,6] With fracture-dislocations of both the ankle and subtalar joints, the incidence of ON increased to 91%.[5]

Nontraumatic Osteonecrosis

Atraumatic talar ON is relatively rare, if osteochondral fractures of the talar dome, osteochondritis dissecans, and juvenile osteochondrosis are excluded. By 1975, only a few cases had been reported and they were associated with either Fabry-Anderson disease,[7] hypercholesterolemia,[8] occlusive vascular disease,[9] alcoholism,[10] or hypercortisonism,[10,11] especially exogenous corticoids for systemic lupus erythematosus.[10-13] For example, in 1979, Klippel and associates[14] reported talar ON in 11 of 55 (20%) patients with systemic lupus erythematosus who were examined with routine radiographs. Recently, magnetic resonance imaging (MRI) studies of talar lesions suggest that they progress through various stages.[15]

Dead Bone Without Repair

ON without any repair occurs with physiologic death of the human skeleton. Irreversible osteocytic necrosis requires a minimum of two hours of complete ischemia with total anoxia.[16] ON appears in paleopathologic specimens that were dehydrated by natural[15] or artificial mummification (Fig. 1, *left*) and not permineralized. Dead bone at this stage is essentially as strong as living bone, and it does not collapse spontaneously.

As expected, in posttraumatic ON following total talar dislocation, once the completely extruded and devascularized talus is replaced in the wound, the initial postoperative radiographs of the talar body appear normal.[6] Although conventional radiographs appear normal in this stage, radionuclide scans will show photo-deficient ("cold") lesions,[17] as apparently involved both tali during a sickle-cell crisis in one case.[18] Conventional MRI studies have limited value at this stage because they may erroneously appear normal (false-negative).[17,19]

Repair Without Collapse

At this stage the patient is usually asymptomatic and has no physical findings. Histologically, progressive autolytic reduction of the necrotic marrow has resulted in amorphous debris. It is impossible to determine to what extent the preexisting marrow vessels had thrombosed unless very early lesions are examined. At the peripheral reparative fronts, dead marrow and trabeculae are partially or completely resorbed by osteoclasts

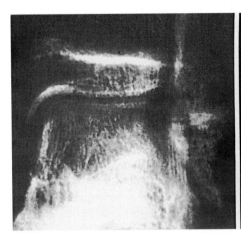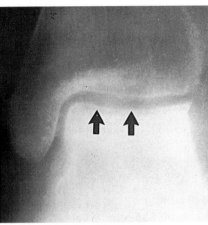

Fig. 1   Left, Anteroposterior radiograph of ankle from the ancient, mummified Egyptian skeleton of a 13-year-old boy, with a remarkably unaltered trabecular and cortical pattern. In physiologic bone death the distal tibia and talar body have similar radiodensity. (Courtesy of the Museum of Natural History, Basel, Switzerland). **Right**, Anteroposterior tomograph of an ankle from a living patient with nontraumatic talar necrosis. There is relative and absolute sclerosis of the talar body in contrast to the viable and more radiolucent distal tibia. A narrow band of subchondral lucency is present in the medial talar dome (arrows), suggesting revascularization with focal resorption.

and are replaced or covered with new appositional bone, resulting in thickened, reinforced trabeculae. After six to eight weeks from a known ischemic event it is possible to detect ON radiographically by a relative and/or absolute increase in radiodensity of the sclerotic-appearing talar body (Fig. 1, *right*), as compared to the viable, but often osteopenic, distal tibia and calcaneus.

However, there is a delay before the repair response of revascularization (resorption) and reossification is activated.[15] It is likely that a combination of platelet-derived growth factor (PDGF), insulin-like growth factor (IGF-1), endothelial cell growth factor (ECGF), and other unknown factors activate angiogenesis. Osteoclast migration may be stimulated by necrotic collagen degradation products. Conceivably, small talar lesions at this stage are not diagnosed because complete healing may occur spontaneously, depending on the size and location of these lesions. In lesions of the dome of the talar body, repair usually begins at the reactive interface of the ischemic zone surrounding the dead area and the viable marrow with intact circulation. Resorption results in vague areas of radiolucency within the sclerotic talar body on conventional radiographs (Fig. 2, *top*) without evidence of late segmental collapse.

Osteoclastic bone resorption is not possible without blood supply. Hawkins[5] described a useful radiographic sign which suggests viability of the talar body. This sign, a band of subchondral radiolucency (Fig. 1, *right*), indicates revascularization and subchondral bone resorption. At this stage, scintigraphy shows either a central area of decreased uptake with a border of increased uptake ("cold/hot" lesion), or diffusely increased radionuclide uptake ("hot" lesion) in the talar body (Fig. 2, *bottom left*).

Once a significant revascularization response has been generated, MRI is the most sensitive and specific noninvasive test for the localization and configuration of the ON lesion.[15,20,21] At this stage, MRI indicates low-intensity bands or rings which represent the revascularization fronts surrounding the necrotic zone on T-1 weighting (Fig. 2, *bottom right*), or the pathognomonic "double-line sign" on T-2 weighting.[15]

Repair With Collapse

The patient is symptomatic with pain, swelling, tenderness, and stiffness of the ankle. Late segmental collapse is a result of the revascularization (resorption) process. In this stage, the reparative front has resorbed and weakened subchondral trochlear and subtalar bone. Shear-induced microfractures of the previously necrotic trabeculae result from impulse loading, beginning at stress risers, which propagate into the talar body, either superiorly (from the ankle joint) and/or inferiorly (from the subtalar joint). Irreversible collapse and depression of the talar dome appear with progressive articular incongruity and secondary osteoarthritis of the ankle (Fig. 3).

At this stage, scintigraphy shows diffusely increased radionuclide uptake (Fig. 4, *left*). Occult segmental collapse with subtle osteochondral fracture of the talar dome is particularly well-visualized with multi-planar or three-dimensional computed tomography or MRI. MR imaging[22] is also useful in diagnosing additional, previously unsuspected, but contiguous ON lesions affecting the tibia (Fig. 4, *right*) and/or calcaneus. Pathologic examination usually reveals trabeculae devoid of osteocytes with a fibrovascular repair response (Fig. 5, *left*), and perinecrotic thromboses may be found (Fig. 5, *right*).

Concept: Final Common Pathway

Nontraumatic ON of the talus may be associated with multiple and symmetrical involvement of addi-

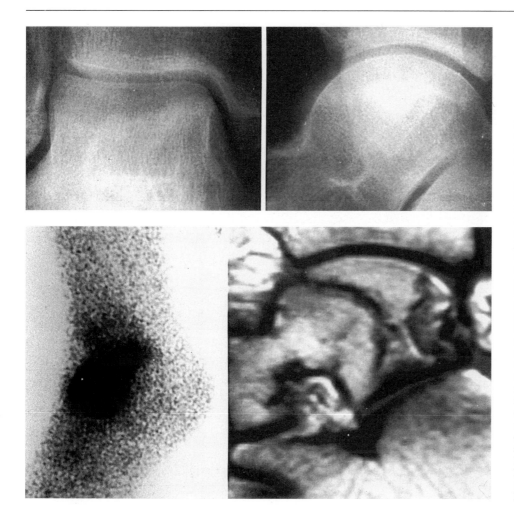

Fig. 2 Top left, Anteroposterior radiograph of right ankle from patient with obesity, diabetes, hyperlipemia, and abnormal liver function tests, but without anticardiolipin antibodies. A precollapse lesion in the talar body has mixed radiolucency and sclerosis. **Top right**, Lateral radiograph of talus with mixed sclerosis and lucency without articular incongruity of either the ankle or subtalar joints. **Bottom left**, Technetium 99m-methylene diphosphonate scintigraphy reveals diffusely increased uptake in the talus. **Bottom right**, Sagittal MR image of talus reveals narrow bands of decreased signal intensity in an hourglass configuration, extending to involve both the ankle and subtalar joints, which represent anterior and posterior revascularization (resorption) fronts surrounding a central area of necrotic talar body. Repair of the dead bone has not resulted in collapse and flattening of the articular surfaces. Additional lesions were found in the talar head and second cuneiform. (Courtesy of Gary L. Baker, Minneapolis, Minnesota.)

tional, and often contiguous, bones (Fig. 4, *right*), suggesting systemic osseous devascularization from an underlying disease process.[11,14,23] Evidence of altered hemostasis was first described in patients with nontraumatic ON by Hamilton and associates[24] in 1965, and reemphasized by Boettcher and associates[25] and Bonfiglio.[26] In 1974, I hypothesized[27] that intravascular coagulation (IC) with fibrin thrombus propagation is the specific intermediary pathophysiology and final common pathway producing ON.

Intravascular Coagulation

It is likely that the same ischemic events that produce microvascular damage and nontraumatic ON in the femoral and humeral heads[28,29] also cause ON of the talar body. Recently, direct histologic evidence of IC has been discovered in humans with intraosseous fibrin-platelet thromboses within prenecrotic femoral and humeral head segments, both 70 minutes,[30] and 18 hours,[31] after a known ischemic event, and *prior* to complete autolytic reduction of the avascular zone. Intraosseous arterial and arteriolar thromboses (Fig. 5,

right) have also been observed histologically within later lesions.[26,29,32-35] Either focal (FIC) or disseminated (DIC), IC appears to be the most likely final common mechanism[15,28,29,31] producing ON in several different conditions (Outline 1). IC would also explain the coexistent ON involvement of bones contiguous to the talus, including the distal tibia (Fig. 4, *right*), calcaneus, and/or navicular.[21,33]

Prethrombotic Factors

A combination of three factors probably produces microcirculatory thrombosis of the talus and other vulnerable bones: (1) stasis, (2) hypercoagulability, and (3) endothelial damage. The initial juxta-articular lesion appears to be localized to the subchondral bone of the dome of the talar body, which has a microanatomy that facilitates vascular stasis. Terminal arteries with few collaterals supply subchondral areas, with long, narrow arcades of end-capillaries, which favors embolic occlusion and thrombosis, especially with vasospasm (Raynaud's phenomenon) or localized arteriolar vaso-

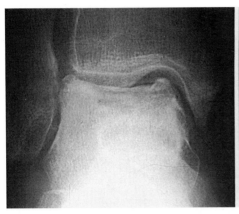
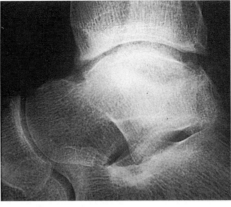

Fig. 3   Left, Anteroposterior radiograph of ankle from a corticoid-treated patient. A sclerotic lesion in the talar body is associated with late segmental collapse and depression of the talar dome. **Right**, Lateral radiograph shows obvious incongruity of the ankle mortise without evidence of necrosis involving the distal tibia.

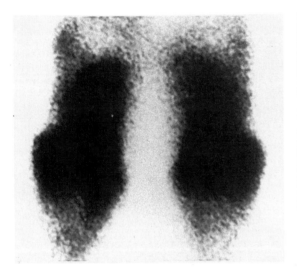
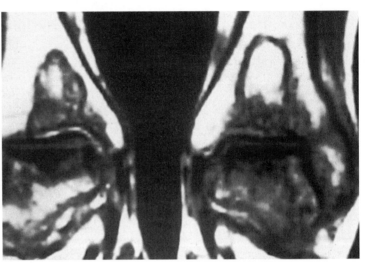

Fig. 4   Left, A scintigraphic scan of both ankles reveals symmetrically increased radioisotope uptake involving both distal tibias and tali. **Right**, Coronal MR images of both ankles demonstrate lesions within both talar bodies with decreased signal intensity, and lesions of both distal tibias extending to the tibial plafonds, surrounded by narrow revascularization bands of decreased signal intensity.

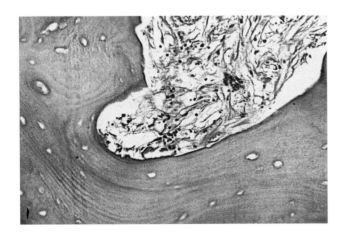
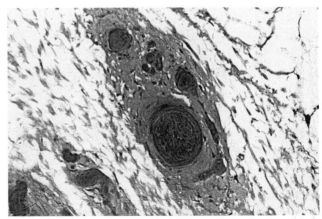

Fig. 5   Left, Photomicrograph of talar lesion showing a bony trabeculum devoid of osteocytes and fibrotic marrow, as evidence of osteonecrosis (hematoxylin and eosin, X 200). **Right**, Photomicrograph of perinecrotic tissue with thromboses and interstitial fibrosis which completely obliterate the lumens of an artery and several arterioles, without evidence of vasculitis (hematoxylin and eosin, X 200).

constriction (neuropeptide Y, endothelin-1, and norepinephrine).[29,31]

Increased procoagulants and activated coagulants (with impaired hepatic and splenic reticuloendothelial clearance), decreased natural anticoagulants (especially proteins C and S), vasoconstriction of the subchondral arteriolar bed, and probably the most important factor, decreased endogenous fibrinolysis[36] result in a hypercoagulable state. The subchondral capillary bed has a high surface/volume ratio which results in a marked increase of endothelial cells in direct contact with blood. Normally, circulating blood does not come in contact with cells expressing surface membrane tissue factor (thromboplastin) activity.

However, endothelial damage to the intraosseous microcirculation (terminal arterioles, capillaries and

---

Outline 1
Conditions potentially activating intravascular coagulation and causing osteonecrosis

Fat Embolism
Alcoholism
Carbon tetrachloride poisoning
Diabetes mellitus
Dysbaric phenomena
Hemoglobinopathies
Hypercortisonism
Hyperlipemia (Types II and IV)
Obesity
Pancreatitis (lipase)
Pregnancy (fatty liver)
Unrelated fractures

Hypersensitivity Reactions
Allograft organ rejection
  kidney, heart, liver, bone marrow
Anaphylactic shock
Antiphospholipid antibody syndrome
Immune complexes
Serum sickness
Systemic lupus erythematosus
  Anticardiolipin antibodies

Infections
Endotoxic reactions
  Neisseria meningitidis
  Haemophilus influenzae
  Escherichia coli
  Others
Bacterial coat lipopolysaccharides
Septic abortion
Toxic shock
  Staphylococcus aureus exotoxin
Viruses
  Cytomegalovirus
  Hepatitis
  Human immunodeficiency virus (HIV)
  Rubella
  Others

Proteolytic Enzymes
Pancreatitis (trypsin)
Snake venom

Thromboplastin (Tissue Factor III) Release
Inflammatory bowel disease
  Crohn's disease
  Ulcerative colitis
Malignancies
  Acute leukemias
  Hodgkin's disease
  Metastatic carcinoma
  Pancreatic carcinoma
  Others

Thromboplastin (Tissue Factor III) Release *(continued)*
Chemotherapy
  L-Asparaginase
  Intra-arterial
Neurodamage
  Brain/Spinal surgery
  Cerebral injury/Tumor
  Ruptured aneurysm
  Spinal cord injury
Pregnancy
  Amniotic fluid embolism
  Fatty liver of pregnancy
  Normal deliveries
  Retained fetus in utero
  Toxemia
    Preeclampsia
    Eclampsia

Other Prethrombotic Conditions
Anorexia nervosa
Anovulatory agents
Anticoagulant deficiencies
  Antithrombin III
  Extrinsic pathway inhibitor
  Heparin cofactor II
  Protein C
  Protein S
Current cigarette smoking
Decompression sickness
Diabetes mellitus
Gaucher crisis
Hemolytic-Uremic syndrome
Hepatic failure
Hyperlipemia (Types II or IV)
Hyperviscosity
Hypofibrinolytic disorders
  Dysfibrinogenemia
  Plasminogen deficiency
  Tissue plasminogen activator deficiency
  Excess plasminogen activator inhibitor activity
Nephrotic syndrome
Polycythemia
Postoperative states
Sickle-cell crisis
Storage diseases
  Fabry-Anderson disease
  Gaucher disease
  Polyvinylpyrrolidone (PVP)
Thrombocytosis
Thrombotic thrombocytopenic purpura
Vascular disorders
  Aortic aneurysms
  Arteriosclerosis
    Leriche syndrome

sinusoids), with exposure of procoagulant subendothelial collagen, is the most likely event triggering platelet aggregation and fibrin thrombosis, with progressive involvement of venules, veins, arterioles, and extraosseous arteries.[20,37] Once circulating blood comes into contact with tissue factor in the outer vascular walls, factor VIIa/tissue factor complexes are formed, which catalyze the activation of factors IX and X to convert prothrombin to thrombin. Fibrinopeptides A[38] and B are split from fibrinogen by thrombin. Fibrin monomer then polymerizes into fibrin clot in the microcirculation, and fibrin-platelet thrombosis may result in localized, ischemic end-organ damage. Subchondral thrombosis may then be potentiated by hypofibrinolysis with delayed and impaired secondary, endogenous fibrinolysis (reperfusion of necrotic vessels with peripheral marrow hemorrhages),[28,29,34] with prolonged ischemic anoxia of the talus.

Intraosseous Hypertension

Although arterial occlusion results in more severe intraosseous hypoxia than venous congestion,[39] intraosseous venography and bone marrow pressure studies indicate extensive medullary venous stasis and intraosseous hypertension in very early ON.[32] However, venous congestion and intraosseous hypertension do not appear to actually cause ON.[40] Increased hydraulic outflow resistance with deficient venous drainage and impaired marrow perfusion probably occur after generalized thrombosis of the marrow vasculature.

Bioactive lipids, including unbound free fatty acids, thromboxanes, leukotrienes, and prostaglandins have also been found in ON,[41,42] particularly in the revascularization (resorption/formation) front.[43] The intraosseous infusion of prostaglandin E_2, especially with coexistent intraosseous hypertension, results in a marked increase in new bone formation in animals.[44] Eicosanoids and cytokines are also capable of stripping capillary endothelium and causing passive congestion, platelet aggregation, vascular hyperpermeability with edema formation, and most likely, additional intraosseous hypertension, which now appears to be a very early secondary, but nonspecific, effect within the postischemic marrow cavity.

Etiologic Risk Factors

Intravascular coagulation is not the primary cause of ON but is only an intermediary event, which is always trigger-activated by some other underlying etiology, including the intravascular release of particulate matter (fat embolism or, perhaps, amniotic fluid embolism, metastatic cancer cell debris, or Gaucher cells), immune (antigen-antibody) complexes, proteolytic enzymes (trypsin), tissue thromboplastin (tissue factor III), and bacterial endotoxins (Outline 1).[45-47]

Endotoxic (Shwartzman) Reactions

Rabbits administered bacterial endotoxins not only develop disseminated intravascular coagulation (DIC), but also hyperlipemia, fatty liver, systemic fat embolism and fibrin thrombosis during the generalized Shwartzman phenomenon.[48,49] Depletion of extrinsic pathway inhibitor[50] also sensitizes rabbits to IC and the Shwartzman reaction. ON can complicate postmeningococcal or posthemophilus DIC (Outline 1).[28,29,51] Fifty-one ON lesions, including the humeral and femoral heads, complicated DIC in eight children.[15,29] Another child (Case 3) developed postmeningococcal DIC with gangrene, requiring amputations of her left fingers and right hand, and was found by Richard Beauchamp to have nine ON lesions, including both distal tibias and tali (Fig. 6). Histologic studies[52] reveal ischemia and fibrin thrombi within the microvasculature adjacent to the necrotic bone, as was observed by John Ogden in his specimen of a partially necrotic talus (Fig. 7) from a postmeningococcal patient with DIC and ON.

Various viral illnesses can also activate DIC,[53] including cytomegalovirus, hepatitis, rubella, rubeola, and varicella. Perhaps children with protein C or S deficiency[29] or with decreased fibrinolytic activity[54] may be more susceptible to developing ON following these viral or bacterial infections, because increases in immunoglobulins (IgG and IgM) are found in Perthes' disease,[55,56] some of which could conceivably represent antiphospholipid antibodies. Moreover, human immunodeficiency virus (HIV) is associated with DIC[45] and ON,[57] as well as hypertriglyceridemia and anticardiolipin antibodies.

A Shwartzman reaction also occurs after human renal homotransplantation.[58] DIC can also be triggered by hyperacute rejection of other organ allografts, with fibrin thrombi and necrosis.[59,60] Exogenous glucocorticoids also contribute to the precipitation of microthrombi in DIC by (1) preparing the vascular system for the generalized Shwartzman reaction[61] by stimulating alpha-adrenergic receptor sites and potentiating the effect of catecholamines on vessels, (2) facilitating hyperviscosity and hypercoagulability,[62] (3) decreasing fibrinolytic activity,[63,64] (4) impairing reticuloendothelial clearance of fibrinogen degradation products, circulating soluble fibrin monomer, or activated coagulation factors, and (5) causing hyperlipemia and fatty liver with intraosseous fat embolism.

Fat Embolism

The association of ON with intraosseous fat embolism was first demonstrated clinically in 1965, and was confirmed experimentally in 1966.[38] Platelet aggregation occurs in vivo over the surface of intravascular fat globules, which is followed within two hours by the appearance of fibrin-platelet microthrombi.[65]

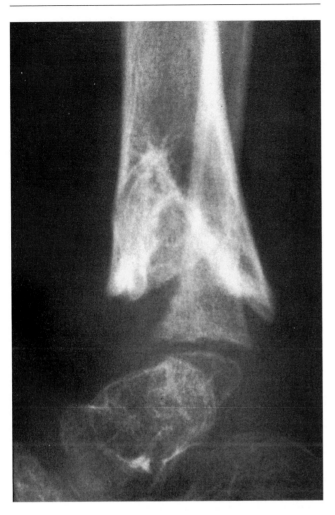

Fig. 6   Lateral radiograph of the right ankle of a 4-year-old child who developed disseminated intravascular coagulation following meningococcemia in infancy which resulted in gangrene and multifocal osteonecrosis with premature physeal closures, limb shortening, and angulatory deformities. A central physeal growth arrest of the distal tibia is apparent, as well as residual necrosis of the talus. (Courtesy of Richard D. Beauchamp, Vancouver, British Columbia.)

In addition to hypercortisonism,[11,66] ON of the talar body has also been reported in alcoholism.[10,67] The author hypothesizes that in these and several other conditions (Outline 1), fat emboli may arise from a fatty liver (Mechanism A), destabilization and coalescence of plasma lipoproteins (Mechanism B), and/or disruption of fatty bone marrow or other adipose tissue depots (Mechanism C).[11,38]

Absolute Fat Overload   The most likely cause of ON in alcoholism and hypercortisonism is an absolute overload[68,69] of intraosseous fat emboli,[31,38,43] which exceed the ischemic threshold, with impaired clearance, and hydrolysis by lipase into unbound free fatty acids which cause endothelial damage and trigger IC and thrombosis. Either exogenous corticoid use (Figs. 2-4) or endogenous hypercortisonism[70] can cause ON. Elevated serum and urine cortisol can also be found in alcoholics with ON.[71] The embolic source is most likely the corticoid- or alcohol-induced fatty liver.[11,38] Intravascular fat can also migrate through canaliculi to become deposited within osteocytic lacunae.[28,38] Lipid accumulates in subchondral osteocytes which subsequently become necrotic, as demonstrated both experimentally by Kawai and associates,[72] and clinically by Muratsu and associates,[73] in both alcoholism and hypercortisonism.

There appears to be a cumulative alcohol/corticoid dose-related ON response.[74,75] In my experience, the exposure threshold for alcohol-associated ON (at a consumption of 400 ml or more of absolute ethanol a week) is about 150 liters of 100% ethanol, and the corticoid exposure threshold is about 2,000 mg of prednisone, continuously administered over a variable time period, for ON to appear in adults. However, the very early detection of acute ON by dynamic contrast-en-

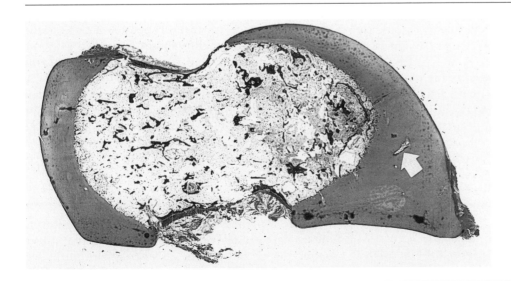

Fig. 7   Sagittal section of a talus from a child who had meningococcemia complicated by disseminated intravascular coagulation. A necrotic lesion is apparent within the posterior talar body, which is adjacent to areas of microthrombus formation within a cartilage canal (arrow). (Courtesy of John A. Ogden, Tampa, Florida.)

hanced MRI[19,76] and the prothrombotic and hypofibrinolytic effects of multiple coexistent factors (Outline 1) (septic shock, for example[77]) will decrease these exposure thresholds, thereby increasing both the incidence rate and relative risk.

Relative Fat Overload A cause of decreased osteoblastic bone formation in glucocorticoid- or alcohol-induced osteoporosis may be a relative overload of intraosseous fat emboli, which is below the ischemic threshold and insufficient to trigger IC.[28,31] For example, Hirohata and associates[78] demonstrated fatty degeneration of osteocytes of the fourth metatarsal head in patients with atraumatic ON of the femoral head. Coexistent osteoporosis was detected by Arlot and associates[79] in histomorphometric studies from 68 (89%) of 77 ON patients. Prolonged heparin therapy with increased lipolytic activity and hyperlipemia prevents IC but causes osteoporosis. Also, Wang and associates[80] showed that lipid-clearing agents can prevent corticoid-induced osteoporosis, perhaps by diminishing the steroid-induced accumulation of lipids within osteocytes, as demonstrated by Maruno and associates.[81]

Relative Fat Underload I theorized[15,31,82] that a relative underload of fat emboli, especially arising from the fatty liver of obesity, could produce sufficient subchondral hypoxia to cause necrosis of calcified chondrocytes and subjacent osteocytes. Cheras[83] has observed intraosseous microembolic lipid and thrombi in ON, and to a lesser extent in primary osteoarthritis. Primary osteoarthritis of aging and obesity could potentially occur when overzealous revascularization (angiogenesis precedes osteogenesis) and chondroclastic resorption, abnormally extending through the (reduplicating and advancing) tidemark and into the progressively thinned noncalcified articular cartilage, is coupled with excessive subchondral osteoblastic new bone formation.[31]

Confirmatory Animal Studies Corticosteroid-treated rabbits were studied in nine laboratories.[20] All instances involved hyperlipemia, fatty liver, pulmonary and systemic fat embolism, subchondral fat embolism of the femoral (and humeral) heads, and osteoporosis. Focal osteocyte death in the femoral heads occurred in six of the eight series studied.

This sequence of intraosseous fat embolism, endothelial cell necrosis, extravascular lipid migration, reduced osteoblastic activity, and fatty osteocytic necrosis has been confirmed in osteopenic space-flight rats with possible endogenous hypercortisonism.[84] Similarly, rat long bones and vertebrae studied with microangiography after six weeks of corticoid treatment showed a partial disappearance of epiphyseal microvascularity.[85]

Hypersensitivity Reactions

Eighteen hours after anaphylactic shock and DIC, very early evidence of nontraumatic ON, affecting both humeral and femoral heads, appeared with subchondral fat embolism and fibrin thrombosis.[31] Peripheral interadipocytic hemorrhage had apparently resulted from secondary fibrinolysis and reperfusion of necrotic vessels.

IC is also suggested in two animal models (type III hypersensitivity, immune-complex mediated). Two to three hours following antigen injection into the rabbit knee, Mahowald and associates[86] showed that focal areas of subchondral bone were devoid of secondary and tertiary branches of epiphyseal arteries. At one to two weeks there were occlusions of subchondral vessels adjacent to avascular subchondral bone. Matsui and associates[87] found that serum sickness and corticoids produced arteriolar interruptions and necrotic lesions in 14 (70%) of 20 femoral metaphyses and diaphyses.

The symmetrical (83%) and polyarticular (90%) involvement of ON in patients with systemic lupus erythematosus (SLE)[14] suggests systemic risk factors in the pathogenesis.[88] DIC was first reported complicating SLE in 1965 by McKay.[89] Although thrombosed vessels have been found adjacent to areas of necrotic bone in SLE,[13,29] usually the local activation of the coagulation system in SLE remains subclinical. However, Resnick and associates[33] found widespread ON involving the distal tibia and fibula, and virtually every bone of the foot, including the talus, in a corticoid-treated SLE patient who had the lupus anticoagulant and occlusion of multiple vessels.

Antiphospholipid Antibody Syndrome

It has also been observed that ON could occur in SLE patients who had never received corticoids. Asherson and associates[90] discovered that antiphospholipid antibodies (aPL) can cause a coagulopathy with venous and arterial thromboses, as well as ON of the femoral heads. ON in the antiphospholipid antibody syndrome has been confirmed in patents with SLE,[91] and without SLE, who have never received corticoids, the so-called primary antiphospholipid antibody syndrome.[92,93] There are three reported cases of widespread microvascular thromboses associated with aPL in patients without connective tissue disease or vasculitis.[94] Protein C deficiency with lupus anticoagulants can also result in arterial occlusions.[95] Thrombocytopenia is associated with aPL, suggesting platelet aggregation, and it is now considered that these antibodies initiate thrombosis by activating platelets.[96] Moreover, Stinson and associates[97] detected recurrent DIC in this syndrome.

Dysbaric Phenomena

I have hypothesized[27] that ON does not result from the primary embolic or compressive effects of nitrogen bubbles alone on the osseous vasculature, but by secondary injury to the marrow adipose tissue by rapidly expanding nitrogen gas which triggers focal, and probably systemic, IC. Following a single hyperbaric air exposure with inadequate decompression, dysbaric ON can appear in humans[98] and sheep.[99] Intravascular fat and tissue factor accelerate DIC after decompression sickness (DCS). Fibrinogen, lipid, and platelet aggregation at the blood-bubble interface are associated with post-dive thrombocytopenia, accelerated platelet and fibrinogen turnover, decreased antithrombin III activity, prolongation of the prothrombin time, and increased fibrin degradation products.[100]

An autopsy[30] of a diver who expired 70 minutes after surfacing with DCS revealed gas bubbles in the fatty marrow of his femoral and humeral heads. Lipid and platelet aggregates were found on the surface of marrow bubbles. Fibrin thrombi occluded dilated sinusoids adjacent to the bubbles (Fig. 8), as well as veins, capillaries, and arterioles. Pulmonary, renal, and intraosseous (subchondral) fat embolism and fibrin thromboses were also observed, and it is suggested that injured marrow adipocytes can release liquid fat, thromboplastin, and other vasoactive substances, which appear to also play a systemic procoagulant role in triggering DIC and additional dysbaric ON. These observations are consistent with Kawashima and associates[101] and Kitano and Hayashi[102] in their studies of diving fatalities.

Hemoglobinopathies

DIC can also occur during sickle-cell crisis.[103,104] Although ON rarely complicates sickle-cell trait, those patients with the hemoglobin SS genotype,[105] especially when associated with alpha-thalassemia,[106] have the highest risk of femoral head ON. Overexertion, hypoxia, acidosis, and hemoconcentration are considered to predispose to sickling in patients with sickle-cell trait, which is capable of triggering IC.[107,108] However, these dense sickled red cells, which are selectively sequestered in the microcirculation during vasoocclusive crises, probably do not cause ON by themselves, because they produce stasis without thrombosis.[109]

Normally, the erythroid hyperplasia of the sickle hemoglobinopathies results in increased marrow blood flow.[110] However, a hypercoagulable state[111] with increased platelet activation, thrombin generation, fibrin deposition, and impaired fibrinolysis occurs at the same time as erythrocyte sequestration.[112] Thrombosis with increased serum fibrinogen degradation products most likely results from activation of the coagulation system[113] in the sickle hemoglobinopathies by a combination of fat and marrow embolism, high hemoglobin levels, thrombocytosis, hyperfibrinogenemia, hyperviscosity, increased factor VIII, plasma B-thromboglobulin, platelet factor 4, and thromboxane B2, and decreased clotting factors V and XIII, plasminogen, tissue plasminogen activator, and proteins C and S.

An increase in circulating endothelial cells in sickle-cell crisis is compatible with local vascular damage.[114] Necrotic marrow can be aspirated from the site of the acutely painful bone crises. The source of the pain is presumed to be an increased intramedullary pressure from the secondary inflammatory response, because

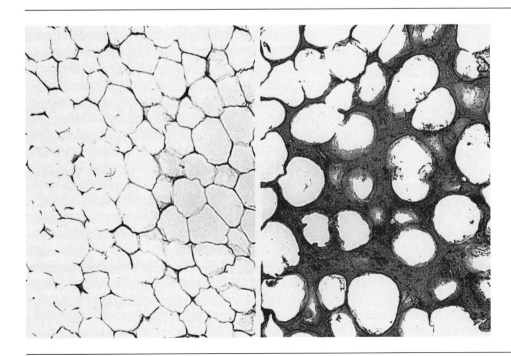

Fig. 8 **Left**, Photomicrograph of an area of normal-appearing fatty marrow from diver with inadequate decompression who expired 70 minutes after surfacing (phosphotungstic acid hematoxylin, X 200). **Right**, Photomicrograph of ischemic fatty marrow from same diver, showing evidence of intravascular coagulation of dilated sinusoids by interadipocytic fibrin thrombi (Masson trichrome X 200).

MRI studies indicate acute infarction with edema in the majority of patients with painful crisis.[115,116] During some painful sickle-cell crises, especially in late pregnancy, systemic fat and marrow embolism may potentiate IC. Recently, antiphospholipid antibodies have also been found to commonly occur in sickle cell disease.[117]

Pregnancy Complications

Hypercoagulability occurs during late pregnancy with hyperlipemia, depression of the fibrinolytic system, and occasionally, decreased anti-thrombin III. ON also occurs in late pregnancy or in the early postpartum period.[32] Although ON can follow normal deliveries, it is also related to fatty liver of pregnancy,[38] retained fetus in utero,[29] toxemia (pre-eclampsia or eclampsia), and several other obstetric problems. These disorders are able to activate DIC[45] because of the rich content of thromboplastin in human placental tissues which may gain access to the maternal circulation.

Malignancies

Tumorous conditions, especially metastatic carcinoma[118] and acute promyelocytic or lymphoid leukemias, may be complicated by DIC[119] and talar ON.[21] Human tumor procoagulants may be associated with DIC, particularly the acute leukemias. Systemic L-asparaginase chemotherapy[120] and intra-arterial cis-platinum chemotherapy can also cause thrombosis and bone infarctions.[121] In addition, the proteolytic enzyme, trypsin, may be systemically released in pancreatic carcinoma and trigger DIC. Talar ON in pancreatitis,[122] without coexistent alcoholism, may also potentially result from trypsin-induced DIC.

Neurotrauma

In addition to the placenta, brain tissue is also rich in thromboplastin, which may gain access to the systemic circulation following trauma or surgery and activate the extrinsic clotting cascade. Head injury has been found to be complicated by DIC,[123] as well as the formation of fibrin microthrombi within bone marrow on postmortem examination.[124,125] An increase in catecholamines and corticosteroids may aggravate this process, as previously mentioned. In my experience, ON may occur when short-term, high-dose glucocorticoids are used for their neuroprotective, anti-inflammatory effects,[29,126] which are to reduce cerebral or spinal cord edema and to inhibit posttraumatic lipid peroxidation.

Inflammatory Bowel Disease

Ulcerative colitis and regional enteritis (Crohn's disease) can cause DIC, which is probably mediated by chronic thromboplastin release.[127] Bilateral ON of the femoral heads may occur in patients with inflammatory bowel disease who have not received any corticosteroid therapy.[128]

Other Prethrombotic and Hypofibrinolytic Conditions

DIC with end-organ damage is enhanced by inhibition or impairment of endogenous fibrinolytic activity. In order to exceed the ischemic threshold and produce a bone infarction, it is likely that significant microthrombi must remain within the intraosseous vasculature for a minimum of two to six hours, and not be immediately dissolved by endogenous fibrinolysis.

Hypofibrinolysis results from increased plasminogen activator inhibitor[54,129] and/or increased alpha-2 plasmin inhibitor in the nephrotic syndrome, hemolytic-uremic syndrome, thrombotic thrombocytopenic purpura, and hypertriglyceridemic syndromes (types II and IV), all of which are associated with ON. Moreover, coexistent protein C and S deficiencies,[29] antithrombin III deficiency, hyperviscosity, hyperfibrinogemia, polycythemia, thrombocytosis,[130] and other unknown factors[54] could also facilitate thrombogenesis and ON. For example, DIC[131] and ON[132] have been found in anorexia nervosa.

The nephrotic syndrome is also associated with several other coagulation abnormalities,[133] including thrombocytosis and platelet hyperaggregability, increased factors V and VIII, increased fibrinogen with hyperviscosity, and decreased protein S and antithrombin III. The hyperlipemia of the nephrotic syndrome may also be exacerbated by corticoid therapy, further increasing ON susceptibility.

Although intraosseous lipomas of the talus do not cause ON,[134] hyperviscosity and the gradual obliteration of vascular lumens by progressive lipid (or polyvinylpyrrolidone)[135] storage within marrow histiocytes or endothelial cells could conceivably cause talar ON in Gaucher disease[23] and Fabry-Anderson disease.[7] However, the painful crises in Gaucher disease, acute leukemia, sickle-cell disease, and decompression sickness result from sudden ischemia and acute infarction, because bone scintigraphy shows decreased uptake ("cold," photopenic lesions) shortly after symptoms appear,[136-139] which suggests acute marrow thrombosis (Fig. 8, *right*) and secondary hemorrhage of IC.

For example, Gaucher disease is associated with thrombocytopenia, hyperviscosity, and decreased levels of a wide spectrum of coagulation factors, including factor IX (hemophilia B) and protein C.[140,141] Bone crises have been reported in 23% to 37% of patients with type I Gaucher disease. At the onset of a crisis, scintigraphy reveals decreased radionuclide uptake at the site of pain as evidence of ischemia.[142] Within 7 to 14 days of the acute bone crisis, intramedullary hemorrhages can be identified by MRI.[143]

Conclusions

Current concepts and hypotheses regarding the pathophysiology of osteonecrosis are reviewed, as exemplified by lesions of the talus. Traumatic ON appears to result from a sudden ischemic event (arterial severance). Intravascular coagulation, an intermediary mechanism, is the most likely final common pathway producing intraosseous thrombosis and nontraumatic osteonecrosis. Etiologic risk factors capable of triggering intravascular coagulation include intraosseous fat embolism, hypersensitivity reactions, bacterial endotoxic (Shwartzman) reactions and various viral infections, proteolytic enzymes, thromboplastin release (inflammatory bowel disease, malignancies, neurotrauma, and pregnancy), and several other prethrombotic and hypofibrinolytic conditions.

References

1. Haliburton RA, Sullivan CR, Kelly PJ, et al: The extraosseous and intra-osseous blood supply of the talus. *J Bone Joint Surg* 1958;40A:1115-1120.
2. Mulfinger GL, Trueta J: The blood supply of the talus. *J Bone Joint Surg* 1970;52B:160-167.
3. Calandruccio RA, Anderson WE II: Post-fracture avascular necrosis of the femoral head: Correlation of experimental and clinical studies. *Clin Orthop* 1980;152:49-84.
4. Brooks CH, Revell WJ, Heatley FW: Vascularity of the humeral head after proximal humeral fractures. *J Bone Joint Surg* 1993;75B:132-136.
5. Hawkins LG: Fractures of the neck of the talus. *J Bone Joint Surg* 1970;52A:991-1002.
6. Mindell ER, Cisek EE, Kartalian G, et al: Late results of injuries to the talus: Analysis of forty cases. *J Bone Joint Surg* 1963;45A:221-245.
7. Pittelkow RB, Kierland RR: Angiokeratoma corporis diffusum. *Arch Dermatol* 1955;72:556-561.
8. Dall D, Macnab I: Spontaneous avascular necrosis of the talus: A report of two cases. *S Afr Med J* 1970;44:193-196.
9. Jaffe HL: *Metabolic, Degenerative, and Inflammatory Diseases of Bones and Joints.* Philadelphia, PA, Lea & Febiger, 1972, pp 674-692.
10. Harris RD, Silver RA: Atraumatic aseptic necrosis of the talus. *Radiology* 1973;106:81-83.
11. Jones JP Jr: Alcoholism, hypercortisonism, fat embolism and osseous avascular necrosis, in Zinn WM (ed): *Idiopathic Ischemic Necrosis of the Femoral Head in Adults.* Baltimore, MD, University Park Press, 1971, pp 112-132.
12. Aptekar RG, Klippel JH, Becker KE, et al: Avascular necrosis of the talus, scaphoid, and metatarsal head in systemic lupus erythematosus. *Clin Orthop* 1974;101:127-128.
13. Ruderman M, McCarty DJ Jr: Aseptic necrosis in systemic lupus erythematosus: Report of a case involving six joints. *Arthritis Rheum* 1964;7:709-721.
14. Klippel JH, Gerber LH, Pollak L, et al: Avascular necrosis in systemic lupus erythematosus: Silent symmetric osteonecroses. *Am J Med* 1979;67:83-87.
15. Jones JP Jr: Osteonecrosis, in McCarty DJ, Koopman WJ (eds): *Arthritis and Allied Conditions: A Textbook of Rheumatology,* ed 12. Philadelphia, PA, Lea & Febiger, 1993, pp 1677-1696.
16. James J, Steijn-Myagkaya GL: Death of osteocytes: Electron microscopy after in vitro ischaemia. *J Bone Joint Surg*

1986;68B:620-624.
17. Ruland LJ III, Wang GJ, Teates CD, et al: A comparison of magnetic resonance imaging to bone scintigraphy in early traumatic ischemia of the femoral head. *Clin Orthop* 1992;285:30-34.
18. Sy WM, Westring DW, Weinberger G: "Cold" lesions on bone imaging. *J Nucl Med* 1975;16:1013-1016.
19. Nadel SN, Debatin JF, Richardson WJ, et al: Detection of acute avascular necrosis of the femoral head in dogs: Dynamic contrast-enhanced MR imaging vs spin-echo and STIR sequences. *AJR* 1992;159:1255-1261.
20. Jones JP Jr: Osteonecrosis, in McCarty DJ (ed): *Arthritis and Allied Conditions: A Textbook of Rheumatology,* ed 11. Philadelphia, PA, Lea & Febiger, 1989, pp 1545-1562.
21. Shahabpour M, Handelberg F, Opdecam M, et al: Magnetic resonance imaging (MRI) of the ankle and hindfoot. *Acta Orthop Belgica* 1992;58:5-14.
22. De Smet AA, Fisher DR, Burnstein MI, et al: Value of MR imaging in staging osteochondral lesions of the talus (osteochondritis dissecans): Results in 14 patients. *AJR* 1990;154:555-558.
23. Drury P, Sartoris DJ: Osteonecrosis in the foot. *J Foot Surg* 1991;30:477-483.
24. Hamilton HE, Bonfiglio M, Sheets RF, et al: Relation of altered hemostasis to idiopathic aseptic necrosis of the femoral head. *J Clin Invest* 1965;44:1058-1065.
25. Boettcher WG, Bonfiglio M, Hamilton HE, et al: Non-traumatic necrosis of the femoral head: Part I. Relation of altered hemostasis to etiology. *J Bone Joint Surg* 1970;52A:312-321.
26. Bonfiglio M: Development of bone necrosis lesions, in Lambertsen CJ (ed): *Underwater Physiology V. Proc. Fifth Symposium Underwater Physiology.* Bethesda, MD, FASEB, 1976, pp 117-132.
27. Jones JP Jr, Sakovich L, Anderson CE: Experimentally produced osteonecrosis as a result of fat embolism, in Beckman EL, Elliott DH, Smith EM (eds): *Dysbarism-related Osteonecrosis.* HEW Pub (NIOSH) 75-153, Washington, DC, U.S. Government Printing Office, 1974, pp 117-132.
28. Jones JP Jr: Etiology and pathogenesis of osteonecrosis. *Semin Arthroplasty* 1991;2:160-168.
29. Jones JP Jr: Intravascular coagulation and osteonecrosis. *Clin Orthop* 1992;277:41-53.
30. Jones JP Jr, Ramirez S, Doty SB: The pathophysiologic role of fat in dysbaric osteonecrosis. *Clin Orthop* 1993;296:256-264.
31. Jones JP Jr: Fat embolism, intravascular coagulation and osteonecrosis. *Clin Orthop* 1993;292:294-308.
32. Ficat RP, Arlet J (eds): *Ischemia and Necroses of Bone.* Baltimore, MD, Williams & Wilkins, 1980, pp 75-103.
33. Resnick D, Pineda C, Trudell D: Widespread osteonecrosis of the foot in systemic lupus erythematosus: Radiographic and gross pathologic correlation. *Skeletal Radiol* 1985;13:33-38.
34. Saito S, Ohzono K, Ono K: Early arteriopathy and postulated pathogenesis of osteonecrosis of the femoral head: The intracapital arterioles. *Clin Orthop* 1992;277:98-110.
35. Spencer JD, Brookes M: Avascular necrosis and the blood supply of the femoral head. *Clin Orthop* 1988;235:127-140.
36. Müller-Berghaus G: Pathophysiologic and biochemical events in disseminated intravascular coagulation: Dysregulation of procoagulant and anticoagulant pathways. *Semin Thromb Hemost* 1989;15:58-87.
37. Atsumi T, Kuroki Y: Role of impairment of blood supply of the femoral head in the pathogenesis of idiopathic osteonecrosis. *Clin Orthop* 1992;277:22-30.
38. Jones JP Jr: Fat embolism and osteonecrosis. *Orthop Clin North Am* 1985;16:595-633.

39. Kiaer T, Dahl B, Lausten G : Partial pressures of oxygen and carbon dioxide in bone and their correlation with bone-blood flow: Effect of decreased arterial supply and venous congestion on intraosseous oxygen and carbon dioxide in an animal model. *J Orthop Res* 1992;10:807-812.

40. Welch RD, Johnston CE II, Waldron MJ, et al: Bone changes associated with intraosseous hypertension in the caprine tibia. *J Bone Joint Surg* 1993;75A:53-60.

41. Gold EW, Fox OD, Weissfeld S, et al: Corticosteroid-induced avascular necrosis: An experimental study in rabbits. *Clin Orthop* 1978;135:272-280.

42. Surat A: Isolation of prostaglandin E2-like material from osteonecrosis induced by steroids and its prevention by kallikrein inhibitor, aprotinin: An experimental study in rabbits. *Prostaglandins Leukot Med* 1984;13:159-167.

43. Tsai CL, Liu TK: Evidence for eicosanoids within the reparative front in avascular necrosis of human femoral head. *Clin Orthop* 1992;281:305-312.

44. Welch RD, Johnston CE II, Waldron MJ, et al: Intraosseous infusion of prostaglandin E2 in the caprine tibia. *J Orthop Res* 1992;11:110-121.

45. Bick RL, Baker WF Jr: Disseminated intravascular coagulation syndromes. *Hematol Pathol* 1992;6:1-24.

46. Halleraker B: Fat embolism and intravascular coagulation. *Acta Pathol Microbiol Scand* 1970;78:432-436.

47. Harigaya K, Watanabe S, Watanabe Y, et al: Multiple bone marrow necrosis and disseminated intravascular coagulation. *Arch Pathol Lab Med* 1977;101:652-654.

48. Allardyce DB, Groves AC: Intravascular coagulation, hyperlipemia, and fat embolism: Their association during the generalized Shwartzman phenomenon in rabbits. *Surgery* 1969;66:71-79.

49. Hirsch RL, McKay DG, Travers RI, et al: Hyperlipidemia, fatty liver, and bromsulfophthalein retention in rabbits injected intravenously with bacterial endotoxins. *J Lipid Res* 1964;5:563-568.

50. Sandset PM, Warn-Cramer BJ, Maki SL, et al: Immuno-depletion of extrinsic pathway inhibitor sensitizes rabbits to endotoxin-induced intravascular coagulation and the generalized Shwartzman reaction. *Blood* 1991;78:1496-1502.

51. Duncan JS, Ramsay LE: Widespread bone infarction complicating meningococcal septicaemia and disseminated intravascular coagulation. *Br Med J* 1984;288:111-112.

52. Grogan DP, Love SM, Ogden JA, et al: Chondro-osseous growth abnormalities after meningococcemia: A clinical and histo-pathological study. *J Bone Joint Surg* 1989;71A:920-928.

53. McKay DG, Margaretten W: Disseminated intravascular coagulation in virus diseases. *Arch Intern Med* 1967;120:129-152.

54. Gregosiewicz A, Okonski M, Stolecka D, et al: Ischemia of the femoral head in Perthes' disease: Is the cause intra- or extravascular? *J Pediatr Orthop* 1989;9:160-152.

55. Joseph B: Serum immunoglobulin in Perthes' disease. *J Bone Joint Surg* 1991;73B:509-510.

56. Matsoukas JA: Viral antibody titers to rubella in coxa plana or Perthes' disease. *Acta Orthop Scand* 1975;46:957-962.

57. Chevalier X, Larget-Piet B, Hernigou P, et al: Avascular necrosis of the femoral head in HIV-infected patients. *J Bone Joint Surg* 1993;75B:160.

58. Starzl TE, Lerner RA, Dixon FJ, et al: Shwartzman reaction after human renal homotransplantation. *N Engl J Med* 1968;278:642-648.

59. Leunissen KML, Ruers TJM, Bosman F, et al: Intravascular coagulation and kidney donation. *Transplantation* 1986;42:307-308.

60. Pardo-Mindán FJ, Salinas-Madrigal L, Idoate M, et al: Pathology of renal transplantation. *Semin Diagn Pathol* 1992;9:185-199.

61. Latour JG, Prejean JB, Margaretten W: Corticosteroids and the generalized Shwartzman reaction: Mechanisms of sensitization in the rabbit. *Am J Pathol* 1971;65:189-202.

62. Cosgriff SW, Diefenbach AF, Vogt W Jr: Hypercoagulability of the blood associated with ACTH and cortisone therapy. *Am J Med* 1950;9:752-756.

63. Bergstein JM, Michael AF Jr: The effect of thorotrast and cortisone on renal cortical fibrinolytic activity in the rabbit. *Am J Pathol* 1973;71:113-118.

64. Gerrits WB, Prakke EM, van der Meer J: Corticosteroids and experimental intravascular coagulation. *Scand J Haematol* 1974;13:5-10.

65. Thompson PL, Willams KE, Walters MN: Fat embolism in the microcirculation: An in-vivo study. *J Pathol* 1969;97:23-28.

66. Adleberg JS, Smith GH: Corticosteroid-induced avascular necrosis of the talus. *J Foot Surg* 1991;30:66-69.

67. Jacobs B: Alcoholism-induced bone necrosis. *N Y State J Med* 1992;92:334-338.

68. Haber LM, Hawkins EP, Seilheimer DK, et al: Fat overload syndrome: An autopsy study with evaluation of the coagulopathy. *Am J Clin Pathol* 1988;90:223-227.

69. Shapiro SC, Rothstein FC, Newman AJ, et al: Multifocal osteonecrosis in adolescents with Crohn's disease: A complication of therapy? *J Pediatr Gastroenterol Nutr* 1985;4:502-506.

70. Alexakis PG, Wallack M: Idiopathic osteonecrosis of the femoral head associated with a pituitary tumor: Report of a case. *J Bone Joint Surg* 1989;71A:1412-1414.

71. Rico H, Gomez-Castresana F, Cabranes JA, et al: Increased blood cortisol in alcoholic patients with aseptic necrosis of the femoral head. *Calcif Tissue Int* 1985;37:585-587.

72. Kawai K, Tamaki A, Hirohata K: Steroid-induced accumulation of lipid in the osteocytes of the rabbit femoral head: A histochemical and electron microscopic study. *J Bone Joint Surg* 1985;67A:755-763.

73. Muratsu H, Shimizu T, Kawai K, et al: Alcohol-induced accumulations of lipids in the osteocytes of the rabbit femoral head. *Trans Orthop Res Soc* 1990;15:402.

74. Felson DT, Anderson JJ: A cross-study evaluation of association between steroid dose and bolus steroids and avascular necrosis of bone. *Lancet* 1987;1:902-905.

75. Matsuo K, Hirohata T, Sugioka Y, et al: Influence of alcohol intake, cigarette smoking, and occupatonal status on idiopathic osteonecrosis of the femoral head. *Clin Orthop* 1988;234:115-123.

76. Lang P, Mauz M, Schorner W, et al: Acute fracture of the femoral neck: Assessment of femoral head perfusion with gadopentetate dimeglumine-enhanced MR imaging. *AJR AM J Roentgenol* 1993;160:335-341.

77. O'Brien TJ, Mack GR: Multifocal osteonecrosis after short-term high-dose corticosteroid theapy: A case report. *Clin Orthop* 1992;279:176-179.

78. Hirohata K, Shimizu T, Toyoda Y: Fatty degeneration of osteocytes of the fourth metatarsus in patients with idiopathic necrosis of the femoral head. *Kobe J Med Sci* 1990;36:127-135.

79. Arlot ME, Bonjean M, Chavassieux PM, et al: Bone histology in adults with aseptic necrosis: Histomorphometric evaluation of iliac biopsies in seventy-seven patients. *J Bone Joint Surg* 1983;65A:1319-1327.

80. Wang GJ, Chung KC, Shen WJ, et al: Preventing steroid induced osteoporosis in the femoral head using lipid clearing agents. *Trans Orthop Res Soc* 1989;14:457.

81. Maruno H, Shimizu T, Kawai K, et al: The response of osteocytes to a lipid clearing agent in steroid-treated rab-

bits. *J Bone Joint Surg* 1991;73B:911-915.

82. Jones JP Jr: Evidence for progressive intraosseous fat overload causing osteoarthrosis, osteoporosis, and osteonecrosis. *J Jpn Orthop Assoc* 1992;66:S16-S17.

83. Cheras PA: The role of thrombosis in ischaemic necrosis of bone (INB) and primary osteo-arthritis (OA). Greenslopes, Australia, University of Queensland, 1993, p 226, Thesis.

84. Doty SB, Morey-Holton ER, Durnova GN, et al: Cosmos 1887: Morphology, histochemistry, and vasculature of the growing rat tibia. *FASEB J* 1990;4:16-23.

85. Alonso MP, Navarrina F, Navarrina JA, et al: Microvascular changes in osteoporotic long bones caused by the action of corticosteroids. *Assoc Res Circ Osseous (ARCO) Newsletter* 1992;4:102-110.

86. Mahowald ML, Majeski PJ, Ytterberg SR: Microvascular pathology of antigen induced arthritis. *Arthritis Rheum (Suppl)* 1988;31:S91.

87. Matsui M, Saito S, Ohzono K, et al: Experimental steroid-induced osteonecrosis in adult rabbits with hypersensitivity vasculitis. *Clin Orthop* 1992;277:61-72.

88. Ono K, Tohjima T, Komazawa T: Risk factors of avascular necrosis of the femoral head in patients with systemic lupus erythematosus under high-dose corticosteroid therapy. *Clin Orthop* 1992;277:89-97.

89. McKay DG: Diseases of hypersensitivity: Disseminated intravascular coagulation. *Arch Intern Med* 1965;116:83-94.

90. Asherson RA, Khamashta MA, Ordi-Ros J, et al: The "primary" antiphospholipid syndrome: Major clinical and serological features. *Medicine* 1989;68:366-374.

91. Nagasawa K, Ishii Y, Mayumi T, et al: Avascular necrosis of bone in systemic lupus erythematosus: Possible role of haemostatic abnormalities. *Ann Rheum Dis* 1989;48:672-676.

92. Seleznick MJ, Silveira LH, Espinoza LR: Avascular necrosis associated with anticardiolipin antibodies. *J Rheumatol* 1991;18:1416-1417.

93. Vela P, Batlle E, Salas E, et al: Primary antiphospholipid syndrome and osteonecrosis. *Clin Exp Rheumatol* 1991;9:545-546.

94. Pérez RE, McClendon JR, Lie JT: Primary antiphospholipid syndrome with multiorgan arterial and venous thromboses. *J Rheumatol* 1992;19:1289-1292.

95. Harrison RL, Alperin JB: Concurrent protein C deficiency and lupus anticoagulants. *Am J Hematol* 1992;40:33-37.

96. Lin YL, Wang CT: Activation of human platelets by the rabbit anticardiolipin antibodies. *Blood* 1992;80:3135-3143.

97. Stinson J, Tomkin G, McDonald G, et al: Recurrent disseminated intravascular coagulation and fulminant intra hepatic thrombosis in a patient with the anti-phospholipid syndrome. *Am J Hematol* 1990;35:281-282.

98. James CCM: Late bone lesions in caisson disease: Three cases in submarine personnel. *Lancet* 1945;2:6-8.

99. Lehner CE, Lin TF, Lanphier EH, et al: Early pathogenesis and detection of dysbaric osteonecrosis induced in sheep. *Undersea Biomed Res (Suppl)* 1992;19:52-53.

100. Philip RB: A review of blood changes associated with compression-decompression: Relationship to decompression sickness. *Undersea Biomed Res* 1974;1:117-140.

101. Kawashima M, Torisu T, Hayashi K, et al: Pathological review of osteonecrosis in divers. *Clin Orthop* 1978;130:107-117.

102. Kitano M, Hayashi K: Acute decompression sickness: Report of an autopsy case with widespread fat embolism. *Acta Pathol Jpn* 1981;31:269-276.

103. Corelli AI, Binder RA, Kales A: Disseminated intravascular coagulation in sickle cell crisis. *South Med J* 1979;72:505-506.

104. Devine DV, Kinney TR, Thomas PF, et al: Fragment D-dimer levels: An objective marker of vaso-occlusive crisis

and other complications of sickle cell disease. *Blood* 1986;68:317-319.

105. Ware HE, Brooks AP, Toye R, et al: Sickle cell disease and silent avascular necrosis of the hip. *J Bone Joint Surg* 1991;73B:947-949.

106. Milner PF, Kraus AP, Sebes JI, et al: Sickle cell disease as a cause of osteonecrosis of the femoral head. *N Engl J Med* 1991;325:1476-1481.

107. Hynd RF, Bharadwaja K, Mitas JA, et al: Rhabdomyolysis, acute renal failure and disseminated intravascular coagulation in a man with sickle cell trait. *South Med J* 1985;78:890-891.

108. Jones SR, Binder RA, Donowho EM Jr: Sudden death in sickle cell trait. *N Engl J Med* 1970;282:323-325.

109. Billett HH, Nagel RL, Fabry ME: Evolution of laboratory parameters during sickle cell painful crisis: Evidence compatible with dense red cell sequestration without thrombosis. *Am J Med Sci* 1988;296:293-298.

110. Thrall JH, Rucknagel DL: Increased bone marrow blood flow in sickle cell anemia demonstrated by thallium-201 and Tc-99m human albumin microspheres. *Radiology* 1978;127:817-819.

111. Francis RB Jr: Platelets, coagulation, and fibrinolysis in sickle cell disease: Their possible role in vascular occlusion. *Blood Coagul Fibrinolysis* 1991;2:341-353.

112. Beurling-Harbury C, Schade SG: Platelet activation during pain crisis in sickle cell anemia patients. *Am J Hematol* 1989;31:237-241.

113. Rickles FR, O'Leary DS: Role of the coagulation system in the pathophysiology of sickle cell disease. *Arch Intern Med* 1974;133:635-641.

114. Sowemimo-Coker SO, Meiselman HJ, Francis RB Jr: Increased circulating endothelial cells in sickle cell crisis. *Am J Hematol* 1989;31:263-265.

115. Rao VM, Fishman M, Mitchell DG, et al: Painful sickle cell crisis: Bone marrow patterns observed with MR imaging. *Radiology* 1986;161:211-215.

116. van Zanten TE, Statius van Eps LW, Golding RP, et al: Imaging the bone marrow with magnetic resonance during a crisis and in chronic forms of sickle cell disease. *Clin Radiol* 1989;40:486-489.

117. Kucuk O, Gilman-Sachs A, Beaman K, et al: Antiphospholipid antibodies in sickle cell disease. *Am J Hematol* 1993;42:380-383.

118. Milgram JW, Gruhn JG (eds): *Radiologic and Histologic Pathology of Nontumorous Diseases of Bones and Joints.* Northbrook, IL, Northbrook Publishing, 1990, pp 1067-1092.

119. Bick RL: Coagulation abnormalities in malignancy: A review. *Semin Thromb Hemost* 1992;18:353-372.

120. Hanada T, Horigome Y, Inudoh M, et al: Osteonecrosis of vertebrae in a child with acute lymphocytic leukaemia during L-asparaginase therapy. *Eur J Pediatr* 1989;149:162-163.

121. Ollivier L, Leclere J, Vanel D, et al: Femoral infarction following intraarterial chemotherapy for osteosarcoma of the leg: A possible pitfall in magnetic resonance imaging. *Skeletal Radiol* 1991;20:329-332.

122. Baron M, Paltiel H, Lander P: Aseptic necrosis of the talus and calcaneal insufficiency fractures in a patient with pancreatitis, subcutaneous fat necrosis, and arthritis. *Arthritis Rheum* 1984;27:1309-1313.

123. van der Sande JJ, Emeis JJ, Lindeman J: Intravascular coagulation: A common phenomenon in minor experimental head injury. *J Neurosurg* 1981;54:21-25.

124. Fujii Y, Mammen EF, Farag A, et al: Thrombosis in spinal cord injury. *Thromb Res* 1992;68:357-368.

125. Kaufman HH, Hui KS, Mattson JC, et al: Clinicopath-

ological correlations of disseminated intravascular coagulation in patients with head injury. *Neurosurgery* 1984;15:34-42.

126. Taylor LJ: Multifocal avascular necrosis after short-term high-dose steroid therapy: A report of three cases. *J Bone Joint Surg* 1984;66B:431-433.

127. Bick RL: Disseminated intravascular coagulation and related syndromes, in Bick RL (ed): *Hematology: Clinical and Laboratory Practice*. St. Louis, MO, CV Mosby, 1993, pp 1463-1499.

128. Freeman HJ, Kwan WCP: Non-corticosteroid-associated osteonecrosis of the femoral heads in two patients with inflammatory bowel disease. *N Engl J Med* 1993;329:1314-1316.

129. Glueck CJ, Glueck HI, Mieczkowski L, et al: Familial high plasminogen activator inhibitor with hypofibrinolysis, a new pathophysiologic cause of osteonecrosis? *Thromb Haemost* 1993;69:460-465.

130. Bunting RW, Doppelt SH, Lavine LS: Extreme thrombocytosis after orthopaedic surgery. *J Bone Joint Surg* 1991;73B:687-688.

131. Katamura K, Ishimoto F, Yamasaki M, et al: Disseminated intravascular coagulation syndrome in anorexia nervosa. *Acta Paediatr Jpn* 1992;34:469-472.

132. Warren MP, Shane E, Lee MJ, et al: Femoral head collapse associated with anorexia nervosa in a 20-year-old ballet dancer. *Clin Orthop* 1990;251:171-176.

133. Kanfer A: Coagulation factors in nephrotic syndrome. *Am J Nephrol* 1990;10(suppl 1):63-68.

134. Döhler R, Poser HL, Harms D, et al: Systemic lipomatosis of bone: A case report. *J Bone Joint Surg* 1982;64B:84-87.

135. Kim YY, Bae DK, Suh DS, et al: Osteonecrosis of the femoral head associated with polyvinylpyrrolidone storage. *Korea J Orthop Surg* 1982;17:598-606.

136. Katz K, Mechlis-Frish S, Cohen IJ, et al: Bone scans in the diagnosis of bone crisis in patients who have Gaucher disease. *J Bone Joint Surg* 1991;73A:513-517.

137. Macleod MA, McEwan AJB, Pearson RR, et al: Functional imaging in the early diagnosis of dysbaric osteonecrosis. *Br J Radiol* 1982;55:497-500.

138. Sebes JI: Diagnostic imaging of bone and joint abnormalities associated with sickle cell hemoglobinopathies. *AJR* 1989;152:1153-1159.

139. Szasz I, Morrison RT, Lyster DM, et al: Bone scintigraphy in massive disseminated bone necrosis. *Clin Nucl Med* 1981;6:97-100.

140. Vreeken J, Meinders AE, Keeman JN, et al: A chronic clotting defect with some characteristics of excessive intravascular coagulation in a patient with Gaucher's disease. *Folia Med Neerl* 1967;10:180-185.

141. Yates P, Morse C, Standen GR: Gaucher's disease and acquired coagulopathy. *Clin Lab Haemat* 1992;14:331-334.

142. Israel O, Jerushalmi J, Front D: Scintigraphic findings in Gaucher's disease. *J Nucl Med* 1986;27:1557-1563.

143. Horev G, Kornreich L, Hadar H, et al: Hemorrhage associated with "bone crisis" in Gaucher's disease identified by magnetic resonance imaging. *Skeletal Radiol* 1991;20:479-482.

Early Diagnosis, Evaluation, and Staging of Osteonecrosis

Marvin E. Steinberg, MD

Our goal in treating osteonecrosis is to preserve, not replace, the femoral head. Without specific treatment, the majority of femoral heads with osteonecrosis will collapse. A number of different methods of treatment have been described. Although the literature is somewhat contradictory about their effectiveness, it is generally agreed that the results are better than with symptomatic treatment alone. Whichever method is selected, optimum results will be obtained if the diagnosis is made early and treatment is instituted promptly. It is thus essential to have a clear understanding of the best means for early diagnosis. Once the diagnosis is made, an effective method of evaluation and staging helps determine the treatment. It also assists in following the progression or resolution of this condition, establishing a prognosis, and comparing the results of various methods of management.

This chapter begins with a review of the modalities that have proven most helpful in making an early diagnosis. It covers the history, physical examination, laboratory tests, and imaging modalities. Awareness of the etiologic factors that lead to osteonecrosis is essential. Good quality anteroposterior and lateral radiographs, together with MRI, are the basic tools that supplement a thorough clinical evaluation. The quantitative system for evaluation and staging, described below, has several advantages over older systems and allows us to determine the extent, as well as the stage, of the lesion. It thus improves our ability to treat patients with osteonecrosis.

Early Diagnosis

In most instances, the definitive diagnosis of osteonecrosis will be made when pathognomonic changes appear on plain films. Figure 1 shows an advanced case of osteonecrosis. The femoral head has already begun to collapse, and this hip is beyond the point where it can be saved. The diagnosis must be made well before this stage, ideally before any changes appear on ordinary radiographs.

History

The symptoms of osteonecrosis are nonspecific and include pain, limp, and decreased motion. In the early stages, and sometimes even in the later stages, this condition may be entirely asymptomatic. An awareness of predisposing factors is essential in making the diagnosis. The most common etiology is trauma, especially when it causes a displaced subcapital or high transcervical fracture, or a dislocation or fracture-dislocation of the hip. The incidence of osteonecrosis following a displaced transcervical fracture is approximately 30%. However, because this chapter deals with nontraumatic osteonecrosis, little more will be said about the posttraumatic variety.

Of the many predisposing factors and conditions associated with osteonecrosis, the most common are corticosteroid administration and excessive alcohol intake. In approximately 15% to 20% of cases, no etiology can be identified, and these are referred to as idio-

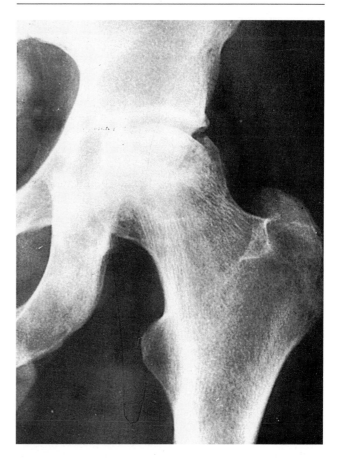

Fig. 1 Plain radiograph showing an advanced case of osteonecrosis with collapse of the femoral head (Stage IV-C)

pathic. Osteonecrosis is bilateral in more than 50% of cases. If one hip, or perhaps another area, has been diagnosed with osteonecrosis, it is essential to examine the opposite hip and perhaps the shoulders and knees as well. In our experience, the femoral head is afflicted more commonly and earlier than other areas, but, when this condition has been diagnosed in the femoral head, the incidence of shoulder or knee involvement is approximately 15%.[1-5]

Physical Examination

The physical examination is nonspecific and is often within normal limits until relatively late. When present, abnormal findings may include pain on motion, decreased range of motion, and a limp. Shortening of the extremity is noted only with advanced disease and is caused either by gross collapse of the femoral head or by flexion contracture.

Laboratory Tests

In most instances, presently available laboratory tests are within normal limits. One exception is in osteonecrosis associated with sickle cell disease. Recent evidence also suggests an increased incidence of elevated anticardiolipin antibody in certain cases of systemic lupus erythematosus. In cases associated with gout, there may be an elevated serum uric acid; however, this is an infrequent etiology for osteonecrosis. In most circumstances, serologic testing is of greatest value to rule out other causes of hip pathology.

Imaging Modalities

The most important diagnostic test is a routine radiographic study, including good quality anteroposterior and lateral films of both hips. In the earliest stages of osteonecrosis, these are within normal limits. Later, diffuse osteopenia may be seen in certain cases. If this is the initial finding, the condition must be differentiated from other causes of osteopenia, such as transitory osteoporosis. More frequently, the radiographic picture is one of mottling composed of areas of sclerosis and radiolucency, sometimes referred to as "cysts". If collapse of the subchondral bone occurs prior to flattening of the articular surface, a crescent sign may be seen. This is usually followed by gross flattening of the articular surface, which eventually leads to joint-line narrowing and secondary changes in the acetabulum.

Occasionally tomograms or computed tomography (CT) may show subtle changes not seen on plain films. At the present time, I rarely rely on these two modalities for early diagnosis, but on occasion I may order one or both studies if it is suspected that the condition may be more advanced than it appears on plain films.

A technetium bone scan is also useful to identify lesions before they appear on plain radiographs. It must be remembered that the bone scan is a nonspecific study and does not distinguish between osteonecrosis and a variety of other conditions. It may be a very useful screening technique if we wish to rule out involvement of a number of areas of bone with a single study. A positive bone scan shows an area of increased uptake in the reactive bone formation that surrounds the necrotic region. If obtained early, there may be an area of decreased isotope uptake over the avascular segment, but this is an uncommon finding. Even less frequently, a "cold" area is seen over the necrotic segment, surrounded by a ring of increased uptake that corresponds to new bone formation. Although there has been some interest in the use of single photon emission computed tomography (SPECT), reports about its sensitivity and specificity have been mixed. To date, this technique has not been developed well enough for it to be used routinely in the evaluation of osteonecrosis.

The best single method for the early diagnosis of osteonecrosis is magnetic resonance imaging (MRI). For maximum effectiveness, it is essential that a good quality, high-powered unit be used, and that the images be interpreted by experienced observers. Images taken in the coronal plane are of more value than those taken in the transverse or axial plane. The use of sagittal sections, surface coils, and other techniques have been helpful. Both T_1- and T_2-weighted images should be evaluated. This field is advancing very rapidly, and a number of special techniques have

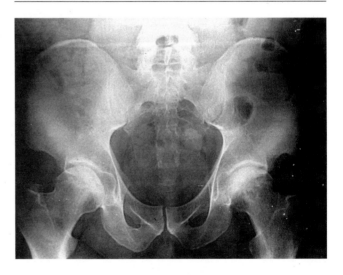

Fig. 2 Plain radiograph of a patient with known alcohol-related osteonecrosis of the left hip and recent pain on the right. Abnormalities in the left femoral head are consistent with osteonecrosis (Stage II-B), whereas the right hip was interpreted as being within normal limits.

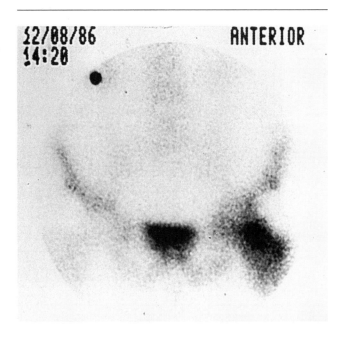

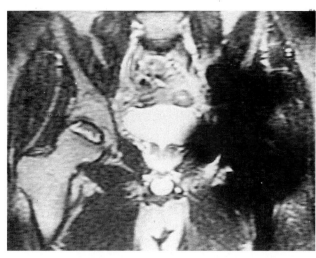

Fig. 5 This MRI of a patient with previous left total hip replacement and active osteonecrosis on the right demonstrates the dramatic picture obtained with a weighted spin-echo image.

Fig. 3 Technetium scan showing increased uptake over the left hip but normal uptake over the right.

been developed that add to the sensitivity and specificity of MRI. These include the use of quantitative MRI, out-of-phase or opposed images, and weighted spin-echo images.

With modern refinements in MRI and increased experience on the part of radiologists, use of MRI frequently allows the diagnosis of osteonecrosis before it can be seen on plain films or bone scans. Figure 2 shows an anteroposterior radiograph of the pelvis of a patient known to have alcohol-related osteonecrosis of the left hip. He recently developed pain in the right

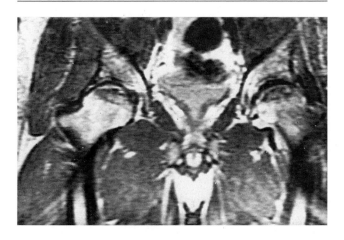

Fig. 4 MRI of the same patient showing a decreased signal intensity in both femoral heads, consistent with bilateral osteonecrosis.

hip; however, both this film and a laminogram of the right hip were interpreted as being within normal limits. Figure 3 shows a technetium scan done a few days later. There is an increased uptake over the left hip but the right is within normal limits. An MRI, however, shows a decreased signal intensity in both femoral heads (Fig. 4). The patient underwent a core decompression on the right side which confirmed the diagnosis.

Special MRI techniques have been developed that demonstrate the lesion of osteonecrosis in a very dramatic fashion. Figure 5 is a weighted spin-echo image of the pelvis in a patient with a total hip replacement done previously on the left for osteonecrosis, and early, biopsy-proven osteonecrosis on the right.

As with any new technique, it is important that MRI be neither over used nor over read. For example, the patient with classic radiographic findings of osteonecrosis in both femoral heads does not need an MRI of the hips. We must also remember that not every abnormality of the MRI signal in the femoral head is caused by osteonecrosis. Other conditions, such as tumor, infection, fracture, and transient osteoporosis, can give an altered MRI signal. Figure 6 shows a decrease in the signal intensity over the femoral head and neck in a young male with mild left hip pain. This was initially diagnosed as osteonecrosis. Plain radiographs, however, showed diffuse osteopenia, and there were no risk factors for osteonecrosis. The patient was treated conservatively and the condition resolved spontaneously. The final diagnosis was transient osteoporosis.

A number of studies have compared the sensitivity and specificity of MRI to various other imaging modali-

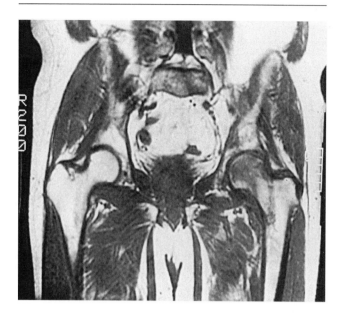

Fig. 6 MRI of a patient with transient osteoporosis showing a decreased signal intensity involving the entire femoral head and neck. This picture can be confused with osteonecrosis.

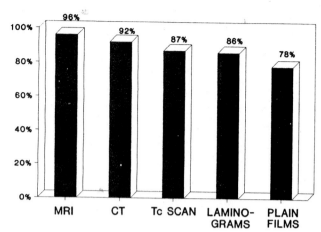

Fig. 7 Graph showing the diagnostic accuracy of various imaging modalities in 55 hips with proven osteonecrosis.

ties in osteonecrosis. The results of a study done at our institution several years ago are shown in Figure 7. This graph shows the diagnostic accuracy of MRI, computed tomography, technetium scans, laminograms, and plain films in 55 hips with biopsy-proven osteonecrosis. As noted, MRI was the most accurate of these techniques. Figure 8 shows the results of a study that compared the accuracy of MRI, technetium scans, and computed tomography in 14 early, pre-radiologic cases of osteonecrosis. Again MRI showed itself to be the most accurate.

At the present time, magnetic resonance imaging is the most effective method for the early diagnosis of osteonecrosis. Although this is an expensive test and is not always readily available, it is without known side effects. It should not be used without specific indications, but should be ordered without hesitation when there is clinical suspicion of osteonecrosis, which cannot be diagnosed by simpler methods, such as routine radiographs. Its sensitivity and specificity are such that we do not hesitate to institute treatment based on the MRI alone, provided that the diagnosis is corroborated clinically.[6-10]

Other Diagnostic Modalities

Other modalities for the early diagnosis of osteonecrosis are available. These include such special angiographic techniques as superselective angiography, intraosseous pressure measurements, intraosseous venography, and biopsy. These tests are invasive or

semi-invasive and, with the development of MRI, are now less useful than they once were. Although in most instances the diagnosis can be made prior to biopsy, histologic material should always be examined carefully if it is available, because in rare instances other conditions, such as tumor, can mimic osteonecrosis.

Evaluation and Classification

Patients with avascular necrosis of the hip should be evaluated both clinically and radiographically. These two techniques provide different information and proper decision making requires that both be employed.

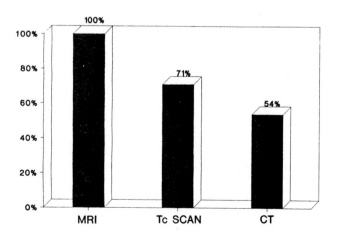

Fig. 8 Graph showing the diagnostic accuracy of MRI, technetium scanning, and CT in 14 cases of early, pre-radiologic osteonecrosis.

Table 1
Criteria for staging osteonecrosis

Stage	Criteria
0	Normal or nondiagnostic X-ray, bone scan, and MRI
I*	Normal X-ray, abnormal bone scan, and/or MRI
II*	Abnormal X-ray ("cystic" and sclerotic changes in the femoral head without collapse)
III*	Subchondral collapse (crescent sign) without flattening of articular surface
IV*	Flattening of femoral head without joint narrowing or acetabular involvement
V*	Joint narrowing and/or acetabular involvement
VI	Advanced degenerative changes

* (The extent of involvement in Stages I through V should also be indicated as "A", "B", or "C" as described in Table 2)

Table 2
Quantitating the extent of involvement

Stages I and II
    Determine percent of head involved on MRI (Stage I) or
    X-Ray (Stage II):
        A. <15%
        B. 15% to 30%
        C. >30%
Stage III
    Determine percent of articular surface under which bone has
    collapsed (crescent sign):
        A. <15%
        B. 15% to 30%
        C. >30%
Stage IV
    Determine percent of surface flattening and extent of collapse:
        A. <15% and <2 mm collapse
        B. 15% to 30% or 2 to 4 mm collapse
        C. >30% or >4 mm collapse
Stage V
    A, B, C. Determine the average of femoral head involvement,
    as in Stage IV, and the acetabular involvement, which is
    estimated.

Radiographic Evaluation and Staging

There are a number of systems currently in use for the classification or staging of osteonecrosis. Probably the most popular and most widely used is the system of Ficat.[11] This system has been modified and updated recently. It is quite useful, and one of its greatest advantages is its simplicity. Unfortunately, neither this nor most other systems provides a method to quantitate the extent of involvement. This is a major drawback, which has led to many erroneous conclusions as to the progression of the condition, particularly following various methods of treatment.

Many systems attempt to incorporate both radiographic and clinical determinants. This is often confusing, because frequently there is poor correlation between the extent of pathology present and the patient's pain and disability.

An effective method for radiographic evaluation and staging must include both the stage of the lesion and the size or the extent of involvement. The stages must be clearly defined and must match closely the documented pathologic changes. It must be objective and quantifiable. Modern imaging techniques, such as MRI, must be included and older invasive techniques, now rarely employed, should be eliminated. Such a system was developed several years ago at our institution and is outlined schematically in Tables 1 and 2. It is based specifically on radiographs, MRI, and other imaging modalities. Although clinical features are carefully recorded and are essential in the final decision making, they do not enter into the staging per se. Initially, the type of change is used to place the hip into stages 0 through VI (Table 1).

Next the extent or degree of involvement is either estimated or measured (Table 2). For routine clinical purposes, this can be estimated simply as "A" (mild), "B" (moderate), or "C" (severe).

When needed, a more precise measurement of the extent of involvement can be done easily and accurately. The area of abnormality seen on the MRI or on plain films is measured either manually with a grid or by a computerized technique and is then expressed as a percentage of the volume of the entire head. If a crescent sign is present, its length is measured in millimeters and expressed as a percent of the entire articular surface. When flattening is present, it is expressed both as a percent of the articular surface and in millimeters at the point of maximum collapse.

This technique has been used on approximately one thousand femoral heads. Small changes can be measured and the resolution or progression of the disease can be determined accurately. This precision allows us to evaluate and compare the effectiveness of various therapeutic measures, aids in establishing a prognosis, and gives us effective guidelines as to which method of treatment should be used.[12,13]

Several different modalities of "prophylactic" treatment have been used during the earlier stages of osteonecrosis to retard or reverse its progression in order to preserve the femoral head. These include osteotomies of the proximal femur, various types of grafting procedures, electrical stimulation, and core decompression. Reports differ as to the effectiveness of and indications for these procedures. This is discussed in more detail elsewhere.

Clinical Evaluation

As mentioned, the method for staging described above does not include clinical factors. In order to determine the optimum method of treatment, however, a variety of clinical factors must be evaluated care-

Table 3
A treatment algorithm for osteonecrosis

Stage	Treatment
I-A	Close observation or prophylactic RX
I-B - II	Prophylactic RX
III - IV-A	Prophylactic RX if signs and symptoms are minimal
IV-B - VI	THR when clinically indicated

fully. One of the standard hip rating systems must be used routinely and diligently both preoperatively and at set intervals following treatment.

In addition, a number of clinical features that do not comprise a part of the traditional hip evaluation must also be thoroughly investigated. Items of interest include the specific etiology of the osteonecrosis, whether the insult was limited or ongoing, determination of other areas of involvement, associated medical diagnoses, the age and general health of the patient, occupational status, and social, environmental, and economic factors. Only after a thorough clinical and radiographic evaluation of the involved hip and the entire patient can an appropriate decision be made as to treatment.

Although detailed discussion of therapy is beyond the scope of this chapter, we have included a simple algorithm based upon the described method of staging and evaluation and the clinical factors discussed above. This algorithm has proven extremely helpful in determining the best method of treatment (Table 3). It discusses treatment only in general terms, because, at present, there are many modalities to choose from, each of which has specific advantages and disadvantages.

Summary and Conclusions

Although we still do not have an optimum method of treatment for osteonecrosis of the femoral head, significant advances have been made during the past decade. A number of newer techniques for prophylactic management have been developed. Whichever technique is selected, for the best results the condition must be diagnosed early and treatment instituted promptly. Thus, it is essential that the reader be familiar with those modalities available for the early diagnosis of osteonecrosis.

Once the diagnosis has been made, an effective method of evaluation and staging must be used to help determine the most appropriate treatment. In addition, the uniform use of a quantitative staging system will allow investigators to speak a common language, will help dispel much of the confusion and contradiction that currently exists in this field, and will allow us to compare the effectiveness of various methods of treatment. Ultimately, this will improve our ability to treat patients with osteonecrosis.

References

1. Glimcher MJ, Kenzora JE: The biology of osteonecrosis of the human femoral head and its clinical implications: III. Discussion of the etiology and genesis of the pathological sequelae; comments on treatment. *Clin Orthop* 1979;140:273-312.
2. Hungerford DS, Lennox DW: Diagnosis and treatment of ischemic necrosis of the femoral head, in Evarts CM (ed): *Surgery of the Musculoskeletal System*, ed 2. New York, Churchill Livingstone, 1990, vol 3, chap 95, pp 2757-2794.
3. Jones JP Jr: Osteonecrosis, in McCarthy DJ (ed): *Arthritis and Allied Conditions: A Textbook of Rheumatology*, ed 11. Philadelphia, Lea & Febiger, 1989, chap 98, pp 1545-1562.
4. Steinberg ME: Early diagnosis of avascular necrosis of the femoral head, in Bassett FH III (ed): American Academy of Orthopaedic Surgeons *Instructional Course Lectures, XXXVII*. Park Ridge, IL, 1988, pp 51-57.
5. Steinberg ME, Steinberg DR: Avascular necrosis of the femoral head, in Steinberg ME (ed): *The Hip and Its Disorders*. Philadelphia, WB Saunders, 1991, chap 30, pp 623-647.
6. Glickstein MF, Burk DL Jr, Schiebler ML, et al: Avascular necrosis versus other diseases of the hip: Sensitivity of MR imaging. *Radiology* 1988;169:213-215.
7. Mitchell MD, Kundel HL, Steinberg ME, et al: Avascular necrosis of the hip: Comparison of MR, CT, and scintigraphy. *AJR* 1986;147:67-71.
8. Mitchell DG, Rao VM, Dalinka MK, et al: Femoral head avascular necrosis: Correlation of MR imaging, radiographic staging, radonuclide imaging, and clinical findings. *Radiology* 1987;162:709-715.
9. Steinberg ME, Thickman D, Chen HH, et al: Early diagnosis of avascular necrosis (AVN) by magnetic resonance imaging (MRI), in Arlet J, Mazieres B (eds): *Bone Circulation and Bone Necrosis*. New York, Springer-Verlag, 1990, pp 281-285.
10. Thickman D, Axel L, Kressel HY, et al: Magnetic resonance imaging of avascular necrosis of the femoral head. *Skeletal Radiol* 1986;15:133-140.
11. Ficat RP: Idiopathic bone necrosis of the femoral head: Early diagnosis and treatment. *J Bone Joint Surg* 1985;67B:3-9.
12. Marcus ND, Enneking WF, Massam RA: The silent hip in idiopathic aseptic necrosis: Treatment by bone grafting. *J Bone Joint Surg* 1973;55A:1351-1366.
13. Steinberg ME, Steinberg DR: Evaluation and staging of avascular necrosis. *Semin Arthroplasty* 1991;2:175-181.

Bone Tumors, Infectious Diseases, and Problem Fractures

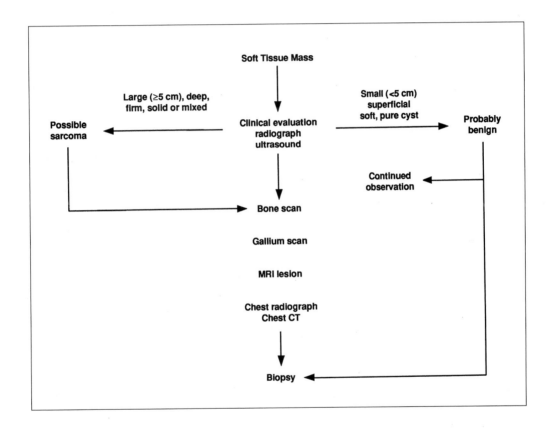

Biopsy of Bone and Soft-Tissue Lesions

Michael A. Simon, MD

J. Sybil Biermann, MD

The biopsy of a soft-tissue mass or of a radiographically apparent bone lesion is usually essential before one embarks on a treatment plan. Whereas biopsy frequently demands relatively few technical skills, the decisions related to the performance of the biopsy require considerable thought and experience.[1] Without appropriate planning or execution, biopsies frequently lead to adverse effects on patient prognosis and on treatment options.[2] Poorly performed biopsies, poorly placed incisions, and biopsy complications can considerably compromise the subsequent local management of bone and soft-tissue tumors.[2]

In order to carry out the biopsy appropriately, the surgeon must first ensure that adequate diagnostic and staging studies were performed.[1,3] These studies include clinical, laboratory, and radiographic assessments to provide the surgeon with knowledge of the extent of the tumor. The surgeon can then develop a differential diagnosis that facilitates decision-making regarding the optimum location of the biopsy site, the performance of closed or open biopsy or an incisional or excisional biopsy, and the processing of the biopsy specimen.

The biopsy has potential prognostic and therapeutic consequences and, therefore, should be undertaken by the surgeon who plans to carry out the definitive treatment of the patient. Lesions that are highly likely to be malignant should be referred promptly to a musculoskeletal oncologist for biopsy or additional staging studies. These lesions include large or deep soft-tissue masses as well as bone lesions that are suspected, on the basis of their radiographic appearance, of being primary malignancies.

Prebiopsy Strategy

The management of musculoskeletal tumors requires a multidisciplinary approach. In addition to the surgeon, radiologists and pathologists play a role in the planning of the diagnostic and staging strategy prior to biopsy. Depending on the prebiopsy differential diagnosis, consultation before biopsy may also have to include radiation oncologists, medical oncologists, or other surgical specialists. Optimum integration of clinical and radiographic information prior to biopsy has special significance for the diagnosis of bone tumors and is a requirement for accurate pathological interpretation. Because the decision to perform a biopsy is based almost exclusively on the initial clinical and radiographic interpretation, the clinician who is ultimately responsible for the care of the patient must be knowledgeable about the clinical and radiographic behavior of tumors.

Bone lesions other than tumors can cause focal abnormalities on conventional radiographs. These lesions include, among others, traumatic defects, metabolic bone disease, circulatory disease of bone, synovial disease, and, most importantly, bone infection. The orthopaedic surgeon must consider these diagnoses at all times in the assessment of focal abnormalities of bone. If a bone tumor is suspected, it may be classified in one of three main diagnostic categories: (1) benign bone tumor, (2) malignant primary bone tumor, and (3) metastatic bone tumor. Each of these groups includes specific subcategories, which may often be diagnosed by careful clinical and radiographic interpretation. At this point, the clinician should decide whether to continue to care for the patient or to refer the patient to a medical center or to another physician with more experience in the management of musculoskeletal tumors.[3] A patient with a malignant-appearing bone tumor should be referred to an experienced orthopaedic oncologist. Biopsy and additional diagnostic studies should then be left to the center or physician to whom the patient is referred.

It is more difficult to make an accurate clinical evaluation of a primary soft-tissue tumor than to evaluate a bone tumor. A conventional radiograph of a soft-tissue mass, unlike that of a bone tumor, usually does not provide any diagnostic information, and there is no simple diagnostic test that helps the physician to distinguish a malignant from a benign tumor. For these reasons, soft-tissue sarcomas are often mistakenly biopsied by a physician who will not ultimately be responsible for the management of the patient. If a mass is 5 cm or larger, especially if it is deep and in the thigh, it is likely to be a sarcoma.[4] A patient who has such a lesion should be referred to an experienced orthopaedic or surgical oncologist before a biopsy or additional diagnostic imaging is performed.

Biopsy Placement

The decision regarding where to place the biopsy is crucial. When a biopsy is being done for a malignant tumor, it should be performed at a site that can be excised en bloc with the lesion during the subsequent local operative procedure or amputation. Because limb-saving operations are now in common use for all types of malignant disease, the placement of the biopsy site is critical. Unnecessary amputation may become necessary if the location of the biopsy precludes excision of the biopsy site en bloc with the tumor when the definitive procedure is performed.[2] The location of the biopsy must be chosen with the realization that several alternative operative plans may have to be considered. Information for the development of the appropriate operative plans is obtained mainly from the differential diagnosis before the biopsy and from the results of the clinical staging studies from which the extent of the primary tumor can be determined. Knowledge of the operative alternatives that are available comes only through operative and diagnostic experience with musculoskeletal neoplasms.

For appropriate placement of the biopsy, the surgeon must be familiar with standard and nonstandard amputation flaps and know which limb-salvage procedures can be performed under what conditions. To accomplish this, the surgeon needs to know the probable diagnosis and the extent of the tumor and to have established an operative plan prior to biopsy. If the surgeon is concerned only with obtaining a tissue diagnosis and does not think about the definitive operative procedure, he or she is likely to place the incision inappropriately, thereby threatening the possibility that a limb-saving procedure can be performed as well as the survival of the patient and vastly complicating the task of the tumor specialist to whom the patient may be referred.[2]

It is difficult to give specific guidelines as to where the biopsy should be placed. Transverse incisions in the extremities are almost always contraindicated because the site of the incision cannot be excised en bloc with the longitudinally directed segments of bone or musculoaponeurotic compartments. Therefore, a longitudinal biopsy incision must almost always be used in the extremities. The major neurovascular structures should be avoided, because if they are contaminated during the biopsy they may have to be sacrificed during the definitive procedure that follows. The biopsy tract also should not traverse a normal anatomic musculoskeletal compartment in order to reach a compartment that is involved by tumor, so that it will not be necessary to remove both compartments at the time of the definitive procedure.

Standard operative approaches employed in orthopaedic procedures may prove inappropriate for a biopsy. For example, a biopsy through the buttock for a bone tumor of the pelvis may cause considerable difficulty when a subsequent hemipelvectomy or local pelvic resection is planned, because the buttock is the standard source of the skin flap for both procedures.

If the buttock skin has to be removed en bloc with the pelvis because of contamination by the biopsy, a limb-saving local pelvic resection becomes impossible. Even in a subsequent hemipelvectomy, the surgeon would have to use an anterior flap, which entails higher morbidity than does the standard hemipelvectomy with a posterior flap. As a second example, a biopsy of the humerus through the deltopectoral interval (a standard exposure for many orthopaedic procedures) causes dissemination of tumor cells at a distance, through normal neurovascular planes. Following such a biopsy approach, local resection of the proximal aspect of the humerus is more prone to be followed by a local recurrence. It would be more appropriate to biopsy the tumor through the anterior deltoid muscle and then to resect en bloc the biopsy-contaminated deltoid with the humerus during the definitive procedure. Such concepts are not widely applied in the education or practice of routine orthopaedic surgery.

Open Biopsy Compared with Closed Biopsy

In a closed biopsy, no incision is required and the tissue specimen is obtained by skin puncture with a needle or trephine. An open biopsy, which requires an incision, has been the more common and conventional method, but closed biopsy is increasing in popularity, particularly for soft-tissue masses.

In an open biopsy, the surgeon can obtain a relatively large amount of tissue for diagnosis. The larger tissue specimen may help the relatively inexperienced pathologist to make a more accurate diagnosis. This is an advantage because primary bone and soft-tissue tumors are rare. An open biopsy also decreases the likelihood that the surgeon will make a sampling error. However, the risks, complications, and consequences of poor placement of the biopsy site increase markedly with an open biopsy, unless it is done skillfully and knowledgeably. An open biopsy is more likely to result in operative hematoma, tumor-cell spillage, operative infection, and, if the bone is entered, pathological fracture. In almost all instances, open biopsy must be performed in an operating suite, with all of the accompanying problems of scheduling, procurement of time, and cost.

Closed biopsy of soft-tissue lesions, particularly deep lesions, may reduce the costs of biopsy and the time required for diagnosis. Additionally, for patients whose skin is compromised because of rapidly expanding tumor, incisional problems are avoided. Closed biopsy of soft-tissue masses can be performed in an outpatient office, which increases the convenience for the patient and surgeon, and it has fewer potential operative risks. Techniques include fine-needle aspiration and Tru-cut needle biopsy.

Fine-needle aspiration of soft-tissue masses can be carried out with a relatively small needle (0.7 mm in diameter). The diagnostic accuracy is 90% for determination of malignancy when the procedure is performed by an experienced surgeon.[5] However, the accuracy rate is lower for the determination of a specific tumor type or histologic grade because of the limited tissue volume obtained and the loss of tissue architecture. Interpretation by a cytopathologist with special knowledge of musculoskeletal lesions greatly enhances diagnostic accuracy. Fine-needle aspiration may be most useful in the determination of local recurrence of soft-tissue tumors and spread to lymph nodes. Fine-needle aspiration of a bone lesion cannot be done unless the cortex has been disrupted, and it is often difficult to obtain cells from some solid soft-tissue tumors.

The Tru-cut needle-biopsy system consists of a cannulated needle with an inner trochar that contains a specimen notch. With this system, it is possible to retrieve a limited amount of tissue from the specimen notch with the original architecture preserved. The biopsy is carried out percutaneously through a stab incision, with the patient under local anesthesia. The diagnostic accuracy for this technique approaches 96%.[6,7] Because the amount of material retrieved is limited, the disposition of the material must be planned carefully before the tissue is processed, and an experienced pathologist must perform the interpretation. It should be emphasized that, despite the high degrees of diagnostic accuracy reported, a nondiagnostic closed biopsy should not be interpreted as reassurance that no tumor exists, because the sample may be from the normal adjacent tissue or from the pseudocapsule surrounding the tumor.

Closed biopsy of bone tumors has been reported to be successful in some centers with extensive experience.[8-10] When performed in the clinical setting on a lesion that is highly suggestive of osteosarcoma, fine-needle aspirations have been reported to have a diagnostic accuracy of as high as 80%.[11] In bone, a closed biopsy, with the resultant smaller defect, reduces the risk of pathological fracture through the biopsy site. Closed biopsy may be preferred particularly for bones such as the pelvis or spine, which are difficult to access.[12,13] Closed biopsy may also be optimum when the diagnosis, such as metastatic disease, infection, or local recurrence, is expected with a high degree of certainty. When used for the diagnosis of heterogeneous tumors, however, closed bone biopsy may present sampling problems. The procedure must be done in a radiology suite or operating room, and it necessitates the use of an image-intensifier. It may present a diagnostic challenge to all except the most experienced pathologist.[14,15] Insufficient tissue for diagnosis has been reported to have been the result of 25% to 33% of the procedures, even in institutions with the most

experienced personnel.[9,10,16] In such institutions, even when sufficient tissue is available, the diagnostic accuracy is only about 80%. The diagnostic accuracy is lower for primary bone tumors and for patients with nondiagnostic radiographs than for homogeneous tumors, including metastases or multiple myelomas.

A closed biopsy should not be performed by any physician who is inexperienced in making operative decisions about malignant tumors. The physician must be aware that the needle tract from the closed biopsy is always contaminated by tumor cells and should be resected en bloc with the tumor. Because neoadjuvant chemotherapy or radiation therapy may delay definitive surgery, it may be difficult to locate the needle tract. The site of entry of the needle can be identified at the time of biopsy by prior tattooing of the adjacent skin with India ink. However, the surgeon who will perform the definitive procedure must also direct the biopsy needle in such a way that the direction and location of the needle tract are known and properly located. Both closed and open biopsies should be done only by an experienced surgeon. Ideally, this is the same surgeon who will be responsible for the operative procedure, if one should be necessary.

Techniques of Open Biopsy

An open biopsy may be incisional or excisional. Incisional biopsy is most common and is the procedure of choice for open biopsy of almost all malignant tumors because, when skillfully done, it involves less local tumor-cell spillage than does an excisional biopsy.

Occasionally, primary excision of a bone lesion is preferable. If the preoperative diagnosis is fairly certain or if a bone tumor is small or radiographically benign, an excisional biopsy can be used for both diagnostic and therapeutic purposes. The diagnosis of osteochondroma or osteoid-osteoma usually is based on an excisional biopsy. If the surgeon is very experienced, excision can be used as the initial operative approach for tumors with the radiographic characteristics of secondary low-grade chondrosarcoma.

The decision to perform a primary excision of a soft-tissue mass is complex. Small subcutaneous masses with a low likelihood of malignancy generally lend themselves well to excision. On the other hand, excisional biopsy of large or deep soft-tissue masses may cause extensive tumor contamination at the time of the biopsy and can subsequently limit treatment options.[17] Primary myectomy with or without antecedent fine-needle aspiration has been described, but such a procedure is not commonly employed in the United States.[18] An excision along the margin of a large, deep mass should rarely, if ever, be performed unless magnetic resonance imaging has shown the distinct characteristics of a lipoma.

During an incisional biopsy, attention to technical details is important for high specimen quality and reduced tumor spread. The incision should be as small as is compatible with the obtaining of an adequate tissue specimen. As the pseudocapsule of a malignant tumor is approached, the color of the muscle changes from red to salmon. A malignant tumor is usually grey or white, and its pseudocapsule alone must not be biopsied. Instead, the pseudocapsule-tumor interface should be included in the biopsy of a malignant tumor, and the host tissue-tumor interface should be included in a biopsy of a benign tumor. The periphery of any malignant tumor is its most viable, representative, and diagnostic portion, whereas the central region is often necrotic. The tissue specimen should not be crushed with forceps. There is rarely a need to obtain multiple samples of tissue; such a procedure results in excessive spillage of tumor cells.

The surgeon selecting the site for an incisional biopsy of bone should assess the radiograph as well as the computed tomography scan or the magnetic resonance imaging scan, or both, to locate the least differentiated or least mineralized portion of the neoplasm, because this is usually the most representative portion. The surgeon should avoid a biopsy in the area of the Codman triangle, because of the risk that the reactive bone will be interpreted as osteosarcoma. It is not necessary to biopsy the bone containing a malignant bone tumor unless there is no soft-tissue extension. Violating the cortex of a bone that contains malignant tumor can lead to pathological fracture, which usually results in the need for an amputation. If the bone must be opened, a small circular hole should be made with a circular saw, so that only minimum stress-risers are created.[19] If a larger window is needed, an oblong opening can be made in the bone by creation of two separate circular cortical holes in the long axis of the bone, followed by connection of the holes by means of parallel cuts with a power saw. Because a rectangular pattern of multiple drill holes connected by an osteotome causes stresses to concentrate at the corners of the rectangle and may result in fracture, this method should not be used.

Meticulous hemostasis is necessary so that substantial postoperative hematoma is prevented. If a hole has been created in the bone, it should be plugged with Gelfoam or methylmethacrylate to prevent bleeding into the soft tissues. The biopsy site must be closed carefully to prevent necrosis or ulceration of the wound, especially if skin nutrition was impaired by pressure from a large tumor or by radiation therapy. Suction drains should not be used if malignant disease is likely, because the drainage-tube tract can be a site for tumor spread and will have to be excised en bloc with the biopsy site. If a drain must be used, the tract should be adjacent to and in line with the biopsy incision. En bloc excision of a biopsy site and a drainage-tube tract may be technically impossible if the drainage-tube tract is at a distance from the site of the biopsy.

The question of whether to use a proximally placed tourniquet during biopsy of a malignant tumor is controversial. Opponents claim, but without substantiation, that the tourniquet causes venous stasis and that tumor embolization is increased upon release of the tourniquet. They also point out that an extensive hematoma may develop if the tourniquet is released after the wound has been closed. The advantage of the use of a tourniquet, however, is that it allows better visualization of the biopsy site, so that the surgeon can operate more quickly and with less blood loss. A theoretical, but scientifically unproved, advantage is prevention of tumor embolization if definitive surgery is performed immediately, before the tourniquet has been released.[20]

Two precautions must be observed if a tourniquet is used. First, the limb should not be exsanguinated by wrapping with a compressive bandage, as this forces tumor cells to enter the bloodstream. Second, if a definitive procedure is not to be performed immediately, the tourniquet should be released and meticulous hemostasis must be obtained before skin closure. If the biopsy wound for a malignant tumor is closed before the tourniquet has been released, a large hematoma may form because of bleeding of large vessels in the pseudocapsule. Large hematomas after biopsy may have a dramatic effect on the operative options, as all areas into which a hematoma has spread must be presumed to be contaminated.

Whenever possible, the surgeon should obtain a specimen for frozen section at biopsy, even if a definitive operation is not to be performed under the same anesthesia. An experienced pathologist should be able to recognize, on frozen section, whether enough viable and representative tissue has been obtained. If not, more tissue can be obtained immediately, so that the operation need not be repeated. A frozen section can be done only on soft tissue; obviously, it cannot be done on well-mineralized tissue. However, almost all malignant tumors of bone have nonmineralized areas that are suitable for frozen-section analysis. By this means, it is often possible to distinguish metastatic tumors from round-cell tumors, infections, and primary bone tumors. The diagnostic accuracy achieved with the use of frozen sections has been claimed to be as high as 90% when the procedure is performed by an experienced surgeon.[21]

An immediate operation must never be performed if there are any doubts about the diagnosis. Only when the preoperative and radiographic information is characteristic, and when the interpretation of the frozen section unquestionably confirms the prebiopsy diagnosis, is it safe to carry out a definitive procedure under the same anesthesia. If there are discrepancies between the clinical and radiographic information and the interpretation of the frozen section, additional tissue must be obtained. The wound must be closed, and a definitive operation must be postponed until permanent sections have been processed and diagnosed.

If a definitive operative procedure is to be carried out immediately after the biopsy of a proved malignant tumor, the following steps must be taken. The biopsy site must be closed meticulously and an adhesive seal applied over the incision. The patient should be redraped, and the instruments and surgical attire that were used during the biopsy must be changed because of possible contamination of the operative site by tumor cells from the biopsy. In a similar fashion, separate sterile instruments, drapes, and gowns must be used when autogenous bone-grafting is performed following tumor removal, to avoid seeding the bone-graft donor site with benign and malignant tumor cells. For this reason, the bone graft may be obtained first and the donor-site wound closed before the tumor operation proceeds. Use of this sequence minimizes the likelihood that the donor site will be contaminated. The other alternative is to have two separate surgical teams and instruments and to perform the procedures simultaneously or sequentially, without cross-contamination.

Examination of the Tissue

The surgeon must discuss radiographic findings and diagnostic possibilities with the pathologist before proceeding with a biopsy. This will allow the pathologist to give more useful interpretations of the frozen sections, and it will ensure that tissue is processed appropriately for necessary tests. Besides the study of sections that have been stained with hematoxylin and eosin and embedded in paraffin, additional studies of the biopsy tissue may be indicated. Because infection is often misinterpreted clinically as a tumor, or the reverse, it is often advisable to obtain biopsy specimens for aerobic, anaerobic, fungal, and acid-fast bacillus culture. Electron microscopy is an important diagnostic tool for the study of round-cell and soft-tissue tumors, and, if these lesions are suspected, a portion of the specimen must be placed in glutaraldehyde, rather than in formaldehyde, for examination with an electron microscope.

Immunohistochemical study has become invaluable for the differentiation among many types of malignancies, and some immunologic markers can be used only on frozen tissues. Tissue examinations that are performed less commonly and that may require special processing include cytologic studies, tissue imprints, tissue cultures, hormone receptors, flow cytometry,

and, most recently, cytogenetics. For these reasons, knowledgeable communication with the pathologist before and during the biopsy procedure is essential.

In summary, biopsy of bone and soft-tissue lesions, although often technically simple, is a complex cognitive skill requiring a thoughtful, knowledgeable, and experienced surgeon. Poorly performed biopsies, inappropriately placed incisions, and biopsy complications compromise the local treatment of sarcomas and, occasionally, the survival of the patient. Because large soft-tissue masses and radiographically aggressive-appearing bone tumors have a high probability of being malignant, patients who have these sorts of tumors should be referred to an experienced musculoskeletal oncologist before additional imaging studies and biopsy are undertaken.

References

1. Simon MA: Biopsy of musculoskeletal tumors. *J Bone Joint Surg* 1982;64A:1253-1257.
2. Mankin HJ, Lange TA, Spanier SS: The hazards of biopsy in patients with malignant primary bone and soft-tissue tumors. *J Bone Joint Surg* 1982;64A:1121-1127.
3. Enneking WF: Editorial: The issue of the biopsy. *J Bone Joint Surg* 1982;64A:1119-1120.
4. Rydholm A, Berg NO: Size, site and clinical incidence of lipoma: Factors in the differential diagnosis of lipoma and sarcoma. *Acta Orthop Scand* 1983;54:924-934.
5. Åkerman M, Rydholm A, Persson BM, et al: Aspiration cytology of soft-tissue tumors: The 10-year experience at an orthopedic oncology center. *Acta Orthop Scand* 1985;56:407-412.
6. Ball AB, Fisher C, Pittam M, et al: Diagnosis of soft tissue tumours by Tru-cut biopsy. *Br J Surg* 1990;77:756-758.
7. Kissin MW, Fisher C, Carter RL, et al: Value of Tru-cut biopsy in the diagnosis of soft tissue tumours. *Br J Surg* 1986;73:742-744.
8. deSantos LA, Murray JA, Ayala AG: The value of percutaneous needle biopsy in the management of primary bone tumors. *Cancer* 1979;43:735-744.
9. Moore TM, Meyers MH, Patzakis MJ, et al: Closed biopsy of musculoskeletal lesions. *J Bone Joint Surg* 1979;61A:375-380.
10. Schajowicz F, Derqui JC: Puncture biopsy in lesions of the locomotor system: Review of results in 4050 cases, including 941 vertebral punctures. *Cancer* 1968;21:531-548.
11. White VA, Fanning CV, Ayala AG, et al: Osteosarcoma and the role of fine-needle aspiration: A study of 51 cases. *Cancer* 1988;62:1238-1246.
12. Craig FS: Vertebral-body biopsy. *J Bone Joint Surg* 1956;38A:93-102.
13. Ottolenghi CE: Aspiration biopsy of the spine: Technique for the thoracic spine and results of twenty-eight biopsies in this region and over-all results of 1050 biopsies of other spinal segments. *J Bone Joint Surg* 1969;51A:1531-1544.
14. Hadju SI, Melamed MR: Needle biopsy of primary malignant bone tumors. *Surg Gynecol Obstet* 1971;133:829-832.
15. Katz RL, Silva EG, deSantos LA, et al: Diagnosis of eosinophilic granuloma of bone by cytology, histology, and electron microscopy of transcutaneous bone-aspiration biopsy. *J Bone Joint Surg* 1980;62A:1284-1290.
16. den Heeten GJ, Oldhoff J, Oosterhuis JW, et al: Biopsy of bone tumours. *J Surg Oncol* 1985;28:247-251.
17. Lawrence W Jr, Donegan WL, Natarajan N, et al: Adult soft tissue sarcomas: A pattern of care survey of the American

College of Surgeons. *Ann Surg* 1987;205:349-359.

18. Rydholm A, Rööser B, Persson, BM: Primary myectomy for sarcoma. *J Bone Joint Surg* 1986;68A:586-589.

19. Clark CR, Morgan C, Sonstegard DA, et al: The effect of biopsy-hole shape and size on bone strength. *J Bone Joint Surg* 1977;59A:213-217.

20. Broström LA, Harris MA, Simon MA, et al: The effect of biopsy on survival of patients with osteosarcoma. *J Bone Joint Surg* 1979;61B:209-212.

21. Dahlin DC: *Bone Tumors. General Aspects and Data on 6,221 Cases,* ed 3. Springfield, IL, Charles C. Thomas, 1978, chap 1, pp 3-16.

Diagnostic Strategy for Bone and Soft-Tissue Tumors

Michael A. Simon, MD

Henry A. Finn, MD

A patient with a bone tumor usually complains of pain and has a change in locomotive or prehensile function, regardless of the presence or absence of a palpable mass. In contrast, a patient with a soft-tissue tumor usually has a palpable mass that produces little or no pain and causes little alteration in function. Both types of symptoms ultimately cause the patient to consult the physician, who, in turn, almost invariably obtains a conventional radiograph of the region in question. This radiograph, when correlated with even sparse clinical information, leads to a differential diagnosis that is remarkably specific for the patient with the bone tumor but is of little diagnostic import for the patient with the soft-tissue tumor. At this point, at least in the hands of a knowledgeable orthopaedic oncologist, the diagnostic and staging process begins.

Clinical and Radiographic Interpretation of Bone Tumors

Clinical Evaluation

In the diagnosis of bone tumors, the patient's medical history usually contributes only limited information. The age of the patient is probably the most important piece of clinical information used in the clinicoradiographic interpretation of bone tumors. Most bone tumors develop in an age-range of about two decades. For example, in a patient with a destructive lesion of bone who is more than 40 years old, the lesion is likely to indicate metastasis to bone, even if information about a known primary focus is lacking. On the other hand, histiocytosis should be considered as a diagnostic possibility in a patient younger than 10 years old who has a destructive lesion in a bone.

Some tumors have a sex predilection (for example, giant-cell tumors are more frequent in female patients and osteosarcomas occur more often in male patients), but the bias is not sufficiently striking to be helpful in the diagnosis. The race of a patient is of limited relevance, except perhaps in the case of Ewing's sarcoma, which is rare in black individuals. The character and intensity of the pain and the presence of altered function are usually of little diagnostic importance. However, unremitting pain or pain that is more severe at rest or at night than during the day is often considered a symptom of malignant disease. A history of activity that could have caused a stress fracture, or of a traumatic event that could have resulted in myositis ossificans, can be of diagnostic value. Information that the patient has been exposed to chemical or physical agents that are known to be carcinogenic may also be useful for the diagnosis.

Findings on physical examination are also nonspecific and are rarely diagnostic. The presence of a soft-tissue mass should make the physician suspect an aggressive bone lesion with an extraosseous extension. Furthermore, a large bone tumor may be accompanied by a locally elevated temperature and, occasionally, by dilation of superficial veins. The presence of café-au-lait spots or hemangiomas can sometimes be helpful in the diagnosis. Neurologic dysfunction is not common, but it may result when the tumor is in an anatomic region in which nerves cannot move freely, such as the sciatic notch or the sacrum. Edema of an extremity may occur unilaterally when a bone tumor has undergone extensive spread to soft tissue.

Laboratory Tests

Except for tests of the presence of immunoglobulins in patients who have multiple myeloma, or of prostate-specific antigen in those who have metastatic prostate cancer, serological, biochemical, and immunological tests of peripheral blood have limited value in the diagnosis and staging of bone and soft-tissue tumors. The erythrocyte sedimentation rate (ESR) is a nonspecific value that is elevated in patients with a bone infection and often in those with a marrow-cell tumor (Ewing's sarcoma, lymphoma of bone, multiple myeloma, histiocytosis, or leukemia) or a metastatic bone tumor.[1] For other primary bone tumors, both malignant and benign, the ESR is almost always normal. For patients with Ewing's sarcoma or lymphoma, an elevated ESR may indicate a poor prognosis. The clinician should be aware that many other conditions, such as infection, pregnancy, or a recent operative procedure, can cause the ESR to be elevated.

The alkaline phosphatase level is high in about one half of patients with osteosarcoma and in a smaller fraction of those with another type of primary malignant bone tumor. Currently, there is disagreement as to the prognostic value of this test before treatment and as to its value for the monitoring of the course of the disease during treatment.[2,3] There is wide variation in normal values because of the unpredictable growth spurts during adolescence, which is a period of peak prevalence of osteosarcoma. In patients whose alkaline phosphatase level is markedly elevated, one should consider the possibility of multicentric (metastatic) osteosarcoma or Paget disease.

Radiographic Interpretation

Conventional biplane radiography is a noninvasive, low-cost technique that provides a gross pathological image of a bone tumor. It is the most effective diagnostic tool in orthopaedic oncology and often can, by itself, provide a correct diagnosis. Certain basic guidelines may be helpful to the clinician who is interpreting conventional radiographic images.[4] The clinician should pay particular attention to (1) the anatomic site of the lesion, (2) the zone of transition between the lesion and the host bone, and (3) the specific internal radiographic characteristics of the lesion.

The anatomic site is crucial to the diagnosis of bone tumors. Some tumors have a predilection for the axial skeleton, whereas others occur mainly in the long bones. The anatomic site within a long bone has diagnostic importance. A tumor located primarily in the epiphyseal region is most likely a giant-cell tumor if the growth plate is closed and it is most likely a chondroblastoma if the growth plate is open. Diaphyseal lesions are infrequent; however, Ewing's sarcoma, histiocytosis, fibrous dysplasia, and adamantinoma are primary neoplasms that often originate in the diaphysis of a long bone. The metaphysis of a long bone is a site for many types of tumors, and, therefore, this site is not diagnostically discriminating.

The most frequent sites for metastases or multiple myeloma are the ribs, pelvis, and spine. Primary bone tumors such as Ewing's sarcoma and chondrosarcoma often occur in the innominate bone, and fibrous dysplasia, Ewing's sarcoma, and chondrosarcoma may occur in the ribs. Any lesion in the anterior elements of the spine in an adult is probably a hemangioma, metastatic bone tumor, or multiple myeloma, whereas a lesion of the body of a vertebra in a child is usually histiocytosis. A lesion in the posterior elements of the spine in a child or adolescent is likely to be a primary bone tumor (osteoid-osteoma, osteoblastoma, or aneurysmal bone cyst). These observations should impress on clinicians that, regardless of the radiographic characteristics of a tumor, the anatomic site of the lesion often has diagnostic importance.

The zone of transition between the lesion and the host bone is a particularly important region for diagnostic observation on a conventional radiograph. If the zone of transition is wide or poorly demarcated, without clear boundaries, or if it has a permeative appearance, then the lesion is aggressive—that is, it is a rapid process in which the host bone did not have time to respond to the disease. Aggressive, in this context, can indicate a malignant tumor, a locally aggressive tumor, or an infection. If the zone of transition is narrow or well demarcated, the host bone has responded by forming new bone in reaction to the lesion and the lesion is likely to be benign.

Occasionally, the internal radiographic characteristics of the lesion can be diagnostic. The distinction between ossification and calcification is of diagnostic importance. Ossification is mineralization of the matrix that confers the appearance of organization or structure. Calcification is unstructured mineralization, which appears on a conventional radiograph to be more haphazard and dense than does ossification. Calcified areas in the substance of a lesion usually indicate a cartilaginous process, whereas ossification in the substance of the lesion indicates bone formation by tumor.

If a tumor destroys the cortex or causes the periosteal formation of new bone (the Codman triangle), the lesion must be considered aggressive. Occasionally, a tumor will cause expansion and thinning of the cortex without destroying it. This pattern is seen with benign tumors, such as aneurysmal bone cysts, fibrous dysplasias, or enchondromas. The terms onion-skinning and sunburst are rarely sufficiently specific to be of diagnostic value. On conventional radiographs of a bone tumor, the outline of an extraosseous extension may be visible and should lead one to suspect a malignancy. The clinician should look carefully at any soft-tissue mass because it is in this area that ossification or calcification in the tumor substance can be identified most reliably, as this process is not shielded from view by the host bone.

The finding that a tumor has arisen on the surface of a bone should immediately lead to a diagnosis of parosteal (juxtacortical) tumor. These tumors cannot be diagnosed without radiographic confirmation of their parosteal location.

Clinical and Radiographic Correlation

There is little disagreement that optimum correlation of clinical and radiographic information is necessary for the most accurate pathological interpretation. Collaboration among the orthopaedic surgeon, radiologist, and pathologist is necessary for appropriate diagnosis and treatment of bone tumors. If any one of the three disciplines is poorly correlated with the others, a misdiagnosis is likely to occur. The clinician who is ultimately responsible for the care of the patient should be well versed in all three areas in order to treat bone tumors successfully.

The clinician makes crucial treatment decisions, which lead to the various possible diagnostic and therapeutic approaches, on the basis of the clinical and radiographic data, before the pathological interpretation becomes available. If the clinical and radiographic data indicate that a tumor is benign, observation may be the chosen option. If malignancy is the most probable

Outline 1
Common Tumors of Bone

Benign primary tumors

    Fibrous/cystic
        Aneurysmal bone cyst
        Giant cell tumor
        Unicameral bone cyst
        Fibrous dysplasia
        Nonossifying fibroma

    Cartilaginous
        Enchondroma
        Osteochondroma
        Chondroblastoma
        Chondromyxoid fibroma

    Osseous
        Osteoid-osteoma
        Osteoblastoma

Malignant primary tumors
    Osteosarcoma
    Chondrosarcoma
    Malignant fibrous histiocytoma
    Adamantinoma
    Chordoma

Parosteal tumors
    Osteosarcoma
    Chondroma

Marrow cell tumors
    Adults
        Lymphoma
        Multiple myeloma
        Plasmacytoma
    Children
        Histiocytosis
        Ewing's sarcoma

Metastases
    Breast
    Prostate
    Lung
    Kidney

diagnosis, a sophisticated diagnostic and staging strategy should be employed. Even the decision to perform a biopsy is based on clinical and radiographic data. Therefore, one cannot stress enough how important these disciplines are in the management of bone tumors.

The orthopaedic surgeon should be aware that disorders other than bone tumors cause focal abnormalities on conventional radiographs. These include, among others: (1) a traumatic lesion (stress fracture and myositis ossificans); (2) metabolic bone disease (Paget disease and brown tumor of hyperparathyroidism); (3) circulatory disease of bone (infarction); (4) synovial disease (for example, synovial chondromatosis and pigmented villonodular synovitis); and, most importantly, (5) bone infection. If non-neoplastic conditions are always considered prior to tumors of bone, major errors in judgment can be avoided.

In the differential diagnosis of a bone tumor, one should consider three major diagnostic categories: (1)

a benign primary bone tumor, (2) a malignant primary bone tumor, and (3) a metastatic bone tumor. Each major category includes several subcategories, which should be considered for each case. The common bone tumors are listed in Outline 1. Specific diagnoses are based on careful clinical and radiographic interpretation. If the interpretation shows that the tumor is benign and self-limiting, the choice may be observation of the patient, unless there are overriding concerns about pathological fracture. If the diagnosis is uncertain or if the lesion appears to be malignant, an evaluation should be undertaken that will ultimately lead to the diagnosis, staging, and treatment of the tumor. The clinician should then decide whether to refer the patient to a medical center or to another physician who has more experience with bone tumors. A malignant bone tumor should be treated by an orthopaedic oncologist. A biopsy or additional staging should not be performed if a referral is planned.

Clinical and Radiographic Interpretation of Soft-Tissue Masses

Clinical Evaluation

There are four major types of soft-tissue masses in the limbs: a malignant soft-tissue tumor, a benign soft-tissue tumor, an inflammatory process, and a traumatic mass such as myositis ossificans or a false aneurysm. The consistency of a mass is an inaccurate indicator of its aggressiveness. The most common malignant soft-tissue tumors are sarcomas, including malignant fibrous histiocytoma, liposarcoma, fibrosarcoma, and synovial sarcoma.[5] Most soft-tissue sarcomas cause little pain and little limb dysfunction. Intramuscular lipoma, desmoid tumor, hemangioma, and nerve-sheath tumor are the most common deep benign tumors. All masses should be evaluated with auscultation and percussion. An aneurysm can be diagnosed by auscultation of a bruit, and Tinel's sign (a tingling sensation in the distal end of a limb on percussion of a lesion involving a nerve) may signify a nerve-sheath tumor. Tumor-registry studies in Scandinavia[6,7] have shown that masses in the extremity that are deep and larger than 5 cm in diameter have a much higher probability of being malignant than do smaller subcutaneous masses. It must be pointed out, however, that almost one third of all sarcomas are subcutaneous, and that they are often small.[8]

Radiographic Interpretation

Radiographic studies are not as diagnostic for soft-tissue tumors as they are for bone tumors. Without additional diagnostic aids, plain radiographs of soft-tissue masses usually show that they are isodense with muscle.[9] Plain radiographs may demonstrate a homogeneous fat density (consistent with a lipoma), calcification, ossification, or extrinsic pressure on the adjacent bone. Calcification and ossification are both important distinguishing findings. Calcification is frequently caused by deposition of calcium in necrotic tissue and is distinct from the ossification seen with soft-tissue osteosarcoma or myositis ossificans. Calcification is often seen in malignant soft-tissue tumors, but it is infrequently seen in benign tumors except for the rounded phleboliths visible in hemangiomas.

The clinical evaluation of a soft-tissue mass is unreliable, and conventional radiographic examination usually does not lead to a diagnosis.[9] Therefore, malignant soft-tissue tumors are often biopsied by a clinician who will not be responsible for the later care of the patient. A biopsy is crucial to the management and care of patients with a soft-tissue sarcoma.[10,11] Poorly performed biopsies, poorly placed incisions, and piecemeal excision of a large mass can have considerable adverse effects on the subsequent local management of such tumors.[10] However, most soft-tissue masses of the limbs are benign,[6] and for this reason the primary physician who diagnoses the mass faces a dilemma: should the probably benign mass be excised or should the patient be referred for staging studies and excision because the lesion may be malignant?

Ultrasound imaging is useful for evaluation of a soft-tissue mass, especially if the mass is adjacent to a joint. With ultrasound, one can document the size and depth of a soft-tissue mass and show whether it is entirely cystic.[12] If the mass is found to be entirely cystic (especially around the knee or any joint), if it is small (less than 5 cm), and especially if it is superficial, it is probably benign. If a mass is 5 cm in diameter or larger, especially if it is deep and in the thigh, it is likely to be a sarcoma. It would then be advisable to refer the patient to an experienced clinician or to a medical center before a biopsy or additional diagnostic imaging is performed.

Diagnostic Strategy for Primary Bone and Soft-Tissue Tumors

The diagnostic strategy of most orthopaedic oncologists includes staging of a tumor before any biopsy is carried out. The selection of diagnostic and staging tests depends on a differential diagnosis that is based on clinical and radiographic information. This approach can be used in a cost-effective manner only if the clinician can make the clinical and radiographic correlation competently and can order appropriate tests (Figs. 1 and 2).

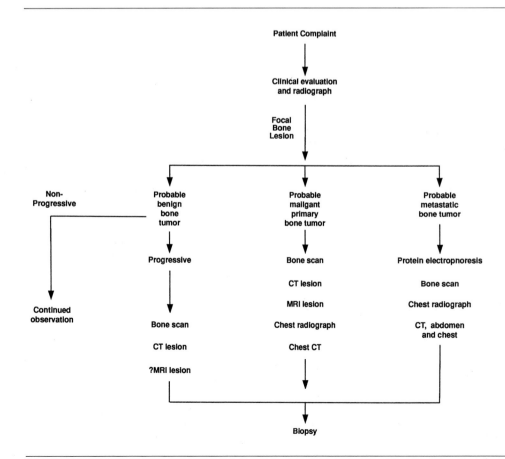

Fig. 1 Diagnostic strategy for a bone tumor. (Modified with permission from Finn HA, Simon MA: Musculoskeletal neoplasms, in Poss R (ed): *Orthopaedic Knowledge Update 3: Home Study Syllabus.* Park Ridge, IL, American Academy of Orthopaedic Surgeons, 1990, pp 115-144.)

The diagnostic and therapeutic advantages of such an approach are twofold. First, appropriate pre-biopsy evaluation may provide information about a tumor that substantially affects the prebiopsy differential diagnosis. A change in diagnosis at this point may also result in a better clinical, radiographic, and pathological correlation, providing a more solid foundation for the final diagnosis. Second, the diagnostic and staging tools for demonstration of the extent of local tumors are much less useful after a biopsy than before it. Skeletal scintigraphy, computed tomography (CT), and magnetic resonance imaging (MRI) each have a limited capacity to show the extent of local disease after a biopsy. Thus, because these tests may be crucial to the operative management of primary tumors, it is necessary to maximize their usefulness by performing them prior to biopsy.

Diagnostic and Staging Tests

The following basic types of information about musculoskeletal tumors need to be obtained prior to treatment: (1) the pathological diagnosis, (2) the local extent of the tumor, and (3) the extent of distant spread of the tumor. The first is obtained by biopsy and the latter two, by clinical staging. For the treatment of most musculoskeletal tumors in the extremities, the surgeon needs to know the intraosseous and extraosseous (soft-tissue) extent of the tumor and if the tumor has metastasized, because treatment of the primary tumor may be modified if disseminated disease is present. The imaging tests that will be described may have either diagnostic or staging value, or both. It is crucial to know the intraosseous extent of a bone tumor if the bone of origin is to be operatively violated. Also, the soft-tissue extent of a malignant tumor needs to be delineated so that the surgeon can determine whether limb preservation is possible. In addition, the surgeon needs to know the location of vital neurovascular structures, so that they can be protected when soft-tissue extension is present. If disseminated disease is present, the treatment of the local tumor may be modified.

Local Extent of the Tumor

Conventional Radiography Conventional radiographs[4] give fairly accurate information about the intraosseous extent of a bone tumor, except when the zone of transition is indistinct. That finding makes it difficult to ascertain the medullary extent of the tumor. A conventional radiograph also can delineate destruction of the

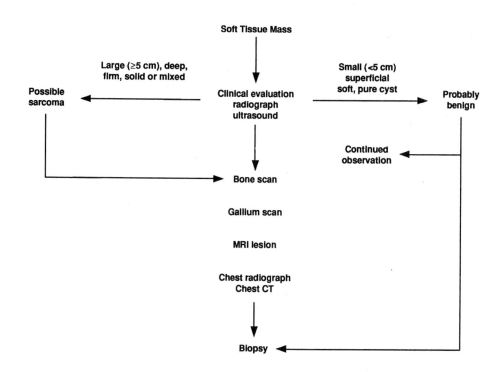

Fig. 2 Diagnostic strategy for a soft-tissue mass. (Modified with permission from Finn HA, Simon MA: Musculoskeletal neoplasms, in Poss R (ed): *Orthopaedic Knowledge Update 3: Home Study Syllabus.* Park Ridge, IL, American Academy of Orthopaedic Surgeons, 1990, pp 115-144.)

cortex and the response of periosteal new bone to aggressive tumors. Conventional radiographs, however, give the surgeon little information about soft-tissue tumors, and they do not accurately delineate the soft-tissue extension of bone tumors.

Ultrasound As stated previously, ultrasound may be used to determine the size and depth of a soft-tissue mass and whether it is solid or cystic.[12] This information is helpful for the prediction of whether a soft-tissue mass is benign or malignant. Ultrasound has no role in the evaluation of bone tumors.

Scintigraphy of Bone Tumors Skeletal scintigraphy is a sensitive but nonspecific tool for diagnosis and staging of bone tumors.[13] The technetium-99m-methylene diphosphonate (^{99m}TcMDP) bone scintigram is the most sensitive, cost-effective test for detection of bone metastases from carcinomas.[14-16] The bone scintigram is more sensitive than the conventional radiograph for most metastatic bone tumors; its sensitivity is reduced, however, in patients with multiple myeloma and histiocytosis X. A normal bone scintigram strongly suggests that a primary bone tumor is benign; however, abnormal bone scintigrams are not very useful for distinguishing of benign from malignant primary bone tumors.[17] They do not reliably define the intraosseous extent of malignant primary bone tumors, partly because of poor resolution and partly, and more importantly, because the scintigraphic intensity increases in the contiguous bone as a result of the increased blood flow.[17] Bone scintigraphy is of value as it reveals additional sites of involvement by benign bone tumors that affect more than one bone, such as fibrous dysplasia, hereditary multiple exostosis, enchondroma, hemangioma, and histiocytosis.[17] Gallium citrate scintigrams are more accurate than ^{99m}TcMDP scintigrams for the demonstration of a primary bone malignancy.[17] If a gallium scintigram of a primary bone tumor is normal, the tumor is likely to be benign. Gallium scans may delineate the local intraosseous extent of a primary bone tumor more clearly than does bone scintigraphy,[17] because increased blood flow leads to a lesser increase in scintigraphic intensity in the contiguous bone compared with that seen on technetium bone scans. At present, because of the superb quality of computed tomography and magnetic resonance images, gallium citrate scintigraphy is not used routinely for primary bone tumors.

Scintigraphy of Soft-Tissue Masses Bone scintigrams are also useful for the initial clinical staging of primary, malignant soft-tissue tumors, because they provide information on the presence of bone metastases.[16] Bone scintigraphy has some but limited value for the diagnosis or local staging of the soft-tissue tumors themselves. If a malignant soft-tissue tumor is vascular, the mass itself may exhibit a diffuse increase in scintigraphic intensity.[18,19] The bone underlying a soft-tissue malignancy may also show increased scintigraphic intensity if the tumor involves the bone or has caused a periosteal response. Such involvement might not be visible on conventional radiographs.[18,19] The gallium scintigram can be a diagnostic aid for soft-tissue tumors. Most soft-tissue sarcomas cause increased activity on gallium scintigrams, whereas non-inflammatory benign tumors usually appear normal.[19] Scintigraphic intensity is almost always increased in sites of infection in bones and soft tissues. Gallium imaging may demonstrate non-pulmonary metastases of soft-tissue sarcomas that are not recognized on routine staging studies and physical examination.[20] However, MRI and CT are more effective than gallium citrate imaging for assessment of the local anatomic extent of a musculoskeletal tumor.

Conventional Tomography Conventional tomography[21] is no longer considered very useful in the evaluation of bone tumors because of the superiority of CT and MRI.

Peripheral Angiography Peripheral angiography may occasionally be useful for the identification of a false aneurysm or an arteriovenous malformation. However, the primary role of angiography is determination of the relationship of a tumor to the vascular structures.[22,23] Arterial embolization of pelvic and axial tumors (especially highly vascular lesions, such as renal-cell carcinoma or aneurysmal bone cysts) or arterial instillation of cytotoxic drugs can be accomplished by angiography.[24-26]

Because CT and MRI provide markedly superior information concerning the relationship of tumors to vascular structures, they are the methods of choice for imaging of the extraosseous and intraosseous extension of bone and soft-tissue tumors.

Computed Tomography of Bone Tumors CT materially enhances the ability of the surgeon to assess not only the extent but also the composition of an abnormal focus in bone. It is an excellent tool for imaging of the local extent of both bone and soft-tissue tumors.[27-30] In addition, it can accurately indicate the intraosseous extent of a primary bone tumor.[31] Because it shows mineralization, CT is superior to MRI for visualization or detection of subtle cortical destruction, subtle fracture, and calcification or ossification. Thus, CT is often of diagnostic importance in the detection of punctate calcifications in cartilage lesions or of a thin rim of reactive bone surrounding an aneurysmal bone cyst.

Computed Tomography of Soft-Tissue Masses CT examination of a soft-tissue mass usually demonstrates an isodense, often heterogeneous mass that is similar to muscle, a finding that is not of diagnostic value. CT is useful for detection of soft-tissue masses, however, and for determination of their size and their relationship to adjacent anatomic structures.[28] A mass with a homogeneous fat density is likely to be a lipoma and one with a heterogeneous fat density, a liposarcoma. The mineralization of a mass, as well as extrinsic cortical invasion, can be visualized better on CT scans than on plain radiographs or MRI. However, CT scanning cannot be used for reliable differentiation between a malignant tumor and a benign soft-tissue tumor in a limb.[32] For soft-tissue tumors, MRI is superior to CT as a diagnostic tool.

Magnetic Resonance Imaging of Bone Tumors MRI is an excellent method for examination of the musculoskeletal system. Axial images as well as coronal and sagittal displays show many features of joints, ligaments, nerves, arteries, and physes. In the evaluation of benign or malignant tumors of bone, MRI is superior to CT for visualization or detection of extraosseous and intraosseous extension,[33,34] joint involvement, skip metastases, and epiphyseal extension. In the presence of metal prostheses, there is less degradation of MRI than is noted on CT scans, and thus MRI allows monitoring for tumor recurrence. MRI is perhaps too sensitive, in that it shows an abnormal signal when there is edema. It is not accurate for distinguishing between malignant and benign bone tumors. In fact, neither CT nor MRI helps the clinician to make an accurate diagnosis as much as conventional radiography does. Because of the low signal emanating from the cortex, MRI cannot delineate fractures or cortical destruction as accurately as does CT. In addition, the signals from regions of mineralization are low and thus make visualization of matrix calcification in cartilaginous or bone-producing osseous tumors more difficult.

Magnetic Resonance Imaging of Soft-Tissue Masses Because of the superior image contrast and because of the capacity to provide sagittal and coronal images, MRI is superior to CT for the demonstration of the size and extent of soft-tissue tumors and their relationships to bone, nerves, and blood vessels.[35-37] Destruction of bone cortex by a soft-tissue sarcoma, however, is best seen with CT. MRI is superior to CT for the definition of the anatomic relationship of soft-tissue masses in the limbs,[33] but it is not reliable for differentiation of malignant from benign masses and it can reliably distinguish only tumors that are composed of fat from those that are not.[35] Lipogenic tumors produce higher signals when compared with muscle on T_1-weighted and T_2-weighted images; other benign or malignant tumors have low signals on T_1-weighted and high signals on T_2-weighted images. Malignant tumors, in contrast to benign tumors, are likely to appear as heterogeneous masses on both pulse sequences, and often edema (with a high signal) is seen to surround the mass on T_2-weighted images; however, this generalization has too many exceptions to be reliable for clinical purposes. Initially, desmoid tumors were thought to have low signals on T_1-weighted and T_2-weighted images, but evaluation of a recent, more extensive series has shown that these tumors often appear similar to other benign and malignant soft-tissue tumors

on MRI scans.[38] Because of the inherently superior contrast of MRI, this technique is preferable to CT for delineation of soft-tissue masses and bone tumors with soft-tissue extension from muscle, vessels, nerves, fat, bone, and joints. There is now little or no need for angiography for the delineation of vascular anatomy. MRI does not show mineralization in these masses, nor does it indicate cortical erosion by an extensive soft-tissue mass. However, it is superior to CT for demonstration of the relationship of a soft-tissue mass to the cortex of a bone. In all studies of soft-tissue tumors, MRI is equal or superior to CT with respect to image quality, detection of the tumor, and clarity of the boundaries of the tumor on the image.

Magnetic Resonance Imaging Versus Computed Tomography In summary, because of the superb quality of MRI, the technique is excellent for delineation of any soft-tissue extension of bone tumors, and it appears to be more useful than CT for imaging of malignant bone tumors when anatomic delineation is of primary importance. CT still appears to be equal to MRI for demonstration of benign bone tumors and of malignant bone tumors that are entirely intraosseous. For the evaluation of soft-tissue tumors, MRI is superior to CT in almost all respects, and it should replace CT as the method of choice when information on the anatomy of a mass is desired. In future investigations, MRI technology may be used for specific diagnoses and for the prediction and definition of the response to chemotherapy and radiation therapy.

Lymph Node Metastases

Lymph node metastases are rare in patients with primary malignant bone tumor and in those with primary soft-tissue sarcoma, except those with childhood rhabdomyosarcoma, epithelioid sarcoma, or synovial sarcoma. However, the true prevalence of regional nodal metastases of even these tumor types at the time of the initial operation is unknown. Much of the available information indicates an increased prevalence of lymph node involvement by those tumors, but the data come from large series that contained many autopsy cases or from operative series that did not include random sampling of the regional lymph nodes.

It is not clear whether, even in the presence of metastases in regional lymph nodes, lymph node dissection has any therapeutic value. However, there is no doubt that the presence of sarcoma in the regional lymph nodes is a bad prognostic sign. Lymphangiography has not proved to be a specific or sensitive method for the detection of regional lymph-node metastases from primary sarcomas of the limb. False-positive findings in the inguinal and femoral lymph nodes are common. Physical examination remains the most reliable method with which to evaluate lymph node involvement in the antecubital fossa, axilla, popliteal fossa, and groin. CT scanning of the mediastinum, abdomen, and pelvis is an excellent way to look for pathological lymph nodes in these locations.

Disseminated Disease

The lung is the most common site of disseminated disease caused by malignant primary bone and soft-tissue tumors. Bone, the second most frequent site, is becoming increasingly common as the life span of patients with primary bone malignancy increases and the disease course is modified by aggressive multidrug chemotherapy. The value of ^{99m}TcMDP scintigraphy in the detection of bone metastases has been discussed previously in this chapter.

The methods of detection of pulmonary metastases have undergone extensive evolution. Lesions can be detected more readily with conventional tomograms than is possible with conventional biplane chest radiographs.[39] CT, in turn, can show more lesions than does conventional tomography, especially if the lesions are located in the periphery of the lungs.[40-43] However, CT is so sensitive that, in many instances, the lesions that it detects are found at thoracotomy to be inflammatory rather than neoplastic.[43]

Diagnostic Strategy for Skeletal Metastases of Unknown Origin

The skeleton is a common metastatic site for several visceral carcinomas. In 3% to 4% of all patients with metastatic disease, the primary site is unknown,[44-48] and 10% to 15% of these patients have skeletal involvement.[44,46,48,49] In patients older than the age of 40 years who have a symptomatic, destructive bone lesion, the diagnosis is most frequently skeletal metastases of unknown origin. Because the search for the primary carcinoma often becomes the task of the orthopaedic surgeon, a rational approach to this challenging clinical problem is needed.

If the lesion, which is usually located in the axial skeleton or in the proximal portion of the appendicular parts of the skeleton, shows a wide zone of transition on a conventional radiograph, a modest search for the primary site is indicated. Prior to biopsy, the physician should design a diagnostic and staging evaluation in order to (1) confirm the impression that the lesion is metastatic; (2) find another, less hazardous, biopsy site; and (3) find the site of the primary tumor.[50,51] The primary malignant growths that most commonly spread to bone are carcinomas of the breast and prostate. However, when the primary carcinoma is unknown, it is usually located in the kidney or lung.[50,51] In addition, screening for multiple myeloma is necessary.

When a metastatic bone tumor is suspected in a patient in whom the location of the primary tumor is unknown, the diagnostic strategy consists of recording of a medical history, physical examination, routine laboratory analysis, plain radiography of the involved bone and chest, whole-body ^{99m}TcMDP bone scintigraphy, and CT of the chest and abdomen (Fig. 1).

Physical examination of the breast, thyroid, and prostate should be performed in conjunction with simple laboratory tests, including guaiac-testing of the stool (gastrointestinal tract), prostate-specific antigen (prostate), urinalysis (kidney), and thyroid function tests, as well as serum protein electrophoresis (multiple myeloma). Other tests, including a complete blood-cell count and determinations of serum calcium and serum alkaline phosphatase, may show some nonspecific abnormalities related to metastatic disease. Conventional radiography and CT of the chest identify primary lung carcinomas. Abdominal CT may identify kidney carcinomas and carcinomas of the gastrointestinal organs, such as the liver.

The breast is an uncommon site of the primary malignancy when the patient has a skeletal metastasis of uncertain origin. Therefore, mammography is not a useful part of the diagnostic strategy unless an abnormality is identified in the history and physical examination. Mammography should be considered as an additional diagnostic test for women in whom the primary malignancy remains unknown after the entire diagnostic strategy has been completed.

A bone scintigram can be used for visualization and confirmation of additional sites of osseous involvement by all types of metastatic tumors, except multiple myeloma. If other sites of involvement are discovered, the diagnosis of metastatic bone disease is secure, and more appropriate sites for biopsy may be found. If the bone scintigram does not show other osseous abnormalities and if the remainder of the just described evaluation for metastases reveals normal results, then the possibility of a primary bone tumor should be considered. If a diagnosis has still not been made, a biopsy of the presenting site is indicated. Even if a biopsy is performed, however, the primary site may not be found, especially when the pathological diagnosis is adenocarcinoma.[50]

By using the described diagnostic strategy, we were able to identify the primary carcinoma in 85% of patients.[51] This diagnostic strategy was more successful than strategies reported in previous studies.[47-50,52-57] The greatest single difference between this strategy and the methods described in previous reports was the increased utilization of CT. With CT, one can identify primary tumors that would not have been identified with the other diagnostic modalities, and suspected primary tumors are confirmed in many patients.[51]

Because most patients in whom the site of the primary lesion is unknown have a short life expectancy,[45,46,54] it may seem appropriate to limit costly staging tests[47] and to proceed directly to the biopsy to begin the search for an occult malignancy. However, there are six reasons for not doing so. First, the lesion may be a bone sarcoma; if so, a poorly planned biopsy will compromise the ability of the surgeon to obtain high-quality images of the bone lesion and to perform a limb-sparing procedure. Second, the remainder of the evaluation may identify another lesion, the biopsy of which could be technically easier and safer for the patient. Third, renal-cell metastases can be very vascular, and it is helpful to know, before the biopsy, that a bone lesion is likely to be renal in origin. This allows the surgeon to consider prebiopsy embolization or the use of a needle biopsy. Fourth, in the case of multiple myeloma, an unnecessary biopsy can be avoided if an appropriate evaluation is carried out. Fifth, in our series,[51] the tissue diagnosis itself identified the primary lesion only in a minority of the patients and, therefore, usually did not direct the search for the occult malignancy. Lastly, the surgeon and pathologist will be more confident with the histologic diagnosis based on frozen section if a primary malignant site is identified before a biopsy is performed. This will allow internal fixation of impending fractures to be carried out at the time of the biopsy, and it will eliminate the need for a second operation after a final histopathological diagnosis has been obtained.

Summary

The diagnostic strategy to be used for a bone tumor depends on the ability of the clinician to make an accurate differential diagnosis on the basis of clinical information and plain radiographs. The clinician must be able to classify the patient as having a non-progressive or a progressive primary benign bone tumor, a primary malignant bone tumor, or a metastatic bone tumor. Only after assignment to one of these four categories can an effective diagnostic strategy ensue. If the clinical and radiographic information favors a diagnosis of malignant or aggressive benign bone tumor, the clinician should refer the patient to an experienced orthopaedic oncologist without performing additional diagnostic tests or a biopsy. If a soft-tissue mass is 5 cm in diameter or larger on physical examination, and especially if it is deep to the fascia, the patient should also be referred to an orthopaedic oncologist, without additional evaluation or biopsy, because of the relatively high probability that the mass is malignant.

References

1. Simon MA, Schaaf HW, Metz CE: Clinical utility of the erythrocyte sedimentation rate in preoperative evaluation of solitary skeletal lesions. *J Orthop Res* 1984;2:262-268.
2. Mosende C, Gutierrez M, Caparros B, et al: Combination chemotherapy with bleomycin, cyclophosphamide and dactinomycin for the treatment of osteogenic sarcoma. *Cancer* 1977;40:2779-2786.
3. Thorpe WP, Reilly JJ, Rosenberg SA: Prognostic significance of alkaline phosphatase measurements in patients with osteogenic sarcoma receiving chemotherapy. *Cancer* 1979;43:2178-2181.
4. Lodwick GS: A systematic approach to the roentgen diagnosis of bone tumors, in *Tumors of Bone and Soft Tissues.* Chicago, IL, Year Book Medical, 1965, pp 49-68.
5. Collin C, Godbold J, Hajdu S, et al: Localized extremity soft tissue sarcoma: An analysis of factors affecting survival. *J Clin Oncol* 1987;5:601-612.
6. Myhre-Jensen O: A consecutive 7-year series of 1331 benign soft tissue tumours: Clinicopathologic data: Comparison with sarcomas. *Acta Orthop Scand* 1981;52:287-293.
7. Rydholm A, Berg NO: Size, site and clinical incidence of lipoma: Factors in the differential diagnosis of lipoma and sarcoma. *Acta Orthop Scand* 1983;54:929-934.
8. Rydholm A, Gustafson P, Rööser B, et al: Subcutaneous sarcoma: A population-based study of 129 patients. *J Bone Joint Surg* 1991;73B:662-667.
9. Martel W, Abell MR: Radiologic evaluation of soft tissue tumors: A retrospective study. *Cancer* 1973;32:352-366.
10. Mankin HJ, Lange TA, Spanier SS: The hazards of biopsy in patients with malignant primary bone and soft-tissue tumors. *J Bone Joint Surg* 1982;64A:1121-1127.
11. Simon MA: Current concepts review: Biopsy of musculoskeletal tumors. *J Bone Joint Surg* 1982;64A:1253-1257.
12. Lange TA, Austin CW, Seibert JJ, et al: Ultrasound imaging as a screening study for malignant soft-tissue tumors. *J Bone Joint Surg* 1987;69A:100-105.
13. Kirchner PT, Simon MA: Current concepts review: Radioisotopic evaluation of skeletal disease. *J Bone Joint Surg* 1981;63A:673-681.
14. Alazraki NP, Davis MA, Jones AG, et al: Skeletal system, in Kirchner PT (ed): *Nuclear Medicine Review Syllabus.* New York, NY, Society of Nuclear Medicine, 1980, pp 539-586.
15. Belliveau RE, Spencer RP: Incidence and sites of bone lesions detected by 99mTc-polyphosphate scans in patients with tumors. *Cancer* 1975;36:359-363.
16. McNeil BJ: Rationale for the use of bone scans in selected metastatic and primary bone tumors. *Semin Nucl Med* 1978;8:336-345.
17. Simon MA, Kirchner PT: Scintigraphic evaluation of primary bone tumors: Comparison of technetium-99m phosphonate and gallium citrate imaging. *J Bone Joint Surg* 1980;62A:758-764.
18. Enneking WF, Chew FS, Springfield DS, et al: The role of radionuclide bone-scanning in determining the resectability of soft-tissue sarcomas. *J Bone Joint Surg* 1981;63A:249-257.
19. Kirchner PT, Simon MA: The clinical value of bone and gallium scintigraphy for soft-tissue sarcomas of the extremities. *J Bone Joint Surg* 1984;66A:319-327.
20. Finn HA, Simon MA, Martin WB, et al: Scintigraphy with gallium-67 citrate in staging of soft-tissue sarcomas of the extremity. *J Bone Joint Surg* 1987;69A:886-891.
21. Norman A: The value of tomography in the diagnosis of skeletal disorders. *Radiol Clin North Am* 1970;8:251-258.
22. Hudson TM, Haas G, Enneking WF, et al: Angiography in the management of musculoskeletal tumors. *Surg Gynecol Obstet* 1975;141:11-21.
23. Levin DC, Watson RC, Baltaxe HA: Arteriography in diagnosis and management of acquired peripheral soft-tissue masses. *Radiology* 1972;104:53-58.
24. Bowers TA, Murray JA, Charnsangavej C, et al: Bone metastases from renal carcinoma: The preoperative use of transcatheter arterial occlusion. *J Bone Joint Surg* 192;64A:749-754.

25. Jaffe N, Robertson R, Ayala A, et al: Comparison of intra-articular cis-diamminedichloroplatinum II with high-dose methotrexate and citrovorum factor rescue in the treatment of primary osteosarcoma. *J Clin Oncol* 1985;3:1101-1104.

26. Wallace S, Granmayeh M, deSantos LA, et al: Arterial occlusion of pelvic bone tumors. *Cancer* 1979;43:322-328.

27. Berger PE, Kuhn JP: CT of tumors of the musculoskeletal system in children. *Radiology* 1978;127:171-175.

28. Bernardino ME, Jing B-S, Thomas JL, et al: The extremity soft-tissue lesion: A comparative study of ultrasound, CT, and xeroradiography. *Radiology* 1981;139:53-59.

29. deSantos LA, Goldstein HM, Murray JA, et al: Computed tomography in the evaluation of musculoskeletal neoplasms. *Radiology* 1978;128:89-94.

30. McLeod RA, Stephens DH: CT of pelvic musculoskeletal neoplasm. *Contemp Orthop* 1979;1:36-41.

31. Schreiman JS, Crass JR, Wick MR, et al: Osteosarcoma: Role of CT in limb-sparing treatment. *Radiology* 1986;161:485-488.

32. Rosenthal DI: CT in bone and soft tissue neoplasm: Application and pathologic correlation. *Crit Rev Diagn Imaging* 1982;18:243-278.

33. Berquist TH: MRI of musculoskeletal neoplasms. *Clin Orthop* 1989;244:101-118.

34. Zimmer WD, Berquist TH, McLeod RA, et al: Bone tumors: MRI versus CT. *Radiology* 1985;155:709-718.

35. Kransdorf MJ, Jelinek JS, Moser RP Jr, et al: Soft-tissue masses: Diagnosis using MR imaging. *AJR Am J Roentgenol* 1989;153:541-547.

36. Petasnick JP, Turner DA, Charters JR, et al: Soft-tissue masses of the locomotor system: Comparison of MR imaging with CT. *Radiology* 1986;160:125-133.

37. Totty WG, Murphy WA, Lee JKT: Soft-tissue tumors: MR imaging. *Radiology* 1986;160:135-141.

38. Quinn SF, Erickson SJ, Dee PM, et al: MR imaging in fibromatosis: Results in 26 patients with pathologic correlation. *AJR Am J Roentgenol* 1991;156:539-542.

39. Miller WE, Crowe JK, Muhm JR: The evaluation of pulmonary parenchymal abnormalities by tomography. *Radiol Clin North Am* 1976;14:85-93.

40. Chang AE, Schaner EG, Conkle DM, et al: Evaluation of CT in the detection of pulmonary metastases: A prospective study. *Cancer* 1979;43:913-916.

41. Muhm JR, Brown LR, Crowe JK: Detection of pulmonary nodules by CT. *AJR Am J Roentgenol* 1977;128:267-270.

42. Muhm JR, Brown LR, Crowe JK: Use of CT in the detection of pulmonary nodules. *Mayo Clin Proc* 1977;52:345-348.

43. Schaner EG, Chang AE, Doppman JL, et al: Comparison of computed and conventional whole lung tomography in detecting pulmonary nodules: A prospective radiologic-pathologic study. *AJR Am J Roentgenol* 1978;131:51-54.

44. Holmes FF, Fouts TL: Metastatic cancer of unknown primary site. *Cancer* 1970;26:816-818.

45. Lleander VC, Goldstein G, Horsley JS III: Chemotherapy in the management of metastatic cancer of unknown primary site. *Oncology* 1972;26:265-270.

46. Moertel CG, Reitemeir RJ, Schutt AJ, et al: Treatment of the patient with adenocarcinoma of unknown origin. *Cancer* 1972;30:1469-1472.

47. Nystrom JS, Weiner JM, Wolf RM, et al: Identifying the primary site in metastatic cancer of unknown origin: Inadequacy of roentgenographic procedures. *JAMA* 1979;241:381-383.

48. Stewart JF, Tattersall MHN, Woods RL, et al: Unknown primary adenocarcinoma: Incidence of overinvestigation and natural history. *Br Med J* 1979;1:1530-1533.

49. Didolkar MS, Fanous N, Elias EG, et al: Metastatic carcinomas from occult primary tumors: A study of 254 patients. *Ann Surg* 1977;186:625-630.

50. Simon MA, Bartucci EJ: The search for the primary tumor in patients with skeletal metastases of unknown origin. *Cancer* 1986;58:1088-1095.

51. Rougraff BT, Kneisl JS, Simon MA: Skeletal metastases of unknown origin: Prospective evaluation of a diagnostic strategy. *J Bone Joint Surg* 1993;75A:1276-1281.

52. Barón MG, de la Gándara I, Espinosa E, et al: Bone metastases as the first manifestation of a tumour. *Int Orthop* 1991;15:373-376.

53. McMillan JH, Levine E, Stephens RH: CT in the evaluation of metastatic adenocarcinoma from an unknown primary site: A retrospective study. *Radiology* 1982;143:143-146.

54. Nottebaert M, Exner GU, von Hochstetter AR, et al: Metastatic bone disease from occult carcinoma: A profile. *Int Orthop* 1989;13:119-123.

55. Nystrom JS, Weiner JM, Heffelfinger-Juttner J, et al: Metastatic and histologic presentation in unknown primary cancer. *Semin Oncol* 1977;4:53-58.

56. Panza N, Lombardi G, De Rosa M, et al: High serum thyroglobulin levels: Diagnostic indicators in patients with metastases from unknown primary sites. *Cancer* 1987;60:2233-2236.

57. Woods RL, Fox RM, Tattersall MHN, et al: Metastatic adenocarcinomas of unknown primary site: A randomized study of two combination-chemotherapy regimens. *N Engl J Med* 1980;303:87-89.

Staging Systems for Musculoskeletal Neoplasia

Dempsey S. Springfield, MD

Introduction

In the late 1950s, the American Joint Committee for Cancer Staging and End Results Reporting (AJC) was formed. This committee was responsible for developing and encouraging the use of staging systems for a variety of malignancies, including those of the musculoskeletal system. The assumption made then and still held was that cancer progresses from a confined solitary malignancy, spreads into local tissue, then to regional lymph nodes, and finally to distant sites and that the state of a cancer at the time of the patient's presentation is an indication of where that cancer is in its natural history. It was thought that by grouping cancer patients who had progressed to similar positions in the natural history of tumor development it would be possible to select an appropriate treatment program more objectively, to predict the patient's outcome more accurately, and to establish protocols to study new methods of treatment. The AJC wanted to develop a language that physicians could use to compare cancer patients. This common language would allow more accurate understanding of an individual patient's prognosis and would assist the physician in making the decision of how to treat that patient. They established the T, N, and M system of grouping cancers as a means of describing how far a cancer had progressed. The T indicates the local extent of the cancer—the primary cancer's size is the measurement used to indicate the extent. The N, which refers to the spread of tumor to local or regional lymph nodes, is either positive or negative. The M, which refers to the presence or absence of non-lymph node sites of metastasis, is also either positive or negative. The staging systems developed by the AJC have been useful in the management of patients with malignant tumors and are used in all settings of cancer management.

In 1977, the first AJC staging system for musculoskeletal neoplasms was published.[1] This system was designed to be used with soft tissue neoplasia only. They had not been able to develop a staging system for primary malignancies of the skeleton. The histologic grade (G) of the tumor was added to the T, N, and M variables, because in sarcomas histologic grade is a critical variant. This system was difficult to use because of uncertainty regarding what "involvement" of bone, vessels, and nerves meant, and in 1988 a revision was published.[2] The revised system is used by many physicians today.

In 1980, Enneking and associates[3] published a staging system that could be used for both skeletal and soft tissue malignancies. This staging system was designed principally as an aid to the surgeon, and they stated, "Although an effective staging system should serve all members of the multidisciplinary team, the biologic behavior of musculoskeletal sarcomas suggest that the most useful staging system will articulate with the surgical procedure." This staging system was developed with the idea that the surgical stage should be an indicator of the type of surgical resection required. This staging system was proposed before the regular use of preoperative irradiation or adjuvant chemotherapy, and although these treatments do not change the stage of a tumor they often change the recommended surgical margin.

Hajdu[4] reminded the reader of what Bucy and Gustafson had said in 1939 when he quoted them: "Classification must be regarded as providing merely arbitrary pockets into which we can place tumors in order that they may be more easily considered." Hajdu was reminding the reader that there are limitations to staging systems and that he was aware of the risk of offering his modification of the previously proposed AJC staging system. He felt, nevertheless, that his modifications were an improvement. His system is simple and uses broad criteria for its divisions. He proposed it, at the same time suggesting that further modification was to be expected.

General Considerations

From their inception staging systems have been developed to assist the physician in a variety of ways.[5] The first, and probably most important, is to assist the physician in understanding a patient's prognosis. The staging system's primary function is to group cancer patients with similar prognoses together. Before staging systems were developed, it was difficult to know whether a patient had a good, fair, or poor chance of survival with the treatments available. At a time when treatment options were limited, it was not as important to know the prognosis, but, as treatment options, and the potential side effects of those treatments increased, it became important to be able to predict the risk that a patient with a cancer faces in order to judge the risk that should be taken with treatment. Additional benefits of staging systems are improved communication between physicians and the ability to design studies to test the effectiveness of a treatment.

If the staging system is to fulfill its purpose, which is to group patients with similar prognoses together, it is necessary to know what factors are critical determinants of a patient's prognosis and to know the relative importance of each prognostic factor. A number of studies have been done to determine the prognostic variables in sarcomas, and, although there remains some controversy, in general, the significant variables are agreed on. They include: (1) the presence of metastatic disease at presentation (N or M); (2) the histologic grade of the sarcoma (G); (3) the size of the sarcoma (T); and (4) the depth of the sarcoma (subcutaneous versus superficial).

The order of the importance of these variables determines how the staging system is arranged. The presence of clinically apparent metastatic disease at the time of presentation, either to lymph nodes or another organ system, is a very poor prognostic factor. All staging systems have separated patients with metastatic disease at presentation into a single poor-prognosis group. The single most significant prognostic factor for patients who do not have clinically apparent metastasis at presentation is the histologic grade of the sarcoma. Therefore, histologic grade is the focal point around which all musculoskeletal staging systems are arranged.

Histologic grade is determined by microscopic examination of representative tissue from the sarcoma.[6] The variables that determine the histologic grade include: (1) number of mitoses per ten high power fields; (2) the degree of cellular pleomorphism; (3) the degree of cell differentiation; (4) the amount of necrosis; (5) the cell-to-matrix ratio; and (6) the local invasiveness of the malignant cells. The more mitoses, the greater the pleomorphism, the poorer the cell differentiation, the greater the necrosis, the greater the cell-to-matrix ratio, and the more invasive a tumor is, the higher the grade and the worse the patient's prognosis.

Sarcomas can be separated into two grades, three grades, or four grades. The most common grading systems use a three-grade system—low (grade 1), medium (grade 2), and high (grade 3). Enneking and associates[3] preferred to use only two histologic grades, low (I) and high (II) grade, because they felt that the surgical operations were best served with a simple system with as few grades and stages as possible.

The next most important prognostic indicator is the local extent of the sarcoma. Size may indicate the rate of growth or length of time the tumor has been present. In either case, size is a predictor of the risk of eventually developing a metastasis. Most physicians believe that size is important because it reflects the rate of growth and that rate of growth is the indicator of

risk. Size is the most common measure of local extent, and size correlates with prognosis. When sarcomas of the same histologic grade are compared, those with a diameter of 5 cm or less are much less likely to metastasize than are larger sarcomas. Enneking and associates[3] chose to indicate local extent by determining whether the primary sarcoma was confined to a single anatomic compartment or had extended beyond the confines of a single compartment. Tumors confined to a single compartment tend to be smaller than those that extend beyond their compartment of origin. Compartments are important in the Enneking staging system because it is a surgical staging system and anatomic compartmentalization is more important than size when deciding between amputation and limb salvage. Whether extent correlates best with size or with compartmentalization remains to be determined, but, either way, local extent is a significant prognostic factor.

Recent publications have established that lesions confined to the subcutaneous tissues are less likely to metastasize than those that are deep to the most superficial fascia.[7-9] The subcutaneous sarcomas should be staged separately.

Specific Staging Systems

The American Joint Committee for Cancer Staging and End Results Reporting The AJC revised their original staging system for soft tissues tumors and developed one for bone tumors (Table 1).[2] These systems use three histologic grades and separate tumors by size—those 5 cm and less and those larger than 5 cm. These staging systems also separate those patients with a lymph node metastasis from those with a metastasis to another site. As is the convention in all staging systems, the lower the number the better the prognosis.

Stage I is for patients with a sarcoma of histologic grade 1 (low grade). The patients are further separated within Stage I into an A subgroup (sarcomas 5 cm or less) and a B subgroup (sarcomas larger than 5 cm). Patients in Stage I do not have clinically apparent metastatic disease.

Stage II is for patients with a sarcoma of histologic grade 2 (medium grade). As with patients in Stage I, a further separation is done within Stage II for patients with grade 2 sarcomas 5 cm or less (subgroup A) and those with sarcomas larger than 5 cm (subgroup B). Patients in Stage II do not have clinically apparent metastatic disease.

Stage III is for patients with a sarcoma of histologic grade 3 (high grade). Again those with sarcomas 5 cm or smaller are separated (subgroup A) from those with a sarcoma larger than 5 cm (subgroup B). Patients in Stage III do not have clinically apparent metastatic disease.

Stage IV is for patients with a sarcoma of any grade and any size with a metastasis at the time of presenta-

Table 1
American Joint Commission staging systems

Soft Tissue Sarcoma

Stage	Grade (G)	Size (T)	Nodes (N)	Mets (M)
IA	1	1	0	0
IB	1	2	0	0
IIA	2	1	0	0
IIB	2	2	0	0
IIIA	3 or 4	1	0	0
IIIB	3 or 4	2	0	0
IVA	any	any	1	0
IVB	any	any	any	1

Bone Sarcoma

Stage	Grade (G)	Size (T)	Nodes (N)	Mets (M)
IA	1 or 2	1	0	0
IB	1 or 2	2	0	0
IIA	3 or 4	1	0	0
IIB	3 or 4	2	0	0
III	not defined			
IVA	any	any	1	0
IVB	any	any	any	1

Histological Grade (G):
- 1 = well differentiated
- 2 = moderately differentiated
- 3 = poorly differentiated
- 4 = undifferentiated

Primary Tumor Size (T):
For soft tissue sarcoma
- 1 = 5 cm or smaller
- 2 = larger than 5 cm

For bone sarcoma
- 1 = confined by cortex
- 2 = extends beyond cortex

Regional Lymph Node Involvement (N):
- 0 = none
- 1 = involved

Distant Metastatic Spread (M):
- 0 = none
- 1 = present

(Reproduced with permission from American Joint Commission on Cancer in Beahrs OH (ed): *Manual for Staging of Cancer*, ed 3. Philadelphia, PA, JB Lippincott, 1988, pp 123-131.)

Table 2
Enneking's surgical staging system for bone and soft tissue sarcomas

Stage	Grade (G)	Site (T)	Mets (N or M)
IA	low	intra	none
IB	low	extra	none
IIA	high	intra	none
IIB	high	extra	none
IIIA	any	intra	present
IIIB	any	extra	present

Histological Grade (G):
- low = well differentiated
- high = all non-well differentiated

Primary Tumor Site (T):
- intra = intracompartmental
- extra = extracompartmental

Metastasis (N or M):
- regional lymph nodes involvement or any distant metastasis

(Reproduced with permission from Enneking WF, Spanier SS, Goodman MA; A system for the surgical staging of musculosketal sarcoma. *Clin Orthop* 1980;153:106-120.)

course but with a low to medium histologic grade would be placed into the high grade category.

Both grades were subdivided by the anatomic extent of the tumor, but instead of using tumor size as the indicator of extent, the tumors were said to be either intracompartmental or extracompartmental. The body

Table 3
Enneking's anatomic compartments

Intracompartmental	Extracompartmental
Intrassoeous	Extraosseous extension
Intraarticluar	Extraarticular extension
Subcutaneous	Extension to deep fascia
Paraosseous	Extension into bone or adjacent soft tissue
Soft tissue:	Soft tissue:
Ray of hand or foot	Mid and hindfoot, palm
Posterior calf	Popliteal space
Anterolateral leg	
Anterolateral thigh	Groin (femoral triangle)
Medial thigh	
Posterior thigh	
Buttocks	Intrapelvic
	Retroperitoneal
Periscapular	Axilla
	Periclavicular
Anterior arm	
Posterior arm	
Volar forearm	Anticubital fossae
Dosal forearm	
	Paraspinous

(Reproduced with permission from Enneking WF, Spanier SS, Goodman MA; A system for the surgical staging of musculosketal sarcoma. *Clin Orthop* 1980;153:106-120.)

tion to either a lymph node or other site. Stage IV is divided into an A and B subgroup, with those patients with a lymph node metastasis in the A subgroup and those with a metastasis to any other site in the B subgroup.

The Enneking or Musculoskeletal Tumor Society System The Enneking or Musculoskeletal Tumor Society (MSTS) staging system was originally proposed by Enneking and associates[3] in 1980 (Table 2). They wanted a surgical staging system that would be easy to use and that would apply to both bone and soft tissue tumors. Histologic grade was used as the primary method to group the tumors, but only two grades were used, high and low. The grade of the tumor was not determined solely by the histologic appearance. Histologic features were the most important determinant of prognosis, but clinical grade was used as well. For example, a tumor which presented with an aggressive clinical

Table 4
Enneking's definitions of surgical margins

Type	Description
Intralesional	Debulking or curettage
Marginal	Removal through tumor's pseudocapsule (reactive zone)
Wide	Intracompartmental removal with cuff of surrounding normal tissue
Radical	Extracompartmental removal of tumor

(Reproduced with permission from Enneking WF, Spanier SS, Goodman MA; A system for the surgical staging of musculosketal sarcoma. *Clin Orthop* 1980;153:106-120.)

Table 5
Hajdu staging system for soft tissue sarcomas

Stage	Size	Site	Grade
0	1	S	L
IA	1	S	H
IB	1	D	L
IC	2	S	H
IIA	1	D	H
IIB	2	S	H
IIC	2	D	L
III	2	D	H

Size:	1 = 5 cm or less
	2 = larger than 5 cm
Site:	S = subcutaneous
	D = deep
Grade:	L = low
	H = high

(Reproduced with permission from Hajdu SI: Pathology of Soft Tissue Tumors, in *History and Classification of Soft Tissue Tumors*. Philadelphia, PA, Lea and Febiger, 1979, chap 1, pp 1-55.)

was divided into anatomic compartments, which were thought to represent compartments that tend to contain a tumor's growth (Table 3). All patients with metastatic disease at presentation were grouped together in a separate stage. Initially the patients with metastatic disease were not further subdivided, but, in a later revision of the staging system, these patients were subdivided into those with intracompartmental and those with extracompartmental primary disease.[10]

This system is used extensively by orthopaedic oncologists and is useful in separating patients into groups with similar prognoses. The major criticism is that too many of the patients fall into the stage IIB category. Stage IIB probably needs to be divided further. Enneking reviewed 219 bone tumors and 178 soft tissue tumors and showed that each stage had a distinct prognosis.[10]

Enneking and associates[3] made another contribution in their 1980 article by offering definitions for types of surgical margins (Table 4). Before this, there had been no generally agreed upon meaning for terms used to describe a surgical procedure. Four types of surgical margins were defined: intralesional, marginal, wide, and radical. These terms have been used with increasing frequency and have improved communications between physicians. An intralesional margin is obtained when the lesion is entered and the tumor removed from within. This usually leaves macroscopic disease in the patient. A marginal margin is obtained when the tumor is removed through its pseudocapsule. This is the margin achieved when a tumor is "shelled out" and leaves microscopic tumor cells behind if the tumor is a benign aggressive or malignant tumor. A wide margin is achieved when the tumor is removed with a surrounding cuff of normal uninvolved tissue. This is also often called an en bloc resection. A resection with a wide margin will remove all tumor cells unless there are local or distant metastasis. This margin is used for the surgical management of most sarcomas and is felt to be an adequate margin for all but the

most locally aggressive sarcomas. A radical margin is achieved when the tumor and the entire compartment(s) are removed. This usually requires an amputation and is the most definitive surgical margin. A resection with a radical margin is occasionally used for the primary treatment of large sarcomas but is usually reserved for locally recurrent sarcomas.

The Hajdu System Hajdu based his system on the three variables that he thinks are the most important: size, site, and histologic grade (Table 5).[4] Each of these three has a good prognosis group and bad prognosis group. Size is divided between those that are small (good) and those that are large (bad) with small meaning 5 cm or less and large meaning larger than 5 cm. Site is divided into lesions that are superficial, meaning subcutaneous (good), and those that are deep (bad). Histologic grade is divided into those that are low grade (good) and those that are high grade (bad). Low grade lesions have minimal necrosis, good maturation, less than five mitoses per ten high power field, are hypocellular, and have a moderate amount of stroma. High grade lesions have extensive necrosis, poor maturation, more than five mitoses per ten high power fields, are hypercellular, and have minimal stroma. The staging system has five major groupings with three subgroupings in two of the stages. Stage 0 lesions are those with three good prognostic signs. Stage I lesions are those with one bad prognostic sign and two good prognostic signs. Stage I is subdivided into three groups, each with a specific single poor prognostic factor. Stage II lesions are those with two bad prognostic signs and one good prognostic sign. Stage II is subdivided into three groups, each with a specific single good prognosis factor. Stage III lesions are those with

Table 6
Intergroup rhabdomyosarcoma staging system

Stage	Site	Size	Nodes (N)	Mets (M)
1	Orbit Head & Neck GU-not bladder or prostate	any	any	none
2	Bladder & Prostate Extremity Cranial parameningeal Other	A	0 or ?	none
3	Bladder & Prostate Extremity	A	1	none
	Cranial parameningeal Other	B	any	none
4	All site	any	any	present

Size: A = 5 cm or smaller
B = larger than 5 cm
Nodes: 0 = none
1 = clinically involved
? = unknown
(Reproduced with permission from Mauer HM, Ortega J: Intergroup rhabdomyosarcoma study. Amendments to IRS-IV protocols, June, 24, 1992.)

three poor prognostic signs. Stage IV is for patients who present with metastatic disease. Hajdu's review of 1,331 patients with soft tissue sarcomas staged with his system revealed a mortality of 8% for patients with a Stage I lesion, of 36% for patients with Stage II lesions, and of 79% for patients with Stage III lesions.

Rhabdomyosarcoma Rhabdomyosarcoma is a small cell malignancy which is almost exclusive to children. It often arises in bladder or prostate, head and neck, or the extremity muscles. In the past, the most common staging system for rhabdomyosarcoma was based on the amount of tumor left after a surgical resection had been done. Recently (June 1992), however, the Pediatric Oncology Group (POG) and the Children's Cancer Group (CCG) Intergroup for the study of rhabdomyosarcoma developed a new staging system for patients with rhabdomyosarcoma (Table 6).[11] This system uses the TNM groupings and is based on the status

Table 7
Enneking staging for benign musculoskeletal tumors

Stage	Definition	Behavior
1	Latent	Remains static or heals spontaneously
2	Active	Slow progressive growth, but limited by natural barriers
3	Aggressive	Rapid growth, not limited by natural barriers

(Reproduced with permission from Enneking WF: Musculoskeletal Tumor Surgery in *Staging Musculoskeletal Tumors*. New York, NY, Churchill Livingstone, 1983, chap 2, vol 1, pp 69-88.)

of the patient at presentation. Anatomic site is important in the prognosis of patients with rhabdomyosarcoma and is used as a major grouping.

Benign Bone Staging System Enneking suggested a staging system in his textbook for benign tumors (Table 7).[10] This system is useful as a means of categorizing benign bone tumors so that an appropriate management plan can be made. It is not intended to dictate the treatment of a specific lesion but rather to provide guidelines for evaluation and treatment. Three stages are designated by name or number: (1) latent, (2) active, and (3) locally aggressive. The clinical presentation and radiographic appearance of the lesion determines its stage. Patients with a Stage 1 lesion have minimal or no symptoms and a lesion that is confined to the bone, usually surrounded by a reactive rim of bone. Stage 1 lesions either remain dormant or heal spontaneously. Patients with a Stage 2 lesion have mild to moderate symptoms and a lesion, which, although confined by the periosteum, deforms the cortex. There is usually active periosteal and/or endosteal reaction, but the lesion is not completely surrounded by a reactive rim of bone. Stage 2 lesions are slowly progressive but usually can be cured with an intralesional curettage. Patients with a Stage 3 lesion have pain and may present with a pathologic fracture. The lesion will have extended through the periosteum and may invade the surrounding soft tissues. There will be an acute periosteal reaction and the border between the tumor and normal bone will be difficult to delineate. Stage 3 lesions require a resection, preferably with a wide surgical margin.

Future

The current staging systems are useful, but improvements are needed. Histologic grading remains subjective, and it is often impossible to obtain consensus. In the future, new diagnostic tools will provide better grading methods for the staging of tumors. It was thought that flow cytometry would offer a method for predicting a tumor's behavior but so far this has not proven to be the case. As a more thorough understanding of molecular biology is gained, intracellular mechanisms are being found that determine how cells behave. It is hoped that an even better understanding of these mechanisms will enable us to predict which tumors have the ability to spread locally and metastasize and which do not. If this goal is realized, it will provide an entirely new means of grading tumors. I suspect that in the future histologic type will play a lesser role in the staging of malignancies, and that staging systems will be unified based on the biologic behavior of a specific tumor. It is possible that there are tumors of completely different histogenesis that behave identically. If this is the case, they should be staged together.

References

1. Russell WO, Cohen J, Enzinger F, et al: A clinical and pathological staging system for soft tissue sarcomas. *Cancer* 1977;40:1562-1570.
2. American Joint Commission on Cancer in Beahrs OH (ed): *Manual for Staging of Cancer*, ed 3. Philadelphia, PA, JB Lippincott, 1988, pp 123-131.
3. Enneking WF, Spanier SS, Goodman MA: A system for the surgical staging of musculoskeletal sarcoma. *Clin Orthop* 1980;153:106-120.
4. Hajdu SI: Pathology of Soft Tissue Tumors, in *History and Classification of Soft Tissue Tumors*. Philadelphia, PA, Lea and Febiger, 1979, chap 1, pp 1-55.
5. Finn HA, Simon MA: Staging systems for musculoskeletal neoplasms. *Orthopedics* 1989;12:1365-1371.
6. Broders AC, Hargrave R, Meyerding HW: Pathological features of soft tissue fibrosarcoma with special reference to the grading of its malignancy. *Surg Gynecol Obstet* 1939;69:267-280.
7. Gaynor JJ, Tan CC, Casper ES, et al: Refinement of clinicopathologic staging for localized soft tissue sarcoma of the extremity: A study of 423 adults. *J Clin Oncol* 1992;10:1317-1329.
8. Rooser B: Prognosis in soft tissue sarcoma. *Acta Orthop Scand Suppl* 1987;225:1-54.
9. Rydholm A, Gustafson P, Rooser B, et al: Subcutaneous sarcoma: A population-based study of 129 patients. *J Bone Joint Surg* 1991;73B:662-667.
10. Enneking WF: Musculoskeletal Tumor Surgery in *Staging Musculoskeletal Tumors*. New York, NY, Churchill Livingstone, 1983, chap 2, vol 1, pp 69-88.
11. Mauer HM, Ortega J: Intergroup rhabdomyosarcoma study. Amendments to IRS-IV protocols, June 24, 1992.

Orthopaedic Surgery on the HIV-Positive Patient: Complications and Outcome

James V. Luck, Jr, MD

Introduction

It has been estimated that 18% to 24% of patients with AIDS require surgery.[1,2] It has also been estimated that 0.5% to 1.0% of the U.S. population is HIV-positive.[3,4] In high endemic areas, trauma centers report up to 10.4% of their emergency trauma patients to be HIV-positive.[5] In anonymous serosurveys conducted by the Centers for Disease Control at multiple institutions, 0.2% to 8.9% of emergency room patients and 0.1% to 7.8% of all hospital admissions were found to be HIV-positive.[6] Orthopaedic surgeons practicing in high endemic areas may anticipate that 5% to 10% of their acute trauma cases are HIV-positive. Elective surgical case rates are highly variable. In an anonymous study, Charache and associates,[7] at Johns Hopkins, found 18 out of 4,087 elective surgical patients to be HIV-positive. Under special circumstances, these percentages may be much higher. Because I have responsibility for orthopaedic care in a large hemophilia center, my elective caseload is 10% HIV-positive.

Surgery on the HIV-positive patient, elective or emergent, involves special risks, which may be divided into two categories: risk to the patient and risk to healthcare personnel. Because of concern about these issues, many orthopaedic surgeons may pursue nonsurgical management of fractures usually treated surgically and are reluctant to recommend elective surgery in the HIV-positive patient. Some authors have expressed special concern about the use of prosthetic implants in HIV-positive patients.[8,9] Both types of risks must be understood and considered when making decisions regarding the appropriateness of surgery for these patients.

Because of documented seroconversion of healthcare personnel following HIV-contaminated puncture injuries[10] and the frequency of parenteral and surface exposure to blood and body fluids in the operating room setting,[11] there has been extensive study of the risks to healthcare personnel. Recommendations of methodologies to reduce this risk in the practice of orthopaedics have been developed and published by the Task Force on AIDS of the American Academy of Orthopaedic Surgeons.[12] In my opinion, if these recommendations are followed closely, the risk to healthcare personnel is real but manageable.

Perhaps, the more crucial and currently uncertain issue is the element of increased risk to the patient because of HIV infection. This risk may be divided into three categories: early and late postoperative complications and acceleration of HIV-related disease. Early postoperative complications of greatest concern in the HIV-positive patient include sepsis and impaired healing. Sepsis may be divided into bacterial surgical site infection and remote opportunistic infection. The late postoperative complication of primary concern in the HIV-positive orthopaedic patient is implant infection. The risk of septic complications is increased because of impaired cellular and humoral immunity which is fairly well understood. The magnitude of increased risk, based on a limited series of reports of the outcome of surgery on HIV-positive patients, is less well delineated than the theoretical basis. These clinical studies also address our ability to successfully prevent complications in the HIV-positive surgical patient.

Pathophysiology of Immunity Impairment

The CD4 lymphocyte, which is responsible for cellular immunity, is the primary target cell in HIV infection. However, differentiation of the B lymphocyte, responsible for humoral immunity, is indirectly impaired.[13] Additional derangements occur in the monocyte/macrophage cell line and the production of gamma interferon and lymphokines.[13]

As the disease progresses, the absolute polymorphonuclear leukocyte count drops to levels that impair phagocytosis.[14] This may be further reduced by as-yet-unspecified humoral factors and aggravated by marrow-suppressing drugs such as AZT, used to treat AIDS. Malnutrition, which is the consequence of both the disease process and therapeutic medications, causes hypoalbuminemia which further impairs both lymphocyte function and phagocytosis.[15,16]

In addition to the crucial role they play in the immune system, CD4 lymphocytes and lymphokines are important in wound healing.[17] Fishel and associates[18] documented the migration, which peaks at 7 days, of CD lymphocyte subsets into healing wounds. Furthermore, Cyclosporine A, which impairs both cellular and humoral immunity, was shown to reduce wound tensile strength to a significant degree at ten days.[19]

The platelet deficiency associated with AIDS is thought in many cases to have an autoimmune basis. Immunodeficiency-associated thrombocytopenic purpura (IDTP) may be the result of an autoimmune globulin directed against platelet antigens similar to the IgG produced in idiopathic thrombocytopenic purpura.[20] It seems somewhat paradoxical that autoimmune afflictions should occur in individuals with reduced immunity but such reactions are common among AIDS patients. Neuropathy on the basis of autoimmune neuritis occurs in about one quarter of AIDS patients. Root-Bernstein[21] has proposed that this phenomenon is the result of multiple antigenic stimuli from heterologous blood products, semen, and a wide variety of infecting microbes. Autoimmune reactions can be produced in experimental animals by the injection of complex foreign antigens or homologous antigen, adjuvant mixtures. These adjuvant materials are usually derived from such bacteria as *Mycobacterium tuberculosis*, a common infecting organism in AIDS.

This platelet deficiency is treated initially with steroids and, if persistent, with splenectomy. The former further reduces host resistance to infection and the latter is associated with an increased risk of septicemia.[20,22]

Types and Prevalence of Bacterial Infection

As a result of this complex and widespread immune system impairment, HIV-positive patients have increased susceptibility to common orthopaedic pathogens as well as to opportunistic infections. Ganesh and associates[23] showed that the carriage rate for *Staphylococcus aureus* in nose, throat, and perineum was double for the asymptomatic HIV-positive individual (49%) compared to HIV-negative controls (27%). Krumholz and associates[24] reported 44 episodes of community-acquired bacteremia in 38 AIDS patients. These cases represented 5% of the AIDS admissions at San Francisco General Hospital. The most common organisms in order were *S aureus*, *Streptococcus pneumoniae*, and *Escherichia coli*.

The most common infections included pneumonia, central line phlebitis, cellulitis, and urinary tract infection. Only about one half (57%) of these patients were febrile, which is typical of the AIDS patient with a bacterial infection including pyarthrosis and other orthopaedic infections. These cases often present with a deceptively benign appearance.

Several groups have studied neutrophil bactericidal capacity in HIV-positive patients. This capacity is dependent on chemotaxis, phagocytosis, and secretion of oxygen dependent and independent microbicides. Using *S aureus* as the target organism, Murphy and associates[25] studied 90-minute bacterial survival in 19 AIDS patients who had no active infections and were on no drugs, and compared them to 17 healthy controls. In addition, they included four seronegative identical twins of four of the AIDS patients. Bacterial

survival in the study group was 32.5% compared to 13.8% in the controls which was highly significant. Reduced bacterial killing against *S aureus* was also demonstrated by Ellis and associates[14] in patients who had AIDS-related complex (ARC) and AIDS patients who had Kaposi's sarcoma. ARC was a term used to describe the HIV-positive patient with depressed CD4 cells and some manifestations of disease but not yet fulfilling the criteria for the diagnosis of AIDS. The recent change in the CDC definition of AIDS would include most of these patients, and the term ARC is no longer in use.[26] Ellis and associates[14] were also able to show that control patient leukocyte chemotaxis was inhibited by serum from the AIDS or ARC patients. Heat treating this serum, which inactivates HIV and certain proteins, reversed the inhibitory effect. Leukocyte phagocytosis was also significantly worse in the AIDS or ARC groups than in the controls. In summary, these two studies suggest impairment of all three leukocyte bactericidal functions, chemotaxis, phagocytosis, and secretion of microbicides.

Surgical Complications and Outcome

Impaired defenses to common surgical pathogens and delayed wound healing are causes for concern about the outcome of orthopaedic procedures on the HIV-positive patient. A moderate number of surgical outcome studies have been published that focus on early complications. The earlier studies involved general surgical procedures on the patient with advanced ARC or AIDS. Later studies included the asymptomatic HIV-positive group of patients. A few orthopaedic studies have also been published.

Robinson and associates[27] reported the outcome of 31 general surgical procedures performed on AIDS patients between 1982 and 1985. Most of the procedures were major, including thoracotomy, laparotomy, and craniotomy, and were performed on patients with advanced disease, including opportunistic infection and malignancy. The 30-day mortality rate for the 24 elective procedures was 43%; for the seven emergent procedures, it was 57%. The authors believed this very high postoperative mortality rate was the result of progression of opportunistic infection, Kaposi's sarcoma, or lymphoma.

A second study by the same authors involved 35 major abdominal procedures on AIDS patients from 1984 to 1988.[28] The 30-day mortality rate for the 22 elective procedures was 9% and for the 13 emergencies was 46%. The dramatic difference in the elective mortality rate between these two studies may reflect the improvement in management of opportunistic infections and preterminal AIDS.

Vipond and associates[29] reported the results of general surgical procedures on 47 HIV-positive and 100

AIDS patients performed between 1985 and 1990. Most of these operations were relatively minor, including anorectal operations, biopsies, and vascular access procedures. Postoperative complications included one death, 24 hours following laparotomy in an HIV-positive patient, 32 wound problems (22 HIV-positive and 10 AIDS), and 10 cases of sepsis (all in AIDS patients, mostly following insertion of vascular access devices). Delayed wound healing for anorectal procedures was about of equal incidence in the HIV-positive (13 of 54) and the AIDS (4 of 24) groups. Burke and associates[30] reported on 80 anorectal operations performed in 52 patients during the same years as the above study. The average time to wound healing in the HIV-positive group was seven weeks. In the patients with more advanced disease (CDC group IV) it was 12 weeks (p < .09).

Diettrich and associates[16] reported a series of 120 major surgical procedures performed between 1986 and 1990. Both elective and emergent groups were studied, and 48% of the procedures were on patients with AIDS. Results were divided into two groups, HIV-positive without AIDS and AIDS. The 30-day mortality for the emergent group was none of 24 in the HIV-positive patients and seven of 30 (23%) in the AIDS patients. For the elective group it was none of 40 in the HIV-positive patients and one of 26 (4%) in those with AIDS. Among the seven surviving cases with postoperative complications there was one wound infection and one delay in healing, both in the HIV-positive group. The risk of morbidity or mortality was higher if the patient had a history of opportunistic infection and a serum albumen level below 25 g/l. This study shows even further improvement in the outcome of general surgical procedures on AIDS patients with lengthened experience in managing this disease. The HIV-positive group had zero mortality and 4% postoperative complications, figures that are comparable to those seen in the HIV-negative population.

Hoekman and associates,[31] in a series from Kigali, Rwanda, compared the rate of postoperative infection after open reduction and internal fixation of fractures in 171 HIV-negative patients, 26 asymptomatic HIV-positive patients, and 17 symptomatic HIV-positive patients. The surgeons did not know the patients' HIV status, and no prophylactic antibiotics were used. The infection rates were 5% in the HIV-negative group, zero in the asymptomatic HIV-positive group, and 23% in the symptomatic HIV-positive group. As in the other studies discussed, the infecting organisms were common surgical pathogens: S aureus in eight, Group A Streptococcus in two, E coli in one, and Pseudomonas aeruginosa in one. All infections resolved with antibiotic management, and there were no deaths.

Buehrer and associates[1] studied wound infection rates in HIV-positive and negative hemophiliacs. A total of 169 procedures, 53 of which were orthopaedic, in 83 patients were reviewed. There were two wound infections but no statistically significant difference in the wound infection rate between the HIV-positive group (1.4%) and the HIV-negative group (0). There were no wound infections in the seven procedures performed on patients with AIDS.

Greene and associates[32] reviewed 26 orthopaedic procedures performed between 1984 and 1988 on HIV-positive hemophiliacs. There were no surgical site infections, but there was one IV-site cellulitis in a patient whose CD4 level was 174 at the time of surgery. Five patients had a protracted postoperative fever but did not develop clinical infection. The outcome or functional result was stated to be similar to the patients treated prior to 1982.

Teeny and associates[33] found the incidence of joint infections in hemophiliacs increased significantly after HIV-1 contamination of the blood pool. In the period between 1973 and 1980 there were three such infections in a stable population of 480 hemophiliacs that varies less than 6% per year. In the subsequent seven-year period, from 1981 to 1988, there were thirteen. In the group of hemophiliacs with a CD4 cell count of less than 250, the incidence of musculoskeletal infection was 11.0%, compared with an incidence of 1.1% in all other hemophiliacs at this center. Both of these differences were statistically significant. All of these infections involved either arthropathic or prosthetic joints. In the six prosthetic joints, the time from implantation to infection was six months to 15 years. In the HIV-positive patient with fewer than 250 CD4 cells, the infected joint appeared deceptively benign and fever was usually low grade or absent.

Effect of Surgery on Disease Progression

To date, there have been very few studies that address this issue, even indirectly. Disease progression of the patients in the surgical outcome studies quoted thus far does not seem to follow an accelerated course. The average CD4 count of the patients in the study by Greene and associates[32] dropped from 336 to 250 from 1984 to 1988, and six patients progressed to AIDS. This rate of disease progression is certainly not beyond the expected range in unoperated patients.

The study by Buehrer and associates[1] took place from 1979 to 1988. During that time 12 of the 43 HIV-positive patients progressed to AIDS. The first two were in 1985. There were two more in 1986, six in 1987, and two in the first third of 1988. This course also follows the usual rate of progression.

Vipond and associates[29] reviewed the literature on this question and suggested the need for a prospective study. The only prospective study of which I am aware that was designed to specifically address this issue was a pilot project by Hopkins and associates.[34] An abstract of this study was published in 1988. The investigators monitored CD lymphocyte subsets and other immune system markers in 15 hemophiliacs undergoing surgery. Patients were studied preoperatively and at two to three weeks and three to five months postoperatively. Average CD4 cell levels actually went up slightly, from 650 preoperatively (range 200 to 1,600) to 670 (with the identical range) at three months postoperatively. IgG also showed a slight rise. Mitogen stimulation, which is an indication of lymphocytic function, significantly improved during the same interval. Platelets remained the same. The white-blood-cell count dropped from 5,500 to 4,700.

It seems likely that the high 30-day mortality rates reported in the early general surgical series reflect the advanced stage of illness of the patients, all of whom had AIDS, and the very limited therapeutic options then available, rather than disease acceleration as a consequence of surgery. Certainly the stress of surgery is a significant factor in the pre-terminal patient, but that is a separate issue from disease progression in the asymptomatic or minimally symptomatic HIV-positive patient.

Recommendations

The clinical studies available to date do not demonstrate an increased incidence of early postoperative complications in the asymptomatic HIV-positive patients compared to the HIV-negative group. Furthermore, most of the orthopaedic studies and the more recent general surgery studies do not show a significantly increased incidence of early complications in the symptomatic HIV-positive patients. However, the basic science work establishes some impairment of defenses against common orthopaedic pathogens and of wound healing as well. As the disease progresses and these impairments increase, the hazard of such late complications as prosthetic implant infection, although not yet quantified, may be somewhat increased. In view of all these factors, special management of the HIV-positive patient undergoing surgery seems warranted.

If the procedure is elective, decision making about the advisability of surgery is crucial. Following a thorough assessment of the patient's medical status, a thoughtful discussion of the risk/benefit ratio should ensue. As in patients with cancer, quality rather than quantity of life is often a principal consideration in the patient's view.

The spectrum of disease in HIV infection is a continuum on which each patient must be positioned to properly assess risk. No single clinical factor is a reliable predictor of longevity or risk of surgery. Several components should be combined in determining a prognosis and assigning risk. The factors that seem to correlate most closely with outcome risk are: history of opportunistic infection, CD4 cell level less than 200, serum albumen less than 25 gm/l, and cutaneous anergy. Greene and associates[32] used four agents to assess anergy—tetanus, tricophyton, mumps, and Candida, which were used in the Walter Reed classification system.[35] More recently, Centers for Disease Control have recommended the use of only two of the delayed type hypersensitivity skin test antigens mentioned, preferably mumps and either Candida or tetanus.[36] Using this information it is possible to construct a surgical risk rating system. A sample system is presented in Table 1. As demonstrated in the articles reviewed, risk of postoperative complication does not correlate precisely with any of these factors, and such a rating system should be used as a general guide in the decision-making process, not as absolute criteria for surgical candidacy. However, the validity of such a system will increase as more data are collected and reported.

Preparation of the Surgical Patient

Once a decision is made to proceed with surgery, several steps can be taken to reduce the risk. Some measures are applicable to an emergent situation, but

Table 1
Surgical risk-rating system

Status	Points
CD4 cell level	
>500	0
200-500	1
<200	2
<100	3
Anergy	
1 test	1
2 tests	2
Platelets	
<60,000	1
Absolute PMNs	
<1000	1
Serum albumen	
<25 grams/liter	1
AIDS defining condition	
Opportunistic infection	1
Neoplasm	2

Risk of postoperative complication for orthopaedic procedures about same as general population, 0 points. Slight increased risk of postoperative complications, 1 point. Moderate increased risk of postoperative complications that may be acceptable for elective procedures if all appropriate measures are taken, 2 to 3 points. Higher risk of postoperative complications making these patients generally candidates only for emergent procedures, 4+ points.

others require more time and are only feasible in elective surgery. The absolute polymorphonuclear leukocyte count should exceed 1,000, and the platelet count should exceed 60,000. In patients for whom surgery is essential, granulocyte-stimulating factor is used to elevate an unacceptably low white-blood-cell count. Platelet transfusions also may be used when needed. If the patient has any treatable opportunistic infections, they are brought under control. Because of anergy, the patient with more advanced disease is at risk for active infection with common childhood viruses. The measles, mumps, and rubella vaccine should be updated two weeks preoperative. Many of the drugs used to suppress HIV and as prophylaxis against opportunistic infections cause various degrees of marrow suppression (Table 2). Furthermore, many symptomatic HIV-positive patients are chronically anemic. When clinically appropriate, these drugs should be stopped a few days preoperatively and resumed after the first postoperative week.

Clinical Examples

The following cases compare, side by side, clinical scenarios for which surgical options are commonly considered to analogous cases involving HIV-positive patients. This exercise should place in perspective the material thus far presented and assist the orthopaedic surgeon in developing guidelines for surgery in the HIV-positive patient.

Both patients A and B (Outlines 1 and 2) are possible candidates for total hip replacement based on their degree of symptomatology and joint destruction and both have higher than normal risk factors. Life expectancy is roughly equal or perhaps greater in case B due to improved ability to extend the disease-free interval by the use of antiviral drugs and opportunistic infection prophylaxis. It is probable that treatment will continue to improve and consequently so might longevity. Based on current knowledge and technology, it is unlikely that either would outlive their prosthesis with the possible exception of infection in Case B. The surgeon and patient must weigh the potential benefit of joint replacement against the unquantified risk of late infection. In my experience, late prosthetic infections in HIV-positive hemophiliacs occur in those patients who do not take good care of themselves in terms of regular medical visits and early treatment of potential foci of infection. Secondary prosthetic joint infections in both HIV-positive and negative hemophiliacs occurred at about the same rate and have followed untreated dental abscesses, sinusitis, dysentery, and pyarthrosis of unoperated joints.

If the patient in Case A (Outline 1) is mentally alert and would be capable of full community ambulation were it not for the arthritic hip, surgery seems a reasonable consideration. If the individual in Case B (Outline 2) is medically reliable, and sees his physician regularly, hip replacement would also seem appropriate.

Case C (Outline 3) is a tragic but not uncommon scenario. The usual approach is to offer the patient internal fixation of the fracture if life expectancy is beyond 6 to 12 weeks. Pathologic fractures tend to be very painful and are unlikely to heal without internal fixation. With internal fixation and, possibly, radio-

Table 2
AIDS medications that can cause marrow suppression

Generic Name	Brand Name	Usage
Zidovudine	Retrovir (AZT)	Anti-retroviral
Didanosine	Videx (DDI)	Anti-retroviral
Zalcitabine	Hivid (DDC)	Anti-retroviral
Acyclovir	Zovirax	Anti-viral (herpes)
Diaminodiphenyl-sulfone	Dapsone (DDS)	Dermatitis herpetiformis
Sulfadoxine and Pyrimethamine	Fansidar	Toxoplasmosis
Sulfamethoxazole	Bactrim/Septra	Pneumocystis prophylaxis
Interferon alfa	Intron A	Kaposi's sarcoma

Outline 1
Case A

84-year-old female HIV–

Advanced osteoarthritis of left hip
    Pain at rest
    Ambulates with cane

History of mental illness 5 years ago

```
Lab: WBC  = 3500
     PMNs = 2500
     Plat = 300,000
     Hct  = 34%
     Creat = 2.4
     Alb  = 32 g/l
```

Med: Lanoxin, lasix, KCl, colase, ibuprofen

Outline 2
Case B

48-year-old male HIV+

Osteonecrosis of left hip, advanced osteoarthritis
    Pain at rest
    Ambulates with cane

```
Lab: WBC  = 3500
     PMNs = 2500
     Plat = 90,000
     Hct  = 32%
     Creat = 350
     Alb  = 38 g/l
```

Med: AZT, steroids

therapy, this patient, assuming she has no other serious musculoskeletal impairments, should be able to resume ambulation and lead a reasonable existence for as long as her disease can be controlled.

Case D (Outline 4) may have a longer life expectancy than Case C. The median survival of AIDS patients after the first episode of Pneumocystis carinii pneumonia is currently 18 months. Due to the effect of his disease on healing and a poor nutritional status, his fracture may not heal without internal fixation. The risks of infection are real but, according to Hoekman and associates,[31] are manageable with antibiotics should it occur. Surgical site infection rates have been negligible to very low when prophylactic antibiotics were used.[1,32] Preoperative preparation would probably include platelet transfusion, because platelets are less than 60,000, and hyperalimentation, because the albumen level is borderline at 25 g/l.

Summary

Orthopaedic surgeons practicing in areas with high prevalence of HIV-infected individuals may anticipate that up to 10% of their emergent cases and a highly variable percentage of elective cases will be HIV-positive. Basic science studies have demonstrated impairment of defenses to routine orthopaedic pathogens as well as opportunistic organisms. Clinical studies show that this impairment has not resulted in an increased incidence of postoperative infections or failure of wound healing in the asymptomatic HIV-positive patient. Current medical management seems adequate to prevent increased risk of early postoperative infection in the symptomatic HIV-positive patient undergoing orthopaedic procedures.

The HIV-positive patient with a prosthetic implant may be at increased risk of late hematogenous implant infection as host defenses diminish. Regular medical attention, prophylactic antibiotics before dental work and any invasive procedures, and early evaluation and treatment of possible infections are especially important in this group.

Because the risk of surgical complications increases with progression of the disease, guidelines for elective surgery should include an assessment of the HIV-positive patient's immune status. The CD4 cell count, history of opportunistic infection, serum albumen, skin anergy, and state of nutrition and general health probably provide the best information regarding the risk of postoperative complications.

Based on current knowledge, orthopaedic surgeons should develop a general philosophy or guideline for elective and emergent surgery on the HIV-positive patient in various stages of disease.

Acknowledgements

The author wishes to thank Mark Begandy, MD, for his contributions to the section on preoperative preparation and Lawrence Logan, MD, for his assistance with the effect of surgery on disease progression.

Outline 3
Case C

33-year-old female HIV–

Fracture left femur (pathologic)
    transverse, midshaft

Metastatic adenocarcinoma

Lab: WBC = 4200
    PMNs = 3800
    Hct   = 32%
    Plat = 160,000
    Alb   = 30 g/l

Outline 4
Case D

28-year-old male HIV+

Fracture right femur
    transverse, midshaft

Hx Pneumocystis pneumonia

Lab: WBC = 2200
    PMNs = 1200
    Hct   = 28%
    Plat = 50,000
    CD4   = 180
    Alb   = 25 g/l

References

1. Buehrer JL, Weber DJ, Meyer AA, et al: Wound infection rates after invasive procedures in HIV-1 seropositive versus HIV-1 seronegative hemophiliacs. *Ann Surg* 1990;211:492-498.
2. Nugent P, O'Connell TX: The surgeon's role in treating acquired immunodeficiency syndrome. *Arch Surg* 1986;121:1117-1120.
3. Centers for Disease Control: Quarterly report to the Domestic Policy Council on the prevalence and rate of spread of HIV and AIDS. *MMWR* 1988;37:551-559.
4. Centers for Disease Control: Update: Acquired immunodeficiency syndrome - United States 1981-1990. *MMWR* 1991;40:358-363.
5. Kelen GD, Fritz S, Qaqish B, et al: Unrecognized human immunodeficiency virus infection in emergency department patients. *N Engl J Med* 1988;318:1645-1650.
6. Ward JW, Janssen RS, Jaffe HW: Recommendations for HIV testing services for inpatients and outpatients in acute-care hospital settings. *MMWR* 1993;42:1-6.
7. Charache P, Cameron JL, Maters AW, et al: Prevalence of infection with human immunodeficiency virus in elective surgery patients. *Ann Surg* 1991;214:562-568.
8. Kjaersgaard-Andersen P, Christiansen SE, Ingerslev J, et al: Total knee arthroplasty in classic hemophilia. *Clin Orthop* 1990;256:137-146.

9. Threats to health-care workers from human immuno-deficiency virus and hepatitis B, in Frymoyer J (ed): *Orthopaedic Knowledge Update 4.* Rosemont, IL, American Academy of Orthopaedic Surgeons, 1993, pp 164-165.

10. Marcus R: Surveillance of health care workers exposed to blood from patients infected with the human immunodeficiency virus. *N Engl J Med* 1988;319:1118-1123.

11. Tokars JI, Bell DM, Culver DH, et al: Percutaneous injuries during surgical procedures. *JAMA* 1992;267:2899-2904.

12. Benson D, Day L, Luck J, et al (eds): *Precautions for the Prevention of Transmission of Human Immunodeficiency Virus in the Practice of Orthopaedics.* Park Ridge, IL, American Academy of Orthopaedic Surgeons, 1989.

13. Grant IH, Armstrong D: Management of infectious complications in acquired immunodeficiency syndrome. *Am J Med* 1986;81:59-72.

14. Ellis M, Gupta S, Galant S, et al: Impaired neutrophil function in patients with AIDS or AIDS-related complex: A comprehensive evaluation. *J Infect Dis* 1988;158:1268-1276.

15. Burack JH, Mandel MS, Bizer LS: Emergency abdominal operations in the patient with acquired immunodeficiency syndrome. *Arch Surg* 1989;124:285-286.

16. Diettrich NA, Cacioppo JC, Kaplan G, et al: A growing spectrum of surgical disease in patients with human immunodeficiency virus/acquired immunodeficiency syndrome experience with 120 major cases. *Arch Surg* 1991;126:860-865.

17. Barbul A, Damewood RB, Wasserkrug HL, et al: Fluid and mononuclear cells from healing wounds inhibit thymocyte immune responsiveness. *J Surg Res* 1983;34:505-509.

18. Fishel RS, Barbul A, Beschorner WE, et al: Lymphocyte participation in wound healing: Morphologic assessment using monoclonal antibodies. *Ann Surg* 1987;206:25-29.

19. Fishel R, Barbul A, Wasserkrug HL, et al: Cyclosporine A impairs wound healing in rats. *J Surg Res* 1983;34:572-575.

20. Schneider PA, Abrams DI, Rayner AA, et al: Immunodeficiency-associated thrombocytopenic purpura (IDTP): Response to splenectomy. *Arch Surg* 1987;122:1175-1178.

21. Root-Bernstein RS: Multiple-antigen-mediated autoimmunity (MAMA) in AIDS: A possible model for postinfectious autoimmune complications. *Res Immunol* 1990;141:321-339.

22. Ravikumar TS, Allen JD, Bothe A Jr, et al: Splenectomy: The treatment of choice for human immunodeficiency virus related immune thrombocytopenia? *Arch Surg* 1989;124:625-628.

23. Ganesh R, Castle D, McGibbon D, et al: Staphylococcal carriage and HIV infection. *Lancet* 1989;2:558.

24. Krumholz HM, Sande MA, Lo B: Community-acquired bacteremia in patients with acquired immunodeficiency syndrome: Clinical presentation, bacteriology, and outcome. *Am J Med* 1989;86:776-779.

25. Murphy PM, Lane HC, Fauci AS: Impairment of neutrophil bactericidal capacity in patients with AIDS. *J Infect Dis* 1988;158:627-630.

26. Castro KG, Ward JW, Slutsker L: 1993 Revised classification system for HIV infection. *MMWR* 1993;41/RR-17:1-3.

27. Robinson G, Wilson SE, Williams RA: Surgery in patients with acquired immunodeficiency syndrome. *Arch Surg* 1987;122:170-175.

28. Wilson SE, Robinson G, Williams RA, et al: Acquired Immune Deficiency Syndrome (AIDS) indications for abdominal surgery, pathology, and outcome. *Ann Surg* 1989;210:428-434.

29. Vipond MN, Ralph DJ, Stotter AT: Surgery in HIV-positive and AIDS patients: Indications and outcome. *J R Coll Surg Edinb* 1991;36:254-258.

30. Burke EC, Orloff SL, Freise CE, et al: Wound healing after anorectal surgery in human immunodeficiency virus-infected patients. *Arch Surg* 1991;126:1267-1271.

31. Hoekman P, Van de Perre P, Nelissen J, et al: Increased frequency of infection after open reduction of fractures in patients who are seropositive for human immunodeficiency virus. *J Bone Joint Surg* 1991;73A:675-679.

32. Greene WB, DeGnore LT, White GC: Orthopaedic procedures and prognosis in hemophilic patients who are seropositive for human immunodeficiency virus. *J Bone Joint Surg* 1990;72A:2-11.

33. Teeny S, Luck JV Jr, Sanders N, et al: HIV and musculoskeletal infection in hemophiliacs, in preparation.

34. Hopkins J, Dietrich S, Boylen L: The effect of surgery on the immune status in HIV+ hemophiliacs. Von Crevald Symposium 1988.

35. Redfield RR, Wright DC, Tramont EC: The Walter Reed staging classification for HTLV-III/LAV infection. *N Engl J Med* 1986;314:131-132.

36. Hinman AR, Snider DE, O'Brien RJ: Anergy and HIV infection. *MMWR* 1991;40:27-32.

Tuberculosis in a Health Care Setting

Theodore Malinin, MD

Introduction

Even a brief glance at the history of tuberculosis, with its sociologic, medical and economic importance, would make the reader aware of the permanent imprint this disease has left on mankind. Tuberculosis is one of the few diseases that has made its way into the arts, both by claiming lives of such noted individuals as Frederic Chopin, Johann Friedrich von Schiller, and physician and writer Anton P. Chekhov and by afflicting the well-known fictional characters of Alexandre Dumas, Thomas Mann, A. J. Cronin, and others.

In the past, tuberculosis occupied an important position in orthopaedic surgery. Manifestations of skeletal tuberculosis were recognized by eponyms of Pott's disease, Jungling's disease, Poncet's disease, Rust's disease, etc. Some surgical procedures devised for the treatment of skeletal tuberculosis are still in use, the most notable of these being bone grafting.[1]

Tuberculosis is not a recent medical entity. Some of the earliest unearthed human skeletons appear to show evidence of tuberculosis of the spine. Accounts of pulmonary tuberculosis were given by Hippocrates. The Greek work *phthisis* (shrivel up and waste away) was used for centuries to describe the disease, and its English counterpart, *consumption*, was until recently a common term.

Tubercle, the principal anatomic lesion of the disease, and source of the word tuberculosis, was first described in 1804 by René Laënnec, the inventor of the stethoscope. His understanding of the disease process was based on clinical observations of hundreds of cases and on postmortem studies. Until the discovery of roentgen rays, his treatise on the auscultation of the chest (1819) was the foundation for the study of the chest disease for nearly a hundred years.[2]

The infectious nature of tuberculosis was demonstrated by Villemin in 1868, 14 years before isolation of the *Mycobacterium tuberculosis* by Robert Koch. Because the control of transmission of tuberculosis was largely a matter of preventing the dissemination of the disease among humans, restrictions were often placed on those who were ill. Isolation of contagious patients remained the cornerstone of tuberculosis control until the introduction of anti-tuberculosis chemotherapy shortly after World War II. In the United States, tuberculosis incidence was gradually reduced by streptomycin, isonicotinic acid hydrazide (isoniazid or INH),

para-aminosalicylic acid (PAS) and viomycin. Chemotherapeutic regimens, although prolonged, were so effective that the perception of public health threat from the disease virtually vanished. Tuberculosis sanatoriums were closed, but the disease itself was never eradicated. Recently, it manifested itself again as multiple drug resistant tuberculosis (MDR-TB).

Pathogenesis and Epidemiology of Tuberculosis

Tuberculosis is caused by the bacteria *Mycobacterium tuberculosis* and, rarely, by *Mycobacterium bovis* and *Mycobacterium africanus*. The *Mycobacterium avium* complex is associated with disease in patients with HIV infections. Tuberculosis is transmitted through the air from an infectious source to the susceptible individual. Most persons who become infected do not experience clinical illness. The only evidence of an infection may be a reaction to an intradermal injection of tuberculin. However, infection can persist for years, and the infected person may remain at risk of developing clinically apparent disease. A compromised immune system favors such a development.

It has been estimated that some 10 to 15 million Americans harbor latent tuberculosis infections. Some 90% of persons who develop clinically apparent disease have had tuberculosis for at least a year.[3] In the remainder, an acquired infection progresses without interruption.

When the tubercle bacilli gain entrance into a susceptible host, they produce either exudative or proliferative changes depending on the number of the microorganisms, their virulence, and the resistance of the host. These events culminate in the necrosis of normal pre-existing structures or of the exudative or proliferative processes. Proliferative changes follow exudation, and start with the appearance of mononuclear cells. Because these cells resemble cells of normal epithelium, they have been termed epithelioid cells. Epithelioid cells form nodules (tubercles), which grow by apposition of new epithelioid cells or by coalescing adjacent nodules. The epithelioid nodule is usually surrounded by a reactive zone composed of lymphocytes, plasma cells, and fibroblasts. In most individuals the initial (primary) infection is self-limited. The tubercles become walled off and eventually calcified. A similar process usually affects regional lymph nodes, which become infected very early. These, too, become calcified. The so-called primary complex, or Ghon complex, remains dormant, and serves only as an indication of a self-limiting infection. Virtually all individuals with a positive skin tuberculin test have a primary TB complex. However, the process of encapsulation and healing may be interrupted. The breaking up of young or inactive tubercles may delay healing and favor further dissemination of the tubercle bacilli. When infection is not arrested in the early stages, the bacilli multiply rapidly and either produce caseation, which later develops into cavities, or they seed the entire organism through a hematogenous route.

In the United States tuberculosis is not evenly distributed. A high incidence of tuberculosis has been recorded in blacks, in American Indians, and in Alaskan natives, and in individuals who have immigrated from geographic areas that have a high prevalence of the disease. Such behavior patterns as chronic alcohol abuse and intravenous use of recreational drugs also predispose to the disease. Tuberculosis is more prevalent in the elderly than in the younger age groups.

Despite various attempts to eradicate the disease, tuberculosis was still prevalent in the United States, even before the onset of MDR-TB among a large population of HIV-infected individuals. In 1988, 22,436 cases of tuberculosis were reported (9.1 per 100,000 population).[4] Tuberculosis mortality data indicate that, in 1987, 1,755 persons died from this preventable and curable disease. At that time, an occurrence of tuberculosis in HIV-infected individuals was already noted.[5] Therefore, the outbreaks of the MDR-TB in the same susceptible population should not have come altogether as a surprise. In 1991, 26,283 new cases (a 23% increase) of TB were reported to the Centers for Disease Control (CDC).

In 1989, CDC's Advisory Committee for the Elimination of Tuberculosis published "A Strategic Plan for the Elimination of Tuberculosis in the United States."[4] This plan established a goal of tuberculosis elimination by the year 2010, with an interim goal of a case rate of 3.5 per 100,000 population by the year 2000. Screening high-risk groups and providing appropriate treatment to the sick were crucial to the plan.[3] Persons infected with HIV, close contacts of persons known or suspected to have tuberculosis, and other high-risk groups of individuals were to be screened. Prophylactic therapy was expected to play an important role in eliminating tuberculosis in the United States. When taken as prescribed, isoniazid was said to be highly effective in preventing latent tuberculosis infections from progressing to clinically apparent disease. However, in practice, fewer than 60% of persons with newly identified risk for clinical infections were treated with isoniazid.[4] When treatment was instituted it reduced the incidence of disease progression by 54% in household contacts and by 88% in children with primary tuberculosis.[6] In addition, reports of adverse reactions to the drug and fatalities led to a call for monthly monitoring of patients taking isoniazid prophylactically.[7] Poor compliance was attributed to the side effects of the drug.[8]

Because the proportion of infected persons within the high-risk group is unknown, it is conceivable that a large number of infected individuals either were not treated at all or were inadequately treated. CDC's Advisory Committee for the Elimination of Tuberculosis (ACET) went on record stating that the percentage of infected persons each year who are screened and treated for tuberculosis must be increased substantially beyond 1% if the disease is to be eliminated by the year 2010. In the present circumstances, it is doubtful these goals can be met.

After a period of decreasing prevalence, tuberculosis has resurfaced as a significant public health problem.[9] Of particular importance was the appearance of multiple-drug resistant *Mycobacterium tuberculosis* strains and their impact on health-care workers.[10] "Multiple drug-resistant" is defined as resistance to two or more of the primary drugs used for the treatment of tuberculosis—isoniazid, rifampin, pyrazinamide, streptomycin and ethambutol. In a recent survey in New York City, 33% of tuberculosis cases were infected with organisms resistant to at least one drug, and 19% had organisms resistant to both isoniazid and rifampin. When organisms are resistant to both drugs, the cure rate decreases from about 95% to 60% or less.[11]

Airborne Transmission of Tuberculosis

Particles that carry tubercle bacilli are expelled by infected individuals when they cough or speak. These particles become aerosolized as droplets.[12] *Mycobacterium tuberculosis* bacilli are rod shaped and are from 0.5 to 4.0 µm long and 0.2 to 0.6 µm wide.[13] The droplets that contain the bacilli measure less than 100 µm in diameter and evaporate readily to form the so-called stable nuclei 1 to 4 µm in size.[11,14] Droplet nuclei can remain airborne for hours, causing those who breathe the contaminated air to become infected.[15] Inhaled droplet nuclei are small enough to reach alveoli of the lungs, where they initiate the infection.

Persons who share the same air with an infectious individual either because of proximity or through a common ventilation system are at the greatest risk of becoming infected.[16] Recently, CDC advised that "Any person who shared the air space with an MDR-TB patient for a relatively prolonged time (for example, household member, hospital roommate) is at higher risk for infection than those with a brief exposure to an MDR-TB patient, such as one-time hospital visitors. Exposure of any length in a small, enclosed, poorly ventilated area is more likely to result in transmission than exposure in a large, well-ventilated space. Exposure during cough-inducing procedures, such as bronchoscopy, endotracheal intubation, sputum induction, or administration of aerosol therapy greatly enhances TB transmission and is more likely to result in infection."[17]

Airborne transmission of tuberculosis has been studied exhaustively and is well documented. One study reports 27 new infections among 67 susceptible office workers who were exposed through air to an infectious office worker in the same building.[18] Rapid transmissions to health-care workers have also been reported under circumstances such as intubation and suctioning with mechanical ventilation, prolonged intubation, and open abscess irrigation.[11] Until recently, relatively little attention was paid to possible TB transmissions in hospitals. When these did occur they may have gone unnoticed, because transmissions did not usually produce large clusters of active TB cases. However, recent TB outbreaks have alerted public health officials to the problem. As a result, surveillance programs were instituted and recommendations for the prevention of transmission of tuberculosis in health-care facilities were made.

Although the exact time of exposure is difficult to determine with precision, active disease commonly develops within six months following infection. The infectiousness of a person with tuberculosis correlates with the number of organisms that are expelled into the air, which in turn correlates with the anatomic site of the disease process. Patients with immunosuppressed status are at a risk of not only acquiring the infection via inhalation of *Mycobacterium tuberculosis*, but also of reactivation of latent tuberculosis infections.

Tuberculosis in Patients with HIV Infections

Details of the first recognized nosocomial outbreak of tuberculosis among the HIV-infected patients in a single hospital were provided by Fischl and associates.[19] Successful control of a hospital outbreak of MDR-TB was described by investigators from the same institution.[20]

Public interest in the MDR-TB was stimulated by the 1991 CDC report on the results of the investigations of nosocomial transmissions of MDR-TB in four hospitals, one in Miami and three in New York City.[21] Similar outbreaks were reported in Puerto Rico,[22] Texas, California, and Pennsylvania.[23] The findings in this report documented the increased susceptibility of HIV-infected persons to life-threatening nosocomially transmitted TB. At the same time, the report underscored the importance of implementing infection-control precautions to prevent transmission of tuberculosis to patients and health-care workers. Although the investigation focused on MDR-TB, the CDC report also reem-

phasized the infectiousness of tuberculosis and, particularly, the susceptibility of HIV-infected patients to infection with *Mycobacterium tuberculosis*.

In the study of 83 patients with HIV infection cited in the preceding paragraph, 76 had a diagnosis of AIDS with advanced immunosuppression. At least two factors were thought to contribute to tuberculosis outbreaks. The diagnosis of TB was delayed because of the uncharacteristic features of clinical presentation and radiologic findings. Recognition of drug resistance was delayed by the time required for the laboratory to determine drug resistance. Thus drug therapy was adjusted empirically when a patient failed to respond to treatment and, as a result, many patients remained infectious for prolonged periods. Because of the prevailing feeling that the isolation of patients was not necessary, isolation procedures were not implemented on admission and readmission of symptomatic AIDS patients with tuberculosis. Because the HIV-infected patients were usually clustered, the spread of airborne infection was accentuated. These outbreaks again emphasized the need for health-care facilities to implement measures to prevent nosocomial transmission of TB.[21]

Further lessons were learned from a detailed analysis of individual hospital outbreaks. Studies documented the frequent occurrence of tuberculosis caused by multidrug-resistant *Mycobacterium tuberculosis* in patients with HIV infections. From the onset the abrupt, rapid increase in tuberculosis cases with resistance to two or more primary antituberculosis drugs suggested nosocomial transmission of the infectious agent. This notion was supported by a subsequent decline in new infections, which occurred in the same institutions after implementation of recommended infection control measures.[20]

Fischl and associates[19] explored factors associated with multiple drug resistance by comparing patients who had tuberculosis caused by single drug-resistant or susceptible bacilli with those whose disease was caused by multiple drug-resistant bacilli. Hospitalization on the HIV ward, clinic visits, intravenous treatments, and use of aerosolized pentamidine in the HIV clinic were associated with multiple drug-resistant organisms.

Recent Tuberculosis Outbreaks in Hospitals and Correctional Institutions

Concomitant with the increased incidence of tuberculosis among HIV-infected individuals, outbreaks of tuberculosis in hospitals and correctional facilities have been reported. Many of these were caused by multidrug-resistant strains. One epidemiologic study concluded that patients with MDR-TB posed a greater risk to health-care workers than did patients with drug-susceptible bacilli.[24]

From 1990 through the first part of 1992, the CDC investigated institutional outbreaks of tuberculosis in New York and Florida totaling over 200 cases.[21] Almost all patients were infected with organisms resistant to both isoniazid and rifampin. However, some were infected with organisms that were resistant to as many as seven antituberculosis drugs.[11,21] Most patients were also infected with HIV. In addition to hospitalized patients and individuals confined to correctional institutions, MDR-TB had also been transmitted to health-care workers and prison guards. At least nine have developed clinically active tuberculosis, and five have died. Of health-care workers who developed active tuberculosis, five were known to be infected with HIV.[21] Virtually all studies showed that the recent emergence of multiple-drug resistant strains of *Mycobacterium tuberculosis* occurred primarily among individuals with HIV infections,[19] which further emphasizes the need for implementation of tuberculosis control initiatives.[9]

Transmission of Tuberculosis to Health-Care Workers

The transmission of tuberculosis to health-care workers is a recognized risk of the medical profession.[25] However, despite the recent outbreaks of MDR-TB in institutional settings, the actual incidence of occupationally acquired tuberculosis remains ill defined. Pathologists have been traditionally singled out as a group most at risk of contracting tuberculosis in a workplace. Sugita and associates[26] reported that the incidence of pulmonary tuberculosis was significantly higher in pathologists than in other hospital employees, including physicians who treated patients with tuberculosis. However, observations by Ussery and associates[27] could document only a small number of tuberculin conversions in pathologists and morgue personnel who had performed autopsies in MDR-TB cases.

Although in the last two years several outbreaks of MDR-TB have occurred in health-care facilities, CDC documented only eight cases of occupationally acquired active tuberculosis among hospital personnel. As previously mentioned, five were infected with HIV. The remaining data on occupationally acquired tuberculosis in health-care workers are based on tuberculin skin tests. Pearson and associates[28] noted that in a New York City teaching hospital, health-care workers assigned to wards housing HIV-infected patients were more likely to have tuberculin skin test conversions than were the health-care workers on other wards.

At Jackson Memorial Hospital in 1989, 124 tuberculin skin test conversions were recorded among the employees, including the house staff. In 1992, after institution of controls to prevent nosocomial transmission of tuberculosis, there were only 22 conversions.

Of these, nine were classified as possible occupationally acquired infections. The employees who seroconverted for a tuberculin positive status worked in different parts of the hospital. None worked on HIV wards or other infection isolation facilities.

Prevention of Transmission of Tuberculosis

Emergence of MDR-TB and recognition of the danger of nosocomial transmission of the same, as well as the frequent association of infectious tuberculosis with HIV infections, were responsible for the formulation of guidelines for preventing transmission of tuberculosis in health-care facilities.[25] The guidelines stipulate: "The prevention of tuberculosis transmission in health-care settings requires that all of the following basic approaches be used: a) prevention of the generation of infectious airborne particles (droplet nuclei) by early identification and treatment of persons with tuberculous infection and active tuberculosis, b) prevention of the spread of infectious droplet nuclei into the general air circulation by applying source-control methods, c) reduction of the number of infectious droplet nuclei in air contaminated with them, and d) surveillance of health-care-facility personnel for tuberculosis and tuberculous infection. Experience has shown that when inadequate attention is given to any of these approaches, the probability of tuberculosis transmission is increased."

Specific actions to reduce the risk of tuberculosis transmission should include: (1) screening patients for active tuberculosis and tuberculous infection; (2) providing rapid diagnostic services; (3) prescribing appropriate curative and preventive therapy; (4) maintaining physical control measures to reduce microbial contamination of the air; (5) providing isolation rooms for persons with, or suspected of having, infectious tuberculosis; (6) screening health-care-facility personnel for tuberculosis; and (7) promptly investigating and controlling outbreaks. Although complete elimination of tuberculosis transmission in hospitals may be impossible, adherence to these guidelines should minimize the risk of infection.

The institution of these measures in our hospital resulted in a dramatic decline of nosocomial transmissions of TB.[20] In this instance, a total of 80 cases of MDR-TB were uncovered in a 44-month period ending in October 1991. After the outbreak was recognized, several measures were instituted to control the transmission of TB. Streptomycin and ethambutol were added to the therapeutic regimens of all HIV-positive patients with suspected TB. The number of patients who were maintained in isolation was increased. Respiratory isolation precautions were strictly enforced. Aerosol treatments were administered only in isolation rooms and Emerson chambers. Adequate numbers of isolation rooms with negative air pressure were constructed and were equipped with high-efficiency particulate air (HEPA) filters. In all high-risk areas, regular surgical masks were replaced with submicron molded masks. In the AIDS clinic and the emergency room, where negative pressure was not available, ultraviolet light fixtures were installed. For outpatient care, a separate TB respiratory clinic was established. Finally, and probably most importantly, respiratory isolation was implemented on all patients as soon as acid-fast bacteriology was requested (J. Otten, personal communication).

After these measures were implemented, no further nosocomial transmission of MDR-TB occurred. In retrospect, probably the most important factors in the curtailment of nosocomial transmission of MDR-TB were respiratory isolation, institution of adequate treatment, and changes in the criteria by which patients were placed in respiratory isolation. The most costly measures were the construction of isolation rooms and purchase of asepter 3M masks. In one year 427,497 of these masks were used, at a cost of almost $500,000.

Clearly an effective means of preventing outbreaks of occupationally acquired tuberculosis is the elimination of the threat of inhalation of infectious nuclei. Isolation facilities with negative pressure and HEPA filtration of contaminated air prevent dissemination of these particles through the buildings. However, health-care workers may be exposed to droplet nuclei from tuberculosis transmitters when infected patients make their first contacts with a health-care facility and its workers. In most cases, definitive states of these patients as potential tuberculosis transmitters are not known. However, high prevalence of MDR-TB in patients with HIV infections, in homeless persons, and in persons from high endemic areas should alert health-care workers to the possibilities of patients harboring tuberculosis. After patients with active TB are isolated, a certain number of health-care personnel inevitably come in contact with the patients to provide patient care. Moreover, patients with infectious tuberculosis must be transported from the isolation or emergency rooms for diagnostic procedures or for treatment. In each case health-care personnel may be exposed to aerosolized droplet nuclei. To prevent inhalation of infectious particles, health-care workers must rely on individual filtering devices. A simple technique of droplet containment is the placement of a surgical mask or a particulate respirator on the patient. Recommendation for patients to cover their mouth and nose with tissue while coughing or sneezing to allow for containment of drops or droplets before evaporation can occur is certainly not practical, bearing in mind the compliance and motivation requirements. Placing of face masks on the patient is practical only in limited circumstances, such as when being transported for diagnostic procedures or treatment. To be effective, masks or respirators must be worn at all times. Patients certainly cannot be expected to do that. Thus to avoid the risk of becoming infected, health-care workers must place barriers between themselves and the hazardous environment. This can be accomplished by wearing masks designed to exclude airborne infectious agents. Although conventional surgical masks protect the wearer from inhaling large particle droplet infectious nuclei, the inevitable filter and face seal leakages present a problem. Because surgical masks cannot be fitted to each wearer's face, leakage of 10% to 20% is possible. Filter leakage has also been reported to occur at 30 L/min. over the size range 1 to 5 µm aerodynamic diameter.[10] The alternatives to surgical masks are respirators, but most respirators do not offer 100% protection.

National Institute for Occupational Safety and Health (NIOSH) evaluated the efficacy and reliability of different types of respirators.[29] Negative pressure respirators have 99.97% filtering efficiency. Therefore NIOSH concluded that negative pressure, non-elastomeric cup-shaped, disposable particulate filter respirators cannot be relied upon to protect workers exposed to infectious tuberculosis. For hazardous locations, when confirmed or potential tuberculosis transmitters are present, NIOSH recommends the use of battery-powered industrial type NIOSH certified, positive pressure, air-line, half-mask respirators.[10] The response of health-care providers and physicians caring for patients with TB to this extreme recommendation was not warm. In the industry, these respirators are worn to prevent inhalation of fumes, gases, and vapors. "In TB droplet dissemination, the size of the droplet is many orders of magnitude larger than a gas molecule. That's the best reason to question the necessity of this recommendation."[30] In October, 1992, the CDC called a meeting on Tuberculosis Prevention in Health Care Facilities to assess the need to revise existing CDC guidelines.[25] A report is pending. In the interim, previously unfamiliar disposable particulate respirators (PR's) are making their way into hospitals. In high-risk areas, these respirators have replaced conventional surgical masks. There are several types of such respirators. Dust/mist respirators filter out particles from 0.4 to 0.7 µm. However, data regarding their efficiency vary, and the CDC notes that "the efficacy of PR's in protecting susceptible persons from infection with tuberculosis had not been demonstrated." High-efficiency particulate respirators, supplied with HEPA filters, provide a 99.7% efficiency at 0.3 µm. Disposable or reusable HEPA filter respirators do not exceed high-efficiency particulate respirators in their filtration efficiency.

Discussion

In the first half of this century, tuberculosis was common. There were no drugs. Patients with tuberculosis were confined to the sanatoriums, where they were treated with diet, rest, and good food. Later pneumothorax and lung surgery were used. Many physicians and nurses fell victim to the disease. In the pre-antituberculosis therapy era this meant confinement at the sanatorium for a year or two. When the disease was diagnosed in its early stages, the recovery rate was high, as was the return to the medical profession. In reviewing medical literature of the period one detects neither fear nor panic.

The doctors and nurses of the present generation entered the medical profession at a time when TB on medical wards was something of a rarity. They did not anticipate the return of a ghost of the previous era, but with the AIDS epidemic tuberculosis has re-emerged as a public health problem. This has stimulated concern, which is fully justified. However, uncontrolled fear of MDR-TB is another matter.

Recent outbreaks of MDR-TB, when viewed in perspective, are clearly linked to patients with HIV infections. However, tuberculosis is not the only infectious disease superimposed on immunodeficient persons. In addition to pulmonary infections with *Pneumocystis carinii*, in some geographic areas histoplasmosis presents a problem.[31] The incidence of hepatitis in HIV-infected individuals is also high.[32] Association of secondary infections with HIV-infected individuals has been noted almost from the beginning of the AIDS epidemic. Until the recent outbreaks of MDR-TB, little was done to apply to these patients public health measures proven effective in dealing with a variety of infectious diseases. Compassionate treatment of AIDS patients should not have precluded taking firm measures to halt its spread.[33] The proponents of the laissez faire attitude towards AIDS asserted that so-called punitive legal remedies have been the most ineffectual means by which to control the spread of infectious disease.[34] This is not entirely correct. Before the advent of effective antituberculosis chemotherapy, placing patients with tuberculosis in isolation facilities prevented the spread of the epidemic and offered the best means of treatment.[35,36] Isolation of patients with MDR-TB, followed by appropriate treatment, has also worked now and has prevented the rampant spread of MDR-TB through the hospitals. But it has been costly. A half a million dollar tab for particulate respirators in a single hospital is but a small example of another burden placed on society by the AIDS epidemic.

For an orthopaedic surgeon, outbreaks of MDR-TB and their effective curtailment by rational measures serve as a reminder that once the medical establishment recognizes the problem in which there are no unknowns and is willing to devote sufficient resources to its solution the solution can be found. MDR-TB today poses little threat to hospitalized patients and to health-care workers in the institutions where recommended procedures for containment of outbreaks of tuberculosis have been implemented and are being adhered to. However, the future is difficult to predict. Tuberculosis is not a new entity; its many clinical manifestations are well known. If the disease becomes more prevalent, patients with tuberculosis of the skeletal system will become more common. Treatment of these patients would present a challenge to present-day orthopaedic surgeons, as it did to their predecessors. In meeting this challenge, knowledge gained from the recent outbreaks of MDR-TB may be especially valuable.

Acknowledgment

The author wishes to express his gratitude to J. Maxwell McKenzie, MD, Chief, Medicine, and Ms. Joan Otten, RN, Tuberculosis Control, Jackson Memorial Hospital for the information and assistance kindly provided to him.

References

1. Albee FH: *Bone-Graft Surgery.* Philadelphia, PA, WB Saunders, 1915.
2. Collins HS: Tuberculosis, in *Encyclopedia Americana,* International ed. New York, NY, Americana Corp, 1964, pp 193-202.
3. CDC: Screening for tuberculosis and tuberculous infection in high risk populations and the use of preventive therapy for tuberculous infection in the United States. *MMWR* 1990;39/NoRR-8.
4. CDC: Update: Tuberculosis elimination, United States. *MMWR* 1990;39:153-156.
5. Bloch AB, Rieder HL, Kelly GD, et al: The epidemiology of tuberculosis in the United States. *Semin Respir Infect* 1989;4:157-170.
6. Comstock GW, Woolpert SF: Preventive therapy, in Kubica GP, Wayne LG (eds): *The Mycobacteria: A Sourcebook Part B.* New York, NY, Marcel Dekker, 1984, chap 44, pp 1071-1082.
7. Moulding TS, Redeker AG, Kanel GC: Twenty isoniazid-associated deaths in one state. *Am Rev Respir Dis* 1989;140:700-705.
8. Addington WW: Patient compliance: The most serious remaining problem in the control of tuberculosis in the United States. *Chest* 1979;76(6 suppl):741-743.
9. Hopewell PC: Impact of human immunodeficiency virus infection on the epidemiology, clinical features, management, and control of tuberculosis. *Clin Infect Dis* 1992;15:540-547.
10. Villarino ME, Dooley SW Jr, Geiter LJ, et al: Management of persons exposed to multidrug-resistant tuberculosis. *MMWR* 1992;41(NoRR11):58-71.
11. NIOSH Recommended guidelines for personal respiratory protection of workers in health care facilities potentially exposed to tuberculosis. Atlanta, GA, United States Department Health & Human Services PHS, CDC, 1992.
12. American Thoracic Society: Diagnostic standards and classification of tuberculosis. 1990;142:725-735.
13. Smith DT: Mycobacterium tuberculosis and tuberculosis, in

Joklik WK, Smith DT (eds): *Zinsser Microbiology*, ed 15. New York, NY, Appleton-Century-Crofts, 1972, chap 35, pp 454-469.

14. Riley RL, O'Grady F: *Airborne Infection Transmission and Control.* New York, NY, Macmillan, 1961.

15. CDC: National action plan to combat multidrug-resistant tuberculosis. *MMWR* 1992;41(RR-11):1-48.

16. CDC: Prevention and control of tuberculosis in facilities providing long-term care to the elderly: Recommendations of the Advisory Committee for Elimination of Tuberculosis. *MMWR* 1992;39(NoRR-10):7-20.

17. Harris HW, McClement JH: Pulmonary tuberculosis, in Hoeprich PD (ed): *Infectious Diseases: A Modern Treatise of Infectious Processes*, ed 3. Philadelphia, PA, Harper & Row, 1983, pp 378-404.

18. Nardell EA, Keegan J, Cheney SA, et al: Airborne infection theoretical limits of protection achievable by building ventilation. *Am Rev Respir Dis* 1991;144:302-306.

19. Fischl MA, Uttamchandani RB, Diakis GL, et al: An outbreak of tuberculosis caused by multiple-drug-resistant tubercle bacilli among patients with HIV infection. *Ann Intern Med* 1992;117:177-183.

20. Otten J, Chan J, Cleary T: Successful control of an outbreak of multidrug-resistant tuberculosis in an urban teaching hospital. Poster presentation, 32nd Interscience Conference on *Antimicrobial Agents and Chemotherapy*, Anaheim, CA, October 11-14, 1992.

21. CDC: Nosocomial transmission of multidrug-resistant tuberculosis among HIV-infected persons—Florida and New York, 1988-1991. *MMWR* 1991;40:585-591.

22. Dooley SW, Villarino ME, Lawrence M, et al: Nosocomial transmission of tuberculosis in a hospital unit for HIV-infected patients. *JAMA* 1992;267:2632-2634.

23. CDC: Outbreak of multidrug-resistant tuberculosis—Texas, California, and Pennsylvania. *MMWR* 1990;39:369-372.

24. Beck-Sague C, Dooley SW, Hutton D, et al: Hospital outbreak of multidrug-resistant Mycobacterium tuberculosis infections: Factors in transmission to staff and HIV-infected patients. *JAMA* 1992;268:1280-1286.

25. CDC: Guidelines for preventing the transmission of tuberculosis in health-care settings, with special focus on HIV-related issues. *MMWR* 1990;39(RR-17):1-29.

26. Sugita M, Tsutsumi Y, Suchi M, et al: High incidence of pulmonary tuberculosis in pathologists at Tokai University Hospital: An epidemiological study. *Tokai J Exp Clin Med* 1989;14:55-59.

27. Ussery XT, Bierman JA, Valway SE, et al: Transmission of multidrug-resistant Mycobacterium tuberculosis among persons exposed at a Medical Examiner's Office. 32nd Interscience Conference on *Antimicrobial Agents and Chemotherapy*, Anaheim, CA, October 11-14, 1992, p 203.

28. Pearson ML, Jereb JA, Frieden TR, et al: Nosocomial transmission of multidrug-resistant Mycobacterium tuberculosis: A risk to patients and health-care workers. *Ann Intern Med* 1992;117:191-196.

29. NIOSH 30 CFR Part 11, Respirator protective devices: Tests for permissibility fees. Code of Federal Regulations. United States Government Printing Office, Washington, DC, 1992.

30. Cugell D: In: R. Voelker. New guidelines prompt debate over TB control. *Am Med News* October 19, 1992.

31. Sarosi GA, Johnson PC: Disseminated histoplasmosis in patients infected with human immunodeficiency virus. *Clin Infect Dis* 1992:14(suppl 1):560-567.

32. Twu SJ, Detels R, Nelson K, et al: Relationship of hepatitis B virus infection to human immunodeficiency virus type 1 infection. *J Infect Dis* 1993;167:299-304.

33. Seale J: Kuru, AIDS and unfamiliar social behaviour. *J R Soc Med* 1989;82:571.

34. Cominos ED, Gottschang SK, Scrimshaw SC: Kuru, AIDS and unfamiliar social behaviour-biocultural considerations in the current epidemic: Discussion paper. *J R Soc Med* 1989;82:95-98.

35. Goldberg B: *Clinical Tuberculosis.* Philadelphia, PA, F.A. Davis Co, 1936.

36. Riley RL: Airborne infection. *Am J Med* 1974;57:466-475.

The Management of Fractures With Soft-Tissue Disruptions

Roy Sanders, MD

Marc F. Swiontkowski, MD

James A. Nunley, II, MD

Phillip G. Spiegel, MD

The purpose of this review is to maximize the reader's understanding of the management of fractures associated with soft-tissue disruption. Although open fractures occupy a predominant place in the subsequent discussion, closed fractures may also be associated with a severe crush component, a vascular lesion, a degloving injury, or a compartment syndrome. It is of paramount importance that the treating physician understand the implications of the potential or actual soft-tissue damage in order to render treatment that will lead to the best possible outcome after these devastating injuries.

Mechanism of Injury

The damage that is associated with a severe soft-tissue injury to an extremity is the result of a high-energy impact between an object and the limb. The amount of energy dissipated during this collision is determined by the equation, $E_k = mv^2/2$, where E_k is the kinetic energy, m is the mass, and v^2 represents the square of the speed.[1] Typically, a low-velocity injury, such as a fall onto the sidewalk, generates approximately 100 foot-pounds of energy, which is dissipated into the forearm. A high-velocity gunshot wound generates approximately 2,000 foot-pounds of energy, and an injury sustained by a pedestrian who is hit by a motor vehicle traveling at 20 miles (34 km) per hour results in the liberation of at least 100,000 foot-pounds of energy.[2] On contacting the object, the limb absorbs energy and then releases it in an explosion that comminutes bone and creates a soft-tissue shock wave. This shock wave strips the periosteum. If the shock wave is substantial, it will tear apart the skin, creating an open fracture as well as a momentary vacuum that sucks adjacent foreign material into the depths of the limb.[1] Therefore, the amount of deep-tissue contamination cannot be determined by the obvious dimensions of the wound. Additionally, loss of skeletal stability may cause stretching, tearing, or laceration of the neurovascular bundle with obvious sequelae, including compartment syndrome.[3-8]

In 1976, Gustilo and Anderson described a prognostic classification scheme for open fractures that was based on the size of the wound.[9] Type-I open fractures are associated with a 1 cm-long or shorter opening in the skin and with minimum stripping of soft tissue, and they are clean. Type-II injuries are associated with a laceration of more than 1 cm in length and with moderate soft-tissue damage. With type-III open fractures, there is extensive soft-tissue damage and crushing, and the injuries are caused by a high-velocity trauma. Gustilo and Anderson defined type-III open fractures as having the worst prognosis, with a high rate of infection, non-union, and secondary amputation. In 1984, Gustilo and associates[10] reported on a subclassification of type-III open fractures, which included type IIIA—adequate soft-tissue coverage of a fractured bone despite flaps or extensive laceration of the soft tissue; type IIIB—extensive soft-tissue injury with periosteal stripping and exposure of bone, usually associated with massive contamination; and type IIIC—an open fracture with an arterial injury requiring repair. This scheme has gained widespread support because it is of prognostic value.[4] Unfortunately, because the scheme is based on an assessment before debridement of a fractured limb with an associated open wound, many surgeons underestimate the severity of the injury, especially if the wound is small. With experience, surgeons have begun to understand that the prognosis for both the fracture and the limb depends more on the injury to the muscle, nerve, and bone in the depths of the wound than on the surface characteristics. Therefore, one should not make any projections regarding outcome until the first debridement has been completed.

Initial Assessment and Resuscitation

In the emergency room, the initial assessment of the entire patient is performed by the trauma team. First, the patient's airway is evaluated and, if necessary, adequate ventilation is established and cardiopulmonary resuscitation is begun. Radiographs of the chest and pelvis and lateral radiographs of the cervical spine are made. Large-bore intravenous access lines are placed; specimens are obtained for laboratory analysis; and, if the patient is hypotensive, fluid resuscitation is initiated and causes for bleeding are evaluated. If military antishock trousers (a MAST suit) were applied, they should be removed at this time, once the patient's blood pressure has been stabilized. This device prevents adequate examination of the extremity, causes limb ischemia and compartment syndromes, and ultimately may produce irreversible tissue necrosis.[11,12]

Once the patient has been stabilized, the pelvis and spine are examined and dressings and splints that were applied at the scene of the accident are gently and partially removed to expose the involved extremities. If active bleeding is present, a compression dressing should be placed. If this is insufficient, a tourniquet may be applied. Vessels should not be clamped, as this can damage the vessels or result in the inadvertent clamping of an adjacent nerve. If there are open fractures, and the patient has been resuscitated adequately, debridement and stabilization should be performed within six hours after the initial injury.[13,14]

The wound is initially assessed and graded according to the criteria of Gustilo and associates.[10,15] It is not irrigated or debrided and specimens are not obtained for culture at this time, as the emergency room is often the most contaminated part of the hospital.[13] Furthermore, adequate treatment cannot be performed without the proper lighting and equipment found only in the operating room. Attainment of a specimen in the emergency room will result in the isolation of only superficial contaminants on culture, and there is a risk of inoculation of deeper tissues with nosocomial organisms.[8,16,17] Finally, removal of culture specimens from the deep tissues may break off clots and cause additional bleeding.

Any obvious joint dislocations or prominent bone fragments causing undue pressure on the soft tissues or neurovascular structures should be reduced.[8] A clinical examination to determine pulses is performed before this is done. If pulses are absent because the displacement resulted in kinking and decreased pulse pressures in an otherwise normal vessel, a reduction may restore blood flow. The benefits of restoration of arterial blood flow after reduction far outweigh the alternatives, which are to leave the contaminated bones displaced or the joints dislocated out of a fear that foreign material will be introduced into the depths of the wound, because the joint or fracture will be subsequently redislocated in the operating room during debridement.

After reduction maneuvers have been carried out, the pulses are rechecked. If palpable pulses were lost or are still not present after these maneuvers, a Doppler examination is required.[18] If pulses are heard or felt, the vascular status of the limb is carefully observed over time. It must be remembered that the restoration of blood flow does not absolve the surgeon of the responsibility to evaluate the vascular tree by other diagnostic methods, as intimal damage often occurs in association with these injuries, creating a delayed vascular occlusion. Angiography should therefore be performed in the radiology suite after the assessment of the patient has been completed. If pulses are still absent after Doppler examination, the vascular status must be evaluated with angiography or direct exploration.[19,20] Although an angiogram may be made in the radiology suite, this often delays definitive treatment because of excessive transport times and delays in procedural set-up. Direct exploration seems to be the most logical and efficient manner of proceeding, as there is little question about the zone of injury. This examination should be performed by a surgeon with experience in this field—for example, a vascular surgeon. Overall assessment of the patient in the emergency room should therefore be curtailed, and transfer to the operating theater should be expedited in coordination with the trauma team. The trauma team will complete the assessment of the patient in the operating room.

With resuscitation of a hypotensive patient, increased blood pressure may lead to increased tissue pressures in traumatized limbs, resulting in compartment syndromes. In a polytraumatized patient, parameters such as pain may be impossible to assess because the patient has been sedated or has lost consciousness. Measurements of compartment pressure in the forearm, tibia, and foot have become increasingly critical, especially in these patients.[3,21-23]

Unfortunately, published criteria for fasciotomy vary depending on the method employed and the patient's diastolic pressure. The older method of continuous infusion monitoring is somewhat cumbersome in a polytraumatized patient. Matsen and associates[23] suggested that, if this system is being used, fasciotomy should be done when the tissue pressure rises to more than 45 mm Hg (6 kPa). More recently, self-contained needle-manometer systems have become popular. Whitesides and associates[24] recommended that, when these devices are used, fasciotomy should be performed when the compartment pressure rises to within 10 to 30 mm Hg (1.3 to 4 kPa) of the patient's diastolic pressure. Thus, many authors have recommended decompression in comatose or hypotensive patients when the compartment pressure exceeds 30 to 35 mm Hg (4 to 4.6 kPa). Because disagreement remains about the correct pressure at which a fasciotomy should be performed, the surgeon must maintain a high index of suspicion and perform fasciotomies as necessary in the operating room during the debridement phase. It is better to err on the side of performing an unneeded fasciotomy than to not do a needed fasciotomy.

After the initial assessment in the emergency room, a sterile dressing is applied to the wound and a splint is applied to the limb. The extent of the wound is drawn in the medical record or a photograph is made, or

Table 1
Guide to tetanus prophylaxis[55]

History of Tetanus Immunization (Doses)	Clean Minor Wounds		All Other Wounds	
	Tetanus/Diphtheria Toxoids	Tetanus Immunoglobulin	Tetanus/Diphtheria Toxoid	Tetanus Immunoglobulin
Uncertain or <2	Yes	No	Yes	Yes
2	Yes	No	Yes	No*
≥3	Not†	No	Not‡	No

* Yes if the wound is more than twenty-four hours old.
† Yes if it was more than ten years since the last dose.
‡ Yes if it was more than five years since the last dose.

both. The dressings are not removed until the patient is in the sterile environment of the operating room.[8] The remainder of the orthopaedic examination is completed, with the examiner noting any areas of pain (if the patient is alert), any obvious deformities, or any lacerations or bruises. Approximately 25% of skeletal injuries are missed in the patient with multiple trauma. These injuries are often in the hand and foot, and these areas should be evaluated carefully.[25] If the patient is stable and there are no vascular injuries, a radiographic examination of all known and suspected injury sites is performed at this time.

It must be remembered that all open fractures are contaminated and that an infection will develop unless necrotic tissue is debrided adequately. *Clostridium tetani*, an anaerobic gram-positive rod, is found in soil, dust, and animal feces. Because it produces a potentially fatal neurotoxin, patients must be given prophylaxis against tetanus[26] (Table 1). Therapeutic antibiotics are also begun at this time.[7,15,17,27] Generally, for low-energy injuries (Gustilo[10,15] types I and II [closed fractures with injury to soft tissues]), a broad-spectrum cephalosporin (Ancef [cefazolin]; loading dose, 1 to 2 g, followed by 1 g every eight hours) is adequate. With increasing wound severity (Gustilo types IIIA, IIIB, and IIIC), an aminoglycoside (gentamicin; loading dose, 1.5 to 2.0 mg per kg, followed by 1 mg per kg every eight hours) may be added. *Clostridium perfringens*, an anaerobic gram-positive bacterium, releases several exotoxins that result in rapid myonecrosis, vessel thrombosis, and, if inadequately treated, rapid death.[28] If the injury is farm or soil-related or has a severe crush component, or if vascular compromise is present, penicillin G (two to four million units given intravenously every four to six hours) must be added as a third antibiotic.

Initial Debridement and Bone Stabilization

Before the patient arrives at the operating room, a preoperative plan should be formulated in coopera-

tion with the trauma team. If the patient has multiple injuries, several procedures will have to be staged or performed simultaneously, often by multiple teams. Patients may require the insertion of an intracranial pressure-transducer, so that intracranial pressure can be monitored, before a long procedure is undertaken. Equipment needs, such as a fracture-table, special instruments, and implants, must be available, and operative strategies must be preplanned to minimize operative time. These initial procedures, performed in a timely manner, are, without doubt, among the most important determinants of the outcome of treatment of a fracture that is associated with serious soft-tissue disruption. Rather than these tasks being relegated to a junior member of the team, the surgeon with the most experience should be present, even if the procedure is done in the middle of the night. Similarly, the surgeon may wish to transfer a patient with a complex injury to a regional trauma center, where the staff has more experience and may be in a better position to manage the patient over the entire course of treatment.

After induction of anesthesia and as soon as the trauma team permits, preparations are made for irrigation, debridement, and stabilization of the extremity in the operating room. All splints and dressings are removed, and final evaluations are made. If previous radiographs of periarticular fractures are less than ideal, traction radiographs are now obtained. Tourniquets are placed, if possible, but they are not inflated unless there is severe bleeding. If a vascular injury is suspected, an angiogram is obtained at this time. Gross debris is removed and the limb is prepared and sterilely draped. If the angiogram reveals an arterial injury, then direct exploration is required, and the vascular and orthopaedic surgeons must decide on the most appropriate treatment sequence. Direct arterial repair is rarely performed before the fracture has been stabilized because attempts at fracture reduction may disrupt the repair. Usually, there is enough time for the orthopaedist to first irrigate, debride, and provisionally stabilize the extremity with a simple fixator. If the vascular surgeon feels that distal flow must be restored immediately, a Javid shunt can be used to reperfuse the limb distal to the arterial lesion.[29,30] Care must be taken to avoid further intimal damage from the shunt.

Gustilo[13] stated that adequate debridement (the removal of unhealthy tissue) is the single most important factor in the attainment of a good result after the treatment of an open fracture. Unfortunately, although this principle is emphasized in books and taught in lectures, experience is required to accomplish this correctly. Failure to adhere to the basic principle will place the patient at an increased risk for infection and its sequelae. Debridement begins with excision of the wound edges. As mentioned earlier, the shock wave creates severe stripping of soft tissue, followed by a momentary vacuum, which sucks debris into the limb. It is not unusual to find a wound of modest size concealing a completely degloved bone with particulate material embedded deep within it. Because the zone of injury cannot be determined by casual inspection, the wound must be enlarged through an extensile incision to preserve skin viability and allow for subsequent skeletal stabilization.[31] Once exposed, the limb is irrigated with a minimum of 9 l of isotonic saline solution delivered through a pulsed lavage system. Antibiotics (50,000 units of bacitracin per liter of irrigating solution) may be added to the middle 3 l of solution, because experimental evidence indicates that doing so lowers infection rates.[32]

As debris and clot are washed away, the specific characteristics or so-called personality of the injury becomes apparent. A systematic debridement is now performed. All necrotic skin, fascia, and tendon are excised. Muscle is evaluated on the basis of the four C's: contractility, color, consistency, and capacity to bleed.[13] The most common error made at the time of the initial debridement is underestimation of the amount of muscle damage.[33] Contractility is best tested by the surgeon squeezing the muscle belly with a pair of forceps or touching it lightly with a cautery tip. Muscle that does not contract, disintegrates to touch, is pale or discolored, or fails to bleed when cut must be excised. Not infrequently, entire muscle bellies have to be removed. Care must be taken throughout the debridement procedure to protect the neurovascular structures. If it had been previously determined that a fasciotomy was needed, it should be performed at this time. Specimens for culture are no longer routinely obtained in the operating room. In the past, this was thought to be the best time to obtain a specimen for culture from a patient who had an open fracture, but Lee and associates[34] showed that there is very little correlation between the findings on these cultures and the actual infecting organism. Should the signs and symptoms of an infection appear later, cultures at that time will be extremely specific and cost-effective.

Finally, the bone must be carefully evaluated.[35] The ends of the principal fragments must be washed and cleaned of debris. Free-floating cortical fragments represent potential sequestra and should be removed. If large, these fragments are kept sterile on the back table and are used to estimate limb length and alignment during the bone stabilization process, but they are rarely, if ever, permanently replaced. Bone fragments that have reasonable soft-tissue attachments should be maintained. Large osteochondral fragments that are important for joint congruence and alignment are preserved if at all possible. Although some authors[1,13] have recommended complete redraping and use of a clean set of instruments after debridement, there are insufficient data to substantiate that this practice actually makes a difference.

Once irrigation and debridement has been completed, the bone is stabilized. Stabilization of the fracture also stabilizes the soft tissues. Immobilization of the bone in its anatomic position restores alignment to the neurovascular and muscular structures. When this has been done, inflammatory responses are decreased, venous return is improved, local neovascularization is enhanced, and further soft-tissue and neurovascular damage from excessive motion is prevented. Stable fixation of the fracture decreases dead space and minimizes problems such as pain, edema, stiffness, and osteopenia.[36] Finally, fixation of the fracture permits mobilization of the patient.[37-39] The absence of motion at the fracture site minimizes pain, and elimination of the need for skeletal traction minimizes respiratory complications and difficulties with regard to nursing care. Stable fixation also permits easier transport of the patient and facilitates access to the wound during subsequent procedures.

Although the exact methods of skeletal stabilization are complex, the basic principles should be understood. It is important to know which bone is injured, what parts of the bone are involved, the true extent of the soft-tissue damage, and what associated medical problems exist (for example, multiple trauma or diabetes). These facts must be integrated into a cohesive plan of action. It must be reiterated that this can be done only after the specific characteristics of the wound have been accurately determined after the initial debridement.

Three broad categories of skeletal fixation are available to the orthopaedic surgeon: intramedullary nails, which may be locked in place; plates and screws; and external fixation.[40-52] Each method can be adapted to the individual injury. Intramedullary nails act as internal splints and are an optimum mechanical means of fixation for diaphyseal fractures of long bones. Because axial alignment is all that is required, exact repositioning of individual fragments is unnecessary.

Recently, the addition of interlocking has extended the indications for nailing to include all but the most proximal and distal portions of the long bones. Articular fractures, in contrast, require exact anatomic restoration and are best treated with lag screws. Plates or external fixators are then added in an attempt to neutralize forces across the joint. Metaphyseal and periarticular fractures fall into a gray zone and may be treated with either plates and screws or intramedullary nails, depending on the preference of the treating surgeon. External fixation is biomechanically less stable compared with either of these methods and is primarily used for injuries with severe soft-tissue damage. In this respect, external fixation should be thought of as a self-contained traction device, which usually is applied for temporary skeletal or joint stabilization. However, some trauma centers continue to employ external fixation as the definitive method of treatment for selected fractures.

The extent of the wound and its location must be considered in the decision-making process. In general, low-velocity type-I injuries can be treated as closed fractures, but wounds caused by higher-velocity impacts require a more specifically detailed analysis.[13,53] Type-II and type-IIIA open fractures are associated with more stripping of soft tissue. Open reduction and application of a plate, if not performed with the use of indirect reduction, result in further soft-tissue stripping and bone devitalization.[54] Both of these techniques, then, increase the risk of infection. If the fracture is in a well-vascularized bone, such as the femur or humerus, these concerns are minimum. If a similar injury occurs in the tibia, concerns about further devitalization are credible, and rods that require reaming of the bone and plates are contraindicated. Type-IIIB injuries are associated with such major destruction of soft tissue that, even in well-vascularized bones, initial placement of an external fixator should be considered. Finally, open and degloved fracture-dislocations may be fixed with internal lag screws and external fixation, placed away from the site of the injury, to stabilize the wound and the joints in an effort to minimize soft-tissue compromise.

After stabilization has been completed, osseous defects may be filled with antibiotic-impregnated methylmethacrylate beads. These are made by the mixing of 1.2 to 2.4 g of tobramycin or 1 to 2 g of vancomycin, or both, with one 40-g package of methylmethacrylate. The antibiotic-impregnated methylmethacrylate is formed into beads, which are pressed onto a braided 26-gauge wire and allowed to harden. These beads provide a local depot administration of antibiotic and maintain a space for subsequent bone graft.[35,55] All wounds, including those created by fasciotomies, should be left open. Surgical incisions may be sutured closed if doing so does not produce undue

tension at the skin edge. Exposed tendons, joints, and bone should be covered with adjacent soft tissue to prevent desiccation. Temporary coverage of exposed tissue was often obtained in the past by placement of sterile dressing sponges soaked in isotonic saline solution over the wound, but this leads to wound desiccation. Other alternatives, such as pigskin, Epigard (Synthes USA, Paoli, Pennsylvania), or another synthetic biologic dressing may be used. This dressing is applied in a manner similar to skin-grafting: it is stapled to the wound edges and then covered with sterile dressings. It is left in place until the next debridement, obviating the need for painful dressing changes in the patient's room and minimizing the risk of contamination with nosocomial organisms. In the past, broad-spectrum antibiotics were given for three to five days.[7,13] However, in many patients, infections developed from resistant organisms, so now a shorter course of therapy (24 to 48 hours) appears to be indicated. Antibiotics, in the form of a single dose given 20 minutes before the incision is made, are used prophylactically during all subsequent operative procedures.

After successful debridement and stabilization of the limb, the patient requires repeated debridements at intervals of 24 to 48 hours, until no necrotic tissue remains. Once the soft-tissue wound is clean, closure within five to seven days after the injury is ideal.[4,8,27,56-58] This can be accomplished with delayed primary closure, split-thickness skin-grafting, local flaps, or vascularized free tissue transfer (most commonly with the latissimus dorsi or serratus anterior muscles). If this treatment is successful, the surgeon has transformed a massively contaminated, open fracture into a clean, closed fracture that requires only bone and joint reconstruction.

The most frequent method for restoration of moderate diaphyseal bone loss (1 to 3 inches [2.5 to 7.6 cm]) is through the use of cancellous iliac-crest bone as a graft.[9,35,59,60] Because most open wounds of the tibia are anteromedial, a posterolateral bone graft placed away from the area of the damaged soft tissue is ideal. This technique, popularized by Harmon,[59] allows union by bridging between the fibula and the remaining part of the tibia. If the fibula is fractured at the same level as the tibia, reduction of the fibula and internal fixation should be performed.[61] Grafting at the time of wound closure is not recommended, because this increases the possibility that the graft will dissolve or become secondarily infected.[13] Rather, posterolateral grafting is recommended at approximately four weeks after wound closure. If flap coverage is required, bone-grafting is delayed until the flap has stabilized, generally six to eight weeks later. The graft may take three to six months to consolidate sufficiently to permit weightbearing. Multiple grafting procedures may be needed if the graft appears inadequate or slow to mature. If a defect is larger than 3 inches (7.6 cm), the surgeon should consider newer alternative techniques, such as free fibular transfer or the Ilizarov method.[58,62,63]

Rehabilitation to regain motion and strength should begin during the hospital stay; weightbearing, however, is delayed until the fracture has united solidly. Realistically, the patient should understand from the outset that the entire process until maximum function is restored will take a minimum of six months if the injuries were simple and as long as two years if they were complex.

Decision-Making with Respect to the Lower Extremity

Skeletal Stabilization of Open Fractures of the Femur

Although an open fracture of the femur poses fewer management problems to the surgeon than other open fractures do, primarily because of the excellent muscle coverage and blood supply of the femur, one should remember that tremendous force is required to break the femur. In the patient with multiple trauma, immediate stabilization of the femur is ideal. When a patient presents with an isolated open fracture of the femur, it is also best to irrigate, debride, and fix the fracture as soon as possible, as irrigation and debridement followed by skeletal traction for several days increase the risk of infection and can result in respiratory complications and difficulties with respect to nursing care.

For type-I, II, and IIIA open fractures, the choice of fixation technique is not affected by the characteristics of the wound.[64-66] Intertrochanteric fractures are best treated with a sliding hip screw. Subtrochanteric fractures may be treated similarly, or interlocking intramedullary or reconstruction nailing can be used. Shaft fractures should be fixed with interlocking intramedullary nailing, with the use of intramedullary reaming of the bone for insertion of the nails, as several authors[63,64] have shown that this technique does not increase the risk of infection. Distal femur fractures may be treated with either interlocking intramedullary nailing (with the use of intramedullary reaming techniques for insertion) or plates and screws, depending on the fracture configuration and the surgeon's preference. Type-IIIB fractures of the femur represent a combination of massive contamination and a high-energy injury, and they are best stabilized with an external fixator until the specific characteristics of the fracture are determined.[66] Usually, a definitive procedure can be carried out seven to ten days after the injury. Type-IIIC fractures should be treated temporarily with external fixation, which requires less operative time and results in less soft-tissue destruction; however, a plate can be applied if the surgeon is comfortable

with this technique. Definitive stabilization is performed when the condition of the wound and the patient permits.

Skeletal Stabilization of Open Fractures of the Tibial Shaft

Because of its tenuous vascular supply and poor soft-tissue coverage, the open fracture of the tibial shaft remains a dilemma to even the most experienced surgeon. Conventional methods of treatment, such as the application of plates and screws and insertion of a rod with the use of intramedullary reaming, are associated with a high rate of infection in patients who have an open fracture. Bach and Hansen[40] randomly assigned 59 Gustilo type-II and III open tibial fractures to two treatment groups—application of a plate or external fixation—and found that the prevalence of infection after plate fixation was 35% compared with 13% after external fixation. This was a significant difference (p<0.05), and the findings were similar to those of Burwell[42] and those of Spiegel and VanderSchilden.[49] Because Bach and Hansen noted acceptable anatomic results in the group treated with external fixation, they concluded that this is the better treatment option for osseous stabilization of open fractures of the tibial shaft. Similarly, several authors have shown that interlocking intramedullary nailing with intramedullary reaming is associated with infection rates as high as 33% when used for the treatment of these fractures.[4,43,68] In these series also, infection rates were markedly lower when external fixation had been employed.

External fixation has, therefore, emerged as the safest method for initial skeletal stabilization of open fractures of the tibial shaft because it protects the remaining blood supply, stabilizes the bone, and allows easy access for wound care with a lower rate of infection than associated with other modalities.[15,40,44,50,68-70] However, external fixation is associated with its own set of complications, including non-union, malunion, pin-loosening, and pin-track infections.[71] A solution to these problems was thought to be the later insertion of an interlocking intramedullary nail with intramedullary reaming for insertion of the nail, but early exchange nailing (within the first three weeks) has been associated with infection rates as high as 44%.[41,47,72,73] As a result, only delayed secondary exchange nailing has been advocated, and this must be done in the uninfected, nutritionally balanced patient. These contraindications severely limit the number of cases that can be converted.

Klein and associates[74] showed experimentally that use of an intramedullary nail without reaming decreased cortical bone blood flow only by an average of 31%. Until very recently, there were only two types of nails that could be used without reaming: the Lottes nail and the flexible nails of Ender.[45,52,75,76] Because the nails were inserted without reaming, it was necessary to use a small-diameter nail to pass across the tibial isthmus. The use of these two nails for the treatment of injuries with unstable fracture patterns was limited, as neither nail could be locked. In 1983, Velazco and associates[51] reported on the use of Lottes nails for the treatment of open fractures of the tibia. Union occurred in 98% of the fractures in their study, with only two superficial and one deep infection. There were only two malunions, although 41 of the fractures were associated with shortening of as much as 1 cm. Holbrook and associates[45] prospectively evaluated 60 open fractures of the tibial shaft that had been randomly assigned to treatment with either Ender nailing or external fixation. With the numbers available, no difference in healing time was found when the fractures were subdivided by Gustilo type. Again, there were more malunions, non-unions, and secondary procedures in the external fixation group. The infection rate was two of 29 in the Ender-nailing group, compared with four deep, one superficial, and six pin-track infections in the 28 patients in the external fixation group.

These studies suggested that nails inserted without reaming have several advantages over plates, intramedullary nails inserted with reaming, and external fixation. The principal disadvantage of the technique is that the ability to control axial rotation of the fracture is limited. In 1991, Howey and associates[46] reported on the use of the technique of Brooker for interlocking intramedullary tibial nailing without reaming for the treatment of both open and closed fractures of the tibial shaft. The advantages of this nail included both insertion without reaming and the possibility of static locking for fracture stabilization. In this series, 35 of 76 fractures were open; these included nine Gustilo type-IIIA, two type-IIIB, and two type-IIIC fractures. A follow-up examination was possible for 77% of the fractures, and it showed a union rate of 93%, an infection rate of 7%, and no malunions.

Whittle and associates[77] followed, for an average of 12 months, 50 open fractures of the tibial shaft that had been treated with nailing without reaming. Type-IIIC injuries were excluded. Of the 50 fractures, 68% were type-IIIA or IIIB injuries. Within seven months, 96% had united; there were no malunions. The overall infection rate was 8%, with all infections occurring at the sites of type-III fractures. Within this group, the rate of infection was 4.5% for type IIIA and 25% for type IIIB. Similarly, in another study, 46 open fractures of the tibial shaft (excluding type IIIC) that had been treated with interlocking intramedullary nailing without reaming were followed for an average of two years. Of those fractures, 55% were type-IIIA or IIIB injuries. Although all but one fracture went on to uneventful healing, 20 exhibited a delay in healing of more than

six months. This appeared to be related to the amount of soft-tissue stripping and nail stiffness. Clinically, all patients had a full range of motion of the knee and ankle unless these joints had also been injured. The patients complained of only occasional pain. Overall, the rate of chronic infection was 4%, with no chronic infections in association with type-I, II, or IIIA open fractures and a 13% rate in association with type-IIIB open fractures. There were no malunions.

On the basis of these recent reports, it appears that interlocking intramedullary nailing without reaming permits excellent union and osseous alignment, with minimum infection rates, and that it is the superior initial technique for osseous stabilization of type-I, II, and IIIA open fractures of the tibial shaft. Although the procedure can be used for the treatment of type-IIIB fractures, a higher rate of infection should be expected. This may be due to the injury and not the implant, but additional data are needed before this question can be answered. Because of the time constraints created by the need to restore blood flow in the management of type-IIIC fractures, intramedullary nailing without reaming may not be possible for the treatment of these injuries. Thus, external fixation may be preferable for both type-IIIB and type-IIIC tibial fractures. It must be reiterated, however, that meticulous wound care is the cornerstone of successful management of all open fractures of the tibial shaft, regardless of the implant employed for tibial fixation.

The Mangled Extremity and Limb Salvage

Occasionally, the orthopaedic surgeon is confronted with a lower extremity that is so mangled that salvage is questionable, even though the arterial supply is intact. While the outcome for some injuries may be fairly predictable, for most it is not. An extremity with disruption of the posterior tibial nerve coupled with severe foot and ankle trauma has a poor prognosis. When injuries involve so much muscle damage that debridement leaves the patient with little if any functional capability, especially when there is associated osseous loss in excess of 6 cm, immediate amputation will probably serve the patient well. Large segmental defects involving the knee joint and the extensor mechanism, coupled with peroneal nerve injury, will, if a salvage procedure is performed, at best result in a knee fusion and the use of an ankle-foot orthosis. The lack of mobility (especially in older patients) and the large energy expenditure required make amputation in this situation desirable. Unfortunately, before a decision regarding limb salvage can be made, the prognosis for the injury must be known. Usually this is not possible, due in part to the unique nature of the injury and the limited amount of personal experience that most orthopaedic surgeons have in this field.

Mangled extremities associated with a vascular injury requiring repair (type-IIIC injuries) have also posed a major quandary to the treating physician, as prospective grading scales are not in widespread use and there have been few outcome studies. In their review of 62 type-III open tibial fractures, Caudle and Stern[4] found the classification of Gustilo to be prognostic. Type-IIIA injuries were associated with a low complication rate; type-IIIB open fractures, with serious complications; and type-IIIC open tibial fractures, with disastrous rates of major complications (100%) and secondary amputation (78%). Lange and associates[78] analyzed 23 cases of open tibial fractures with limb-threatening vascular compromise. Fourteen patients (61%) underwent amputation, and none had complications or functional disability at the one-year follow-up visit. In contrast, all of the patients who underwent limb salvage required several operations and had persistent wound or tibial healing problems at the one-year follow-up examination. The authors suggested that functional outcome be appraised realistically before a decision is made in favor of salvage for limbs with a type-IIIC injury, as the overall amputation rate after these injuries has approached 60% in the more recent literature.[79]

Bondurant and associates[80] reported on the financial cost of limb salvage in patients who had an open type-IIIB or IIIC tibial fracture. Of 263 patients, 43 ultimately underwent amputation. Fourteen patients had a primary amputation and, on the average, were hospitalized for 22 days, had 1.6 operative procedures, and incurred $28,964 in hospital costs. Those who had attempts at limb salvage averaged 53 days in the hospital, seven surgical procedures, and $53,462 in hospital costs. Another study evaluated the results of a salvage protocol for the treatment of eleven grade-IIIB ankle and talus injuries.[81] All patients were hospitalized on a minimum of three separate occasions and had at least five surgical procedures, with an average of eight procedures per patient. The total inpatient hospital stay averaged 62 days (range, 20 to 107 days), and inpatient costs averaged $62,174 (range, $33,535 to $143,847). Although all injuries healed, the majority of the patients were dysfunctional with respect to physical activities and family interactions. Both of these studies suggested that, if early amputation is performed on the basis of appropriate criteria, it improves function, shortens hospitalization, and lessens the financial burden on both the patient and the institution. Similarly, Hansen[82,83] noted that when patients who had had post-traumatic limb-salvage procedures were candid, they frequently stated that although their limbs had been saved, their lives had been ruined by the prolonged and costly attempts at reconstruction. Hansen characterized this approach as "triumphs of technique over reason." Several authors have recently suggested that early amputation and prosthetic fitting is preferable to salvage of a questionably functional lower limb.[78-80,82-86]

To determine when amputation is not only justified but also beneficial, a predictive scale with objective criteria is required. Well-designed, prospective, controlled, multicenter studies with large patient populations are needed to obtain these data. Although several investigators have attempted to develop objective criteria, to date we know of no predictive scale that can be used with confidence to make decisions regarding amputation. Long-term functional outcome studies on patients with salvage procedures are needed as well.

Decision-Aiding Scales

Daines evaluated 26 lower-extremity fractures with vascular injuries with regard to four variables: (1) extent of soft-tissue damage, (2) duration and severity of ischemia, (3) presence of shock, and (4) age of the patient (M. Daines, personal communication). He defined a score that was predictive of amputation and had no overlap in data. He felt that soft-tissue grading was the most important variable. Gregory and associates[85] proposed a mangled extremity severity index (MESI). A point system was developed for grading of the severity of the injury to four major organ systems of the extremity (integument, nerve, vessel, and bone), and overall injury severity, lag time between the injury and treatment, age of the patient, pre-existing disease, and shock. They found a dividing line at 20 points, below which limb salvage was predictable and above which the chance of amputation having to be performed was 100%. This initial series was limited to only 12 cases, the type of fracture was not identified, and an unspecified number of primary amputations was included. Lange and associates[78] proposed a protocol based on absolute and relative indications for amputation (Outline 1). The occurrence of one absolute indication or two relative indications warranted amputation. Unfortunately, only a minority of cases fit these criteria, and the relative indications were extremely subjective and required considerable experience to determine.

Recently, Helfet and associates[86] combined most of the above studies into a modified version of the mangled extremity severity index (MESI) to predict amputation rates (Table 2). Their version is called the mangled extremity severity score (MESS). This system was used only for documented type-IIIC open tibial fractures, first retrospectively in 26 cases and then prospectively in an equal number of cases. The scoring was performed after the salvage-versus-amputation decision had been made. In both groups, there was a marked difference in the mean MESS scores between the limbs that were eventually amputated and those that were salvaged. For both, a score of 7 points or more was

Outline 1
Criteria According to Lange et al.[78, 79]

Protocol for primary amputation (type-IIIC tibial fracture)
  A. Absolute indications
    1. Anatomically complete disruption of the posterior tibial nerve in adults
    2. Crush injuries with warm ischemia time >6 hrs.
  B. Relative indications
    1. Serious associated polytrauma
    2. Severe ipsilateral foot trauma
    3. Anticipated protracted soft-tissue and osseous reconstruction

Decision-making variables in limb salvage
  A. Patient
    1. Age
    2. Chronic disease
    3. Occupational considerations
    4. Patient and family desires
  B. Extremity
    1. Mechanism of injury
    2. Fracture pattern
    3. Arterial/venous injury (location)
    4. Neurologic status (anatomic)
    5. Injury status of ipsilateral foot
    6. Ischemia zone after revascularization
  C. Associated
    1. Magnitude of associated injury (injury severity score)
    2. Severity and duration of shock
    3. Warm ischemia time

100% predictive of amputation. Although the preliminary data base is small, this system holds promise as the first objective scoring method that can predict poor outcome and thereby justify primary amputation.

At the present time, the basis on which to make a sound, defensible, and reasonable decision for primary amputation is still insufficient. Lange[79] has recently identified certain variables that are important, but feasibility variables (those that indicate that the limb is technically salvageable) and advisability variables (those that indicate that salvage is in the best interest of the patient) create a complex interplay. A crush injury in a young laborer is very different from the same injury in a 60-year-old diabetic. Similarly, a tibial injury may need a different approach when severe ipsilateral foot trauma exists. It should be obvious, therefore, that the majority of cases will fall into a gray zone of indeterminate prognosis. In these cases, an experienced decision-making team and a tertiary-care facility are almost mandatory.[87] Lange[79] stated that: "Inexperience in evaluating these injuries and the lack of multidisciplinary consultation may render it ethically impossible for a surgeon to recommend a primary amputation and, as well, may make successful limb salvage unrealistic."

Table 2
The Mangled Extremity Severity Score[86]

Type	Characteristics	Injuries	Points	Score
Skeletal and soft-tissue group				
1	Low energy	Stab wounds, simple closed fractures, small-caliber gunshot wounds	1	____
2	Medium energy	Open or multiple-level fractures, dislocations, moderate crush injuries	2	____
3	High energy	Shotgun blast (close range), high-velocity gunshot wound	3	____
4	Massive crush	Logging, railroad, oil-rig accidents	4	____
			Subtotal	_____
Shock group				
1	Normotensive	Blood pressure stable in field and op. room	0	____
2	Transient hypotension	Blood pressure unstable in field, but responsive to intraven. fluids	1	____
3	Prolonged hypotension	Systolic blood pressure <90 mm Hg in field and responsive to intraven. fluids only in op. room	2	____
4	Advanced	Pulseless, cool, paralyzed, and numb	3	____
			Subtotal	_____
Ischemia group (points double if ischemia >6 hrs.)				
1	None	Pulsatile leg without signs of ischemia	0	____
2	Mild	Diminished pulses only	1	____
3	Moderate	No pulse by Doppler, sluggish capillary refill, paresthesias, diminished motor activity	2	____
4	Advanced	Pulseless, cool, paralyzed, and numb	3	____
			Subtotal	_____
Age group				
1	<30 yrs.		0	____
2	30-50 yrs.		1	____
3	>50 yrs.		2	____
			Subtotal	_____
Total mangled extremity severity score			**Total**	_____

The MESS score and Lange's absolute and relative indications should be used to determine possible need. Limb and wound photographs should always be obtained, and several surgeons should be consulted. Patient and family conferences (perhaps with an amputee present) are required, and a frank discussion should take place. Then a joint decision can be made in the best interests of the patient.

Conclusions

In summary: (1) The patient should be stabilized and the open fracture should be evaluated but not definitively treated in the emergency room. Patients with vascular injuries should be transported to the operating room as soon as possible to minimize ischemia time. (2) In the operating room, meticulous irrigation and debridement are the cornerstone of success. The open fracture is graded, as it is only then that a more realistic appraisal of the injury is possible. Stabilization of the fracture stabilizes the soft tissues. Fixation choices depend on the bone involved, the fracture site, the location of the wound, and the condition of the patient. Operative extensions of the wound may be closed, but open wounds are never closed primarily. (3) Repeat irrigation and debridement should be performed every 24 to 48 hours until the wound is clean and necrotic tissue is no longer present. The open wound ideally is closed within five to seven days after the injury, with the use of skin grafts or local or free vascularized flaps. Once the limb is clean, closed, and stabilized, definitive reconstruction can be performed, if needed.

References

1. Gregory GF, Chapman MW, Hansen ST Jr: Open fractures, in Rockwood CA Jr, Green DP (eds): *Fractures in Adults*, ed 2. Philadelphia, PA, JB Lippincott, 1984, vol 1, pp 169-218.
2. Chapman MW: Role of bone stability in open fractures, in Frankel VH (ed): American Academy of Orthopaedic Surgeons *Instructional Course Lectures XXXI*. St. Louis, MO, CV Mosby, 1982, pp 75-87.
3. Blick SS, Brumback RJ, Poka A, et al: Compartment syndrome in open tibial fractures. *J Bone Joint Surg* 1986;68A:1348-1353.
4. Caudle RJ, Stern PJ: Severe open fractures of the tibia. *J Bone Joint Surg* 1987;69A:801-807.
5. DeBakey ME, Simeone FA: Battle injuries of arteries in World War II: An analysis of 2,471 cases. *Ann Surg* 1946;123:534-579.
6. DeLee JC, Stiehl JB: Open tibia fracture with compartment syndrome. *Clin Orthop* 1981;160:175-184.
7. Dellinger EP, Miller SD, Wertz MJ, et al: Risk of infection after open fracture of the arm or leg. *Arch Surg* 1988;123:1320-1327.
8. Tscherne H, Gotzen L: *Fractures with Soft Tissue Injuries*. New York, NY, Springer-Verlag, 1984.
9. Behrens FD: Bone grafting: General principles and use in open fractures, in Murray DG (ed): American Academy of Orthopaedic Surgeons *Instructional Course Lectures XXX*. St. Louis, MO, CV Mosby, 1981, pp 152-156.
10. Gustilo RB, Mendoza RM, Williams DN: Problems in the management of type III (severe) open fractures: A new classification of type III open fractures. *J Trauma* 1984;24:742-746.
11. Christensen KS: Pneumatic antishock garments (PASG): Do they precipitate lower-extremity compartment syndromes? *J Trauma* 1986;26:1102-1105.
12. Mattox KL, Bickell W, Pepe PE, et al: Prospective MAST study in 911 patients. *J Trauma* 1989;29:1104-1112.
13. Gustilo RB: *Management of Open Fractures and Their Complications*. Philadelphia, PA, WB Saunders, 1982.
14. Robson MC, Duke WF, Krizek TJ: Rapid bacterial screening in the treatment of civilian wounds. *J Surg Res* 1973;14:426-430.
15. Gustilo RB, Anderson JT: Prevention of infection in the treatment of one thousand and twenty-five open fractures of long bones: Retrospective and prospective analyses. *J Bone Joint Surg* 1976;58A:453-458.
16. Gustilo RB: Use of antimicrobials in the management of open fractures. *Arch Surg* 1979;114:805-808.
17. Patzakis MJ, Harvey JP Jr, Ivler D: The role of antibiotics in the management of open fractures. *J Bone Joint Surg* 1974;56A:532-541.
18. Johansen K, Lynch K, Paun M, et al: Non-invasive vascular tests reliably exclude occult arterial trauma in injured extremities. *J Trauma* 1991;31:515-522.
19. Feliciano DV: Evaluation and treatment of vascular injuries, in Browner BD, Jupiter JB, Levine AM, et al: (eds): *Skeletal Trauma: Fractures; Dislocations; Ligamentous Injuries*. Philadelphia, PA, WB Saunders, 1992, vol 1, chap 12, pp 269-284.
20. Sibbitt RR, Palmaz JC, Garcia F, et al: Trauma of the extremities: Prospective comparison of digital and conventional angiography. *Radiology* 1986;160:179-182.
21. Allen MJ, Stirling AJ, Crawshaw CV, et al: Intracompartmental pressure monitoring of leg injuries: An aid to management. *J Bone Joint Surg* 1985;67B:53-57.
22. Lieb FJ, Perry J: Quadriceps function: An anatomical and mechanical study using amputated limbs. *J Bone Joint Surg* 1968;50A:1535-1548.
23. Matsen FA III, Winquist RA, Krugmire RB Jr: Diagnosis and management of compartmental syndromes. *J Bone Joint Surg* 1980;62A:286-291.
24. Whitesides TE, Haney TC, Morimoto K, et al: Tissue pressure measurements as a determinant for the need of fasciotomy. *Clin Orthop* 1975;113:43-51.
25. Ward WG, Nunley JA: Occult orthopaedic trauma in the multiply injured patient. *J Orthop Trauma* 1991;5:308-312.
26. Wassilak SGF, Brink EW: Tetanus, in Last JM, Chin J, Fielding JE, et al (eds): *Maxcy-Rosenau Public Health and Preventive Medicine*, ed 12. Norwalk, CT, Appleton-Century-Crofts, 1986, pp 429-471.
27. Patzakis MJ, Wilkins J, Moore TM: Considerations in reducing the infection rate in open tibial fractures. *Clin Orthop* 1983;178:36-41.
28. Darke SG, King AM, Slack WK: Gas gangrene and related infection: Classification, clinical features and aetiology, management and mortality: A report of 88 cases. *Br J Surg* 1977;64:104-112.
29. Johansen K, Bandyk D, Thiele B, et al: Temporary intraluminal shunts: Resolution of a management dilemma in complex vascular injuries. *J Trauma* 1982;22:395-402.
30. Rich NM, Metz CW Jr, Hutton JE Jr, et al: Internal versus external fixation of fractures with concomitant vascular injuries in Vietnam. *J Trauma* 1971;11:463-473.
31. Brumback RJ: Wound debridement, in Yaremchuk MJ,

Burgess AWR, Brumback RJ (eds): *Lower Extremity Salvage and Reconstruction: Orthopedic and Plastic Surgical Management.* New York, NY, York Elsevier Science, 1989, chap 6, pp 71-80.

32. Rosenstein BD, Wilson FC, Funderburk CH: The use of bacitracin irrigation to prevent infection in postoperative skeletal wounds: An experimental study. *J Bone Joint Surg* 1989;71A:427-430.

33. Heppenstall RB, Scott R, Sapega A, et al: A comparative study of the tolerance of skeletal muscle to ischemia: Tourniquet application compared with acute compartment syndrome. *J Bone Joint Surg* 1986;68A:820-828.

34. Lee J, Goldstein J, Madison M, et al: The value of pre- and post-debridement cultures in the management of open fractures. *Orthop Trans* 1991;15:776-777.

35. Christian EP, Bosse MJ, Robb G: Reconstruction of large diaphyseal defects, without free fibular transfer, in grade-IIIB tibial fractures. *J Bone Joint Surg* 1989;71A:994-1004.

36. Müller ME, Allgöwer M, Schneider R, et al: *Manual of Internal Fixation. Techniques Recommended by the AO-ASIF Group,* ed 3. Berlin, Germany, Springer-Verlag, 1991.

37. Bone LB, Johnson KD, Weigelt J, et al: Early versus delayed stabilization of femoral fractures: A prospective randomized study. *J Bone Joint Surg* 1989;71A:336-340.

38. Goris RJ, Gimbrére JS, van Niekerk JLM, et al: Early osteosynthesis and prophylactic mechanical ventilation in the multitrauma patient. *J Trauma* 1982;22:895-903.

39. Johnson KD, Cadambi A, Seibert GB: Incidence of adult respiratory distress syndrome in patients with multiple musculoskeletal injuries: Effect of early operative stabilization of fractures. *J Trauma* 1985;25:375-384.

40. Bach AW, Hansen ST Jr: Plates versus external fixation in severe open tibial shaft fractures: A randomized trial. *Clin Orthop* 1989;241:89-94.

41. Blachut PA, Meek RN, O'Brien PJ: External fixation and delayed intramedullary nailing of open fractures of the tibial shaft: A sequential protocol. *J Bone Joint Surg* 1990;72A:729-735.

42. Burwell HN: Plate fixation of tibial shaft fractures: A survey of 181 injuries. *J Bone Joint Surg* 1971;53B:258-271.

43. Chapman MW: The role of intramedullary fixation in open fractures. *Clin Orthop* 1986;212:26-34.

44. Court-Brown CM, Wheelwright EF, Christie J, et al: External fixation for type III open tibial fractures. *J Bone Joint Surg* 1990;72B:801-804.

45. Holbrook JL, Swiontkowski MF, Sanders R: Treatment of open fractures of the tibial shaft: Ender nailing versus external fixation: A randomized, prospective comparison. *J Bone Joint Surg* 1989;71A:1231-1238.

46. Howey TD, Helfet D, Dipasquale T, et al: Treatment of open and/or unstable tibial fractures with an unreamed double locked tibial nail. *Orthop Trans* 1992;16:826.

47. McGraw JM, Lim EV: Treatment of open tibial-shaft fractures. External fixation and secondary intramedullary nailing. *J Bone Joint Surg* 1988;70A:900-911.

48. Merritt K: Factors increasing the risk of infection in patients with open fractures. *J Trauma* 1989;28:823-827.

49. Spiegel PG, VanderSchilden JL: Minimal internal and external fixation in the treatment of open tibial fractures. *Clin Orthop* 1983;178:96-102.

50. Velazco A, Fleming LL: Open fractures of the tibia treated by the Hoffmann external fixator. *Clin Orthop* 1983;180:125-132.

51. Velazco A, Whitesides TE Jr, Fleming LL: Open fractures of the tibia treated with the Lottes nail. *J Bone Joint Surg* 1983;65A:879-885.

52. Whitelaw GP, Wetzler M, Nelson A, et al: Ender rods versus external fixation in the treatment of open tibial fractures. *Clin Orthop* 1990;253:258-269.

53. Davis AG: Primary closure of compound-fracture wounds: With immediate internal fixation, immediate skin graft, and compression dressings. *J Bone Joint Surg* 1948;30A:405-415.

54. Mast J, Jakob R, Ganz R: *Planning and Reduction Technique in Fracture Surgery.* New York, NY, Springer-Verlag, 1989.

55. Wahlig H, Dingeldein E, Bergmann R, et al: The release of gentamicin from polymethylmethacrylate beads: An experimental and pharmacokinetic study. *J Bone Joint Surg* 1978;60B:270-275.

56. Cierny G III, Byrd HS, Jones RE: Primary versus delayed soft tissue coverage for severe open tibial fractures: A comparison of results. *Clin Orthop* 1983;178:54-63.

57. Weiland AJ, Moore JR, Daniel RK: The efficacy of free tissue transfer in the treatment of osteomyelitis. *J Bone Joint Surg* 1984;66A:181-193.

58. Yaremchuk MJ, Brumback RJ, Manson PN, et al: Acute and definitive management of traumatic osteocutaneous defects of the lower extremity. *Plast Reconstr Surg* 1987;80:1-14.

59. Harmon PH: A simplified surgical approach to the posterior tibia for bone-grafting and fibular transference. *J Bone Joint Surg* 1945;27A:496-498.

60. Sanders R, DiPasquale T: A technique for obtaining bone graft. *J Orthop Trauma* 1989;3:287-289.

61. Brumback RJ: Open tibial fractures: Current orthopaedic management, in Eilert RE (ed): *Instructional Course Lectures XLI.* Park Ridge, IL, American Academy of Orthopaedic Surgeons, 1992, pp 101-117.

62. Paley D, Chaudray M, Pirone AM, et al: Treatment of malunions and mal-nonunions of the femur and tibia by detailed preoperative planning and the Ilizarov techniques. *Orthop Clin North Am* 1990;21:667-691.

63. Tucker HL, Kendra JC, Kinnebrew TE: Tibial defects: Reconstruction using the method of Ilizarov as an alternative. *Orthop Clin North Am* 1990;21:629-637.

64. Klemm KW, Börner M: Interlocking nailing of complex fractures of the femur and tibia. *Clin Orthop* 1986;212:89-100.

65. Lhowe DW, Hansen ST: Immediate nailing of open fractures of the femoral shaft. *J Bone Joint Surg* 1988;70A:812-820.

66. Patzakis MJ, Wilkins J, Wiss DA: Infection following intramedullary nailing of long bones: Diagnosis and management. *Clin Orthop* 1986;212:182-191.

67. Dabezies EJ, D'Ambrosia R, Shoji H, et al: Fractures of the femoral shaft treated by external fixation with the Wagner device. *J Bone Joint Surg* 1984;66A:360-364.

68. Clancey GJ, Hansen ST Jr: Open fractures of the tibia: A review of one hundred and two cases. *J Bone Joint Surg* 1978;60A:118-122.

69. McAndrew MP, Lantz BA: Initial care of massively traumatized lower extremities. *Clin Orthop* 1989;243:20-29.

70. Marsh JL, Nepola JV, Wuest TK, et al: Unilateral external fixation until healing with the dynamic axial fixator for severe open tibial fractures. *J Orthop Trauma* 1991;5:341-348.

71. Rommens P, Gielen J, Broos P, et al: Intrinsic problems with the external fixation device of Hoffmann-Vidal-Adrey: A critical evaluation of 117 patients with complex tibial shaft fractures. *J Trauma* 1989;29:630-638.

72. Fischer MD, Gustilo RB, Varecka TF: The timing of flap coverage, bone-grafting, and intramedullary nailing in patients who have a fracture of the tibial shaft with extensive soft-tissue injury. *J Bone Joint Surg* 1991;73A:1316-1322.

73. Maurer DJ, Merkow RL, Gustilo RB: Infection after intramedullary nailing of severe open tibial fractures initially treated with external fixation. *J Bone Joint Surg* 1989;71A:835-838.

74. Klein MP, Rahn BA, Frigg R, et al: Reaming versus nonreaming in medullary nailing: Interference with cortical cir-

culation of the canine tibia. *Arch Orthop Trauma Surg* 1990;109:314-316.

75. Howard M, Zinar D: The use of the Lottes nail in the treatment of tibial fractures. *J Orthop Trauma* 1989;3:175.

76. Lottes JO: Medullary nailing of the tibia with the triflange nail. *Clin Orthop* 1974;105:53-66.

77. Whittle AP, Russell TA, Taylor JC, et al: Treatment of open fractures of the tibial shaft with the use of interlocking nailing without reaming. *J Bone Joint Surg* 1992;74A:1162-1171.

78. Lange RH, Bach AW, Hansen ST Jr, et al: Open tibial fractures with associated vascular injuries: Prognosis for limb salvage. *J Trauma* 1985;25:203-208.

79. Lange RH: Limb reconstruction versus amputation decision making in massive lower extremity trauma. *Clin Orthop* 1989;243:92-99.

80. Bondurant FJ, Cotler HB, Buckle R, et al: The medical and economic impact of severely injured lower extremities. *J Trauma* 1988;28:1270-1272.

81. Sanders R, Pappas J, Mast J, et al: The salvage of open grade IIIB ankle and talus fractures. *J Orthop Trauma* 1992;6:201-208.

82. Hansen ST Jr: Editorial: The type-IIIC tibial fracture: Salvage or amputation. *J Bone Joint Surg* 1987;69A:799-800.

83. Hansen ST Jr: Overview of the severely traumatized lower limb: Reconstruction versus amputation. *Clin Orthop* 1989;243:17-19.

84. Border JR, Allgöwer M, Hansen ST Jr, et al: *Blunt Multiple Trauma: Comprehensive Pathophysiology and Care*. New York, NY, Marcel Dekker, 1990.

85. Gregory RT, Gould RJ, Peclet M, et al: The mangled extremity syndrome (M.E.S.): A severity grading system for multisystem injury of the extremity. *J Trauma* 1985;25:1147-1150.

86. Helfet DL, Howey T, Sanders R, et al: Limb salvage versus amputation: Preliminary results of the mangled extremity severity score. *Clin Orthop* 1990;256:80-86.

87. Sanders R, Helfet DL: Trauma, in Bowker JH, Michael JW (eds): American Academy of Orthopaedic Surgeons *Atlas of Limb Prosthetics: Surgical, Prosthetic, and Rehabilitation Principles*, ed 2. St. Louis, MO, Mosby-Year Book, 1992, pp 19-24.

Publishing and Presenting

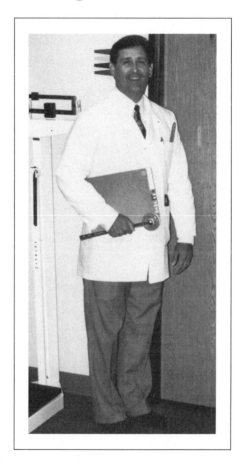

Preparing Manuscripts for Publication in *The Journal of Bone and Joint Surgery*: A View From the Former Editor of the British Volume

A. Graham Apley, MB BS, FRCS

Writing is like having a baby; the gestation period is long and the labor is painful, but in the end you have something to show for it. Since you are reading these words, I assume that you have a worthwhile message and that you intend to submit it to *The Journal of Bone and Joint Surgery* for publication. I hope that the following pages will help you to achieve that aim. In them, I will discuss the stages of preparation and outline what is involved in each; the question of style is outside my remit.

First Steps

The Different Kinds of Article

Before you begin, you should decide what kind of article you are planning to write. Is it about research, or a case report, or a clinical study? Each has its own special problems.

Studies in basic research tend to be very long and to be overloaded with technical jargon. If you think that your subject is so important that only a long article will do, it is worth remembering that the original account of the double helix by Watson and Crick[1] (an article that changed the thinking of the scientific world) occupied only one page of the journal *Nature*. As for technical jargon, the trouble is that you know so much about your subject that you are liable to forget that the average reader is less well informed. It is a mistake to suppose that long words are better than short ones. There's no need to refer to a group of old women with few teeth as "an oligodentulous female cohort." A good way of getting into the right frame of mind is to assume that you have been commissioned by *The New York Times* or *Newsweek* to write a brief account of your work using only words that the intelligent layperson will understand.

Single case reports are not usually difficult to write, but even they need to have a message. If you are merely claiming that yours is the first published report of an osteoid osteoma in the navicular bone of a left-handed basketball player with six toes on each foot, your chances of acceptance are not very high. Incidentally, I must warn you that the phrase "this is the first published report" often attracts angry letters from authors claiming priority and demanding to know why you

don't read the literature even if their article was published in a Mongolian journal of pediatric neurology or whatever.

A series of three or four cases has a rather better chance of acceptance, providing the similarities between them are not simply that they have the same sex or political affiliation. Even with a small series of cases, you need to scour the literature to make sure that the combination of features you are describing has not been published before; if you really have an interesting "first," you may be lucky enough to find your name attached to a syndrome.

Whether you are describing one or a handful of cases, you may feel that you would like to embellish your report by adding a "Review of the Literature." However, while your discussion should certainly mention any published cases similar to yours, a detailed review is of little value unless it sheds fresh light on the subject. I am not referring to comprehensive review articles; these are usually commissioned by the Editor, so their discussion here would be out of place.

Clinical studies, by which I mean articles dealing with a substantial number of patients or operations, are usually described under headings that have the well-known formula IMRAD. This acronym stands for Introduction, Material (or patients) and Methods, Results, and Discussion. These will be considered in detail a little later, but meanwhile it is useful to think of them in simple terms: Introduction—why did I start? Material and Methods—what did I do, and to whom? Results—what did I find? Discussion—what does it matter, or who cares?

Before Starting to Write

Before putting pen to paper (or hand to word processor), you need to take three steps: read widely, summarize your message, and arrange your material.

It goes without saying that you must scan the literature thoroughly. Good sources of reference can be found in Medline, *Index Medicus*, and review articles on related topics. Also remember that good librarians are worth their weight in gold. It is useful to keep a separate card or sheet for each important article. Note carefully the exact title, the names of the authors and of the journal, and the volume and page numbers, and include a two- or three-line summary of the article.

This will save a lot of time later. Discussion with knowledgeable colleagues also is worthwhile—fears that they may steal your ideas are usually groundless.

Summarizing your message is not the same as writing the abstract, which comes later. It means compressing into as few words as possible (preferably less than 50) the essence of your message and then, with a felt-tip pen, printing these words on a large piece of cardboard, which you display prominently in your place of work. Its purpose is to keep you on the rails and to prevent you from straying into irrelevancies, which waste your time and distract the reader.

This summary should tell you if you have something important to say. If not, it is worth recalling the injunction attributed to T. S. Eliot: "Blessed is the man who, having nothing to say, refrains from saying it." Provided your contribution is useful, go ahead and assemble your material. Collect every scrap of information that you have, including your illustrations, pathology reports, graphs, and references. Leave nothing out. Then sort everything into heaps, each under the appropriate heading and each heap arranged and filed in date order. Headings are vital; they are the signposts that tell readers where they are. Thus, they must be disciplined: you must include, under each heading, every item that belongs there—and, equally important, you must exclude every item that does not belong there.

Individual Headings

Introduction

In this section, you tell the reader what shortcomings in our present knowledge, or inadequacies in our results, prompted you to study this particular subject. You will probably need to quote from previous publications, but this does not mean that you need to cite every conceivable article ever written on anything even remotely connected with your subject. Try not to get carried away; choose only those articles that are important and strictly relevant, and only enough of those to convince readers and reviewers that you really have studied the literature. Selectivity is important because this opening section is where you grab your readers and make them want to go on reading. A dreary catalog of 88 previous publications is merely soporific. Try to start with a bang and try not to go on and on; if you don't strike oil quickly, stop boring.

Material and Methods

The object here is to give enough information for others to be able to repeat your work, if they so wish, and to be able to compare their findings with yours. You need to be explicit in detailing your methods; it is, however, unnecessary to describe something that everyone knows, like how to measure the Cobb angle.

You also need to specify numbers: how many patients or animals were involved? If you are dealing with patients, how were they selected? Do not say they were chosen at random, because randomized has a precise statistical meaning and to use the word without specifying the process is to invite the suspicion that your choice was biased. If you were using animals and you killed them, please don't say that you sacrificed them unless you actually performed a ritual killing to propitiate the gods.

You may need to divide the population that was studied into groups and subgroups according to age, sex, or the particular procedure that was done. Make sure that the basis on which these subdivisions were made is clearly specified, and then ask yourself if the number in each subgroup is sufficient to justify your conclusions, or indeed any conclusions. Don't ask only yourself; ask a statistician if necessary. Words like good, fair, and poor should of course be defined with precision. As for controls, their number and the method of selection need to be specified; if you are not using controls, you may need to justify their omission.

Illustrations

Because illustrations are usually first required in the Material and Methods section, this is a convenient place to discuss them. Most papers need illustrations, and readers like them, but you can have too much of a good thing. One paper on injuries sustained during parachute-jumping was sent in with 72 illustrations, all showing severe injuries. However, since the message of the paper was that if you jump out of an airplane and your parachute fails to open you may hurt yourself quite badly, one or two pictures would have been enough. Don't send more than you really need, leaving it to the Editor to choose the best; it is your article and it is up to you to do the selection. If you are illustrating a sequence, such as the radiographic changes during union of a fracture, you may have radiographs of ten or 12 sequential stages. Don't include them all, however beautiful they are. Lay them in a row and see how many you can leave out without spoiling the story. With a sequence of clinical photographs, it is best if they were all made from the same angle.

Quality is important. It is no good hoping that the printer will produce a beautiful picture from an underexposed, uncentered, foggy radiograph of a fat man's spine. Methods for the reproduction of illustrations are excellent nowadays, but at each stage of the process a little definition may be lost, so the originals that you send in must be of the highest quality. Lack of clarity is unacceptable (even if accompanied by a note to the Editor claiming justification). Glossy prints are required.

Operative photographs have to be exceptionally good to be worth printing; often it is difficult to see which part of the body is involved, let alone what is being done. Line drawings are usually much clearer, because the extraneous tissues have been omitted, but they do require skilled draftsmanship. Color is very attractive when projected from a transparency, but a color print needs to be a lot better than black and white before the additional difficulties and expense are justified.

Remember also that the purpose of illustrations is not merely to give "artistic verisimilitude to an otherwise bald and unconvincing narrative" (W. S. Gilbert). They must make their point more clearly than can be done in words. If you are in doubt as to whether a particular picture is good enough, try showing it to a colleague and see whether, without being told, he or she can appreciate its significance.

Results

Under this heading, we need to consider how the results are assessed, how they are presented, and problems that may arise with the use of numbers. Do not include the results of your preliminary work unless they are strictly relevant.

Assessment is of paramount importance in any article about a new operation or about any modification of an old one. If you are using a known scoring system, it is important that you specify which one and acknowledge its drawbacks. If you have devised a new scoring system, you need to justify it. It is worth reading the comments on scoring systems in *The Journal of Bone and Joint Surgery.*[2,3]

Errors of arithmetic are astonishingly common. They seem to slip in unobtrusively and they diminish the author's credibility. For example, the population of the patients described in the Material and Methods section may consist of 11 men and 17 women, but the results (usually on another page) may be assessed in terms of 29 patients. No less disturbing is when the total number is less than the sum of its constituent parts; the reader is left wondering whether the missing patients are dead, defaulters, or have results opposed to the author's thesis. It is always important to account for any discrepancy between the number of patients who were entered into a study and the number at its termination. One maddening error concerns bilateral procedures. The author is perhaps describing the results of 78 knee replacements in 50 patients and states that 47 were successful. Forty-seven patients or 47 knees?

Numbers need careful handling, and it is wise to ask an independent person (not necessary medical) to check them. Percentages also, despite the availability of electronic calculators, are not always correct, and even those that are correct may be used wrongly. It is a mistake and possibly misleading to apply them to very small numbers; would you say, "50% of two patients survived"? With large numbers, excessive detail is a common mistake; to say that, of 100 patients, 79.612% had a satisfactory result makes no sense. Nor does a 75% success rate of 79 cases tell us how many succeeded. As for means and averages, does it really help anyone to be told that a man and his dog possess an average of three legs each?

You may decide, at this point, that you need to consult a statistician, but unless you sought such advice much earlier, as I suggested, the statistician may tell you that your entire methodology is worthless. If you do seek expert help, remember that consultation is not the same as co-authorship—an article by a surgeon and a statistician may not combine the virtues of each. When a famous beauty suggested to George Bernard Shaw that, with her looks and his brain, they should have a child, he replied, "Suppose it had my looks and your brain?"

Results are sometimes expressed in long continuous sentences, such as: in men who were older than 70, the mean range of motion was 72.5° (range, 64.3 to 77; standard deviation, ± 3.5) and the mean fixed flexion was 15.3° (range, 5.6 to 22.7; standard deviation, ± 5.8); in men who were younger than 70, the mean range of motion was 81.9° (range, 74.3 to 93.6; standard deviation, ± 8.2) and the mean fixed flexion was 12.8° (range, 10.2 to 15.5; standard deviation, ± 28); in women who were older than 70, the mean range of flexion was...and so on, for line after line. This is almost unreadable, even early in the morning after a good night's sleep and a cup of strong coffee. Tables or charts are much easier to take in.

Tables, however, are by no means easy to construct. They need considerable craftsmanship if one is to steer a middle course between excessive simplicity and excessive complexity. The information that, of five patients, three did well and two did poorly is better expressed as a sentence in the text; it would look pretentious as a table. On the other hand, it is overwhelming to tabulate so much information that you need a battery of asterisks and daggers as well as a column crammed full of additional comments. Admittedly, some journals welcome tables that include everything, but I think most readers of *The Journal of Bone and Joint Surgery* prefer something a little simpler.

Bar charts, pie charts, and graphs make it easier for the eye to take in results at a glance. If these are prepared manually, it is important that you check that the measurements tally with the figures. It is better to use a word processor with facilities for graphics; supplied with the figures, this can construct charts with total accuracy. As with illustrations, charts and tables should not merely repeat the information in the text; the written descriptions should be a commentary, highlighting notable features.

An account of the complications is, of course, essential to a description of the results of any clinical study; indeed, it may merit a section to itself. You should not assume that readers will regard the omission of any mention of complications as meaning that none occurred; they may wonder if the existence of complications has been suppressed. Always admit, or even parade, your complications; this will enhance your credibility, especially if you can provide a reasonable explanation for them.

Conclusions

Under this heading, you should not simply repeat all that you have said in the earlier sections. This is where you discuss the significance of your findings. If, for example, you have found that, in patients who are more than 60 years old and have osteoarthrosis of the knee, replacement is better than osteotomy, say this boldly and without listing, yet again, all of the figures that led to that conclusion.

You may, however, need to justify any unusual aspect of your methods and, if your results differ from those of other people, to explain these differences. It is also worth indicating what useful work could follow from your studies. These various aspects of your discussion should not be over-elaborated; as with needless repetition, this merely diminishes their impact. The simpler your conclusions, the more memorable they are.

Final Stages

Assembling

This means putting together what you have written, ensuring that the arguments and statements follow one another in a logical sequence and that the total product adds up to a single, comprehensible article. This is also the stage at which to write the abstract, unless you are submitting a case report, which does not need one. Go back to the summary of your message that you wrote earlier. It will probably need to be expanded from its 50 words to as many as 150, but not more. It is best to avoid details and precise statistics; these belong in the body of the article. The reader who is sufficiently interested by your abstract will know where to find the details. Too lengthy an abstract may be so indigestible that readers never finish it and, if they do, they may feel that they no longer need to read the article itself.

The title is best left until last. You will probably have thought of a half-dozen titles while writing the article and, if you are wise, you will have written them down; but now you must make your final selection. You may prefer a long title, such as "The Effect of Combinations of Dihydroergotamine and Heparin on the Incidence of Calf Vein Thrombosis and Pulmonary Embolism fol-

lowing Total Hip Replacement in Normotensive Patients Aged Over 70 Years," or a short one, such as "Fractures at Football." The first makes an impressively long addition to your curriculum vitae, but many people find the simplicity of the second more attractive, especially as it can always be amplified by a subtitle. I remember reading that an article dealing with psychological disturbances associated with thyroid deficiency was repeatedly rejected while it bore an excessively lengthy title; the unchanged article was instantly accepted when entitled "Myxoedematous Madness."

Polishing and Pruning

Every article needs polishing. When you think that you have finished, put the article away in a drawer and forget about it. After two or three weeks, take it out and read it straight through. You are sure to find passages with which you are dissatisfied. If you don't, you are not being sufficiently self-critical. Who can write words that are perfect the first time, as Mozart wrote music? Even Beethoven repeatedly revised the early drafts of many of his compositions.

Pruning also is important. Aim to make the article shorter and simpler. All physicians are busy people, and in medical writing brevity is the kiss of life. The best way to shorten an article is to omit irrelevancies and to cut out needless repetition. It is impossible to specify what is, or is not, relevant but, with any doubtful passage, ask yourself whether your message would be weakened if it were omitted. If you are not sure, follow the old general surgical maxim: "When in doubt, cut it out." Repetition of certain points is, of course, necessary, but in excess it is counterproductive; we are liable to feel that the writer, in Hamlet's words, "doth protest too much." I said that the rewritten version should also be simpler; this is because a number of readers of *The Journal*, thought to be about 11,000, do not speak English as their mother tongue. You and I prefer simplicity; they need it.

You will probably find that, by now, you have virtually rewritten the article. This new version should be sent to each of your co-authors for their revision or approval. After you have incorporated their amendments, it is prudent to put the article back in the drawer for another two or three weeks before again rereading and revising it and then pausing and revising yet again—and again. How many times should the process of rewriting be repeated? I cannot say, but Sir Reginald Watson-Jones, probably the finest surgical writer of this century, once told me that six rewrites was his minimum. I doubt if many surgeons alive today are such perfectionists.

Between two of the rewrites, I strongly advise you to read the paper aloud to a small but select audience. Your listeners need not be expert in your subject because the object of this exercise is not criticism of your material. However, they do need to be medically literate and attentive to the flow of words. Reading aloud brings to light strange phrases that may have seemed sensible when they were written but whose absurdity is revealed by being spoken. Examples include: "under general anesthesia in the prone position the surgeon makes a vertical incision" (would you like to be operated on by an anesthetized surgeon who was lying down?) and "the growth charts of children produced by Anderson and Green." These are not mythical examples. Both were submitted in manuscripts and one was published unchanged, although not by *The Journal of Bone and Joint Surgery.* The most striking example I know—and I cannot vouch for its authenticity—is "If the baby fed on milk fails to thrive, boil it."

Checking

You have already checked your facts, your arithmetic, and your phrases, so you have nearly finished, but not quite. You still need to check your references. A considerable number of papers submitted contain errors such that the reader would fail to find the listed articles. In an editorial, I once compared references

with insulin: when appropriate, both are essential, but in excess they induce coma, and impurities are disastrous. That is why I suggested earlier that you limit the number of your references and that you note their details with great care; photocopying of the title pages is very useful.

Finally, check the page of *The Journal* headed Instructions to Authors or, in the British volume, Guide to Authors. You may have read it in the past, but it is worth reading again. I am not suggesting that acceptance of your paper will depend on your having fulfilled the requirements to the letter, but a sweet-tempered Editor is a splendid ally.

References

1. Watson JD, Crick FHC: Molecular structure of nucleic acids: A structure for deoxyribose nucleic acid. *Nature* 1953;171:737-738.
2. Johnston RC, Fitzgerald RH, Harris WH, et al: Clinical and radiographic evaluation of total hip replacement: A standard system of terminology for reporting results. *J Bone Joint Surg* 1990;72A:161-168.
3. Apley AG: Editorial: An assessment of assessment. *J Bone Joint Surg* 1990;72B:957-958.

Preparing Manuscripts for Publication in *The Journal of Bone and Joint Surgery*: Responsibilities of Authors and Editors: A View From the Editor of the American Volume

Henry R. Cowell, MD, PhD

The responsibilities of preparing a manuscript for publication do not start with writing; they begin long before the first word is put on paper. Nor is the process a simple one involving the placement of words on paper and then correction and improvement of the material before transmission to *The Journal*. Research, observation, recording, and writing are all involved, as is an adherence to ethical and moral standards. The process of writing and editing thus not only requires basic skills, but also involves responsibilities on the part of both the authors and the editor.

The authors must provide complete, accurate data in the manuscript. After all, the reader will make decisions regarding a patient on the basis of these data and the authors' conclusions. The authors also must provide new material that does not waste the reader's time with the repeated rehashing of old ideas. As an Editorial in the July 21, 1900, edition of *The Journal of the American Medical Association* noted: "Two thirds of the American medical literature is not especially valuable."[1] The same is true today.

The editor's responsibility to authors is to help them to present their material clearly, concisely, and accurately. The editor serves as a facilitator and an assistant to the authors. However, the editor has a greater responsibility to the reader. Each day, many more articles are added to the literature than anyone can hope to read. The editor must serve as a gatekeeper, stemming the flow of worthless jargon that besieges the reader each day and making sure that only valid, accurate articles that will benefit readers and be worth their time will be published. The editor, as a guardian of the truth, must do everything possible to ensure that what is published is, indeed, valid. Finally, the editor's ultimate responsibility is to the patient, and to society in general. Only articles that will serve to enhance patient care deserve a place in the literature. Both the authors and the editor must be certain that these responsibilities are taken into account through every step in the process of preparing a manuscript for publication.

Preliminary Planning

The first step of any study is to define a problem that needs to be addressed or to conceive a question that needs to be answered. A study that is undertaken without a goal seldom achieves a goal. Put another way, authors who begin a study without insight rarely gain insight into the problem during the study. It is seldom appropriate for a would-be author to investigate a number of patients just to see how those patients have fared. While the literature is full of such studies, and while such studies do, on occasion, answer critical questions, most investigations that have been done without previous definition of a problem or formulation of a question result in a manuscript that is unlikely to be accepted for publication. This is a waste of valuable time and resources. Instead, once a problem or a question has been defined, the study should be performed in such a fashion as to address that problem or to answer that question.

The cost of performing a study should be established, and the study should be done only if it is anticipated that the benefits to be derived from solving the problem or answering the question outweigh the cost of the study itself.

Review of the Literature

A complete search of the literature is the first part of any clinical study. Before embarking on a study, the authors should read the full text of all of the pertinent literature. All literature should be read at the source. If a reference is used, it must be cited correctly, a dictum alluded to almost 100 years ago in another Editorial in *The Journal of the American Medical Association*: "Much annoyance and loss of time are caused by errors in the references to the literature cited in articles."[2]

Authors should maintain a record of the information that they glean from the literature. The easiest way to do this is to obtain a xerographic copy, or a full-text computer printout, of all of the material that is evaluated. The pertinent information in the reference should be underlined or noted on an index card. The full and correct citation should be included at the top of the copy of the text or at the top of the index card. If an electronic notepad is used, the full citation should be entered, followed by notes relating to the article. Selection of the final material for the references is a matter of inclusion and exclusion. Only references that have been read at the source should be included in the bibliography. Many references that were originally evaluated will not prove to be of value, and these should be excluded from the final list appended to the manuscript. Authors must be certain that they understand the complete reference and that they cite the material in the reference correctly in the manuscript.

The major reason why authors should read the pertinent literature is to see if others have addressed the defined problem. Authors should remember that manuscripts are published for three major reasons: addition of information to the literature in support of an old idea, correction of information that is already in the literature by the addition of new and different data obtained from a study, and presentation of a new idea. Thus, by reading the literature, the authors can establish whether others have performed similar studies. If they have, and the literature is extensive, it is unlikely that the performance of the conceived study will be of value. On occasion, a longer period of follow-up or the identification of new problems after a particular procedure will benefit the reader. If others have written extensively on a problem, the authors must consider whether, in their judgment, the previously presented material is correct or whether their proposed study would correct erroneous information. If the authors think that the information in the literature is not correct, then the study design should include a mechanism whereby the information in the literature can be tested by the null hypothesis. Formation of the appropriate question to test the null hypothesis and obtaining of the necessary data in an accurate and valid fashion is the most appropriate way to proceed in the study of a problem.

Once the authors have read all of the literature, they must decide whether the study will be worthwhile and cost effective. The proposed study must advance science, not simply place an additional article in the literature. Man's ideas are infinite; the space available in the literature is finite. Thus, the authors must recognize, at an early stage, that only valid material has a good chance of being accepted for publication.

Protection of Patients' Rights

The authors should design the study in such a way that no patient's rights will be violated. The study must be done for the benefit of the patient; a single patient's rights cannot be sacrificed in the hope that a study will help society in general. The authors should obtain the approval of the institutional review board, or human rights committee, before embarking on a study. If such permission was not obtained, and if informed consent was not given by the individuals who participated in the study, the material will not be accepted for publication in *The Journal*.[3]

Statistics

The authors should consult a statistician at the onset of a study if they think that a statistical analysis should be performed on the data that they have obtained. The authors and statistician should review the suggestions of *The Journal* regarding the use of statistics.[4] Often, however, there is no reason to do a statistical analysis. At other times, statistically significant data are not clinically relevant. For example, an author may be able to show a statistically significant difference between a hospital stay of 10.4 days with one procedure and a stay of 10.8 days with another procedure, but this difference is hardly clinically relevant. Thus, it is important to involve a statistician at the onset, to be sure that the collected data are appropriate and the proposed statistical methods are valid. *The Journal* receives many articles from authors who have attempted to validate their study by statistical means when they did not have sufficient data, or the correct data, for statistical analysis. Even the most capable statistician cannot resurrect such a manuscript.

Performance of the Study

Once the authors have made sure that the study will be worthwhile, that the approval of the institutional review board has been obtained, and that the data will be sufficient for a valid statistical analysis (if a statistical analysis is to be used), they may proceed with the study. All data on all patients should be recorded systematically and accurately, with individual sheets used for each patient and the information summarized on tally sheets for the population as a whole. This will help to ensure that data will be available at all points in time for every patient. It will also facilitate accurate tabulation of the data and the subsequent creation of appropriate tables for the manuscript. When the information has been accurately recorded in tabular form, there is much less chance that an error regarding the numbers will occur when the manuscript is written.

Preparation of an Outline

The next step before writing is the preparation of an accurate outline. An outline ensures an organized approach to the problem and decreases the possibility that unnecessary information will be included. Once the outline has been completed, material that cannot be placed under an appropriate heading in the outline has no place in the manuscript. Regrettably, it is obvious that most authors do not create an outline before writing an article. More than half of the manuscripts received by *The Journal* for publication reflect this.

Writing of the Manuscript

Instructions to Authors

Before writing the manuscript, the authors should read the "Instructions to Authors," which appear immediately after the title page in each issue of *The Journal*. The Instructions should also be read by the individual who is going to prepare the manuscript for submission, and both the authors and their assistants should adhere to these Instructions.

Style

The authors should convey their ideas clearly, concisely, and accurately. While styles of writing differ, the easiest sentence to understand generally starts with a noun followed by a verb. Each sentence should express an idea, and one idea should follow another, sentence by sentence. Each paragraph should contain a complete concept, and each paragraph should lead logically to the next paragraph. The previously prepared outline will lead the authors logically through the manuscript.

Authors must guard against two major pitfalls: the use of jargon and the use of a shorthand style. *The Journal* is read by orthopaedists throughout the world, and a number of its readers may need a dictionary to learn the meaning of certain terms. Placement of jargon in quotes makes it no easier for the foreign reader to understand the word. Any word that has a meaning different than that found in the dictionary, or that would not be found in the dictionary, should be defined. Similarly, many specialties employ a jargon that is known only to the practitioners of that specialty. Manuscripts replete with such jargon are difficult for the general reader. If such terms are used at all, they should be defined the first time that they appear in the text.

The authors of an article have a much greater knowledge of their subject than the reader has, and they will often describe an operative procedure or the findings in a patient in a type of shorthand. While authors should be concise, they must remember that the general reader who does not have a specific knowledge of the subject matter will be lost if each step of an operative procedure is not presented in detail.

The Parts of the Manuscript

Introductory Paragraph Each section of the manuscript should include certain information. The introductory paragraph should begin with a concise statement of the problem, with brief reference to the pertinent literature (extensive citing of the literature should be left for the Discussion), and end with the purposes of the study. In simplest form, the final sentence in the introductory paragraph should state that the study was done to provide additional information regarding a particular clinical entity or operative procedure, or that the study was done to refute information in the literature.

Materials and Methods The Materials and Methods section should provide demographic data on the study population and state the period of time during which the study was performed, where the study was done, who supervised the treatment of the patients, and who evaluated the patients at the time of the follow-up. The section should also include specific reasons for the selection and exclusion of patients, the specific indications for an operative procedure, the details of how that operation was performed, how long the patients were followed before and after an operative procedure, and any special studies that were performed on the patients. If a standard procedure was done, a simple reference to that procedure may be all that is necessary. However, if the operation involved modifications of a previously described procedure, these modifications should be given in detail. If a new procedure was done, or if there were major modifications, a detailed description of the entire procedure should be included. Similarly, laboratory studies may be simply alluded to if they are common, but they should be described in detail if they are not. All parameters involved in the use of magnetic resonance imaging should be described in detail, as should all statistical methods.

Attention should be paid to the accurate recording of data. The manuscript that notes that 29 patients, including 11 men and 17 women, were examined causes an editor to wonder how carefully the data were evaluated. A paper that states that 78 knee replacements were performed in 50 patients, of which 47 were successful, leaves open the question as to whether success was obtained in 47 knees or 47 patients. When dealing with bilateral procedures, authors must be especially careful to be sure that the data are accurate.

Results The Results section should be a detailed report of all of the data obtained during the study. The data should be consistent throughout the text and between the text, the tables, the figures and legends, and the Abstract. Again, authors must be careful to avoid the confusion that can result when bilateral procedures are being reported on.

Data should be reported accurately, but not to several decimal places. It makes little sense to state that the average duration of hospitalization was 10.48 days, that the average transfusion was 320.24 ml, or that the average progression of a scoliotic curve was 1.27° per year. Percentages, too, can be overly accurate. It is inappropriate to note that 29 patients represented

48.33% of a population of 60 patients. All percentages should be rounded off to whole numbers. Percentages should not be used with numbers less than 20.

Discussion The Discussion section should serve several functions. The literature should be summarized and the authors' findings should be related to the literature. The strengths and weaknesses of the study should be described in detail, and the pertinent findings of the study should be summarized. The Discussion should not repeat the results; rather, it must justify the conclusions that may be drawn from the results.

Illustrations Photographs and radiographs serve the purpose of illustrating important points in the text. They should not be mere add-ons, included simply to break up the text. The use of illustrations should be considered as the study is being undertaken. As the authors find points that they wish to emphasize, appropriate illustrations should be selected. It is inappropriate, and almost impossible, to select illustrations after the study has been completed.

The illustrations must be of the highest quality, or they cannot be reproduced well. Any lines drawn to measure angles on radiographs, and any identifying material such as dates or initials, should be removed before the radiographs are photographed. Information that the authors wish to convey should be placed in the legend. Arrows or lines forming angles may be placed on the print by an artist, or on an overlay.

Authors should select illustrations with care, remembering that *The Journal* is not a photo album. Authors should also recognize that a radiograph of the normal side is seldom necessary, as most readers of *The Journal* will know what the normal side looks like.

Tables Tables take up a great deal of space and should be used only to add information that cannot be included in the text. Generally, a table should list the patients in the study and provide detailed information regarding each patient. The use of a table with only two or three columns is seldom warranted, unless it is appropriate for emphasis of a specific important finding. If the information in the table can be stated in two or three lines in the text, there is no reason to include the table. Tables that are simply lists, such as those derived from slides, are inappropriate.

There are several electronic versions of *The Journal*, one of which does not include tables. Therefore, when tables are used to present detailed information, averages and ranges should be summarized briefly in the text to give the reader who does not have access to the tables a sense of what is included in them.

References For manuscripts submitted for publication in *The Journal*, the references should be listed alphabetically. They should be included only if the reference has been read at the source and the information has been used in the text. Each reference must be referred to in the text. The full citation of all authors

and complete pagination should be included.

Title The title, which should be composed after the manuscript has been completed, should summarize the study as completely as possible, in as few words as possible. The authors should remember that words such as treatment and operation will not aid an individual who is attempting to retrieve the manuscript from a database.

Abstract The Abstract should also be written after the manuscript has been completed. The Abstract should state the problem, what was done, the results, and the conclusion. The purpose of the Abstract is to convey the authors' findings as concisely as possible. The authors should not attempt to induce the reader to read the full paper by supplying incomplete information in the Abstract; rather, the Abstract should provide complete information regarding the manuscript.

Preparation of the Manuscript

The manuscript should be printed double-spaced, and the pages should be numbered. A dot-matrix printer should not be used, because *The Journal* scans manuscripts electronically during the production process and a dot-matrix print-out is extremely difficult to scan.

The authors should check the manuscript to be sure that it adheres to the "Instructions to Authors" before the manuscript is sent to *The Journal*. The manuscript also should be proofread. Authors should remember that, while word processors have a spell-check function, they do not know the difference between seen and scene or between cite, site, and sight. Moreover, the word processor cannot select the appropriate references for the manuscript. In the past, *The Journal* received a manuscript on the hip accompanied by a set of references relating to the shoulder. When questioned, the author responded, "For reasons which are not entirely clear to me, the references for this paper and another book chapter were inadvertently mixed up on the word processor." Such a response hardly leaves the editor with a good feeling regarding the contents of the manuscript. When reviewing a manuscript before submission, authors must make sure that they have used appropriate terms and that they have used them consistently. One manuscript submitted during the last year contained the word allograft when the correct words were autologous graft. When questioned, the author responded, "Unfortunately, the word allograft was used on two occasions [actually, he meant twice in the same paragraph] instead of autograft." The author went on to state, "I apologize for overseeing this mistake." Such inattention to detail and inappropriate use of words does little to enhance the publishable quality of a manuscript.

The Peer-Review Process

Once received in *The Journal* office, the manuscript will be evaluated and sent out for peer review to two or three consultant reviewers, or associate editors, who have been selected on the basis of their knowledge and of their interest in reviewing material for *The Journal*. Reviewers come both from academic institutions and from the clinical practice of orthopaedics. It is the editor's responsibility to select the reviewers as a group, and to select the specific reviewer for each manuscript. In order to do this, the editor must be aware of the abilities and expertise of the consultant reviewers. A manuscript is often sent to one reviewer who has a special interest in the subject of the manuscript, and to a second reviewer who does not, so that *The Journal* can obtain an opinion regarding the interest of the manuscript to the general orthopaedic audience. The editor must show no bias in the selection of reviewers and must evaluate each review to make sure that it contains no bias. *The Journal* provides a handout to instruct reviewers about how to evaluate manuscripts. When the reviews have been returned, and the decision regarding the acceptance of the manuscript has been made, each reviewer receives a copy of all of the reviews regarding that particular manuscript and a copy of the decision letter. Thus, the reviewer is informed of the opinions of others and obtains feedback regarding the decision process.

The editor has the responsibility of choosing new reviewers, and of retiring individuals who do not provide helpful reviews. Each review is graded, and the time that was required for the return of the review is noted. Individuals who consistently take more than three weeks to return a review are retired, as are those who do not provide consistently excellent reviews or who are found to be biased. *The Journal* has a group of approximately 400 consultant reviewers at any one time, and this group is constantly changing. Approximately 1000 manuscripts are reviewed, on first submission, each year, and approximately 16% of them are accepted for publication. The reviewers evaluate more than 100 of these manuscripts a second time and, on occasion, a third time, before a final decision is made regarding publication. During the peer-review process, the editor's responsibility is to be fair and to be prompt in returning a decision letter to the authors.

The Selection Process

During the selection process, the editor has a responsibility to the reader and to the author. For the reader, the editor must select valid and accurate material that will help physicians to care for their patients. At the same time, the editor must stem the tide of worthless jargon that crosses his or her desk. Authors should remember that only one of six manuscripts will be accepted for publication. The reasons for rejection relate to the high quality sought by *The Journal*; they are not dictated by the space available for publication in *The Journal*. Authors must be aware that manuscripts are submitted to *The Journal* "because of its reputation and editorial standards" and should take pride in the fact that their manuscript, if accepted, "helps to maintain those standards and adds to that reputation."[5]

The editor also has the obligation to be as fair as possible to the authors. Additional reviews may be obtained if they are necessary for an impartial decision, and it must be ensured that no bias was introduced into the selection process by either the editor or a reviewer. On occasion, reviewers will disagree about whether a study should be published. When this occurs, a third reviewer may be consulted, or the manuscript may be discussed at a workshop of the Board of Associate Editors. These workshops are held every two months, and approximately 18 manuscripts are discussed at each one. The manuscripts are sent to associate editors before the workshop, so any manuscript that is discussed at a workshop has been evaluated by at least two consultant reviewers, one or more editors in *The Journal* office, and three associate editors before the workshop. A decision is reached by consensus, or by a vote if necessary. The majority rules. While the editor concurs with the decision made at the workshop, it should be recognized that, in all other instances, the final decision is the editor's responsibility. Authors sometimes question reviewers' comments, with the suggestion that it was the reviewer who rejected the manuscript. In fact, the editor makes the final decision after taking into account all of the reviewers' comments.

Major Reasons for Rejection

Authors should be aware of the primary reasons why articles are not accepted for publication and make an effort to address these concerns before submitting a manuscript to *The Journal*. First, authors should take into account the selection of the patients for the study. Only patients who have the specific disease entity or the specific procedure under study should be included. If, for example, the manuscript is to deal with the findings in patients who have been managed with resection of bone and replacement with a segmental allograft because of a malignant tumor, the authors should not attempt to increase the series by including patients who had a giant-cell tumor of the distal part of the radius or another non-malignant lesion. The authors should select as homogeneous a group of patients as possible. If patients who are not suitable for the series are included, and if, by chance, the manuscript is determined to have sufficient information to warrant publication, the authors will have the onerous task of eliminating patients from the study and redoing all of the calculations and statistical analysis used in the manuscript.

A second major reason for rejection of a manuscript is the lack of adequately detailed indications for the selection of patients for an operative procedure. The authors should have specific indications in mind before performing a procedure. To say that a procedure was done for a leg-length discrepancy is inappropriate. A specific amount of leg-length discrepancy should be required for a particular operation.

Manuscripts are also rejected when they do not provide sufficient data regarding the patients or complete detail regarding the results. If the study deals with the results of an operative procedure, complete preoperative and postoperative data on all patients should be provided. This is almost always impossible when a study involves a retrospective review of charts, because much of the needed information is not included in the charts. This is one reason why a prospective study has a much greater chance of producing meaningful data than does a retrospective study.

A fourth reason for rejection is an inaccurate description of the operative procedure or of the patients. For example, a manuscript dealing with a procedure on the foot that notes that the pin was placed through the heads of the third, fourth, and fifth metatarsals reveals that the authors have a poor understanding of the anatomy of the foot. It is virtually impossible to pass a pin through the heads of these three bones; the pin must be placed through the shaft, rather than the head, of at least one of these metatarsals. Similarly, a description of a patient as having tight hamstrings and a normal lumbar lordosis suggests to the editor that an incomplete physical examination was done.

Next, the conclusions must be consistent and must be drawn from the data included in the manuscript. A manuscript that states that seven patients had a wound infection, four had non-union of the osteotomy site, and three had peroneal palsy, and yet asserts that the grades of all but two of the results of the procedure were excellent, reflects a poor understanding of the evaluation of patients.

Finally, the most common reason for rejection of a clinical manuscript is that the duration of the follow-up was less than two years. While a follow-up period of less than two years may be indicated if the manuscript deals with poor results that were seen early after a procedure, and while a short follow-up may also be permissible when certain fractures are dealt with, a two-year period is mandatory after reconstructive procedures and after the treatment of any fractures that might be associated with long-term complications. *The Journal* prefers a five-year follow-up for many reconstructive procedures. Follow-up until the patient reaches maturity is ideal for any study of reconstructive procedures done in children, but this is rarely possible.

Authors should also be aware that there are certain reasons for the rejection of a Case Report. In order to be publishable, a Case Report should have educational value.[6] The documentation of a rare lesion in a rare location seldom meets this criterion. Similarly, a report on a fracture or a condition that is easy to diagnose and amenable to standard treatment seldom is accepted for publication. A second reason for the rejection of a Case Report is that the material — again, albeit rare — is available in standard texts. A third reason for rejection is that the report documents obviously inappropriate treatment. A Case Report that states that a poor result was obtained after a patellar ligament was removed inadvertently or inappropriately, and reattached improperly, does not warrant publication. Similarly, a Case Report about a patient who had normal radiographs preoperatively and no indications for total knee arthroplasty does not warrant publication even though the patient had an untoward complication after the arthroplasty. While it is not the editor's place to suggest how authors should practice medicine, the editor cannot accept inane material for publication. Finally, many Case Reports are submitted because they are the so-called first published report of the condition. Rarely, however, are they actually the first. There is even less reason to publish a Case Report that begins: "This is only the eleventh case of this lesion reported in the English literature."

The Editing Process

During the editing of a manuscript, it is the editor's responsibility to be prompt, to be helpful, to correct the data in the manuscript, and to not be pejorative to the authors. All editing involves an exchange between the authors and the editor. The editor makes suggestions for the authors to act on. If the authors disagree with the editor's suggestions, then an exchange must take place to resolve these concerns.

The editor attempts to correct outlandish grammar and syntax but leaves most of this work to the copy editors, who receive the manuscript once revision has been completed. Rather, it is the function of the editor to identify problems that interfere with the author presenting the material in the best fashion possible. The editor identifies discrepancies in the data, eliminates jargon, identifies questions that the authors should address, and makes sure that the authors have provided all of the data necessary to support appropriate conclusions.

It is at this time that the editor often determines that the authors did not use an outline in the preparation of the manuscript. Frequently, it is necessary for the editor to create this outline for the authors, so that the manuscript will flow in a logical fashion.

Together, the editor and authors should determine what the reader will want to know and how to supply this information. The editor asks questions that he or she thinks will be asked by the reader, with the hope that the answers will result in a comprehensive text. The editor must often take the position of the average reader and ask the authors to provide the details left out from a shorthand description of their operative procedure or experimental approach. The authors should answer the editor's questions in the text of the manuscript, with the explanations in an accompanying letter. Authors must remember that their ultimate goal is to satisfy the reader rather than the editor. They should also remember that there is a permanence to material published in *The Journal*, that it is difficult if not impossible to correct errors once they have appeared in print, and that the editor is attempting to save them from the embarrassment that would result from the publication of inaccurate material.

After the manuscript has been edited, it will contain numbers in the margin referring to a detailed, numbered series of concerns in an accompanying letter. An edited manuscript will, on the average, be accompanied by a six- or seven-page letter, detailing 50 to 60 concerns that need to be addressed by the authors.

The Revision Process

The revision process is designed to enhance the value of the manuscript to the reader and to make it easier to read. When the authors receive the acceptance letter, they should review the manuscript along with the letter. The questions should not be answered without checking the editing that has already been done. The authors should realize that the questions were asked in an effort to improve the manuscript, and they should revise the manuscript in response to the detailed concerns expressed by the editor. When they return the revised manuscript, it must be accompanied by a letter noting, in detail, how each of the concerns was addressed and, if any concerns were not addressed, providing an adequate reason why they were not. The authors must realize that if they cannot address certain concerns, the manuscript may not be accepted for publication. On the other hand, an author should not blindly accept the editor's suggestions. If the authors truly think that a suggestion is inappropriate, then the reasons should be conveyed to the editor. The process of editing and revising should involve a friendly exchange, with both the authors and the editor realizing that the goal is a clear, concise, and accurate manuscript. After the authors have made all of the necessary corrections, they should read the manuscript again instead of merely asking an assistant to retype it.

While the editor's aim is to identify all concerns during the first editing of the manuscript, and while the authors' aim should be to answer all of the editor's questions during the first revision, the editor frequently will identify additional concerns or those that the authors did not deal with adequately, when the revised manuscript is returned. On occasion, so little has been done to address the concerns that the manuscript cannot be accepted for publication, but usually any remaining or additional problems can be resolved with a second revision.

Responding to Rejection

The editor recognizes that the receipt of a rejection letter is a tremendous blow, because the authors have devoted a great deal of time to the preparation of a manuscript. However, the editor, while distressed at having to reject manuscripts, has a responsibility to provide quality material to the reader. Also, authors should remember that if they have fulfilled their responsibilities, the chances of acceptance are high. Authors should also remember that rejection of a manuscript that does not meet the standards of *The Journal* serves to protect their reputation as well.

The authors should read and understand the entire rejection letter before replying. Rejection letters take three basic forms. If the editor and the reviewers think that, with extensive work, the manuscript might be publishable, the authors are invited to revise and resubmit the manuscript. The reviewers' comments must be taken into account before the manuscript is resubmitted. If there is a good chance such a manuscript will be accepted for publication, the editor often supplies a personal set of comments for the authors. On the other hand, if extensive revision is required, the editor does not supply a series of comments at this time, but, rather, offers the possibility of a second review of the manuscript after the revision. A second type of rejection letter includes the reviewers' comments but also the suggestion that the manuscript not be revised and resubmitted. A third type of rejection letter details the two or three major reasons why the manuscript cannot be accepted for publication. It is not appropriate for the authors to revise and resubmit a manuscript if they have received either of these latter types of letters.

A final appeals mechanism is available to authors who totally disagree with the editor for what they think are valid reasons. The authors can send the editor a letter noting the specific reasons for the disagreement. If the reasons seem valid, the manuscript will be evaluated at a workshop of the Board of Associate Editors. However, authors should be aware that the editor's decision has been made after a careful evaluation and that, while it is possible that the workshop will reverse the editor's decision, this rarely happens.

Responsibilities When Manuscripts Have Multiple Authors

The Journal has been concerned about the increase in the number of authors listed on a manuscript.[7,8] For this reason, *The Journal*, in its "Instructions to Authors," suggests that no more than six authors be included in a byline. In reality, most manuscripts should list only two or three authors. If an article has more than one author, each must have had a part in the planning of the project, must have worked on the project, must have helped in the writing of the manuscript, must have read the entire manuscript, must have helped in the revision process, and must be responsible for the content of the manuscript—that is, each should be able to defend the entire contents of the manuscript in a public forum. Having supplied the statistical analysis or having evaluated the radiographs does not qualify one as an author. It should be remembered that the purpose of scientific publication is to disseminate accurate information to readers, not to enhance an author's curriculum vitae. It is hard for the editor to understand how eight authors can be listed on a single Case Report, but this has happened.

In the past, *The Journal* has occasionally received a note that a manuscript was sent in without the knowledge of one of the coauthors. Thus, *The Journal* requires that each author sign a statement that he or she has read and approved the final manuscript.

Detection of Fraud

It has been suggested that one of the responsibilities of the editor is to detect fraudulent material. While every effort is made to do so during the editoral process, it is much easier to detect errors in data or in the description of an operative procedure than it is to detect outright fraud. Nevertheless, the editor is aware of such problems,[9] and each manuscript is scrutinized carefully with this possibility in mind.

Final Thoughts

Both the authors and the editor have responsibilities that they must be aware of when preparing manuscripts for publication. While the responsibilities of each are similar, the nature of the process dictates that each will approach their responsibilities from a different perspective. First, authors approach the project of preparing a manuscript for publication as a task that has a definite completion time, and they think more of the present than of the future. They see publication as the completion of the project. The editor recognizes that publication is also, in a sense, a beginning. The reader, and future authors, will use the published material as the basis for future work. Thus, the editor is aware of a permanence not always appreciated by the author.

Second, authors devote a great deal of time to the performance of the study and the preparation of the manuscript and thus have a vested interest in the project. The authors' interest is focused on the specific material in the manuscript and they want to see this manuscript published. The editor, on the other hand, has a broad perspective and no vested interest. The editor focuses more on how the manuscript will add to medical knowledge than on the publication of specific facts.

Both, however, have an interest in the manuscript and hope that the personal investment on the part of the authors and editor will produce dividends: the advancement of science, recognition, praise for a job well done, and, perhaps, academic advancement. As both the authors and the editor share most of these concerns, it is apparent that they all should put their best effort into fulfilling their individual responsibilities in preparing a manuscript for publication.

The practice of medicine depends on accuracy in the scientific literature. The ultimate goal of the editorial process is the presentation of accurate and valid data to the reader. For authors to produce less, or for the editor to accept less, would signify a shirking of the authors' and the editor's responsibility to society.

References

1. Editorial: A Plea for conciseness in writing. *JAMA* 1900; 35:164-165.
2. Editorial: Medical literature and medical writing. *JAMA* 1900;35:626-627.
3. Cowell HR: Editorial: Informed consent. *J Bone Joint Surg* 1992;74A:639-640.
4. Senghas RE: Editorial: Statistics in The Journal of Bone and Joint Surgery; Suggestions for authors. *J Bone Joint Surg* 1992;74A:319-320.
5. Curtiss PH Jr: Writing for The Journal of Bone and Joint Surgery. *J Bone Joint Surg* 1979;61A:799-804.
6. Cowell HR: Editorial: The case report. *J Bone Joint Surg* 1987;69A:639.
7. Cowell HR: Editorial: Responsibilities of authors. *J Bone Joint Surg* 1987;69A:1311.
8. Cowell HR: Editorial: Multiple authorship of manuscripts. *J Bone Joint Surg* 1989;71A:639-640.
9. Broad W, Wade N: *Betrayers of the Truth, Fraud and Deceit in the Halls of Science.* New York, NY, Simon and Schuster, 1982.

Challenging the Validity of Conclusions Based on P-values Alone: A Critique of Contemporary Clinical Research Design and Methods

Edward Ebramzadeh, MS

Harry McKellop, PhD

Frederick Dorey, PhD

Augusto Sarmiento, MD

Introduction

In the last few decades, clinical investigators have become increasingly aware that the use of statistical methods to assess the reliability of the outcome of a study forms an essential part of the scientific decision-making process. Unfortunately, among clinical researchers, there is a widespread misunderstanding of the meaning of the term, "statistical significance." Despite a consistent and emphatic outcry from statisticians and epidemiologists, the widely held misconceptions that $P \leq 0.05$ is synonymous with statistically significant, and that statistically significant is synonymous with clinically significant or scientifically significant, have permeated the community, and are responsible for serious, ongoing damage to the scientific literature.

Several articles have been published in the medical, statistical, and epidemiologic literature in which the authors have attempted to clarify the meaning of P-values and statistical significance for the biomedical researcher.[1-7] In spite of these efforts, many investigators, as well as editors and reviewers of medical journals, continue to misinterpret the meaning of the P-value and the role it plays in the overall decision-making process.

This chapter seeks to convince the reader of two concepts. First, we will demonstrate that a P-value considered alone does not distinguish important from unimportant results and, second, that phrases such as "a statistically significant difference was observed" or "no significant difference was measured" would best be eliminated from the clinical and biomedical literature altogether. To accomplish our goal, we will need to discuss some issues involved in research design and data analysis.

Throughout the chapter, we will assume that the scatter in the measurements in our examples results primarily from the natural variation in the subject population from which the samples were drawn, rather than from error caused by inadequate precision of the measuring instruments, mistakes in calibrating machines or in logging the data, or other types of measurement error that might lead to bias. Therefore, the P-value reflects the probability that the observed difference occurred by chance, that is, that we randomly selected subjects from the experimental and/or control groups that were not representative of the parent populations from which they were drawn.

Shortcomings of P-values

A Hypothetical Study

We will begin with a simple example to demonstrate one of the most common decision-making processes using statistical methods. A clinical investigator was interested in comparing the effectiveness of a newly developed drug to treat a specific fatal type of infectious disease. This investigator conducted a randomized, prospective study, comparing the outcome for two similar groups of patients, one treated with drug A (the experimental drug), and the other with drug B, a conventional drug that had been used with limited success over the last few years. Assume for the moment that drug A costs somewhat more, and that neither drug produces any significant side effects.

The investigator found that the rate of recovery from the infection was 30% higher in the group treated with the experimental drug A than in the group treated with the conventional drug B. However, a large variation in the grade and progression of the infection among patients and the relatively small number of patients in each group caused the corresponding P-value for the measured difference in recovery rates to be 0.11, well above the level of 0.05 that is often used to designate statistical significance.

A Wrong Decision Based on the P-value

In the subsequent publication of the above study, the investigator reported simply that "There was no statistically significant difference in mortality between patients treated with drug A and those treated with drug B (P > 0.05)." The investigator proceeded to recommend the continued use of the conventional drug B over the new drug A for three reasons: (1) because no significant difference was found, (2) because the new drug costs more, and (3) because use of the conventional drug was standard, routine procedure. Based on this published information, several other institutions abandoned development of the experimental product.

The reader will surely appreciate that something is seriously wrong with the above application of the concept of statistical significance. Although the above form of decision-making is common practice, it represents a serious misuse of statistics that, nevertheless, is often encouraged or even required by the reviewers and editors of prominent medical journals. Clearly, if treatment with drug A has the potential to save the lives of more of the patients who have this disease, and there are no apparent side effects, then these results should not be dismissed in such an absolute way. Reporting simply that "no significant difference in mortality was noted between the two groups" would be a serious disservice to the medical and scientific community and, most importantly, to those patients whose lives might be saved by treatment with the new drug.

Unfortunately, this is precisely the type of interpretation, and terminology, that has come to permeate the clinical literature. For example, as a result of commonly held misconceptions regarding statistical significance, some journals have misguidedly come to require that the word "significance" be used *only* in relation to a *statistically* significant result, without regard to clinical or scientific significance,[8] and many journals allow the word significant only in association with P-values of less than 0.05.[9] Many have taken this type of confusion a step further by implying that the lower the P-value, the more important or valid the result. For example, an editorial in a prominent psychology journal[10] stated that, while results associated with a significance level of 0.05 may qualify for symposia and handouts, in order to qualify for archival journal publication, generally a P-value of 0.01 would be required.

For many investigators, having an associated P-value greater than 0.05 is considered to indicate that the observed difference is somehow an illusion, and that the statistical calculations fortunately save us from erroneously accepting the results as real. This is an absolutely wrong interpretation of the meaning of the P-value. In our example, as long as the result of the study is the only information that we have on the effect of drug A, the best estimate of the rate of recovery in a group of patients taking drug A is that it will be 30% higher than in the control group. Conversely, a P-value exceeding 0.05, or any other fixed value, does not mean that the rate of recovery will be the same for the two groups, or any difference other than 30%. As we shall discuss later on, in order to determine the stability and precision of this estimate, we need to calculate the confidence interval surrounding the 30% differ-

ence. While the consequences of such erroneous interpretations in the medical literature are typically more subtle than in our intentionally dramatic example, they nevertheless represent many misleading conclusions and serious loss of potentially important research knowledge.

Objective Conclusions and Reporting of the Results

To further clarify this issue, the reader should imagine being among those clinicians who are desperately in search of a more effective treatment for the infectious disease in our example and should consider which of the four following reports represents the proper, logical deduction from the information at hand, and which is the most complete and accurate for reporting the results of the above study. (1) There was no significant difference in the recovery rate between the group taking drug A and the control group taking drug B ($P > 0.05$). (2) The group taking drug A showed a statistically insignificant greater recovery rate ($P > 0.05$). (3) The group taking drug A had a 30% greater rate of recovery, although this was not statistically significant ($P > 0.05$). (4) The group taking drug A had a 30% greater recovery rate, with associated 95% confidence limits of –15% to 75% ($P = 0.11$). Because this represents a potentially large and important clinical improvement, because there are no known deleterious side effects of taking drug A in this dosage, and because there was just over one chance in ten that the 30% difference occurred by accidental selection, we feel that it is justified to accept the results as true and to recommend the administration of drug A to patients with this disease while further studies are taking place.

The fourth statement clearly represents the most sound interpretation and conclusion. It also conveys the essence of the findings to the reader, and demonstrates how these findings are not overshadowed by the P-value in arriving at the decision to accept the results. Rather than an oversimplified statement of whether the results were "statistically significant" or not, the data, along with a range of likely values as well as the associated P-value, are presented, followed by an assessment of the scientific or clinical importance of the results.

In contrast, the first two statements provide virtually no useful information to the reader and, in fact, serve to hide the fact that a cure for the disease may be at hand. The third statement, while an improvement over the first two, still fails to address those issues that are more important than the P-value, such as what constitutes a scientifically or clinically important increase in the rate of recovery from the disease, what the potential benefits are of accepting the study's result as real, and what the potential losses are in rejecting it as false. Only after such issues are addressed can one decide whether the certainty of the results, represented by the confidence interval and/or the P-value, is small enough to justify accepting or rejecting the results.

More on Decision-Making Based on P-values

There are historical reasons why results with P-values of 0.05 or less have mistakenly come to be taken as synonymous with statistically significant in so many studies today. The significance level of 0.05 was originally devised as an arbitrary convention by Sir Ronald Fisher,[9,11] who also laid the foundation for the formal process of testing for significance (hypothesis testing), which we will describe in some detail. Fisher, who has been called the greatest statistician who ever lived,[12] along with a number of most influential statisticians of our century, later denounced the widespread practice of considering any single significance level as always indicating statistical significance. Similarly, Kendall and Stuart,[13] writing in *The Advanced Theory of Statistics*, avoided the use of the word "significance" altogether, perhaps to prevent confusion between clinical and statistical significance.[9] In his book on clinical epidemiology, Feinstein[9] cites these and other eminent statisticians and mathematicians, including Yates,[14] Box,[15] and others, who have vigorously complained about how researchers commonly misuse statistical significance. Feinstein notes that in this regard, Box[15] referred to such researchers as being "overawed by what they do not understand" and who "mistakenly distrust their own common sense and adopt inappropriate (mathematical) procedures." As elaborated by Feinstein:[16]

"The [faulty] method of making statistical decisions about 'significance' creates one of the most devastating ironies in modern biological science...a clinician investigator will usually go to enormous efforts in mensuration. He will get special machines and elaborate technologic devices to supplant his old categorical statements with new measurements of 'continuous' dimensional data. After all this work in getting 'continuous' data, however, and after calculating all the statistical tests of the data, the investigator then makes the final decision about his results on the basis of a completely arbitrary pair of dichotomous categories. These categories, which are often called 'significant' and 'nonsignificant,' are usually demarcated by a P-value of either 0.05 or 0.01, chosen according to the capricious dictates of the statistician, the editor, the reviewer, or the granting agency. If the level demanded for 'significant' is 0.05 or lower, and the P-value that emerges is 0.06, the investigator may be ready to discard a well-designed, excellently conducted, thoughtfully analyzed, and scientifically important experiment, because it failed to cross the Procrustean boundary demanded for statistical approbation."

Elsewhere, Feinstein[9] writes:

"Because clinicians have a long tradition of avoiding any specifications for quantitative judgements....there are no medical standards for quantitative significance....The absence of standards of quantitative significance...has been a boon for investigators, pharmaceutical companies, editors, and regulatory agencies.... It has enabled the accomplishments....to be appraised exclusively according to standards of....[statistical]....significance....If P is < 0.05, the investigator is granted approval for the claim that the observed distinction is significant....Because the desideratum of P < 0.05 can always be obtained [by studying a larger sample], no matter how trivial the quantitative importance of the observed distinction, investigators who were wise enough (or fiscally supported enough) to study large groups have been able to achieve significance and to gain editorial or regulatory approval for claiming a significant action for agents that had minor importance in science or in clinical therapy. Conversely, however, an investigator who has found an agent of major quantitative importance may have his paper rejected for publication or his drug disapproved for marketing because one or two of patients dropped out of the study, thereby raising the P value above 0.05 to the disastrous height of 0.06. This policy continues to be applied....even though [it] has been disclaimed or condemned by Fisher himself and other prominent leaders in...statistics."

Bias in the Literature

In addition to preventing publication of potentially important, clinically significant research, these misguided policies have created a systematic bias in the literature. This occurs because only those papers that have shown a particular difference at a "statistically significant" level (commonly $P \leq 0.05$) are published, even though a larger number of studies may have used the same method and measured the same type of difference, but obtained a lower level of statistical significance, indicated by a larger P-value. Thus, when one conducts a survey mathematically combining the results of several studies (technically called a meta-analysis),[17] the prior selection of those studies with low P-values for publication creates a false impression of the overall level of certainty associated with the observed difference.

Conversely, if several investigators, working independently and using similar methods on similar samples, each observe a particular difference, but with P-values that, individually, would not justify accepting the results, the combined results (obtained by a meta-analysis) may provide an acceptable level of certainty. The reason for this combined difference may be clarified by referring to the fundamental principles of probability.[17] Each time that a particular apparent result is obtained in independent investigations, the combined probability of the difference having occurred by chance selection is decreased. It is through this process that the scientific method is used to increase progressively our confidence in an observed difference when that difference represents a true effect, particularly when the number of samples included in each individual study is small and the inherent scatter is large. This illustrates yet another important reason for not adopting a significance level of 0.05, or any other specific value, as a criterion for publishing scientific results.

Scientific Deduction Versus Decision Making

In order to understand how we generally come up with decisions following observation of a particular difference, we need to clarify our thinking process. Consider an everyday occurrence in clinical practice; to select between two or more methods of treatment for a particular case. Suppose that you are faced with making such a decision, and that you have just read the results of a study, such as our initial example above, that appears to show an advantage with one of two treatments. Rather than a single decision, there are now two distinct considerations at hand. First, you need to assess what can be learned from the information obtained with the sample, and whether you believe the results of the study to be an accurate representation of the true difference in effectiveness of the treatments in the general population. To assist in making this first decision, you may use statistical methods such as a P-value, confidence intervals, or other measures, as we will discuss later on. Once you have made the decision on whether or not you accept the results of the study, the second decision is what course of action you should take. This decision is made partly based on whether or not you believed the results to be representative of the differences, but also on risk-benefit assessments and other practical considerations. As Edwards and associates[18] stated, "Sometimes the.... definition of [statistical] testing is expressed as a decision to act as though one of the two hypotheses were believed, and that has apparently led to some confusion. What action is wise of course depends in part on what is at stake. You would not take the plane if you believed it would crash, and would not buy flight insurance if you believed it would not." Choosing to take a course of action other than what the results of the study suggested is not necessarily equivalent to believing that the results of the study are false. In short, we need to distinguish between our judgment on the data on the one hand, and our decision regarding an action on the other.

To clarify this point, consider an example of a mountaineer descending a glacier and faced with the choice of either jumping across a narrow but very deep crevasse, or of walking several tiring miles around the crevasse to arrive at his camp. The mountaineer has no rope, so failing to jump completely across the crevasse will result in his death. However, he has practiced such jumps wearing a rope in the past and knows that his mean jumping distance is twice the width of the crevasse, with an associated P-value of 0.001. Thus, while he is almost certain that he can jump across the crevasse (he believes his data to be a true representation of his jumping skill in general), because there is a small probability that his data was obtained by chance, combined with the severe penalty of death if it is wrong, he chooses to walk around the crevasse.

Now consider a second mountaineer faced with the same decision. He is not quite as consistent a jumper as the first, such that, although his mean jumping distance is also twice the width of the crevasse, the associated P-value is 0.1. Although he at first also chooses to walk around the crevasse, a nearby television crew offers him one million dollars to make the jump on camera. With this in mind, the second mountaineer now chooses to attempt the jump.

Comparable situations arise in medical science when an apparent experimental difference is demonstrated with a very low P-value that, if correct, would cause a major change in current theory or organizational policies. That is, if the results are accepted, then it will be necessary to rewrite textbooks, to redesign experimental equipment to take the effect into account, and to reallocate millions of dollars of research funds in this area. Because this would be a major disaster if it was subsequently learned that the apparent difference occurred by chance, the scientific community may justifiably choose to reject the results, despite a P-value of, say, 0.001, until several independent investigators have obtained similar results with comparably low P-values. Once again, however, rejecting such results is not the same as believing them to be false, in spite of whether the associated P-value is 0.001 or 0.1. Conversely, if an apparent measured difference is consistent with present theory (or, if there are no contradictory results or theory) and the penalties for a wrong decision are minor, it may be appropriate to accept results that have potential scientific or clinical importance, despite a relatively high P-value.

In the above examples, the mountaineers used the P-value to assess the risk of being wrong in concluding that they could jump over the crevasse. For the first mountaineer, there was a one in a thousand chance of being wrong in concluding that he could jump successfully; for the second mountaineer this chance was one in ten. Obviously, in order to arrive at a decision, it was more useful for the mountaineers to know the actual P-value, which represents the risk that they are taking, rather than only if the P-value was less or more than

0.05, or some other specific value, which is all they would know if they were only told the result was "significant" or "not significant."

The Controversy Over Hypothesis Testing

Hypothesis testing was adopted as an indispensable tool for industrial applications and quality control. For instance, in factory assembly lines, a decision needed to be made regarding the quality control based on a small sample of the day's lot. The choices were distinct: accept the day's lot or reject it. Therefore, a standard, routine, simple and relatively thought-free[19] way of making this decision needed to be developed. The answer was to measure a critical value with the sample, and base the decision on whether the difference between the measurement obtained with the sample and a control value was statistically significant or not. This facilitated making many decisions that would, in the long run, produce a controlled amount of variation in the outcome.

In contrast to industrial applications, in the scientific world, measurements are performed primarily to further our knowledge and understanding of how the world works.[19] Although we certainly use this knowledge in our daily decision making, we must distinguish between the process of making judgments about the data and decision making. The distinction is subtle but important, because it affects the way we interpret our observations and decide on the consequent course of action.[19,20] To clarify the issue, consider once more the example of the mountaineers who were faced with either jumping the crevasse or walking a long, tiring distance. Each one made a decision which was partly influenced by the knowledge gathered from previous experience but was primarily based on practical issues that had little to do with statistical significance. Because we are human, our decisions are to a large degree governed by our desire to obtain the benefits and by our fear of the penalties, and, therefore, they can at times be far from objective.

These considerations have led to two schools of thought regarding scientific research design and data analysis. Some statisticians still believe that, as in the factory setting described above, hypothesis testing is a useful tool for research.[21] That is, if we set up the study appropriately, we can and should determine our course of action, such as which treatment to use, based on the scientific and statistical significance of the data. These statisticians still recommend hypothesis testing, arguing that a standard method of decision making is required. This point of view, while apparently held by very few statisticians today, unfortunately still remains the dominating viewpoint among the majority of clinical researchers.

The more popular perception among statisticians, one that is not yet fully recognized by many researchers, is that scientific research design and data analysis should not necessarily include a strict decision on accepting or rejecting a hypothesis. Statisticians have long argued that the process of data evaluation by hypothesis testing is so erratic and subjective and can be so misleading and deceptive that it would best be abandoned entirely in scientific applications.[1,2,22] Rather, the goal in scientific research should be to extract as much useful information as possible from the sample data to assess meaningful judgment on the general population.

Even statisticians who encourage hypothesis testing agree that it has been subject to misinterpretation, and therefore may be misleading, in at least some situations. For example, Fleiss, who wrote in defense of the use of significance tests,[21] nevertheless started his article with the following: "There is no doubt that significance tests have been abused.... statistically significant associations have, in error, been automatically equated to substantively important ones, and statistically nonsignificant associations or differences have, in error, been automatically equated to ones that are zero." Unfortunately, alternative solutions, such as data evaluation using confidence intervals, have also been subject to misuse, as will be described. Regardless of whether one decides to conduct a formal hypothesis test or not, one must understand the underlying principles involved in risk-benefit assessment, which is the only way to select a proper sample size for a given study.

In the next sections, we will discuss the issues involved in risk-benefit assessments and in estimating the precision of our measurements. For thoroughness, we will describe the issues involved with and without a formal hypothesis test. It must be emphasized that mathematically the procedures are very similar, whether or not a formal hypothesis test is performed; the difference lies mostly in the interpretation of the results and in the deriving of conclusions.

Assessing the Uncertainty in Our Data

Generalizing Conclusions From Experimental Study Groups

Consider our initial hypothetical study again, which compared the effectiveness of two drugs for the treatment of a particular disease. This study evaluated the difference in the recovery rate with the two drugs in an experimental sample, but its final goal was to estimate the difference in the effectiveness of the drugs in the general population. In other words, we would like to use the difference obtained with our selected group of patients to predict the difference that would be obtained if we used the same treatment in all patients with the disease, now and in the future.

Because we found a 30% difference in recovery rate between patients treated with the two drugs, we estimate that the difference in the general population will also be 30%. This remains the best estimate of the outcome in the general population, regardless of the associated P-value. Similarly, in the example of the mountaineers, the best estimate of how far either one would jump remained twice the width of the crevasse, and having a higher or lower P-value did not change what was the best estimate of the outcome.

While the sample provides us with the best estimate of the difference in the larger population, this is still only an estimate. The investigator in the drug study should not expect to see an improvement of exactly 30% with the new drug in the general population, and neither mountaineer should expect to jump exactly twice the width of the crevasse in subsequent attempts. The fluctuation of distance for various attempts might be extremely small or very large. While a large P-value suggests (but does not show unequivocally) that there is perhaps more of this type of fluctuation, it provides no indication of the magnitude of this fluctuation. We use confidence intervals to determine the possible magnitude of fluctuation of treatment effects.

Confidence in Our Estimation

Just how precise is our estimate of a difference (in ratios or means) obtained from an experimental sample? Surely, if a difference of 30% is obtained between two groups of 1,000 patients each, it is more reliable than the same difference if it were obtained with ten patients in each group. The P-value provides us with the probability that our difference was obtained by accident, but does not provide us with a measure of variation for the obtained difference.

The confidence interval can be used to estimate a range of numbers within which the true difference (the difference in the general population) lies. In order to calculate the confidence interval, we must first decide what level of certainty we require. Suppose, in our drug test example, that we calculate the 95% confidence intervals for the difference in recovery from infection, and we obtain a range of between 15% and 45%. This would mean that we can be 95% certain that the true difference in recovery rate in the general population will be between 15% and 45%. If a lower level of certainty is acceptable, such as 90%, then one could calculate the 90% confidence interval. The lower the level of certainty that is required, the smaller the confidence interval.

Confidence intervals, which give a range of likely values for the true difference, provide more insight into the nature of the data than do P-values.[2,4,6,22] Statisticians have encouraged researchers to use confidence intervals for comparisons in addition to or instead of assessing statistical significance using P-values. Whether one uses P-values or any other statistical measure, confidence intervals can always provide more

useful information. However, one must bear in mind that each confidence interval is based on a fixed probability level. Making a comparison using 95% confidence intervals will point to the same conclusion as if the comparison were made using $P \leq 0.05$ to indicate statistical significance. The investigator must consider the difficult yet important question of what confidence level to use for a given study.

Estimating the Appropriate Sample Size

As demonstrated with our examples, the decision-making process in a scientific study is much more complex than simply inspecting whether the P-value is smaller or greater than some reference value such as 0.05. A firm understanding of each of the steps in this process is fundamental to arriving at sound conclusions. Most investigators are advised that they must establish a clear, unambiguous statement of a hypothesis. However, too few researchers pay sufficient attention to other vital questions that need to be answered in advance of the study, regardless of whether they want to establish a formal hypothesis test or not. Specifically, before each study, an investigator must answer the following questions:

(1) What is the smallest observed difference (for example, difference in survival rate for patients taking drug A or B) that one could consider to be of scientific, clinical, or practical importance? This value is referred to as δ (delta). This value may be difficult to assess, but if one cannot state before the study begins how much of a measured difference one will consider to be clinically significant, this is not likely to be a simpler matter after the results are obtained, and one should question whether the study should be conducted in the first place.

(2) What will be the scientific or clinical benefits of correctly accepting the observed difference as representative of the general population, and what will be the penalties for incorrectly accepting the difference as real?

(3) What will be the benefits of correctly rejecting an observed difference as having occurred by chance? What will be the penalties of incorrectly rejecting the observed difference as having occurred by chance?

(4) With what certainty does one need to know the difference, and what magnitude of error in the difference would be acceptable?

The required certainty is called the confidence level. For example, we may need to know the increase in serum glucose in patients following a treatment with a particular type of oral hypoglycemic. If we select a 90% confidence level and an error of 25 mg/dL², we are stating that we would like to be in error by no more than 25 mg/dL², with an associated assurance of 90%. Mathematically, selection of the error is equivalent to the selection of the smallest clinically or scientifically significant difference, δ, which was the answer to the first question. Stated differently, if we select an error of 25 mg/dL^2, we would like to know the serum glucose to within 25 mg/dL^2, which in turn would mean that a difference of smaller than 25 mg/dL^2 would not be clinically significant. Therefore, δ and the error are practically the same parameter, and these cannot be selected independently, though they have different interpretations.

(5) If a formal hypothesis test is to be performed, one must answer the following. Given the above assessments, for a given magnitude of observed difference, what is the maximum probability that the observed difference occurred by chance selection that one is willing to allow and still accept that the difference is representative of the general population?

The answer to this fifth question is called the significance level, α (alpha), and is the number to which we later compare our obtained P-value. As discussed earlier, based on traditional but misleading terminology, if the obtained P-value is smaller than alpha, then the measured difference is referred to as statistically significant, whereas, if the P-value exceeds alpha, the results are called not statistically significant. Also based on tradition, the alpha level is widely, but often inappropriately, chosen as 0.05, implying that the investigators are willing to accept no greater than a one-in-twenty probability that the observed difference occurred by chance alone. However, for a given study, the appropriate level of certainty may be above or well below 0.05.

Mathematically, selecting a significance level α of 0.05 is equivalent to selecting a 95% confidence level. Therefore, α and the confidence level cannot be selected independently, although they have somewhat different interpretations.

The considerations in the assessment of the above risk may include whether the apparent results contradict established scientific principles or the results of earlier studies, whether there are dangerous side effects of a drug or treatment, the cost of the treatment, and others. Thus, depending on the consequences of accepting results that may have occurred by chance, the investigators may choose to require a very small significance level, such as 0.01, or they may be comfortable with a higher probability that the apparent difference occurred by chance such as 0.25, or one chance in four. Equivalent statements to these would be to select a high confidence level, such as 99%, or a low confidence level, such as 75%, respectively.

Unless the significance level (α) is selected in advance, and is based on careful assessment of risk-to-benefit ratios, there is little point in dividing results into categories of statistically significant and not statistically significant after the study has been conducted. Particularly in such cases, it is most appropriate to report the difference obtained along with the associated confidence interval and P-value, rather than simply to report whether the result was statistically significant or not. By the same token, it is inappropriate for the editors of a scientific journal to designate a single significance level, such as 0.05, or a single confidence level, such as 95%, as a universal designation of statistically significant results, because, in effect, the implementation of this significance level may be occurring well after the results are obtained from the study.

(6) Given the above assessments, for a given magnitude of observed difference, what is the maximum probability that one is willing to allow that one will fail to detect a clinically significant difference when in fact there is one? The answer to this question is called β (beta), the probability of a type II error. The importance of type II errors in clinical research has been emphasized by many authors.[3,7,23] The probability of not making a type II error is called the power of the test. Suppose, in our example of the comparison of the effectiveness of two drugs, that the power of the test was 83%. This would mean that there is an 83% probability that the 30% difference that we obtained with the sample was truly representative of the difference in the general population.

When one selects the significance level (α), the tendency may be to select the smallest value that the sample study allows. An equivalent practice is to select the confidence level as high as possible. However, the investigator must realize that, for a given sample size, selecting a smaller significance level means increasing the probability of type II error. In other words, the smaller the chances one chooses to take in erroneously concluding that there is a difference, the larger the chances that one would fail to detect a difference when in fact there is one. The investigator, then, must wisely consider the seriousness of each type of error, and select α and β accordingly. In addition to answering the above questions, the investigator must either measure or somehow estimate the variance(s) in the groups being considered.

It should be obvious by now that the selection of the smallest outcome that would be considered clinically important (the first question) and the assessment of the risk-to-benefit ratios that lead to the selection of the required levels of certainty (α and β) are not arbitrary, although they may be subjective. These decisions must be made taking into account all of the available relevant information, including fundamental theory, existing literature on the subject, prior experience of the investigators, and, above all, common sense.

The answers to all six questions must be provided by the investigators, with the collaboration of a qualified statistician, who may then apply the appropriate mathematical formulas for each case in order to select the minimum sample size (number of patients) that would be required to detect the magnitude of the difference in question at the required level of statistical certainty. Note that the sample size can be selected to limit the error (based on confidence intervals), or to obtain the desired power.

Selection of the appropriate sample size is perhaps the most important part of the preparation for a study. If the sample size is too small, even very large measured differences may have associated P-values greater than the alpha level, such that the result would be considered statistically insignificant. Conversely, with an excessively large sample size, even small differences with little or no scientific or clinical importance may, nevertheless, be measured with a very high level of statistical significance. In addition to being misleading, the latter event may represent a major waste of scarce research funds.

Evaluation of Data Using Confidence Intervals

Statisticians have been advocating the use of confidence intervals instead of (or in addition to) P-values,[2,4,6,22] because they can be more informative, illustrative, and less misleading than P-values. As a first step, given the confidence level that was determined before the study, such as 90%, we can calculate the confidence interval of the difference that was obtained with our sample. This confidence interval provides us with a range of likely values for the difference. Technically, we could use the confidence interval to evaluate the statistical significance of the difference. That is, if the confidence interval of the difference includes zero, the obtained difference is not statistically significant; and on the other hand, if the confidence interval is on one side of zero only, the result can be considered statistically significant. Mathematically, if we had selected a 90% confidence interval, this comparison would be the equivalent of selecting a significance level of 0.1. However, it would be a waste of resources if we only used confidence intervals to assess statistical significance. As indicated, the range of numbers provides us with the proper perspective of the likely values for the difference. Thus, we should consider the entire range of values of the confidence interval, rather than simply the end points. In contrast, considering the P-value alone is similar to looking at only one end of the confidence interval.

Because the confidence interval includes a range of likely values for the difference, it can be used to evaluate clinical or scientific significance along with statistical significance. That is, if the lower end of the confidence interval of the obtained difference is larger than the magnitude of smallest difference that we consider clinically significant, then the obtained difference is clinically significant; and on the other hand, if the confidence interval of the obtained difference is entirely below this value, then the result is clinically insignificant. If the minimum value that we consider to be clinically significant lies somewhere within the confidence interval, we require further study. In addition, the confidence interval of the difference provides us with some indication of the power of the test. However, as with the assessment of statistical significance, the entire range of values that the confidence interval represents must be considered, and not simply the end points.

Unfortunately, in the literature, analysis with confidence intervals is plagued with problems similar to those with P-values.[19,24] Most authors use only 95% confidence intervals, rather than 75%, 80%, 90% or any other value, without regard to the risk-benefit considerations that we have already discussed. In order for the conclusion to be valid, the level of confidence must be selected, on the basis of risk-benefit assessment as described above, before conducting the study. Furthermore, rather than paying attention to the approximate range of values that the confidence interval provides, and where the larger portion of the ranges lie, many simply inspect whether zero is inside or outside of the confidence interval of the difference. This oversimplified practice, as described, may lead to many misleading conclusions. Technically, this would be no different from concluding that, say, a P-value of 0.051 indicates an insignificant result.

Evaluation of Data for Hypothesis Testing

Evaluation of Clinical Significance

As mentioned in the previous section, the first step in the planning of a study should be to select δ, which is the smallest difference that would be of medical, practical, or clinical importance. After the study has been conducted, the first step in the evaluation of the results should be to compare the obtained difference to δ, in order to assess whether the observed difference should be considered of scientific or clinical importance. Unless confidence intervals are used, this may be the only step in which one considers the consequences and thinks directly about the magnitude of the obtained differences.

If the observed difference is larger than δ, the result is considered clinically or scientifically significant, and we may proceed with the calculations of statistical significance in order to assess the reliability of our assessment. If, on the other hand, the observed difference is smaller than δ, then the result is likely clinically insignificant. In this case, the data suggest that the groups being compared are similar, at least for practical purposes. Again, we need to assess the statistical reliability of this assessment, as explained below.

Although the evaluation of the clinical significance is the most important step in the interpretation of the results of a study, this is commonly ignored entirely in studies published in the medical literature. For example, if one has measured the blood cholesterol level in patients following a certain diet, is the magnitude of the measured decrease or increase in the level of cholesterol large enough to make a considerable difference in the risk of heart disease? If one is comparing the longevity of a new design of total joint replacement with that of conventional designs, is an increase (or decrease) in longevity of a month or two important enough to justify recommending the new design? If not, would an increase of one year be sufficient? How about two years? The only way to objectively answer these types of questions is to decide on and document what would constitute a clinically significant outcome before starting the study. Otherwise, once the study is done, the investigator may be compelled to exaggerate the importance of small (though perhaps statistically significant) differences in order to justify the time and money spent on the study.

Considerations in Accepting That a Difference Exists

If the magnitude of a difference obtained in a study is determined to be of scientific or clinical significance, then one should evaluate the reliability of this difference. In other words, we should evaluate the risk of making the assessment that the difference with our observed sample is representative of the true difference in the general population. This is commonly done using P-values. A difference that is clinically significant should never be dismissed, regardless of the P-value.

Supposing that the difference is clinically significant, let us consider the possible outcomes. If the P-value is smaller than the predetermined significance level, then the result is considered statistically significant. Most investigators manage this type of result quite well, particularly if they are using the traditional significance level of 0.05. On the other hand, if the P-value is larger than 0.05 (say, 0.08), there is much confusion among investigators regarding how to interpret and report the results, or even what kind of conclusions to make from the finding. Some regard the reporting of differences associated with P-values of larger than 0.05, however large and important, as "controversial," "liberal," "weak," or "lowering the (established) statistical standard." However, the only objective way of reporting such results is to report the obtained difference along with the associated P-value. There are strong reasons to thoroughly consider the likelihood that such results are true representations of the general populations from which they were drawn.

When the obtained difference is clinically or practically significant, and the associated P-value is too large to indicate statistical significance, the most likely reason is that the sample size was too small. In other words, other investigators may repeat the study with larger samples and eventually obtain statistical significance. On the other hand, if the result was obtained only by chance, that is, if the difference does not exist in reality, that, too, will be determined by other, perhaps larger, studies. The important point is that not reporting obtained differences because the P-value was larger than what is considered statistically significant may hinder the progress of science by hiding potentially important results from other investigators.

Establishing That Groups are Similar

When the obtained difference is smaller than what is considered clinically significant, it suggests that the groups being compared are samples from functionally similar populations. To validate this, it is common for investigators to erroneously use P-values alone. In doing so, investigators run a potentially high risk of arriving at the wrong conclusion that no difference exists in the general populations, when in fact there is a large difference (a type II error). This erroneous type of deduction is quite common among clinical investigators, despite clear warnings against it in the literature.[7,23]

As an example, Freiman and associates[23] analyzed the results from 71 clinical trials, published in well-known international medical journals, all of which had reported "no significant difference, $P > 0.05$" between the study and the control groups. Freiman and associates demonstrated that 67 of the 71 trials had a greater than 10% chance of failing to detect a true 25% therapeutic improvement with the study group compared to the control group, and that 50 of the trials had a greater than 10% chance of failing to detect a true 50% improvement. When these authors calculated the 90% confidence intervals for the true improvement in each trial, 57 of the treatments had a potential for 25% improvement over the control, and 34% had a potential for 50% improvement. Despite these potential improvements, only one of the studies had mentioned that both α and β were considered prior to the start of the trial. In short, Freiman and associates concluded that it is quite likely that a large number of the studies included in their survey would reveal a true benefit with the treatment they were studying, had they continued the clinical trial longer. This study vividly demonstrated the potential risks in making conclusions based on P-values alone. Such incorrect analyses account for substantial loss of scientifically and clinically important information.

To illustrate the proper analysis when the results indicate similarity rather than difference, and when a hypothesis test is necessary, consider the following. A study published in 1981 compared the risk of death as a result of lung cancer among wives of over 175,000 smoking and nonsmoking men.[25] In this 12-year study, it was found that, compared to the wives of nonsmokers, there was 10% higher mortality from lung cancer among wives of heavy smokers (≥ 20 cigarettes per day), but the difference was not statistically significant. (Diamond and Forrester[26] have reanalyzed the data from this and several other studies using posterior probability based on Bayes' theorem, and have demonstrated some additional shortcomings of P-values beyond those discussed here. The discussion of posterior probability is beyond the scope of this article, as is the discussion of the literature on passive smoking. The purpose of citing Garfinkel's study is to demonstrate the underlying concepts of clinical significance, delta and power.) Suppose that, at the outset, the investigators had decided that any increase (or decrease) greater than 5% in the risk of lung cancer should be considered clinically significant. In other words, they set δ to be 5%. In this case, the difference of 10% increase in lung cancer obtained in the sample would be clinically significant. However, they reported the result as not statistically significant, that is, they obtained a P-value that was larger than the significance level they had selected. When the result is clinically significant but not statistically significant, as discussed in the previous section, further study is required to determine whether the difference was obtained by chance, or whether it can be attributed to the general population. In any case, the difference cannot and should not be ignored based on the fact that it was not statistically significant. The most likely reason for this type of result (clinically significant but not statistically significant) is having a sample size that is too small. In such cases, the value of β becomes critical in determining what conclusion can be made from the study.

On the other hand, suppose that the investigators had decided at the outset that a difference in mortality from lung cancer has to be at least 20% before it can be considered clinically significant, that is, δ = 20%. (In reality, such a decision should have a reasonable basis, the purpose here is to demonstrate a different condition of the evidence using the same example). In this case, a 10% difference is not large enough to be considered clinically or practically significant. Therefore, because we have not observed a sufficiently large difference with the wives of smokers and nonsmokers that we happened to study, the data suggests the conclusion that the wives of smokers and nonsmokers are at similar or the same risk of lung cancer in the general population. The result in this case is neither clinically nor statistically significant. Again, we must consider the likelihood that this result was obtained because we had too few samples. We thus turn to other statistics to arrive at a conclusion.

What we need to evaluate in this case is the probability that a larger difference exists between wives of smokers and nonsmokers, which we failed to detect by studying this particular sample. This type of error, as

mentioned earlier, is called a type II error, and the chances we are willing to take in making such an error is called β (beta). As indicated, we must decide on β before beginning the study. However, unlike α, which can and should be set exactly before the study, β can only be approximated in advance. When we have the results, we can calculate β. In practice, we more commonly deal with the power of the statistical comparison, which is the probability of not making such an error, and therefore correctly concluding that there is no difference. For instance, if β = 15%, then the power is 100%–15% = 85%.

Hypothesis Testing Versus Confidence Intervals

We have described two methods of evaluating the data observed in a study and making conclusions about the general population. As indicated, the mathematical calculations are similar. However, as demonstrated, confidence intervals offer a straightforward, simple way of evaluating data, whereas analysis of data for hypothesis testing can become quite complex. One must recognize that even if we do not conduct a hypothesis test, and even if we only use confidence intervals to describe our data, we still need to select α, β, and δ before the study in order to select the proper sample size.

Comparing two analyses of the same problem, one with 95% confidence intervals of the obtained difference and the other with the P-value compared to 0.05, the conclusion will technically be the same. If the difference is marginally approaching significance, the confidence interval of the difference will barely cross zero, indicating that most of the likely values of the difference will be larger than zero. In contrast, for the same analysis, P = 0.053 does not convey a range of values for the difference, but rather just one probability value. Therefore, confidence intervals are more informative and less misleading, as long as they are presented in their entirety, and not the conclusion of significant or not significant, which will essentially be the same no matter which method is used.

Guidelines for Proper Description and Interpretation of Results

It would be naive to imagine that any single solution would solve the problems of misuse of statistical analysis within a short period of time. However, the authors feel that, as indicated, hypothesis testing inevitably leads to incomplete description of the data. In order to encourage complete reporting of the results, and to help minimize some of the problems we have outlined in this chapter, we propose that the orthopaedic community adopt the following guidelines for evaluating and publishing the results of an investigation.

First and foremost, the terms statistically significant and not statistically significant should be avoided entirely in the literature. Editors should not allow authors to describe the results of comparisons simply as being either significant or not significant. Rather, the investigators should report the data obtained by the measurements (tabulated, plotted along with standard deviations, etc.) along with the actual values of the associated confidence intervals and P-values. In discussing the observed differences, the authors should address the following issues: (1) What magnitude of difference was measured? (2) How does the magnitude of the observed difference compare to one that constitutes a scientific or clinically important difference? (3) If the measured difference is large enough to be scientifically or clinically important, what was the associated level of certainty for the measurement? In particular, what is the corresponding confidence interval of the difference obtained? (4) What will the benefits be if the investigator is correct in accepting the results? What are the penalties if the investigator is wrong? (5) Considering the above assessments, and based on the results, what conclusion can be made regarding the general population? In addition to the above, it is always beneficial to indicate the associated P-value, but report the P-value itself rather than comparing it to a significance level.

Conclusions

Sound research practice requires a great amount of preparation. While some researchers mistakenly consider statistical analysis as a task that needs to be performed after the study is concluded to see if the result was significant or not, the correct way to design a study is to appraise the risk-to-benefit ratio and estimate the required sample size before the study is commenced. In particular, the smallest difference that would be considered scientifically, practically, or clinically significant should be specified in advance of the study.

In reaching a conclusion regarding the outcome of a study, the researcher must take into account all of the facts, figures, and evidence available and, above all, must apply common sense. For example, if the results directly contradict long-established scientific principles, then they may be viewed with justified skepticism, even though very strong statistical significance is obtained, at least until the same results have been obtained by further research or by other independent investigators. It should be kept in mind that, even at P = 0.05, one out of every 20 observations will have occurred by chance. On the other hand, if an observed difference is consistent with previously established scientific principles, follows logical deduction, and/or has been demonstrated in similar studies by others, it may be reasonable to accept the difference as real,

regardless of a relatively large P-value for an individual study. Finally, sound research requires a fundamental understanding of the statistical methods that are used. Most importantly, whether the investigator chooses to accept or reject the results, all of the results of the study should be reported along with the associated confidence intervals and P-values, regardless of whether these meet one's criterion of statistically significant.

Acknowledgements

This study was supported in part by the Los Angeles Orthopaedic Foundation. The authors wish to thank Patricia Normand for her contribution.

References

1. Walker AM: Reporting the results of epidemiologic studies. *Am J Public Health* 1986;76:556-558.
2. Rothman KJ: Editorial: A show of confidence. *N Engl J Med* 1978;299:1362-1363.
3. Rennie D: Editorial: Vive la difference (P less than 0.05). *N Engl J Med* 1978;299:828-829.
4. Thompson WD: Statistical criteria in the interpretation of epidemiologic data. *Am J Public Health* 1987;77:191-194.
5. Altman DG: Statistics and ethics in medical research: VII. Interpreting results. *Br Med J* 1980;281:1612-1614.
6. Dorey F, Amstutz H, Nasser S: The need for confidence intervals when presenting orthopaedic data. *J Bone Joint Surg,* in press.
7. Lieber RL: Statistical significance and statistical power in hypothesis testing. *J Orthop Res* 1990;8:304-309.
8. Ingelfinger FG: Editorial: Significance of significant. *N Engl J Med* 1968;278:1232-1233.
9. Feinstein AR: *Clinical Epidemiology: The Architecture of Clinical Research.* Philadelphia, PA, WB Saunders, 1985.
10. Melton AW: Editorial. *J Exp Psychol* 1962;64:553-557.
11. Fisher RA: *Statistical Methods and Scientific Inference,* ed 2. Edinburgh, Oliver and Boyd, 1959.
12. Brown BW: Statistics, scientific method, and smoking, in Tanur JM, Mosteller F, Kruskal WH, et al (eds): *Statistics: A Guide to the Unknown,* ed 2. San Francisco, Holden Day, 1978, p 66.
13. Kendall MG, Stuart A: *The Advanced Theory of Statistics,* ed 4. New York, Hafner Press, 1977, vol 1, 1979, vol 2, 1983, vol 3.
14. Yates F: Theory and practice in statistics. *J R Statist Soc* 1968;131:463-475.
15. Box GEP: Science and statistics. *J Am Statist Assoc* 1976;71:791-799.
16. Feinstein AR (ed): *Clinical Biostatistics.* St. Louis, MO, CV Mosby, 1977, chap 5, pp 54-70.
17. Rosenthal R: Combining results of independent studies. *Psychol Bull* 1978;85:185-193.
18. Edwards W, Lindman H, Savage LJ: Bayesian statistical inference for psychological research. *Psychol Rev* 1963;70:193-242.
19. Poole C: Beyond the confidence interval. *Am J Public Health* 1987;77:195-199.
20. Cox DR, Hinkley DV: *Theoretical Statistics.* London, Chapman and Hall, 1974.
21. Fleiss JL: Significance tests have a role in epidemiologic research: Reactions to AM Walker. *Am J Public Health* 1986;76:559-560.
22. Gardner MJ, Altman DG: Confidence intervals rather than P values: Estimation rather than hypothesis testing. *BMJ* 1986;292:746-750.

23. Freiman JA, Chalmers TC, Smith H Jr, et al: The importance of beta, the type II error and sample size in the design and interpretation of the randomized control trial: Survey of 71 "negative" trials. *N Engl J Med* 1978;299:690-694.

24. Poole C: Confidence intervals exclude nothing. *Am J Public Health* 1987;77:492-493.

25. Garfinkel L: Time trends in lung cancer mortality among nonsmokers and a note on passive smoking. *J Natl Cancer Inst* 1981;66:1061-1066.

26. Diamond GA, Forrester JS: Clinical trials and statistical verdicts: Probable grounds for appeal. *Ann Intern Med* 1983;98:385-394.

Outcomes Research in Orthopaedics

Robert B. Keller, MD

Sally A. Rudicel, MD

Matthew H. Liang, MD, MPH

Outcomes Research

The concept of outcomes research is relatively new, but it should be understood that this set of research methodologies really represents an evolution and extension of the kind of clinical research that is familiar to all physicians. There are, however, important differences that characterize outcomes research.

Outcomes research, in its most complete form, may contain a number of different components. These include analysis of large databases (Outline 1), such as the Medicare database; organized or structured reviews of the literature, known as meta-analysis; small-area analysis of health-care utilization; prospective clinical studies emphasizing patient-oriented outcomes of care; and development of decision-making analytical models, cost-effectiveness studies, and practice guidelines.

There are important factors that have clarified the need to develop these new methods. In this chapter, we will discuss the conditions in medical practice and research that have led to the need to redefine clinical research and to move rapidly into the field of outcomes research. We will also describe the various elements that constitute outcomes research.

Outline 1
Examples of large data sets for research

United States Census
National Center for Health Statistics
    National Hospital Discharge Survey
    National Ambulatory Medical Care Survey
    National Health Examination Survey
    Health and Nutrition Examination Survey
    National Health Interview Survey
    National Death Index
Registries:
    National Tumor Registry
    Total Joint Arthroplasty Registries
        Brigham and Women's Hospital
        Mayo Clinic
        Stanford Medical Center
Third-party payers
    Medicare Part A
    Medicare Part B
Veterans Administration Hospitals
Health Maintenance Organizations
Kaiser
Harvard Community Health Plan

Three important factors have stimulated the emergence of this concept: the rapidly rising cost of health care, variations in practice patterns, and deficiencies in clinical research methods.

The Cost of Health Care

As we approach the end of the 20th century, one of the major social and political issues confronting this nation and others is the rapidly rising cost of health care. While the United States may have the biggest problem, other industrialized nations are facing, or soon will face, similar difficulty.

Few would disagree with the statement that the United States has been the world's leader in biomedical research and in the development of new technologies and treatments. We also recognize that most of the population has access to medical care of the highest quality. However, an estimated 37 million Americans do not have access to adequate care, and there is evidence that we may provide and utilize more of certain kinds of care than is necessary or beneficial to patients.

There is a strong belief that we spend too large a portion of our national resources on health care and still do not provide adequate care for all of our citizens. Spending 14% of the gross domestic product on health care, the United States far outspends its economic competitors, whose health-care expenditures are well under 10%.

Further analysis of the cost and the economic issues of health care is beyond the scope of this chapter, but it is important to keep in mind that the cost of health care and its apparent inefficiencies underlie the need of the profession to analyze carefully the practice of medicine and to invest in outcomes research. Beyond any economic imperatives, it has become evident that outcomes research is an important concept with respect to the assessment of the quality and appropriateness of medical care.

Variations in Practice Patterns

The first step down the road to outcomes research came about as the result of work by Wennberg and Gittelsohn.[1] Their development and delineation of the concept of small-area variations revealed major deficiencies in what the medical profession might have viewed as well conceived and established medical practice patterns.

Small-area analysis permits us — for the first time — to calculate population-based rates of medical-care utilization by patients, hospitals, and health-care providers. Before implementation of this methodology, only overall numbers of procedures, treatments, and tests could be ascertained. For example, knowledge of the total number of disk-excision procedures performed in each of two hospitals does not indicate anything about the per capita rate of the operation among the residents served by those institutions.

If utilization rates were essentially the same in every geographic area, this information would be of limited value. What Wennberg and Gittelsohn discovered, however, was that rates of utilization of almost all kinds of medical care are strikingly different. Moreover, the variations appeared to be almost exclusively the result of differences in beliefs among physicians about the best way to treat various conditions.

The massive degree of uncertainty underlying variations does not indicate whether low, medium, or high rates of utilization are the most appropriate, but all who have studied variations in practice patterns agree that not all of the rates can be right. From the perspective of cost and quality, the study and resolution of variations in practice patterns deserve prompt attention.

Problems in Clinical Research and the Literature

In recent years, it has become increasingly evident that the clinical research literature in orthopaedics (and all fields of medicine) has a number of deficiencies. Gartland,[2] as well as Gross,[3] analyzed the literature on total hip arthroplasty. Both found the quality of the reports to be lacking for major reasons, including the lack of prospective studies, the absence of comparisons of alternative treatments, inadequate and inconsistent definitions of terms and measures, a focus on the process of care rather than on functional and quality-of-life measurements, and poor statistical methodologies and analyses. On the basis of his critical review of ten papers on hip arthroplasty, Gartland stated, "All ten articles were found to be deficient in terms of design, to be flawed by confusing data, and to contain results of doubtful validity."

In attempting to conduct structured reviews of the literature, other investigators have found similar problems. Meta-analysis is a relatively new concept of structured literature review. It permits data from a number of studies to be combined into a large pool of information, resulting in improved statistical accuracy and power. Ideally, meta-analysis should be conducted only on reports of randomized clinical trials. However, under specific conditions, the technique can be modified for use on other types of reports. What is required, at a minimum, is high-quality data with consistent defi-

nition of terms, patient groups, and outcome data. Structured literature reviews of the treatment of spinal stenosis,[4] lateral epicondylitis,[5] femoral neck fractures,[6] and spinal arthrodesis[7] have revealed serious deficiencies in the quality of the literature on those conditions.

Clearly, weaknesses in the literature make it very difficult for orthopaedists to decide how to select the most appropriate, highest-quality care for their patients. Clinical practice is completely dependent on the knowledge base created by those who carry out research, develop new ideas and technologies, and teach and report this information. Thus, if the research and literature are deficient, so too will be the clinical practice of the specialty.

There is evidence that these problems are being recognized and addressed both by scientific journals[8,9] and by physicians. A number of musculoskeletal specialty societies and The American Academy of Orthopaedic Surgeons have developed committees and programs to develop standardized language and definitions as well as outcomes measurements. These instruments should focus not only on the process of care (radiographic results, range of motion, and laboratory findings), but also on patient-oriented outcomes, such as function, quality of life, and patient utilities (the usefulness of a specific outcome in the life of a given patient).

In the following sections, we will describe the various elements of outcomes research, concentrating on the methods that are specifically related to clinical research.

Small-Area Variations

In developing the concept of small-area analysis, Wennberg and Gittelsohn[1] adapted classic epidemiologic principles to study the utilization of health-care services on the basis of population. With the advent of computers and hospital-discharge databases, they were able to calculate per capita rates of medical and surgical care for patients at hospitals. While hospitals and physicians have long known their own volume or numbers of procedures, they have not been able to calculate the rate of those interventions because they have not known the denominator of the formula — the population served. The work of Wennberg and Gittelsohn solved that problem. By defining what they called hospital service areas, defined by the zip codes within which most patients seen at one or more hospitals resided, they were able to establish rates of utilization for all diagnoses and procedures as they were recorded by hospitals, on insurance claim forms, and in other data sources. The patient's utilization of a service was always recorded according to the place of residence. In other words, a patient traveling outside of his or her hospital service area for treatment was counted in the geographic area of residence.

The methodology also permits analysis by hospital

and physician as well as by service areas created on the basis of a specific procedure. As an example, most hospitalizations for medical conditions involving the back occur in local hospitals. In this case, the per capita admission rates within the service area would be relevant. If, however, patients being managed with total joint arthroplasty were treated only in a regional or tertiary hospital, the activity in local hospitals would not be relevant. New hospital-service areas can be developed by consolidation of zip codes to analyze utilization patterns in the geographic areas served by the larger centers.

Prior to this type of analysis being done, most physicians believed that, once adjustments for age, sex, and other potential variables have been made, rates of utilization for a procedure such as a lumbar disk excision or total hip arthroplasty would be similar and consistent across regions. On the contrary, the practice of medicine and surgery in the United States and other countries is characterized by a remarkable degree of inconsistency.

Through small-area analyses, we have learned that there are statistically significant variations in almost all areas of medical and surgical care studied. In orthopaedics, we do not see variations in rates of admission to hospitals or of surgical treatment for conditions such as hip fracture and polytrauma, but variations are seen in these rates for essentially all elective orthopaedic procedures that have been analyzed.[10]

To illustrate the problem, consider operations on the lumbar spine. There are large differences in the rates of spinal procedures between the four large geo-

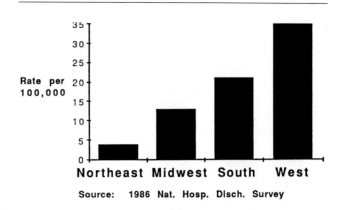

Fig. 1 This graph illustrates that there are major differences in the rates of spinal arthrodesis between four large geographic regions of the United States. The rate in the western region is nearly nine times that in the northeast. (Reproduced with permission from Deyo RA: Non-surgical care of low back pain. *Neurosurg Clin N Am* 1991;2:851-862.)

graphic regions of this country (Fig. 1). It does not seem logical that the probability of being managed with a spinal arthrodesis in the western United States should be nearly nine times that in the northeast, but that is what the data tell us. Likewise, there are statistically significant differences with respect to use rates between selected states (Fig. 2). Finally, there are marked differences even within states. The likelihood of a resident of the state of Washington being managed with a spinal operation varies by a factor of 15, depending on the county of residence (Fig. 3).[11]

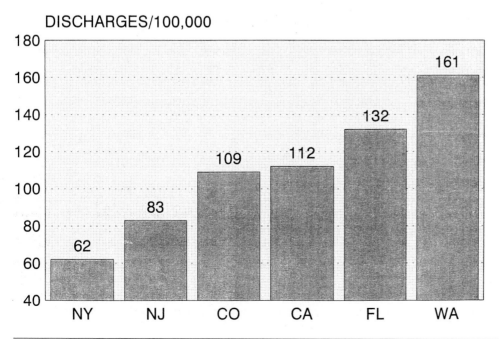

Fig. 2 This graph illustrates that rates for spinal operations vary between states. New York has a rate of 62 per 100,000; Washington's rate is 161 per 100,000. (Reproduced with permission from D. Cherkin, MD.)

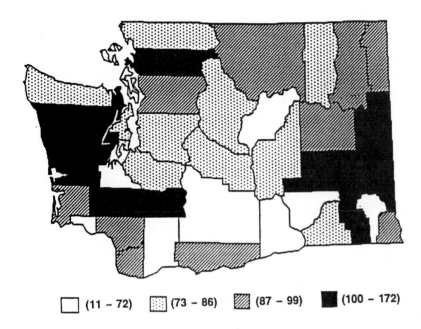

Fig. 3 This graph illustrates that there have been marked differences in the rates of spinal operations between counties in the state of Washington. The probability of having an operation ranges from as low as 11 procedures per 100,000 to as high as 172 per 100,000. (Reproduced, with permission from Volinn E, Mayer J, Diehr P, et al: Small area analysis of surgery for low-back pain. *Spine* 1992;17:575-581.)

☐ (11 – 72)   ▦ (73 – 86)   ▨ (87 – 99)   ■ (100 – 172)

Similar variations have been seen for many procedures and conditions in every location where they have been studied. These variations suggest that despite similarities in residency training, board certification, and continuing education, orthopaedists and their patients have very different perceptions about the value and outcomes of various kinds of treatment. In addition, we do not know which rate is the right rate. It does appear that variations in practice patterns are more clearly related to uncertainty about the best way to treat clinical problems than to financial incentives for physicians to do more.

Until the concept and methodology of small-area analysis were developed and widely adopted, physicians had no idea how their practice styles compared with those of their peers; even now, there is no wide, routine, and timely dissemination of this kind of information. Experience in Maine has demonstrated that when doctors are appropriately provided with information about practice patterns, they respond in responsible ways.[12] For example, orthopaedists and neurosurgeons in Maine carried out analyses of rates of lumbar disk excision. Not unexpectedly, statistically significant variations in practice patterns were discovered. A study group was developed to carry out detailed analyses of the variation data, and it concluded that the rapidly increasing rates of diskectomy in several service areas were best explained by the relocation of three surgeons into the community where all of the procedures were performed. Feedback of this information to those concerned produced a prompt decrease in the rates of performance of the operation (Fig. 4).

Variation analyses are important for several reasons. First, they clarify the remarkable degree of difference in utilization of services across small and larger areas. While we might disagree about which rate is right, few, if any, would argue that widely varying rates represent cost-efficient, appropriate, and high-quality care. Second, the elucidation, analysis, and informed debate about variations in practice patterns can lead to changes in practice patterns — a useful result in and of itself. Third, and perhaps most important, the revelation of variations in practice patterns stimulates us to try to understand the problem and helps us to define an agenda for additional research.

Our experience with several medical specialties in Maine confirms that, in a confidential, educational setting, practitioners will become active in the process of small-area analysis, the feedback of information, the change in practice behavior, and the participation in outcomes research.[12] For example, having been through the process of analysis of variations in the performance of disk procedures, orthopaedists and neurosurgeons in Maine became active participants in a prospective outcome study of patients receiving medical and surgical treatment of herniated lumbar disks and spinal stenosis.

Once they understand the problem, clinicians are eager to participate in the solution. Knowledge of variations in practice patterns has thus led to the definition of the need for outcomes research, helped to set the agenda for it, and engaged the profession in the process.

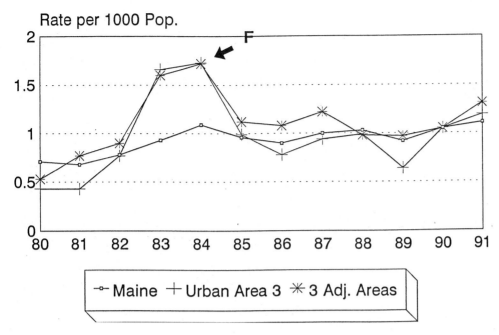

Fig. 4 This graph indicates the change in the rates of lumbar disk excision in one Maine city and three surrounding communities. Before 1982, the rates for these areas were equal to or less than the overall rate for the state. In 1983, the rates began to rise rapidly. The entrance into practice of three surgeons was the only explanatory variable. After feedback of information through the study-group methodology, the rates decreased to the state average, where they have remained.

Study Designs and Implementation in Orthopaedics

Clinical research questions can be designed and answered in various ways. All studies, whether they involve the administration of a drug or the performance of an operation, have some of the same basic research architecture. The methods of answering questions or the difficulties encountered may be different, but the overall design and structure are similar. We will first define the various types of study design and then focus on the randomized clinical trial and discuss various components of this form of research design.

Observational and Experimental Studies

First, the study question must be posed clearly before the investigator can determine the best design or method to answer that question. Some research is observational — that is, the investigator observes events rather than altering them. A review of the prevalence of pulmonary emboli after total hip replacement is an example of an observational or descriptive study.

In other instances, research is experimental: the investigator applies a maneuver and then observes the outcome. For example, a surgeon may conduct a randomized trial comparing the effects of warfarin and heparin on the prevalence of deep venous thromboses in patients managed with a total hip replacement. This is experimental research that is done in an attempt to answer a question through a maneuver.

Cross-Sectional Studies

In a cross-sectional study, patients or events are examined at one point in time. All measurements are made at once, without the need for follow-up. Such studies may be used to describe variables and their distribution, or they may be carried out to examine associations. Cross-sectional studies can be conducted relatively quickly. They may suggest causal links between variables, but one must be careful when drawing conclusions. Rare diseases are difficult to study with this method.

This type of study is rarely done in orthopaedics, but it can occasionally be useful. Staheli and associates[13] employed cross-sectional methodology in their study of the longitudinal arch of the foot. They examined the arches of children and adults of various ages at a single point in time and described the general progression and development of the arch with age. The same individual was not followed over time, as would have been done in a longitudinal study. The results of a cross-sectional study may be useful in that they give a general overview of a condition or a specific finding, such as the development of the longitudinal arch.

Retrospective and Prospective Cohort Studies

A cohort is a group of patients. A cohort study, therefore, follows a group of patients longitudinally over time. Such studies may be observational or experimental, and they may be either prospective or retrospective. A prospective cohort study follows patients forward in time. The outcomes of interest occur after the study has begun. In a retrospective study, the outcomes of interest have already occurred, and the investigator follows a cohort of subjects forward from some point of time in the past.

Prospective studies are stronger than retrospective studies because the investigator can determine what outcomes to observe and can record them in a standard fashion. The data to be recorded are determined before the study. Retrospective studies, on the other hand, depend on records and previously recorded data or on the memory of the patients. The investigator has no control over what was recorded or how it was recorded. The data are more reliable in a prospective study because the investigator controls those data, and the same information can be recorded reliably for all patients.

Case-Control Studies

A case-control study is a retrospective form of cohort study in which patients with an outcome of interest and a control group without that outcome are followed backward from some point in time to ascertain whether some earlier treatment or other exposure had a relationship to that outcome. For example, suppose we want to know whether the duration of diabetes has an effect on the development of a Charcot foot. From a group of insulin-dependent diabetics, we would select the patients who had a Charcot foot (cases) and a group of patients who did not have a Charcot foot (controls) and determine how long they had had the diagnosis of diabetes. The study is retrospective in that we are going backward in time, and the determination of the data depends on information recorded in the past. Investigators have no control over how and when the data were recorded. Patients do not have specified, periodic visits to physicians for determination of the presence or absence of diabetes, so there are inherent weaknesses in the design of the study. However, it still may be possible to get some idea as to whether or not having diabetes longer increases the chances of a Charcot foot developing. Case-control series, although rarely used in orthopaedics, can provide some clinically relevant information if they are carefully constructed. Important information has been gained from the medical literature with the use of this study design.[14]

Control Groups

Control groups enhance the validity of a study. Many studies, however, are uncontrolled and merely present a series of patients who had a particular treatment or maneuver applied to them. The case series is an all-too-frequent study design in the orthopaedic literature. It is often very difficult to know how to interpret the results of such studies and, therefore, what conclusions to draw from them. These studies may be either prospective or retrospective.

Some type of control group is preferable to no control at all. Historical controls can be used. A previous study describing patients with no treatment (or a different treatment) may serve as a historical control group and provide comparative information about the treatment under study. We know the prevalence of death from pulmonary emboli for patients who had a fracture of the proximal part of the femur and had received no prophylaxis for deep venous thromboses,[15] so we can compare that historical control group with a current group receiving a specific prophylactic treatment. In this case, the comparison will not prove that the treatment used is better than another, but it may demonstrate that the treatment is better than no treatment at all.

There are difficulties involved in the use of historical controls because the studies are not done concurrently. Patients may have received different types of adjunctive treatment, and this can confound the results. The historical trial may have been conducted years before, when over-all medical care was quite different. While a historical control may be better than no control, the use of historical controls requires that the study subjects be similar. The methods used to determine outcome must be the same, or similar enough for the investigator to make valid comparisons. The appropriate use of historical controls in clinical research is very difficult.

A concurrent control group is obviously the best choice. Similar types of patients being treated during the same time period and by the same investigator can be compared with the group under study. It is important that the two groups be the same and have similar comorbidities. This may be difficult to accomplish. Patients may be given one treatment in preference to another, for example, depending on how sick they are. Less sick patients may have surgical treatment, while those with more severe disease or other medical problems may be considered unfit for surgery and end up as so-called controls. Biases are easily interjected into the study without the investigator realizing it.

To summarize, studies may be either observational or experimental. Investigators may use different approaches. Timing determines whether the investigators will look at patients at one point in time (a cross-sectional study) or follow patients over a period of time (a cohort study). In cohort studies, patients may be followed forward from some point in the past or may be tracked forward prospectively from the present. A case-control study is a particular type of retrospective cohort study that may help to answer questions of cause and effect. Control groups, either historical or concurrent, improve the validity of the study.

Randomized Clinical Trials

The randomized clinical trial is a prospective cohort study with concurrent controls. It is the gold standard of scientific studies and was developed to avoid the flaws discussed with regard to the other study designs.

In a randomized clinical trial, patients are randomly allocated into two (or more) study groups, each of which receives a different treatment option. A strict protocol, determined prior to randomization, defines criteria for study participants. The protocol determines exactly how the study will be conducted; what information will be recorded; and how the maneuver will be enacted, the data will be gathered, and the outcome will be measured. Nothing is left to the vagaries of the medical record or the patient's memory. Rather, the maneuver is performed and data are gathered prospectively, according to the specified protocol. Similarly, outcomes are evaluated in a uniform, predetermined fashion.

Treatment, however, is allocated randomly. No patient factors allow one treatment to be preferred. It is this random allocation that differentiates a randomized clinical trial from any prospective, concurrently controlled study. This feature makes it the strongest possible study design and the one that is advocated as the most reliable way to gain accurate scientific information.

Blinding

Blinding can make the performance of the maneuver and the determination of the outcomes even better. It is best if the person applying the maneuver (the surgeon in a surgical trial) and the patient do not know which maneuver is being applied. This is easily done in drug trials in which two different drugs are administered, but obviously a surgeon cannot be blinded to the procedure being performed.

Blinding of the outcome assessment also strengthens study results. Neither the assessor nor the patient should be aware of which maneuver was performed. If this is the case, the result is a double-blind trial, which further eliminates bias in a study. It is obvious that some of this blinding is impossible in a surgical trial. However, if the assessor of the outcome is not the individual who provided the maneuver and can be blinded to the nature of that maneuver, the assessment will be less biased. For example, a covering bandage can be placed on all patients being evaluated, in an attempt to blind the assessor with regard to whether or not a patient was managed with an operation. The difficulty involved in carrying out double-blind surgical studies is obvious; thus, such studies rarely can be accomplished.

Bias

Several forms of bias can occur in prospective study designs. Although randomized clinical trials may reduce the chances of biases occurring, they cannot totally eliminate the possibility. There may be more difficulties with biases with surgical trials than with medical trials.[16] Biases are any systematic errors arising from the design or conduct of a study that may affect the validity of the study. Of the study designs discussed, randomized clinical trials have the fewest potential biases, although biases may not be completely avoidable even in those studies.

Susceptibility bias occurs if the two groups under investigation are dissimilar in terms of their initial state; that is, if they have any feature that results in a prognosis for a better or worse outcome. A randomized clinical trial is valuable in that it should preclude the possibility of susceptibility bias because the alternative treatment groups are randomly selected. Theoretically, all comorbidities and other factors should be evenly distributed so the outcomes in both groups will be equally affected by those factors.

In any randomized clinical trial, the maneuver in both arms (groups) of the trial must be performed similarly. A dissimilar level of skill in the performance of a procedure is called performance bias. While performance bias may be easy to avoid in a trial of drug therapy, it may be difficult to control in a surgical trial. Surgeons must be equally proficient in the performance of both study operations, and all comaneuvers must be similar. A surgeon who is asked to perform procedure A in some patients and procedure B in others may not be equally proficient in both. Similarly, if two different surgeons are performing the two procedures, comparisons of surgical skill and their impact on outcome will be difficult to make.

Detection bias occurs when the means for the detection of the outcome are dissimilar. If the outcomes in two groups are measured by different people or in different ways with different criteria, the measurements cannot be compared. This problem can also occur if surgeons assess their own outcomes and are influenced, perhaps inadvertently, by what they want that outcome to be. Ideally, outcome evaluators should be blinded to protect against this form of bias. It is preferable for patients to be blinded as well, but this may be impossible in a surgical trial, because patients may agree to be randomized to alternative treatments but they generally must be informed of the treatment that they will receive. In the ideal situation, double-blinding (blinding of both the physician and the patient) or, at a minimum, single-blinding (blinding of either the physician or the patient) is the best protection against detection bias.

Transfer bias, which can also occur in a randomized clinical trial, results when there is a differential loss to follow-up. Not all patients return for follow-up. If their reasons for not returning are unknown (as is usually the case), this lack of follow-up can bias the study. Perhaps all of the patients who had procedure A and did not return had poor results and sought care from different physicians. Alternatively, suppose that all of the patients who had procedure B and did not return had good results and felt no need for follow-up. The study that considers only the patients who were followed will be biased because of this differential loss. A randomized clinical trial does nothing to protect against this potential problem. Only vigorous attempts to follow all patients, as one should make in any study, can prevent this bias.

In summary, the randomized clinical trial is a prospective, concurrently controlled study that has a specified protocol for inclusion and exclusion criteria, that randomly allocates patients to both arms of the trial, and that specifies the mechanics of the trial and the method of outcomes measurements. Its great achievement is its avoidance of susceptibility bias. Other biases can occur, however, and the investigator must take as many precautions as possible to prevent them.

Problems with Surgical Trials

Surgical trials, and orthopaedic trials in particular, may present other difficulties, as already mentioned. Because the medical model of the randomized clinical trial cannot always be applied to surgery, it is important that studies in surgery be carefully constructed and that protocols be diligently specified in order to avoid bias whenever possible. Still, randomized clinical trials can have particular problems when used to study surgical interventions.[16]

Ethical Issues

Surgical trials raise ethical issues that are not necessarily faced in medical trials. A randomized clinical trial requires that the investigator not believe that one treatment method in the trial is superior to the other. This may be difficult in a trial comparing two operations. A surgeon may have more experience with, or a greater belief in, one operation. Surgeons become familiar, adept, and comfortable with certain operations, and they have personal experience with the results. It may, therefore, be difficult to get them to participate in a randomized study.[16,17]

Performance Issues

As noted, it may be impossible for surgeons to perform two different operations with equal skill and enthusiasm, as might be required in a randomized clinical trial. The surgeon may not want to open the envelope in the operating room and do either procedure A or procedure B. It also may be difficult for the physician to convince the patient to participate in such a trial. Patients may find it much easier to accept alternative medications from their physician than to accept the thought of being managed with a different operation (or none at all).[16-19]

Another difficulty with surgery is that it is irreversible. A drug trial can be stopped, and the patient may not have any after-effects from the trial. This is not the case with surgery. The alternative maneuver cannot be tried. There can be no escape clause as in a drug trial.

Outcome Issues

Long-term studies are often needed to determine clinically important outcomes in orthopaedic trials. For instance, orthopaedists may need five, ten, or even more years to determine the outcomes of hip replacement procedures. The results of a drug trial often can be evaluated in months. The blinding of outcomes for years is difficult but may be necessary.

Philosophical Issues

We have alluded to the differences in surgical philosophy that add to the difficulties of surgical trials compared with medical ones. Surgeons take responsibility for the results of an operation in a different fashion than an internist feels responsible for the results of a drug. Society also draws these lines clearly. A rash from a drug is generally considered to be related to the drug, not to the individual who prescribed it. A wound infection, a dislocated prosthesis, or a broken implant is more often seen as the surgeon's failure than as an inherent risk of the procedure. Both patients and physicians may view bad outcomes in drug trials differently from those in surgical trials. The very nature of surgical intervention creates different aspects of participation on the part of the investigator. The surgeon is not merely an investigator but is an active participant in the determination of the outcome. This sets the stage for very different attitudes on the part of investigators participating in a randomized clinical trial of surgical treatment.

Alternative Study Designs

For all of these reasons, alternative study designs and other methods of randomization may be necessary for surgical trials. While no one denies the credibility and usefulness of the randomized clinical trial, revisions in study design may maintain a high level of credibility and yet allow for participation by more surgeons and patients. Orthopaedic and surgical studies need to be better constructed. With some alterations of the medical model, this may be possible.

Randomization of studies by surgeon rather than by patient (as proposed by Rudicel and Esdaile[16]) is one such possibility. This method randomizes patients to either surgeon A, who will perform procedure A, or to surgeon B, who will perform procedure B. Patients are thus randomized primarily to the surgeon and only secondarily to the procedure. The net result is the same as in a classic randomized clinical trial, but the mechanics of the design are different. This method of randomization solves some of the problems of different skill levels that may occur in a classic randomized clinical trial, but it maintains the surgeon-patient relationship, which is inherently different than the physician-patient relationship in a medical trial. The strengths of the randomized clinical trial are maintained. However, the randomized-by-surgeon design solves some but not all of the possible concerns of surgeons about randomized clinical trials.

We need to develop and evaluate other possibilities for the conduct of high-quality outcomes research while still maintaining the necessary adherence to appropriate protocols for the study design. It will then be possible for surgical procedures to be evaluated with the rigorous clinical investigations that are required to obtain information that is accurate, meaningful, and useful to physicians and patients. While the randomized clinical trial remains the most scientific method available for the conduct of research, other approaches, if well thought out, well designed, and well conducted, may effectively answer questions of clinical importance.

Survey and Measurement Methodologies

There are two large categories of clinical research. Efficacy research is done to determine if a procedure or treatment works at all. For example, the investigator wishes to determine whether a new spinal fixator will provide stable fixation, whether the implant is strong enough, and whether the spine will fuse. Effectiveness or outcomes research is done to find out whether the procedure works well when applied to the general population and what the patient-oriented outcomes of the treatment are. Both questions are important. Frequently, procedures and technologies are widely disseminated and used solely on the basis of their efficacy, even though the essential effectiveness studies have never been conducted. This section outlines the various method and measurement concepts that have been developed in order to conduct outcomes research.

In the selection of clinical endpoints and the measurement of results, the investigator needs to have a clear idea of the questions being asked. Clinical studies done in the 1990s must also recognize the variety of decision-makers who may be using the study results. Health-care administrators, clinicians, and patients will all be looking for information to guide their judgment of an intervention's worth. Although each is concerned about whether the intervention works, the need for other information varies. The administrator, for example, may be particularly interested in the cost of one procedure compared with other options, its

cost-effectiveness, its potential to satisfy patients, and the opportunity costs lost (the cost lost by failure to apply a resource to its most productive use) because one procedure or strategy was picked over another. The patient may be more concerned about the risks versus benefits, the recovery time, and the long-term results. The clinician may be particularly interested in selecting patients who would do the best and in assessing refinements of the intervention or co-interventions that might improve the results.

Outcomes research, then, is characterized by an expanded view of end-results, from measures of technical success to patient-oriented outcomes, including physical, psychological, and social function as well as quality of life and patient satisfaction.

Measurement of Function

Impaired physical, social, and emotional function is an end result of all acute and chronic conditions. Over the last 15 years, methods to assess physical function by self-administered questionnaires have improved tremendously, with a wide number of instruments becoming available.

The new survey instruments build on a model of how illness affects the individual, distinguishing between impairment and disability. Impairment is demonstrable anatomic loss or damage, a physiologic state. Examples include a reduced grip strength or radiographic evidence of structural joint damage. Impairment may not cause functional limitations; for instance, a patient with joint-space narrowing of the hip may not have a problem with walking. Disability is functional limitation caused by impairment or impairments limiting what a patient needs or wants to do, such as carry out the tasks of daily living, employment, recreation, and sexual activity. Instrumental activities of daily living are those activities required for independent living, such as using a telephone or shopping for groceries. The inability to perform these activities suggests a need for special services.

Physical function is complex and is dependent on the integrity of the joint and the neuromuscular system, cognitive ability, and motivation. Disability arises when there is a discrepancy between physical ability and need; it is dependent on whether there is an actual or perceived need to perform a specific function and on the patient's expectations, motivation, and support system. In addition, function changes over the course of a person's development because one's capabilities, wishes, and needs change.

Numerous self-administered questionnaires quantitatively measure function and quality of life[20] and have excellent measurement properties for evaluation research; these properties include validity (the ability to measure what the instrument is supposed to measure), reliability (reproducibility between raters and by one rater from one administration to another), and sensitivity to clinically important changes.

Work Status

Work status, which may be related to the severity of the disease or to individual motivation, is an important outcome, reflecting both the improved function and the increased economic productivity that may result from an intervention. Work status is a critical factor in the economic evaluation of an intervention. However, the effect of orthopaedic procedures on the ability to work is not the only criterion for success, because many patients with musculoskeletal disease are not in the workforce. Work status depends, in part, on one's physical capacity to do the task, but also on motivation, availability of work, and the ability to control the pace of work. An inability to work must be differentiated from voluntary retirement, and an inability to work because of the orthopaedic problem under study must be distinguished from an inability resulting from more important, coexistent conditions, such as cardiovascular disease.

Health Status

Health status, or quality of life, a more difficult concept, embodies physical, social, and emotional function. In outcome studies, a person's health status is both an outcome and a factor that may affect treatment results. Self-administered questionnaires that measure a patient's general health status and quality of life are as reliable, valid, and sensitive as traditional measures of outcome.[21,22] These kinds of measures are particularly important in the evaluation of patients with chronic diseases whose life expectancy is not markedly decreased and for whom morbidity and quality of life are the principal concerns. Such questionnaires have been used to evaluate general health among populations and individuals as well as the effectiveness of a wide variety of medical and surgical interventions, including total joint arthroplasty, back surgery, and carpal tunnel surgery. Health status and quality-of-life measures can be generic or disease-specific. Generic instruments permit comparisons across interventions and diagnostic conditions and are better suited to capture the impact of toxicity of treatment and comorbid conditions. Disease-specific measures can be useful for those who wish to focus on particular functional areas, and such measures may be more responsive to specific interventions. Recently developed short instruments can discriminate changes in clinical status as effectively as the longer instruments can.[23]

Pain

The relief of pain is one of the primary reasons for the performance of orthopaedic procedures. Pain can be measured with a variety of techniques. There is no gold standard, and many techniques are interchangeable. For patients who have musculoskeletal disease, assessment of pain that limits function of a specific joint may be a reliable measure. A simple numerical or adjectival scale is easy to administer and analyze in a standardized format. Visual analogue scales are less convenient to score, and respondents tend to use only a portion of the range. The use of analgesics or anti-inflammatory agents and assistive devices affects the level of pain and function, and this variable should be captured to assist in the interpretation of the patients' responses.

Patient Satisfaction and Expectation

While objective measures of pain and function are critical parameters in the assessment of orthopaedic procedures, the extent to which an operation meets the patients' expectations or goals is also important. Measurement of patients' expectations; their priorities for relief of a particular symptom such as pain, a limp, or the use of assistive devices; and their satisfaction with the operation provide the surgeon with parameters with which to select patients for treatment. While patient satisfaction can be measured, there is no agreement on the best way to measure patients' preferences and the resultant priorities determined by them. Patient preferences have been measured on a variety of bases (willingness to pay, time trade-off, and standard gamble). There has been little work comparing different ways of assessing preferences and how the method used may influence the response. About 10% to 15% of people cannot deal with or interpret questions regarding preferences for management. These may be the same people whose points of view are not represented in social and health-care policy; such groups may include certain ethnic groups, the economically disadvantaged, and the elderly. The priorities and preferences of a group may not be those of an individual. Also, values change with time and with the experiences of illness because people learn, adjust, or accommodate. No system of gauging patients' preferences takes these factors into account.

Complications

Outcomes assessment should evaluate both positive and negative aspects of an intervention to determine the net benefit to the patient. Perisurgical complications may be defined generally as complications occurring during the operation and up to two weeks after the operation. Complications must be assessed actively by explicit procedures and algorithms to judge whether the event was directly related to the operation.

Cost-Effectiveness and Cost-Benefits

The cost of health care is an increasingly important factor in modern medical practice and should be considered in any evaluation of effectiveness. Costs of medical services (such as those incurred for equipment, supplies, and professional labor) involved in the provision of care are called direct medical costs. Indirect medical costs include lost income due to illness, as measured by the difference between expected and actual earnings. The opportunity cost of a resource is the funds or benefits lost by a failure to apply the resource to its most productive use.

Cost-effectiveness and cost-benefit analyses are related but different approaches to the evaluation of an intervention. Cost-benefit analysis compares expenditures for different programs or interventions and expresses all outcomes, including morbidity and death, in economic or monetary terms. An example would be an estimation of the economic value of lives saved or hospitalizations avoided. The major problem with the cost-benefit model is that it suggests that lives saved or quality of life should be valued in monetary units. This is a challenge methodologically and it raises major ethical issues. Cost-benefit analysis allows costs to be subtracted from benefits to express the net benefit for each intervention or program evaluated. Cost-effectiveness evaluation, in contrast, requires that all health outcomes be measured in some quantitative way and be expressed in commensurate units. One example of a unit of cost-effectiveness measurement is the quality-adjusted life-year. Quality-adjusted life-years are the number of years of expected survival, adjusted by weight for any morbidity during those years. Typically, perfect health would be assigned a weight of 1 and a state of health approaching death, a weight near 0.

Covariates That Affect Outcome

The previous discussion outlined the major endpoints or outcomes that should be measured in clinical trials of orthopaedic interventions. Documentation of results without identification of the characteristics that might be associated with a poor outcome may lead to incorrect conclusions. In biostatistics, these characteristics are called covariates, and they include a variety of elements that describe the patient's condition, the surgeon, or the institution.

Patient Characteristics

Age Age is an important factor in terms of a patient's general health. Medicare data show increased mortality rates with increasing age after all types of elective operations, including total hip arthroplasty. This is probably related to the case mix of patients who receive Medicare benefits and to the severity of disease associated with advanced age.

Race Being a member of a racial minority is associated with increased morbidity and mortality, decreased utilization of health-care facilities, and decreased access to health care. These relationships are complex and may be confounded by the patient's socioeconomic status.

Socioeconomic status Health is influenced by socioeconomic factors, including family income, educational level attained, and occupation. A low socioeconomic status may affect access to health care, recognition that care is needed, communication with health-care professionals, nutrition, housing conditions, educational opportunities, employment skills, and resourcefulness in the face of adversity. It appears that lower levels of education, income, and occupation are strongly associated with poor health in people of all ages. Poverty has been associated with a worse outcome for virtually every medical condition and surgical treatment that has been studied.

Operative Factors

Surgeon The surgeon's expertise, training, and specialization in the procedure or condition being studied has an important effect on the result of the operation. A profile of the surgeon can be ascertained by the number of procedures that he or she has performed each year and by his or her specific training in the trial procedure.

Operative Technique and Type of Implant The technical aspects of various orthopaedic procedures differ, and this difference is frequently difficult to capture. Examples of variations include the type of implant, the surgical exposure, the adequacy of the bone stock, and whether the operation is a primary procedure or a revision of a failed operation.

Institutional Characteristics The characteristics of the hospital influence the result of an operation and correlate, to a degree, with some characteristics of the surgeon. The volume of operations performed in an institution is a strong determinant of mortality from total hip arthroplasty. Volume may also correlate with differences in other surgical results and complications, but the relationship between volume and outcome is not altogether clear. For example, patients may be referred to a large-volume practice because they had complications after a primary operation. This would create a different patient mix for the high-volume practice that might lead to poorer outcomes. Functional results may also be affected by the availability of a skilled rehabilitation staff as well as by the length of time that the patient stays in the hospital. Resources such as laminar air-flow and isolator systems may reduce the rate of postsurgical infections.

Medical Conditions

Comorbidity Concurrent medical or surgical problems may be associated with pain or with a loss of function, and this association can confound the outcome of an orthopaedic procedure such as a total hip arthroplasty. Several instruments, probably interchangeable, are available for quantification of comorbid conditions. Often a trained person or a physician is needed to make a judgment about the importance of comorbid conditions.

Risk of Infection Factors predisposing to postoperative infection should be documented. These include previous operations, rheumatoid arthritis, poor nutrition, steroid therapy, diabetes mellitus, and pre-existing infection in such sites as carious teeth or the urinary tract.

Current Medications Data about medications used by the patient relate to the severity and activity of the underlying disease. Medications can also predispose to complications. Corticosteroids increase the fragility of the skin, predispose to infection, and impair healing of the wound. It has been suggested that penicillamine impairs healing and that methotrexate predisposes to infection, but these relationships have not been proved.

General Considerations

Whether one is a reader of a study or an investigator, some general points should be kept in mind during the evaluation of a study or the planning of data collection.

The endpoints should measure impairment or disability. In general, although impairment does not correlate perfectly with disability, measures of impairment (such as range of motion or alignment) may be more sensitive and more easily obtained over the short term.

The determination of the outcome should include both the benefits and the risks of the procedures. Most studies demonstrate benefits well but pay less attention to the rigorous measurement of complications or side effects. At a minimum, the study should include a standardized way of defining and ascertaining these complications.

The outcomes and complications should be documented according to a protocol. Collection of information on problems only when patients report them or make a return visit may lead to an underestimation of the frequency and severity of complications.

The techniques used should be tested for their reliability, validity, and sensitivity. As discussed, the options for measurement of both impairment and patient-centered outcomes are numerous, and although ad hoc measures can be used, standardized instruments permit more accurate comparisons. Testing of whether a questionnaire is reproducible is particularly important in multicenter studies. Use of self-administered questionnaires has the additional advantages of reducing the time spent by the physician and eliminating the bias of the person who performed the procedure.

When multiple end-points are determined, statistical corrections should be used to examine these end-points. Performance of multiple tests of statistical significance on many end-points increases the chance that statistically significant but spurious or irrelevant results will be found. This can be adjusted, in part, by the setting of higher levels of statistical significance or by correction for multiple significance testing.

There should be a sufficient number of subjects. The finding of an unusual event, whether it be an outcome or a complication, requires a sample that is large enough and has been followed long enough for rates to be ascertained reliably. The required sample size can be estimated before the study is constructed, by use of standard statistical methods, or, when the information is not known beforehand, it can be estimated retrospectively.

Conclusion

We have defined outcomes research, discussed several factors underlying its development, and discussed a number of specific components of this methodology. In closing, we would like to emphasize that it is imperative for orthopaedists (and all specialists) to understand and participate in the outcomes agenda. Reform of health care in this country will occur. The precise form that it will take and the time span necessary to produce change are not evident, but there is no doubt that major restructuring is urgently required.

Regardless of the method of financing and the structural form of health care that results, outcomes research should be a central element of the process. The need to understand more about utilization rates and real outcomes of care, to develop accurate and comparable databases, and to learn what works for individual patients is paramount. The deficiencies in current medical practice are widely known by policymakers, payers, and the public. If the medical profession does not play the key role in this element of reform, it will lose both credibility and its ability to play a role in the other issues at stake.

Beyond that, outcomes research presents an exciting opportunity for orthopaedists. Improvements in the quality of clinical research will result in better information. Through the use of standardized measures and definitions, investigators will be able to compare results of new technologies and procedures accurately. Better information about patient-oriented results of treatment will be available, and large databases will enable individual researchers to pool data to gain increased power and statistical validity of studies.

Two other elements should be mentioned. Many aspects of outcomes research will need to involve community-based orthopaedists, because the value of procedures and technologies that have been developed at the research or medical-center level needs to be confirmed as these procedures are widely adopted in clinical practice. The opportunity to participate in effectiveness research of this kind will stimulate the interest and participation of all orthopaedic surgeons in the concept of continuous quality improvement and education.

Finally, outcomes research will result in increased participation of patients in decision-making about the kind of care that they want. Most orthopaedic procedures and treatments are elective. Outcomes research has shown that, when they are given accurate and unbiased information about the risks and benefits of various treatments, patients will make very different choices about the care that they desire. For many years medical decision-making has been largely delegated to doctors. For example, two patients with identical symptoms and findings would likely receive (and accept) the same treatment recommendation from their physician. Just as we have learned that individual physicians differ in terms of the recommendations that they make to patients, outcomes research has taught us that patients also vary in the value and utility that they place on different treatment alternatives. Thus, the two patients just described, who appear so similar to their physician, may choose quite different types of treatment. Outcomes research will provide information and technologies that inform and empower patients. The end result will be that patients, in partnership with their physicians, will be able to make decisions that are best for them.

References

1. Wennberg J, Gittelsohn A: Variations in medical care among small areas. *Sci Am* 1982;246:120-134.
2. Gartland JJ: Orthopaedic clinical research: Deficiencies in experimental design and determinations of outcome. *J Bone Joint Surg* 1988;70A:1357-1364.
3. Gross M: A critique of the methodologies used in clinical studies of hip-joint arthroplasty published in the English-language orthopaedic literature. *J Bone Joint Surg* 1988;70A:1364-1371.
4. Turner JA, Ersek M, Herron L, et al: Surgery for lumbar spinal stenosis: Attempted meta-analysis of the literature. *Spine* 1992;17:1-8.
5. Labelle H, Guibert R, Joncas J, et al: Lack of scientific evidence for the treatment of lateral epicondylitis of the elbow: An attempted meta-analysis. *J Bone Joint Surg* 1992;74B:646-651.
6. Lu-Yao GL, Littenberg B, Keller RB, et al: Outcomes of internal fixation and arthroplasty among elderly patients with displaced femoral neck fractures, unpublished data.
7. Turner JA, Ersek M, Herron L, et al: Patient outcomes after lumbar spinal fusions. *JAMA* 1992;268:907-911.
8. Chalmers IG, Collins RE, Dickersin K: Editorial: Controlled trials and meta-analyses can help resolve disagreements among orthopaedic surgeons. *J Bone Joint Surg* 1992;74B:641-643.
9. Senghas RE: Editorial: Statistics in the Journal of Bone and Joint Surgery: suggestions for authors. *J Bone Joint Surg* 1992;74A:319-320.
10. Keller RB, Soule DN, Wennberg JE, et al: Dealing with geographic variations in the use of hospitals: The experience of the Maine Medical Assessment Foundation Orthopaedic Study Group. *J Bone Joint Surg* 1990;72A:1286-1293.
11. Volinn E, Mayer J, Diehr P, et al: Small area analysis of surgery for low-back pain. *Spine* 1992;17:575-581.
12. Keller RB, Chapin AM, Soule DN: Informed inquiry into practice variations: The Maine Medical Assessment Foundation. *Qual Assur Health Care* 1990;2:69-75.
13. Staheli LT, Chew DE, Corbett M: The longitudinal arch: A survey of eight hundred and eighty-two feet in normal children and adults. *J Bone Joint Surg* 1987;69A:426-428.
14. Horwitz RI, Feinstein AR, Harvey MR: Case-control research: Temporal precedence and other problems of the exposure-disease relationship. *Arch Intern Med* 1984;144:1257-1259.
15. Salzman EW, Harris WH, DeSanctis RW: Anticoagulation for prevention of thromboembolism following fractures of the hip. *N Engl J Med* 1966;275:122-130.
16. Rudicel S, Esdaile J: The randomized clinical trial in orthopaedics: Obligation or option? *J Bone Joint Surg* 1985;67A:1284-1293.
17. Taylor KM, Margolese RG, Soskolne CL: Physicians' reasons for not entering eligible patients in a randomized clinical trial of surgery for breast cancer. *N Engl J Med* 1984;310:1363-1367.
18. Lacher MJ: Patients and physicians as obstacles to a randomized trial. *Semin Oncol* 1981;8:424-429.
19. Spodick DH: The randomized controlled clinical trial: Scientific and ethical bases. *Am J Med* 1982;73:420-425.
20. Liang MH, Katz J, Ginsburg KS: Chronic rheumatic disease, in Spilker B (ed): *Quality of Life Assessments in Clinical Trials.* New York, NY, Raven Press, 1990, pp 441-458.
21. Liang MH, Fossel AH, Larson MG: Comparisons of five health status instruments for orthopedic evaluation. *Med Care* 1990;28:632-642.
22. Liang MH, Larson MG, Cullen KE, et al: Comparative measurement efficiency and sensitivity of five health status instruments for arthritis research. *Arthritis Rheum* 1985;28:542-547.
23. Katz JN, Larson MG, Phillips CB, et al: Comparative measurement sensitivity of short and longer health status instruments. *Med Care* 1992;30:917-925.

Practical Implementation of the Computer-Based Medical Record in Orthopaedic Surgery

Philip J. Branson, MD
Roy A. Maxion, PhD

Overview

The foundation of modern orthopaedics was crafted with simple tools. Patients were treated, offices were managed, and studies were published based on hand-written records and plain x-ray films. In today's world, an orthopaedist who had only these tools would face denial of procedures, rejection of manuscripts, and legal peril.

In a typical office, medical record activities now consume 38% of physician time. Errors or omissions can occur in up to 70% of paper-based records.[1] The computer-based medical record (CMR) provides a modern tool to cope with the increased complexity of orthopaedic practice and documentation. The CMR can be used to improve the accuracy and efficiency of medical records. The analysis required to structure and implement the CMR is likely to identify problems with availability, dependability, and accuracy of medical information in most orthopaedic offices. Implementation of the CMR should improve patient care and increase office efficiency.

The CMR is presented as a practical means to streamline the clinical and financial aspects of medical records in orthopaedic practice. Emphasis is placed on the organization necessary to improve accuracy, availability, and reliability of information in the medical chart. A plan for implementation of CMR technology is discussed based on a four-year, 20,000 chart experience with CMR in private practice. A survey of commercial CMR products is provided as a starting place.

Benefits of CMR

Both academic and clinical orthopaedic practices can benefit from a properly structured computerized record. The CMR can improve availability of records on a physical and logical level. Office tasks can be streamlined for improved efficiency and accuracy. The CMR can be used to improve collection of data for clinical decision making and research.

In addition to the familiar chronologic presentation of data in the paper-based medical record (PMR), the CMR permits reorganization of data based on such medical goals as the establishment of trends or causal mechanisms. Access to information in the medical record is not constrained by the physical location of

the chart or the format used to enter the data.[2] The fact that some data is missing becomes obvious when it is viewed as a defect or anomaly in an otherwise orderly presentation.

The CMR is a tool to improve the availability and reliability of information contained in the patient record on a physical and logical level. At the physical level, the CMR allows instantaneous filing and retrieval of charts. CMR information is immediately and simultaneously available to all staff handling calls, patient care, and billing.

At the logical level, the CMR allows grouping of data by problems, causality, context, and problem activity. Data collected across periods of weeks or years can be viewed as an organized aggregate. Reliability, legibility, and accuracy of data are enhanced by systematic data entry and computer shorthand techniques.

As a practical aid to dealing with increased paperwork load, the CMR enhances office productivity by allowing staff to work smarter instead of working harder. Records and reports can be structured to satisfy peer review organization, and utilization review requirements. Pre-certification and other office activities require less staff time. Less transcription is required, because common office correspondence can be constructed by automated assembly of data previously entered into the CMR. The system can track ordered tests and interventions noting absent and abnormal results. Many office tasks can be completed more quickly and reliably than on a paper-based system.

In clinical research, the CMR facilitates structured collection of data. Information can be efficiently recorded and retrieved from multiple patient records. Lack of standardization remains a significant barrier to realizing the full potential of the CMR in multicenter studies. As progress is made in data collection techniques and standardization of nomenclature, the CMR will become an invaluable tool in clinical research.

Goals of the CMR

A CMR can provide many services to its users. A properly structured CMR should (1) represent clinical priorities accurately at any given time, irrespective of evolving conditions; (2) provide to medical records the level of accuracy and dependability accorded to billing records; (3) manage clinical data flow across time; (4) present medical data at an appropriate level of detail; (5) make charts and the information contained in them available in a timely fashion; and (6) present data in a format that facilitates good clinical decision making.

The CMR can enhance confidence that the record contains information that is complete, timely, accurate, and legible. CMR structures and processes make identification of missing or incomplete data reliable. The electronic format ensures legibility.

The idiosyncratic aspects of clinical cases often provide subtle clues to guide pattern recognition and clinical decision making. The temptation to reduce patient contacts to a fill-in-the-blank or multiple-choice record is a common pitfall in implementing the CMR. Forms tidy up the annoying problems in record automation and clinical research presented by the variability of real life clinical practice. Unfortunately, tidiness may be obtained at the expense of introducing systematic error and inaccuracy into the record. Form-based entry can result in incomplete, inaccurate, or erroneous representation of clinical events.

Clinical or statistical methods must be used to validate form or instrument-based data collection. In clinical validation, the form is used as a clue or aid for the physician. Each use of the form is reviewed and edited by the physician for accuracy.

Statistical validation involves detailed analyses of the order, wording, and interpretation of questions and available responses presented by the form or data-collection instrument. Validation requires extensive testing of the instrument. Statistical validation is probably beyond the scope of most academic practitioners and is impractical for the general orthopaedist. To preserve record accuracy, fill-in-the-blank and multiple-choice data collection must be used with caution in clinical practice and research. The same CMR tools that provide efficiency in completing repetitive tasks can introduce systematic error and inaccuracy into the record.

Recording and Presenting Data

The CMR can present data grouped by process, topic, and causality. Pattern and problem recognition is enhanced by viewing data in logical aggregates. Few physicians would consider mixing billing information randomly into the narrative text of patient records. Yet in the paper-based medical record, physicians routinely "mix statements about symptoms, signs, and diagnoses at various levels of abstraction and detail."[3] Billing processes are more efficient and accurate when information about charges, payments, and accounts are grouped on a ledger card. The process of prescribing medications would be more efficient and accurate if prescriptions and allergies were listed in ledger card form. The CMR should make it possible to group medical data. In the CMR, the processes that achieve accuracy and reliability in billing can be applied to all information contained in the medical chart.

The second major difference that distinguishes the CMR is the ability to control data flow within the record across time. Although all detail in the medical record must be preserved for archival purposes, detail relevant to clinical decisions should be most evident in the record. The chronologic entry format of the paper-based record does not allow presentation of clinically relevant data apart from archival detail. The CMR provides a practical means to manage shifts in emphasis and detail in the record across time. Appropriate data can be selected and presented at the level of detail needed to support clinical decision making. Archival detail can be stored in a manner that allows easy retrieval and preserves the integrity of the record, without clouding clinical priorities. The CMR provides simple, powerful tools that allow the physician to direct the flow of data to best represent and support clinical decision making.

Availability

Availability must be defined in terms of content and time. For information to be considered in a clinical decision, it must be relevant to the decision and present when the decision is made. The format of data presentation can significantly influence what and when data is considered in clinical decisions.

In a paper-based system, information is available only to the bearer of the chart. Charts may be unavailable for up to 30% of patient visits.[4] Although most offices probably do better than this, few could achieve a 99% availability level. Consider a practice of two physicians and a 17 man-year history of clinical practice. The practice contains 120,452 charts and 60,880 radiographs. With a 99% availability, 1,204 of the charts and 608 of the radiographs are unavailable at any given time.

Patient visits account for only a small number of the requests for medical records. Availability should be defined in terms of all requests for and reports of data. Phone calls and correspondence outnumber office visits by more than ten to one. In every patient contact, medical record information is either reported or requested. In a typical call to schedule an appointment, a patient reports a medical problem to the receptionist. The person answering the call requires access to medical record information to respond appropriately, and access to the medical record to document the transaction. Non-visit data, obtained when a patient is not physically in the office, is typically recorded on notes outside the official patient record if it is recorded at all. A single example—after-hours requests for inappropriate narcotic prescriptions—suggests that the problem of record availability is obvious to both physicians and patients.

The CMR enhances availability of medical record information at the physical level and the data level. Physical availability is improved by providing rapid access to record information independent of the location of the physical chart. Access to information at the logical level is enhanced by the CMR through organized entry, retrieval, and data-tracking functions.

Reliability

Reliability, along with accuracy and dependability, comprises the third major service that the CMR provides. Accuracy refers to how faithfully the written document reflects the patient contact. Inaccuracy results when information is incomplete or incorrect. Misrepresentation of involved side (right versus left) and date are common examples of inaccuracy in many orthopaedic medical records. The PMR requires that every word contained in the medical record be written or transcribed. In the CMR, only unique information is dictated and entered in full text. Common problems, examinations, and histories can be carefully structured once and transferred many times to different records using computer shorthand techniques. Consistency in documentation of such details as right/left, site, and date can be achieved by computer entry structure. Given the same transcription effort, less time is spent documenting common findings and more time can be devoted to documenting characteristic or idiosyncratic aspects of the case.

Implementation of the CMR

The most critical step in implementation of the CMR is analysis of office needs and information flow. Analysis should proceed from the top down, looking at total information flow. The analysis should be translated into a functional specification of the services required for the office. A system is then selected to supply the necessary services. A master plan of implementation is formulated to allow for gradual transition from the paper-based record to the CMR. Plans must be made to match information flow with the physical location of patients, staff, and computer hardware. Finally, the transition from paper-based to computer-based records occurs from the bottom up. The CMR is implemented in a small subset of the patient records. Implementation problems are identified, resolved, and other patient subsets are added. This iterative process continues until conversion is complete.

Analysis of Information Flow

In the CMR, patient records and correspondence documents are constructed by assembling component parts. The parts are segregated at the time clinical information is entered into the system. Implementation involves description of the component parts and rules for entering and assembling these parts into purposeful forms and documents.

Analysis of information flow is the most challenging aspect of CMR implementation. Clinical information must be divided to allow simultaneous evolution and tracking of multiple clinical problems. Shifts in relative importance of clinical data must be possible. Diversity in the correspondence generated by the office drives the process towards finer and more detailed divisions. Ease of entry and readability drive the process toward fewer, broader categories. The goal is a division scheme detailed enough to allow construction of common correspondence and logical presentation of clinical information, while keeping data entry simple.

Correspondence

The division of data required to generate office correspondence without additional dictation is straightforward. Samples of office correspondence should be broken down to form a list of unique component topics. If the list is properly constructed, most office documents can be generated by assembling topics from the list. Topics and items already accessible from the financial or scheduling software should not be duplicated. The actual correspondence letter or document is constructed by a report generator that assembles appropriate component topics from the medical record with standard text.

Because the automated correspondence document may contain data elements collected across a wide date range, date information should be recorded in absolute terms. Relative date references (three weeks ago) can be corrupted when presented out of chronological context. This problem can be solved by using absolute dates (12/23/93) or by using a variable that allows the computer to calculate a relative date appropriate to the time context of the document.

Clinical Information

Clinical information must be divided so that all information relevant to a given medical problem is readily available and is presented in a format that facilitates good decisions. The requirements for managing clinical data are numerous and complex. The records should allow rapid and easy identification of active problems and relevant data apart from archival data. Incomplete or missing data should be easy to identify. Data may be pertinent for a short time, or the same data may be relevant over a longer period of time, as part of a trend or disease process. For example, a single low hematocrit value may be relevant for a few weeks within the context of surgery, or it may be relevant for many months in the context of the anemia of chronic disease.

As the record evolves, active problems that have been resolved must be assimilated into the past medical history. At any given time, single data elements may be relevant to one or many active problems. As a disease evolves, the same data element may become related to different active problems.

The ability to assign relationships and priorities between data elements and disease processes is the essence of clinical judgment. No CMR system to date is capable of performing these functions automatically. The desired outcome, however, can be achieved with a simple schema of division, summary, and transfer of data.

Division of Clinical Data

Clinical data is divided by topics. Topics generally contain data related by content. Topics are further grouped or subdivided by temporal relationships.

Topics such as present illness are active topics. The content of active topics relates to the evolution of a problem. Active topics contain such information as symptoms, observations, or values used to infer importance and relatedness of clinical data (clinical judgment). Periodically, active topics undergo significant change to reflect new priorities assigned by clinical insights.

In the CMR these changes can be termed "information flow within a topic." A simple way to handle this flow is to divide active topics into two topics, a main topic and a worksheet subtopic. At the inception of clinical investigation, data is entered into the main topic. A basic clinical history or baseline examination is recorded. Interval events related to the problem are stored in the worksheet subtopic. At junctures of significant clinical insight, data from the subtopic is summarized and appended to the main topic, and the revised main topic replaces the initial main topic. The original version of the main topic is stored unaltered for archival purposes. The interval information is cleared from the subtopic. The entire process of summary, addition, and revision is repeated until the problem is resolved. At any time during the clinical course, active patient status is represented by a combination of the most recent main topic and the subsequent occurrences of the worksheet subtopic.

At major clinical junctures, such as the resolution of a problem, information from the active topic flows to an archival topic. Archival topics grow by the process of addition, and serve as a chronologic log. Past illness is an example of an archival topic. Information from several active topics may be summarized to an archival topic as a statement of a process, an outcome, and date within the archival topic.

For example, when a wrist fracture heals, the history, radiographs, and treatment details are summarized as a process: fracture treatment outcome (healed with casting); and date (12/29/93). Entries in archival topics like past illness are sufficient to identify trends, and

they provide an index to archival detail stored in the record for future reference. At the time of summary, archival detail is moved out of the active problem area, allowing remaining data related to active problems to increase in relative importance.

The summary and transfer procedure would be time consuming and difficult in a paper-based record. In the CMR, the existing information is copied, archived, and edited with a few keystrokes. For routine case management, only the most recent entry of each topic needs to be seen. Archival detail is easily retrieved by a directed search, following the map of the summary statements contained in summary topics.

Outside Information

A large part of the data stored in a paper-based record consists of consultation, surgery reports, and discharge summaries. Conversion of the full text of these documents to electronic format is impractical and cumbersome. Instead, the information is summarized for on-line access. For example, a surgical report can be summarized to the CMR as the date of operation, operation performed, site of operation, and significant findings. Infrequently accessed information can be retrieved from the source document if necessary.

Consultations and other hospital information are summarized into the record either before or at the first post-hospital office visit. Surgical reports can be entered on a daily basis. The average time required to enter summary information from an operation into the record is 15 seconds.

Tracking

The CMR provides the capability to track laboratory data, tests, and consultations. The CMR can generate reports of abnormal or unreported items, just as a billing system can identify incorrect payments or past-due accounts. For a tracking system to be reliable, the act of ordering the item to be tracked must also initiate the tracking process. For a single entry to both order the test and initiate tracking, the data needed to process the test order must be entered on-line. The order document must be printed while the patient is in the office. Information required to requisition laboratory or test orders includes diagnosis, tests ordered, and other information present in the database. Computer shorthand can be used to streamline the entry process. Laboratory tests, for example, are commonly ordered as a panel or group of tests. After the diagnosis and reason for testing are entered, a single keystroke can produce the order form, including the panel of tests, no matter how lengthy. Demographic and billing information required by the facility performing the test can be added to the requisition form without further operator entry. When the form is printed, the tracking system is initiated to ensure that results are reported and addressed. The average time required to enter and print a request for services is approximately 20 seconds.

Abnormal test results can be handled when results are entered. The system should be configured to handle normal ranges and flag abnormal results. The process of result entry is likely to be automated in the near future. Currently, the diversity and proprietary nature of laboratory databases make manual entry of results more practical.

The details of surgery scheduling can be tracked in a similar manner. Preoperative consultations, authorizations, and certifications can be recorded. Incomplete items are identified with routine queries, so that deficiencies can be identified and addressed before they result in problems with scheduled surgeries.

Non-Visits

The telephone is a primary source of non-visit patient contacts. The CMR makes the chart available to every staff member for each patient contact. Common patient contacts, like calls with questions or problems, should be handled promptly and efficiently. Ready access to record information decreases the number of messages by allowing many calls to be handled on the spot. The telephone interaction is easily documented in the electronic chart while the patient is still on the phone. The non-visit category, suggested by our medical record vendor, has been a valuable tool for handling patient problems and streamlining phone messages.

System Selection

A commercial medical records package is probably the most practical place to start in implementing the CMR. The benefits of a commercial CMR package include stability, service, and clear definition of the cost of the project. The tradeoff is that the commercial package will not fit 100% of your needs. A package created specifically for your needs has the benefit of being built to order, but this approach has significant risks. CMR software development costs can range from hundreds of thousands of dollars for an office system to over 25 million dollars for a hospital-based CMR. Generic database programs can experience significant degradation in performance when the database reaches a critical size. Few physicians have the time or inclination to deal with software or hardware problems. In practice, even large groups will be hard-pressed to afford the initial cost and ongoing support required to maintain reliability and performance in a custom-made CMR.

Table 1
Vendor Comparison

Services	Vendor					
	AN1	EP2	MC3	MD4	MT5	WL6
Systems Installed						
CMR	200	4	11	NA	12	5
Orthopaedic CMR	15	1	11	NA	4	1
Financial	900	1,000	3,600	NA	72	150
Years in Business	8	14	10	5	8	15
Type*	TPM	TPM	TPM	CAD	MR	TPM
Approximate Cost-$†	35,000	40,000	35,000	33,000	49,500	42,000
Input	Keypad Menu	Mouse Template	Mouse Template	Keypad Template	Keypad	Keypad
Scanning	–	–	–	+	–	–
Images	–	+	–	–	–	–
Prints Rx	+	+	+	+	–	?
Integration w/Financials	+++	+	++	–	–	++
Speed	+++	++§	++§	NA	NA	NA
Labs	+‡	++	–	+	NA	–
Fixed Fields	–	++	++	+	NA	–
Problem List Maintenance	+	++1/2	++1/2	–	NA	+
Spell Check	–	–	+	–	NA	–

* TPM = total practice management, includes CMR, financials and scheduling; CAD = computer assisted dictation and transcription; MR = medical records package, no financials or scheduling.

† Approximate cost - 5 stations, storage for 15,000 pts, 2 laser printers, installation and training. Costs may vary significantly for all vendors based on exact configuration.

‡ Lab values stored as text. Manual evaluation of abnormals required.

§ New products. Insufficient data to determine speed.

Outline 1 Vendor Summary

ANI
  Best integration of scheduling financial and CMR functions
  Largest installed base of CMR users
  Numeric keypad entry: Rapid
  Query structure simple and powerful
  Reporting functions powerful
  Support excellent; Replacement of fully configured machines
  CMR and financial run on the same hardware platform
  Handling fixed field data like labs: Poor
  Major revision due next release

EP2
  Stores graphic drawings
  Problem list works well
  Handles fixed fields well
  "Mini" program: Data collection algorithms
  Lab system: Minor errors in logic
  Graphic trend display
  Templates require definition of maximum length of text entry
  Financials must be exited to enter medical records package
  Demographic data are duplicated
  CMR and financials require different hardware
  Support: On-site service contracts
  Imaging and scanning next release

MC3
  Workable integration of scheduling financial and CMR function
  Problem list works well
  Interface to drug/disease interaction program
  Scanning and labs in next release
  CMR and financials require different hardware
  Support: On-site service contracts
  Work in progress file
  Many innovative features

MD4
  No site visit: Demo disk

MT5
  No site visit/No evaluation of program

WL6
  No site visit

An increasing number of commercial vendors offer medical records packages. Products range from a modified word-processing system to full capability medical-record packages. Both types of packages provide methods for shorthand entry of frequently used data. The full capability medical record system is distinguished by its ability to divide and index medical information for access and retrieval. The best packages offer seamless access to all patient information, including scheduling, financial, and clinical information.

Surveys were sent to 32 vendors who had advertised at the American Academy of Orthopaedic Surgeons meetings and courses in 1991. Six of the 32 responded, and three arranged for on-site evaluation of product. The results of the product evaluations are presented in Table 1 and Outline 1. Factors that should weigh heavily in the selection of a vendor include financial stability, software functionality, client support, and medical records client base.

Vendors that responded completed a detailed 12-page questionnaire and furnished samples of medical records formats. Four of the vendors who responded provide total practice management (TPM) solutions. A TPM package includes medical records, financials, and scheduling. Only one TPM vendor has had an orthopaedic installation on line for more than one year. Entry level costs for a system are approximately 35,000 to 40,000 dollars. There is significant upward cost variation based on system size and configuration.

Most commercial medical records packages furnish an application for the non-programmer to construct an office record database. Rudimentary word-processing functions provide the ability to insert and delete text from the record. Most packages provide a computer shorthand function and provide for multiple office and multiple terminal access to the medical record. Important differences exist in how easily one can switch between financial, scheduling, and medical information, and the mechanisms to organize and regulate data flow within the record.

Interestingly, none of the commercial systems surveyed provided proper methods for editing records after the fact. Most legal sources recommend that retrospective record corrections be performed by placing a single line through text to be deleted. Additions should be underlined, or otherwise distinguished from unaltered text. All deletions or additions should be clearly identified with the time, the date, and the identity of the person performing the modification. Authentication of the record currently requires archived backup tapes to prove data integrity.

Some new and innovative ideas are coming to the market. Vendors EP2 and MC3 offer a feature that helps to maintain a problem list. MC3 has an option for automated cross-reference of prescription orders with disease processes and allergies. Warnings can be generated for possible interactions. EP2 offers a feature that allows the user to define a mini-program that will direct data entry based on some user responses. It is beyond the scope of this discussion to enumerate these special features in detail.

Software Evaluation

Software evaluation is the key to determining if a given system will accomplish the specified goals. Software is far more important than hardware in determining how the system will perform on a day-to-day basis. System selection should be undertaken after the needs of the office are clearly defined.

Interface

The end-user and setup interfaces should be evaluated. Interface refers to all of the aspects concerning how the operator and system interact. The end user interface is what the operators will use on a day-to-day basis in the office. It should be easy to use and easy to look at. In general, functions that are complex to understand and use will not be used. Interfaces that require the use of special characters and computer syntax should be avoided if possible. Mice and other pointing devices should be considered in terms of functional considerations of speed and availability of desk space in the area where entry will occur. Voice recognition has not yet proved to be reliable or practical enough for general use.

Operator entry devices supported in the commercial packages include the numeric keypad, mouse, barcode reader, and keyboard. In our experience, the numeric keypad, located at the right hand side of the keyboard, is the most efficient input device for experienced operators. Patient eye contact can be maintained while entering data, and the hand returns easily to the correct position after interruptions.

A good system will allow extensive control over what is displayed on the computer screen and how it is displayed. The time between the keypress and display of common information should be less than one second. The look, feel, and operation of the medical record package should resemble the operation of the financial system as closely as possible. Switching between financial and medical record data should occur as easily and quickly as switching from one patient to another. Operation should be self-evident to simplify training. The user should be able to define scripts or macros that allow a single keystroke to accomplish a complex set of repetitive tasks.

The end-user interface contains the computer shorthand function that simplifies data entry. Most systems use a combination of menus and templates to assist data entry. The shorthand function provides a way to enter frequently dictated words, phrases, or paragraphs with a single keystroke. Selection of an item on a menu or template list copies a block of pre-defined text into the record. The purpose of menus and templates is to decrease transcription work and to facilitate entry. The system should provide a structure that will accommodate the data flow and format used in your office.

The setup interface allows customization of the system on an office-by-office basis. It is used to create, modify, and fine-tune the user interface. The setup interface allows the user to create menus and templates, define the topics the system will use, and compose the text that will be copied to the record by the shorthand mechanism provided by the program. The setup function should be evaluated for ease of use, simplicity, and flexibility.

Data Entry

Menus and templates provide structure for data entry and access to the computer shorthand function. Both structures exist in most CMR systems. Menus are computer screens that contain lists of choices. Choices are selected with keystrokes or a mouse. Selection of a choice performs a function or adds text to the record. Menus are used in both systems to provide computer shorthand.

Templates are blank forms or outlines for data collection. Templates usually provide some ability to access menus to perform operations, or append text to the record. In a menu-based system, information is entered and is later combined by a set of rules to create a form. In a template-based system, the menu-based collection of information is driven by definition of the form. The end result of both systems is similar. Menu- or template-based operation should be evaluated for the best fit in your particular office.

A good system should handle narrative text and numeric entry from both direct keyboard entry and computer shorthand. The system should handle both numeric and text data in an efficient manner. Some systems require definition of the number of characters or lines that will be reserved for a given topic or data element. While this works well for numeric entry, it is a disadvantage for text-based entry. Systems that do not require advance reservation of space allowed for keyboard text entry are superior.

Computer shorthand, or menu-based entry, should be used to enter text that is commonly typed more than three times per day. It is also useful for unusual terms and words that are difficult to spell. The system should allow easy keyboard entry of information that is infrequently used or idiosyncratic in nature. Text added to the record by the shorthand technique should be easily edited in the individual record to meet specific needs.

If typed entry is faster than menu or template entry, the structure is wrong. Numeric organization and selection of menu choices tends to be the fastest. Acronyms or the use of a mouse for choice selection may be too slow to be useful.

Numeric data should be handled with fixed fields that allow for numeric calculation and comparison. A means should be provided to verify accuracy of entry where possible. For example, if a hospital record number is supposed to have six numeric digits, entry of a five-digit number or use of alpha characters would not be accepted. Calculations and logical comparisons allow for efficient manipulation of numeric data, such as laboratory results or measurements.

Data Flow

Significant differences exist between vendors in how information flows within the record. Only two of the six vendors surveyed understood the requirement for data flow in the record. In evaluating a system, it is essential for the prospective user to understand how evolution of problems will be handled. Problems with data flow will become manifest after several visits, when documents generated yield surprising or inappropriate results.

The system should provide ready access to the information commonly used in your office. It should be able to display a listing of prescriptions, allergies, and diagnoses in less than a second after the enter key is pressed. A structure that requires queries of the data to answer common questions is too slow to be useful.

Correspondence

The system should be capable of generating correspondence. Most systems do this with some form of merge. In a merge, a form letter contains variables that pull in specific information from a patient record. A good system will allow merge letters to pull information from scheduling, financials, and medical records. A general practice may require in excess of 175 different form letters. On demand, the system should be able to generate rapidly a single letter for an individual patient. Letters for multiple selected patients should be produced for batch mailing. Letters should reformat automatically to omit blank spaces if information is absent in the record. The printed output should not look or read like a form letter. All correspondence generated should be automatically logged in the individual patient record with date, time, and contents.

Maintenance

Maintenance is one of the key benefits of a commercial package. Maintenance contracts vary widely in scope. The annual cost ranges from 5% to 15% of the initial purchase price. Services should include hardware and software support. New or updated versions of the software are usually included in the cost of the contract. The best contracts offer 7-day, 24-hour access to phone software support. Hardware problems are managed with on-site service or prompt hardware replacement. It is our experience that a single source responsible for both hardware and software is the best approach. Same-day or next-day replacement service on computer hardware has proven to be superior to the on-site service contracts we hold on other office equipment. On-site service in many cases lacks sufficient inventory and expertise to achieve the same turnaround time possible with same-day or next-day replacement service.

Offices using systems AN1, EP2, and MC3 were selected at random from a list of installations and interviewed by phone. Three offices for each vendor were contacted. Only AN1 practices were using medical records. All nine practices contacted were satisfied with the level of service provided. Downtime was not reported as a significant problem by any installation.

Security

Security is a major topic for most CMR discussions. Most systems require security authorization in the form of passwords to access the records. Unauthorized modification of the record is a major concern. Modifications can be difficult to identify in an electronic record. Unauthorized modification of records could result in existence of different versions of the record. The security and medical records audit-trail features of every commercial package could be improved. Nonetheless, access to the information contained in the records is probably better controlled in the CMR than it is in charts on the shelves and desks of a paper-based office.

Getting Started

Once a vendor is selected, the physical constraints of how and where the information will be entered must be considered. Major changes in current office procedures can be disruptive. Conversion must occur through a process of gradual transition. The process should be orderly, and run in parallel with paper records until sufficient dependability, confidence, and competence are demonstrated. The conversion should be expected to take three to six months after the hardware is on-line, configured, and tested.

Menus and Templates

Construction of menus and templates is part of system setup. It is a time-consuming process that is required for every commercial package. Ideal menus contain from three to 14 items per column, and up to two columns.[5] Menus should be no more than three layers deep. Menu layering, or branching, occurs when selection of a menu choice results in the presentation of another menu. Use of more than three branches results in confusion and significantly slows entry. Options that appear at more than one place in the program should be presented in a consistent manner in every case. Items that are difficult to spell or that are typed more than three times per day should be added to a menu or template. Entries that are used infrequently should be removed. In our experience, organizing menus to correspond to common dictation patterns is more effective than anatomic or functional classifications.

Records should meet peer review organization, precertification, and level-of-service reviews. Menu- or template-assisted record entry can be used to help records pass checklist quality and utilization reviews. The work spent in careful wording and design of menus and templates will be evident in all subsequent records generated.

Data Entry

Data entry can be performed in a number of ways. Checklists, forms, on-line entry, or batch transcription may be used. Many ophthalmologists successfully enter all information during office visits (on-line entry). For each examination station, a transcriptionist and terminal will be required. This consumes significant resources in terms of staff and machines. Batch entry from dictation is traditional in many orthopaedic offices. It decreases initial hardware requirements, but does not provide for on-line entry of laboratory tests or other orders.

A combination of data entry methods, (forms, batch, and on-line) can result in a good compromise of economy and function. On-line entry can be used for information that is required to generate laboratory test orders or other documents required before the patient leaves the office. Other information can be entered into the record after the fact by traditional batch dictation and transcription.

An example of patient and information flow in an office using a combination of data entry methods is presented diagrammatically in Figure 1. Patients complete a form detailing basic past medical information in a checklist fashion (Fig. 2). The information is transcribed on-line from the checklist by the receptionist, who uses menus that correspond to the paper forms. The receptionist enters a brief narrative chief complaint. A document is printed that contains a combination of the transcribed checklist, chief complaint, and demographic information. This information accompanies the patient to the examination room. Information

entered by the receptionist is verified and edited by the physician as needed. History of present illness, examinations, and other information are dictated to tape and are transcribed into the record later.

In our experience, information necessary to generate orders for drugs, tests, and supplies can be entered on-line by the one or two staff members who coordinate examination room patient flow. A single terminal and printer can service eight active exam rooms efficiently. Because all information is on-line, overflow entry can be handled by staff at any of the front-office terminal locations, even though this is not within their normal scope of activities.

On return visits, medical record summaries can be shown on the screen or printed as hard copy from the CMR to avoid pulling charts. The reception staff can review the summaries, making note of any new problems.

A major benefit of the CMR is that information relevant to patient visits can be presented based on predictable practice patterns. Well-defined reasons for appointments in a computerized scheduler can be used to automate what and how information from the medical record will be presented to the physician at the time of the office visit. For example, follow-up fracture care patients would display the most recent radiograph report, date, and a brief history of injury and treatment. A chronic back patient may display MRI, bone scan, and neurologic examinations. Identi-

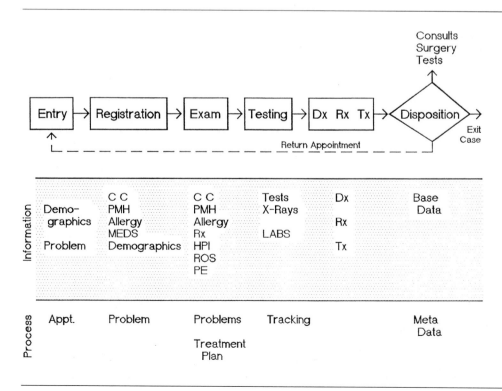

Fig. 1 Office information flow-chart.

Please mark those that apply to you under "patient", and those that apply to blood relatives under "family"

PAST MEDICAL PROBLEMS

	Patient	Family		Patient	Family
High blood pressure			Bleeding problems		
Heart Murmur			Blood Clots		
Heart Attack			Stroke		
Angina (chest pains)			Cancer		
Shortness of Breath			Anemia		
Asthma			Thyroid		
Black lung			Seizures/ epilepsy		
Diabetes			Anesthesia Problem		
Ulcers			Sinus trouble		
Arthritis			Jaundice / Hepatitis		
Stroke			Pregnancy		
Aids, ARC			Other		
Osteoporosis			Other		

PAST SURGERIES

SURGERY	DATE	SURGERY	DATE
Tonsils		Gall Bladder	
Hysterectomy		Prostate	
Ovaries left?		Cancer Surgery	
Hernia		Kidney R L	
Appendectomy		Other:	
Arthroscopy R L		Back Surgery	
Total Hip R L		Fracture/Break	
Total Knee R L		Other	

ALLERGIES: Note reaction (nausea, hives etc.)
Codeine   . . . .
Antibiotic   . . . .
Arthritis pill   . . . .
Aspirin   . . . .
Environment   . . . .
Other   . . . .
                  . . . .

MEDICINES: Please List:
Medicine   Name / Dose   Last taken
Insulin   . . . .
Blood pressure   . . . .
Heart
Blood Thinner   . . . .
Pain Pill   . . . .
Nerve Pill   . . . .
                  . . . .
                  . . . .
                  . . . .
MEDICAL DOCTOR: . . . .

SMOKING
    Packs / day ..
    Cigar/pipe   ..
    Chew Tobacco

ALCOHOL:
__ None __ Occasional __ Frequent

DATE OF INJURY: _____

COMPENSATION: YES NO
AUTO ACCIDENT: YES NO
OTHER LIABILITY: YES NO

ATTORNEY: _____

PRIOR DISABILITY: YES NO

Fig. 2 Orthopaedic Center of the Virginias' patient medical history form.

Signature_____

fication of predictable information requirements and good logical structure will allow efficient management of the flow of both patients and information.

Transition

Transition from the paper-based system to the CMR should be carefully planned. Errors in logic and entry structure should be identified on a small group of pilot records. The master plan must allow for gradual conversion of existing paper records. New patients should be given higher priority, because attrition will decrease the number of existing charts that will require conversion. Simultaneous use of electronic and paper records should be considered until the dependability and reliability of the system is verified. In many cases, this duplication can be accomplished by printing and filing a copy of the electronic record.

In our experience, entry of a limited number of new patients, presenting with a single common complaint is a good place to start. The initial CMR entries should be critically reviewed and corrected by the physician.

Hard copy should be kept until several cycles of return visits can be handled efficiently. When the structure appears to be working well, more records of the same type can be added. The scope of the CMR is then expanded to include new patients with other problems. Structures to handle common problems can be refined one at a time until all new patients are handled on the CMR system. It is a challenge to handle the special requirements for each problem while maintaining a simple, consistent menu system.

Existing patients with extensive history on the PMR will require a transition period during which both records are used. At the first visit of an established patient, appropriate past history is summarized into the CMR from the paper chart. On a small number of extensive or thick charts, summary may be impractical. In these cases, the paper chart can be used unless the benefit of conversion justifies the work required to summarize the chart. As the physician gains proficiency, conversion of old records becomes simple and rapid.

Conclusion

The CMR offers significant benefits to the orthopaedic surgeon. It is possible and practical to implement the CMR in orthopaedic practice. The major benefit of the CMR is improved availability, reliability, and dependability of medical records. The keys to successful implementation are a solid logical structure for recording data and meticulous management of data flow. The CMR is practical as long as the physician understands its benefits and shortcomings.

Implementation of the CMR requires clinical insight and extensive physician participation. Decisions required to structure clinical data and evaluate the accuracy of the system cannot be delegated to non-physician personnel.

As progress is made in standardization of nomenclature, the CMR will become a valuable tool in clinical research. Technologic advances in hardware and software engineering are making powerful tools available and practical for clinical practice. It is the opinion of these authors that collaborative effort on the part of organized orthopaedics could result in substantial advances and benefits from this technology.

References

1. Institute of Medicine, in Dick RS, Steen EB (eds): *The Computer Based Patient Record, An Essential Technology for Health Care.* Washington, DC, National Academy Press, 1991.
2. Barnett GO: The application of computer-based medical-record systems in ambulatory practice. *N Engl J Med* 1984;310:1643-1650.
3. Rector AL, Nowlan WA, Kay S: Foundations for an electronic medical record. *Methods Inf Med* 1991;30:179-186.
4. Winslow: Putting it on paper. *Wall Street Journal*, Monday, April 6, 1992.
5. Drews: Medical Record Keeping NOW. *Administrative Ophthalmology.* Winter 1993.

Research Communication Media: Creating An Outstanding Impression With Abstracts, Poster Exhibits, and Slides

Jeffrey A. Russell, MS
G. William Woods, MD

Introduction

At no time is one's appearance to one's peers under greater scrutiny than when he or she is addressing them in the context of a professional society. Whether submitting an abstract of a study or proffering research conclusions in a poster exhibit or slide presentation, an individual is judged not only by the content of the message, but also by how it looks. Often the caliber of these interactions is the only tool the audience can use to formulate their opinions of the author. We have developed our thoughts on this topic (although not all the concepts are originally ours) after much introspection, self-criticism, and experimentation. We have also made careful analyses of medical writing and audiovisual tendencies over our years of involvement in research and professional conferences. Our purposes for writing are several. Primarily, we want others to benefit from our collection of information and references. If one goes away from this manuscript without a desire to raise his or her standard of quality in communicating, then we have failed miserably.

We hope that novice researchers and presenters can learn many techniques that will help them project themselves and their work favorably. Veterans at writing and presenting will find new methods and refine old ones. We strive to blend long-standing successful procedures with the innovation of technology. In this way, everyone can, in some measure, feel they are on the cutting edge without being overwhelmed by insurmountable learning curves and upwardly spiraling equipment and supply costs. We do not believe that one must be a professional writer or graphic designer to do high quality work. A little ingenuity, a careful eye, and an unrelenting desire to give the best effort possible will equip you for attaining new heights with your research communication media. The following two premises form the basis for our paper: (1) the ability to produce impressive research communications is not an innate attribute; and (2) the orthopaedic professional should be intimately involved in the preparation of his or her research communications because he or she is ultimately responsible for their quality. The corollary to these is: you are what you present (or, at least, that is what the audience thinks). Practically speaking, whether in the audience's eyes you conform to the image in Figure 1 or in Figure 2 depends largely on the merit of your communication media!

Why Improve?

Because producing high-quality communication media typically requires more effort and time than does a substandard approach, the question for time-constrained professionals is, "Why should I expend such effort to improve above the norm?" The best answer to this relates to the nature of the medical field. Medicine is a profession of high standards: physicians routinely make decisions that affect people's function, appearance, emotional well-being, even whether they live or die. Although research communication media do not possess the same critical overtones, they should, in their own way, demand a physician's careful attention.

Also, presenters have a unique opportunity to affect their colleagues by exerting a positive influence with their media. Each medium should be an orchestrated model of skillfully crafted segments. Furthermore, the mere fact that one prepares a communication suggests importance of the material; therefore, it should be delivered without the detraction of deficient preparation. All of the foregoing reasons, then, substantiate that projecting a favorable research communication image and projecting a favorable personal image are inseparable.

The Initial Steps

There are five basic steps that will immediately affect the quality of research communications, no matter what the medium. If presenters analyze their work with regard to these five points and act on their analysis with diligence, they will realize significant improvement.

Know your audience. If you do not know to whom you will be sending an abstract, presenting a poster exhibit, or giving a slide lecture, how can you expect to perform well in preparing it? Like it or not, any audience is made up of critics. Whether they are abstract reviewers, poster viewers, or lecture attendees, the fewer

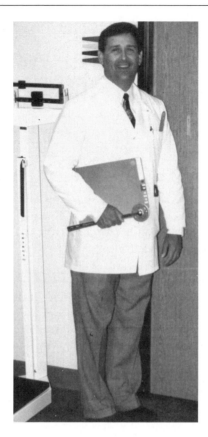

Fig. 1 The image of the consummate professional is fostered by excellent work.

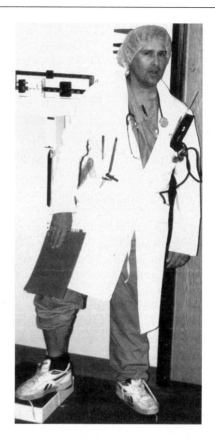

Fig. 2 Members of an audience who do not know a speaker will have no reason to believe he or she is anything but a buffoon unless the speaker demonstrates otherwise.

opportunities you give them for destructive criticism, the better chance you have of gaining acceptance of your message. To accomplish this, however, you must know the audience members' wants and needs and meet them!

Resolve to make your work better than everyone else's. "Better than everyone else's" is another way of saying "best." If you want to be the best, you have to think and act like the best. We are not proposing arrogance and conceit. The concept is more a refusal to accept in yourself less than excellent performance; you must push yourself to execute well. From the perspective of an audience member, consider the joy in partaking of exclusively superlative work!

Declare war on misspellings and poor grammar. This step is closely aligned with the previous one. You must adopt zero tolerance for errors of this sort. There is no excuse for such blunders. In addition to a dictionary, a medical dictionary, and a thesaurus, there are numerous reference books to assist the process of writing, proofreading, and correcting.[1-6] In addition, for those who use computers to prepare their communications (and we highly recommend this approach), several software products are available that point out errors in spelling and grammar. There are also thesaurus programs, which provide synonyms for those well-worn words that frequent your text.

Plan ahead. Prevention is a much better modus operandi than repair. Prevention comes with thorough planning. True, planning takes time, but not nearly as much time as trying to fix the result of inadequate planning. Remember, someone very smart once said, "If you don't have time to do a job right, how are you going to find time to do it again?" Not only does planning help you, it also is beneficial to those who assist your media preparation process because they will not have to work under the undue stress of tight (or impossible) deadlines.

Do not assume that your staff and service providers will do your work correctly. That is to say, do not think that your assistants will accurately read your mind. Although one of the best political moves you can make is to be kind to your service providers,[7] the presenter has the ultimate responsibility for content and quality. Poor work created the materials.

Abstracts

We will start our discussion of the specific types of media by addressing abstracts, because if a society does not accept your abstract, you will not even have the opportunity to present your work as a poster or slide program. The American College of Sports Medicine, on its abstract submission forms, lists several reasons why abstracts are rejected. Among these are: (1) Authors failed to include any objective results and data. (2) The abstract did not clearly indicate the purpose of the study and the significance of the findings. (3) Conclusions were not stated or the phrase "the results will be discussed" was used as a concluding sentence. These errors, and others, are correctable and we will discuss how as we proceed.

Mechanics

Reading the abstract preparation instructions several times and following them is the first and most important step one can take. This will eliminate the majority of mechanical errors in your abstract writing. Most professional organizations will not even allow the review of abstracts that do not meet their specific appearance criteria. Since directions are printed on every form, there is really no excuse for not adhering to them.

All abstract forms have a common factor: a box into which one must squeeze a lot of information. Some societies specify a maximum number of words. As a general rule, try to keep the word total at or below 200, and certainly not more than 250. Count them by hand or with a word processing program, if yours has this capability. However, it is more important that the abstract fit legibly into the box than for it to have an exact word count.

Different societies use different size boxes and some are easier to use than others. One key is to practice fitting everything onto a photocopy of the form before ruining your only copy of the form two days before its receipt deadline. Do your abstract on a word processor or desktop publishing program. Then, laser print it onto a practice photocopy of the form and, when your final draft is ready, onto the original form. The advantage of a desktop publishing program over a word processing program is that it tends to be much easier to set up a text holder of the exact dimensions of the abstract form's box and to place the text holder at the exact location needed to print onto the form.

If you use a computer for your writing, there are several ways of fitting a maximum amount of text into a given space (Fig. 3). (The qualification of that, however, is that legibility, readability, and the guidelines of the receiving society must be of prime importance.) Some fitting functions can be done more easily with a desktop publisher than with a word processor. Optical, or proportional, spacing allows more characters per line than does mechanical, or typewriter style, spacing. Optically spaced type is also easier to read.[8]

Changing the point size of the text is another technique. Twelve points is a fairly standard and readable size, but ten points is usually acceptable. Where the desktop publisher shines over the word processor is when there are a few final, and crucially important, words to fit into the box. Eleven points may be too large and ten points may be too small; an odd point size like 10.645 assigned by the software may afford your abstract the best visual appearance.

Another way to squeeze an extra line or two into the abstract box is by altering the line leading, the space between the lines of text. A fraction less than standard single spacing may be perfect. Again, the desktop publishing package may be preferable, because it allows these minor adjustments in the leading. Be cautioned that a leading value which is too small is unacceptable: the descenders of letters like p and y must not overlap the ascenders of letters such as d and b on the line below (Fig. 3).

This is an example of optically spaced letters.
This is an example of mechanically spaced letters.
There is a large difference in the number of characters that can fit on a line.
There is a large difference in the number of characters that can fit on a line.

A decrease in leading can allow more lines in a given vertical space.
A decrease in leading can allow more lines in a given vertical space.
A decrease in leading can allow more lines in a given vertical space.
A decrease in leading can allow more lines in a given vertical space.
A decrease in leading can allow more lines in a given vertical space.
A decrease in leading can allow more lines in a given vertical space.
A decrease in leading can allow more lines in a given vertical space.
A decrease in leading can allow more lines in a given vertical space.

Fig. 3 Tricks for fitting a little more text into an abstract box include using optically spaced instead of mechanically spaced letters and decreasing the leading measurement.

Writing

Abbreviations generally are acceptable in an abstract, except in the title. At the first occurrence of a word or phrase that you want to abridge, the abbreviation should follow in parentheses. This is fundamental in scientific writing. A few standard abbreviations, however, need not be preceded by an unabbreviated form. These include scientific units and such notations as: Ss (subjects), yr (year or years), d (day or days), ANOVA (analysis of variance), and certain common anatomic abbreviations like AP (anteroposterior). Of course, the guidelines of the society to which you are submitting the abstract must supersede all other rules.

While abbreviations can save valuable abstract space, they can also be very annoying. Using too many, especially ones that are uncommon or are author-devised, can break a reader's concentration. If the reader happens to be a society's reviewer, the chances of the abstract being accepted are probably diminished. We caution you to use abbreviations very judiciously in an abstract.

Avoid misspellings and poor grammar by careful proofreading. Computer spelling and grammar analyzers are useful, but do not rely exclusively on these. Most medical terms are not contained in standard computer-based composition tools. Additionally, there are several possible instances of correctly spelled words not intended for use in a particular spot in one's writing. Consider if the previous sentence was written: "Addition ally, the are several possible in stances of correct spelled word no in tended for us in a particular pot in ones wring." A computer will find no incorrectly spelled words, but it is obvious that the sentence is replete with misspellings! Homonyms (words that sound the same, but that are spelled differently and have different meanings) can create further problems for an inattentive author.

Manually proofreading your material yourself is the most reliable method. Become conversant with three books which are foreign to many professionals: a standard dictionary, a medical dictionary, and a thesaurus! A valuable rule to follow is, if you are not willing to bet fifty dollars on the spelling of a word, look it up. We recommend certain tricks to assist your proofreading. One is to put your abstract away for several days after you write it, and then read it again. The time delay will provide a new outlook on your writing. Reading the abstract backwards is also a good technique. Although it is useless for analyzing grammar, it does require extra attention to the spelling of each word. A third proofreading method is to allow your colleagues to read your work.

The title of an abstract must be chosen carefully so the reader will want to read the body of the abstract. It must describe the research, but it cannot be lengthy. Conciseness is important, but clarity is even more essential. Here are two actual examples of titles of research (presented in a spirit of education, rather than one of maliciousness) that, while somewhat amusing, underscore the point about lucidity: "Major *Orthopaedic Surgery on* the Leg and *Thromboembolism*"[9] and "Long Segment Coronary Ulcerations in *Survivors of Sudden Cardiac Death*"[10] (emphases added). The title is your only opportunity for a good first impression; it must be well written.

State the purpose of the study in the first sentence of the abstract so there is no confusion about what the study was designed to accomplish. "The purpose of this study was to..." is a simple, tried, and true initial line.

The next part of the abstract describes the subjects and should give basic information about them, especially the number, the gender composition of the group, and the mean age with a variation statistic. Other characteristics about the subjects that are pertinent to the study should be included, as well. The methodology should briefly discuss what you did and how you did it. Continue the abstract in single paragraph form, rather than in a sectional format with subtitles. This makes it more fluid and readable and is consistent with typical scientific style.

The results portion should contain the important data you collected, reported as means and deviation statistics. Some societies allow the insertion of tabular data in abstracts. Confine this technique to data that benefit from such presentation, and include only indispensable data. Also, name the statistical procedures used and their results: significance status, trends of the data, important correlational coefficients, and the appropriate probability values are examples.

An abstract's conclusions should *suggest* what the data and the statistical analyses seem to show, that is, your interpretation of the data. A basic tenet of the scientific method is that a hypothesis cannot be proven or disproven, only supported or refuted. Thus, it is presumptuous and technically incorrect to state that an investigation found, discovered, showed, indicated, or proved an answer to its research question.

An abstract does not contain discussion; there is not room for that. In its place, at least in clinically oriented research, the clinical relevance is very important and may make or break the abstract. Reviewers and clinicians alike will ask "So, what?" about your research. The answer should be found at the end of your abstract.

Poster Exhibits

The poster exhibit is a very valuable form of research communication because it allows extended periods of viewing and, if desired, audience and author interaction. Oral presentations, being six to 15 minutes in length, depending on the society, do not provide this kind of opportunity. A poster may actually show the results of a complex experiment better than an oral presentation.[3] A poster must be carefully planned and produced, so it will attract a viewer's interest and provide the desired message.[3,11]

Design

The space a society usually allots for a poster exhibit is a 4 by 8 foot or 4 by 6 foot bulletin board. The American Academy of Orthopaedic Surgeons provides 4 by 8 boards. Use the entire space that you are allotted. Remember that a viewer will not stand still for long. If his or her attention is not seized within three seconds of an initial glance, it will probably not be secured at all. If he or she actually stops to observe your work, it will usually be for less than 30 seconds. It is crucial, therefore, that you provide the viewer with a visually exciting and important message in that short period by using color, pictures and graphs, and short phrases.

The main sections to present on a poster are: abstract, purpose, methods, results, conclusions, and, usually, clinical relevance. A poster is like a visual journal article in many ways. However, one section that should be absent is discussion. Discussion does not lend itself well to succinctness, a main quality of an effective poster exhibit. The three most important parts of an exhibit are the title, purpose, and conclusions, because these provide the salient points of an investigation. Hence, they should stand out from everything else.

When designing your poster, remember that people will pass at least four feet from it as they walk by. Large, easy-to-read lettering is critical to the success of information transfer. Minimum capital letter sizes for the various types of wording are: title, 1.5 inches; authors, institution(s), and section titles, 1 inch; section subtitles and labels, 0.5 inch; and narratives, statements, and phrases, three eighths inch.

Production

The application of poster lettering must be neat. Stencils and magic markers certainly lack professionalism. One of the best products for large-format lettering is die-cut vinyl. It is neat and easy to apply to a lightly penciled baseline, which is erased after completion of the lettering. Current technology in computer guided die-cutting, such as that found at commercial sign and graphics shops, even allows preparation of the entire title in adhesive strips. The lettering is peeled from its backing, applied to the surface, and pressed down firmly. The front facing of the letters is then peeled away, leaving an attractive display. This method allows a wide selection of vinyl colors, typefaces, and point sizes.

A laser printer produces high quality output—acceptable both for large titles and narratives—using a printer language like Postscript. The large point sized titles can be printed on single sheets of standard 8½ by 11 inch paper, mounted to poster board or foam board, and "tiled," or fastened to the poster in small sections that fit together to create a large image. Printing also can be done on colored paper for pleasing effects.

Obviously, some verbiage is necessary, but too many words make a poster exhibit tedious. When describing methods, nongraphable results, and conclusions, use phrases instead of complete sentences so viewers can get your message in a minimum amount of time. Generally, it is best to show, rather than tell, viewers what you did. Use photographs, drawings, and graphs whenever possible. These must be of high quality. Color production of your graphics will greatly enhance the overall poster. There are numerous ways to produce these, and an exhaustive discussion of them is beyond the scope of our paper. Basic concepts of taking photographs and creating graphics are presented in a subsequent section about slide production.

If high technology excites you and you have a healthy audiovisual budget, a very intriguing and impressive way of creating a poster exhibit is first to design a computer scale model of it on a freehand graphics or desktop publishing program. Then, a graphics service bureau can output it in a large color plotter format and laminate it. There is virtually no limit to the ways you can present research with this method. A little creativity can make for a very striking poster. Perhaps the main benefit of this is the poster's transportability. It is simply rolled up and carried in a mailing tube, a much less cumbersome form than the large artist's portfolio used to carry the usual tiled format poster exhibit.

The key to an effective poster exhibit is to create an atmosphere of visual excitement for the viewers. If it is gaudy or if too much information is presented, it will not have the desired effect. In short, plan your poster carefully, prepare it neatly, and make sure it is viewer friendly.

Slide Presentations: Planning

The rest of this paper pertains to slide presentations. We have broken the topic into three P's: Planning, Producing, and Presenting. There is more information about this medium than the other two because it is more complicated and because, unquestionably, it is the one most commonly used. However, accompanying its familiarity is a susceptibility to many errors that are unique to slides.

One of the first decisions you must make is whether to use one carousel or two. Two carousels may be overkill for a research presentation. Bear in mind that doubling the number of projectors and carousels also doubles (at least) the potential for mechanical problems and presentation errors.

For instance, consider the presentation of data about the subjects in a study. In a side-by-side format, the left slide might say,"Subjects," and the right slide would give the mean age of the subjects and, perhaps, their mean height and weight, along with the number of males and females. Using two carousels does not provide any advantage because a single slide can have the title, "Subjects," at the top and the data underneath.

On the other hand, two carousels can be very helpful when discussing methods, because they allow you to present a written description and show a picture. For example, with only one carousel, if you want to show the technique of performing a knee ligament exam while you discuss your methods, the picture would have to follow the title slide. Side-by-side slides allow you to show the test while you present text about the specific method used. Perhaps the best approach for slide presentation of research is to use two carousels, but to load one of them with dark slides (opaque plastic squares) except where side-by-side slides are really needed. This effectively allows one to take advantage of the benefits of both single- and double-carousel lectures.

The number of slides in a presentation can be difficult to plan, because it depends on many factors, some concrete and others nebulous. The length of time a society allots for research presentations is easily determined, as is the number of sections contained in the lecture. However, the technicality of your procedures, the depth of your descriptions, the extent of your statistical analysis, and the breadth of your conclusions are flexible elements of your presentation that challenge your time constraints. And, obviously, two-

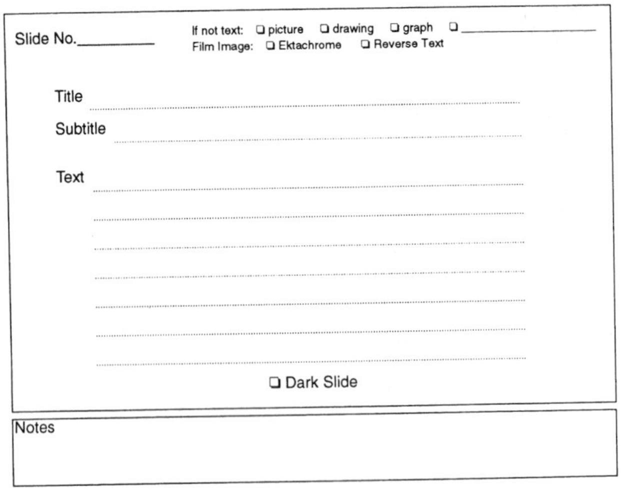

Fig. 5 A sample lecture storyboard.

carousel lectures require up to twice as many slides as a one-carousel talk. Garson and associates[12] recommend one minute per slide, with alterations made for slides that show or describe new techniques (1.5 to 2 minutes) and for slides that are similar in format and data (30 seconds). They specify a total of 13 or 14 slides per ten-minute talk.

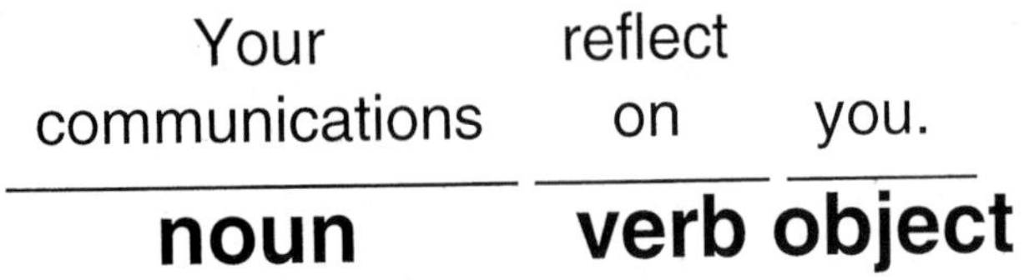

Actually, because of the frequency with which side-by-side slides are used, the key variable of interest is the number of projector advances. Based on our experience, we have developed a general formula for all talks: Number of Projector Advances = Presentation Minutes x 1.5. This is equivalent to one slide change every 40 seconds. The formula is merely a guide; you are strongly cautioned that good sense must prevail. Customization of the slide talk to your style and how much you are going to say about each slide should define your projector advance total.

As you begin to create slides you must have a single concept in mind, so direct your energy at developing your critical message. Eastman Kodak presents an excellent way of narrowing your focus.[13] Reminiscent of sentence diagramming in grade school, it proposes that you outline your main message as a noun, verb, and object using three to six words. Figure 4 shows the conceptual diagram for the instructional course on which this manuscript is based. Using this scheme, the essence of the course is, "Your communications (noun) reflect on (verb) you (object)." This was the framework for everything we prepared.

An excellent means to eliminate stress from planning a slide show is to use lecture storyboards (Fig. 5) to map your thoughts initially. Storyboards will help you visualize how each slide will appear, how the pre-

Fig. 4 A technique for focusing the message of your research presentation.[13] (Adapted with permission from Eastman Kodak: Just what did you have in mind? in *How to Be a Knockout with AV!* Rochester, NY, Eastman Kodak Company, 1989, p 3.)

Repetition	Mean Torque	Mean Work	Mean Power
1	602.0 N·m	253.0 J	159.0 J/s
2	615.0	262.0	161.0
3	627.0	279.0	176.0
4	611.0	258.0	160.0
5	619.0	275.0	163.0
6	610.0	257.0	160.0
Grand Mean n = 32	614.0 N·m	264.0 J	163.2 J/s

Mean Performance Values
(6 repetitions, n = 32)

Torque: 614.0 N·m
Work: 264.0 J
Power: 163.2 J/s

Fig. 6 The slide format on the left contains too much data and fails the Nelson Slide Test.[14,15] The format on the right contains the important parts of the same data set, but is designed specifically for a slide. It passes the Nelson test.

sentation sequence flows, and how consistent the formatting is across your series of slides. These handwritten models also simplify the entry of the slides' text into the computer that will generate the actual slides or into the computer or typewriter that will produce copy sheets from which the slides are to be photographed.

Once you actually begin to put words or graphics to the slides, limit the amount of information you present on each slide. Here are two tricks to prevent wordiness and to maintain one main thought per slide. Use a large point size for your text, or place a confining box around your text area. These techniques will force you to remove unnecessary words from text slides. Either technique places a premium on space and trains you to state your points efficiently. A third way, progressive revelation, is a method of incrementing information across a group of slides. In this scheme, each point made about the general topic of your slide series is highlighted. Points already discussed are then darkened on subsequent slides of the series as successive points are introduced. The idea is to control the rate of information flow to the audience.

Nelson[14,15] postulates that the way information is presented on a slide is vastly different from the way information is presented in other visual media, especially print. His Nelson Slide Test helps the presenter evaluate slides on the basis of whether or not the information on each slide is appropriate for a slide format by asking,"Has the information to be presented been prepared specifically for a slide?"[14] Day[3] provides what might be considered a corollary to the Nelson Slide Test: "If a slide cannot be understood in four seconds, it is a bad slide." Legibility in one form is not equivalent to legibility in another form;[16] simplification is the key. Compare the two slides shown in Figure 6. The one on the left, which resembles a table taken from a journal article, has a surplus of data. The data in the right-hand slide were prepared from the same information, but specifically for a slide; the slide only presents the data of interest.

The Arm's Length Rule will help you immensely in designing slides, too. Capital letters should be readable on a slide held out in front of you at arm's length. If they are not, redo the slide.

Slide Presentations: Producing

The production of slides can fall anywhere in a gamut from simplistic to complex. There are many choices to consider and decisions to make. Our intent is not to provide the epitomized reference source of slidemaking. Bear in mind that for every idea we have, there are many more equally sensible and useful ideas. We will share methods in which we are experienced, that we know are sound, and that most individuals with basic knowledge and equipment can successfully incorporate.

Color

Because color is so important to the appearance of slides, we will discuss it first. Creating slides on a computer has become very popular. Remember, though, that the color seen on a computer screen is usually much different from what is projected on a screen. Additionally, the powerful presentation graphics software available today has created a unique problem. Software provides too many options and promotes poor judgment on the part of the user. One result of this is what we call Salad Bar Slides, those slides composed of so many colors that they look like a myriad of fruits and vegetables on a salad bar. Four bit computer color capability allows the use of sixteen colors on a monitor. Eight bit color provides 256 colors. Sixteen bit technology escalates those choices to about 32,000 different colors. A twenty-four bit video card placed in a computer rockets the number of colors to almost 17,000,000! For some high end graphics applications, that variety is very important. For making research presentation slides, it is not! The majority of color computers in use today are either eight or sixteen bit. As a general guideline, avoid using more than four colors on a slide, including the background color.

Another pitfall when choosing colors is picking colors that are not agreeable, or are downright ugly. This often happens because, again, the colors look better on the computer monitor than they do on the screen and because there are so many colors from which to choose. Select slide backgrounds from the set of dark and rich colors, such as black, dark blue, medium blue, dark green, teal, and carmine red. The blues and black, always good choices, are the ones most commonly used.

Gradient, or linear blended, backgrounds are gaining popularity. They look good when the blending is smooth, but some film recorders are not capable of recording smooth blends. The banding that results is caused by software technology being ahead of hardware technology and it detracts from the appearance of the slides. The only solutions to this problem are to purchase a higher quality (and usually more expensive) recorder, have your slides recorded at a commercial output bureau, or use plain, instead of gradient, backgrounds.

Light colored lettering should be chosen for display on dark backgrounds because dark colored letters do not contrast well and are difficult to read. White, yellow, golden yellow, and light blue all provide the necessary readability on the backgrounds suggested above. Once more, avoid using several different colors and applying unusual colors to text. We recommend that you use one layout and color scheme per talk. It is routine at conferences to see slides of varying colors and formats in a series. One particularly troublesome type of slide is the old and faded classic. A presentation that contains a variety of mismatched slides looks exactly like what it is: a patchwork of miscellaneous slides thrown together because a speaker did not put out the effort necessary to create a new presentation. If including information from a previous presentation is a must, a minimum effort consists of transposing the text and data from old slides onto a new set of slides. Consistency is a mark of an effective presenter.

There are two plans that one can follow in trying to initiate and maintain slide consistency. If creating entirely new presentations is simply too much effort, always use the exact same color and layout scheme in your slides so you can trade back and forth, when necessary. The other means of protecting against an incongruous appearance is to use completely different colors and layouts for every talk. This forces one to create each lecture as stand-alone communication, without sharing slides.

Design

Word slides tend to be easier to read and understand when the title and text are separated visually.[7,12] Most commonly, the separator is simply a line. Other ways of accomplishing the same task are to place the slide's title in a rectangular space that contrasts with the background or to use a different color for the title lettering. The purpose of this separation, no matter how it is performed, is to orient the audience to the contents of each slide as it is projected.

There are several common pitfalls of designing slides, not the least of which is the typeface used. Sans serif typefaces, like Helvetica, are preferable because they tend to be easier to read than serif typefaces, such as Times Roman. (Serifs are the small decorative lines on certain typefaces, usually at the tops and bottoms of letters.) Using entirely uppercase letters also makes text difficult to read. Confine completely capitalized words to short titles only, or do not use them at all.

Vast differences in letter sizes among your slides also detract from the overall presentation. Choose a type size that will fit the slide that contains the most information and then use this size for all the slides. Of course, this will require that you carefully plan what appears on each slide, which is really the point. Replan slides that either (1) contain very little information compared to other slides in the presentation, or (2) contain much more information than the other slides in the presentation. Note that small differences in type sizes are acceptable when necessary for fine tuning the amount of the slide frame that is filled. It is also permissible to use larger titles for section headings.

Graphs are an excellent way of presenting data for maximum impact, but they do have limitations. When you use bar graphs, make sure that the bars are wider than the space between them. Three-dimensional bar graphs are attractive but can be difficult to read accurately if it is important for the viewer to obtain specific values from the graph. Limit a single graph to six individual bars or three series of two bars each. Line graphs should have no more than four individual lines to maintain readability and comprehensibility.

One other slide design pitfall bears mentioning; we call it Burma Shave Slides. Perhaps you have seen, or at least heard of, Burma Shave Signs, the sequential signboards that used to dot the country's roads. Each successive board provided an additional piece of the message. When applied to slides, however, this technique is annoying. Audiences resent being tagged along in this way. Do not split a single thought among several slides.

The best solution for slide design pitfalls is to review a printed output of your slides before spending time and money putting them on film. Use the printouts to preview your presentation as if you were actually delivering it. Critically evaluate your work. This technique is a revealing exercise that will assist the solidification of your talk.

Photography

Following the design portion of slide production, the slides must be processed to film. The previous discussion dealt with text and graph slide production. This section focuses on methods of creating text slides from black and white printed output and on picture photography. All the techniques discussed are the "do-it-yourself" variety. Using a 35 mm camera and a copystand, there are many ways to produce high quality, visually pleasing text and line art slides. Each of the numerous types of film has different characteristics and uses. We refer the reader to Kodak's publications, *Guide to Kodak 35 mm Films: How to Choose the Right Film*,[17] and *Kodak Vericolor Slide and Print Films*,[18] for information that falls beyond the scope of this paper.

The Kodak Legibility Calculator[19,20] determines the dimensions and type size of the copy you will be photographing based on the size of the lecture room's screen and how far the screen is from the back row of the audience. The calculator is a pair of different diameter circular cut-outs fixed together through their centers. Calculations are made by rotating the inner (smaller) circle upon the outer one. As an example, we will assume you are able to determine from a meeting organizer that your research presentation will be in a room where the back row of the audience is 96 feet from the screen and the height of the screen is approximately eight feet. The Legibility Calculator indicates that if you use a piece of paper with a copy area of six inches by nine inches—the same proportion as a camera viewfinder—the letters of the copy to be photographed should be at least three sixteenths of an inch tall in order for the audience to see them easily when the copy is projected as a slide. (The letter height measurement, by the way, is the height of a lower case letter's body.)

Reverse Text Films. For text slides and line drawings, reverse text films are very effective, easy to use, and economical. The name "reverse text" refers to these films' negative slide image: black or dark areas of your text or artwork will be white or light-colored on the slide, while white or light areas (for example, the paper on which the copy is printed) will be dark on the slide.[18, 21]

Kodak High Contrast Ektagraphic (or, Ektagraphic HC) Film gives an opaque black background with clear (white when projected) text or artwork. A reverse text color film is Kodak SO-279 Vericolor Slide Film, which delivers different colored backgrounds and text depending on the shutter speed, F stop, and color filter used (Table 1).

The advantage of SO-279 over Ektagraphic HC is its ease of processing. It requires the same C-41 process provided for print film at any one-hour photo lab. Specify processing only—no prints. When your film is returned, simply cut the frames and put them in slide mounts. Ektagraphic HC processing usually must be done by a professional laboratory and, in our experience, labs that routinely perform this are hard to find. Medical graphics departments should be able to handle it, however.

A benefit of Ektagraphic slides is the opacity of the black background. These slides can be enlivened by the application of color to the clear lettering or artwork areas. There are two main ways to do this. A piece of color transparency placed in the mount with the Ektagraphic film will alter the text or art to that color. Or, transparency felt-tip markers can be used to color certain portions of the slide. Both of these techniques are effective because any coloration not coincident with the clear text or image part of the slide is blocked from projection by the opaque black.

There are some simple guidelines to follow when preparing the copy for reverse text slide photography. A poor quality original will result in poor quality slides. Correction fluid blotches, tape edges, and black photocopier specks all detract from the appearance of a reverse text slide. It is best if text and line art are boldly stroked (Fig. 7) to keep the background color from bleeding into the text or art. Artwork for reverse text slides should not contain grey tones or halftones because reverse text films are essentially very high contrast negative images, and grey tones tend to reproduce erratically. Necessary shading in artwork for reverse text slides should be done with a percentage screen of black, or a percentage density of black dots. The shaded area will appear grey, but close inspection will reveal the dot pattern (Fig. 7).

Chrome Films. The chrome films (for example, Kodak Kodachrome, Kodak Ektachrome, Fuji Fujichrome) produce color picture slides. There are different types for use with different lighting conditions and different applications.[17,20]

Kodachrome produces excellent quality slides with very pure coloration and high sharpness, but its processing is complex and must be performed by a Kodak

---

Table1: Kodak SO-279 slide color results with different filters

Filter	Slide Color	Text/Art Color
None	Brown	Golden Yellow
Blue (80A)	Carmine to Maroon	Golden Yellow to Orange
Yellow	Violet	White
Orange	Diazo Blue	White
Red	Turquoise	White
Green	Dark Blue	White to Light Blue
Sepia	Teal	White to Light Green

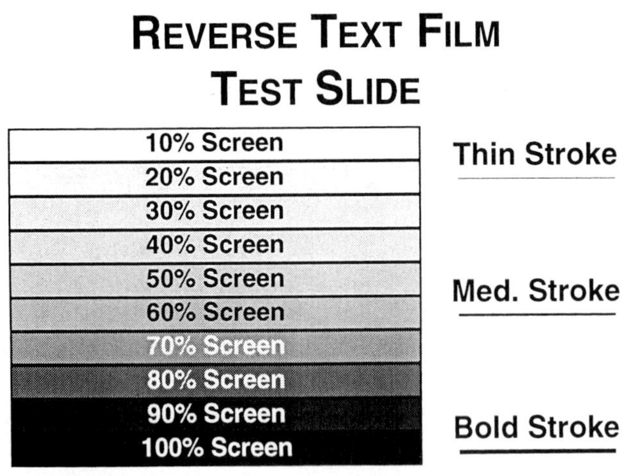

REVERSE TEXT FILM
TEST SLIDE

10% Screen	**Thin Stroke**
20% Screen	
30% Screen	
40% Screen	
50% Screen	**Med. Stroke**
60% Screen	
70% Screen	
80% Screen	
90% Screen	**Bold Stroke**
100% Screen	

Fig. 7   This shows the variations among different line stroke weights. The graphic also shows the proper means of applying shading to reverse text slide artwork. Note that there are no halftones; the grey effects are produced by varying the density of black dots.

lab or other high-end commercial facility. Because shipping involved lengthens the processing time, Kodachrome may not be the proper choice of film when you must meet a deadline.

Ektachrome is probably the most commonly used slide film. Like Kodachrome, it produces sharp, richly colored images. Its processing time is much shorter, however; two to three hours at many labs. As expected, there are different types of Ektachrome for different types of lighting.

We have found Ektachrome 100HC to be the best all-purpose color slide film. Fujichrome 100 is similar. Ektachrome 100HC is balanced for daylight or flash photography. Under fluorescent lighting, such as is found in x-ray viewboxes, special filters like an FL-1A or 85B may help avoid a greenish-blue film tinge. (This may require some experimentation, because there are many different types of fluorescent tubes.[17,22]) If you use Ektachrome 100HC under tungsten lighting without a correction filter like an 80A, your slides will exhibit a brownish-yellow tint.

Special Films. There are other special types of Ektachrome. Use Ektachrome 160T when the lighting is tungsten or another 3200 Kelvin source, such as quartz copystand lamps. It is color balanced to alleviate the brownish-yellow tinge seen in standard Ektachrome slides taken in tungsten light. Ektachrome Slide Duplicating Film (Kodak 5071) is designed for an obvious application. It is corrected for tungsten lighting. It also is well suited for photographing radiographs, because the slides it produces retain most of the contrast of the originals. Creasey and Warren-Smith[22] performed a study of different film types and

fluorescent tubes to find the best and easiest films and tubes for achieving acceptable radiographic slides. They found that duplicating film combined with an 85B filter gave the best results, although Agfachrome 200 film with 81C and FL-1A filters was the most *convenient* way of rendering good quality slides using a variety of fluorescent tube types.

Kodak Rapid Process Copy, or RPC, film is often used by medical presenters to make slides of radiographs because it is very easy to process in a standard x-ray developing apparatus available in all orthopaedic departments. The use of RPC involves two risks; one is annoying, the other is disastrous. The annoying one first: RPC usually requires very long exposure times (30 seconds to two minutes or more, depending on the contrast of the original and the strength of the light source). Obviously, your photography sessions will be extended if you have a quantity of radiographs to reproduce. Additionally, you cannot hand-hold your camera with such long shutter speeds, an inconvenience at best. Most importantly, RPC does not tolerate well the high temperature of projector bulbs. If you use it, you may watch helplessly from the podium as your only copy of that rare radiograph melts before your eyes.

The most germane advice we can provide about using different films is to experiment with the films and with your photography equipment to attain the effects you want. We have based much of our discussion on years of carefully controlled photography research. You will quickly discover that you must follow a few hard and fast rules, but, after that, there is a wealth of room for error, customization, and creativity. In the end, triumph comes to those who persevere.

Picture Composition. Composing picture slides is at least as important as planning title slides. Fill the camera frame with the subject and do not include unnecessary, disquieting backdrops. This requires both moving toward the subject during photography and redirecting shots initially composed against windows, mirrors, loud wallpaper, and similar surfaces. Closely related to this is the caution to remove distracting, nonessential, irrelevant items from the area around the subject before taking the shot. Finally, human subjects should be dressed neatly and discreetly.

Computerized Film Recorders

The presence of computerized film recorders in medical centers has become routine and, even, necessary. Orthopaedic private practitioners are embracing these high quality slide producers, too. Although film recorders are capable of generating slides of very high complexity, we will only comment on their application to the usual multicolored text and graph transparencies. Slide quality generally is far above that obtainable with other techniques, but recorders cost several thousand dollars. If you use a lot of slides, purchasing a film recorder can be very cost effective and you will have maximum control over your slide production. When using equipment like this, you first create your slides, remembering the planning and design tips presented in this paper. Then, the computer outputs the slide files to the film recorder, which uses a camera, a light beam, and a series of color filters to produce the slide on film.

A system of this type requires a computer, specialized graphics software, and a film recorder. For advice about the best type of computer platform and system configuration to use for slidemaking, we refer you to the guidance of someone you trust who has been successful doing this type of work. Your institution's medical graphics department or an exemplary colleague will be of the most service to you. An introductory article by Hurt[23] may also be helpful.

Parenthetically, a computer, a color monitor, and a camera tripod provide a simple, less costly means of producing color text and graph slides. With a camera mounted on a tripod in front of the computer monitor, one can photograph images on the monitor's screen using Ektachrome 100HC film. Consideration must be given to proper shutter speed (to avoid screen refresh banding), F stop (to obtain satisfactory color and proper depth of field), and lens focal length (to avoid peripheral image distortion). Refer to technique articles by Chew[24] and Hunter and Brewer[25] for specific guidance.

Slide Presentations: Presenting

The third of our three P's is presenting. This is where all of your hard work pays off. Your exquisite professional image is preserved until you reach the podium and press the slide advance button for the first time. Then, you either uphold the favorable portrait or shatter it.

Lecture Preparation and Delivery

There is no advice more timely, and timeless, than to practice your presentation. In fact, an excellently polished delivery using marginal slides is far more effective than superb slides accompanied by a mangled, ill-prepared speaking performance.

There are two approaches for presenting a slide program. The first is a cue script, a narrative outline of what you intend to say at each film advance with the comments enumerated according to their corresponding slides. A cue script easily can be prepared by situating your computer/word processor near your slide projector, or vice versa, and writing notes as you advance your slides. As you present your talk, refer to the outline for assistance in maintaining fluidity and for remembering all the points you intend to make. There is a pitfall to using this method, however. Do not bury yourself in your script. Reading directly from your notes not only shows a lack of preparation, but the audience will not, and should not, tolerate being ignored. (There is one exception to the directive not to read your notes verbatim, but it applies to longer presentations that are audiotaped and which are scripted specifically for oral delivery—a completely different type of composition than technical writing.[26] Even then, however, rehearsal is critical and frequent visual surveys of the audience are mandatory.)

The other approach is to use cue slides. In this approach, each slide, when it is projected, serves as a reminder of what you are to say. Slides should augment your lecture. The main pitfall, reading the slides to the audience,[3] can be avoided by using only key words on your slides. You should mention the key words as you speak,[12,27] but it is unlikely you will read from a slide when the main grammatical parts of a sentence are missing from it.

Your demeanor in front of the audience greatly dictates the appeal of your subject matter. You should demonstrate a level of expertise, without cockiness, about your research. After all, you are the one who did the investigation and the audience rightly expects your complete conversance with the protocol and findings. Co-authors who present in place of lead authors, note: you are responsible for a knowledgeable, cogent presentation as the lead author would be. A second (but, not secondary) aspect of a good presenter's demeanor is enthusiasm.[28] If you are not excited about your work, no one else will be the least bit stimulated by it.

Never point out errors in your slides or mention the poor quality of your slides.[28] Doing so only draws further attention to a problem. Let's say 60% of an audience recognizes a blunder you project on the screen. Your admission that the slide is unreadable or that it contains a spelling error brings that percentage up to 100%. There is a real solution for errors in slides or poor quality slides: exorcise them from your programs. The all too frequent "Forgive the misspelling" and "I know you can't read this, but," slides are useless and do not belong in the careful presenter's carousel.

Another common practice is the use of rest slides. This technique is acceptable, especially during particularly intense presentations, but there is some accompanying advice. Such slides should be of a fun or pleasing nature. Use them sparingly or they will be a distraction rather than a relief. Most importantly, rest slides should be tasteful—there is no place for naked photographs or off-color cartoons. Using this sort of rest slide will detract from the professional image you have tried so hard to cultivate.

Mechanics

There are a few points about delivering an oral presentation that should, but often cannot, go unsaid. Do not regard these lightly because, as soon as you label them ridiculous, you fall prey to one or more of them. Each of these miscues has happened to someone we know. On the day of your lecture make sure that it actually is the correct day and that you get out of bed early enough (if you have a morning speaking slot). Set the alarm clock in your hotel room and register for a wake-up call with the hotel operator. Be certain that you have plenty of time to spare. It is better to arrive very early for your presentation than to have to rush to squeak in under the wire. If you are late, most moderators will, and should, go on without you.

Research paper presentations are normally anywhere from six to 15 minutes in length. Do not go longer than your alloted period. Abiding by this cardinal rule will save you the embarassment of having the moderator halt your lecture before you are finished in order for the program to remain on schedule. If you are unsure what the proper duration is, ask your moderator before the session begins. If a question-and-answer period is to follow your lecture, leave ample time for this. A speaker light system at the podium is a tremendous help, but you cannot always expect to have one. If you do not have such a system, take off your watch and place it down in front of a group. Overcome timing problems by carefully planning and designing your slides and by practicing!

Audiovisual Equipment and Procedures. Familiarity with audiovisual equipment can save your lecture. The first step, of course, is to insert your slides into the carousel. This is not nearly as difficult as some speakers apparently think it is. Simply look at a slide so it reads properly, then turn is upside down and place it into a carousel slot with its back toward the slots with the smaller numbers. A useful trick is to place a red dot in the upper right-hand corner when the slide is oriented correctly for insertion into the carousel. This allows for easy slide manipulation and for fast future loading because the dots on all the slides will be in the same position when the slides are correctly installed in the tray. Once the slides are loaded, visit the speaker preparation room. Not only can you check your slide orientations, you will gain an amazing amount of reassurance by going through your slides before your presentation.

Become acquainted with the controls for the projector, pointer, and lights.[29] Some podium consoles can be confusing for the first time user, so visit your room ahead of time and find out how everything works. We also recommend that whenever possible you actually project some of your slides in your lecture room prior to your session. Early in the morning before the meetings start, after they are over for the day, or during the lunch hour are good times to do this. Additionally, listen to someone's lecture in the same room in which you will be speaking to acclimate yourself to the acoustics, the lighting, and the audience seating. For some reason, microphones scare people. Speak clearly and into the microphone. But, do not place your mouth so close to the mike that you transmit feedback pings. Use the electronics to your advantage.

Finally, if you use a light pointer, avoid flashing the pointer all over the screen, walls, and ceiling. Use the pointer for its intended purpose: turn it on to point at a specific spot and, having highlighted that spot, turn it off.

Conclusion

Research communication media can be as effective or ineffective as you want to make them. However you can create them will reflect on you. Be attentive to the fact that you are what you present. Although professional expertise in writing or the graphic arts is not a requirement, dedication and significant effort are. Excellent labor begets excellent results. The image and message you present to an audience member, whether it be an abstract reviewer, a poster exhibit spectator, or an oral presentation attendee, depends on your preparation of the medium. Perhaps a quote by Willa A. Foster best expresses the work ethic we hope to promote with this paper: "Quality is never an accident; it is always the result of high intention, sincere effort, intelligent direction, and skillful execution. It represents the wise choice of many alternatives."

References

1. Bernstein TM: *The Careful Writer: A Modern Guide to English Usage.* New York, NY, Atheneum, 1965.
2. Blauvelt CT, Nelson FRT: *A Manual of Orthopaedic Terminology,* ed 4. St. Louis, MO, CV Mosby, 1990.
3. Day RA: *How to Write and Publish a Scientific Paper,* ed 3. Phoenix, AZ, Oryx Press, 1988.
4. Iverson C, Dan BB, Glitman P, et al: *The American Medical Association Manual of Style,* ed 8. Baltimore, MD, Williams & Wilkins, 1989.
5. Kilcoyne RF, Farrar EL: *Handbook of Orthopaedic Terminology.* Boca Raton, FL, CRC Press, 1990.
6. Strunk WJ Jr, White EB: *The Elements of Style,* ed 3. New York, NY, Macmillan, 1979.
7. Kohl HW: Big screens and tiny numbers: Tips for effective slide presentations. Presented at the 39th Annual Meeting of the American College of Sports Medicine. Dallas, TX, 1992.
8. Casciero AJ, Roney RG: *Audiovisual Technology Primer.* Littleton, CO, Libraries Unlimited, 1988.
9. Parker-Williams J, Vickers R: Major orthopaedic surgery on the leg and thromboembolism. *Br Med J* 1991;303:531-532.
10. Lo Y-S, Cutler JE, Wright A, et al: Long segment coronary ulcerations in survivors of sudden cardiac death. *Am Heart J* 1988;116:1444-1447.
11. *How to Prepare a Scientific or Poster Exhibit.* Park Ridge, IL: American Academy of Orthopaedic Surgeons, 1990.
12. Garson A Jr, Gutgesell HP, Pinsky WW, et al: The 10-minute talk: Organization, slides, writing, and delivery. *Am Heart J* 1986;111:193-203.

13. *How to Be a Knockout with AV!* (Publ. S-31). Rochester, NY, Eastman Kodak Co, 1989.

14. Nelson RC: Are your presentations sliding away? *Sports Med Bull* 1978;13:8-9.

15. Nelson RC: Are your presentations still sliding away? *Sports Med Bull* 1990;25:14.

16. *Effective Lecture Slides* (Publ. S-22). Rochester, NY, Eastman Kodak Co, 1988.

17. *Guide to Kodak 35 mm Films.* (Publ. AF-1). Rochester, NY, Eastman Kodak Co, 1990.

18. *Kodak Vericolor Slide and Print Films* (Publ. E-24). Rochester, NY, Eastman Kodak Co, 1990.

19. *Legibility—Artwork to Screen* (Publ. S-24). Rochester, NY, Eastman Kodak Co, 1988.

20. Bishop A: *Slides: Planning and Producing Slide Programs* (Publ. S-30). Rochester, NY, Eastman Kodak Co, 1989.

21. *Reverse Text Slides* (Publ. S-26). Rochester, NY, Eastman Kodak Co, 1985.

22. Creasey MG, Warren-Smith CD: Reproduction of radiographs for 2 x 2 transparencies. *J Audiov Media Med* 1987;10:138-141.

23. Hurt W: Introduction to film recorders for computer-generated slide production. *J Audiov Media Med* 1991;14:67-70.

24. Chew FS: The use of a microcomputer to make rapid and inexpensive lecture slides. *Am J Roentgenol* 1989;152:185-188.

25. Hunter TB, Brewer M: Production of text and graphics slides on a personal computer. *Am J Roentgenol* 1985;144:1309-1312.

26. Kenny M: *Presenting Yourself* (Eastman Kodak Publ. S-60). New York, NY, John C. Wiley and Sons, 1982.

27. Kroenke K: The 10-minute talk. *Am J Med* 1987;83:329-330.

28. Kroenke K: The lecture: Where it wavers. *Am J Med* 1984;77:393-396.

29. Findley LJ, Antczak FJ: Commentary: How to prepare and present a lecture. *JAMA.* 1985;253:246.

Index